FASCIA

The Tensional Network of the Human Body

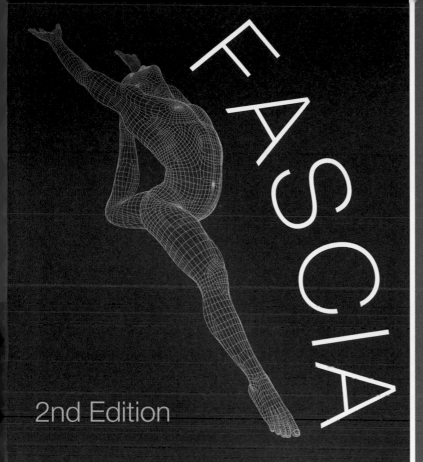

FASCIA

2nd Edition

The Tensional Network of the Human Body

The science and clinical applications in manual and movement therapy

Edited by
Robert Schleip, PhD, MA
Director, Fascia Research Project, University of Ulm, Ulm, Germany; Research Director European Rolfing Association; Vice President of the Fascia Research Society; Visiting Professor IUCS Barcelo; Certified Rolfing & Feldenkrais Teacher

Carla Stecco, MD
Orthopedic Surgeon; Professor of Human Anatomy, University of Padua, Padua, Italy; Certified Fascial Manipulation® Teacher

Mark Driscoll, Eng, PhD
Professor, Department of Mechanical Engineering, McGill University, Montreal, Quebec, Canada; Canada NSERC Chair, Design Engineering for Interdisciplinary Innovation of Medical Technologies; Director, Musculoskeletal Biomechanics Research Lab, McGill University; Codirector, Orthopaedic Research Lab, Montreal General Hospital; Associate Member, Biomedical Engineering, McGill University; Professional Engineer with the Order of Engineers of Quebec, Canada

Peter A. Huijing, PhD
Professor Emeritus, Department of Human Movement Sciences, Faculty of Behavioural and Movement Sciences, Amsterdam Movement Sciences, Vrije Universiteit, Amsterdam, The Netherlands

Foreword by
Professor Andry Vleeming, PhD
Chairman, 11th Interdisciplinary World Congress on Low Back and Pelvic Girdle Pain, Melbourne, Australia, 2022

ELSEVIER

London New York Oxford Philadelphia St Louis Sydney 2022

Notices

Practitioners and researchers must always rely on their own experience and knowledge in evaluating and using any information, methods, compounds, or experiments described herein. Because of rapid advances in the medical sciences, in particular, independent verification of diagnoses and drug dosages should be made. To the fullest extent of the law, no responsibility is assumed by Elsevier, authors, editors, or contributors for any injury and/or damage to persons or property as a matter of products liability, negligence or otherwise, or from any use or operation of any methods, products, instructions, or ideas contained in the material herein.

ISBN: 978-0-7020-7183-6

Content Strategist: Poppy Garraway
Content Development Manager: Laurie Gower
Content Development Specialist: Sally Davies, Helen Leng
Project Manager: Julie Taylor
Design: Brian Salisbury
Illustration Manager: Muthukumaran Thangaraj
Marketing Manager: Ed Major

Printed in Scotland

Last digit is the print number   9   8   7   6   5   4   3   2

CONTENTS

FOREWORD

I am honored to welcome you to the second edition of *Fascia: The Tensional Network of the Human Body.*

The first edition was readily met with anticipation and was translated into five languages. If this was such a success, why then is a second edition necessary you may ask?

In the not so distant past, the world of fascia was, for the better part, neglected. If musculoskeletal research was comparable to moon exploration, then fascia research was not dissimilar to exploring the rest of the universe. Perhaps too focused on the moon, our predecessors failed to realize the importance of the poorly understood universe of this matrix. A continuous connective tissue matrix expanding and connecting every cell in the human body.

To be fair, much of this short-sightedness was not out of disinterest, but due to the lack of sophisticated techniques and equipment. As the scientific literature grew so did our enthusiasm to learn more. It is thanks to the collaboration of these authors who have devoted their time to uncover this observable universe and bring it to you neatly organized into this 2nd edition for us to enjoy.

While this edition will revisit the functional anatomy, physiology, biomechanics and neurology, it will also investigate more recent topics in the quest to connect the evidence-based science and its application. The addition of this new research gives an even deeper understanding into the multiple interactions this matrix has within the living human body. After all, the human body relies upon its *total* function and not the functions of single parts in isolation from others.

Our deepest appreciation is extended to all the authors who have helped in the contribution of this book. It will help us gain a better understanding into this once inadequately explored universe and it should further inspire us to enter dialogue and continue its investigation.

Prepare to broaden your horizons as you dive deeper into its fundamental secrets, I really hope you enjoy this book and above all, appreciate the beauty and the complexity of its architecture.

Professor Dr Andry Vleeming

ONLINE VIDEO RESOURCES

Besides the printed pages that you hold in your hands, this book goes along with an extensive data bank of video material that is available via Expert Consult. A number of the authors have used this website for posting instructive video sequences related to their chapter. Many of these videos include demonstrations and educational sequences of therapeutic applications, such as specific manual therapies or tool-assisted therapies directed at different fasciae. Other videos are in support of the basic science chapters related to the anatomy, physiology, and biomechanical properties of the fascial net. We happily invite all readers to access these videos early on during their orientation through the wealth of information and inspiration that this book provides. For full access to this website please register at Expert Consult using the details provided on the inside front cover.

Video contributors
Thomas W. Findley
Chris Frederick
Warren I. Hammer
Yasuo Kawakami
Thomas W. Myers
Andrzej Pilat
Robert Schleip
Antonio Stecco

VIDEO CONTENTS

CONTRIBUTORS

Amit Abraham, BPT, MAPhty, PhD
Assistant Professor,
Department of Physical Therapy,
Faculty of Health Sciences,
Ariel University,
Ariel, Israel

Marwan F. Abu-Hijleh, MD, PhD, MHPE
Head of Basic Medical Sciences,
Professor of Anatomy and Medical Education,
College of Medicine, Qatar University,
Doha, Qatar

Sue Adstrum, PhD, MSc
Integrative Anatomist, author and speaker,
Self-employed,
Auckland, New Zealand

Mariane Altomare, PT, MSc
CEO,
Physiotherapist/Manual Therapy,
ETRS Member,
Mariane Altomare Institute,
Rio de Janeiro, Brazil

Ricardo J. Andrade, PhD, PT
Research Fellow,
Menzies Health Institute Queensland,
Griffith Centre of Biomedical and Rehabilitation
    Engineering,
School of Health Sciences and Social Work,
Griffith University,
Brisbane and Gold Coast, Queensland, Australia

Katja Bartsch, BBA, BSc, MBA, BCSI
Yoga Teacher and Sports Scientist,
Kalamana Yoga and Fascia Research Charity
    Association,
Wendelstein, Bavaria;
PhD candidate,
Department of Sport Science and Sport, Exercise
    and Health,
Friedrich–Alexander University Erlangen–Nürnberg,
Erlangen, Bavaria, Germany

Carlo Biz, MD
Assistant Professor,
Orthopedic Clinic,
Department of Surgery, Oncology and
    Gastroenterology (DiSCOG),
University of Padua, Padua, Italy

Marie-José Blom, BA
Movement Educator and Pilates Master Teacher,
International Presenter and Lecturer,
Founder and Director of Somasom Inc.,
Breda, The Netherlands

Michele Bond, BA, MS
Published Fascia Researcher, Presenter, and Event Host,
Lead Biomechanical Analyst and Exercise Program
    Developer,
Michele Bond Enterprise,
Los Angeles, CA, USA

Benjamin S. Boyd, PT, DPTSc
Adjunct Associate Professor,
Department of Physical Therapy,
Samuel Merritt University,
Oakland, California, USA

Sicco A. Bus, PhD
Associate Professor,
Amsterdam University Medical Center,
University of Amsterdam,
Department of Rehabilitation Medicine,
Amsterdam Movement Sciences,
Amsterdam, The Netherlands

Joeri Calsius, PhD, MSc, MA, DO
Clinical Psychologist,
Body-Oriented Psychotherapist,
Osteopath, Physical Therapist,
Faculty of Rehabilitation Sciences,
University of Hasselt, Belgium

Monica Caspari, BN, RS
Certified Advanced Rolfer,
Rolf Movement Integration Practitioner,
Sao Paulo, Brazil;
Faculty member (retired),
Dr. Ida Rolf Institute of Structural Integration,
Boulder, Colorado, USA

Kelly Clancy, OTR/L, LMT
Educator and Rehabilitation Specialist,
Clinical Faculty,
University of Washington,
Rehabilitation Department,
Seattle, Washington, USA;
Occupational Therapist,
Colorado State University,
Fort Collins, Colorado, USA;
Structural Integrator,
Institute of Structural Medicine,
Twisp, Washington, USA;
International Bowen Instructor,
Bowtech Association of Australia

Bernie Clark, BSc
Yoga Educator and Author,
Vancouver, British Columbia, Canada

Michel W. Coppieters, PhD, PT
Menzies Foundation Professor of Allied Health
    Research,
Menzies Health Institute Queensland,
Griffith University,
Brisbane and Gold Coast, Australia;
Adjunct Professor,
Faculty of Behavioural and Movement Sciences,
Vrije Universiteit Amsterdam,
Amsterdam, The Netherlands

Kyra De Coninck, PhD
Lecturer in Sports Therapy and Rehabilitation,
School of Sport and Exercise Sciences,
University of Kent,
Canterbury, Kent, UK

Jean-Paul Delage, PhD
Laboratoire de Physiopathologie Mitochondriale,
Inserm U 1034 (Adaptation cardiovasculaire
    à l'ischémie),
Université Victor Segalen,
Bordeaux, France

Amol Sharad Dharap, MBBS, MS
(Former) Assistant Professor,
Department of Anatomy,
College of Medicine & Medical Sciences,
Arabian Gulf University, Manama, Bahrain

Jan Dommerholt, PT, DPT
Physical Therapist,
Bethesda Physiocare,
Bethesda, Maryland, USA;
Lecturer,
School of Medicine,
University of Maryland,
Baltimore, Maryland, USA

Mark Driscoll, Eng, PhD
Professor, Department of Mechanical Engineering,
McGill University,
Montreal, Quebec, Canada;
Canada NSERC Chair, Design Engineering
    for Interdisciplinary Innovation of Medical
    Technologies;
Director, Musculoskeletal Biomechanics Research Lab,
    McGill University;
Codirector, Orthopaedic Research Lab, Montreal
    General Hospital;
Associate member, Biomedical Engineering, McGill
    University;
Professional Engineer with the Order of Engineers of
    Quebec, Canada

Khaled El-Monajjed, JEng, PhD
Researcher,
Department of Mechanical Engineering,
McGill University,
Montreal, Quebec, Canada

Chenglei Fan, MD, PhD
Doctor,
Department of Neurosciences,
Institute of Human Anatomy,
University of Padua,
Padua, Italy

Caterina Fede, PhD
Postdoctoral Researcher,
Department of Neurosciences,
Institute of Human Anatomy,
University of Padua,
Padua, Italy

The late Thomas W. Findley, MD, PhD
Associate II Member, Cancer Institute of New Jersey;
Professor, Physical Medicine,
New Jersey Medical School,
Rutgers, the State University of New Jersey,
Newark, New Jersey, USA

Johannes Fleckenstein, Priv.-Doz., MD
Senior Researcher,
Sports Medicine and Exercise Physiology,
Goethe University Frankfurt,
Frankfurt, Germany

Eric Franklin, BFA, BS
Director,
Movement Education,
Institute for the Franklin Method,
Wetzikon, Switzerland

Chris Frederick, PT
Director,
Stretch to Win Institute,
Chandler, Arizona, USA

Roland U. Gautschi, MA, DipPT
Physiotherapist;
Senior Instructor in Triggerpoint Therapy IMTT®
    and Dry Needling Therapy IMTT®,
Baden, Switzerland

Federico Giordani, MD
Resident Doctor,
Institute of Physical Medicine and Rehabilitation,
Department of Neurosciences,
University of Padua,
Padua, Italy

Ling Guan, PhD
Professor,
Acupuncture and Moxibustion,
PLA General Hospital,
Beijing, China

Jean-Claude Guimberteau, MD
Plastic Surgeon and Hand Surgeon,
Cofounder and Scientific Director,
Institut Aquitain de la Main,
Pessac, France

Warren I. Hammer, DC, MS, DABCO
Adjunct Professor,
Postgraduate Faculty, Soft Tissue,
University of Bridgeport Department of Chiropractic,
Bridgeport, Connecticut, USA;
Adjunct Professor,
Certified instructor for Fascial Manipulation
    Association®
Instructor for www.handsonseminars.com

Elizabeth A. Hankinson, MPH, MHS, PA-C
Physician Assistant II,
Brigham & Women's Hospital,
Boston, Massachusetts, USA

**Mary Therese Hankinson, MBA, MS, RD, EDAC,
FACHE**
Adjunct Professor/Internship Coordinator,
Master of Healthcare Administration Program,
School of Health and Medical Sciences,
Seton Hall University,
Nutley, New Jersey, USA

Mohammad Haroon, MSc
PhD candidate,
Department of Human Movement Sciences,
Faculty of Behavioural and Movement Sciences,
Amsterdam Movement Sciences,
Vrije Universiteit Amsterdam,
Amsterdam, The Netherlands

Georg Harrer, MD
Past President,
European Fascial Distortion Model Association
    (EFDMA);
FDM Instructor, Private Practice;
Consultant in Anesthesiology and Intensive Medicine
Vienna, Austria

Philip F. Harris, MD, MSc, MBChB, FAS
Emeritus Professor of Anatomy,
University of Manchester,
Manchester, UK;
Teacher in Anatomy,
University of Nottingham Medical School,
Nottingham, UK

Katharina Helbig, BSc, MD
Assistant Doctor,
Department of Anesthesiology, Emergency Medicine,
    Intensive Care and Pain Therapy,
SRH Hospitals Sigmaringen,
Sigmaringen, Germany

Boris Hinz, PhD
Professor,
Laboratory of Tissue Repair and Regeneration, Faculty
    of Dentistry,
University of Toronto,
Toronto, Ontario, Canada

Ulrich Hoheisel, Dr. rer. nat.
Postdoctoral Researcher
Department of Neurophysiology,
Medical Faculty Mannheim,
University of Heidelberg,
Mannheim, Germany

Peter A. Huijing, PhD
Professor Emeritus,
Department of Human Movement Sciences,
Faculty of Behavioural and Movement Sciences,
Amsterdam Movement Sciences,
Vrije Universiteit Amsterdam,
Amsterdam, The Netherlands

Hidetaka Imagita, PhD, PT
Professor,
Basic Science & Biomechanics Laboratory,
Graduate School of Health Sciences,
Kio University,
Nara, Japan

Dominik Irnich, MD
Professor,
Multidisciplinary Pain Centre,
Department of Anesthesiology,
LMU University Hospital Munich,
Munich, Germany

Natasha Jacobson, BSc, P.Eng
PhD Candidate,
Department of Mechanical Engineering,
McGill University,
Montreal, Quebec, Canada

Marek Jantos, PhD
Director,
Behavioural Medicine,
Behavioural Medicine Institute of Australia,
Adelaide, South Australia, Australia

Heike Jäger, PhD
Institute of Applied Physiology,
University of Ulm,
Ulm, Germany

Richard T. Jaspers, PhD
Professor,
Department of Human Movement Sciences,
Faculty of Behavioural and Movement Sciences,
Amsterdam Movement Sciences,
Vrije Universiteit Amsterdam,
Amsterdam, The Netherlands

Yasuo Kawakami, PhD
Professor,
Faculty of Sport Sciences,
Waseda University,
Saitama, Japan

Christl Kiener
Doctor, Publisher, Editor, and Translator,
Kiener Press,
Munich, Germany

Hiroaki Kimura, MD
Director,
Medical Corporation Fascia Research Group and
    Kimura Pain Clinic;
President of Japanese Non-Surgical Orthopedics
    Society (JNOS),
Gunma, Japan

Hollis H. King, DO, PhD
Professor,
Department of Family Medicine and Public Health,
University of California San Diego School of Medicine,
San Diego, California, USA

Werner Klingler, MD, PhD
Physiologist and Anaesthesiologist;
Chair Department of Anesthesiology,
Emergency Medicine, Intensive Care, and Pain Therapy
  Academic SRH Hospitals Sigmaringen,
Germany;
Professor,
University of Ulm,
Germany;
Adjunct Professor,
Queensland University of Technology,
Brisbane, Australia

Tadashi Kobayashi, MD, PhD
Medical Lecturer,
Department of General Medicine,
Hirosaki University School of Medicine and Hospital,
Aomori, Japan;
Director, Head of Academic Department,
Japanese Non-Surgical Orthopedics Society (JNOS),
Gunma, Japan

Tiina Lahtinen-Suopanki, BHSc, PT
PT Lecturer,
Physiotherapy Department,
Orton Oy,
Helsinki, Finland

David Lesondak, BCSI, ATSI, FST
Fascia Specialist, Structural Integrator,
Center for Integrative Medicine,
University of Pittsburgh Medical Center (UPMC),
Pittsburgh, Pennsylvania, USA

Stephen M. Levin, BS, MD, FACS, FACOS
Director,
Ezekiel Biomechanics Group,
McLean, Virginia, USA

Torsten Liem, DO, MSc Ost, MSc Paed Ost
Academic Director,
Osteopathie Schule Deutschland GmbH,
Hamburg, Germany

Heidi Massa, BA, JD
Certified Advanced Rolfer, Rolf Movement Practitioner,
Dr. Ida Rolf Institute,
Boulder, Colorado, USA;
Registered Movement Educator,
International Somatic Movement Education and
  Therapy Association,
Chicago, IL, USA

Guido F. Meert, Dip PT
Physical Therapist,
Private Practice,
Schorndorf, Germany

Siegfried Mense, Prof. Dr. med.
Professor of Anatomy (retired),
Department of Neurophysiology,
Medical Faculty Mannheim,
Heidelberg University,
Mannheim, Germany

Divo G. Mueller, HP
Director,
Movement Education,
Somatics Academy GbR,
Munich, Germany

Hannes Müller-Ehrenberg, MD, PhD
Orthopedic Doctor,
Private Practice, Orthopädische Privatpraxis,
Münster, Germany

Thomas W. Myers, LMT
Director,
Anatomy Trains,
Walpole, Maine, USA

Ian L. Naylor, BPharm, MSc, PhD
Senior Lecturer in Pharmacology,
School of Pharmacy,
University of Bradford,
Bradford, UK

Robert J. Nee, PT, PhD, MAppSc
Professor,
Department of Physical Therapy,
Samuel Merritt University,
Oakland, California,
USA

Arya Nielsen, PhD
Assistant Clinical Professor,
Family Medicine & Community Health,
Icahn School of Medicine at Mount Sinai,
New York, New York, USA

Nathan Nyamsi Hendji, MSc
Laboratory of Innovation and Analysis of
    Bioperformance,
Mechanical Engineering,
Polytechnique Montréal,
Montreal, Quebec, Canada

James L. Oschman, BS, PhD
President,
Nature's Own Research Association,
Dover, New Hampshire, USA;
Professor,
Energy Medicine University,
Mill Valley, California, USA

Stephanie Otto, PhD
Sport Scientist (Diploma), Clinical Exercise
    Physiologist,
Exercise Oncology Service, Comprehensive Cancer
    Center Ulm (CCCU),
Ulm University Hospital,
Ulm, Germany;
Founding Member of the National Expert Group for
    Sports Therapy and Physical Activity in Oncology
    (NEBKO);
Speaker on the Hematology Panel;
Member of the German Cancer Society;
Section Editor, Exercise Oncology, Scientific Advisory
    Board, Competence Network Complementary
    Medicine in Oncology (KOKON);
Founding Member of the International Prehabilitation
    Society

Andrzej Pilat, PT
Physiotherapist and Manual Therapist;
International Lecturer;
Anatomy Researcher;
Director,
Tupimek Myofascial Therapy School,
Madrid, Spain

Carmelo Pirri, MD, PT
Medical Doctor, Physical and Rehabilitation Medicine;
    Physiotherapist;
PhD Student in Regenerative Medicine (Molecular
    Medicine),
Department of Neurosciences,
Institute of Human Anatomy, University of Padua,
Padua, Italy

Peter P. Purslow, BSc, PhD
Professor,
Departamento de Tecnología y Calidad de los Alimentos,
Universidad Nacional del Centro de la Provincia de
    Buenos Aires,
Tandil, Buenos Aires, Argentina

Jeni Saunders, MBBS, PhD, FACSEP, CCPU
Adjunct Associate Professor UNDA,
Sport and Exercise Physician,
Spine and Sportsmed,
Sydney, Australia

Graham Scarr, CBiol, FRSB, DO
Chartered Biologist,
Independent Researcher, UK;
Affiliate, Ezekiel Biomechanics Group,
McLean, Virginia, USA

Robert Schleip, MA, PhD
Director,
Fascia Research Project,
University of Ulm,
Ulm, Germany;
Research Director, European Rolfing Association;
Vice President of the Fascia Research Society;
Visiting Professor IUCS Barcelo;
Certified Rolfing & Feldenkrais Teacher

Fabiana Silva, PT, MSc
Professor of Physiotherapy,
Cirklo Health Education,
Porto Alegre, Rio Grande do Sul, Brazil;
Fascia Research Society Board Member,
Director of Fascia Research Center Brazil

**Jane Simmonds, MA, PGDip (Man Ther), BAS,
MCSP MMACP SFHEA**
Associate Professor,
Programme Lead: MSc Paediatric Physiotherapy,
Great Ormond Street Institute of Child Health,
University College London,
London, UK;
Physiotherapy Clinical Lead: London Hypermobility
    Unit,
Central Health Physiotherapy,
London, UK

Antonio Stecco, MD, PhD
Assistant Professor,
Rusk Rehabilitation,
New York University School of Medicine,
New York, New York, USA;
Certified Fascial Manipulation® Teacher

Carla Stecco, MD
Orthopedic Surgeon;
Professor of Human Anatomy,
University of Padua,
Padua, Italy;
Certified Fascial Manipulation® Teacher

Toru Taguchi, PT, DSc
Professor,
Department of Physical Therapy,
Institute for Human Movement and Medical Sciences,
Niigata University of Health and Welfare,
Niigata, Japan

Jörg Thomas, MD
Senior Physician,
Department of Anesthesiology,
University Children's Hospital Zurich,
Zurich, Switzerland

Frans van den Berg, PT, MT, OMT, BSc
Senior Instructor,
Orthopedic Manual Therapy,
Straßwalchen, Salzburg, Austria

Jaap van der Wal, MD, PhD
Retired Associate Professor in Anatomy & Embryology,
Maastricht University,
Maastricht, The Netherlands

Leonardo Sette Vieira, PT, CO
Postgraduate Physiotherapist and Osteopath,
School of Fascia,
Academia Brasileira de Fascias,
Juatuba, Minas Gerais, Brazil

Anna Maria Vitali, MD
Fascial Manipulation Therapist, Fascial Training Master
    Trainer, Pilates Master Teacher,
CEO and Founder,
Fisicamente Formazione,
Movement Education School,
Rome, Italy

Professor Andry Vleeming, PhD
Chairman,
11th Interdisciplinary World Congress on Low Back
    and Pelvic Girdle Pain,
Melbourne, Australia, 2022

Rainer Wander, MD
General Practitioner and Specialist in Chirotherapy,
    Manual Medicine, Specific Pain Therapy, Holistic
    Medicine, Acupuncture, and Neural Therapy,
Elsterberg, Germany;
Profesor Distinguido de la Universidad
    Mesoamericana, Guatemala

Frank H. Willard, MS, PhD
Professor of Anatomy,
University of New England,
Biddeford, Maine, USA

L'Hocine Yahia, PhD
Professor,
Department of Mechanical Engineering,
Polytechnique Montréal,
Montreal, Quebec, Canada

Tomasz Zagorski, MSc, MT, SB, CAFS
Senior Therapist and Researcher,
Senior Sports Physiotherapist,
International Lecturer,
Hands-On Training Institute,
Krakow, Poland;
Director,
European Watsu Centre,
Dobrociesz, Poland

Yoshihiro Zenita, MSc
Physiotherapist and Acupuncture Therapist;
CEO, Zenita Co. Ltd.;
Vice-President of Japanese Non-Surgical Orthopedics
    Society (JNOS),
Gunma, Japan

WELCOME TO THE WORLD OF FASCIA!

This book gives a comprehensive overview into a new field in musculoskeletal therapy and research: the fascinating world of fascia. Fascia forms a continuous tensional network throughout the human body, covering and connecting every single organ, every muscle, and even every nerve and tiny muscle fiber. After several decades of severe neglect, this "Cinderella of orthopedic science" is developing its own identity within medical research. The number of research papers on fascia in peer-reviewed journals has shown a steady rise. The first International Fascia Research Congress, held at the Conference Center, Harvard Medical School, in October 2007 was followed by a series of subsequent events of the same lineage in Amsterdam (2009), Vancouver (2012), Washington (2015), and Berlin (2018), attracting a multidisciplinary international audience of researchers and clinicians and reaching up to 1000 attendants per congress. Like the rapidly growing field of glia research in neurology, this underestimated contextual tissue—fascia—is being found to play an important role in health and pathology.

Hypotheses that accord myofascia a central role in the mechanisms of therapies have been advanced for some time in the fields of acupuncture, massage, structural integration, chiropractic, and osteopathy. Practitioners in these disciplines, especially those who do not have the longevity of osteopathy or chiropractic, are generally unaware of the scientific basis for evaluating such hypotheses. Many practitioners are unaware of the sophistication of current laboratory research equipment and methods. Laboratory researchers, in turn, may be unaware of the clinical phenomena that suggest avenues of exploration. Several decades ago, the study of physical medicine and rehabilitation included muscle strengthening, anatomy, exercise physiology, and other aspects of therapeutic modalities. What was notably less present in the scientific and medical literature was how to understand and treat disorders of the fascia and connective tissues. Since then, much additional information has been developed, particularly during recent years (Fig. 0.1).

The purpose of this book is to organize relevant information for scientists involved in the research of the body's connective tissue matrix (fascia) and for professionals involved in the therapeutic manipulation of this body-wide structural fabric. Though it grew out of materials presented at the International Fascia Research Congress series (www.fasciacongress.org), this book reflects the efforts of almost 100 scientists and clinicians.

NOT ONLY A PACKING ORGAN

As every medical student knows and every doctor still remembers, fascia is introduced in anatomy dissection courses as the white packing stuff that one first needs to clean off in order "to see something." Similarly, anatomy books have been competing, in how clean and orderly they present the locomotor system, by cutting away the whitish or semitranslucent fascia as completely and skillfully as possible. Students appreciate these appealing graphic simplifications, with shiny red muscles, each attaching to specific skeletal points. However, these simplified maps do not fully describe how the real body feels and behaves, whether it be in medical surgery or during therapeutic palpation.

To give an example, in real bodies, muscles hardly ever transmit their full force directly via tendons into the skeleton, as is usually suggested by textbook drawings. They, rather, distribute a large portion of their contractile or tensional forces onto fascial sheets. These sheets transmit the forces to synergistic and antagonistic muscles. Thereby they stiffen not only the respective joint but may even affect regions several joints away. The simple questions discussed in musculoskeletal textbooks—"which muscles" are participating in a particular movement—thus become almost obsolete. Muscles are not functional units no matter how common this misconception may be. Rather, most muscular movements are generated by many individual motor units that are distributed over some portions of one

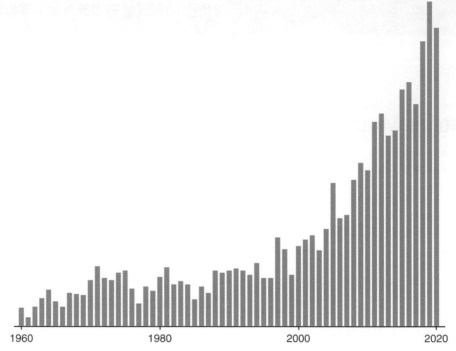

Fig. 0.1 Number of peer reviewed scientific publications on fascia. Papers indexed in PubMed with the word "fascia" in the title have grown from 10 to 20 per year in the 1960s to over 200 in 2020.

muscle, plus other portions of other muscles. The tensional forces of these motor units are then transmitted to a complex network of fascial sheets, bags, and strings that convert them into the final body movement.

Similarly, it has been shown that fascial stiffness and elasticity play a significant role in many ballistic movements of the human body. First discovered by studies of the calf tissues of kangaroos, antelopes, and later by horses, modern ultrasound studies have revealed that fascial recoil plays, in fact, a similarly impressive role in many of our human movements. How far you can throw a stone, how high you can jump, how long you can run, depends not only on the contraction of your muscle fibers; it also depends to a large degree on how well the elastic recoil properties of your fascial network are supporting these movements.

If the architecture of our fascial network is indeed such an important factor in musculoskeletal behavior, why has this tissue been overlooked for such a long time? There are several answers to this question. The development of new imaging and research tools now allows us to study this tissue in vivo. Another reason is

that this tissue resists the classical method of anatomical research: that of splitting something into separate parts that can be counted and named. You can reasonably estimate the number of bones or muscles, yet any attempt to count the number of fasciae in the body will be futile. The fascial body is one large networking organ, with many bags and hundreds of rope-like local densifications, and thousands of pockets within pockets, all interconnected by sturdy septa and by looser connective tissue layers.

WHAT IS FASCIA?

This varied nature of fascia is reflected in the many different definitions of which exact tissue types are included under the term "fascia." The International Anatomical Nomenclature Committee (1983) confirmed the usage of previous nomenclature committees and used the term "fascia superficialis" for the loose layer of subcutaneous tissue lying superficial to the denser layer of "fascia profunda." While most medical authors in English-speaking countries followed that terminology, it was not congruently adopted by authors in other countries. The nomenclature proposed by the Federative Committee on Anatomical Terminology (1998) therefore attempted to lead toward a more uniform international language (Wendell-Smith 1997). It suggested that authors should no longer use the term fascia for loose connective tissue layers, such as the former "superficial fascia," and should instead apply it only to denser connective tissue aggregations.

However, this attempt failed significantly (Huijing and Langevin 2009). Many anatomical textbooks continued to use the term "superficial fascia" to describe subcutaneous tissues. Similarly, there has been confusion on the question of which of the three hierarchical muscular tissue bags—epimysium, perimysium, and endomysium—could be included as fascia. While most authors would agree to consider muscular septi and the perimysium (which is often quite dense, particularly in tonic muscles) as fascial tissues, there is less consensus on the endomysial envelopes around single muscle fibers based on their much looser density and higher quantity of collagen types III and IV. However, almost all authors emphasize the important continuity of these intramuscular connective tissues. So where does fascia stop?

Another area, still to be resolved, is the visceral connective tissues. For some authors the term fascia is restricted to muscular connective tissues. Visceral connective tissues—no matter if they are of loose composition like the major omentum or more ligamentous like the mediastinum—are often excluded. In contrast, more clinically oriented books have placed a lot of emphasis on the visceral fasciae (Paoletti 2006; Schwind 2006).

As valuable as these proposed anatomical distinctions within soft connective tissues are, their very detail may lead to unwitting exclusion of important tissue continuities that are only perceived on the larger scale. For example, the clinical significance of the continuity of the fascia of the scalene muscles of the neck with the pericardium and mediastinum inside the thorax is often surprising in our discussions with orthopedic surgeons, although less so to osteopaths or general surgeons. Figure 0.2 shows another example of perceptual tissue exclusion based on terminological distinction. Here one of the sturdiest portions of the iliotibial tract has been excluded from this important tissue band, because it did not fit the distinct nomenclature defined by the authors of this paper.

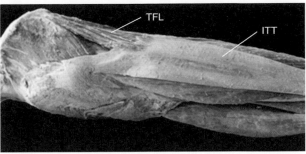

Fig. 0.2 Example of a fascia dissection based on specific terminology. This dissection was used in an otherwise excellent treatise on the iliotibial tract (ITT). Following the proposal of the Federative Committee on Anatomical Terminology (1998) to distinguish between aponeuroses and fasciae, the authors chose to describe this tissue as an aponeurosis. Congruent with this decision, their dissection and illustration therefore excluded all tissue portions with a nonaponeurotic character. Unfortunately this included one of the most dense and most important portions of the iliotibial tract: the connection to the lateral iliac crest, posterior of the anterior superior iliac spine. Notice the common thickening of the iliac crest at the former attachment of this ligamentous portion (located at a straight force transmission line from the knee over the greater trochanter), reflecting the very strong pull of this tissue portion on the pelvis. TFL, tensor fascia lata. Reproduced with permission from Benjamin, M., Kaiser, E., Milz, S., 2008. Structure–function relationships in tendons: a review. J. Anat. 212, 211–228.

Based on this background, the Fascia Research Society established a Fascia Nomenclature Committee in 2013 to advance related discussions and clarifications. This committee conducted a Delphi process, as an interactive structured communication technique among international experts to facilitate a potential consensus agreement over several years. This process culminated in the recommendation of two different usages of the term fascia. While the first one is recommended for description of histological details and of small-scale topographical relationships, the second usage is recommended for the description of larger functional properties, such as muscular force transmission, fibrotic processes, or sensory capacities (such as proprio-, intero-, or nociception) within the fascial net.

A fascia is a sheath, a sheet, or any other dissectible aggregations of connective tissue that forms beneath the skin to attach, enclose, and separate muscles and other internal organs (Stecco and Schleip 2016).

The fascial system consists of the three-dimensional continuum of soft, collagen-containing, loose, and dense fibrous connective tissues that permeate the body. It incorporates elements such as adipose tissue, adventitiae and neurovascular sheaths, aponeuroses, deep and superficial fasciae, epineurium, joint capsules, ligaments, membranes, meninges, myofascial expansions, periostea, retinacula, septa, tendons, visceral fasciae, and all the intramuscular and intermuscular connective tissues, including endo-, peri-, and epimysium. The fascial system surrounds, interweaves between, and interpenetrates all organs, muscles, bones, and nerve fibers, endowing the body with a functional structure and providing an environment that enables all body systems to operate in an integrated manner (Stecco et al. 2018).

Note that the first usage is largely congruent with the *Terminologia Anatomica* of the Federative International

Programme for Anatomical Terminology (FIPAT). In contrast, the second recommendation has been largely adopted by an increasing number of researchers and clinicians in the fascia field to permit the discussion of larger functional relationships within the fascial system (Fig. 03). This wider understanding of the term "the fascial net" then describes those tissue expressions within the larger category of connective tissues whose architecture appears to be primarily shaped by tensional rather than compressive loading demands (Fig. 0.4). This textbook has undertaken the task of serving both perspectives, the one more narrow and focused perspective of a histologist looking at "a fascia," and also the wider and more functional perspective of a yoga or dance instructor talking about tensional force transmission within "the fascial net." Even if sometimes microscopic details of collagenous tissues are explored, an effort will be made to always relate these findings to the body as a whole. The reader will easily recognize the various perspectives taken by the authors of the following chapters.

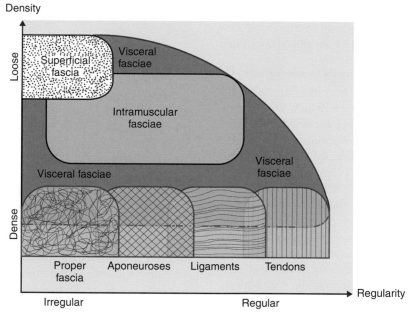

Fig. 0.3 Different connective tissues considered here as fascial tissues. Fascial tissues differ in terms of their density and directional alignment of collagen fibers. For example, superficial fascia is characterized by a loose density and a mostly multidirectional or irregular fiber alignment; whereas in the denser tendons or ligaments the fibers are mostly unidirectional. Note that the intramuscular fasciae—septi, perimysium, and endomysium—may express varying degrees of directionality and density. The same is true—although to a much larger degree—for the visceral fasciae (including soft tissues like the omentum majus and tougher sheets like the pericardium). Depending on local loading history, proper fasciae can express a two-directional or multidirectional arrangement. Not shown here are retinacula and joint capsules, whose local properties may vary between those of ligaments, aponeuroses, and proper fasciae.

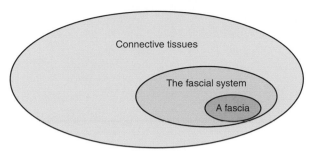

Fig. 0.4 The terminology of the Fascia Nomenclature Committee recommends the term "the fascial net" (also called "fascial system" by some authors) for a subset of tissues belonging to the connective tissue system of the body. Additionally, the phrase "a fascia" (also called "proper fascia" by some authors) describes a subset of tissues within the larger category of "the fascial system."

Note that the current second edition of this textbook contains many additions and revisions compared with the first edition published in 2012. This is because of rapid development in this newly established life science field within the time span of nine years between these editions. This is reflected in many new and completely revised chapters, both within the theoretical foundation section of the book and within the description of clinical applications.

This textbook, as have the fascia congresses, has taken the difficult role of being oriented toward both the scientist and the clinician. Material presented spans anatomy and physiology of fascia in Section I, through clinical conditions and therapies in Section II, to recently developed research techniques in Section III. We have pointed out the definitional struggles the researcher faces surrounding fascia: Which tissue? Which fiber directions? What is connected to what? These research tools will allow the extension of this debate to more clinical areas as well, to help define which tissues are affected and in which directions forces are applied in the clinical therapies. It is our hope that clinicians and scientists, both together and separately, will rise to these challenges to advance our basic understanding and our clinical treatment of fascia.

REFERENCES

Benjamin, M., Kaiser, E., Milz, S., 2008. Structure–function relationships in tendons: a review. J. Anat. 212, 211–228.

Federative Committee on Anatomical Terminology, 1998. Terminologia Anatomica. Thieme, Stuttgart.

Huijing, P.D., Langevin, H.M., 2009. Communicating about fascia: history, pitfalls and recommendations. Int. J. Ther. Massage Bodywork. 2, 3–8.

International Anatomical Nomenclature Committee, 1983. Nomina Anatomica, fifth ed. Williams & Wilkins, Baltimore.

Paoletti, S., 2006. The Fasciae: Anatomy, Dysfunction and Treatment. Eastland Press, Seattle.

Schwind, P., 2006. Fascial and Membrane Technique: A Manual for Comprehensive Treatment of the Connective Tissue System. Elsevier, Edinburgh.

Stecco, C., Schleip, R., 2016. A fascia and the fascial system. J. Bodyw. Mov. Ther. 20, 139–140.

Stecco, C., Adstrum, S., Hedley, G., Schleip, R., Yucesoy, C.A. 2018. Update on fascial nomenclature. J. Bodyw. Mov. Ther. 22, 354.

Wendell Smith, C.P., 1997. Fascia: an illustrative problem in international terminology. Surg. Radiol. Anat. 19, 273–277.

SECTION I

Scientific Foundations

Robert Schleip and Peter A. Huijing

PART 1

Topographical Anatomy

Evolution of Fascia-Focused Anatomy

Sue Adstrum

CHAPTER CONTENTS

INTRODUCTION

History shows that the construction of knowledge is an incremental process accomplished by many people over an extended period of time. One example of this happening is the evolving anatomical knowledge of fascia.

Present-day understandings of fascia, as in this book's chapters, are built on a platform assembled from our fascia-relating forebears' premises and discoveries. From a historical perspective, these ancestors are some of the "giants" upon whose shoulders we metaphorically now stand. If we hope to see as much, more, or even farther than they did, it makes sense to review what they knew, especially as their work is rarely acknowledged by contemporary writers.

Progress is part of a continuum. It depends on the past in order to move forward. Otherwise, as George Santayana warns, "there remains no being to improve and no direction is set for possible improvement" (1905, 284). This chapter summarizes some of what was written about fascia prior to the 21st century in the hope that it may help us understand it more fully, now and into the future.

ANATOMY

Anatomy is the study of the body's physical structure. The word *anatomy* is etymologically derived from Greek ἀνατομία (*anatomia*), meaning a cutting up, or dissection.

Human bodies are complex and extremely difficult to describe in their naturally whole condition. Anatomists have therefore needed to subdivide them, both literally and figuratively, into manageable pieces, all of which can be recognized and explained within certain lived-world settings. In practice, anatomization (the hypothetical and physical deconstruction of animal and human bodies) makes it possible to comprehend the structure, topographic positioning, physical properties, and concerted workings of the body's constituent "parts."

Anatomical knowledge is created and interpreted by people. Different sets of anatomical knowledge (anatomies) are shaped by many factors, including: their proponents' theoretic assumptions, methodological standpoint, selection of research methods and materials, and manner of publishing their findings, together with the sociocultural (e.g., political, epistemic, disciplinary, professional) and time-based environments in which the research is performed and utilized. Consequently, there are many ways of describing human anatomy that are not always entirely commensurable or in agreement and are likely to change over time.

Anatomy is important. Anatomical information about the structure, location, and architectural arrangement of the body and its parts is a prerequisite to explaining how those parts work, separately and together, and how they are associated with injury and disease. From ancient times to the present, anatomy has been an important cornerstone of medical and surgical theory and praxis. Even though the connection between anatomy and medicine is accompanied by intermediary understandings of physiology and pathology, this does not diminish the fact that anatomical knowledge is extremely useful to humanity.

KEY POINTS

- Anatomy is the evolving study of the body's physical structure.
- Present-day knowledge of fascia relies on a scaffold of earlier anatomical discoveries.
- Progress depends on remembering and then continuing to build on previous learning.

ANCIENT AWARENESS OF FASCIA

Medical writers have referred to the body's fascial parts since the Egyptian pyramid age, approximately 3000–2500 years before the Common Era (BCE). The first documented reference to fascia[a] appears in an ancient

---

[a]*Fascia* is a generic anatomical term that, within this chapter, broadly refers to the body's soft fibrous connective tissue parts (Adstrum et al. 2017; Stecco et al. 2018).

Egyptian manuscript, which observes that meningeal membranes can rupture when the skull is badly fractured (Breasted 1930). Around 600 BCE, fascia was identified as a type of connective tissue in an Ayurvedic text on medicine and surgery (Susruta and Bhishagratna 1911). Fascia's anatomical depiction has continued to develop since then (see Table 1.1.1).

Ancient Greek writers (including Hippocrates, Aristotle, Diocles, Herophilus, and Erasistratus) were anatomically acquainted with, and distinguished between, ligaments, tendons, and the membranes that covered and surrounded, for example, the brain, the heart, and the unborn fetus (Adstrum 2015a; Adstrum and Nicholson 2019). Much of their writing was subsequently lost, unfortunately obscuring how much they knew about these body parts, the methods they used to study them, and the terminology they used to describe them.

English translations of Roman physician Galen of Pergamon's (Fig. 1.1.1) writing reveal his familiarity with *aponeuroses*, *membranous aponeuroses*, *membranous fasciae*, *fascial tendons*, *membranes*, *membranous processes*, and *membranous tendons*, as well as his possible use of the term *fascia* when discussing the origins and insertions of muscles (Adstrum 2015a; Adstrum and Nicholson 2019).

Historical Era	Anatomy Research Context	A Few of "The Giants" Who Helped Develop Anatomical Knowledge of Fascia in the Past
TABLE 1.1.1 Fascia's Anatomical Depiction has Evolved in Conjunction with Advances in Research Technology and Time-Based Change in the Human Environments in Which the Research is Conducted and Applied		
Ancient Greece c. 800–150 BCE	• Spiritual and secular medical doctrine. Body's constitution and functioning related to humoral theory. • Anatomical observation of body interior via wounds, surgery, and occasional anatomical dissection. • Anatomical information recorded in handwritten/copied manuscripts. Many later lost.	• **Hippocrates of Kos** (c. 460–370 BCE) Physician. Established medicine as a clinical profession, separate from religion and philosophy. Hippocratic corpus of medical literature contains numerous references to the membranes surrounding organs, ligaments, and tendons. • **Aristotle** (384–322 BCE) Philosopher and scientist. Established anatomy as a distinct branch of knowledge.
Ancient Rome c. 750 BCE– 480 CE	• Spiritual and secular medical doctrine. Humoral theory. • Anatomical dissection mostly used animal subjects. Human dissection forbidden after c. 200 CE.	• **Claudius Galenus** (aka **Galen of Pergamon**) (130–210 CE) Greek-born Roman physician and anatomist. Dissected animals. Writing routinely mentioned aponeuroses, fasciae, membranes, tendons. (Fig. 1.1.1)

Continued

TABLE 1.1.1   Fascia's Anatomical Depiction has Evolved in Conjunction with Advances in Research Technology and Time-Based Change in the Human Environments in Which the Research is Conducted and Applied—cont'd

Historical Era	Anatomy Research Context	A Few of "The Giants" Who Helped Develop Anatomical Knowledge of Fascia in the Past
Medieval or Middle Ages c. CC 5–15	• Spiritual and secular medical doctrine. Humoral theory. • Medicine practiced by academic physicians. By the 13th century, bloodletting, scarification, pulling of teeth, treatment of war wounds, amputations, and surgeries usually performed by barber-surgeons. • Classical (Hippocratic-Galenic) anatomy— philosophical and congruent with Christian church beliefs. • Memorizable aphorisms extracted from classical texts were used to verbally transmit medical knowledge, as books were not widely available. • Emperor Frederick II (1238) required surgeons to study anatomy and ordered a public dissection be performed every 5 years at the Salerno medical school.	• **Rabbi Moshe ben Maimon** (aka **Maimonides** Abü Imrān Müsā ibn Maymün ibn Ubayd Allāh) (1135–1204) Spanish-born Jewish philosopher and physician. Compiled approximately 1,500 medical aphorisms based on Galen's teachings, some of which mention and distinguish between membranes, ligaments, and tendons.
European Renaissance c. CC 14–17 14th–16th centuries associated with refreshed interest in studying classical texts and testing their doctrinal accuracy. 16th–17th centuries characterized by emerging confidence in experimental and mathematical evidence.	• Spiritual and secular medical doctrine. Humoral theory. • Human dissection by certified anatomists increasingly used to augment medical education. Dissection initially performed by a 3-member team—a lector/lecturer, a sector/ dissector, and an ostensor who pointed to relevant body parts. Reinforced classical anatomy doctrine. • Invention of mechanical moving type printing press (c. 1440) enabled mass production of vernacular language publications at a reasonable cost and speed. Helped boost scholarly and public discussion about anatomy. • Galen's and Mondino's anatomical authority began to be empirically tested and improved upon during 17th century, notably by Vesalius. • Increasingly accurate illustrations (e.g., as commissioned by Vesalius) helped disseminate anatomical information. • Emergence of secular trade guilds (e.g., Company of Barber-Surgeons, 1540) and academic societies (e.g., Lincean Academy, 1603; Royal Society of London, 1660; French Academy of Sciences, 1666) fostered scientific anatomical knowledge development.	• **Mondino de Luzzi** (aka **Mundinus**) (c. 1270– 1326) Italian physician, surgeon, and anatomist. Restored study of anatomy as a distinct discipline. Performed first public dissection in Italy in 1315. Wrote first modern anatomy text in 1316, reiterating classical (Hippocratic-Galenic) anatomical knowledge. • **Guy de Chauliac** (aka **Guido de Cauliaco**) (c. 1300–1368). French physician, surgeon, and classical anatomist. Maintained that surgeons required a thorough knowledge of anatomy. Innovatively combined anatomical, medical, and surgical information in his writing. • **Jacapo Berengario da Carpi** (aka **Carpus**) (c. 1460–1530) Italian physician and classical anatomist. His *Isagoge brevis* (1535, 6–10) diagrammatically displays the membranous layers beneath the abdominal skin. • **Thomas Vicary** (1490–1561) English physician, surgeon, and classical anatomist. Compiled first English-language anatomy textbook/dissection guide (1577/1586). Differentiates between membranes (*cotes, pannicles, skinnes*), ligaments, and tendons (*cordes*).

TABLE 1.1.1 Fascia's Anatomical Depiction has Evolved in Conjunction with Advances in Research Technology and Time-Based Change in the Human Environments in Which the Research is Conducted and Applied—cont'd

Historical Era	Anatomy Research Context	A Few of "The Giants" Who Helped Develop Anatomical Knowledge of Fascia in the Past
	• René Descartes's mid-17th century philosophical distinction between body and mind supported strengthening belief in an empirically explainable physicochemical-biological body form. • Robert Hooke (mid-17th century) discovered microscopic empty compartments (*cells*) in cork bark. This term was in time used to describe the tiny spaces in *cellular substance*. • Improving design of optical lenses, and late 17th century development of rudimentary microscopes, enabled closer examination of human tissue.	• **Andreas Vesal** (aka **Andreas Vesalius**) (1514–1564) Flemish anatomist. Founder of modern scientific human anatomy. Used human dissection as research tool. Corrected several of Galen's incorrect animal-dissection-based anatomical assumptions. Pioneered use of accurate anatomical illustrations (1543/1998). • **Helkiah Crooke** (1576–1648) English physician and anatomist. Conceivably the first English medical writer to use the term *fascia* (1615, 1631/1651). Related body's membrane system to a set of taxonomic categories. Described the universal touch-sensitive membrane system as the body's *organ of touching*. • **Francis Glisson** (1597–1677) English physician. Anatomically exposed the fibrous tissue endoskeleton within, and fibrous capsule surrounding (ep. Glisson's capsule), the liver (1654). • **Thomas Bartholin** (aka **Bartholinus**) (1616–1680) Danish physician and scholar. Anatomical illustrations show membranes that cover and surround several parts of the body (1655). • **Samuel Collins** (1618–1710) English physician and anatomist. Comprehensively described membranes and their rudimentary tissue structure (1685). (Fig. 1.1.2) • **Marcello Malpighi** (aka **Malpighius**) (1628–1694) Italian physician, physiologist, and biologist. Founder of microscopic anatomy. Microscopy helped him make many original anatomical discoveries, including the very thin membranes inside the lungs, spleen and liver, and areolar spaces in omental connective tissue.

Continued

TABLE 1.1.1 Fascia's Anatomical Depiction has Evolved in Conjunction with Advances in Research Technology and Time-Based Change in the Human Environments in Which the Research is Conducted and Applied—cont'd

Historical Era	Anatomy Research Context	A Few of "The Giants" Who Helped Develop Anatomical Knowledge of Fascia in the Past
Age of Enlightenment c. C 18 Increasing appreciation of empiricism and rational thought. Popularization of science beyond educated elite.	• Medical humoralism declining. Rise in secular medical doctrine. Disease progressively linked to microbial rather than humoral causation (germ theory). • Progressively more powerful microscopes enable discovery of miniscule fibers and living cells within human tissue; advancing description of *cellular* (loose connective) *tissue*. • Human anatomical dissection became an expected part of medical and surgical education, contributing to expanding demand for suitable cadavers.	• **Frederik Ruysch** (1638–1731) Dutch botanist and anatomist. Developed methods for preparing and embalming body parts and corpses that enabled lengthier anatomical examination of cadaveric fascia. • **Jacob Benignus WinslØw** (aka **Jacques-Bénigne Winslow**) (1669–1760) Danish-born French anatomist. Famously distinguished between *fascia lata* (a ligamentary covering) and *musculus fasciae latae* (a small muscle), thus rectifying ambiguous interpretation of *fascia lata*. • **Bernhard Siegfried Albinus** (1697–1770) German-born Dutch anatomist. Used injection and inflation techniques developed by Swammerdam and Ruysch to show areolar spaces in cellular substance. • **Albrecht von Haller** (aka **Albertus de Haller**) (1708–1777) Swiss anatomist and physiologist. Comprehensively described the constitution and structure of soft fibrous connective tissue through use of microscopy and physiological experimentation (1754). • **Antonio Scarpa** (1752–1832) Italian surgeon and anatomist. Anatomically described membranous layer of fascia investing abdominal wall (ep. Scarpa's fascia) and cremasteric fascia (ep. Scarpa's sheath). Many highly detailed anatomical plates in his books show evidence of fascia and/or myofascial connectivity. (Fig. 1.1.3) • **Marie-François Xavier Bichat** (1771–1802) French anatomist, pathologist. Father of histology. Explored links between body's structure, functioning, and pathology. His treatise on membranes (1800/1813) was ostensibly the first book explicitly devoted to the scientific description of membranes (i.e., fascia). (Fig. 1.1.4)

TABLE 1.1.1 **Fascia's Anatomical Depiction has Evolved in Conjunction with Advances in Research Technology and Time-Based Change in the Human Environments in Which the Research is Conducted and Applied—cont'd**

Historical Era	Anatomy Research Context	A Few of "The Giants" Who Helped Develop Anatomical Knowledge of Fascia in the Past
Age of Science and Technology c. CC 19–20 Prevailing belief that systematic scientific inquiry is the best way of obtaining reliable knowledge, in tandem with continual advances in research technology. Late C 20 Hypothetically disembodied scientific objectivity, and its hegemonic authority, beginning to be questioned in poststructural scholarly environments.	• Secular medical doctrine. • Development of formaldehyde-containing anatomical embalming fluids linked to description of many newly identified sections of fascia (fasciae), and an attendant expansion in fascia-relating terminology. • Emergent science of histology (along with innovation of tissue fixation and specimen-mounting techniques, high precision microtome, hematoxylin and eosin staining) enabled closer examination of fascial tissue, yet also dehydrated, distorted, and damaged it. • X-rays used for medical imaging since 1895. Highlighted bones, yet generally failed to show fascial body parts. • 20th-century emergence of new medical and surgical specialisms (e.g., physiatry, reconstructive and cosmetic surgery), with varying fascia-related anatomical knowledge requirements. • Advent of anatomy subdisciplines (e.g., microscopic anatomy, clinical anatomy, radiological anatomy). Relatively declining emphasis on traditional gross (i.e., macroscopic) anatomical description. • Invention of medical ultrasonography (1953), computed tomography (1971), and magnetic resonance imaging (1971); subsequently used as fascia research tools. • More powerful microscopes, intracellular and biomolecular imaging instruments enable body's structural complexity to be explained in an increasingly reductive manner. • Fascia usually "cleaned" away in dissection lab as obscured view of other, seemingly more important body parts. Minimally described (if at all) in preregistration anatomy training of health professionals (e.g., doctors, dentists, physiotherapists, nurses). Barely mentioned in undergraduate anatomy textbooks. Rarely related to professional principles and practices.	• **Jean Cruveilhier** (1791–1874) French anatomist and pathologist. Wrote at length about fascia under heading of *Aponeurology* (1844, 294–320). Ep. Cruveilhier's fascia (superficial fascia of perineum). (Fig. 1.1.5) • **John Davidson Godman** (1794–1830) American anatomist. Wrote *Anatomical Investigations Comprising Descriptions of Various Fasciæ of the Human Body* (1824). Ep. Godman's fascia (clavipectoral fascia). (Fig. 1.1.6) • **Jean-Baptiste Marc Jean Bourgery** (1797–1849) French physician and anatomist. His eight-volume human anatomy atlas was famed for its highly detailed illustrations, some of which explicitly portray fascia. • **Henry Gray** (1827–1861) English anatomist and surgeon. Wrote first edition of *Anatomy: Descriptive and Surgical* (1858), which influentially bracketed description of muscle and fascia. • **Andrew Taylor Still** (1828–1917) American physician and anatomist. Founded osteopathic medicine. Emphasized universality of fascia and its centrality to life (1899). • **Bern Gallaudet** (1860–1934) American anatomist and surgeon. Described fascial planes in abdomen, pelvis, and perineum based on his own research (1931). Ep. Gallaudet's fasciae (superficial investing fasciae of abdomen and perineum). • **Giuseppe Sterzi** (1876–1919) Italian anatomist, neuroanatomist, and medical historian. Author of the first anatomical report dedicated to describing superficial fascia (1910). Explains subcutaneous tissue is divided into two (superficial and deep) layers. • **Herbert Charles Orrin** (1878–1963) British plastic surgeon. Described emergent use of fascial grafting to treat war and orthopedic injuries (1928). • **Edward Singer** (–1982) American anatomist. Wrote *Fasciæ of the Human Body and Their Relations to the Organs They Envelop* (1935).

Continued

TABLE 1.1.1   Fascia's Anatomical Depiction has Evolved in Conjunction with Advances in Research Technology and Time-Based Change in the Human Environments in Which the Research is Conducted and Applied—cont'd

Historical Era	Anatomy Research Context	A Few of "The Giants" Who Helped Develop Anatomical Knowledge of Fascia in the Past
	• Emergence/empowerment of manual, exercise, and movement therapy–based health professions (e.g., massage therapy, osteopathy, physical therapy, yoga teaching), with varying fascia-related anatomical knowledge requirements. • Emergence of fascia-relating bodywork modalities, including structural integration, myofascial release therapy, trigger point therapy, craniosacral therapy (and many others). • Late 20th C, anatomy textbooks shift from gross anatomical description of separate body systems (where fascia was assumed to be largely redundant) toward description of interlocking systems (i.e., fascia-inclusive body regions), as the latter is more applicable to medical and surgical care of the bodies of living, rather than dead, people. • Fascia increasingly being discussed by nonmedical scientific and clinical writers employing holistic/heuristic (as well as, or instead of) reductionist/descriptive ideological perspectives.	• **J Walter Wilson** (1896–1969). American biologist. Comprehensively explained evolving anatomical understanding of *cellular* (fascial) *tissue* (1944). • **International Anatomical Nomenclature Committee** (1903–). Helped rationalize fascia-relating anatomical language via a series of democratically developed nomenclature lists and is continuing to do so. • **Donald L Stilwell, Jr.** (20th century) American anatomist. Seminally described innervation of deep fasciae and aponeuroses (1957). • **Frank H Netter** (1906–1991) American surgeon and medical illustrator. Many of his pictures (Netter, 1997; first published in 1989) show evidence of fascial tissue that was then regularly obliterated during dissection. • **RJ (Bill) Heald** (20th–21st century) English colorectal surgeon. Described "Holy Plane" (ep. Heald's Holy Plane), a colorectal surgical plane—that is, "a potential space between contiguous organs which can be reproducibly created by dissection" (1988). • **Colin Wendell-Smith** (1942–2015) Australian anatomist. Emphasized importance of accurately naming, and scientifically distinguishing, between fasciae (1997). • **Ted E. Lockwood** (1945–2005) American plastic surgeon. Described anatomy of human superficial fascial system (1991).

Abbreviations: aka, also known as; BCE, before Common Era; CE, Common Era; c., circa, approximately; C/CC, century/centuries; Ep., eponym.

There was a general slowing in anatomical knowledge development during the European Middle Ages. A number of important Greco-Roman medical texts were preserved in monasteries and convents, and also within the Indian and Islamic medical worlds, yet many others were lost. Galen's were possibly the only, out of the many formerly written, anatomy texts that survived through this era, which helped protract his anatomical authority for the next 1500 years (Cunningham 2010).

The 12th-century establishment of the first European universities heralded a widespread reawakening of interest in intellectual knowledge development that eventually resulted in realization that anatomy is best taught in conjunction with human dissection. During the following 200 years, several European countries legalized the dissection of judicially executed criminals to augment the education of surgeons. In the 14th century, some universities began to sponsor public anatomy exhibitions, where an unembalmed corpse was dissected over three consecutive, cold wintertime days. The standard abdomen-chest-head dissection sequence followed the order that these cavities' contents were corrupted by decay and generally ignored the limbs.

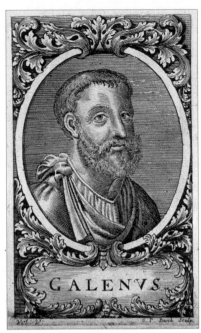

Fig. 1.1.1 Galen of Pergamon (130–210). An 18th-century engraved portrait by Georg Paul Busch. Available at: https://en.wikipedia.org/wiki/Galen#/media/File:Galenus.jpg (public domain).

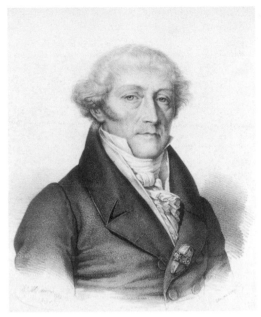

Fig. 1.1.3 Antonio Scarpa (1752–1832). Portrait engraved in 1801 by F. Anderloni. Available at: https://commons.wikimedia.org/wiki/File:Antonio_Scarpa._Line_engraving_by_F._Anderloni,_1801,_after_Wellcome_V0005253.jpg. Courtesy of Welcome Images, licensed under https://creativecommons.org/licenses/by/4.0/deed.en.

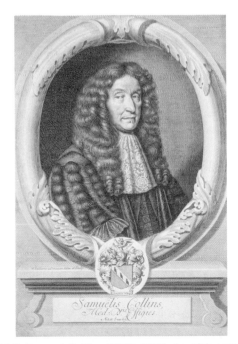

Fig. 1.1.2 Samuel Collins (1618–1710). An 18th-century engraved portrait by William Faithorne (Senior). Available at: https://en.wikipedia.org/wiki/Samuel_Collins_(physician)#/media/File:Samuel_Collins.jpg (public domain).

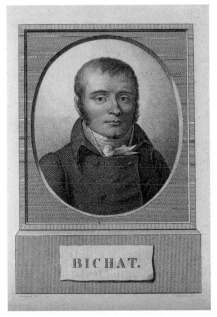

Fig. 1.1.4 Portrait of Marie-Francois Xavier Bichat (1771–1802). Stipple in oval portrait by A. Coupe after Choquet. Courtesy of Wellcome Collection, Attribution 4.0 International (CC BY 4.0), available at: https://wellcomecollection.org/works/n3t5k5cw.

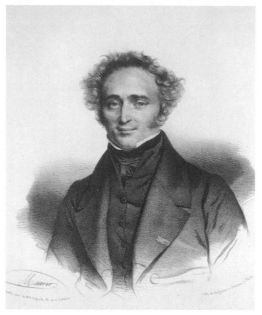

Fig. 1.1.5 Jean Cruveilhier (1791–1874). Lithographic portrait created in 1837 by François-Séraphin Delpech. Available at: https://en.wikipedia.org/wiki/Jean_Cruveilhier#/media/File:CRUVEILHIER.jpg (public domain).

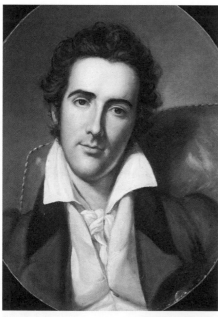

Fig. 1.1.6 John Davidson Godman (1794–1830). Painting by Rembrandt Peale. Available at: https://commons.wikimedia.org/wiki/File:Rembrandt_Peale_-_Dr._John_Davidson_Godman_-_43.136_-_Museum_of_Fine_Arts.jpg (public domain).

THE ILLUMINATION OF FASCIA

17th Century

The word *fascia* most likely entered English medical writing early this century, with Crooke's (1615, 1651) references to the *fasciam* (thoracolumbar fascia) and *fasciam latam* (Adstrum 2015a; Adstrum and Nicholson 2019). Crooke's deployment of these terms was followed and gradually extended by others, although the body's membranous parts were usually identified as *membrana, integuments, coats, strata, skinnes, tunicles,* and *pannicles*. Membranes were then distinguished from bones, cartilage, ligaments, and tendons by their softer consistency and, according to Collins (1685; Fig. 1.1.2), their constitution from "minute nervous Filaments, finely spun, and curiously interwoven in right [vertical], oblique, and transverse positions" This internal structure, he explained, allows membranes to "be several ways extended in length, breadth, and obliquely, without any laceration," and to collectively form a universal body-investing garment (Collins, 1685, p. iii).

Membranes were anatomically described as an interconnected assemblage of soft tissue layers that cover and encircle the body's numerous parts, including: the *fatty membrane* or *adipose membrane* (also named the *fleshy membrane* or *membrana carnosa* for muscle embedded within it in some regions); the *common coat of the muscles;* the *proper coat of* each *muscle;* the *periosteum;* the *pleura;* and the *membranes of the brain* or *meninges.* Crooke taxonomically arranged them in hierarchically ordered categories (Adstrum and Nicholson 2019), explaining that the differences between them are "manifold and taken from their substance, magnitude, site, figure, conformation or texture, & from the nature of the parts which they invest or contain." Despite their solid appearance, he continued, "every membrane is double; through which duplicature runs veins for nourishment, arteries to convey life, and Nerves to convey sense". Consequently, membranes, unlike the muscles and organs they invest, are sensitive to touch and function as the body's "Organ of the sense of touching" (Crooke 1651, 694).

18th Century

Fascia was more frequently mentioned in 18th-century medical writing, alongside the coining of about 10 *fascia*-containing anatomical terms (Adstrum 2015a; Adstrum and Nicholson 2019). The word *fascia* was, however, and possibly more often, applied to the naming of surgical bandages (e.g., *fascia heliodori*, *fascia nodosa*, and *fascia spiralis repens*).

Lacking detailed anatomical explication, fascia was varyingly identified as:
1. A general type of tissue (e.g., aponeurotic fascia, membranous fascia, tendinous fascia);
2. Certain types of fibrous body parts (e.g., aponeuroses, membranes, fibrous sheaths); and
3. Several specific sections of fascia (e.g., fascia lumborum, the fascia of the annular ligament, and the fascia covering a particular muscle, such as temporalis) (Adstrum 2015a; Adstrum and Nicholson 2019).

Anatomists were by then also interested in determining what the body and its membranes are fundamentally made of (Wilson 1944). Both lines of inquiry converged into the discussion of *cellular substance* (also known as *cellular organ*, *cellular texture*, *tela cellulosa*, *cellular membrane*, and *cellular tissue*). Named for the many miniscule *cells* (open areas, or *areolae*) within its open-weave fabric, this *primitive* tissue was portrayed as a universal medium that condenses into membranes, amasses between body parts, surrounds nerves and vessels, and infiltrates muscles and organs, merging from one specifically modified form into another as functionally necessary.

Cellular substance, according to Haller (1754), is generally made up from a combination of "simple fibrils" (now known as type 1 collagen), an "infinite number of little plates or scales, which, joined in various directions intercept small cells and web-like spaces," and the glutinous "*concretum glutinosum chondroides*" that fills the spaces between them. So,

> by extending round every, even the least moving solid parts of the body, [cellular substance] conjoins them altogether in such a manner as not only sustains, but allows them free and ample motion at the same time. But in different parts of the body we observe a great variety of this web-like substance, in respect of the proportion betwixt the membranous sides and the intercepted cells, as well as the breadth and strength of those sides, and the nature of the contained liquor, which is sometimes more watery, and sometimes more oily. . . . Out of this net-like cellular substance, compacted by a concretion of the membranous plates or partitions, and pressed together by the force of the incumbent muscles and distending fluids, arise other broad and flat plates or

> skins in various parts of the body, which being generally disposed in one and the same direction, seem to have a better right to the title of membrane, than the former; and these being convoluted into cones and cylinders, pervaded by a flux of some juice or liquors brought to them, put on the name of vessels, or else being expended round some space that is in a plane parallel to itself, we call it a tunic or coat . . . in the human body [cellular substance] is found throughout the whole; namely, where any vessel or moving muscular fiber can be traced, and this without the least exception. (1754, 10–13).

KEY POINTS
- Medical writers have referred to the body's membranous parts for several millennia.
- The word *fascia* probably entered English medical writing in the early 17th century but was not used very often, as the body's membranous parts were then known by several other names.
- Fascial tissue, then known as *cellular substance*, became a subject of anatomical interest during the 18th century.

FASCIA IN THE AGE OF SCIENCE

19th Century

Fascia came to the fore during this century, attracting an unprecedented amount of anatomical attention. Bichat (Fig. 1.1.4) began his groundbreaking treatise on membranes by observing,

> The membranes have not hitherto been a particular object of research among anatomists. This kind of organs, disseminated as it were through all the others, contributing to the structure of most of them, and having rarely a separate existence, have never been separately examined by them. Their history has been associated with that of the organs over which they are spread. The pericardium and the heart, the pleura and the lungs [etc.]. . . . For description, this is doubtless the best and most simple progress; but in following it, anatomists, struck with the different structure of the organs, have forgotten that their respective membranes could possess any analogy; they have neglected to establish any relation between them, and this leaves an essential chasm. (1813, 21)

The development of more powerful microscopes and histological research methods made it possible to examine fascial (connective) tissue in more detail. These technological advances helped divert anatomists' attention away from the macroscopic cellular spaces toward the fibers, and hence they discovered nucleated cells embedded within its delicate substance. This microscope-assisted change in perspective coincided with the nucleated cell, rather than cellular substance, being perceived as the body's fundamental unit of structure. Cellular substance was rebranded as a cell-containing loose connective tissue (syn. *areolar tissue, cellular texture, cellular tissue, fibrocellular tissue, mucous texture, cellular system,* or *cribriform body*) and typecast as a stroma that supported the parenchymal cells, where the body's real work was then thought to take place (Wilson 1944). Fasciae were, afterward, usually classified in accordance with their tissue type and their relative proximity to the skin—namely, the *fibro-areolar fascia* or *superficial fascia* and the *aponeurotic fascia* or *deep fascia* (as in Gray 1858).

The development of specialized cadaver-embalming fluids, particularly those containing formaldehyde, expedited the examination of fascia (Warwick and Williams 1973). The newly discovered physicochemical preservation processes, along with prolonged exposure to air in the dissection environment, dehydrated and condensed fascial (particularly areolar) tissue, making it unnaturally easier to see and inspect. This artificial accentuation of fascia's visibility almost certainly affected the ways the body and its fascia were perceived by anatomists. On one hand, it enabled the discovery and naming of many previously unspecified sections of fascia. Yet on the other, the unnaturally opaque fascial tissue frequently got in the way and obscured what anatomists most wanted to examine. The latter routinely resulted in fascia being "cleaned away" (removed and discarded) in the dissection laboratory, and then, in many instances, conceptually ignored by medical educators, researchers, and writers.

Most of the newly identified fascial parts were descriptively named for their topographic location (e.g., *superficial fascia, fascia lumborum*), physical appearance (e.g., *cribriform fascia, triangular fascia*), tissue type (e.g., *areolofibrous fascia, fascia adiposa renum*), perceived propriety (e.g., *fascia propria*), or function (e.g., *fasciae of origin*) (Adstrum 2015a; Adstrum and Nicholson 2019). The resultant expansion in recognized fasciae, together with extensive use of synonyms (including eponyms), and the publication of anatomy texts in vernacular languages (rather than just Latin) contributed to a manyfold expansion in fascia-relating terminology (Adstrum 2015b).

20th Century

Advances in the anatomy research environment continued to change the ways fascia was structurally, functionally, and clinically perceived, described, and valued (see Table 1.1.1). For example:

- New and improving research technology (e.g., high-power microscopes, X-rays, histological and immunohistochemical know-how, better embalming fluids and cadaver storage procedures)
- Anatomy branching out into a range of subdisciplines (e.g., microscopic anatomy, radiological anatomy, clinical anatomy, developmental anatomy, structural biology)
- Emergence of new medical and surgical specialisms (e.g., physiatry, rheumatology, plastic surgery, vascular surgery)
- Emergence of fascia-relating bodywork modalities (e.g., connective tissue massage, structural integration, myofascial release therapy)
- Advent of peer-reviewed journals where fascia was varyingly discussed (e.g., *Journal of Anatomy, Acta Anatomica, Connective Tissue Research*)
- Computers and Internet-enabled information and communication technology document storage and retrieval systems that helped disseminate fascia-relating information globally to specialist and lay audiences.

Fascia-related terminology continued to expand due to a variety of factors, including: ongoing research discoveries; the increasingly specific naming of some fasciae (e.g., *hypothenar fascia, pharyngobasilar fascia*); the identification of fasciae terms in English and Latin; and a late-century coining of terms (e.g., *endopelvic fascia/fascia endopelvina, investing fascia*) associated with nomenclatural standardization (Adstrum 2015a; Federative Committee on Anatomical Terminology 1998). New expressions also emerged from clinical literature (e.g., *surgical fascial planes, fascial systems, myofascia*).

By then *fascia* was an internationally recognized anatomical word, yet a long-term lack of precise definition was linked to some confusion about which body parts were recognized as fasciae and their associated names (Wendell-Smith 1997). Medical dictionaries customarily defined *fascia* as a sheet or band of fibrous tissue that covers the body under the skin and invests the muscles and organs. Yet as Hollinshead explained, "there is no generally accepted definition as to how dense connective tissue must be before it can be regarded as forming a fascia" (1954, 282). Some anatomists, including Le Gros Clark, thought of all loose connective tissue as fascia; Clark observed that this "material varies considerably in its consistency, in some places forming a very delicate retinaculum of loose texture, and in other places becoming condensed into a firmly woven feltwork or into tough fibrous sheets" (1945, 31). The customary application of "a specific local term to any aggregation of connective tissue, sizeable enough to dissect" (Warwick and Williams 1973, 490) was challenged by anatomists who contended "the existence of a certain fascia may largely be a question of semantics . . . [since] all connective tissue is continuous with all other connective tissue . . . [hence] a fascia has no beginning and no end" (Rosse and Goddum-Rosse 1997, 21).

From a topographic anatomical viewpoint, fascia was generally comprehended as a relatively unimportant body part that merely "covers and invests all the so-called higher structures" (Gallaudet 1931, 1). Individual exceptions notwithstanding (e.g., Gallaudet 1931; Singer 1935; Sterzi 1910; Stilwell 1957), few anatomical reports explicitly pertained to the description of fascia. Fascia's structure and physical properties were instead more often discussed in relation to their medical and surgical importance (e.g., Orrin 1928; Bogduk and Macintosh 1984).

KEY POINTS

- Fascia attracted an unprecedented amount of anatomical and clinical attention during the 19th and 20th centuries.
- The development of more powerful microscopes changed the way anatomists perceived fascial tissue.
- The development of specialized cadaver embalming fluids, particularly containing formaldehyde, changed the way anatomists perceived fascia.
- Anatomists had mixed views about the importance of fascia.

COMBINED PORTRAYAL OF FASCIA

During the past 400 years, anatomists have unevenly epitomized fascia as: (1) an inconstant range of body parts; (2) the tissues that form them; and (3) a composite body system (see Table 1.1.2). As a result, the word *fascia* has been unusually related to three taxonomically distinct anatomical categories (i.e., tissue, organ, and

TABLE 1.1.2 **Fascia's Anatomical Identity has been Unevenly Related to Three (Organ, Tissue, and Organ System), Rather than the Standard One, Taxonomic Categories During the Past 400 years**

Structure	Alternative Names & Examples
(1) Fascial Organs	
(a) General Fascial Layers	Fascial sheets, fascial planes
Superficial fascia (*fascia superficialis*)	Subcutaneous tissue (*tela subcutanea, hypodermis, subcutis*), fatty membrane (*membrana adiposa, panniculus adiposus*), fleshy membrane (*membrana carnosa*)
Deep fascia (*fascia profunda*)	Investing fascia, aponeurotic fascia, proper fascia, muscular fascia (*fascia musculorum*), fascia of muscles
Appendicular fascia	Fascia of limbs, *fascia membrorum*
Axial fascia	Fascia of trunk (*fascia trunci*). Three sublayers: parietal fascia (*fascia parietalis*), extraserosal fascia (*fascia extraseroalis*), visceral fascia (*fascia visceralis*)
Meningeal fascia (*meninges*)	
Pachymeninx (*dura mater*)	e.g., cranial dura mater (*dura mater cranialis, dura mater encephali*), cerebral falx (*falx cerebri*)
Leptomeninges (*arachnoid mater, pia mater*)	e.g., spinal arachnoid mater (*arachnoidea mater spinalis*)
Terminal filum (*filum terminale*)	e.g., dural part (*pars duralis*, coccygeal ligament, *filum terminal externum*)

Continued

TABLE 1.1.2   **Fascia's Anatomical Identity has been Unevenly Related to Three (Organ, Tissue, and Organ System), Rather than the Standard One, Taxonomic Categories During the Past 400 years—cont'd**

Structure	Alternative Names & Examples
Visceral fascia (*fascia visceralis*) Fascia surrounding individual organs Fascial layer underlying peritoneum & pleura Fascia forming neurovascular sheaths	Splanchnic fascia, subserous fascia, e.g., pharyngobasilar fascia (*fascia pharyngobasilaris*), endothoracic fascia (*fascia endothoracica*)
Muscle fascia (*fascia musculorum*) Investing layer (*fascia investiens*) Muscle sheath (*fascia propria musculi*)	Epimysial fascia
Somatic fascia	Superficial and deep fascia
Fascial planes Regional fascial planes Surgical fascial planes	 Regional sheets of fascial tissue Areolar tissue planes of surgical dissection
(b) Fascial Body Parts Adventitia (*tunica adventitia*)	 e.g., outermost layer (*tunica externa*) of artery wall
Aponeuroses	e.g., bicipital aponeurosis (*aponeurosis bicipitalis*, *lacertus fibrosus*, Grace of God fascia)
A fascia (plural, fasciae)	e.g., axillary fascia (*fascia axillaris*), dorsal fascia of foot (*fascia dorsalis pedus*)
Fibrous Capsules (Capsula Fibrosa, Tunica Fibrosa) Gland capsules	 e.g., fibrous capsule of thyroid gland (*capsula fibrosis glandula thyroidea*)
Organ capsules	e.g., fascial sheath of eyeball (bulbar sheath, *vagina bulbi*, bulbar fascia, Tenon's capsule, Tenon's fascia)
Articular capsules (*capsula articularis*)	e.g., capsular ligament of knee joint (*ligamentum capsularia genu*)
Ligaments Somatic ligaments Visceral ligaments	 e.g., coraco-acromial ligament (*ligamentum coracoacromiale*) e.g., round ligament of the liver (*ligamentum teres hepatis*)
Membranes (membrana) Fibrous membranes (*membrana fibrosa*) Fibroelastic membranes (*membrana fibroelastica*) Interosseous membranes (*membrana interossei*) Universal (enveloping body) membranes Invest whole body Invest same type of body parts	 e.g., aponeuroses, articular capsules e.g., fibroelastic membrane of larynx (*membrana fibroelastica laryngis*) e.g., interosseous membrane of forearm (*membrana interossei antebrachia*) e.g., subcutaneous tissue (*tela subcutanea*), fatty membrane (*membrana adiposa*), superficial fascia (*fascia superficialis*) e.g., common membrane of the muscles (muscle fascia [*fascia musculorum*]), periosteum
Particular Membranes (Enveloping Body Parts) Invest a body region Invest a body part Embryonic membranes	 e.g., intracranial meninges, pleura, peritoneum e.g., pericardium, sclera Fetal fascia, e.g., chorion, amnion

Structure	Alternative Names & Examples
Myofascia	Endo-/peri-/epimysial and epimuscular connective tissue matrix that surrounds muscle cells, muscle fascicles, and muscles
Myofascial expansions	e.g., bicipital aponeurosis extending between biceps brachii and medial region of antebrachial fascia
Myofascial organs	e.g., urinary bladder, gall bladder, stomach, uterus
Nerve fascia	Endo-/peri-/epineurial connective tissue matrix that surrounds myelinated peripheral nerve fibers, fascicles, and nerves
Retinacula	e.g., extensor retinaculum of hand (*retinaculum musculorum extensorum*, dorsal carpal ligament, posterior annular ligament)
Septa	e.g., anterior intermuscular septum of leg (*septum intermuscularae cruris anterius*)
Sheaths (vaginae)	
Muscle sheaths	Fascia surrounding an individual muscle (*fascia propria musculi*), e.g., sartorius sheath
Neurovascular sheaths	e.g., axillary sheath, carotid sheath
Tendons (tendinum)	e.g., calcaneal tendon (*tendo calcaneus*, Achilles tendon)
Tendon sheaths	e.g., tendinous sheath of tibialis posterior (*vagina tendinis musculi tibialis posterioris*)
(2) Fascial Tissue	
Connective Tissue Proper	Connective and supporting tissue proper
Loose connective tissue	Areolar tissue, fibroareolar fascia, cellular tissue, e.g., endomysium, endothoracic fascia
Dense connective tissue	e.g., thoracolumbar fascia, iliotibial tract, periosteum, tendons, ligaments, capsule around liver
Fusocellular connective tissue	Embryonic connective tissue that contains small spindle-shaped cells. Present in developing embryo, e.g., amnion, chorion
Adipose connective tissue	e.g., superficial and deep adipose layers of subcutaneous tissue
(3) Fascial System	A three-dimensional continuum of fascial tissue and organs spread throughout the body. Subsystem: superficial fascial system (superficial musculoaponeurotic system)

TABLE 1.1.2 Fascia's Anatomical Identity has been Unevenly Related to Three (Organ, Tissue, and Organ System), Rather than the Standard One, Taxonomic Categories During the Past 400 years—cont'd

organ system). Fascia's ambiguous portrayal appears to embody a tension between fascia's primary apperception as an assortment of macroscopically discernible body parts *and/or* a chameleon-like soft-tissue network that adopts a variety of functionally determined structural formats—that is, whether fascia is *incidentally* or *essentially* a connective tissue construct. History suggests that both viewpoints, those in-between, and those constructed by joining them together are legitimate and potentially of value—especially as they each segue into different, and sometimes dissimilar, downstream assumptions about fascia's material properties, physiological roles in the body, involvement in mechanisms of injury and pathology, and relative clinical prominence. Understanding this is important if we want to see more and possibly farther than our astute fascia-aware forebears.

Summary

Anatomists have learned a considerable amount about fascia over several millennia, although the ways they have conceptualized and explained it have always been (and still are) inseparable from, and in accordance with, the "how, why, and when" it was studied. Fascia's varying anatomical description through the ages has been powerfully shaped by advances in research technology, as well as by what clinicians have needed to know about it in order to perform their work effectively and safely. Each and every set of fascia-relating anatomical knowledge developed over time has contributed to a cumulative understanding of this pervasive body part. None on their own can entirely explain fascia; however, learning more about them may be useful in developing more complex, and perhaps richer, future understandings of it.

REFERENCES

Adstrum, N.S., 2015a. The Meaning of Fascia in a Changing Society. PhD thesis. University of Otago, Dunedin, New Zealand.

Adstrum, S., 2015b. Fascial eponyms may help elucidate terminological and nomenclatural development. J. Bodw. Mov. Ther. 19, 516–525.

Adstrum, S., Hedley, G., Schleip, R., Stecco, C., Yucesoy, C.A., 2017. Defining the fascial system. J. Bodw. Mov. Ther. 21, 173–177.

Adstrum, S., Nicholson, H., 2019. A history of fascia. Clin. Anat. 23 (7), 862–870.

Bartholin, T., 1655. Anatomia . . . reformata. Available from: <https://archive.org/details/bub_gb_Reo-AAAAcAAJ/page/n7>.

Berengario da Carpi, J., 1535. Anatomia carpi: Isagoge breves: perlucide . . . usitatum. (First published in 1522) Available from: <https://archive.org/details/2222036R.nlm.nih.gov/>.

Bichat, X., 1813. A treatise on the membranes in general and on different membranes in particular (J.G. Coffin, Trans.). Cummings and Hilliard, Boston (First published in 1800).

Bogduk, N., Macintosh, J.E., 1984. The applied anatomy of the thoracolumbar fascia. Spine J. 9, 164–170.

Breasted, J.H., 1930. The Edwin Smith Surgical Papyrus, vol. 1. The University of Chicago Press, Chicago.

Collins, S., 1685. Systeme of anatomy, vol. 1. Robert Midgley, London.

Crooke, H., 1615. Mikrokosmographia: A Description of the Body of Man. William Iaggard, London.

Crooke, H., 1651. A Description of The Body of Man Together with The Controversies and Figures Thereto Belonging. John Clarke, London (First published in 1531).

Cruveilhier, J., 1844. The Anatomy of the Human Body, the first American Edition, from the Last Paris edition (W.H. Madden, G.S. Pattison Trans.). Available from: <https://archive.org/details/anatomyofhumanbo00cruv/>.

Cunningham, A., 2010. The Anatomist anatomis'd: An Experimental Discipline in Enlightenment Europe. Ashgate Publishing Ltd, Farnham, UK.

Federative Committee on Anatomical Terminology (Eds.), 1998. Terminologia Anatomica: International Anatomical Terminology. Thieme, New York.

Gallaudet, B.B., 1931. A Description of the Planes of Fascia of the Human Body: With Special Reference to the Fascia of The Abdomen, Pelvis and Perineum. Columbia University Press, New York.

Glisson, F., 1654. Anatomia Hepatis. Available from: <https://archive.org/details/bub_gb_9lJkAAAAcAAJ/>.

Godman, J.D., 1824. Anatomical Investigations Comprising Descriptions of Various Fasciæ of the Human Body. HC Carey & I Lea, Philadelphia.

Gray, H., 1858. Anatomy: Descriptive and Surgical. John W Parker and Son, London.

Haller, A.V., 1754. Dr. Albert Haller's Physiology; Being a Course of Lectures upon the Visceral Anatomy and Vital Oeconomy of Human Bodies, vol. 1 (S. Mihles Trans.). Available from: <https://archive.org/details/dralberthallersp01hall/>.

Heald, R.J., 1988. The 'Holy Plane' of rectal surgery. J. R. Soc. Med. 81, 503–508.

Hollinshead, W.H., 1954. Anatomy for Surgeons: the Head and Neck, vol. 1. Cassell and Company Limited, London.

Le Gros Clark, W.E., 1945. The Tissues of the Body: An Introduction to the Study of Anatomy. Clarendon Press, Oxford.

Lockwood, T.E., 1991. Superficial fascial system (SFS) of trunk and extremities: a new concept. Plast. Reconstr. Surg. 87, 1009–1018.

Netter, F.H., 1997. Atlas of Human Anatomy, second ed. Novartis, East Hanover, NJ.

Orrin, H.C., 1928. Fascial Grafting in Principle and Practice: An Illustrated Manual of Procedure and Technique. Oliver and Boyd, Edinburgh.

Rosse, C., Goddum-Rosse, P., 1997. Hollinshead's Textbook of Anatomy, fifth ed. Lippincott-Raven Publishers, Philadelphia, PA.

Santayana, G., 1905. The Life of Reason: The Phases of Human Progress, vol. 1. Available from: <https://archive.org/details/lifeofreasonorph01sant/page/284>.

Singer, E., 1935. Fasciæ of the Human Body and their Relations to the Organs they Envelop. Williams & Wilkins, Baltimore.

Stecco, C., Adstrum, S., Hedley, G., Schleip, R., Yucesoy, C.A., 2018. Update on fascial nomenclature. J. Bodw. Mov. Ther. 22, 354.

Sterzi, G., 1910. Il tessuto sottocutaneo (tela sottocutanea). Arch Ital Anat e di Embr IX:1-172.

Still, A.T., 1899. Philosophy of Osteopathy. Academy of Osteopathy, Kirksville, MO.

Stilwell, D.L., 1957. Regional variations in the innervation of deep fasciae and aponeuroses. Anat. Rec. 127, 635–653.

Susruta, Bhishagratna, K.K.L., 1911. An English translation of the Sushruta Samhita, based on original Sanskrit text, vol. 2. Available from: <https://archive.org/details/englishtranslati02susr/>.

Vesalius, A., Richardson, W.F., Carman, J.B., 1998. On the fabric of the human body. Book II, The ligaments and muscles/ Andreas Vesalius, (W.F. Carman Trans.). Norman Publishing, San Francisco.

Vicary, T., 1586. The Englishemans treasure, or treasor for Englishmen with the true anatomye of mans body. John Perin, London (First published in 1577).

Warwick, R., Williams, P.L. (Eds.), 1973. Gray's Anatomy, thirty-fifth ed. Longman, London.

Wendell-Smith, C.P., 1997. Fascia: an illustrative problem in international terminology. Surg. Radiol. Anat. 19, 273–277.

Wilson, J.W., 1944. Cellular tissue and the dawn of the Cell Theory. Isis 35, 168–173.

General Anatomy of the Muscle Fasciae

Peter P. Purslow and Jean-Paul Delage

INTRODUCTION

The soft connective tissues associated with muscle tissue can be referred to as muscle fasciae (MF). A description of MF structure and function in skeletal muscle (Purslow 2014) lists 17 previous reviews in addition to a great deal of original source material, and the reader is referred to these substantial sources for detailed information. Here we shall summarize the main features of their structure, composition, and functional properties. There is a tendency in previous literature to call MF "tubes" or "sheaths" that surround each fiber or fasciculus. The concept of muscle fasciae as continuous connective tissue networks provides a better understanding of the functional anatomy of these structures. MFs form a three-dimensional matrix that is continuous throughout the entire organ, providing connections between fibers and fascicles rather than separating them.

GENERAL STRUCTURE AND COMPOSITION OF MUSCLE FASCIAE

The following description of the general structure of fasciae associated with striated muscles summarizes the consensus of several sources and is schematically shown in Fig. 1.2.1.

Each individual muscle is surrounded by the **epimysium,** a connective tissue layer that is continuous, with the tendons attaching the muscle to the bones. The **perimysium** is a continuous network of connective tissue that divides the muscle up into fascicles or muscle fiber bundles.

KEY POINT

The division of each muscle into fascicles by the perimysium allows flexible movement between the fascicles as the muscle contracts and changes shape. Great variability in the size, shape, and number of muscle fascicles exists between functionally different muscles.

The perimysial network merges into the tendons and into the epimysium at the surface of the muscle and is mechanically connected to them. Within each fascicle or muscle fiber bundle, the **endomysium** is a continuous network of connective tissue that separates individual muscle fibers.

Generally speaking, these connective tissue layers are composed of collagen fibers (and occasionally also elastin fibers) in an amorphous matrix of hydrated proteoglycans (PGs), which mechanically links the

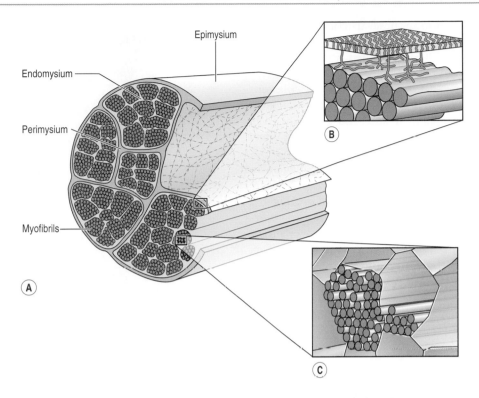

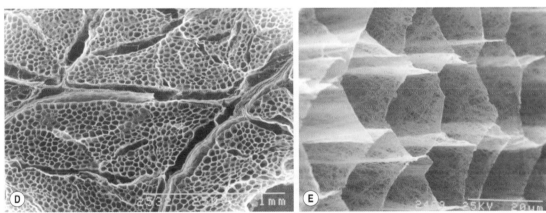

Fig. 1.2.1 General Anatomy of the Fasciae Associated With a Skeletal Muscle. (A) Schematic view of the general arrangement of the epimysium, perimysium, and endomysium within muscle. (B) Schematic depiction of junction zones between the thick perimysium and the endomysium of muscle fibers in the surface layer of the fascicle. Although a gap is shown between the perimysium and endomysium to illustrate the connections, no gap occurs in living muscle. (Separation of the endomysium from the perimysium is seen in some fixed tissue due to shrinkage artefacts; see Fig. 1.2.2). (C) Schematic depiction of myofibrils of an individual muscle cell residing in the honeycomb network of the endomysium. (D&E) Micrographs of IMCT structures in muscle treated with NaOH to digest away myofibrillar proteins and PGs. (D) The spatial arrangement of the thicker perimysium surrounding the honeycombed endomysial network within a fascicle. (E) A higher magnification view of the endomysial network. Abbreviations: IMCT, intramuscular connective tissue; PGs, proteoglycans. Figure reproduced with permission from Purslow, P. P., 2014. New developments on the role of intramuscular connective tissue in meat toughness. Annual Review of Food Science and Technology 5, 133–153.

collagen fiber networks in these structures. Listrat and colleagues (Listrat et al. 1999; Listrat et al. 2000) and Passerieux et al. (2006) identified seven molecular types of collagen in muscle (types I, III, IV, V, VI, XII, and XIV). Types I, III, and V are fibrillar collagens (fiber-forming types). Types I and III are the most prevalent in mammalian striated muscle. Light et al. (1985) found that type III collagen (containing intermolecular disulphide cross-links) comprised approximately 40% of the total of type I and III collagens in a range of bovine muscles. Types XII and XIV are thought to act as molecular bridges connecting the fibrillar collagens to other components in the amorphous matrix. The basement membrane layer of the muscle fibers contains nonfibrous type IV collagen, together with proteoglycan components such as laminin and fibronectin and heparin sulfate–containing PGs, and forms the boundary between the phospholipid cell membrane and the collagen fiber networks of the "reticular layer" of the endomysium.

Collagen fibers are mechanically stabilized by the formation of covalent crosslinks (Eyre and Wu 2005). The formation of crosslinks is essential for the mechanical strength and stiffness of collagen fibers, as without them the collagen molecules slide past each other under load and the fibers have no strength. Throughout gestation and during postnatal maturation there are substantial changes in the types and amounts of covalent crosslinks that mechanically stabilize the collagen molecules in muscle fasciae. The subject of cross-link formation during maturation and aging of connective tissues is reviewed in excellent detail by Avery and Bailey (2008). Here we shall just note that muscle fasciae are rich in covalent crosslinks, that these crosslinks are known to undergo maturation changes in both endomysial and perimysial connective tissue, and that compounds promoting glycation crosslinks can be incorporated into the body from dietary sources and from tobacco smoke. Thus diet and lifestyle may conceivably affect the mechanical properties of some connective tissues, including muscle fasciae, via crosslinking of collagens.

The amounts and composition of muscle fasciae vary among different muscles in the body. A comparison of transverse sections through different muscles from the same species (Purslow 2005; Fig. 1.2.2) shows that the continuous perimysial network surrounds or separates fascicles of very different sizes and shapes in different muscles. This

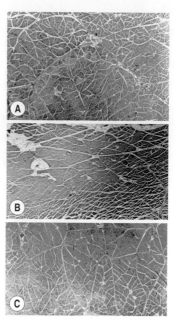

Fig. 1.2.2 Comparison of the fascicular architecture in cross-sections of three muscles from the same (bovine) animal: rhomboideus cervicus (A), sternocephalicus (B), and pectoralis profundus (C). Clear differences in fascicle size, shape, and perimysial thickness can be seen among them and within each muscle. The white gaps between fascicles (separating perimysium from the endomysium of surface muscle fibers) are shrinkage artefacts produced by fixation. Reproduced with permission from Purslow, P.P., 2005. Intramuscular connective tissue and its role in meat quality. Meat Sci. 70, 435–447.

difference also results in different thicknesses of perimysial connective tissue. These variations, especially in the amount and spatial organization of the perimysium, have long been attributed to variations in mechanical roles of different anatomical muscles. If this is correct, then the muscle fasciae must play strong roles in the normal physiological functioning of each muscle. Some possible explanations of these roles are emerging but are far from complete.

FUNCTIONAL ANATOMY OF THE ENDOMYSIUM

There are three distinct structures separating the surface of one muscle fiber (cell) from its adjacent neighboring fiber:

1. At the surface of the fiber is the plasma membrane (plasmalemma) of the muscle cell, which is approximately 9-nm thick.

2. Outside the plasma membrane is the endomysial basement membrane. It is approximately 50 to 70 nm thick and is composed of two layers: the lamina lucida (or lamina rara) next to the plasma membrane and an outer lamina densa.

KEY POINT

The endomysium forms a continuous network binding together all the muscle fibers in a muscle fascicle.
  Load sharing by shear through the endomysium coordinates deformations between muscle fibers and can transmit contractile forces.

Each muscle fiber has its own plasmalemma and basement membrane surrounding it. Filling the space between the basement membranes of two adjacent muscle fibers is the third layer:

3. The collagen fiber network (or reticular) layer, comprised of a network of collagen fibrils and fibers in a proteoglycan matrix. Schmalbruch (1974) reported reticular layer thicknesses of 0.2 to1.0 μm in frog sartorius muscle.

As shown by classical transmission electron microscopy images of longitudinal muscle sections (Trotter and Purslow 1992), the thickness of the endomysium varies with muscle length, becoming thicker at short muscle lengths and thinner as the muscle is extended. The fibrous reticular layer is a common structure shared between adjacent muscle cells and forms a continuous network that runs across the whole muscle fascicle. Muscle cells (with their individual plasma membranes and basement membranes) occupy the polygonal "holes" in the endomysial network, as shown in Fig. 1.2.1(D & E).

The reticular region of the endomysium is often described as a random or quasirandom network of irregularly wavy fine collagen fibers, which lie in the plane parallel to the muscle fiber surface. The network is not truly random. There is a preferred direction in the wide distribution of collagen fiber orientations, and this preferred orientation changes with muscle length (Purslow and Trotter 1994).

A large number of muscles in animals from many phyla contain intrafascicularly terminating muscle fibers, i.e., muscle fibers that are not continuous along the entire length of fascicles and do not run from tendon to tendon. Trotter (1993) lists 28 studies on a wide range of muscles

from humans, amphibians, mammals and birds, showing series-fibered architecture. Muscle fibers in series-fibered muscles are relatively short compared with the length of the fascicle, particularly so in avian species where individual fibers can be as short as 0.4 to 2.6 cm. The endomysium is the only structure that links these muscle fibers together in the fascicle. Transmission of tension generated in intrafascicularly terminating fibers to the tendons at the ends of the fascicles necessitates transmission of force through the endomysial network, as this is the only structure continuously linking the fibers. The endomysium is very compliant to tensile forces acting within the plane of the network and so can easily deform to follow the length and diameter changes of muscle fibers in contracting and relaxing muscles. However, the transmission of force between adjacent muscle fibers by shear through the thickness of the endomysium (translaminar shear), as first described by Street (1983), is an efficient force transduction pathway (Purslow and Trotter 1994; Trotter and Purslow 1992; Trotter et al. 1995). Any linkage that transmits force from intrafascicularly terminating muscle fibers to tendinous attachments must not deform too much in order to be efficient. Particularly in isometric muscle contractions, any significant stretching in the length of the fascicle due to stretchy connections would result in a very poor transmission of contractile force. Purslow (2002) showed that transmission of force by translaminar shear of the endomysium fulfils this criterion; the displacements along the long axis of the muscle due to translaminar shearing of the endomysium are insignificant. The functional significance of this is that the endomysium provides a shear linkage of force from one muscle cell to its neighbors, which is highly efficient while still being able to deform easily in the plane of the network so as to allow the muscle fibers to change length and diameter as they contract and relax.

The architecture of the endomysium linking adjacent muscle fibers in continuous fibered muscles appears identical to that of endomysium in series-fibered muscles. The obvious inference is that load sharing between adjacent muscle cells is a common function in both continuous-fibered and series-fibered striated muscles and even cardiac muscle (Purslow 2008). The endomysium, therefore, forms a continuous three-dimensional connecting matrix that tightly shear-links adjacent fibers together to coordinate force transmission in a fascicle and keep fibers in uniform register.

FUNCTIONAL ANATOMY OF THE PERIMYSIUM

The amounts and spatial distribution of perimysium vary much more between muscles in the body than do those of endomysium (Purslow 1999). Using two pennate muscles from the cow and the rat, Passerieux et al. (2007) showed that the perimysium is a well-ordered structure that lies throughout the muscles. Thick amounts of perimysium enclosing large fascicles of myofibers form tubes in a honeycomb arrangement in the direction of myofibers, the walls of the tubes in continuity with tendons at their ends and in continuity with epimysium at the outer surface of the muscle. The walls of the tubes are made of two (or even more) flat layers of long wavy collagen fibers running in the same direction in each layer. The direction of collagen fibers from each layer crosses the direction of myofibers at $\pm 55°$ at muscle rest length. Long, flattened bundles of collagen fibers can overlap between adjacent walls of tubes so that the assembly of tubes is a very coherent structure. Many of the wide flat cables of collagen fibers diverge into secondary sheets of perimysium, dividing the primary fascicles into secondary fascicles of myofibers, then separate successively as thinner cables separating smaller fascicles. (This is possible in the case of the muscle of the cow because the collagen fibers are up to 5 cm in length.) At the end of the process, small cables join the surface of the myofibers so that the small cables form a rather regular network of long collagen fibers (Passerieux et al. 2007) and rather regular numerous contacts with each myofiber.

The perimysial layers separating two fascicles are comprised of two or more crossed-plies of wavy collagen fibers in a proteoglycan matrix. The long axis of each set of collagen fibers lies at $\pm 55°$ to the longitudinal axis of the fascicle when the muscle is at its relaxed (resting) length. This angle increases as muscle shortens and decreases if it is passively stretched out (Purslow 1989). The waviness of the collagen fiber bundles also changes with muscle length, being maximal at the resting length of relaxed muscle. Perimysium is easily deformed in tension and does not exhibit a high tensile stiffness until it has been stretched far enough that the collagen fibers have become aligned along the stretching direction and the waviness in the fibers pulled out straight (Lewis and Purslow 1989). Thus the perimysium can show a high tensile stiffness and carry large loads in tension, but only at very large extensions well beyond the range of working lengths in living muscle.

The tensile properties of the perimysium are therefore similar in nature to the endomysium, and it is tempting to suppose that the perimysium could also act to transmit the forces generated in fascicles to their adjacent neighbors by translaminar shear. Although it is undoubtedly the case that force transmission by such a mechanism can be invoked in extreme circumstances of muscle damage or surgical disconnection of the tendinous attachments to some fascicles, there are two considerations that weigh against this mechanism under normal working conditions in living muscle. First, an analysis shows that simply because perimysium is so much thicker than endomysium, deformations caused by shear through its thickness would be of orders of magnitude greater than in the endomysium, and so perimysium would represent a rather sloppy and inefficient force transmission pathway at physiologically relevant muscle lengths (Purslow 2002). Second, why should perimysial content and architecture vary so much more than the endomysium if it is fulfilling the same kind of functional role?

Schmalbruch (1985) cites an old model by Feneis (1935) supposing that perimysial structures provide "neutral" connections between muscle fascicles that allow muscle the fascicles to slide past each other, as the geometry of a muscle changes upon contraction. Measurements of "borders" between fascicles in ultrasonic images of human muscles in clinical and sports studies and their rotation on contraction allow these shear strains to be estimated. Using the values in the literature from seven such clinical studies (Purslow 2002), it is possible to show that shear strains within actively contracting human muscles are substantial and vary considerably between quadriceps, vastus lateralis, gastrocnemius, and tibialis muscles. The theory that division of muscle into fascicles facilitates shear deformations explains why fascicle shape and size vary so much from muscle to muscle. However, until detailed quantitative assessment of any relationship between perimysial architecture, fascicle size, and the distributions of shear strains in working muscles has been carried out, this theory remains just an interesting possibility. Using supersonic shear imaging (SSI), Lacourpaille et al. (2012) measured the shear modulus of 9 muscles in 30 human subjects, reporting values of shear modulus in the range 2.99 to 4.50 kPa. A review of in-vivo measurements using the same SSI techniques

(Lima et al. 2018) reported nonlinear shear modulus values in the range 15 to 70 kPa. The longitudinal modulus of the muscles increased as the degree of contraction increased, but values at maximal contractions of 258 kPa (tibialis anterior), 225 kPa (gastrocnemius medialis), and 55 kPa (soleus) were reported. So, in general, the shear stiffness of human muscles in vivo appears to be up to almost one order of magnitude lower than the maximum longitudinal stiffness of contracting muscle. This again argues that, although transmission of force by shear in the perimysium may be possible, it provides a rather flexible connection between adjacent fascicles.

PERIMYSIAL–ENDOMYSIAL JUNCTION ZONES

The endomysium surrounding muscle fibers is connected to the perimysium by intermittent perimysial junctional plates (PJPs), described by Passerieux et al. (2006).

KEY POINT

Perimysial–endomysial junction zones: the perimysium is only sporadically connected to the endomysium at the surface of a muscle fascicle by sparse junction zones. These junctions are infrequent, which may limit their ability to efficiently transmit contractile forces of the muscle, but they probably act as sites of mechanotransduction (input of mechanical signals into the muscle cells).

If, like the endomysial network, the perimysium principally acts to transmit muscle force, then the perimysial–endomysial junction must necessarily be mechanically strong and noncompliant. Alternatively, if the perimysium has only a limited role in myofascial force transmission under normal physiological conditions but is more involved in relieving shear displacements between fascicles during muscle contractions, then the connections could be expected to be more tenuous.

PJPs are staggered at the surface of each myofiber and separated by a distance of approximately 300 μm. They are made of a set of branches of collagen fibers at the end of cables (Fig. 1.2.3) that arise from the tubes separating fascicles. The branches cross the perimysial layer of myofibers and reach their surface on the top and between costameric structures, with attachments on the reticular work of perimysium and the basement membrane of myofibers.

Fracture procedures (as seen in Fig. 1.2.3) show that the perimysium remains present only in the regions where perimysial plexi are attached to myofibers, which leads to the conclusion that these points of attachment between perimysium and myofibers are rather strong and therefore allow transmission of contractile force in synergy with the endomysium. However, the long dimensions of these collagen fibers suggest that the perimysium is stressed after the endomysium and acts under large intramuscular displacements or eccentric contractions produced during downhill exercises. Measurement

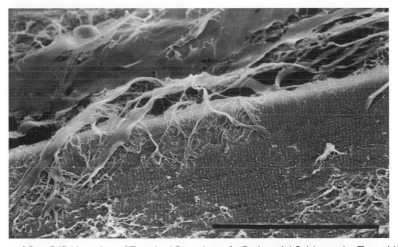

Fig. 1.2.3 View of One PJP (Junction of Terminal Branches of a Perimysial Cable on the Top with the Surface of One Myofiber at the Sarcomeric Level). Note the presence of some endomysium at the bottom of the myofiber. Bovine muscle; scanning electron microscopy; bar = 100 μm. Abbreviation: PJP, perimysial junctional plates.

of the strength of intramuscular connective tissue networks perpendicular to the muscle fiber direction showed that the force required to separate these structures connecting the perimysium and endomysium was low compared with the strength of the perimysial layer (Lewis and Purslow 1990).

PERIMYSIUM AND INTRACELLULAR SUBDOMAINS

Among the main cytoplasmic components of myofibers, nuclei and mitochondria are of importance because they control, respectively, metabolism and energetic production of myofibers, and it can be considered that their position in myofibers is of particular interest. Regarding nuclei, it was thought that they are distributed at the same distance along the myofibers, each of them at the control of a surrounding "myonuclear domain." However, Roy et al. (1999) found that nuclei have a clustered distribution along the myofibers and the number of nuclei in clusters varies with exercise. The case of mitochondria is somewhat different: they are distributed with a great regularity at the level of sarcomeres except for large subsarcolemmal accumulations. Nuclei and subsarcolemmal accumulations of mitochondria are linked to the cytoskeleton in regions where myofibers are crossed by capillaries (Ralston et al. 2006) that are embedded into the perimysium, and Passerieux et al. (2006) found that they are statistically colocalized with PJPs (Fig. 1.2.4).

In addition, the lack of the collagen VI component of perimysium is associated with apoptosis of nuclei and mitochondria of myofibers (Irwin et al. 2003), so it can be expected that the terminal branches of perimysial cables play an important role in mechanotransduction when they are stressed under myofiber contraction.

CONCLUSIONS

Muscle fasciae are important to the functioning of muscle tissues. Load transmission between tightly linked adjacent muscle fibers within fascicles allows for coordination of forces and protection of damaged areas of fibers against overextension, and, in series-fibered muscle at the very least, is a major pathway for the transmission of contractile force. Substantial evidence exists to show that perimysium and epimysium can also act as pathways for myofascial force transmission.

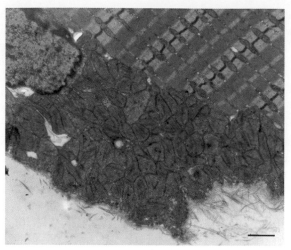

Fig. 1.2.4 View of a PJP-Associated Intracellular Subdomain. Perimysium as thin filaments at the borders of the myofiber is in the vicinity of a nucleus and a large subsarcolemmal accumulation of mitochondria. Rat muscle; transmission electron microscopy; bar = 1 µm. Abbreviation: PJP, perimysial junctional plates.

However, definition of boundaries between muscle fascicles by the perimysium may also have a role in allowing the whole tissue to accommodate large shear displacements. As detailed elsewhere in this book, muscle fasciae are in a continuous dynamic balance between synthesis and remodeling so as to be continually adapted for their mechanical roles in working muscles.

Summary

Each individual muscle is an organ, surrounded and defined by its external fascia, the epimysium. Internally, the muscle is divided into fascicles by another fascia, the perimysium, which forms a continuous network across the muscle and is joined to the epimysium. The division of the muscle into fascicles allows shape changes to occur as the muscle contracts. Within each fascicle a continuous network (the endomysium) integrates and coordinates the forces and deformations of individual muscle cells. There are sporadic junctions between the endomysium and perimysium at the surface of the fascicles that may possibly serve as pathways for force transmission but probably act as pathways for mechanotransduction, i.e., for external mechanical signals to be passed into the muscle cells to affect their expression.

REFERENCES

Avery, N.C., Bailey, A.J., 2008. Restraining cross-links responsible for the mechanical properties of collagen fibers; natural and artificial. In: Fratzl, P. (Ed.), Collagen: Structure and Mechanics. Springer, New York, pp. 81–110 (Chapter 4).

Eyre, D.R., Wu, J.J., 2005. Collagen cross-links. Top. Curr. Chem. 247, 207–229.

Feneis, H., 1935. Uber die Anordnung und die Bedentung des Bindegewebes für die Mechanik der Skelettmuskulatur. Morph Jb 76, 161–202.

Irwin, W.A., Bergamin, N., Sabatelli, P., et al., 2003. Mitochondrial dysfunction and apoptosis in myopathic mice with collagen VI deficiency. Nat. Genet. 35, 367–371.

Lacourpaille, L., Hug, F., Bouillard, K., Hogrel, J.Y., Nordez, A., 2012. Supersonic shear imaging provides a reliable measurement of resting muscle shear elastic modulus. Physiol. Meas. 33 (3), N19–N28.

Lewis, G.J., Purslow, P.P., 1989. The strength and stiffness of perimysial connective-tissue isolated from cooked beef muscle. Meat Sci. 26, 255–269.

Lewis, G.J., Purslow, P.P., 1990. Connective tissue differences in the strength of cooked meat across the muscle fibre direction due to test specimen size. Meat Sci. 28 (3), 183–194.

Light, N., Champion, A.E., Voyle, C., Bailey, A.J., 1985. The role of epimysial, perimysial and endomysial collagen in determining texture in six bovine muscles. Meat Sci. 13 (3), 137–149.

Lima, K.M.M.E, Júnior, J.F.S.C., de Albuquerque Pereira, W.C., de Oliveira, L.F., 2018. Assessment of the mechanical properties of the muscle-tendon unit by supersonic shear wave imaging elastography: a review. Ultrasonography 37, 3–15.

Listrat, A., Picard, B., Geay, Y., 1999. Age-related changes and location of type I, III, IV, V and VI collagens during development of four foetal skeletal muscles of double muscles and normal bovine muscles. Tissue Cell 31, 17–27.

Listrat, A., Lethias, C., Hocquette, J.F., et al., 2000. Age related changes and location of types I, III, XII and XIV collagen during development of skeletal muscles from genetically different animals. Histochem. J. 32, 349–356.

Passerieux, E., Rossignol, R., Chopard, A., et al., 2006. Structural organisation of the perimysium in bovine skeletal muscle: junctional plates and associated intracellular subdomains. J. Struct. Biol. 154, 206–216.

Passerieux, E., Rossignol, R., Letellier, T., Delage, J.P., 2007. Physical continuity of the perimysium from myofibres to tendons: involvement in lateral force transmission in skeletal muscle. J. Struct. Biol 159, 19–28.

Purslow, P.P., 1989. Strain-induced reorientation of an intramuscularconnective tissue network: Implications for passive muscle elasticity. J. Biomechanics. 22, 21–31.

Purslow, P.P., 1999. The intramuscular connective tissue matrix and cell/matrix interactions in relation meat toughness. In: Proc. 45th Intl. Cong. Meat Sci. Technol., 1999 (Yokohama, Japan), Available from: <http://icomst-proceedings.helsinki.fi/papers/1999_04_01.pdf>.

Purslow, P.P., 2002. The structure and functional significance of variations in the connective tissue within muscle. Comp. Biochem. Physiol. A Mol. Integr. Physiol. 133, 947–966.

Purslow, P.P., 2005. Intramuscular connective tissue and its role in meat quality. Meat Sci. 70, 435–447.

Purslow, P.P., 2008. The extracellular matrix of skeletal and cardiac muscle. In: Fratzl, P. (Ed.), Collagen: Structure and Mechanics. Springer, New York, pp. 325–358 (Chapter 12).

Purslow, P. P. (2014). New developments on the role of intramuscular connective tissue in meat toughness. Annu. Rev. Food. Sci. Technol. 5, 133–153.

Purslow, P.P., Trotter, J.A., 1994. The morphology and mechanical properties of endomysium in series- fibred muscles; variations with muscle length. J. Muscle Res. Cell Motil. 15, 299–304.

Ralston, E., Lu, Z., Biscocho, N., et al., 2006. Blood vessels and desmin control the positioning of nuclei in skeletal muscle fibers. J. Cell. Physiol. 209, 874–882.

Roy, R.R., Monke, S.R., Allen, D.L., Edgerton, V.R., 1999. Modulation of myonuclear number in functionally overloaded and exercised rat plantaris fibers. J. Appl. Physiol. 87, 634–642.

Schmalbruch, H., 1974. The sarcolemma of skeletal muscle fibres as demonstrated by a replica technique. Cell Tissue Res. 150, 377–387.

Schmalbruch, H., 1985. Skeletal Muscle. Springer, Berlin, pp 20–21.

Street, S. F.,1983. Lateral transmission of tension in frog myofibers: a myofibrillar network and transverse cytoskeletal connections are possible transmitters. J. Cell. Physiol. 114, 346–364.

Trotter, J.A., 1993. Functional morphology of force transmission in skeletal muscle. Acta Anat. (Basel) 146, 205–222.

Trotter, J.A., Purslow, P.P., 1992. Functional morphology of the endomysium in series fibered muscles. J. Morphol. 212, 109–122.

Trotter, J.A., Richmond, F.J.R., Purslow, P.P., 1995. Functional morphology and motor control of series fibred muscles. In: Holloszy, J.O. (Ed.), Exercise and Sports Sciences Reviews, vol. 23. Williams & Watkins, Baltimore, pp. 167–213.

Somatic Fascia

Frank H. Willard

GLOBAL ORGANIZATION OF FASCIA IN THE BODY

Overview of the Organization of Somatic Fascia in the Body

When we think about the somatic portion of the body, images of skeletal muscle, bones, and joints usually come to mind. However, none of these structures can suffer much direct contact without developing significant pathology. For protective reasons, most of the somatic structures are embedded in a matrix of soft connective tissue termed fascia—the bandage or packing substance of the body. Muscles develop in a matrix of connective tissue such that the adult organ is surrounded by an epimysium; bone arises in a matrix of embryonic fascia termed mesenchyme, which in the adult form becomes the periosteum; and joint capsules consolidate out of a thickening in mesenchyme (Gardner 1963) that ultimately forms a fascial covering over the dense layers of the capsule. In each case, the fascial sheet embracing the somatic structure protects it from direct abrasion by surrounding structures while also providing a conduit through which neurovascular bundles can easily penetrate. By surrounding the components of the somatic system, fascia creates complex and continuous planes or sheets of connective tissue that unite all portions of the body

and present continuous planes along which anatomists tend to dissect (Huber 1930).

The functions of fascia tend to dictate its structure. Fascia must be capable of significant distortion in multiple planes of direction and return rapidly to its native shape. This type of action is best met by constructing fascia out of irregular connective tissue where the fibrous component is interwoven; thus proper fascia is defined as connective tissue with an irregular distribution of fibrous elements as opposed to those tissues containing parallel or well-oriented arrays such as are seen in tendons, ligaments, aponeuroses, and some joint capsules (Clemente 1985; Standring 2008). The irregular weave of the fibrous component allows for easy movement and resistance in all directions but is master of none. Thus tearing fascia apart can be difficult in all planes of dissection. Conversely, because of the highly regular arrangement of collagen fibers in a tendon, ligament, or aponeurosis, these structures can provide maximal resistance of stretch in one or a limited number of directions but can easily be shredded with fingertips when stressed in orthogonal planes.

The density of the fibrous component of fascia will vary tremendously with is location and function. Thus fascia underlying the skin must be very movable and therefore has a lower density of collagenous fibers; this is often given the term *superficial fascia* (Clemente 1985;

Singer 1935; Standring 2008; Stecco 2015). Alternatively, the fascia that invests muscle, ligament, tendon, or joint capsule is providing a stronger support role and is often termed *investing fascia* or *deep fascia*, the density of its collagen fibers being considerably higher; however, they are still irregular in weave (Clemente 1985; Singer 1935; Standring 2008, Stecco 2015).

Finally, unlike the highly differentiated structures of the somatic system—muscle, tendon, ligament, and aponeurosis—fascial planes tend to lack precise borders. Muscles have fairly recognizable origins and attachments, and where they joint with tendons a precise line can be seen even in the microstructure. Attachments of muscle-tendon complexes to bone are definitive, forming an enthesis. However, the lack of precise borders seen in the fascial tissue facilitates the formation of long planes spanning multiple organ systems or compartments surrounding multiple muscles. When entering fascial compartments, neurovascular bundles—which themselves are surrounded by irregular, dense, connective tissue fascial wrappings called an adventitia—course along or through fascial planes that would otherwise represent obstacles if composed of highly organized, regularly arranged fibrous elements such as seen in an aponeurosis, tendon, ligament, or most joint capsules. Lymphatic flow, which would be quickly interrupted if forced through tissue with precise boundaries, can flow easily through lymphatic vessels distributed in the irregular tissue of the fascial plane. From this discussion it is evident that the function of fascia in the somatic body is closely associated with its structure.

A recently discovered function of fascia focuses on its role in guiding the development of limb muscles (Kardon et al. 2003). The myogenic mesenchymal cells migrate from the somites located along the lateral margins of the neural tube. Some of the migrating cells differentiate into myoblasts and give rise to myocytes, whereas others form the fascial matrix into which the myoblasts develop. Evidence supports the concept that the muscle connective tissue is required for the normal development of the muscle.

This chapter divides the fascial system of the body into four primary layers, emphasizing the somatic component, and then describe our initial understanding of the role played by somatic fascia in the development of the musculoskeletal system.

 KEY POINT

Fascia is distinct from the more specialized connective tissue such as tendons, ligaments, aponeuroses, bone cartilage, and blood by its irregular organization and its function as a universal support tissue. It is also apparent that the cells of primitive fascial tissues play a significant role in guiding the initial development of more specialized tissues such as skeletal muscle.

ARCHITECTURE OF FASCIA—THE FOUR PRIMARY LAYERS

General Approach

Several attempts at characterizing the fascia system of the body have been published (Benjamin 2009; Gallaudet 1931; Singer 1935; Stecco 2015). This chapter focuses on irregular connective tissue or "proper fascia" and will describe a system of four primary layers that cover the axial portion of the body. These layers are arranged as a series of "tubes within tubes." Modification of this fundamental plan will allow accommodation of the limbs.

The four primary layers in the torso are arranged as a series of concentric tubes (Fig. 1.3.1). Starting with the outermost layer of fascia, it is best termed the **panniculus** or panniculus adiposus, a term used by Singer (1935) in his treatise on fascia and strongly recommended for general usage by Last (1978) in his textbook of anatomy. Deep to the pannicular layer is the **axial fascia** of the torso (deep fascia described in Stecco 2015). This layer gives rise to the investing fascia or epimysium of the axial muscles; peridentium and periligamentum of tendons, ligaments, and aponeuroses; and the periosteum of bone and perichondrium of cartilage. The axial layer of fascia is continuous with the **appendicular** (deep or investing) **fascia** in the extremity at the shoulders and the hips. As with the pannicular layer, the axial layer can be subdivided; however, again, in this chapter it will be treated as a primary layer. Internal to the axial fascia are two additional layers: the first surrounds the neural structures and can be termed **meningeal fascia,** and the second surrounds all body cavities and is best termed **visceral (splanchnic) fascia.** In considering the limbs, the pannicular layer extends outward covering the entire surface of the limb. Under the pannicular layer, a fascial layer of similar composition to the axial fascia is present, surrounding the muscles of the extremity, and can be termed

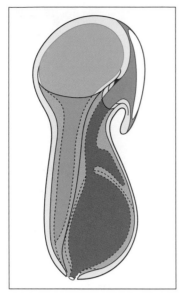

Fig. 1.3.1 The "Fascunculus". This is a schematic diagram of the fascial layers of the human. The whole diagram is covered by a panniculus of fascia (pale gray layer). The axial fascia covers the torso of the body (blue layer) but does not extend to the head. Visceral fascia extends from the naso-oro-pharyngeal region to the aboral (anal) region (red layer). Meningeal fascia surrounds the brain and spinal cord (green layer). Finally, a thin black line in the center of the body represents the notochord separating the meningeal fascia from visceral fascia. In the adult, the notochord would be replaced by portions of the vertebral column. From the Willard/Carreiro Collection, with permission.

appendicular fascia. It lies deep to the pannicular fascia and invests the appendicular muscles. Regional names often relate the fascia to a specific muscle, i.e., deltoid fascia, pectoral fascia, etc. Internal to the appendicular fascia is the intramuscular septum housing the neurovascular bundles; this septal layer is most likely to be derived from the axial fascia at the base of the limb.

> ### ⚡ KEY POINT
>
> The fascial systems create a series of "tubes within tubes" that define the construction of the body. The outermost tube is the pannicular or superficial fascia within which is a complex tube of axial investing fascia in the torso and appendicular investing fascia in the extremities. Central to the axial fascia are two tubes separated by the notochord in the embryo and the vertebral column in the adult. These latter tubes represent the meningeal fascia posteriorly and the visceral fascia anteriorly.

Four Primary Layers of Fascia
Pannicular Fascia

The outermost layer is the pannicular fascia (Singer 1935) and is often termed superficial fascia (Clemente 1985; Standring 2008). This layer can be subdivided into several sublayers. The pannicular layer is derived from the somatic mesenchyme and surrounds the entire body, with the exception of its orifices, such as the orbits, nasal passages, and the oral and aboral openings. It is composed of irregular connective tissue with marked regional variation in collagen fiber density as well as variation in adipose cell density (Fig. 1.3.2). Whereas the outermost portion of this layer is typically invaded by much adipose tissue, the inner portion is more membranous in nature and generally very adherent to the outer portion, except over the abdomen where the two can be easily separated by blunt dissection. The thickness of the pannicular layer is highly variable in the human population. In the region of the head and neck, humans have several thin muscles embedded in the pannicular fascia; these are the platysma and associated facial muscles innervated by the facial nerve. Pannicular fascia covers both the axial and appendicular body.

Axial Fascia

The second layer is the axial or investing fascia (deep fascia, as described in Clemente [1985], Standring [2008], and Stecco [2015]). Axial fascia is fused to the panniculus peripherally and extends deep into the body, surrounding the hypaxial and epaxial muscles. This layer, like the pannicular layer, is derived from mesenchyme and forms the primitive matrix in which skeletal muscles, tendons, ligaments, aponeuroses, and joints develop. The mesenchymal matrix then contributes to the epimysium of skeletal muscle, the periosteum of bone, the peritendon of the tendons, and the investing layer surrounding the joint capsule. The peritendon subdivides into an epitenon, which grasps the regular collagenous fiber bundles of the tendon, and a paratenon, which surrounds the entire tendon; both layers form the peritendon and are constructed of irregular collagenous bundles (Jozsa and Kannus 1997). The arrangement of fascia around an aponeurosis is similar to that of a tendon or ligament; however, the terminology used has created some confusion. In the older literature, two terms exist: "aponeuroses of

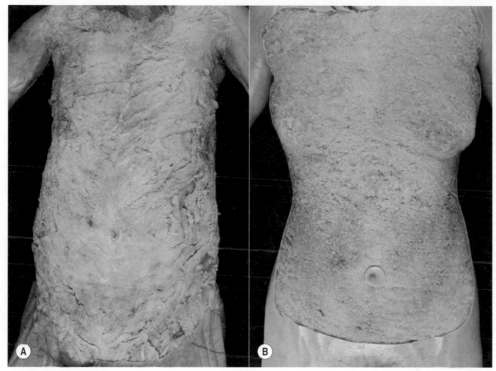

Fig. 1.3.2 The Pannicular Layer of Fascia. This is an anterior view of the thorax and abdomen of a male and female cadaver. The body on the left (A) is that of a 54-year-old male and on the right (B) a 54-year-old female. Both specimens have had the dermis removed to reveal the pannicular layer of fat and fascia. From the Willard/Carreiro Collection, with permission.

attachment" and "aponeuroses of investment" (Singer 1935). Aponeuroses of attachment referred to the well-organized bands of dense connective tissue that made up the true aponeuroses that attached the muscle to its target, whereas those "of investment" made up the irregular connective tissue composing the investing or axial fascia surrounding the true aponeuroses.

The axial fascia can be described as being composed of two, parallel, connective tissue tubes and course anterior and posterior to the vertebral column (Fig. 1.3.3A–C). Developmentally, these two tubes would be separated by the notochord, which is approximated by the vertebral column in the adult. The anterior tube surrounds the hypaxial muscles and attaches to the vertebral column at the transverse process. The hypaxial muscles include the longus and scalene muscles in the cervical region, the intercostal muscles in the thoracic region, and the oblique and rectus muscles in the abdominal region. The posterior tube of the axial fascia surrounds the epaxial muscles

and is attached to the transverse processes. The spinous process of each vertebra divides the epaxial fascial tube into two "half-tubes" (Fig. 1.3.3C). The paraspinal muscles of the back are contained in the "half-tubes" of the epaxial fascia.

Complex fascial relationships exist where the extremities meet the axial portion of the body. Axial fascia extends into the extremities as the intermuscular septum and the appendicular fascia investing individual muscles (Fig. 1.3.4). The fascial sheath that surrounds the neurovascular bundles such as the brachial plexus and lumbosacral plexus extends outward to form the intermuscular septum, in which branches of the neurovascular bundle will course as they progress distally in the extremity. In the upper extremity, the axial fascia surrounding the brachial plexus is regionally termed the axillary sheath; however, it represents an extension of the axial fascia—specifically, it extends from a portion of the axial fascia regionally termed the "prevertebral

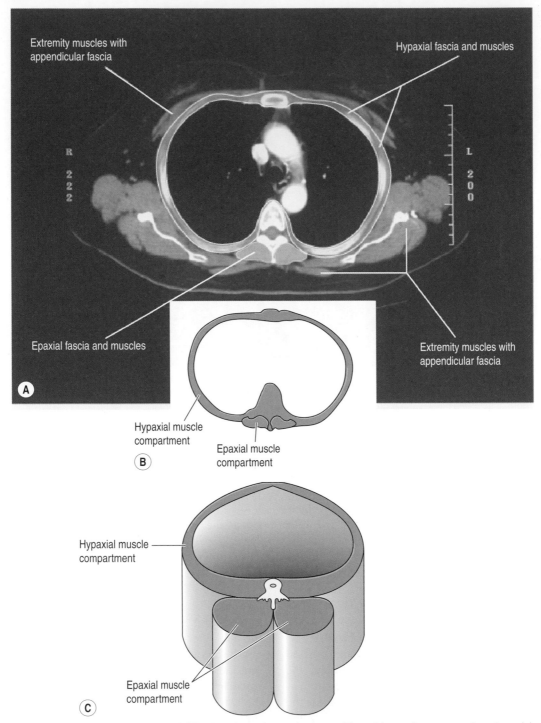

Fig. 1.3.3 (A) An axial plane spiral CT taken through a male thorax. The white outline surrounding the axial muscles—hypaxial and epaxial—marks the course of the axial fascia. (B) Shading representing the hypaxial and epaxial muscle compartments taken from the section in A. (C) A diagram illustrating the epaxial and hypaxial fascial column. From the Willard/Carreiro Collection, with permission.

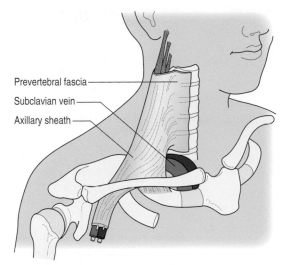

Prevertebral fascia
Subclavian vein
Axillary sheath

Fig. 1.3.4 The fascia surrounding the neurovascular bundle in the axial portion of the body extends outward to the extremity. Reproduced from Mathers, L.H., Chase, R.A., Dolph, J., Glasgow, E.F., 1996. Clinical Anatomy Principles. Mosby, St Louis, with permission.

fascia" (Fig. 1.3.4). The use of the term "axial fascia" as a primary descriptor for all these layers places an emphasis on their common developmental origin and their similarity in microstructure as well as their structural continuity in the adult.

The arrangement of fasciae on the body wall is made very complex by the attachment of the limbs. The muscles of the upper extremity, such as the pectoralis, trapezius, serratus anterior, and latissimus dorsi muscles, form long wing-like expansions that wrap over the torso to attach to the spinous processes on the midline of the body or to structures that ultimately attach to the midline, such as the thoracolumbar fascia. Although some of these muscles are located on the back, they are not paraspinal muscles; instead they migrate from the proximal extremity reaching over the body wall to attach to such structures as the spinous process on the back or to the sternum or clavicle anteriorly. In development, these migrating extremity muscles are moving in a plane internal to the panniculus of fascia and external to the axial fascia as they embrace the axial body wall. Each muscle is surrounded by a layer of investing or appendicular fascia. As the muscle settles on the body wall, its investing fascia fuses with the investing fascias of surrounding structures, thus creating complex relationships.

The arrangement of the investing fascia sheets of migrating extremity muscles can be seen in the two dissections illustrated in Fig. 1.3.5. In Fig. 1.3.5(A) the epidermis and dermis have been removed to expose the underlying pannicular fascia. An elongated rectangular window (outline) was opened into the pannicular fascia to expose the investing fascia (appendicular fascia) of the pectoral muscles, a muscle that migrated onto the thoracic wall. In Fig. 1.3.5(B) the window was enlarged and divided into two portions; the medial portion still has appendicular fascia covering the muscle, but in the lateral portion the investing appendicular fascia has been removed to expose the pectoralis muscle. With the inferolateral border of the pectoral muscle elevated (Fig. 1.3.5 inset), the investing (appendicular) fascia separating it from the serratus anterior can be visualized. To expose the axial-investing fascia of the intercostal muscles, the pectoral major and serratus anterior muscles and their investing appendicular fascia must be removed (Fig. 1.3.6A). In this figure, the pectoralis major and serratus anterior muscles have been removed to expose the intercostal muscles and their thin layer of axial-investing fascia (note that the pectoralis minor muscle is still attached). Finally, Fig. 1.3.6(B) exposes the intercostal muscles by carefully dissecting away all axial fascia.

> ### ⚡ KEY POINT
> During the formation of the body wall, numerous proximal upper extremity muscles migrate onto the body seeking attachment site. Each muscle is contained within its own investing fascia. As the muscles settle onto the thoracic wall they create complex fascial arrangement, such as those seen around the clavicle and pectoral muscles of the adult.

Meningeal Fascia

The third fascial layer is meningeal fascia, which surrounds the nervous system. This layer includes the dura as well as the underlying leptomeninges; it derives from the primitive meninx that surrounds the embryonic nervous system. Specifically, the spinal meninges are most likely derived from the somatic mesoderm, whereas the brainstem meninges arise from cephalic mesoderm and the telencephalic meninges from the neural crest (Catala 1998). Meningeal fascia terminates with the development of the epineurium that surrounds the peripheral nerve.

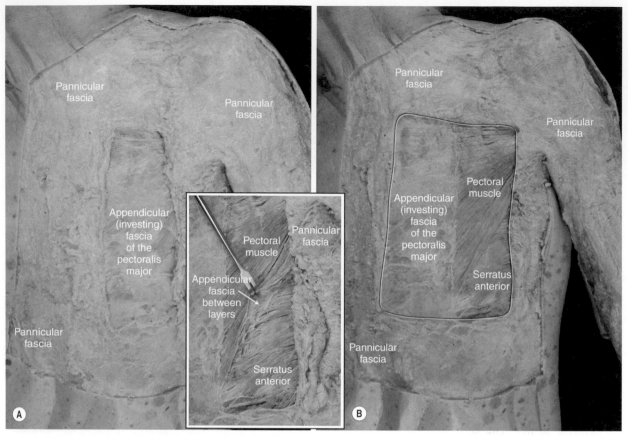

Fig. 1.3.5 (A) Photograph of a male with the epidermis and dermis removed to expose the pannicular fascia on the chest wall. A vertical window has been cut in the pannicular fascia to expose the underlying appendicular fascia. (B) The same specimen with the appendicular fascia cleaned off the pectoralis major and serratus anterior muscles in the right side of the window. In the inset (lower middle) the lateral margin of the pectoralis muscle has been elevated to expose the appendicular fascia that separates the pectoralis major from that of the serratus anterior. Elevating the serratus would reveal a fusion of appendicular fascia on the inner aspect of the serratus and axial fascia on the underlying intercostal muscles and ribs. From the Willard/Carreiro Collection, with permission.

Visceral Fascia

The fourth fascial layer is visceral fascia and is by far the most complex of the four main layers of fascia. Embryologically, this layer of fascia is derived from the splanchnic tissue and thus surrounds the body cavities—pleural, pericardial, and peritoneal. The visceral layer follows the visceral pleura and peritoneum and provides the conduit for neurovascular bundles entering the visceral organs as well as a drainage route out of the organ. On the midline of the body, the visceral fascia forms a thickened mediastinum that extends from the cranial base into the pelvic cavity. This layer of fascia will be discussed in a separate chapter.

The Role of the Somatic Fascial Matrix in Development of the Musculoskeletal System

The functional relationship between somatic axial or appendicular-investing fascia and the development of the musculoskeletal system is relatively unexplored. Of the little that is known, the relationship between the development of muscles and their associated connective tissue (fascia) is best understood for the muscles of the limbs. Each muscle is surrounded by a covering composed of irregular connective tissue, termed the epimysium, from which septae, termed perimysium, extend inward in the body of the muscle. Individual myocytes are embedded in a delicate network of connective tissue

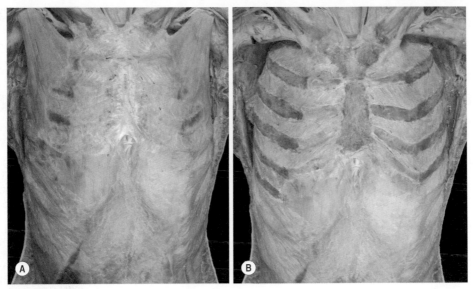

Fig. 1.3.6 Anterior Views of the Thoracic Wall of a 54-Year-Old Female. In (A) the axial (investing) fascia of the thoracic wall is present and it is difficult to visualize the underlying structures. In (B) the axial fascia has been removed to reveal the underlying intercostal muscles and the ribs. From the Willard/Carreiro Collection, with permission.

fibers, termed endomysium, that is anchored to the perimysium. In this way the myocytes are encased in a connective tissue matrix that integrates the muscle with surrounding tissues. The connective tissue cells that form this fascial matrix typically arise from the lateral somatic mesoderm (somatopleure), whereas the myoblasts for skeletal muscle arise from somites. Somites form from the paraxial mesoderm lying along the lateral aspect of the neural tube and notochord from about day 20 to day 30 of gestation (Fig. 1.3.7). Shortly after forming as a dense mass of cells, somites segment into an outer dermomyotome and inner scerotome (Schoenwolf et al. 2015).

Initially, the dermamyotome of the somite splits to form an underlying, medially positioned epaxial portion precursor of the paraspinal muscles and a more laterally positioned hypaxial portion that gives rise to all other muscles of the body (Fig. 1.3.8). The precursor cells destined to form the muscles of the limb delaminate from the ventral surface of the hypaxial region of somite in the lower cervical and lumbosacral region and begin their migration toward their respective limbs (Fig. 1.3.9). Whereas the ventrolateral hypomere (hypaxial mesoderm) gives rise to the limb muscle precursors, the lateral mesoderm in the newly formed body of the embryo gives

rise to the connective tissues (fascia), tendons, ligaments, and skeletal elements of the limb. These later mesenchymal cells join the presumptive myoblasts as they migrate toward the limb bud. It is during this process of migration that an interaction occurs, leading to the differentiation of the limb muscles.

Myoblasts from any somite can form limb muscle in either the upper or lower extremity, thus patterning of limb muscle formation appears to occur after the myoblast precursors leave the somite and enter the limb bud. Evidence suggests that it is the associated connective tissue cells (fascia) of the muscle that pattern the myoblasts to form the appropriate muscle (Kardon et al. 2003). Although many regulatory factors are involved in the process (Schoenwolf et al. 2015), the function of the transcription factor Tcf4 appears to be necessary for the establishment of the cellular connective tissue matrix into which myoblasts develop (Kardon et al. 2003). The Tcf4 transcription factor is seen to be expressed in the fascia surrounding muscle and in the perimysium, but not in the myocytes themselves, further supporting the concept that this transcription factor is distinct for muscle connective tissue (Blasi et al. 2015). Muscle connective tissue patterns will form normally, even in the absence of myoblasts, whereas myoblasts will form abnormal muscles

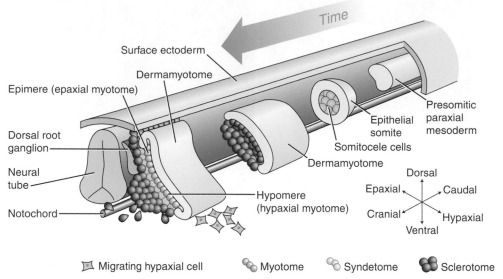

Fig. 1.3.7 This is a diagram illustrating the development of the somite. Mesenchymal cells of the paraxial mesoderm coalesce into bilaterally symmetrical masses located along the lateral margin of the neural tube. The cell mass laminates such that the outer or dorsolateral layer forms the dermamyotome and the inner or ventromedial layer forms the sclerotome. Subsequently, the dermamyotome layer forms an inner layer, the myotome, that separates into a dorsomedial region termed the epimere and a ventrolateral region termed the hypomere. The epimere ultimately gives rise to the paraspinal muscles whereas the hypomere gives rise to the hypaxial muscles and the appendicular muscles. Reproduced with permission from Schoenwolf, G.C., Bleyl, S.B., Brauer, P.R., Francis-West, P.H. (2015) Larsen's Human Embryology, 5th ed., Churchill Livingstone Elsevier, Edinburgh.

when the expression of Tcf4 is suppressed (Kardon et al. 2003). For these reasons, the Tcf4-expressing muscle connective tissue cells have been proposed as playing a key role in establishing the muscle patterns seen in the limb.

The development of the thoracoabdominal diaphragm in the mouse (Merrell et al. 2015) further emphasizes the concept that the fascial tissue supporting skeletal myocytes provides the necessary pattern to allow development of the muscle. Using mouse genetics, the authors demonstrate that both the muscular connective tissue and the connective tissue of the central tendon of the costal diaphragm develop entirely from the pleuroperitoneal folds (PPFs). It is into this matrix of connective tissue that the myoblasts, derived from somites, migrate and establish residency. Using special staining techniques it was possible to demonstrate that the migrating myoblasts ended up surrounded by cells that express Tcf4, a connective tissue cell marker. In a mouse mutant model where the myoblasts fail to migrate into the diaphragm, the Tcf4-expressing cells migrated and formed a muscleless diaphragm. Finally, using a genetic construct that specifically damage connective

tissue–forming cells in the PPFs, it was possible to demonstrate that the absence of muscle connective tissue cells lead to the formation of multiple hernias in the diaphragm. These remarkable results clearly emphasize the role of the connective tissue fascial matrix in the development of normal muscles.

> ### KEY POINT
>
> During development, the extremity muscles are derived from mesenchymal cells that delaminate from the ventrolateral hypaxial region of the somite and migrate outward into the limb bud. At least two populations of mesenchymal cells are involved in this migration, one that ultimately differentiates into myoblasts and forms skeletal muscle and a second cell group that forms the associated muscle connective tissue that then differentiates into the investing fascia. The latter can form a well-defined model of the muscle in an environment devoid of the myoblasts, whereas the former will not form a normal muscle without its connective tissue framework. This suggests that the investing fascias most likely establish the patterns that ultimately shape specific muscles.

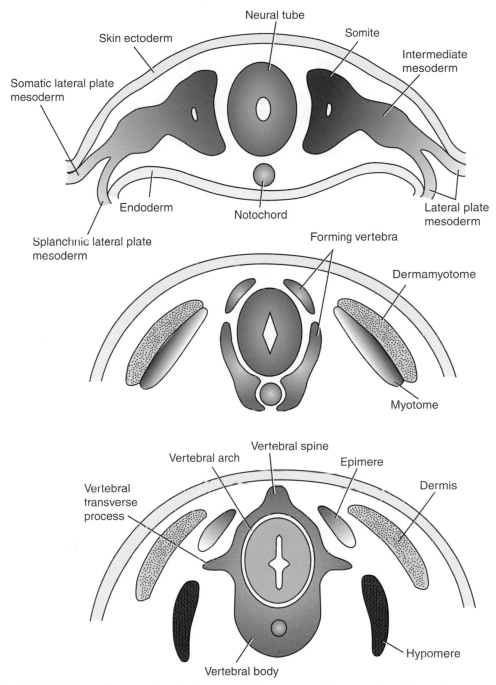

Fig. 1.3.8 This diagram illustrates the development of the epimere and hypomere from the myotome as seen in axial plane sections of a week 4 embryo. The somite forms from the paraxial mesoderm (upper section), which then splits to form the dermamyotome and myotome (middle section). In the lower section, the myotome is seen dividing to form the epimere from which the paraspinal muscles will arise and the hypomere from which the hypaxial muscles and the appendicular muscles will arise . Reproduced with permission from Schoenwolf, G.C., Bleyl, S.B., Brauer, P.R., Francis-West, P.H. (2015) Larsen's Human Embryology, 5th ed. Churchill Livingstone Elsevier, Edinburgh.

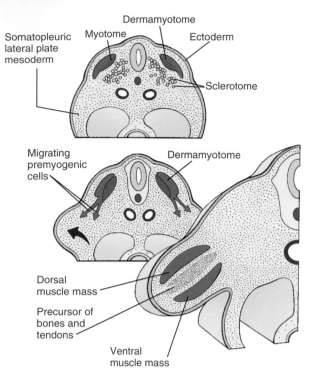

Somatopleuric lateral plate mesoderm

Myotome

Dermamyotome

Ectoderm

Sclerotome

Migrating premyogenic cells

Dermamyotome

Dorsal muscle mass

Precursor of bones and tendons

Ventral muscle mass

Fig. 1.3.9 This diagram illustrates the migration of mesenchymal cells from the ventrolateral portion of the dermamyotome into the developing limb bud. Once in the limb bud the myogenic precursor cells separate into dorsal and ventral muscle mass, defining the muscular compartments of the limb. Reproduced with permission from Schoenwolf, G.C., Bleyl, S.B., Brauer, P.R., Francis-West, P.H. (2015) Larsen's Human Embryology, 5th ed. Churchill Livingstone Elsevier, Edinburgh.

torso and extremities except over the exposed orifices. Next there is a complex arrangement of **axial fascia** (deep or investing fascia) composed of denser, irregular connective tissue–investing muscles, tendons, ligaments, and aponeuroses. Axial fascia also extends into the extremities (appendicular fascia), where it has similar composition and function to its axial counterpart. This network of fascia provides protection and lubrication for the elements of the musculoskeletal system and most likely also transmits some force transduction during muscle contraction. The axial fascia is arranged in two sleeves or tubes separated by the vertebral column, from which extensions into appendicular fascia occur. The final two layers are encased within the axial fascia; these are the meningeal and visceral fascia, both specializations designed to protect the nervous system and the visceral organs, respectively. Limiting the presentation to the primary layers rather than their subcomponents helps emphasize the continuity of fascial planes in the body. Finally, there is evidence that the mesenchymal cells that form the investing fascias of skeletal muscles play a critical role in establishing the form and shape of that muscle.

REFERENCES

Benjamin, M., 2009. The fascia of the limbs and back – a review. J. Anat. 214 (1), 1–18.

Blasi, M., Blasi, J., Domingo, T., Perez-Bellmunt, A., Miguel-Perez, M., 2015. Anatomical and histological study of human deep fasciae development. Surg. Radiol. Anat. 37, 571–578.

Catala, M., 1998. Embryonic and fetal development of structures associated with the cerebro-spinal fluid in man and other species. Part I: the ventricular system, meninges and choroid plexuses. Arch. Anat. Cytol. Pathol. 46 (3), 153–169.

Clemente, C.D., 1985. Gray's Anatomy of the Human Body. Lea & Febiger, Philadelphia.

Gallaudet, B.B., 1931. A Description of the Planes of Fascia of the Human Body with Special Reference to the Fascias of the Abdomen, Pelvis and Perineum. Columbia University Press, New York.

Gardner, E.D., 1963. The development and growth of bones and joints. J. Bone Joint Surg. Am. 45 (4), 856–862.

Huber, G.C., 1930. Piersol's Human Anatomy, ninth ed. J.B. Lippincott, Philadelphia.

Jozsa, L., Kannus, P., 1997. Human Tendons. Anatomy, Physiology and Pathology. Human Kinetics, Champaign, IL.

Kardon, G., Harfe, B.D., Tabin, C.J. 2003. A Tcf4-positive mesodermal population provides a prepattern for vertebrate limb muscle patterning. Dev. Cell. 5, 937–944.

Summary

The term **fascia** represents a form of connective tissue that is widely distributed throughout the body and composed of irregular, interwoven collagenous fiber bundles of varying density. Fascia plays multiple roles in the body; it invests most structural elements, being highly protective in nature, and can also provide a lubricating function. Its network of interconnections between skeletal elements appears to provide a mechanism for limited force transduction, and its cellular composition strongly suggests both an immune function and a neurosensory role as well.

Although many regional names exist for specific fascia, this chapter has attempted to present only four primary layers of fascia for consideration. The outermost or **pannicular layer** (superficial fascia) is mainly composed of loose connective tissue and fat and surrounds the entire

Last, R.J., 1978. Anatomy: Regional and Applied, sixth ed. Churchill Livingstone, Edinburgh.

Mathers, L.H., Chase, R.A., Dolph, J., Glasgow E. F., 1996. Clinical Anatomy: Principles. Mosby, St Louis.

Merrell, A.J., Ellis, B.J., Fox, Z.D., et al. 2015. Muscle connective tissue controls development of the diaphragm and is a source of congenital diaphragmatic hernias. Nat. Genet. 47: 496–504.

Schoenwolf, G.C., Bleyl, S.B., Brauer, P.R., Francis-West, P.H., 2015. Larsen's Human Embryology, fifth ed. Churchill Livingstone Elsevier, Philadelphia, p. 554.

Singer, E., 1935. Fascia of the Human Body and their Relations to the Organs they Envelop. Williams & Wilkins, Philadephia.

Standring, S., 2008. Gray's Anatomy, the Anatomical Basis of Clinical Practice, fortieth ed. Elsevier Churchill Livingstone, Edinburgh.

Stecco, C., 2015. Functional Atlas of the Human Fascial System. Elsevier Churchill Livingstone, Edinburgh.

Fascia Superficialis

Marwan F. Abu-Hijleh, Amol Sharad Dharap, and Philip F. Harris

CHAPTER CONTENTS

INTRODUCTION

Skin, comprising epidermis and dermis, covers the whole surface of the body and is its largest organ. Immediately subjacent is an enveloping layer of dense and areolar connective tissue and fat called the superficial fascia (synonyms: fascia superficialis, hypodermis, subcutaneous tissue, tela subcutanea) (Langevin and Huijing 2009; Standring 2016). Being coextensive with the skin, it too comprises a very considerable tissue mass that conveys blood vessels and nerves to and from the integument.

The subcutaneous tissue connects the skin to the underlying dense deep fascia that invests muscles and aponeuroses throughout the body. Skin, with the subjacent superficial fascia, provides a protective cushion for the musculoskeletal framework over which they slide. Sheets of collagen fibers coupled with elastin facilitate this mobility (Kawamata et al. 2003). The spaces between the collagen sheets facilitate sliding, while stretching results in realignment of collagen fibers within the sheet. Skin shape and position are restored by elastic recoil. The tortuosity of blood vessels and nerves through superficial fascia allows them to accommodate stretching.

Van der Wal (2009) considers fascia as a connective tissue continuum throughout the body. Thus subcutaneous connective tissue provides a unique general pathway through and between regions that blood vessels, nerves, and lymphatics can traverse (Wood Jones, 1946; Benjamin, 2009).

Its widespread distribution, its mechanical role, and the ability of fibroblasts to communicate via their gap junctions suggest fascia may form a mechanosensitive integrating signaling system throughout the body analogous to that of the nervous system (Langevin 2006) and a possible basis for interpreting fibrositis.

KEY POINT

Fascia, which lies just below the skin, serves as a protective cushion for the musculoskeletal framework. It is flexible and consists of elastic connective tissue composed of collagen fibers and elastin.

GROSS STRUCTURE AND DISTRIBUTION

Fiber bundles (retinaculae cutis) traverse the subcutaneous layer from dermis to deep fascia, strengthening their connection. The subcutaneous tissue can be differentiated into a bulky superficial fatty layer, *panniculus adiposus*, and a deeper, mostly vestigial layer, *panniculus carnosus* (McGrath et al. 2004). Within the fatty layer itself, a membranous component can also be recognized. This is commonly seen in the lower abdominal wall as the fascia of Camper (superficial fatty layer) and of Scarpa (deeper membranous layer) (Standring 2016; Pisco et al. 2020). Recent studies (Abu-Hijleh et al. 2006) indicate that the membranous layer has a much wider distribution in the body than suggested by earlier studies (see below).

The fat cells are aggregated into clumps or lobules by fibrous septa (see Fig. 1.4.3). In the adult human the vast majority of the fat is of the white type, with only a very small amount of the energy-rich brown fat. About 20% of body weight in a healthy adult male is white fat but it comprises more in females, being as much as 25%. Subcutaneous fat accounts for about 50% of total fat storage in the body. The storage is dynamic, with the fat itself within the cells being renewed every 2 to 3 weeks. The amount and distribution of the fat varies with age, sex, and site. In infants and young children its distribution is quite uniform through all regions (except for the suctorial pad in the cheek). Fat increases steadily in amounts throughout early childhood. In adults the number of fat cells remains constant, the actual number being established during childhood and adolescence and under genetic control. Nevertheless, it has been found that approximately 10% of fat cells are renewed annually in adults (Spalding et al. 2008). However, in old age fat notably decreases.

Concerning the sexes, subcutaneous fat is thicker in females, as evidenced by their smoother body contours. Measurements of subcutaneous tissue in the anterolateral aspect of the thigh recorded a depth of 0.74 cm in males but it was deeper in females, being 1.74 cm (Song et al. 2004). Using an objective assessment of limb subcutaneous tissue elasticity by an indentation technique, Zheng et al. (1999) noted that the tissue thickness increases by 26% when the underlying muscle contracts. With regard to site differences, fat is particularly thick in the buttocks, hips, waist, thighs, soles, palms, breast, and cheeks. It is thinnest or absent in eyelids, lips, pinna (excluding the lobule), external nose, penis, scrotum, and labia minora.

A distinct membranous layer in the superficial fascia in confined areas of the body, including the lower anterior abdominal wall (Scarpa's fascia) and perineum (Colles' fascia), is well-documented (Carney et al. 2017; Pisco et al. 2020). A membranous layer is also present in relation to the saphenous veins (Caggiati 2000, 2001). More recently, a well-defined membranous sheet was found in the superficial fascia of many regions of the body (Abu-Hijleh et al. 2006; Fig. 1.4.1), its arrangement and thickness varying according to gender, region, and the surface studied. This sheet is more prominent on the posterior aspects of the trunk and extremities than on the anterior. In certain regions, such as the periphery of the female breast, arm, back, and thigh, there may be more than one membranous layer separating the fat into two or more layers (Fig. 1.4.2).

The superficial fascia in the face differs from other regions. Hwang and Choi (2018) have shown that the superficial fascia has a laminar connective tissue layer (the superficial musculoaponeurotic system [SMAS]; Mitz and Peyronie 1976). It is interposed between superficial and deep fibroadipose layers. The superficial layer connects the dermis with the superficial aspect of the SMAS. The deep layer connects the deep aspect of SMAS to the parotid–masseteric fascia. Adipose lobules occur within both layers.

> ### 🛈 KEY POINT
>
> Subcutaneous tissue is divided into a superficial fatty layer and a deep vestigial layer. The subcutaneous fatty layer contains a variable network of membranous connective tissue layers. Subcutaneous fat accounts for half of the total body fat storage, and its amount and composition varies according to age, sex, and site, among other differences.

COMPONENTS AND THEIR RELATION TO FUNCTION

1. *Interstitial fluid:* Subcutaneous tissue contains a rich plexus of lymphatics and lymphatic capillaries. There is a dynamic balance between production of tissue fluid from blood capillaries and its absorption into subcutaneous lymphatics. Drainage is assisted by contraction in underlying muscles. Normally there is a negative pressure of –2 or –3 mmHg (Sven and Josipa 2007), which is influenced by external atmospheric pressure acting on the skin surface. Disturbances in the normally balanced dynamics of tissue fluid formation and absorption may increase the pressure, with fluid accumulating and resulting in edema, the distribution of which is influenced by posture. It may be seen by "pitting" of the skin in response to locally applied pressure. Conversely, fluid may be lost, as in severe dehydration, resulting in wrinkled dry skin and sunken eyes.

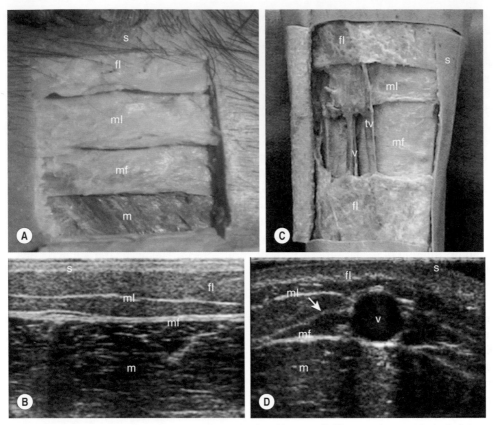

Fig. 1.4.1 (A) Layered dissection of the male breast region (chest wall). The membranous layer (ml) forms a single continuous layer in this dissection and the corresponding ultrasonogram (B), where it is sharply demarcated from the surrounding hypoechogenic fatty tissue layer (fl). (C) Layered dissection of the anterior leg region. Two superficial veins are seen: a tributary vein (tv) lies superficial to the membranous layer, and the main (saphenous) vein (v) is enclosed in a compartment formed by the muscular fascia (mf) deeply and by the membranous layer (ml) superficially. These two fascial layers fuse peripherally, delineating a compartment resembling an "Egyptian eye" shape using ultrasonography (D). In panel (D), the main vein is anchored to the fibrous wall of its compartment by a connective tissue lamina (arrow). Abbreviations: s, skin; m, muscle.

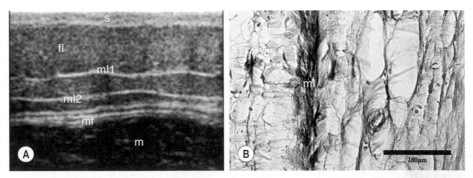

Fig. 1.4.2 (A) Ultrasonogram of the anterior thigh region. At least two membranous layers (ml1 and ml2) can be identified within the superficial fascia. (B) Histological appearance of an excised membranous layer (ml) between two fatty layers in the superficial fascia. Abbreviations: fl, fatty tissue layer; s, skin; m, muscle; mf, muscular fascia.

2. *Force absorption:* Subcutaneous mixtures of "fibro-adipose tissue" function as important pressure absorbers withstanding compressive and shearing forces on the body surface (Benjamin 2009). The best examples are seen in the palm of the hand and sole of the foot, particularly the fat-pad of the heel where strong fibrous septa pass from the dermis deeply to the plantar aponeurosis, dividing the fat into clearly defined compact lobules (Fig. 1.4.3).

3. *Thermal insulation:* Subcutaneous fat insulates the body against heat loss. The greater the thickness of fat, the more effective the insulation. This is particularly important in warm-blooded terrestrial animals.

4. *Energy source:* Subcutaneous fat provides a very significant reserve of stored energy (Marks and Miller 2006). The source of energy is triglycerides, which contain oleic and palmitic acids present in the fat droplets of the adipocytes. Brown fat, which is more abundant in newborns, provides a rapid source of energy and heat.
   a. In severe starvation the body's subcutaneous fat is utilized, resulting in tissue shrinkage, with wrinkling of the skin.

5. *Vascular arrangements:* Superficial veins lying in the subcutaneous tissues may be quite large and easily visible, especially in limbs, where they are available for intravenous injection, transfusions, or blood sampling. Studies on the saphenous veins in the lower extremities indicate that they lie interfascially rather than subfascially (Papadopoulos et al. 1981; Caggiati 2001). Each vein lies within a compartment delimited by two fasciae: the muscular fascia that lies deeply and the membranous layer that lies

superficially. The two fuse peripherally, forming a deep compartment of the hypodermis, resembling an "Egyptian eye" shape when viewed by ultrasonography (Fig. 1.4.1) (Caggiati 2000; Abu-Hijleh et al. 2006). Within their compartments the veins are anchored by a connective tissue lamina. Tributaries of the saphenous veins course superficial to the membranous layer in the subdermal fatty layer (Fig. 1.4.1) (Caggiati 2001; Abu-Hijleh et al. 2006), lacking fascial wrapping in contrast to the main veins. A similar arrangement exists along the cephalic vein and its tributaries in the upper extremity (Abu-Hijleh et al. 2006). There are also fascial canals in the fingers (Doyle 2003), containing digital vessels and nerves.
   a. The fascial relationships of superficial veins, particularly the saphenous system, have important clinical implications for hemodynamics and the pathophysiology of varicosities. Muscular contraction stretches the membranous compartment in which the main vein lies, diminishing the vein's caliber and therefore blood flow. The interfascial course of the main vein could constrain its excessive dilatation, thus diminishing the risk of varicosities. In contrast, the absence of any fascial sheathing of the more superficial tributaries could explain why varicosities more commonly affect them, because they lie outside the saphenous compartment (Caggiati 2000; Abu-Hijleh et al. 2006).

6. *Temperature regulation:* Because it is a ready source of energy, subcutaneous fat has a very rich blood supply and this plays a part in temperature regulation. Small arteries supply two plexuses (Young et al. 2006). The more superficial is the subpapillary plexus lying in the dermis close to the hypodermis. The second deeper plexus is the cutaneous plexus, and it lies in the hypodermis. The two plexuses freely communicate. Their state of distension or constriction determines the skin temperature and skin color in light-skinned races. Marked pallor of the skin, which is seen in acute shock, results from vasoconstriction in the arterial plexuses in the hypodermis. The smaller veins accompany the arteries and are similarly arranged into two plexuses. This arrangement provides rich arteriovenous communications, allowing shunts to occur that control blood flow through the skin and are used in thermoregulation of body temperature.

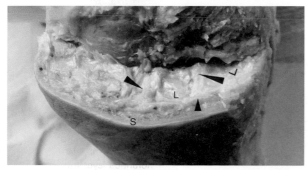

Fig. 1.4.3 Heel Fat Pad. Thick fibrous septa (arrows) beneath the skin (S) enclose fat lobules (L).

7. *Muscle:* In quadrupeds such as horses and cattle there are extensive sheets of subcutaneous muscle forming a distinct layer, the *panniculus carnosus*, in the deeper part of the hypodermis. This has a protective function, enabling the animal to dislodge skin irritants such as insects. In humans this layer is only vestigial, with remnants of smooth muscle in the scrotum, penis, anus, nipples, and labia majora. In the face, subcutaneous striated muscles are more organized, with a protective function, being arranged as sphincters and dilators around the orifices, particularly the eye and mouth. In the neck, the platysma muscle is usually well-defined, extending across the mandible into the upper neck.

8. *Fibers:* Fibers control the biomechanical properties of subcutaneous tissue, particularly its tensile and elastic properties as reflected in the overlying skin. They are dispersed as fine nets (Fig. 1.4.4) throughout the subcutaneous space. Three types of fibers are present in the hypodermis, principally collagen and elastin but also reticulin, a type of collagen. Collagen provides tensile strength when the overlying skin is stretched. The principal form of collagen is type I but types III and V are also present. The fibers surround fat cells, grouping

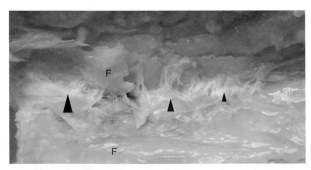

Fig. 1.4.4 Fine White Fibers in Subcutaneous Fat. The fibers (arrows) lie between the fat cells (F).

them into lobules. They also connect the dermis with underlying deep fascia. Elastic fibers are concerned with stretching and elastic recoil of the overlying dermis and epidermis. These fibers are in the form of a continuous network that contains mostly mature elastin (but also immature elaunin and oxytalan) fibers. In mechanical tests of skin and subcutaneous tissue, the response to uniaxial tension shows linear and viscoelastic characteristics (Iatridis et al. 2003).

9. *Cells:* Excluding adipocytes that store fat and form the majority of cells, a very important group of cells in subcutaneous tissue are fibroblasts. Besides synthesizing the proteins that form collagen and elastin fibers and other matrix proteins in subcutaneous tissue, they take part in degradation of collagen and other fibers. Fibroblasts are integral to mechanotransduction. They communicate with each other via gap junctions and respond to tissue stretch by shape changes that influence tension within the connective tissue, mediated via the cytoskeleton (Langevin 2006). These responses to mechanical load could result from changes in cell signaling and cell–matrix adhesion. Cell-shape changes may influence tension within the connective tissue itself. Brief stretching decreases transforming growth factor-beta 1 fibrillogenesis, which may be pertinent to development of manual therapy techniques for reducing the risk of scarring/fibrosis after an injury (Langevin 2006; Benjamin 2009; Correa-Gallegos et al. 2019).

Macrophages, derived from blood monocytes, are significant cell components because they are phagocytic for cell debris and also process and present antigen to immune-responsive lymphocytes that enter the hypodermis from blood capillaries. Other blood cells found in subcutaneous tissues are neutrophils. These also are protective and, as part of their normal, life-cycle leave the capillaries to circulate through the interstitial fluid before returning to the blood, irrespective of participating in inflammatory responses.

Mast cells, which have some of the features of blood basophils in the appearance of their granules, are also present in subcutaneous tissue. They produce heparin, serotonin, and histamine, which act on small blood vessels affecting their permeability. They mediate immunoglobulin E (IgE)-dependent forms of inflammation. Finally, plasma cells form IgE in the hypodermis.

10. *Extracellular matrix-ground substance:* The matrix contains glycoproteins (including fibrillin and fibronectin, which are necessary for the stretching and recoil properties of elastin, and fibronectin, which controls the deposition and orientation of collagen fibers. Other substances are glycosaminoglycans and proteoglycans, also hyaluronic acid, chondroitin, and dermatan sulfates.

11. *Other components:* The deeper parts of the coiled sweat glands extend down into the hypodermis. The roots of hair follicles are also located in the subcutaneous tissue.

Numerous nerve fibers traverse the subcutaneous tissue to reach the dermis and epidermis. While most of the specialized and nonspecialized nerve endings terminate in the dermis, there is one specialized ending that is normally located in the hypodermis. This is the lamellated Pacinian corpuscle, which mediates vibration and pressure sensations.

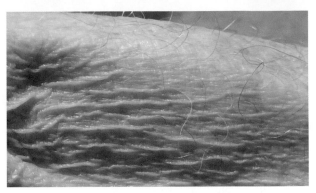

Fig. 1.4.5 Wrinkles in Aging Skin.

 KEY POINT

Subcutaneous tissue also contains many other important components: remnants of smooth muscle, elastic nets of fiber containing collagen and elastin, matrix ground substances, sweat glands and hair follicles, nerve fibers, and a variety of cells such as fibroblasts, mast cells, neutrophils, and macrophages, each with their own respective function.

AGING CHANGES IN SUBCUTANEOUS TISSUE

Age changes in the hypodermis are reflected on the surface of the body in the appearance and properties of the skin. Wrinkles and creases (Fig. 1.4.5) appear with increasing age. A decrease in the number of fibroblasts is accompanied by a decrease in the number of collagen fibers, which also become disorganized. The fibers disrupt and lose shape. Elastic fibers also decrease and become misshapen, appearing thickened and frayed. Using an indentation technique and measuring rebound it was noted that in both males and females there was a progressive decrease in elastic recoil through succeeding decades, starting from the third decade (Kirk and Chieffi 1962). The relationship was nonlinear. The amount of fat gradually declines as the fat cells atrophy. Quantitative and qualitative characteristics of the fibroadipose connective

system are changed, and its viscoelastic properties become reduced. The skin and underlying superficial fascia relax and stretch, resulting in ptotic soft tissues, pseudo fat deposit deformity, and cellulite (Lockwood 1991; Macchi et al. 2010). There is also atrophy of sweat and sebaceous glands, leading to drying of the overlying skin. Overall, these age changes result in less support for the small blood vessels and may be one reason why skin bruises more easily in old age.

 KEY POINT

Over time, changes in subcutaneous tissue result in visible wrinkles and changes in contour. These changes include loss of subcutaneous fat, a decrease in collagen and elastin fibers, and laxity of fascia.

Summary

Fascia superficialis is very extensive and lies deep to the skin, which itself covers the whole body. It has fatty, fibrous, and membranous components, the latter being more extensive than previously described. It particularly supports traversing blood vessels. Its diverse biochemical, cytological, and biomechanical components combine to provide the body with a wide spectrum of processes necessary to normal body stability. The cytology is diverse. Adipose cells produce and store fat, and fibroblasts produce a variety of fibers, all with mechanical properties. Macrophages and other types of leukocyte with protective functions migrate from the bloodstream and patrol through fascia superficialis. Evidence of advancing age is manifest in the skin by folds and wrinkles, but the cause lies in the subjacent superficial fascia and is due to atrophy in fat cells and fibers.

REFERENCES

Abu-Hijleh, M.F., Roshier, A.L., Al-Shboul, Q., Dharap, A.S., Harris, P.F., 2006. The membranous layer of superficial fascia: evidence for its widespread distribution in the body. Surg. Radiol. Anat. 28, 606–619.

Benjamin, M., 2009. The fascia of the limbs and back – a review. J. Anat. 214, 1–18.

Caggiati, A., 2000. Fascial relations and structure of the tributaries of the saphenous veins. Surg. Radiol. Anat. 22, 191–196.

Caggiati, A., 2001. Fascial relationships of the short saphenous vein. J. Vasc. Surg. 34, 241–246.

Carney, M., Matatov, T., Freeman, M., et al. 2017. Clinical, biomechanical, and anatomic investigation of Colles fascia and pubic ramus periosteum for use during medial thighplasty. Ann. Plast. Surg. 78, S305–S310.

Correa-Gallegos, D., Jiang, D., Christ, S., et al., 2019. Patch repair of deep wounds by mobilized fascia. Nature 576, 287–292.

Doyle, J.R., 2003. Hand. In: Doyle, J.R., Botte, M.J. (Eds.), Surgical Anatomy of the Hand and Upper Extremity. Lippincott, Williams & Wilkins, Philadelphia, pp. 532–641.

Hwang, K., Choi, J.H., 2018. Superficial fascia in the cheek and the superficial musculoaponeurotic system. J. Craniofac. Surg. 29, 1378–1382.

Iatridis, J.C., Wu, J., Yandow, J.A., Langevin, H.M., 2003. Subcutaneous tissue mechanical behaviour is linear and viscoelastic under axial tension. Connect. Tissue. Res. 44, 208–217.

Kawamata, S., Ozawa, J., Hashimoto, M., Kurose, T., Shinohara, H., 2003. Structure of the rat subcutaneous connective tissue in relation to its sliding mechanism. Arch. Histol. Cytol. 66, 273–279.

Kirk, J.E., Chieffi, M., 1962. Variation with age in elasticity of skin and subcutaneous tissue in human individuals. J. Gerontol. 17, 373–380.

Langevin, H.M., 2006. Connective tissue: a body-wide signaling network? Med. Hypotheses 66, 1074–1077.

Langevin, H.M., Huijing, P.A., 2009. Communicating about fascia: history, pitfalls, and recommendations. Int. J. Ther. Massage Bodywork 2, 3–8.

Lockwood, T.E., 1991. Superficial fascia system (SFS) of the trunk and extremities: a new concept. Plast. Reconstr. Surg. 87, 1009–1018.

Macchi, V., Tiengo, C., Porzionato, A., et al., 2010. Histotopographic study of fibroadipose connective cheek system. Cells Tissues Organs 191, 47–56.

Marks, J.G., Miller, J., 2006. Lookingbill and Marks' Principles of Dermatology, fourth ed. Elsevier Inc, Oxford.

McGrath, J.A., Eady, R.A., Pope, F.M., 2004. Rook's Textbook of Dermatology, seventh ed. Blackwell Publishing, Oxford.

Mitz, V., Peyronie, M., 1976. The superficial musculo-aponeurotic system (SMAS) in the parotid and cheek area. Plast. Reconstr. Surg. 58, 80–88.

Papadopoulos, N.J., Sherif, M.F., Albert, E.N., 1981. A fascial canal for the great saphenous vein: gross and microanatomical observations. J. Anat. 132, 321–329.

Pisco, A., Rebelo, M., Peres, H., Costa-Ferreira, A, 2020. Abdominoplasty with Scarpa fascia preservation: prospective comparative study of suction drain number. Ann. Plast. Surg. 84, 356–360.

Song, T.T., Nelson, M.R., Hershey, J.N., Chowdhury, B.A., 2004. Subcutaneous tissue depth differences between males and females: the need for gender based epinephrine needle. J. Allergy Clin. Immunol. 113, S241.

Spalding, K.L., Arner, E., Westermark, P.O., et al., 2008. Dynamics of fat cell turnover in humans. Nature 453, 783–787.

Standring, S., (Ed.), 2016. Gray's Anatomy: The Anatomical Basis of Clinical Practice, forty-first ed. Elsevier, New York, pp. 28, 81, 141, 1562.

Sven, K., Josipa, F., 2007. Interstitial hydrostatic pressure: a manual for students. Adv. Physiol. Educ. 31, 116–117.

Van der Wal, J., 2009. The architecture of the connective tissue in the musculoskeletal system - an often overlooked functional parameter as to proprioception in the locomotor apparatus. Int. J. Ther. Massage and Bodywork 2, 9–23.

Wood Jones, F., 1946. Buchanan's Manual of Anatomy, seventh ed. Baillière, Tindall & Cox, London.

Young, B., Lowe, J.S., Stevens, A., Heath, J.W. (Eds.), 2006. Wheater's Functional Histology, fifth ed. Churchill Livingstone Elsevier Limited, Philadelphia, p. 183.

Zheng, Y., Mak, A.F.T., Lue, B., 1999. Objective assessment of limb tissue elasticity: development of a manual indentation procedure. J. Rehabil. Res. Dev. 36, 1–25.

Deep Fascia of the Limbs

Antonio Stecco, Carmelo Pirri, and Carla Stecco

CHAPTER CONTENTS

INTRODUCTION

With respect to the trunk, the limbs present a completely different myofascial organization, as the muscles are arranged in compartments and not in layers. Consequently, the relationship between fasciae and muscles also differs: in the trunk, the fasciae are totally adherent to the muscles, and only a few aponeurotic fasciae are present, placed in series with the muscles. In the limbs, each muscle is enveloped in an epimysial fascia, and there is an aponeurotic fascia in parallel that covers all the muscles and defines the various compartments (Table 1.5.1). Such a fascia is totally free to glide over the underlying muscles and can also act as a bridge, connecting the various muscles involved in the same movements. The fasciae of the upper limbs may be imagined as similar to a woman's elegant glove, and those of the lower limbs like elasticated "stay-up-on-their-own" stockings, the former supported by myofascial expansion of the pectoral, deltoid, and latissimus dorsi muscles, and the latter by the gluteus maximus and external oblique muscles and the tensor of the fascia lata muscle. In this way, the fasciae of the limbs are clearly in continuity with the superficial myofascial layer of the trunk and thus play a key role in connecting the upper limbs with the lower ones.

Studies have reported the unifying role of connective tissue in the limbs. In particular, they have not only demonstrated the serial continuity of the various fasciae (e.g., Krause et al. 2016; Wilke and Krause 2019) but also that the deep fasciae blend with the periosteum, tendons, and ligaments (Benjamin 2009). The many functions of the deep limb fasciae include their role as ectoskeletons for muscle attachments, the creation of osteofascial compartments for muscles, and also their role in venous return, in the dissipation of tensional stress concentrated at the site of entheses. They also serve to protect underlying structures. Modern studies (Langevin 2006; C. Stecco et al. 2019) have shown the primary role played by the fasciae in the proprioception and coordination of movement, as caused by their unique mechanical properties and dense innervation. The deep fasciae are in fact able to perceive contractions of underlying muscles and movements of bones thanks to these myofascial connections, as described in the topographical sections of this chapter. Thus every time a muscular contraction takes place, part of its force is transmitted to the bone through the tendon to perform the movement and part is transmitted to the fascia through myofascial expansions. This is important for perception of movements and maintenance of basal

TABLE 1.5.1.   Differences Between Aponeurotic Fascia and Epimysial Fascia

	Aponeurotic Fascia	Epimysial Fascia
Terminology	Refers to all the well-defined fibrous sheaths that cover and keep in place a group of muscles or generate origins/insertions for wide muscles.	Refers to all the thin but well-organized collagen layers that are strongly connected with the muscle.
Topographical examples	Thoracolumbar fascia, rectus sheath, all the deep fasciae of the limbs.	Deep fascia of trunk muscles, such as pectoralis major, latissimus dorsi, and deltoid muscles, but also the epimysium of the muscles of the limbs.
Relationship with muscles	Envelops groups of muscles and connects them, forming the various compartments of the limbs.	Specific for each muscle and defines their form and volume.

tension in the deep fascia (C. Stecco et al. 2009a). At the points where the mechanical forces acting in the fasciae are stronger, the latter thicken and become more fibrous. These reinforcements around the joints are called retinacula.

Classically, the deep fasciae of the limbs are described as irregular, dense, connective tissues, with the mere function of enveloping muscles. More current studies provide important evidence of a definite microscopic organization of the deep fasciae of the limbs. On microscopic evaluation, the deep fasciae of the limbs and the retinacula are formed of collagen fiber bundles in a slightly undulating arrangement. In the retinacula, the fibrous bundles are more densely packed and there is less loose connective tissue. The fibrous bundles are regularly arranged in two or three distinct layers of parallel collagen fiber bundles. There is normally complete independence among the various layers due to a thin lining of loose connective tissue (mean thickness 43 ± 12 mm), which allows sliding between and among the layers. Throughout the body, the role of loose connective tissue is to cushion and separate differing structures. The specific orientation of the collagen fibers, with an initial crimp at rest; irregular distribution of elastic fibers; and the variable presence of loose connective tissue all imply great complexity in the biomechanical behavior of the deep fasciae of the limbs.

THE DEEP FASCIA OF THE SHOULDER

The deep fasciae of the shoulder present characteristics that are similar to both those of the trunk and the extremities. The pectoralis major, deltoid, trapezius, and latissimus dorsi muscles are enveloped only by their epimysial fasciae, which are relatively thin, collagen fiber layers. All these fasciae adhere firmly to their respective muscles due to a series of intramuscular septa that extend from the internal surface of these fasciae, dividing the muscle itself into many bundles. Several muscular fibers originate not only from the inner sides of these fasciae but also directly from the intramuscular septa.

The fasciae of the pectoralis major, deltoid, trapezius, and latissimus dorsi muscles form a single layer, enveloping all these muscles and passing over the serratus anterior, which is/has a strong fascial lamina. This myofascial arrangement matches the description of the trunk reported by Sato and Hashimoto (1984), who state that the pectoralis major, latissimus dorsi, and trapezius muscles form an additional myofascial layer with respect to the muscular planes of the rest of the trunk.

Although the pectoral fascia originates from the clavicle, only its deep layer adheres to the clavicular periosteum; its superficial layer continues upward with the superficial lamina of the deep cervical fascia, which surrounds the sternocleidomastoid and trapezial muscles. Medially, the deep layer of the pectoral fascia is inserted in the sternal periosteum, whereas the superficial layer extends beyond the sternum to continue with the pectoral fascia on the other side. Distally, the pectoral fascia is reinforced by fibrous expansions originating from the rectus abdominis sheath and from the fascia of the contralateral external oblique muscles. In particular, the pectoral fascia has a mean thickness of 151 μm, which increases in a craniocaudal direction to reach a mean thickness of 578 μm in the mammary region. Over the xyphoid process, the pectoral fascia forms a clearly visible, interwoven pattern of fibers (A. Stecco et al. 2009b). Laterally, the superficial and deep layers of the pectoralis major fascia fuse, passing over the serratus anterior muscle to envelop the latissimus dorsi posteriorly. This fascia also continues with the deltoid fascia. All these fasciae have the same characteristics, adhering strongly to the muscles. Thus when the muscles are relaxed, mechanical forces are transmitted through the connective tissue component connecting the lower and upper limbs. Instead, when these muscles contract, they can stop transmission from the limbs. This means, for example, that we can walk without moving our upper limbs, although this requires a muscular contraction and is more energy demanding. Instead, if we run, it is also easier to move the upper limbs and head, because our fasciae dissipate the energy coming from the lower limbs. On the basis of this anatomical statement, reinforcement of the muscles of this myofascial layer could easily alter any physiological fascial connection between the upper and lower limbs.

Dissections in the shoulder region of unembalmed cadavers (C. Stecco et al. 2008) have shown the constant presence of specific myofascial expansions originating from the pectoralis major, latissimus dorsi, and deltoid muscles, all of which merge into the brachial fascia. The lateral part of the deltoid, mainly involved in abduction of the arm, shows a myotendinous expansion toward the lateral intermuscular septum and the overlying brachial fascia. Lastly, expansions originating from the main adductor muscles (i.e., the latissimus dorsi and the costal portions of the pectoralis major) extend toward the medial intermuscular septum. This means that, during adduction, the synchronous contraction of the latissimus dorsi and the costal fibers of the pectoralis major muscles produces tension in the medial portion of the brachial fascia. In effect, the brachial fascia also stretches toward other more distal points, creating specific lines of forces along it. For example, during antepulsion of the upper limb, contraction of the clavicular fibers of the pectoralis major stretches the anterior region of the brachial fascia, and contraction of the biceps stretches the anterior region of the antebrachial fascia by virtue of its bicipital aponeurosis, whereas the palmaris longus pulls on the flexor retinaculum, palmar aponeurosis, and thenar fascia (Fig. 1.5.1). In the same way, during extension of the upper limb, the latissimus dorsi stretches the posterior portion of the brachial fascia through its myofascial expansion, the medial head of the triceps extends distally into the antebrachial fascia, and the extensor

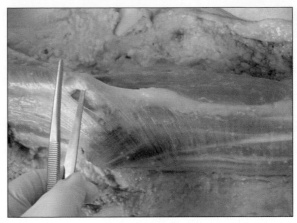

Fig. 1.5.1 Dissection of the anteromedial region of the elbow showing the lacertus fibrosus or the fibrous expansion of the biceps brachii muscle onto the antebrachial fascia.

carpi ulnaris moves into the fascia of the hypothenar muscles. Lastly, the abductor digiti minimi sends a tendinous expansion into the extensor aponeurosis.

In the region of the clavicle, below the superficial muscular layer, there is the second myofascial clavipectoral plane, which is specifically for the stability and movement of the scapula. There is an ample plane of cleavage between the pectoralis major muscle and this fascia due to the presence of loose connective tissue, which allows the deep layer of the pectoral fascia to glide autonomously with respect to the clavipectoral fascia. The latter is a strong connective layer arising from the clavicle and extending distally to enclose the subclavius and pectoralis minor muscles. Laterally, the clavipectoral fascia continues with the axillary fascia and that of the coracobrachialis muscle. Distally, this fascia envelops the serratus anterior muscle and then moves posteriorly to envelope the scapula with all its muscles. Lastly, it envelops the rhomboid muscles and the levator scapulae muscle. In this way, the axillary region contains a superficial fascia and two layers of deep fascia: the former connects the pectoralis major and latissimus dorsi, and the latter corresponds to the coracoclavicular fascia. This topographical region contains many lymph nodes between the superficial and deep fasciae. It is similar to the cribriform fascia of the thigh and, likewise, is filled with a plug of fibrous tissue and fat. This structure is maintained in a healthy state to ensure proper lymphatic return.

THE DEEP FASCIA OF THE ARM AND FOREARM

KEY POINT

The brachial fascia and the antebrachial fascia form the deep fasciae of the arm. The superficial fascia in the arm is clearly evident within the subcutaneous adipose tissue, and it is easily detached from the deep fascia.

The brachial fascia is a strong, semitransparent, laminar sheet of connective tissue covering the arm muscles. It has a mean thickness of 863 μm (SD ± 77 μm), being thinner in the anterior region with respect to the posterior region. Collagen fiber bundles, in different directions, are easily identifiable within this fascia. They have a prevalently transverse course with respect to the long axis of the arm, although longitudinal and oblique collagen bundles are also present. The brachial fascia is easily separable from the underlying muscles, as it is attached to the lateral and medial intermuscular septa and the epicondyles (Fig. 1.5.2). Proximally, it is continuous with the axillary fascia and the fasciae of the pectoralis major, deltoid, and latissimus dorsi muscles.

The antebrachial fascia appears as a thick, whitish layer of connective tissue, sheathing the flexor and

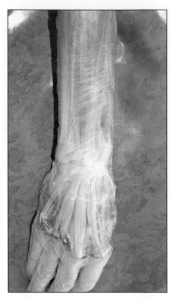

Fig. 1.5.3 Dissection of the Posterior Region of the Forearm. The antebrachial fascia shows a strong reinforcement at the wrist, corresponding to the extensor retinaculum of the wrist.

extensor muscle compartments and extending septa between them from its internal surface. The mean thickness of the antebrachial fascia is 0.75 mm, although this increases (mean value 1.19 mm) in the wrist region, forming the flexor and extensor retinacula of the wrist (Fig. 1.5.3). In the palm, the antebrachial fascia continues laterally and medially with the thenar and hypothenar fasciae and with the thick, transversal fiber bundles between the eminences. In the midpalm region, this thickening is continuous with the deep layer of the palmar aponeurosis. Muscular fibers of the thenar and hypothenar muscles are also inserted in the inner surface of their fascia.

THE PALMAR APONEUROSIS

The palmar aponeurosis adheres closely to the skin because of the presence of thick fibrous septa (retinacula cutis). Two main fibrous layers characterize the palmar aponeurosis: a superficial one, with longitudinal disposition of fibers closely adhering to the skin, which may be considered as a local specialization of the superficial fascia, and a deeper one, distal over the heads of the metacarpal bones, with fibers arranged transversely. The transverse layer, which may be considered as a local specialization of the deep fascia, adheres to the longitudinal layer, which is more superficial.

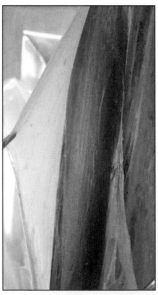

Fig. 1.5.2 Dissection of the Anterior Region of the Arm. The brachial fascia has been detached from the biceps brachii muscle.

Vertical septa detach from the deep aspect of the palmar aponeurosis to form the flexor tendon compartments of the last four digits and to anchor the deep aspect of the palmar aponeurosis to the metacarpal bones. The superficial longitudinal layer is stretched proximally by the palmaris longus muscle, which pierces the deep fascia in the distal part of the forearm. This muscle should be considered as a proper tensor of the palmar aponeurosis. If the palmaris longus muscle is absent, the palmar aponeurosis is nevertheless present, but its superficial macroscopic appearance demonstrates clear-cut disarrangement. This indicates the active role of the palmaris longus muscle, through mechanical tension, in determining the longitudinal disposition of the fibers of the superficial layer.

This fusion between superficial and deep fascia may play a specific role: it combines exteroception, usually related to the superficial fascia, and proprioception, related to the deep fascia. In this way, the shape of the hand is adapted for a perfect grasp. The same thing occurs in the foot, with the plantar aponeurosis.

DEEP FASCIAE OF THE LOWER LIMBS: FASCIA LATA AND CRURAL FASCIA

 KEY POINT

The fascia lata and the crural fascia form the deep fasciae of the lower limb. The deep fascia is easily separable from the underlying muscle due to the presence of the epimysial fascia of the underlying muscles.

The deep fascia of the lower limbs consists of a lamina of connective tissue that can generally be easily separated from both the underlying muscles and the overlying superficial fascia. There is in fact a virtually uninterrupted plane of gliding between the deep fascia and the muscles surrounded by their epimysium, with only a small layer of interposing loose connective tissue to facilitate gliding. This loose connective tissue appears as a pliable, gelatinous substance. Histological studies demonstrate that fibroblasts are widely dispersed within the tissue and that collagen and elastic fibers are arranged in an irregular mesh.

A few strong intermuscular septa originate from the inner surface of the deep fascia of the lower limbs and extend between the belly muscles, dividing the thigh into several compartments and providing an origin for some lower limb muscle fibers (Fig. 1.5.4).

It is important to note that, although the deep fascia of the lower limbs in the thigh is called the fascia lata and in the leg the crural fascia, it is actually the same structure. This fascia appears as a thick, whitish layer of connective tissue, similar to an aponeurosis, with an average thickness of 1 mm. In general, the deep fascia of the lower limbs is also thicker in the posterior regions of the limbs. However, studies on variations in thickness of the lower limb fasciae have revealed some regional differences. In particular, the deep fascia of the anterior thigh has a mean thickness of 944 ± 102 mm. It is thinner in the proximal region (541 ± 23 mm) and thicker near the knee (1419 ± 105 mm) but has a mean thickness of 874 ± 62 mm in the middle third of the

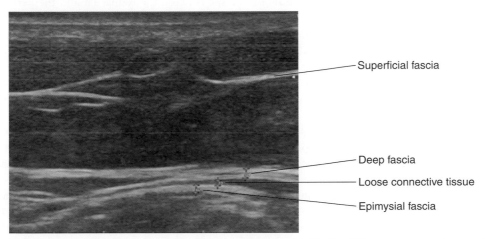

Fig. 1.5.4 Ultrasound Imaging of the Fascial Layers of the Limbs. The fascial layers appear as hyperechoic lines and the loose connective tissue between the layers of deep fascia like hypoechoic lines.

thigh. It is reinforced by the iliotibial tract in the lateral region. The iliotibial tract cannot be separated from the deep fascia by dissection. Anatomically, therefore, it cannot be considered as a separate entity but rather as a reinforcement of the lateral aspect of the fascia lata, probably due to the constant action of the tensor fascia latae muscle and the superficial fibers of the gluteus maximus muscle that are inserted in this fascia and work to maintain bipedal posture. Distally, the iliotibial tract is attached to Gerdy's tubercle at the upper end of the tibia, but it also has an expansion into the antero-lateral portion of the crural fascia. Fairclough et al. (2007) suggest that the iliotibial band syndrome is not caused by frictional forces created by movement forward and backward over the tibial condyle during flexion and extension of the knee but by tensional changes within the iliotibial tract itself. Similarly, the sartorius, gracilis, and semitendinosus muscles form the pes anserinus in the medial portion of the knee (Murlimanju et al. 2019), but they also expand into the medial aspect of the crural fascia. In this way, both the medial and lateral sides of the knee are stabilized by myofascial expansions of the biarticular muscles, which coordinate the movements of the hip with those of the knee. In addition, the quadriceps muscle has several obliquely directed fascial expansions arising from the vastus medialis and lateralis muscles, which pass anterior to the patella and reinforce the fascia lata, called the anterior knee retinaculum. The popliteal area also has some fascial reinforcements: one is due to the mechanical forces of the semimembranosus muscle; others are due to the proximal portions of the gastrocnemius muscle, which is not inserted only into the epicondyles but also into the overlying fascia, thus also working as fascial tensors (Fig. 1.5.5). Anteriorly, the tibialis anterior and flexor hallucis longus muscles are inserted in the overlying fascia and the intermuscular septum. In this way, around the knee it is quite difficult to separate the deep fascia from the underlying muscles and tendons.

The crural fascia has an average thickness of 880 mm, which progressively decreases from 1 mm in the popliteal region to 700 mm in the distal third of the leg. Around the knee and the ankle, the deep fascia is reinforced by more fibrous bundles, commonly called retinacula; however, it should be emphasized that all the fasciae have many fibrous bundles running in different and macroscopically visible directions.

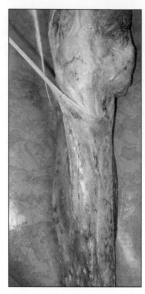

Fig. 1.5.5 Dissection of the Inferior Limb, Anteromedial View of the Knee Region. The expansion of the semitendinosus muscle into the crural fascia is evident.

THE RETINACULA

The retinacula are typically regional specializations of the deep fascia; in particular, they are thickenings of the deep fasciae and, as such, are not separable. They appear as strong fibrous bundles with a mean thickness of 1372 mm and a crisscross arrangement of the collagen fibers. The retinacula have many bone insertions, and these entheses may be fibrocartilaginous. At other points, they can glide over the bones thanks to interposing loose connective tissue between the retinacula and the periosteum. From a functional point of view, the retinacula have classically been considered as a pulley system, maintaining the tendons adherent to the underlying bones during movements of the tibiotarsal joint, and as important elements for ankle stability, connecting various bones. However, in 1984, Viladot et al. stated that they may play an important role in proprioception, and this was confirmed by C. Stecco et al. in 2010. In fact, all the retinacula work to stabilize tendons, reducing movement near the enthesis and, consequently, minimizing the stress that concentrates at bony insertion sites, but they also perceive selective stretching of the fascia, which can activate specific proprioceptor patterns during movement. For example, the peroneal retinacula may be stretched by inversion of the ankle joint, activating reflex contraction of the peroneal muscles. The ankle retinacula can easily be evaluated by magnetic resonance imagery, as they appear as low-signal-intensity bands, sharply defined in the subcutaneous tissue in T1-weighted sequences, with a mean thickness of 1.25 mm (SD: 0.198). The retinacula may also be subject to traumatic rupture, sometimes resulting in subluxation of the underlying tendons.

The knee retinacula can also be easily evaluated by MR imaging (A. Stecco et al. 2011), clearly appearing as low-signal-intensity bands. In patients with patellar femoral malalignment or anterior knee pain, differences in thickness, innervations, and vascularization are all visible. These alterations may also have implications in terms of the observed loss of equilibrium with aging.

Summary

The myofascial expansions showed a quite constant course with a specific spatial organization. During the various movements of the limbs, these expansions stretch selective portions of the deep fascial layers, with possible activation of specific patterns of fascial proprioceptors.

REFERENCES

Benjamin, M., 2009. The fascia of the limbs and back – a review. J. Anat. 214, 1–18.

Fairclough, J., Hayashi, K., Toumi, H., et al., 2007. Is iliotibial band syndrome really a friction syndrome? J. Sci. Med. Sport. 10, 74–76.

Krause, F., Wilke, J., Vogt, L., Banzer, W., 2016. Intermuscular force transmission along myofascial chains: a systematic review. J. Anat. 228, 910–918.

Langevin, H.M., 2006. Connective tissue: a body-wide signalling network? Med. Hypotheses 66, 1074–1077.

Murlimanju, B.V., Vadgaonkar, R., Kumar, G.C., et al., 2019. Morphological variants of pes anserinus in South India. Muscles Ligaments Tendons J. 9, 372–378.

Sato, T., Hashimoto, M., 1984. Morphological analysis of the fascial lamination of the trunk. Bull. Tokyo Med. Dent. Univ. 31, 21–32.

Stecco, A., Masiero, S., Macchi, V., et al. 2009b. The pectoral fascia: anatomical and histological study. J. Bodyw. Mov. Ther. 13, 255–261.

Stecco, A., Stecco, C., Macchi, V., et al., 2011. RMI study and clinical correlations of ankle retinacula damage and outcomes of ankle sprain. Surg. Radiol. Anat. 33, 881–890.

Stecco, C., Macchi, V., Porzionato, A., et al., 2010. The ankle retinacula: morphological evidence of the proprioceptive role of the fascial system. Cells Tissues Organs 192, 200–210.

Stecco, C., Pavan, P.G., Porzionato, A., et al., 2009a. Mechanics of crural fascia: from anatomy to constitutive modelling. Surg. Radiol. Anat. 31, 523–529.

Stecco, C., Pirri, C., Fede, C., et al., 2019. Dermatome and fasciatome. Clin. Anat. 32, 896–902.

Stecco, C., Porzionato, A., Macchi, V., et al., 2008. The expansions of the pectoral girdle muscles onto the brachial fascia: morphological aspects and spatial disposition. Cells Tissues Organs 188, 320–329.

Viladot, A., Lorenzo, J.C., Salazar, J., Rodriguez, A., 1984. The subtalar joint: embryology and morphology. Foot Ankle 5, 54–66.

Wilke, J., Krause, F., 2019. Myofascial chains of the upper limb: a systematic review of anatomical studies. Clin. Anat. 32, 934–940.

The Thoracolumbar Fascia

Andry Vleeming, Frank H. Willard and Robert Schleip

CHAPTER CONTENTS

INTRODUCTION

To stabilize the lumbar vertebrae on the sacral base requires the assistance of a complex myofascial and aponeurotic girdle surrounding the torso (Bergmark 1989; Cholewicki et al. 1997; Willard 2007). On the posterior body wall, the central point of this girdling structure is the thoracolumbar fascia (TLF), a blending of aponeurotic and fascial planes that forms the retinaculum around the paraspinal muscles of the lower back and sacral region (Singer 1935; Romanes 1981; Clemente 1985; Vleeming and Willard 2010; Schuenke et al. 2012).

What is traditionally labeled as TLF is in reality a complex arrangement of multilayered fascial planes and aponeurotic sheets (Benetazzo et al. 2011). Portions of this dense connective tissue structure were described as a "functional composite" of structures (Vleeming and Willard 2010). This complex structure becomes especially notable at the caudal end of the lumbar spine where multiple layers of aponeurotic tissue unite and blend to form a thickened brace between the two posterior superior iliac spines (PSIS) and extending caudalward to reach the ischial tuberosities. Various myofascial structures with differing elastic moduli contribute to the formation of this thoracolumbar composite (TLC).

Currently, several models of this TLF exist, and various authors tend to use somewhat different nomenclature, resulting in confusion that hampers the interpretation of biomechanical studies (for a discussion, see Goss 1973). In this overview, new and existent material on the fascial organization and composition of the TLF will be reviewed, and a geometric structure of the TLF will be proposed.

Abbreviations	Structures
GM	Gluteus Maximus
GMed	Gluteus Medius
IAP	Intra-abdominal Pressure
LD	Latissimus Dorsi
LIFT	Lumbar Interfascial Triangle
LR	Lateral Raphe
MLF	Middle Layer of Thoracolumbar Fascia
IO	Internal oblique
EO	External oblique
PLF	Posterior Layer of Thoracolumbar Fascia
PRS	Paraspinal Retinacular Sheath
QL	Quadratus Lumborum
SIJ	Sacroiliac Joint
slPL	Superficial Lamina of Posterior Layer

Abbreviations	Structures
SPI	Serratus Posterior Inferior
STL	Sacrotuberous Ligament
TLC	Thoracolumbar Composite
TLF	Thoracolumbar Fascia
TrA	Transversus Abdominis

THE THORACOLUMBAR FASCIA

The TLF is a complex of several layers that separates the paraspinal muscles from the muscles of the posterior abdominal wall, quadratus lumborum (QL) and psoas major. Numerous descriptions of this structure have presented either a two-layered model or a three-layered model (Goss 1973). Both models are summarized here, and a consensus approach attempted. Fig. 1.6.1 presents a summary diagram illustrating the two- vs. three-layered model of the TLF.

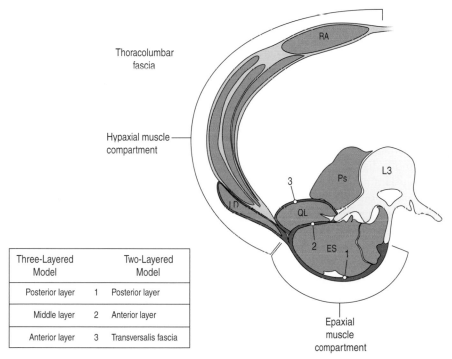

Three-Layered Model		Two-Layered Model
Posterior layer	1	Posterior layer
Middle layer	2	Anterior layer
Anterior layer	3	Transversalis fascia

Fig. 1.6.1 A tracing of the hypaxial and epaxial myofascial compartments, illustrating the comparison between the two-layered and three-layered models of the TLF. The latissimus dorsi (LD) is seen lying on the external wall of the hypaxial compartment and extending over the epaxial compartment to reach its attachments on the midline. In doing so, the aponeurosis of the LD contributes to the superficial lamina of the PLF.

THE TWO-LAYERED MODEL

The two-layered model of TLF recognizes a posterior layer surrounding the posterior aspect of the paraspinal muscles and an anterior layer lying between the paraspinal muscles and the QL (Fig. 1.6.1). The two-layered model has been presented in the early English versions of Henry Gray's work (Gray 1923) and from the first American edition (Gray 1870) to the 30th (Clemente 1985). Other proponents of the two-layered model of TLF include such authorities as Spalteholz (1923), Schaeffer (1953), Hollinshead (1969), and Clemente (1985).

The two-layered model presents a posterior layer that attaches to the tips of the spinous processes of the lumbar vertebrae as well as the supraspinous ligament and wraps around the paraspinal muscles reaching a raphe on their lateral border. The posterior layer is typically described as being composed of two sheets, a deep lamina that invests the paraspinal muscles and a superficial lamina that joins the deep lamina in the lower lumbar region. The superficial lamina is derived in large part from the aponeurosis of the LD. The serratus posterior inferior (SPI) and its very thin, aponeurosis inserts, when it is present, between the aponeurosis of the LD and the deep lamina (Fig. 1.6.2). This latter structure fuses to the outer surface of the deep lamina more so than it does to the superficial lamina.

In a cranial direction, the deep lamina of the posterior layer continues cranially along the thoracic paraspinal muscles. However, here it is thin and can easily be missed; its lateral attachments reach out to the angle of the ribs, and its medial attachments are to the spinous processes and interspinous ligaments. Finally in the cervical region, the deep lamina of the posterior layer continues to cover the paraspinal muscles (all the muscles innervated by the posterior primary ramus) including the splenius capitis, as it blends with surrounding cervical fascias; eventually this paraspinal fascial sheath fuses to the cranial base (Wood Jones 1946).

The trapezius, LD, and rhomboid muscles (all derived from limb buds) are positioned external to the posterior layer and contained in their own envelope of epimysial fascia (see Fig. 1.6.3; Stecco et al. 2009). These bridging extremity muscles pass external to the paraspinal muscles, eventually reaching their attachments on midline structures, such as the spinous processes and supraspinous ligament, or they attach to the outer portion of the investing layer of epaxial fascia surrounding the paraspinal muscles. In the lumbar region, the aponeurosis of the LD crosses diagonally over the deep layer, thus creating the superficial lamina.

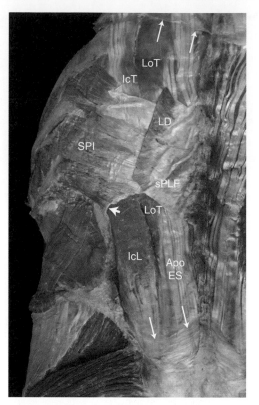

Fig. 1.6.2 A posterior view of the lower thoracic and lumbar spine illustrating the construction of the superficial and deep lamina of the PLF. The LD has been sectioned to expose the underlying SPI. The aponeuroses of these two muscles combine to form the sPLF. The sPLF attaches to the deep lamina of PLF; both of these laminae have been removed over the lumbar region to expose the erector spinae muscles. The short arrow points to the curvature of the deep lamina as it wraps around the erector spinae muscles laterally forming the epaxial myofascial compartment. The paired long arrows, top and bottom, point to the sectioned edge of the deep lamina. Note that the deep lamina is thick and aponeurotic in nature at the lower lumbar level, but thin and fascial in nature in the upper thoracic region. Apo ES, aponeurosis of the erector spinae; IcL, iliocostalis lumborum; IcT, iliocostalis thoracis; LD, latissimus dorsi; LoT, longissimus thoracis; sPLF, superficial lamina of posterior layer of thoracolumbar fascia; SPI, serratus posterior inferior.

In the two-layered model, what is termed the anterior layer of TLF is a thick band of regularly arranged collagen bundles separating the paraspinal muscles from the QL (Fig. 1.6.1). Thus, this layer really represents an aponeurosis. It is attached medially to the tips of the transverse processes of the lumbar vertebrae, and laterally it joins the posterior layer along a thickened seam, termed the lateral raphe. Note that this anterior layer is described in most current textbooks that use the three-layered model as the middle layer (MLF) of TLF.

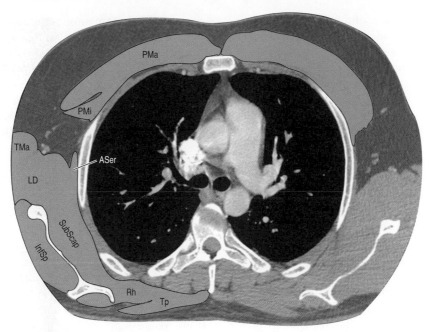

Fig. 1.6.3 An axial plane CT with contrast taken through the chest at the level of the pulmonary trunk. The bridging muscles (muscles that cross between upper extremity and torso) have been shaded white. These muscles are in a common fascial sheath that extends from the extremity medially to surround the upper portion of the torso. This sheath reaches as far caudalward as the sternum anteriorly and the sacrum posteriorly. Inside the sheath are the hypaxial and epaxial muscle compartments of the thorax and abdomen, each surrounded by its own fascial sheath. ASer, anterior serratus; IntSp, intraspinatus; LD, latissimus dorsi; PMa, pectoralis major; PMi, pectoralis minor; Rh, rhomboid; SubScap, subscapularis; TMa, teres major; Tp, trapezius.

Finally, in the two-layered model, the fascia on the anterior aspect of the QL has been depicted to be an extension of the transversalis fascia from the abdominal wall (Fig. 1.6.1; Hollinshead 1969).

THE THREE-LAYERED MODEL

The three-layered model has been endorsed by numerous authors (Testut 1899; Huber 1930; Singer 1935; Green 1937; Wood Jones 1946; Anson and Maddock 1958), including some of the recent authors (Bogduk and Macintosh 1984; Vleeming et al. 1995; Barker and Briggs 2007; Standring 2008). Of interest, Grant's *Atlas of Anatomy* presented the three-layered model of TLF at least up to the 2nd edition, then changed to a two-layered model by the 6th edition (Grant 1972).

The three-layered model has strong similarities with the previously described model containing two layers (Fig. 1.6.1). The posterior layer consists of two laminae: superficial (the aponeurosis of the LD); and deep lamina. In between these laminae above the L4 level, the aponeurosis of the SPI is present. The MLF is the fascial band that passes between the paraspinal muscles and the QL. The anterior layer is defined as passing anterior to the QL and ending by turning posterior to pass between the QL and the psoas. The anterior layer has been described as being an extension of the transversalis fascia.

The three-layered model is the most commonly used model in most research studies (Bogduk and Macintosh 1984; Vleeming et al. 1995; reviewed in Barker and Briggs 2007). This review will use the terminology of the three-layered model with the understanding that the anterior layer may be little more than a thin transversalis fascia and as such may not be able to transmit tension from the abdominal muscles to the thoracolumbar spine.

COMPARTMENTALIZATION OF THE PARASPINAL MUSCLES

In both models of the TLF, the paraspinal muscles are depicted as being contained in a fascial compartment (Fig. 1.6.2); however, terminology and descriptions concerning the layers of this compartment vary considerably. Some authors consider the compartment to be a continuous sheet of fascia wrapping around the paraspinal muscles and attaching to the spinous process posteromedially and transverse process anterolaterally (Spalteholz 1923; Schaeffer 1953; Hollinshead 1969; Bogduk and Macintosh 1984; Clemente 1985; Tesh et al. 1987; Gatton et al. 2010). Others conceive of the anterior and posterior walls of the compartment as arising from a split of the aponeurosis of the transversus abdominis (TrA; Anson and Maddock 1958; Barker and Briggs 1999). Regardless of the approach, it is clear that the paraspinal muscles are contained in a sealed osteofibrous compartment attached to the spinous processes on the midline and the transverse processes anterolaterally (see Standring 2008, pp. 708–709). On the lateral extreme of the compartment, it is joined by the thick aponeurosis of the TrA; this junction point is termed the lateral raphe (Bogduk and Macintosh 1984). A number of texts and reports described or illustrated the aponeurosis of the TrA as simply joining the lateral border of the compartment of the paraspinal muscles (Spalteholz 1923; Tesh et al. 1987; Gatton et al. 2010) or as continuing medially to form the anterior wall (MLF) of the compartment (Romanes 1981). However, a new study confirms that the fascia covering the paraspinal muscles forms a continuous sheath to which the aponeurosis of the TrA contributes laterally (Schuenke et al. 2012).

Although the aponeurosis of the TrA appears to contribute to both the posterior and anterior walls of the paraspinal compartment, based on the increased thickness of the anterior wall (or MLF) it is likely that most of the aponeurosis joins the anterior wall. This dual arrangement supports the work of Tesh et al. (1987) who described the MLF as having two layers. Thus, in the most common terminology, the compartment is made up of the deep lamina of the PLF (Bogduk and Macintosh 1984) that extends continuously from the spinous processes to the transverse processes. When opened, this compartment presents a smooth, curved lateral boundary with no indication of a seam or split.

PROPOSED MODEL OF THE THORACOLUMBAR FASCIA

The TLF is a structural composite built out of aponeurotic and fascial planes that unite together to surround the paraspinal muscles and stabilize the lumbosacral spine. Approaching this composite from the posterior

aspect finds the aponeurotic attachments of two muscles: the LD and the SPI combining to form a superficial lamina of the PLF (Fig. 1.6.4). However, the central component of the TLF is not the superficial lamina of the posterior layer, but the deep lamina of the PLF forming a fascial sheath, coined the paraspinal retinacular sheath (PRS), which lies directly beneath it (Schuenke et al. 2012). The anterior wall, blended to this retinaculum, has been termed the MLF. The compartment arrangement, created by this retinaculum, has been noted or illustrated by numerous authors (Spalteholz 1923; Schaeffer 1953; Hollinshead 1969; Grant 1972, plate 481; Bogduk and Macintosh 1984; Clemente 1985; Tesh et al. 1987; Barker and Briggs 1999; Gatton et al. 2010). Of special note is its designation as an osteofascial compartment (Standring 2008), as the anteromedial portion is made up by the lumbar vertebrae and the remainder by a fascial sheet. Further research is needed to analyze the fiber direction of the PRS. The description of the PRS is best approached from inside out; thus, beginning with the muscles contained in the compartment. Three large paraspinal muscles of the lumbosacral region are present in the compartment in the lumbar region, from lateral to medial: iliocostalis; longissimus; and multifidus (Bogduk 1980; Macintosh et al. 1986; Macintosh and Bogduk 1987; Bogduk and Twomey 1991; Fig. 1.6.5). In the older literature, the two lateral-most muscles of the erector spinae group are often fused in the lower lumbar and sacral levels, where they are termed the sacrospinalis muscle (Gray 1870). Medial to the erector spinae muscles lies the lumbar multifidus, a member of the transverso-spinalis group. This pyramidal shaped, multi-layered muscle begins at L1 and expands caudalward to occupy most of the sacral gutter on the posterior aspect of the sacrum (the region that lies between the lateral and medial sacral crests; Macintosh et al. 1986; Bogduk et al. 1992).

In the lower lumbar region, the paraspinal muscles are completely covered by the dense erector spinae aponeurosis (Fig. 1.6.4F). Laterally, this aponeurotic band extends upward to approximately the inferior border of L3, while medially the aponeurosis extends cranially well into the thoracic region. Thus, the lumbar multifidus is completely covered by this structure (Macintosh and Bogduk 1987). Although this band of regular dense connective tissue is named the aponeurosis of the erector spinae, the lumbar multifidus as well as both of the erector spinae muscles in the lumbar region have strong attachments to its inner surface, making it a common aponeurosis for these three muscles.

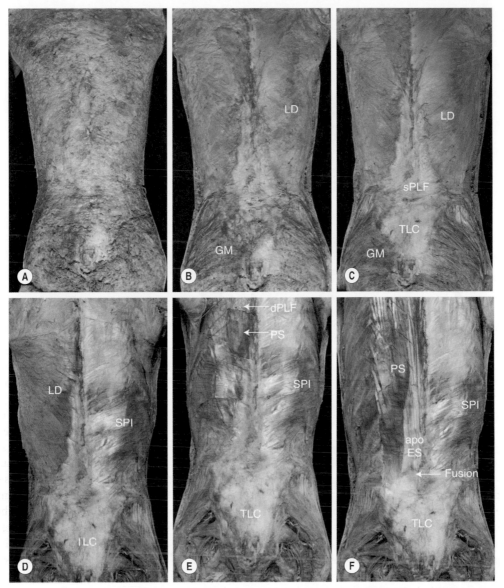

Fig. 1.6.4 A series of photographs illustrating a superficial-to-deep dissection of the lower thoracic and lumbar region. (A) The panniculus of fascia following removal of the skin. (B) The panniculus has been removed to display the underlying epimysium of the latissimus dorsi (LD) and the gluteus maximus (GM). (C) The epimysium of the LD has been removed to display the underlying muscles and the aponeurotic attachments of the LD forming in part the superficial lamina of the PLF (sPLF). (D) The LD has been removed for the right side to reveal the underlying serratus posterior inferior (SPI) and its aponeurosis. (E) The LD and rhomboid muscles have been removed bilaterally and a window placed in the aponeurosis of the serratus posterior superior to expose the underlying paraspinal muscles (PS) and their investing fascia. Note the thin sheet of the deep lamina (dPLF) seen above the window. Finally, (F) the posterior serratus muscles remain on the right side, whilst the left side has had the dorsal aspect of the PRS removed to expose the paraspinal muscles and the aponeurosis of the erector spinae (apo ES) caudally. The apo ES first fuses with the overlying deep and then with the superficial laminae of the PLF to form a tough composite of dense connective tissue that extends over the sacrum and to which the GM is attached. The thoracolumbar composite (TLC) is seen in the last four photographs (C–F).

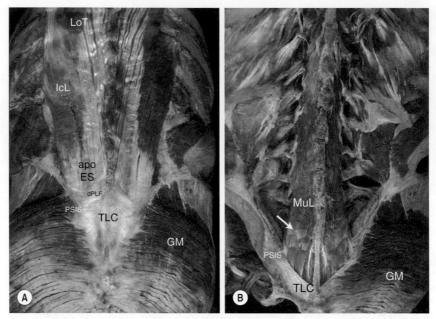

Fig. 1.6.5 Posterior views of the paraspinal muscles in the lumbosacral region. (A) The PLF has been removed to expose the iliocostalis lumborum (IcL) and the longissimus thoracis (LoT), as well as the aponeurosis of these two muscles (apo ES). A narrow rim of the deep lamina (dPLF) is seen at the point where the apo ES and the overlying TLF fuse to form the thoracolumbar composite (TLC). This fusion occurs at or slightly above the level of the posterior superior iliac spine (PSIS). (B) Erector spinae muscles of the lumbar region, IcL and LoT, have been removed to expose the more medially positioned multifidus lumborum (MuL). The opaque white bands (arrow) on the posterior surface of the MuL represent regions where the muscle bands fused with the inner aspect of the overlying apo ES. GM, gluteus maximus.

Beginning at approximately L5 and below, the aponeurosis of the erector spinae muscles and all of the more superficial layers overlying it fuse tightly together making one very thick aponeurotic structure, which attaches laterally to the iliac crest at PSIS (Fig. 1.6.6). It then spreads caudolaterally to join the gluteus maximus and finally ends by covering the sacrotuberous ligament (Bogduk and Macintosh 1984; Vleeming et al. 1995; Barker and Briggs 1999). This combined structure also can receive an attachment from the biceps femoris (Vleeming et al. 1989; Barker and Briggs 1999), and semimembranosus and semitendinosus muscles (Barker and Briggs 1999). It is this combined structure with its multiple sheets of aponeurotic tissue to which the term "TLC" has been applied (Vleeming and Willard 2010).

The PRS is made of dense connective tissue reinforced on the anteromedial wall by the transverse and spinous processes of the lumbar vertebrae (Standring 2008; Schuenke et al. 2012). Older names for this retinaculum include the lumbar aponeurosis (Gray 1870).

More recent terminology utilizes the deep lamina of the PLF to describe the posterior wall of the retinaculum and the MLF to describe the anterior wall. However, these descriptions are based on the assumption that the deep layer is a longitudinally oriented, flat fascial sheath, instead of a circular fascia encapsuling the paraspinal muscles. For that reason, Schuenke et al. (2012) recently described the deep layer as PRS. Laterally, this ring-like retinaculum creates a triangular structure where it meets the anterior and posterior laminae of the TrA aponeurosis (Fig. 1.6.7). This triangulum is named the lumbar interfascial triangle (LIFT).

Posteriorly, on the midline, the PRS is attached to the lumbar spinous processes and the associated supraspinal ligament. This cylindrical sheath then passes laterally around the border of the paraspinal muscles, coursing between these muscles and the QL to reach the tips of the transverse processes of the lumbar vertebrae L2–L4. As the PRS enters the space between the QL and the paraspinal muscles, it is joined by the aponeurosis of the

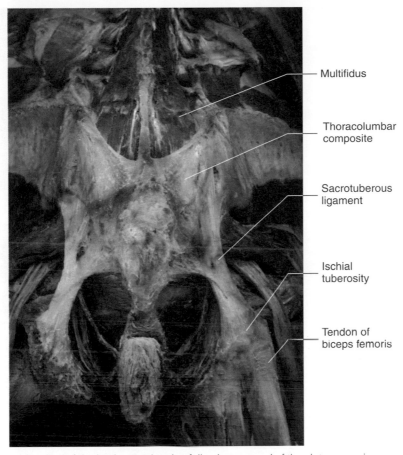

— Multifidus

— Thoracolumbar composite

— Sacrotuberous ligament

— Ischial tuberosity

— Tendon of biceps femoris

Fig. 1.6.6 Posterior view of the lumbosacral region following removal of the gluteus maximus and the erector spinae muscles. Multifidus lumborum is seen inserting into the TLC. The composite extends caudally to cover the sacrotuberous ligaments and reach the ischial tuberosities.

TrA; in addition, these two thickened bands (PRS and aponeurosis of TrA) fuse with the posterior epimysium of the QL. Thus, the structure termed the MLF, in actuality is derived of three separate layers of connective tissue, at least two of which are aponeurotic in nature. These observations are in keeping with the suggestion of Tesh et al. (1987) that the MLF is multilayered.

Anteromedially, the PRS ends on the transverse processes of the lumbar vertebrae (see illustrations in Spalteholz 1923; also see description in Hollinshead 1969; Grant 1972, plate 481; Bogduk and Macintosh 1984; Tesh et al. 1987). Superiorly, the anterior wall of the PRS (at this point fused with the middle layer of fascia) ascends cranially only so far as the 12th rib where it attaches firmly. Above the 12th rib, the anterior wall of the PRS is composed of the posterior aspect of the ribs and associated fascia, to which the paraspinal muscles attach.

The posterior wall of the PRS becomes markedly thinner as it enters the thoracic region and is termed the vertebral aponeurosis (Gray 1870; Spalteholz 1923; Anson and Maddock 1958). The thinness of this layer of fascia in the lower thoracic region has led some authors to report it as absent (Bogduk and Macintosh, 1984), only to describe its reappearance in the cervical region; however, the continuity of this portion of the retinaculum has been demonstrated by its careful isolation and removal as a single entity (Barker and Briggs, 1999). As the posterior layer of the PRS (deep layer of TLF) extends into the cervical region, it becomes the investing fascia of the cervical paraspinal muscles (Gray 1870; Wood Jones 1946), including the splenius muscles as noted by Barker and

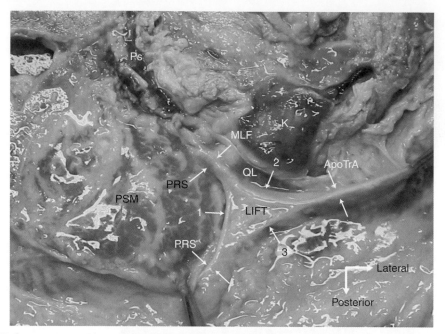

Fig. 1.6.7 A transverse section taken approximately at level L3 and illustrating the fascial structures lateral to the paraspinal muscles. The specimen was embalmed using the Thiel method. This method maintains the non-linear load-deformation characteristics of biological tissue (Wilke et al. 2011). LIFT, lumbar interfascial triangle (Schuenke et al. 2012). The deep lamina of the PLF actually forms an encapsulating sheath around the multifidi and paraspinal muscles (PSM), this is the paraspinal retinacular sheath (PRS). In this image, the LIFT is under tension from forceps pulling laterally (far right side of the figure) and posteriorly (bottom of the figure). The aponeurosis of the transversus abdominis (ApoTrA) is seen to divide into a posterior (3) and anterior (2) layer before joining the PRS. The sheath is seen to form a continuous layer wrapping around the paraspinal muscles (1). This arrangement strongly suggests that the aponeurosis of the TrA and IO does not solely form the PLF and MLF, but splits to contribute to these layers by joining the PRS (a more detailed description of the composition of the fascial layers can be found in Fig. 1.6.9). Note in this specimen that the quadratus lumborum (QL) and the psoas muscle (Ps) are both strongly atrophied. Anteriorly of the QL a small part of the kidney (K) can be seen (specimen kindly supplied by the Medical faculty Ghent Belgium, Department of Anatomy).

Briggs (1999). In essence, the PRS, including that portion of which is termed the deep layer of the PLF, represents the original epaxial fascial sheath into which the paraspinal muscles formed during embryogenesis.

The inferior border of the PRS is more complicated (Fig. 1.6.8). The anterior wall of the sheath (blended with the aponeurosis of the TrA in the MLF) terminates by fusing with the iliolumbar ligament at the level of the iliac crest. Below this level, the anterior wall of the PRS is replaced by the iliolumbar ligament and the sacroiliac joint capsule. The posterior wall of the PRS (deep lamina of PLF) attaches to the PSIS then descends over the sacrum, blending laterally with the attachments of the gluteus maximus and inferiorly with the sacrotuberous ligament (Gray 1870; Bogduk and Macintosh 1984; Vleeming et al.

1995; Barker and Briggs 1999). Attachment of the paraspinal muscles to the inside wall of the sheath is accomplished through very loose connective tissue fascia posteriorly. Below the level of L5, the erector spinae aponeurosis (the common tendon of the erector and multifidi muscles) fuses with the PRS (synonymous with the deep lamina of the PLF; Fig. 1.6.9) and the superficial lamina of the PLF to form one, very thick, aponeurotic composite covering the sacrum, termed the "TLC."

The PRS receives the aponeurotic attachments of several muscle groups. Superficially, the aponeurosis of the LD lies across the retinaculum passing from craniolateral to caudomedial in a broad flat fan-shaped aponeurosis (Fig. 1.6.10). Laterally, above the L4 / L5 levels, the PRS and the aponeurosis of the LD are separated by

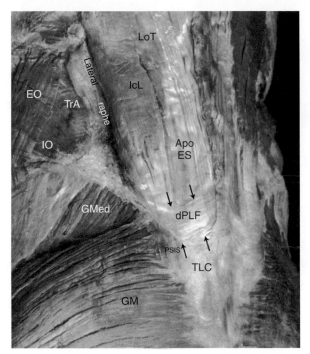

Fig. 1.6.8 A posterior oblique view of the lumbosacral region illustrating the aponeurosis of the erector spinae muscles (Apo ES), the deep lamina (dPLF) and the thoracolumbar composite (TLC). The Apo ES and dPLF fuse with the overlying posterior lamina (not shown) to form the TLC. Laterally, the dPLF will wrap around the border of iliocostalis lumborum (IcL) forming the PRS. This sheath creates a strong fascial compartment around the paraspinal muscles. On the lateral border of the IcL the dl is joined by the aponeurosis of the transversus abdominis (TrA) to form the lateral raphe. Also attached to the raphe in this specimen is the internal oblique (IO); the external oblique (EO) in this specimen did not reach the lateral raphe. The gluteus maximus (GM) attaches to the TLC beginning around the level of the posterior superior iliac spine (PSIS) and below. The gluteus medius (GMed) does not make an attachment to the TLC.

the SPI and its thin aponeurotic attachments. From approximately L5 and below, the PRS and the LD aponeurosis begin fusing together. The attachment of the aponeurosis of the SPI begins on the lateral border of the posterior wall of the PRS (deep lamina of the posterior TLF) and extends medially to reach the spinous processes and supraspinal ligament of the lumbar vertebrae. Whilst the lateral-most connections of the SPI to the PRS can be separated bluntly, those of the medial two-thirds of the sheath cannot be broken by blunt dissection (Fig. 1.6.11).

The major lateral attachment to the PRS arises from the abdominal muscles. Most prominent amongst these is the TrA aponeurosis, which joins the border of the PRS at the lateral raphe (Bogduk and Macintosh 1984; Vleeming et al. 1995; Schuenke et al. 2012) and then continues medially, fused to the retinaculum, to reach the tips of the transverse processes (Fig. 1.6.9; Tesh et al. 1987; Barker et al. 2007). This combined layer has an unusual medial border. Between the transverse processes, this layer is relatively free from attachment giving it a dentate appearance; through this arrangement, the posterior primary rami pass as they depart the spinal nerve and gain access to their epaxial muscular targets in the PRS.

Cranially, there is another specialization involving the middle layer. Because the fibers of the TrA are horizontally oriented and pass inferior to the subcostal margin to reach the vertebral transverse processes, this leaves a small region superior to the aponeurosis of the TrA and inferior to the arch of the 12th rib that would not be covered by thickened aponeurotic tissue. This area is reinforced by thickened bands of collagen fibers derived from the transverse processes of L1 and L2 and extending to the inferior border of the 12th rib. These bands form the lumbocostal ligament (Testut 1899; Spalteholz 1923; Anson and Maddock 1958; Clemente 1985).

What emerges from this discussion is an osteofibrous retinacular sheath surrounding the large paraspinal muscles of the lumbosacral region. The medial wall of the cylinder is made up of the posterior arch elements of the cervical, thoracic and lumbar vertebrae as well as the ribs in the thoracic region, while its base is composed of the sacrum and the ligaments supporting the sacroiliac joint. The posterior, lateral and anterior walls are composed of the PRS. Attached to this structure are several muscles that can influence the tension in the sheath. Given this construction, it is necessary to examine the possible role of the PRS in the stability and movement of the lumbosacral spine. In the following sections, we will examine the details of the construction of specific parts of the TLF and then consider their biomechanical properties.

THE POSTERIOR LAYER OF THE THORACOLUMBAR FASCIA

Superficial Lamina of the PLF

The superficial lamina of the PLF "itself" divide into sublayers (Benetazzo et al. 2011). In this study, the

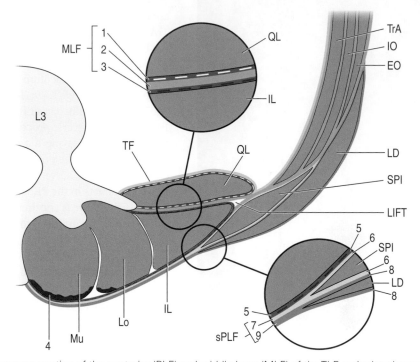

Fig. 1.6.9 A transverse section of the posterior (PLF) and middle layer (MLF) of the TLF and related muscles at the L3 level. Fascial structures are represented such that individual layers are visible, but not necessarily presented to scale. Please note that the serratus posterior inferior (SPI) often is not present caudal to the L3 level. The transversus abdominis (TrA) muscle is covered with a dashed line on the peritoneal surface illustrating the transversalis fascia (TF). This fascia continues medially covering the anterior side of the investing fascia of the quadratus lumborum (QL). Anteriorly and medially, the TF also fuses with the psoas muscle fascia (not drawn). The internal (IO) and external obliques (EO) are seen external to TrA. SPI is highly variable in thickness and, more often than not, absent on the L4 level. Latissimus dorsi (LD) forms the superficial lamina of the PLF together with the SPI, when present. The three paraspinal muscles, multifidus (Mu), longissimus (Lo) and iliocostalis (IL) are contained within the PRS. The aponeurosis (tendon) of the paraspinal muscles (4) is indicated by stippling. Please note that the epimysium of the individual spinal muscles is very thin and follows the contours of each separate muscle within the PRS. The epimysium is not indicated in the present figure but lies anteriorly to the aponeurosis (4). The upper circle shows a magnified view of the different fascial layers contributing to the MLF. This shows that MLF is made up of three different structures: (1) this dashed line depicts the investing fascia of QL; (3) this dashed line represents the PRS, also termed the deep lamina of the PLF encapsulating the paraspinal muscles; (2) the thick dark line between the two dashed lines 1 and 2 represents the aponeurosis of the abdominal muscles especially deriving from TrA. Numbers 1, 2 and 3 form the MLF. The lower circle shows a magnified view of the different fascial layers constituting the PLF. This shows that on the L3 level the PLF is also made up of three layers, as the fascia of SPI is normally present on this level. (5) This dashed line depicts the PRS or deep lamina of the PLF encapsulating the paraspinal muscles; (6) the investing fascia of SPI is seen blending medially into the gray line marked (7) and representing the aponeurosis of SPI – posteriorly to the PRS; (8) this dark line represents the investing fascia of LD blending medially into the black line representing the LD aponeurosis (9) posteriorly to the SPI aponeurosis. Numbers 5, 7, and 9 form the PLF. Numbers 7 and 9 form the superficial lamina of the posterior layer (sPLF). LIFT is the lumbar interfascial triangle, as described by Schuenke et al. (2012). As indicated, the PRS encapsulates the paraspinal muscles; together with PLF and MLF and the lateral border of PRS, a triangle is formed normally also visible on axial lumbar MRIs. For further specification, see Fig. 1.6.7.

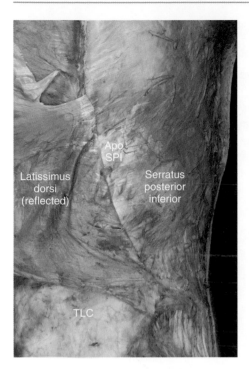

Fig. 1.6.10 A posterior oblique view of the right lumbar region illustrating the removal of the LD to expose the serratus posterior inferior (SPI) and its associated aponeurosis (ApoSPI). Although the LD is firmly adhered to the SPI, it can be separated by careful dissection. These two aponeurotic structures combine to form the PLF. In this specimen, muscle fibers of the LD reach caudalward to the crest of the ilium. TLC, thoracolumbar composite.

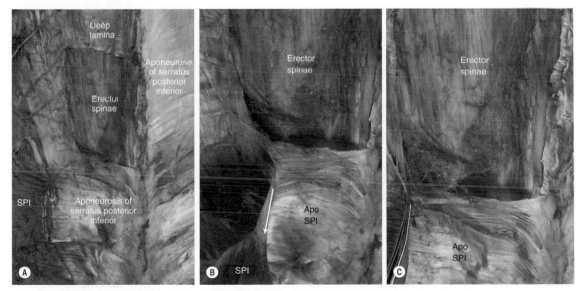

Fig. 1.6.11 A posterior view of the left thoracolumbar region illustrating the relationship of the serratus posterior inferior (SPI) and the deep lamina of the PLF covering the paraspinal muscles. (Note that the deep lamina represents the posterior wall of the PRS.) The bridging muscles from the extremity, such as the LD, trapezius and rhomboids have been removed in this specimen. (A) A window has been opened in the deep lamina to expose the erector spinae muscles. (B) The SPI has been elevated laterally and is being tensioned on the medial attachment of its aponeurosis. (C) The deep lamina (PRS) and aponeurosis of the SPI (ApoSPI) are being elevated with forceps to illustrate the loose connective tissue located between the paraspinal muscles and the surrounding PRS.

authors show that the superficial layer of the PLF (680 μm in their specimen) can be divided into three sublayers based on the organization of collagenous fiber bundles. The superficial sublayer has a mean thickness of 75 μm with parallel undulating collagen fibers and with few elastic fibers. This layer derives of the thin epimysium of the LD. The intermediate sublayer (152 μm) is made of packed straight collagen bundles, dis- posed in the same direction without elastic fibers, deriving from the apo- neurosis of the LD. The deepest sublayer is made of loose connective tissue (450 μm) separating the superfi- cial lamina of the PLF from the deep lamina of the PLF or, on higher lumbar levels, the aponeurosis of the SPI lying between the superficial and deep lamina of the PLF. This deepest sublayer allows for gliding between the superficial and deep lamina of the PLF. The three sublayers form the superficial lamina of the PLF as a multidirectional construct with the same characteristics as the crural fascia also studied by the same authors (Benetazzo et al. 2011).

DISPOSITION OF THE LATISSIMUS DORSI

The LD is a broad, fan-shaped muscle, the aponeurosis of which contributes to the superficial lamina of the PLF (Fig. 1.6.12). The aponeurosis of the LD has been divided into several regions based on its distal attach- ments (Bogduk et al. 1998). The upper border (or thoracic attachment) involves the lower six thoracic spinous processes and supraspinous ligaments. Next are the "transitional" fibers that reach the first and second lumbar spinous processes and supraspinous ligaments. This is followed by the "raphe" fibers of the aponeurosis that attach to the lateral raphe and then continue on to reach the third–fifth spinous processes and intraspinous ligaments. Finally, the "iliac" fibers attach to the iliac crest, and the lower border (or costal fibers) attach to a variable number of the lower first–third ribs. Although much of the aponeurosis is fused to the underlying structures, such as the lateral raphe and the SPI, it can be separated from the sheath by blunt dissection.

FIBER ORIENTATION FOR THE LATISSIMUS DORSI

Bogduk and Macintosh (1984) were the first to carefully analyze the orientation of collagenous fibers within the laminae of the posterior layer. Since then, the trajectory

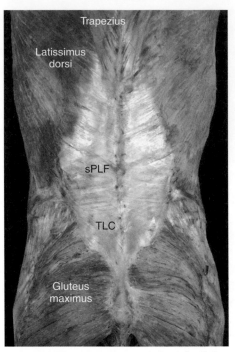

Fig. 1.6.12 A posterior view of the back illustrating the attach- ments of the LD, trapezius and gluteus maximus to the TLF and thoracolumbar composite (TLC). The LD is the major compo- nent of the superficial lamina of the PLF (sPLF).

of collagenous fibers has been examined by several au- thors with relatively good agreement (Barker and Briggs 1999, 2007; Fig. 1.6.13). Fiber angles are described as varying from horizontal superiorly to approximately 20–40° sloping craniolateral-to-caudomedial and pro- gressing from a shallower angle superiorly to a steeper angle inferiorly. These collagen fiber angles should not be confused with the angles described for the muscles fibers that are attached to the TLF. The thickness of this aponeurosis was found to be approximately 0.52–0.55 mm in the lumbar region (Barker and Briggs 1999), but to become significantly thinner in the thoracic portion.

Bogduk and Vleeming separately describe the extension of fibers from the superficial lamina across the midline at the L4–L5 levels and below (Bogduk and Macintosh 1984; Vleeming et al. 1995; Bogduk et al. 1998). Finally, it was noted that the superficial lamina attaches firmly to the lateral raphe only near the iliac crest. Above this level, the SPI intervenes, and the attachment of the LD is less firm and, in some cases, may not exist at all (Bogduk and Macintosh 1984).

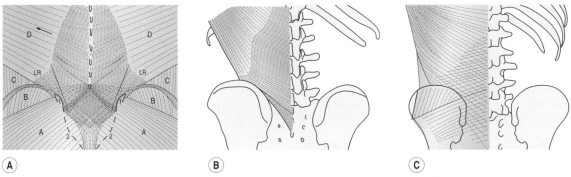

Fig. 1.6.13 A comparison between drawings of three studies of the superficial lamina of the PLF: (A) Vleeming et al.; (B) Bogduk et al.; (C) Barker et al. (A–C) The same fiber direction of the superficial lamina. (A and C) A crosshatched appearance and the connections to the gluteus maximus fascia. (A) Along with variation in fiber direction there are changes in fiber density in the superficial lamina as well. Where the abdominal muscles join the paraspinal muscles, the orientation of the fibers change and they become denser. From the level of L4 to the lower part of the sacrum, the fiber density markedly increases. This density change corresponds to the area where the different fascial layers fuse to form the TLC.

ATTACHMENTS OF THE SERRATUS POSTERIOR INFERIOR

The SPI normally consists of four thin rectangular sheets of muscle attached to the inferolateral margin of the 9th–12th ribs (Fig. 1.6.4). Medially, this muscle gives way to a thin aponeurosis that reaches deep to the aponeurosis of the LD to attach to the lower two thoracic and upper two or three lumbar spinous processes and associated interspinous ligaments. Bogduk and Macintosh (1984) found that the SPI attached to the aponeurosis of the LD, but Vleeming et al. (1995) found some attachments only to the deep lamina.

Superior and inferior borders of the superficial lamina the existent descriptions of the superior and inferior borders of the superficial lamina have significant variation. Wood Jones (1946), who did not distinguish superficial or deep laminae in his text, described the posterior layer as extending upward to cover the splenius capitis in the cervical region. Bogduk and Macintosh (1984) found that superiorly the superficial lamina of the posterior layer passes under the trapezius and rhomboids. Inferiorly, it attaches to PSIS, fusing with the underlying aponeurosis of the SPI and with the origin of the gluteus maximus. Vleeming et al. (1995) describe the posterior layer as extending upward to the fascia nuchae. Barker and Briggs (1999) also commented on the extension of the superior layer to fuse with that of the trapezius and rhomboids while the deep layer reaches the splenius muscles. Barker also noted that the superficial lamina of

the posterior TLF (LD fascia) is continuous with that surrounding the rhomboids.

UNIFYING THEORY OF THE SUPERFICIAL LAMINA

Both the LD and the SPI are innervated by branches from the ventral rami; thus, neither of these muscles are epaxial in origin. Specifically, the LD is innervated by thoracodorsal nerve (C6, 7 and 8), which arises from cords of the brachial plexus (Clemente 1985). The SPI is innervated from branches of the thoracoabdominal intercostals nerves (T9–T12). Therefore, both of these muscles, the aponeuroses of which contribute to the superficial lamina, are not original components of the back but have to migrate posteriorly during development to achieve this position. In this sense, these two muscles are part of a group of bridging muscles that extend from the upper extremity to the torso. This arrangement (LD positioned superficially, and SPI positioned deep in the posterior layer) can be understood from embryological principals. Based on innervations patterns, the SPI is most closely related to the thoracic hypaxial muscles and has to migrate over the intermuscular septum to attach to the outer side of the epaxial compartment containing the paraspinal muscles. The LD, a bridging extremity muscle, then has to migrate over the serratus (a hypaxial muscle) to gain its attachment on the iliac crest and lumbar spine. In a related fashion, the superior extension of the superficial lamina to involve the rhomboid muscles and trapezius is consistent from a developmental standpoint as these two muscles share a similar origin as with the LD. Thus, the superficial lamina can be seen as part of a continuous sheet of fascia containing several muscles that bridge the junction between the extremity and the torso (Sato and Hashimoto 1984; Stecco et al. 2009).

DEEP LAMINA OF THE POSTERIOR LAYER OF THE THORACOLUMBAR FASCIA

Posterior Presentation

Removal of the LD exposes the SPI and its thin aponeurosis, this latter structure is closely applied to an underlying sheet of fascia (the PRS) and the two cannot be separated by blunt dissection (Fig. 1.6.8). Numerous studies have examined this deep fascial structure, grouping it with the posterior layer and giving it the term "deep lamina of the PLF" (Bogduk and Macintosh 1984; Vleeming et al. 1995; Barker and Briggs 1999).

Bogduk described the deep lamina as having alternating bands of fibers based on density; fibers run at an angle of 20–30° below horizontal and are best seen in the lower lumbar levels, becoming scant in the upper lumbar region (Bogduk and Macintosh 1984). The authors termed these bands accessory ligaments and

state that the deep lamina is most likely the crossed fibers of the aponeurosis of the LD. Vleeming et al. (1995) and Barker and Briggs (1999) found the same fascial orientation, typically characterizing the deep lamina of the PLF, but no differentiated accessory ligaments. Fig. 1.6.14 is a comparison of the fiber orientation as depicted by the two major groups studying this area; the similarity in fiber trajectory is obvious in the three diagrams, although there is a discrepancy in the clustering of fibers as illustrated in the Bogduk and Macintosh diagram.

The aponeurosis of the SPI fuses with both the LD (Bogduk and Macintosh, 1984) and the posterior surface of the deep lamina (Vleeming et al. 1995) as it projects toward the midline of the back. This fusion with the deep lamina occurs approximately half the distance across the lateral-to-medial expanse of the deep lamina. Lateral to the fusion with the aponeurosis of the SPI, the deep lamina curves around the lateral border of the paraspinal muscles to form the PRS. For embryological reasons, the deep lamina cannot represent a posterior extension of fascia derived from either the LD, PSI, or any abdominal muscle; as a component of the PRS, developmentally the deep lamina is completely separated from the abdominal (hypaxial) muscle fascia by an intermuscular septum (Bailey and Miller 1916; Fig. 1.6.15).

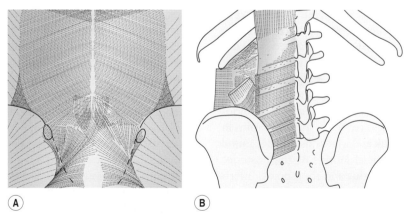

(A)   (B)

Fig. 1.6.14 A comparison between drawings of two studies of the deep lamina of the PLF: (A) Vleeming et al.; (B) Bogduk et al. (A and B) The same fiber direction; however, in (B) the dense parts of the deep lamina are coined as accessory ligaments. (B) The lateral raphe is indicated as a dotted vertical line, indicating the area where the abdominal muscles join the paraspinal muscles. (A) An increase of density in the same area. More caudally, it can be noticed that the sacrotuberous ligament partially fuses to the deep lamina. The fiber characteristics show increased density and an altered pattern in the region over the sacrum. This pattern is another indication that the various layers of the TLF and aponeurosis fuse into the TLC, as referred to in the text.

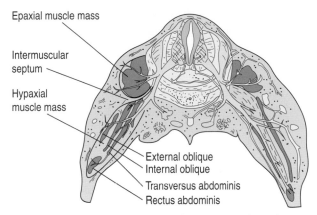

Epaxial muscle mass

Intermuscular septum

Hypaxial muscle mass

External oblique
Internal oblique
Transversus abdominis
Rectus abdominis

Fig. 1.6.15 A schematic diagram of a human embryo demonstrating the epaxial and hypaxial myofascial compartments. The spinal nerve is seen dividing into its dorsal and ventral ramus. The dorsal ramus innervates the epaxial compartment, whilst the ventral ramus innervates the hypaxial compartment. Between the two compartments lies the intermuscular septum of connective tissue from which the middle layer of the TLF will develop (figure modified from: Bailey and Miller, 1916).

INFERIOR BORDER OF THE DEEP LAMINA

The inferior border of the TLF was succinctly described by Henry Gray in 1870 as blending with the "greater sacrosciatic" (sacrotuberous) ligament; more recent authors have elaborated on these arrangements. At L5–S1 level, Bogduk found the superficial lamina of the TLF to fuse inseparably with the underlying aponeurosis of the paraspinal muscles and continuing caudalward to blend with the gluteal fascia (Bogduk and Macintosh 1984). This being the case, the deep lamina would be trapped between these two thick aponeurotic sheets as they fuse. A similar observation was made by Vleeming who found the superficial and deep laminae fusing with the aponeurosis of the erector spinae and the combined structure (TLC) attaching laterally to the PSIS and progressing caudally, to become continuous with the sacrotuberous ligament (Vleeming et al. 1995).

The relationship with the gluteal fascia is complex. Laterally, the deep lamina fuses over the iliac crest with the aponeurosis of the gluteus medius. More medially, the deep and superficial laminae fuse together at the level of PSIS. Below PSIS, this combined aponeurotic structure extends laterally to create an intermuscular septum to which the gluteus maximus attaches in a bipennate arrangement (reviewed in Willard 1995).

SUPERIOR BORDER DEEP LAMINA

Wood Jones (1946) described the PLF (what he terms the layer deep to the attachments of the LD and SPI) as becoming very thin and passing upward under the serratus posterior superior to eventually blend with the fascia surrounding the splenius muscles in the cervical region; thus, he seems to be describing what is currently termed the deep lamina of the PLF. Bogduk found the upper portions of the deep lamina to be poorly developed. In fact, they lost the deep lamina transiently above the superior border of the SPI, only to see it return at higher levels as a thin membrane (Bogduk and Macintosh 1984). Vleeming traced the deep lamina upward into the thoracic region where it thinned significantly and was joined by the aponeurosis of the SPI (Vleeming et al. 1995). Barker was able to trace the superior border of the deep lamina cranially to where it blended with the border of the splenius cervicis and capitis muscles (Barker and Briggs 1999). Taken together, these descriptions suggest that the deep lamina extends from the sacrum cranially to the splenius capitis and eventually fuses to the cranial base at the nuchal line with the cervical fascia. This would be the expected arrangement of the investing fascia (PRS) surrounding the paraspinal muscles.

LATERAL BORDER OF THE DEEP LAMINA

The lateral border of the deep lamina lies along the lateral raphe and has been described by numerous authors (Schaeffer 1953; Bogduk and Macintosh 1984; Tesh et al. 1987; Vleeming et al. 1995; Barker and Briggs 2007). Spalteholz (1923) clearly illustrates the lateral border as curving continuously around the lateral margin of the paraspinal muscles to participate in the formation of the middle layer separating paraspinal muscles from QL. Schaeffer (1953) described the TLF as being continuous around the lateral margin of the erector spinae muscles and forming the ventral or deep layer that creates an intermuscular septum separating QL from the sacrospinalis muscles. Tesh et al. (1987) illustrate the lateral border of the TLF as having a deep lamina that continues uninterrupted around the lateral border of the erector spinae muscles to become what they describe as an inner lamina of the middle layer. In addition, Carr et al. (1985) verified the presence of a retinacular sheath surrounding the paraspinal muscles both anatomically and physiologically using dissection and intracompartmental pressure recordings in various postures. Thus, the PRS is formed by the deep lamina creating a compartment for the paraspinal muscles in the lumbar region.

THE MIDDLE LAYER OF THE THORACOLUMBAR FASCIA

The MLF is situated between the QL and the paraspinal muscles. This aponeurotic structure has been suggested as being the primary link between the tension generated in the abdominal muscle band and the lumbar spine (Barker et al. 2004, 2007). This layer is viewed by many authors as a medial continuation of the aponeurosis of the TrA (Romanes 1981; Clemente 1985; Standring 2008) or, alternatively, a lateral continuation of the intertransverse ligaments (Bogduk 2005). In their study of this layer, Bogduk and Macintosh (1984) found it to be a thick, strong aponeurotic structure arising from the tips of the transverse processes. The upper border of the middle layer of fascia is the 12th rib. However, between T12 and the first two lumbar transverse processes the middle layer is re-enforced by arcuate collagenous bands termed the lumbocostal ligament. From L2 caudally, the MLF is described as giving rise to the aponeurosis of the TrA laterally. The lower border of the MLF is the iliolumbar ligament and the iliac crest.

The abdominal muscles form the primary attachment to the MLF, but their arrangement has proven to be somewhat contentious (Urquhart and Hodges 2007). The TrA and the internal oblique connect in an aponeurosis that becomes the MLF as it passes internal to the lateral border of the erector spinae muscles (Fig. 1.6.9). In the area where the aponeurosis joins the deep lamina of the posterior layer (PRS) on the lateral border of the erector spinae, a thickening in the tissue forms that is termed the lateral raphe (Fig. 1.6.8; Bogduk and Macintosh 1984). The TrA attachment to the PRS extends from the iliac crest to the 12th rib, whilst the attachment of the internal oblique is much more variable and occurs principally in the inferior portion of the lateral raphe (Bogduk and Macintosh 1984; Tesh et al. 1987; Barker et al. 2007). Typically, the lateralmost slips of the external oblique muscle form an attachment to the 12th rib; however, this muscle has been reported to also gain access to the upper boundary of the aponeurosis of the TrA (Barker et al. 2007).

Barker et al. (2007) demonstrated that the precise attachment of the MLF is to the lateral margins of the transverse processes; it was noted that measuring

the MLF as it approached the tip of the transverse process yields a thickness of approximately 0.62 mm, but elsewhere varied from 0.11 to 1.34 mm. Because the average thickness of the superficial lamina of the PLF near the spinous processes was reported to be 0.56 mm (Barker and Briggs 1999), it appears that the MLF is thicker than the PLF. In marked contrast, the anterior layer of TLF is thin (0.10 mm, range 0.06–0.14 mm; Barker and Briggs 1999) and membranous; it extends from the lateral raphe, passing anterior to the QL to attach towards the distal end of each transverse process between the attachments of the psoas and QL.

The attachment of the MLF to the transverse process is quite strong. This was demonstrated in older specimens by applying elevated tension (average: 82 N in the transverse plane and 47 N in the anterior–posterior plane) to the transverse process, which typically fractured before the MLF or its osseous attachment failed (Barker and Briggs 2007).

Most of the collagenous fibers in the middle layer are oriented slightly caudolaterally (10–25° below the horizontal) until they reach the transverse processes (Barker and Briggs 2007). As they approach the lumbar spine, the collagen bundles focus on the tips of the transverse processes, leaving a less well-organized zone between each transverse process (Tesh et al. 1987). It is through this intertransverse region that the posterior primary ramus gains access to the compartment of the PRS (Fig. 1.6.16).

The middle layer appears to derive from an intermuscular septum that separates the epaxial from the hypaxial musculature. This septum develops during the fifth and sixth weeks of gestation (Hamilton et al. 1972). The intermuscular septum represents a consolidation of mesenchyme that not only separates the two components of the myotome but also participates in forming the investing fascia that surrounds both of these muscle masses. Thus, it is speculated that from this mesenchymal wrapping, the PRS and the MLF are formed. Furthermore, the authors would like to pose that the middle layer itself, due to the dual origin, is most likely composed of at least two sublayers of separate embryologic origin—the most posterior sublayer deriving from the epaxial mesenchyme, whilst the more anterior sublayer deriving from the hypaxial mesenchyme. The presence of at least two-layers in the MLF was previously suggested by Tesh et al. (1987) based on histological preparations. In this case, the aponeurosis of the TrA would be representing the hypaxial muscle investment, and the posterior wall of

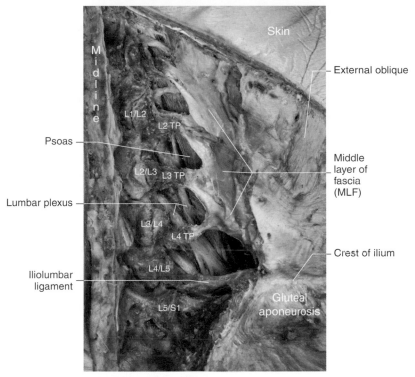

Fig. 1.6.16 A posterior view of a deep dissection of the middle layer (MLF) of the TLF. The erector spinae muscles and the multifidus have been completely removed to expose the facet joints, transverse processes (TP) and the MLF. The MLF is composed of the aponeurosis of the TrA and the PRS, as well as the epimysium of the QL. The ventral rami of the lumbar plexus and the psoas muscle can be seen deep to the arches of the MLF. It is through these arches that the dorsal ramus gains access to the paraspinal muscles in the epaxial compartment.

the PRS would represent the epaxial muscle investment. In addition, Schuenke et al. (2012) observed that the epimysial fascia of the QL represents a third component of the MLF (Figs. 1.6.7 and 1.6.9).

Summary

The posterior layer of TLF is divided into superficial and deep laminae. The superficial lamina is derived from the union of two aponeuroses from the LD and the SPI, whilst the deep lamina of the PLF actually is a retinacular sheath surrounding the paraspinal muscles. This latter structure has been termed the PRS.

ACKNOWLEDGMENTS

This article is an excerpt from Willard F.H., Vleeming, A., Schuenke, M.D., Danneels, L., Schleip R. 2012. The thoracolumbar fascia: anatomy, function and clinical considerations. J. Anat. 221(6), 507–536. For a more extended version of this article (including additional references), see: https://onlinelibrary.wiley.com/doi/full/10.1111/j.1469-7580.2012.01511.x. The following coauthors contributed significantly to this longer article version: Mark D. Schuenke and Lieven Danneels.

REFERENCES

Anson, B.J., Maddock, W.G., 1958. Callander's Surgical Anatomy, fourth ed. W.B. Saunders, Philadelphia.

Bailey, F.R., Miller, A.M. 1916. Textbook of Embryology, 3rd edn. New York: William Wood.

Barker, P.J., Briggs, C.A. 1999. Attachments of the posterior layer of the lumbar fascia. Spine 24, 1757–1764.

Barker, P.J., Briggs, C.A., Bogeski, G. 2004. Tensile transmission across the lumbar fasciae in unembalmed cadavers: effects of tension to various muscular attachments. Spine 29, 129–138.

Barker, P.J., Briggs, C.A., 2007. Anatomy and biomechanics of the lumbar fascia: implications for lumbopelvic control and clinical practice. In: Movement, Stability & Lumbopelvic Pain: Integration of Research and Therapy, second ed. (Eds Vleeming A, Mooney V, Stoeckart R), pp. 63–73. Elsevier, Edinburgh.

Barker, P.J., Urquhart, D.M., Story, I.H., et al. 2007. The middle layer of lumbar fascia and attachments to lumbar transverse processes: implications for segmental control and fracture. Eur Spine J 16, 2232–2237.

Benetazzo, L., Bizzego, A., De Caro, R., et al., 2011. 3D reconstruction of the crural and thoracolumbar fasciae. Surg. Radiol. Anat. 33, 855–862.

Bergmark, A.,1989. Stability of the lumbar spine: a study in mechanical engineering. Acta Orthop. Scand. Suppl. 230, 1–54.

Bogduk, N. 2005. Clinical Anatomy of the Lumbar Spine, 4th edn. Edinburgh: Elsevier Churchill Livingstone.

Bogduk, N., Johnson, G., Spalding, D. 1998. The morphology and biomechanics of latissimus dorsi. Clin Biomech (Bristol, Avon) 13, 377–385.

Bogduk, N., Macintosh, J.E. 1984. The applied anatomy of the thoacolumbar fascia. Spine 9, 164–170.

Bogduk, N., Macintosh, J.E., Pearcy, M.J. 1992. A universal model of the lumbar back muscles in the upright position. Spine 17, 897–913.

Bogduk, N., Twomey, L.T. 1991. Clinical Anatomy of the Lumbar Spine, 2nd edn. Melbourne: Churchill Livingstone, p. 1.

Carr, D., Gilbertson, L., Frymoyer, J., et al. 1985. Lumbar paraspinal compartment syndrome. A case report with physiologic and anatomic studies. Spine (Phila Pa 1976) 10, 816–820.

Cholewicki, J., Panjabi, M.M., Khachatryan, A., 1997. Stabilizing function of trunk flexor-extensor muscles around a neutral spine posture. Spine 22, 2207–2212.

Clemente, C.D., 1985. Gray's Anatomy of the Human Body. Lea & Febiger, Philadelphia.

Gatton, M.L., Pearcy, M.J., Pettet, G.J., et al. 2010. A three-dimensional mathematical model of the thoracolumbar fascia and an estimate of its biomechanical effect. J Biomech 43, 2792–2797.

Goss, C.M., 1973. Gray's Anatomy of the Human Body. Lea & Febiger, Philadelphia.

Grant, J.C.B., 1972. An Atlas of Anatomy, sixth ed. Williams & Wilkins, Baltimore.

Gray, H. 1870. Anatomy, Descriptive and Surgical, 5th edn. Philadelphia: Henry C. Lea.

Gray, H. 1923. Anatomy Descriptive and Applied. Longmans, Green, London.

Green, R.M., 1937. Warren's Handbook of Anatomy. Harvard University Press, Cambridge.

Hamilton, W.J., Boyd, J.D., Mossman, H.W. 1972. Human Embryology, 4th edn. Cambridge: W. Heffer.

Hollinshead, W.H., 1969. Anatomy for Surgeons: The Back and Limbs, second ed. Hoeber-Harper, New York.

Huber, G.C., 1930. Piersol's Human Anatomy, ninth ed. J.B. Lippincott Philadelphia.

Macintosh, J.E., Bogduk, N. 1987. The morphology of the lumbar erector spinae. Spine 12, 658–668.

Macintosh, J.E., Valencia, F.P., Bogduk, N., et al., 1986. The morphology of the human lumbar multifidus. Clin Biomech 1, 196–204.

Romanes, G.J., 1981. Cunningham's Textbook of Anatomy, twelfth ed. Oxford University Press, Oxford.

Sato, T., Hashimoto, M. 1984. Morphological analysis of the fascial lamination of the trunk. Bull Tokyo Med Dent Univ 31, 21–32.

Schaeffer, J.P., 1953. Morris's Human Anatomy, eleventh ed. McGraw-Hill, New York.

Schuenke, M.D., Vleeming, A., Van Hoof, T., Willard, F. H., 2012. A description of the lumbar interfascial triangle and its relation with the lateral raphe: anatomical constituents of load transfer through the lateral margin of the thoracolumbar fascia. J. Anat. 221 (6), 568–576.

Singer, E., 1935. Fascia of the Human Body and Their Relations to the Organs they Envelop. Williams and Wilkins, Philadelphia.

Spalteholz, W. 1923. Hand Atlas of Human Anatomy. J.B. Lippincott, Philadelphia.

Standring, S., 2008. Gray's Anatomy, The Anatomical Basis of Clinical Practice, fortieth ed Elsevier Churchill Livingstone, Edinburgh.

Stecco, A., Macchi, V., Masiero, S., et al., 2009. Pectoral and femoral fasciae: common aspects and regional specializations. Surg Radiol Anat 31, 35–42.

Tesh, K.M., Dunn, J.S., Evans, J.H. 1987. The abdominal muscles and vertebral stability. Spine (Phila Pa 1976) 12, 501–508.

Testut, L., 1899. Traite D'Anatomy Humaine. Octave Doin, Paris.

Urquhart, D.M., Hodges, P.W. 2007. Clinical anatomy of the anterolateral abdominal muscles. In: Movement, Stability & Lumbopelvic Pain, 2nd edn. (eds Vleeming, A., Mooney, V., Stoeckart, R.), pp. 76–84. Edinburgh: Churchill Livingstone Elsevier.

Vleeming, A., Pool-Goudzwaard, A.L., Stoeckart, R., van Wingerden J.P., Snijders, C.J., 1995. The posterior layer of the thoracolumbar fascia: its function in load transfer from spine to legs. Spine 20, 753–758.

Vleeming, A., Stoeckart, R., Snijders, C.J. 1989. The sacrotuberous ligament: a conceptual approach to its dynamic role in stabilizing the sacroiliac joint. Clin Biomech 4, 201–203.

Vleeming, A., Willard, F.H., 2010. Force closure and optimal stability of the lumbopelvic region. In: 7th Interdisciplinary World Congress on Low Back & Pelvic Pain. (Ed. Vleeming A), pp. 23–35. Worldcongress LBP Foundation, Los Angeles.

Willard, F.H. 1995. The lumbosacral connection: the ligamentous structure of the low back and its relation to pain. In: Second Interdisciplinary Congress on Low Back Pain. (eds Vleeming, A., Mooney, V., Dorman, T., et al.), pp. 31–58. San Diego, CA: University of California.

Willard, F.H., 2007. The muscular, ligamentous, and neural structure of the lumbosacrum and its relationship to low back pain. In: Movement, Stability & Lumbopelvic Pain, second ed. (Eds Vleeming A, Mooney V, Stoeckart R), pp. 5–45. Churchill Livingstone Elsevier, Edinburgh.

Wood Jones, F., 1946. Buchanan's Manual of Anatomy, seventh ed. Bailliere, Tindall and Cox, London.

Deep Fascia of the Neck and Deep Inner Fascia of the Anterior Wall of the Trunk

Fabiana Silva and Leonardo Sette Vieira

CHAPTER CONTENTS

INTRODUCTION

Fascial structures do not act or function in isolation because they constitute a body connection system. The head and neck fascia plays a clinically relevant role in various disorders, such as neck pain, shoulder pain, chewing, visual changes, vertigo, and tinnitus (Stecco 2015). The thoracic fascia participates in various functions and may be altered by abdominal surgery and scarring in the region (Killens 2018). Thus knowledge of the particularities of these structures is very relevant in clinical practice.

Cervical fasciae present distinct characteristics in the embryonic formation and consequently morphology, innervation, and function. We can divide the cervical and thoracic fascia into superficial, deep, visceral, and neural fascia according to the tissues to which they report (Serge 2002). We analyze these fasciae beginning with the time of their formation and discussing the embryological, anatomical, physiological, and phylogenetic interactions and their clinical repercussions.

Mechanical vision is addressed through the physical interactions of the fasciae, where the connective tissue has an anatomical and biomechanical continuity (Stecco and Day 2010; Stecco et al. 2008a, 2008b, 2009, 2013), such as the relationship of the joint capsules and ligaments in continuity with the formation of the movement fasciae in the limbs (Schleip 2017; van der Wal 2009). To Myers, this area encompasses the superficial back line and superficial and deep front lines (Myers 2014). We also address the neurofasciogenic model, proposed by Tozzi in 2015, where biotensegrity occurs through the interaction between the neural component and all body systems through connective tissue (Tozzi 2015a). Fascial tissues have a higher concentration of neural receptors with specific neural functions, as specified by Schleip (2017), showing that the fascia can be defined as a sensory organ. The physical and metabolic relationships of tissues, with their functional demand, play a fundamental role in the constitution of receptors and the extracellular matrix (ECM) composition of the corresponding fascial tissue (Blechschmidt 2004).

> ### KEY POINT
>
> Knowing the anatomy and structure of the deep fascia of the neck and anterior chest is extremely relevant clinically, as this region is involved in several pathologies.

SUPERFICIAL FASCIA OF THE NECK

The superficial fascia layer derives from the mesoderm, more precisely from the somatopleure (Stecco 2009), which consists of the interaction of the mesenchymal cells with the ectoderm, mainly relating the formation of the skin with the epidermis and dermis layers. This superficial layer is important to circulation because they contain a large part of the venous and lymphatic superficial circulation (Stecco 2015). The galea capitis, or superficial fascia of the head, connects various superficial muscles of the head such as the frontalis muscles, occipitalis, and auricular muscles. It continues through the face and neck through the platysma muscle that inserts cranially into the muscle of the mimic expression (Stecco 2015). It then continues with the superficial neck fascia that adheres to the nuchal ligament. It has innervation from the spinal cutaneous nerves and also from the autonomic nervous system, with potential for spinal cord sensitization at the respective spinal levels. It is linked to deep neck muscles that are rich in proprioceptors, particularly in muscle spindles, and act to regulate the head position along with gauze and labyrinthine functions (Stecco 2015).

Clinically it is an entryway for addressing body circulation and activating areas that possibly inhibit cortical perception and the emotional dimension of pain. The light and soft touch in the skin region, mainly by dermal and superficial fascia information, promote parasympathetic activation by stimulation of the left insular cortex and left hypothalamus (Olausson et al. 2008). This generates a modulation of vascular control by sympathetic system, with potential increase in vascular flow.

DEEP FASCIA OF THE NECK

Just below the superficial fascia layer is the deep fascia, which is not very elastic. It is rich in proprioceptive, but also interoceptive, neural receptors (Schleip 2003a, 2003b; Stecco et al. 2008a). About 80% of the receptors are free polymodal endings that make synapses in the lamina 1 and 5 of the posterior horn of the spinal cord carry nociceptive information (Schleip 2017). The deep fasciae derive from the paraxial mesoderm (Schoenwolf et al. 2015), which results from the rapid development of the tube and neural crest, with great relation to the formation of somites, thus constituting the musculoskeletal movement system (Blechschmidt and Gasser 2012).

Part of the cervical fasciae is derived from mesenchymal cells coming from the cranial neural crest (Standring 2016). As the main objective is force transmission to promote allostatic load reduction, its histology presents a small amount of elastin and extracellular matrix with a very organized collagenous disposition. In a histological study by Stecco and colleagues, three macroscopic layers were identified with fibers arranged at an angle of 78 degrees (Stecco et al. 2008b). Subdivisions are named according to their depth: the superficial layer of the deep fascia involves the superficial muscles, sternocleidomastoid, and trapezius; the middle layer of the deep fascia involves the infrahyoid muscles and the scapula elevator; and the deep layer of the deep fascia involves the deep axial, suboccipital, and scalene muscles. In the base of the skull, there is a fascial connection with the dura mater (Enix et al. 2014). This is clinically important because several neurovascular structures are located in this region. The deep scalp fascia of the skull is anteriorly continuous with the tenon fascia, which surrounds the structures of the eyeball from the posterior corneal ciliary margin to the optic nerve entrance and is continuous with the dura via the II cranial pair. It acts together with the eye muscles by redistributing tensions (Stecco 2015).

The deepest part of the middle layer is derived from somatopleure, thus having features of the insertional fascia. It starts in the hyoid bone and descends, involving the trachea and the thyroid and parathyroid glands. It crosses the thoracic inlet and helps to form the suspensory ligaments of the pleura and pericardium (Serge 2002; Stecco 2015).

In the region of the mouth, we have the masseteric fascia, which is continuous with the pterygoid fascia and the buccopharyngeal fascia. The latter involves the buccinator, the upper pharyngeal constrictor, and is continuous with the insertional esophageal fascia. This fascia ascends to the basilar apophysis of the occipital bone, where it becomes continuous with the deep fascia of the deep cervical flexor muscles and the dura of this region. Between the bucofaringea fascia and the deep layer of deep fascia, we have a virtual space for food passage, known as retropharyngeal space (Warshafsky et al. 2012). Clinically, it is important to evaluate these relationships in individuals with swallowing difficulties (Fig. 1.7.1).

The pharynx region is linked to the suprahyoid fasciae, which is influenced by the tongue musculature, which is the final tip of the digestive tract. The tongue also has innervation from the hypoglossal nerve that

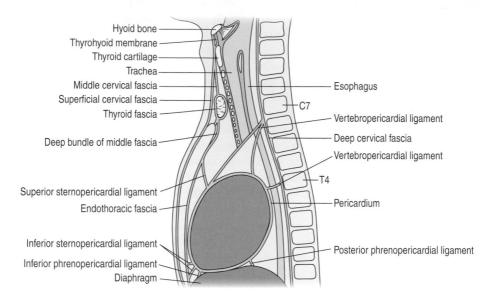

Fig. 1.7.1 Sagittal section showing the fascial relations of the cervical region to the thoracic spine. The middle and deep layers of the deep fascia form the suppository structures of the heart.

also innervates the afferent part of the dura mater located in the anterior region of the foramen magnum (Schleip 2017) and may influence the decrease in cervical range of motion. The tongue is formed by the four pharyngeal arches presenting innervation of cranial nerves V, VII, IX, and X in its sensory part and XII and X in the motor part (Parada et al. 2012). The relationship of the tongue with the infrahyoid area and the upper cervical can present significant clinical alterations regarding range of motion and pain in the neck, associated with digestive difficulties.

The tracheal and pharyngeal insertional fasciae present insertions into the hyoid bone and communicate with the middle cervical fascia (Serge 2002). Clinically this tissue responds very well to techniques that improve mechanical force transmission using a light affective touch. This also is used to promote centrally regulated modulation of the telencephalic (insular) and diencephalic (hypothalamus) pathways of the extracellular matrix together with a modulation of the autonomic nervous system.

The visceral fascia macroscopically is subdivided into a more rigid outer layer, the insertional fascia, and another innermost, lining fascia, which is more flexible

to adapt to volume changes in the digestive and respiratory system (Stecco and Stecco 2014).

The insertional fasciae form from the development of the somatopleure, which consists of the lateral part of the mesoderm that has a metabolic relationship with the development of the ectoderm, mainly due to the rapid growth of the medullary neural system that forms the sympathetic nerves (Blechschmidt 2004). Thus it has a great relationship with the sympathetic autonomic nervous system, with the potential for sensitization of the T1 to L2 medullary levels.

In a study of visceral fascia by Stecco et al. (2017), the insertional fasciae were found to present very little elastin fibers in the ligaments between visceral organs and also between visceral organs and the musculoskeletal system. However, they are filled with nociceptive and movement receptors (Schleip 2017), which have synapses at the spinal cord. The insertional esophageal fascia, which is continuous with the buccopharyngeal fascia, is inserted into the basilar apophysis of the occipital bone where it is continuous with the fascial rings that protect the neurovascular structures that penetrate the skull in the temporal and occipital regions (Warshafsky et al. 2012). A sequence of the middle layer of the deep neck fascia originate, the suspensory ligaments of the heart and lungs.

Sequentially we have the pleura and the pericardium (Stecco 2015) (Fig. 1.7.2). These have a great influence on the development of the transverse septum and thus carry with them a phrenic innervation, where adverse tension of these tissues may present the potential for sensitization on the C3–C5 levels in the cervical spine. This situation presents a direct anatomical relationship between visceral fasciae and movement fasciae. At the clinic we can potentially use deep breaths that alter the intracavitary pressure gradient, increasing visceral movements and their respective mechanosensitive afferences. Adding musculoskeletal movements to the evaluation and treatment system may have a good response due to the connection of the insertional fascia with the musculoskeletal system.

The lining fasciae are developed from the splanchnopleuric mesenchyme, which is a mesodermal structure resulting from the interactions of the mesenchyme with the rapid development of the digestive tract. The development of the digestive tract influences the formation of I, II, III, and IV pharyngeal arches (Schoenwolf et al. 2015).

The development and consequent descent of the digestive tract arises from a region of the head where it will form the submesencephalic septum, dragging the vagus nerve.

The vagus nerve, X cranial pair, accompanies the IV pharyngeal arch and all the viscera that develop from foregut and midgut. The X nerve is the main innervation of the lining fasciae of these same organs. The digestive and respiratory systems also innervate the enteric autonomic nervous system (ANS). This part of the ANS innervates the muscular and mucous layers of these organs and is related to the lining fasciae (Schoenwolf et al. 2015; Standring 2016).

About 80% of vagal axons carry visceral afferent information (Howland 2014). Since 5% of these fibers enter the cervical C1–C2 levels, they can generate sensitization of these levels (Foreman 1999). Histologically, these fasciae present a high concentration of elastin fibers (Stecco et al. 2017), allowing constant volume changes in the digestive and respiratory tract. The kidney

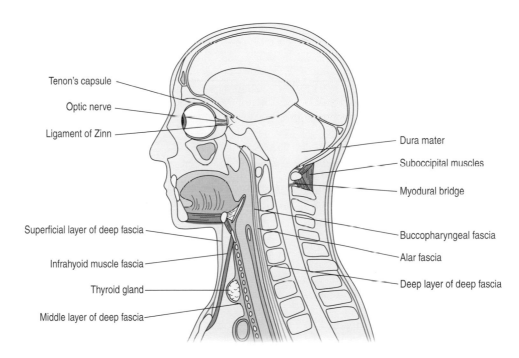

Fig. 1.7.2 Sagittal section of the head and neck with the fascial relations between the dura mater and the fascia of Tenon, between the dura mater and the fascia of the suboccipital muscles, and between the skull base and buccopharyngeal fascia.

and heart lining fasciae are exceptions, containing a lower percentage of elastin in their composition (Stecco et al. 2017) to allow a better adaptation of the fluidic function of these organs.

Vascular fasciae present a similar pattern of behavior to that of the visceral fascial system, presenting a more external, insertional, and internal layer that forms the adventitia of the vessels. An example is the carotid sheath, which is formed by the junctions of the three layers of the deep fascia of the neck and forms a protective layer and a guide for the insertional fascia, the jugular vein, carotid artery, and vagus nerve. The vagus nerve serves as a connection from the base of the skull to the thoracic entrance (Stecco et al. 2013). Between the two carotid sheaths, there is a fascial communication across the neck, creating a pillar of structural, mechanical, and sensory information called the alar fascia (Serge 2002). According to Willard (2018), vascular fasciae are rich in free nerve endings, which are nociceptors with the potential to generate central sensitization through sympathetic pathways at the T1 to L2 medullary levels and may be involved in nociplastic pain in structures innervated by the respective medullary levels (Fig. 1.7.3)

The deep layer of the deep cervical fascia forms a special protective sheath for the brachial plexus, which dampens possible compressions in the cervical to the thoracic path (Meert 2012; Willard 2018). Peripheral neural fasciae are continuous with the central neural fascia, particularly with the dura mater being continuous with the epineurium, the arachnoid layer with the perineurium, and the pia mater with the endoneurium (Standring 2016). These nerves present nociceptive innervation, which connects to the spine via the sympathetic nerves that also innervate the vessels supplying the nerves themselves, thus generating a central sensitization potential at the sympathetic medullary levels (Meert 2012). The sympathetic paravertebral ganglia are surrounded by the deep layer of the deep fascia (Stecco 2015). This is clinically relevant because the densification of this fascia can lead to a ganglion compression or a decrease in motion between adjacent structures when moving the head. This factor could trigger a change in sympathetic function and an increase in nociceptive information.

THORACIC FASCIAE

According to the *Functional Atlas of Human Fascial System*, by Carla Stecco (2015), the three layers of deep fasciae in the cervical region have continuity with the

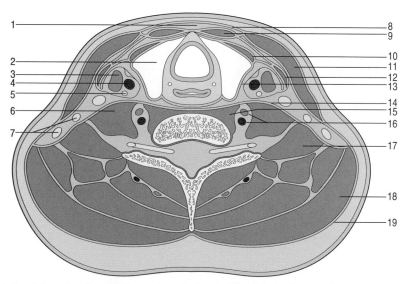

Fig. 1.7.3 Horizontal section through the neck at the level of the first tracheal cartilage. Note how the infrahyoid muscles (9, 10, and 12) are enveloped by the fascia colli media. 1, Spatium suprasternale; 2, thyroid gland; 3, internal jugular vein; 4, arteria carotis communis; 5, vagus nerve; 6, anterior scalene muscle; 7, branches of brachial plexus; 8, fascia colli superficialis; 9, sternohyoid muscle; 10, sternothyroid muscle; 11, sternocleidomastoid muscle; 12, omohyoid muscle; 13, thyroid capsule; 14, fascia colli profunda; 15, prevertebral muscles; 16, vertebral artery and vein; 17, scalenus medius muscle; 18, trapezius muscle; 19, fascia nuchae.

three layers of deep fasciae in the thoracic region. The superficial layer of the deep thoracic fascia surrounds the pectoralis major muscle, the trapezius, latissimus dorsi, and teres major, linking the external oblique muscle fascia. The middle layer of the deep fascia surrounds the scapular muscles, except for the teres major, including rhomboids, anterior serratus, rotator cuff muscles, superior posterior serratus, inferior posterior serratus, and levator scapulae muscles, connecting also with the internal oblique fascia. The endothoracic side of the sternum is covered by the sternalis muscle that would be an intrathoracic expansion of the transverse abdomen. The deep layer of the deep trunk fascia surrounds the intercostal muscles, where they are continuous with the diaphragm and the transverse abdominis muscle in the region of the lower ribs (Stecco 2015).

The deepest lamina of the middle layer of the deep cervical fascia together with the deep layer of the deep fascia gives rise to the suspensory ligaments of the pleura and pericardium, which support these structures and have C7-T1 and first rib fixations (Stecco 2015). The parietal pleura or insertional fascia of the lung fuses with these ligaments at the upper edge of the lungs forming the so-called suprapleural fascia or Sibson's fascia (Kitamura 2018). This thoracic entrance is a very important region because of the passage of various neurovascular structures. Clinically, the release of thoracic inlet tensions may favor the functionality of the movement system, of the brachial plexus passage, and body fluids. Elevation of negative pressure during inspiration may generate a concomitant increase in venous and lymphatic fluid flow to this region. The entire lymphatic system drains into the subclavian venous region (Meert 2012). In the mediastinal region, there are very important fascial scaffolds. The fascial tissue forms the pleura, the pericardium, and various ligaments for the vasculature and respiratory structures and also forms the esophageal fasciae (Standring 2016).

The parietal pericardium or insertional fascia of the heart forms the superior and inferior sternopericardial ligaments and the frenicopericardial ligaments. They also present an insertion in the middle thoracic region where it is continuous with the deep layer of the deep chest fascia at the T4 level (Serge 2002). From a phylogenetic point of view, the parietal pleura fuses with the deep layer of the deep thorax fascia, forming the endothoracic fascia (Stecco and Stecco 2014). This mechanical evolution—coupled with the brainstem neural evolution, especially the vagus nerve—allows the breathing, speech, and trunk movements to function independently (Porges 2011).

The posterior region of the mediastinum between the cardiac, pulmonary hilum, and esophageal fasciae presents an important concentration of loose connective tissue, allowing the passage of the vagus nerve and the formation of the cardiorespiratory and pulmonary plexuses (Janig 2006).

The deep trunk fasciae promote stability while at the same time a greater possibility of movement with less energy expenditure. The most superficial layers of the deep trunk fascia promote dynamic stability, such as the superficial layer of the thoracolumbar fascia, between the gluteus and the latissimus dorsi, with the transmission of force and synchronization of the pelvic girdle to scapular for walking and running. The movement occurs without the participation of the central nervous system but by the distribution of dynamic tension through the extracellular matrix of the connective tissues of the whole body and their relationships with other tissues (Bordoni et al. 2018a; Turvey et al. 2014). The deeper layers of the deep trunk fasciae promote stability for the spine. The previous layer of the thoracolumbar fascia surrounds the lumbar area and the psoas. It assists in the control of the trunk and lower limb movements. At the same time, it presents an interface with the renal fascia, with its origin in the intermediate mesoderm. According to Tozzi et al. (2012) there exists a direct relationship between the lack of sliding mobility between the renal fascia and the psoas fascia and the pain pathology in individuals with chronic low back pain. Tozzi suggests the lack of movement between the visceral fascia of the kidney concerning the previous layer of the thoracolumbar fascia as one of the possible causes of certain low back pain. He describes changes in the stimulation of fascial nociceptors as a possible generator of central sensitization at lumbar spinal cord levels. Clinically it is important to maintain sliding mobility between the musculoskeletal system and the visceral fasciae.

The deep layer of the deep fasciae has a strong relationship with the paravertebral sympathetic ganglia, which are responsible for a part of the cardiorespiratory system innervation (Janig 2006). This is clinically relevant information for the treatment of chest pain because compression of these ganglia can alter the afferent nociceptive information carried by the sympathetic nerves to the medulla. The stimulation of chest mobility with manual therapy associated with breathing patterns can have a major impact on pain perception (Linderoth and Meyerson 2013). There are several fascial links of all thoracic fascia that report the diaphragm to the abdominal and thoracic contents and also to the bone structure linking respiration to vertebral stability.

DIAPHRAGM DEVELOPMENT

The diaphragm is formed by the joining interaction of several different embryological tissues that results in different innervations and additional functions besides the respiratory action (Schoenwolf et al. 2015). It actively participates in reflux control (Bordoni et al. 2018c), stimulates venous and lymphatic return (Byeon et al. 2012; Meert 2012), aids in postural control and in upper limb movement control (Bordoni and Marelli 2016), assists in visceral function (Helsmoortel et al. 2010) and in lumbar stabilization (Hodges et al. 2005), and actively influences adaptations in the emotional sphere (Bordoni et al. 2016) as well as in pain control (Bordoni et al. 2018b).

The diaphragm is anatomically inserted into the T12, L1, L2, and L3 vertebrae on the right side and the T12, L1, and L2 on the left side, as well as into the last six ribs and at the central tendon of the diaphragm (Standring 2016). The diaphragmatic fascia is continuous with the deep trunk fascia and the insertional fascia and is directly related to various thoracic and abdominal organs, forming their ligaments and the omentum (Standring 2016). It connects with the anterior layer of the thoracolumbar fascia and forms the median arcuate ligament and is continuous with the Psoas major fascia, the lateral arcuate ligament, and the quadratus lumborum.

According to Strigo and Craig, slow and deep breaths influence the left insular cortex by increasing the activation of the left hypothalamus with a consequent increase in the parasympathetic tone. With this, we can balance the activation of cortical and subcortical areas related to chronic pain and emotional disorders (Strigo and Craig 2016). The authors suggest the use of specific breathing patterns and touches to enhance the outcome by neurofascial system modulation (Tozzi 2015b).

The embryological development of the digestive tract leads to the formation of the esophageal part of the diaphragm. The growth of the digestive tract in the region of the mesencephalic septum in the skull then pulls the vagal innervation along much of the subsequent length of the digestive tract (Hinrichsen 1990). It plays an important role in the control of reflux, along with the cardiac portion of the stomach, which is also innervated by the vagus (Greenwood-Van Meerveld et al. 2016).

The lumbar part of the diaphragm follows the development of the digestive tract and aorta, receiving vagal and phrenic innervation. It is closely related to lumbar stabilization. In the region of the aortic passage, it presents a fascial thickening called the edial arcuate ligament, protecting the aorta from the contractions of the diaphragm (Ozel et al. 2012). In the aortic hiatus, there also passes the thoracic duct, an important structure for the lymphatic return of the abdominal organs and lower limbs (Hinriebsen 1990; Mirjalili et al. 2012). The authors of this chapter suggest that tension release in this region may function as a fundamental basis for the lymphatic return of the abdominal organs and lower limbs, given that it is through the aortic opening of the diaphragm that the lymph from the cisterna chyli moves to the thoracic duct (Chikly 2001; Meert 2012).

The central tendon of the diaphragm develops from the transverse septum, a mesodermal structure that is formed by the rapid development of the heart and liver (Blechschmidt 2004; Fitzgerald and Fitzgerald 1994). This structure forms in the cervical region of the embryo and thus pulls the phrenic innervation along with itself, which leads to afferences of the insertional fascia and ligaments in the region near the diaphragm. This region has several important functions besides respiratory function, including visceral movement, cardiac function, and changes in cavity pressures and fluid flow (Drews 1995). The posterior part of the diaphragm is influenced by the formation of the pleural sac with its related phrenic innervation (Gilbert and Barresi 2016). The coastal part of the diaphragm develops from the formation of the rib cage and has innervation of the T7 to T12 intercostal nerves, which are mostly related to afferent regulation because the motor part of the costal diaphragm is innervated by the phrenic nerve (Wallden 2017).

The diaphragm is considered a transition point between reptilian and emotional limbic functions in our mammalian body (Wallden 2017). In 2017, McCoss et al. demonstrated that techniques performed in the coastal region of the diaphragm are reflected in the central tendon, altering spinal cord responses at levels C3 to C5 in addition to thoracic levels from T7 to T12 (Willard 2018).

FINAL CONSIDERATIONS

Most fascial structures have a mesodermal origin, except for the fasciae and muscles of the cervical and facial regions that originate from the mesenchymal cells of the cranial neural crest (Hinriebsen 1990).

Differences between the morphologies and histology of these fasciae occur according to the metabolic relationships of the mesodermal tissue with the surrounding tissue (Blechschmidt 2004). Connective tissue is responsible for forming the medium through which metabolic changes will take place throughout the body from embryo to adulthood. Fascial tissue frequently allows movement between structures and helps maintain their allostatic state with the lowest possible energy expenditure (Lunghi and Baroni 2019). The cervical region permits the passage of important structures for the maintenance of life. Any change in movement between them can physiologically alter important body functions. The rib cage allows important protection for life-essential structures such as the heart and lungs and all circulatory framework. A change in rib cage mobility is usually associated with alteration in the histological composition of the fasciae of this region, very common in chronic pathologies such as chronic obstructive pulmonary disease (COPD) and chronic heart disease (Bordoni et al. 2018a; Fukui et al. 2013). Maintaining movement and also good breathing efficiency is therefore critical to the health of the entire body. Knowledge of the anatomy and neurophysiology of the fasciae of the region is fundamental for good evaluation and treatment.

 KEY POINT

The fascia of the cervical and thoracic region has specific characteristics compared with other regions of the body, mainly by its base in three layers. It stays connected to the autonomic nervous system through a large number of proprioceptors and interoceptors that have the sensitivity potential of related spinal systems.

Summary

The cervical region is composed of the superficial surface (linked to the subcutaneous layers) and the deep fascia. The deep cervical fascia is made up of three layers that relate directly to the surrounding muscles and three layers of the deep chest fascia. There is a visceral influence of the fascia on various physiological functions of the body. These fasciae permeate the neurovascular structures and also influence stability and body movement.

Knowing the structures and their interrelationships is fundamental for clinical practice and affects both the evaluation and the treatment of various dysfunctions.

REFERENCES

Blechschmidt, E., 2004. The Ontogenético Basis of Human Anatomy, first ed. North Atlantic Books, Berkeley, CA.

Blechschmidt, E., Gasser, R.F., 2012. BioKinectics and Biodynamics of Human Differentiation, second ed. North Atlantic Books, Berkeley, CA.

Bordoni, B., Marelli, F., 2016. Failed back surgery syndrome: review and new hypotheses. J. Pain. Res. 9, 17–22.

Bordoni, B., Marelli, F., Bordoni, G., 2016. A review of analgesic and emotive breathing: a multidisciplinary approach. J. Multidiscip. Healthc. 9, 97–102.

Bordoni, B., Marelli, F., Morabito, B., Castagna, R., 2018a. Chest pain in patients with COPD: the fascia's subtle silence. Int. J. Chron. Obstruct. Pulmon. Dis.13, 1157–1165.

Bordoni, B., Marelli, F., Morabito, B., Sacconi, B., 2018b. Depression and anxiety in patients with chronic heart failure. Future Cardiol. 14, 115–119.

Bordoni, B., Marelli, F., Morabito, B., et al. 2018c. Low-back pain and gastroesophageal reflux in patients with COPD: the disease in the breath. Int. J. Chron. Obstruct. Pulmon. Dis. 13, 325–334.

Byeon, K., Choi, J.O., Yang, J.H., et al. 2012. The response of the vena cava to abdominal breathing. J. Altern. Complement. Med. 18, 153–157.

Chikly, B., 2001. Silent Waves: Theory and Practice of Lymphatic Drainage Therapy, first ed. International Health and Heline, Inc, Scottsdale, AZ.

Drews, U., 1995. Colour Atlas of Embryology. Thieme, NY.

Enix, D.E., Scali, F., Pontell, M.E., 2014. The cervical myodural bridge, a review of literature and clinical implications. J. Can. Chiropr. Assoc. 58, 184–192.

Fitzgerald, M., Fitzgerald, M., 1994. Human Embryology: A Human Approach. Bailliere Tindall, London.

Foreman, R.D., 1999. Mechanisms of cardiac pain. Annu. Rev. Physiol. 61, 143–167.

Fukui, A., Takahashi, N., Nakada, C., et al., 2013. Role of leptin signaling in the pathogenesis of angiotensin II-mediated atrial fibrosis and fibrillation. Circ. Arrhythm. Electrophysiol. 6, 402–409.

Gilbert, S.F., Barresi, M.J.F., 2016. Developmental Biology, eleventh ed. Sinauer Associates, Sunderland, MA.

Greenwood-Van Meerveld, B, Moloney, R.D., Johnson, A.C., Vicario, M., 2016. Mechanisms of stress-induced visceral pain: implications in irritable bowel syndrome. J. Neuroendocrinol. 28 (8). doi:10.1111/jne.12361.

Helsmoortel, J., Hirth, T., Wuhrl, P., 2010. Visceral Osteopathy, first ed. Eastland Press, Seattle.

Hinrichsen, K.V., 1990. Humanembryologie, first ed. Verlag, Berlin.

Hodges, P., Eriksson, A.E., Shirley, D., Gandevia, S., 2005. Intra-abdominal pressure increases the stiffness of the lumbar spine. J. Biomech. 38, 1873–1880.

Howland, R. H., 2014. Vagus nerve stimulation. Curr. Behav. Neurosci. Rep. 1, 64–73.

Janig, W., 2006. The Integrative Action of The Autonomic Nervous System, first ed. Cambridge University Press, New York.

Killens, D., 2018. Mobilizing the Myofascial System, first ed. Handspring, Pencaitland, East Lothian, Scotland.

Kitamura, S., 2018. Anatomy of the fasciae and fascial spaces of the maxillofacial and the anterior neck regions. Ana. Sci. Int. 93, 1–13.

Linderoth, B., Meyerson, B.A., 2013. Spinal cord and brain stimulation. In: Wall & Melzack's Textbook of Pain, sixth ed. Elsevier, Philadelphia.

Lunghi, C., Baroni, F., 2019. Cynefin framework for evidence-informed clinical reasoning and decision-making. J. Am. Osteopath. Assoc. 119, 312–321.

McCoss, C.A., Johnston, R., Edwards, D.J., Millward, C., 2017. Preliminary evidence of Regional Interdependent Inhibition, using a 'Diaphragm Release' to specifically induce an immediate hypoalgesic effect in the cervical spine. J. Bodyw. Mov. Ther. 21, 362–374.

Meert, G.F., 2012. Venolymphatic Drainage Therapy, second ed. Elsevier, Munich, Germany.

Mirjalili, S.A., Hale, S.J., Buckenham, T., Wilson, B., Stringer, M. D., 2012. A reappraisal of adult thoracic surface anatomy. Clin. Anat. 25, 827–834.

Myers, T.W., 2014. Anatomy Trains. Myofascial Meridians for Manual and Movement Therapists, third ed. Churchill Livingstone Elsevier, Edinburgh.

Olausson, H., Cole J., Vallbo A., et al., 2008. Unmyelinated tactile afferents have opposite effects on insular and somatosensory cortical processing. Neurosci. Letters 436, 128–132

Ozel, A., Toksoy, G., Ozdogan, O., Mahmutoglu, A.S., Karpat, Z. 2012. Ultrasonographic diagnosis of median arcuate ligament syndrome: a report of two cases. Med. Ultrason. 14, 154–157.

Parada, C., Han, D., Chai, Y., 2012. Molecular and cellular regulatory mechanisms of tongue myogenesis. J. Dent. Res. 91, 528–535.

Porges, S., 2011. The Polyvagal Theory, first ed. Norton Company, Chicago.

Schleip, R., 2003a. Fascial plasticity – a new neurobiological explanation: Part 1. J. Bodyw. Move. Ther. 7, 11–19.

Schleip, R., 2003b. Fascial plasticity – a new neurobiological explanation: Part 2. J. Bodyw. Move. Ther. 7, 104–116.

Schleip, R., 2017. Fáscia as a sensory organ: clínical applications. In: Liem, T., Tozzi, P., Chila, A. (eds.), Fascia in the Osteopathic Field. Handspring Publishing, Edinburgh, UK.

Schoenwolf, G.C., Bleyl, S.B., Brauer, P.R., Francis-West, P.H., 2015. Larsen's Human Embryology, fifth ed. Elsevier, Philadelphia.

Serge, P., 2002. The Fasciae, second ed. Eastland Press, Seattle, WA.

Standring, S., 2016. Gray's Anatomy, forty-first ed. Elsevier. London.

Stecco, A., Masiero, S., Macchi, V., et al. 2008a. The pectoral fascia: Anatomical and histological stud. J. Bodyw. Mov. Ther. 13, 255–261.

Stecco, A., Macchi, V., Stecco, C., et al., 2009. Anatomical study of myofascial continuity in the anterior region of the upper limb. J. Bodyw. Move. Ther. 13, 53–62.

Stecco, C., 2015. Functional Atlas of The Human Fascial System, first ed. Elsevier, Churchill Livingstone, London.

Stecco, C., Corradin, M., Macchi, V., et al., 2013. Plantar fascia anatomy and its relationship with Achilles tendon and paratenon. J. Anat. 223, 665–676.

Stecco, C., Day, J.A., 2010. The fascial manipulation technique and its biomechanical model: a guide to the human fascial system. Int. J. Ther. Massage Bodywork 3, 38–40.

Stecco, C., Porzionato, A., Lancerotto, L., et al., 2008b. Histological study of the deep fasciae of the limbs. J. Bodyw. Move. Ther. 12, 225–230.

Stecco, C., Sfriso, M.M., Porzionato, A., et al., 2017. Microscopic anatomy of the visceral fasciae. J. Anat. 231, 121–128.

Stecco, L., Stecco, C., 2014. Fascial Manipulation for Internal Dysfunctions, first ed. Piccin, Padova, Italy.

Strigo, I.A., Craig, A.D.B., 2016. Interoception, homeostatic emotions, and sympathovagal balance. Philos. Trans. R. Soc. Lond. B. Biol. Sci. 371, 1–9.

Tozzi, P., 2015a. A unifying neuro-fasciagenic model of somatic dysfunction – Underlying mechanisms and treatment – Part I. J. Bodyw. Move. Ther. 19, 310–326.

Tozzi, P., 2015b. A unifying neuro-fasciagenic model of somatic dysfunction – Underlying mechanisms and treatment – Part II. J. Bodyw. Mov. Ther. 19, 526–543.

Tozzi, P., Bongiorno, D., Vitturini, C., 2012. Low back pain and kidney mobility: local osteopathic fascial manipulation decrease pain perception and improves renal mobility. J. Bodyw. Mov. Ther. 16, 381–391.

Turvey, M.T., Fonseca, S.T., 2014. The medium of haptic perception: a Tensegrity hypothesis. J. Mot. Beha. 46, 143–187.

van der Wal, J., 2009. The architecture of the connective tissue in the musculoskeletal system-an often overlooked functional parameter as to proprioception in the locomotor apparatus. Int. J. Ther. Massage Bodywork 2, 9–23.

Wallden, M., 2017. The diaphragm – More than an inspired design. J. Bodyw. Mov. Ther. 21, 342–349.

Warshafsky, D., Goldenberg, D., Kanekar, S.G., 2012. Imaging anatomy of deep neck spaces. Otolaryngol. Clin. North Am. 45, 1203–1221.

Willard, F., 2018. Foundations of Osteopathic Field, fourth ed. Lippincott Williams & Wilkins, Philadelphia.

Visceral Fascia

Frank H. Willard

CHAPTER CONTENTS

INTRODUCTION

The organ systems of the body, whether visceral or somatic in nature, are composed of highly differentiated tissue and require an elaborate support system for their maintenance. This sustentacular system is constructed from a connective tissue network comprised of irregularly arranged collagen and elastin fibers, with their supporting cells embedded in a matrix of glycoproteins, all of which is termed fascia. The density of fibrous elements is highly regionally variable as well as individually variable. The role of fascia as a packing or investing tissue, surrounding and protecting organ systems, seems well-accepted in the anatomical literature (Drake et al. 2010; O'Rahilly 1986; Standring 2015).

Although fascia has been described in several academic treatises (Gallaudet 1931; Singer 1935), there still remains much confusion regarding distribution and naming surrounding the visceral fasciae of the body cavities (Skandalakis et al. 2006). Chapter 1.3 of this text suggested that there are four primary fascial layers in the body: (1) *pannicular* (often termed superficial), (2) *axial and appendicular* (often termed deep or investing or muscular fascia), (3) *meningeal* fascia surrounding the central nervous system, and (4) *visceral* (or splanchnic)

fascia surrounding the body cavities and packing around the internal organs. This current chapter will examine this last category, the visceral fasciae of the body, and attempt to present a unifying concept concerning their organization and continuity. The approach will begin with the development of visceral fascia then proceed to a consideration of its adult form.

DEVELOPMENT OF VISCERAL FASCIA

Visceral fascia develops out of the mesoderm that lies in close approximation with the yolk sac. This tissue is composed primarily of mesenchymal cells in a loose meshwork extracellular matrix and represents the embryonic version of irregular connective tissue. Mesenchymal cells can develop to form fibroblasts as well as several other closely related cell types, such as osteoblasts, chondroblasts, smooth muscle cells, and adipocytes. O'Rahilly and Muller (1996) refer to mesenchymal tissue as the primitive "packing tissue" of the embryo in a close analogy to fascia, and it is from this mesenchymal tissue that the adult form of fascia is derived. The inward folding movements of the lateral walls of the embryo in the third week of gestation compressed some of this midline mesenchymal tissue between the newly forming gut and the developing sclerodermal tissue directly anterior to the notochord. This medially placed sclerodermal tissue will contribute to forming the vertebral bodies and the anterior longitudinal ligament.

FORMATION OF THE INTRAEMBRYONIC COELOM AND SURROUNDING VISCERAL FASCIA

By the end of the third week, the lateral plate mesoderm cleaves into two layers separated by a newly formed cavity (Fig. 1.8.1A). The outer layer or somatic mesoderm

is adherent to the overlying ectoderm; the combined structure is termed the somatopleure and gives rise to the somatic body wall. The inner layer or visceral mesoderm is adherent to the underlying endoderm and the combined structure is termed the splanchnopleure. The splanchnopleure, or visceral mesenchyme, will contribute to the visceral fascia surrounding the organs of the thoracoabdominopelvic cavity. The cavity formed between somatopleure and splanchnopleure will become the intraembryonic coelom and form the body cavities in the fourth week. The cavity will be lined with a squamous cell layer forming a mesothelium; where it lines the cavity opposite the body wall it is referred to as a

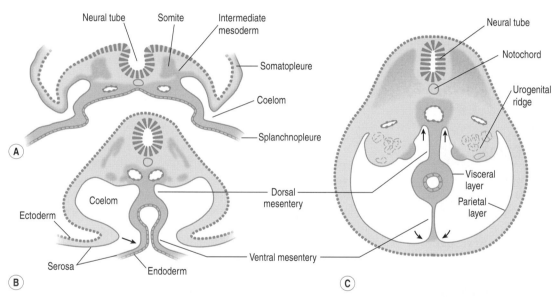

Fig. 1.8.1 The Formation of a Mediastinum. This is a series of drawings of axial plane sections taken through the human embryo in the third, fourth, and fifth weeks of gestation. Modified with permission from Arey, L.B., 1965. *Development Anatomy.* Philadelphia: W.B. Saunders Company. (A) In the end of the third week the neural tube is forming, and directly below lies the notochord. The somite and intermediate mesoderm and lateral plate mesoderm are arranged linearly, and the lateral plate has divided into somatopleure (parietal mesoderm) and splanchnopleure (visceral mesoderm). The two dorsal aortic vessels are positioned directly under the somite. (B) Toward the end of the fourth week, the lateral walls of the embryo sweep ventromedially to fuse on the midline. The intermediate mesoderm expands ventrally to form the urogenital ridge and compress the visceral fascia on the midline. At this level, the two dorsal aortic vessels are closer to the midline, embedded in visceral fascia. The left and right layers of splanchnopleure are fusing on the midline (arrow) to form the gut tube surrounded by visceral fascia. Dorsally the gut tube remains in contact with the body wall through the dorsal mesentery, a conduit for vessels and nerves. Ventrally in the foregut region a mesentery persists into adult life; however, in the midgut and hindgut a ventral mesentery never forms. (C) In the fifth week, the coelom is now completely formed and lined by a serosa. Where the serosa is in contact with the somatic body wall, it is termed *parietal peritoneum*; where it lines the mesenteries and organ walls, it is termed *visceral peritoneum*. (Note that panels B and C are histological sections taken through a mesentery, demonstrating its composition of two thin fibroelastic fascial layers lined with a mesothelium and sandwiching a thick layer of adipose tissue containing vessels, nerves, and lymph nodes.)

parietal mesothelium, and where it lines the body cavity covering the future visceral organs or their suspensory ligaments it is termed a *visceral mesothelium*.

FORMATION OF THE MIDLINE MESODERMAL COLUMN AND ITS RELATIONSHIP TO THE ORGANS OF THE BODY

The visceral mesoderm that is located under the notochord is forced toward the midline as the posterior body wall adapts to its new curved shape. The midline mesoderm surrounds the dorsal aorta as this artery courses parallel to the notochord along the longitudinal axis of the body (Fig. 1.8.1C). On the lateral margins of this visceral mesenchymal column lie the two cardinal veins. The visceral mesoderm surrounding the newly formed gut tube remains attached to this midline mesoderm, thus maintaining an attachment between the organ systems and the posterior body wall, thereby forming the mesenteries and the mesocolons of the abdominal cavity (Fig. 1.8.1C). Within this column of visceral mesoderm will develop the vascular tree, lymphatic drainage, and the nerve plexus that ultimately will supply the organ systems. On either side of the midline mesoderm, the intermediate mesoderm begins to form the kidneys and the gonadal tissues (Fig. 1.8.2A&B)

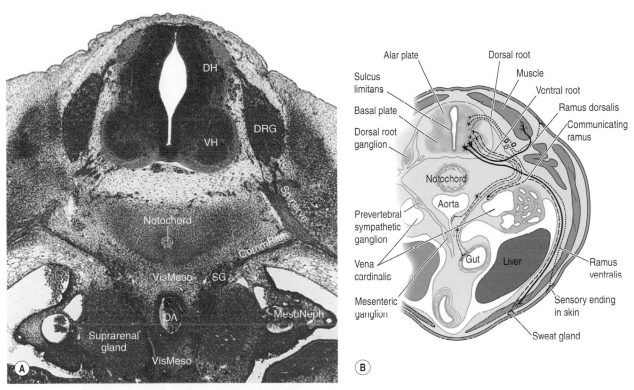

Fig. 1.8.2 Innervation of the Visceral Fascia. (A) This is an axial plane section taken through a stage-17 (41-day) embryo, illustrating the ingrowth of nerves into the visceral fascia. Images modified with permission from The Virtual Human Embryo hosted by the Endowment for Human Development. (B) A drawing of a 6-week-old embryo illustrating the growth of nerves into the mediastinum and through the mesenteries to reach the abdominal organs. Note that the finely dotted line indicates a sensory fiber whose peripheral process lies in the viscera, its cell body in the dorsal root ganglion, and its central process in the deep portions of the dorsal horn. The area of the gut tube innervated by fibers related to a specific dorsal root ganglion is termed a *viscerotome*. Reproduced with permission from Patten, B.M., 1946. *Human Embryology*. Philadelphia: The Blakiston Company, McGraw-Hill Education. Abbreviations: CommRam, communicating ramus; DA, dorsal aorta; DH, dorsal horn; DRG, dorsal root ganglion; MesoNeph, mesonephros; SG, sympathetic trunk ganglion; Sp nerve, spinal nerve; VH, ventral horn; VisMeso, visceral mesoderm.

FORMATION OF THE SPINAL NERVE AND THE VISCEROTOME

During the fourth week of development, the spinal nerves begin to form from the dorsal and ventral rootlets and subsequently grow outward into the body wall from the region of the neural tube (Fig. 1.8.2A&B). Although these nerves are often portrayed as solely efferent in nature, many are afferent or sensory and will provide the spinal cords with significant visceral afferent information. The visceral fascia comes to form a conduit for both the vascular system and the nervous system to reach the organs of the thoracoabdominopelvic cavity. The area of skin innervated by a specific dorsal root ganglion forms a *dermatome*, the muscles innervated by the axons in a specific ventral root constitute a *myotome*, the hard tissue innervated by a specific dorsal root ganglion represent a *sclerotome*, and the viscera innervated by fibers associated with a specific dorsal root ganglion constitute a *viscerotome* (Hazarika et al. 1964).

SUMMARY

As can be seen from the previous description, the visceral mesenchyme forms a midline column of extraperitoneal (extraserosal) fascia that extends from the cranial base to the pelvic basin, coursing parallel with the notochord and positioned directly anterior to the vertebral column (Fig. 1.8.3). Throughout the length of

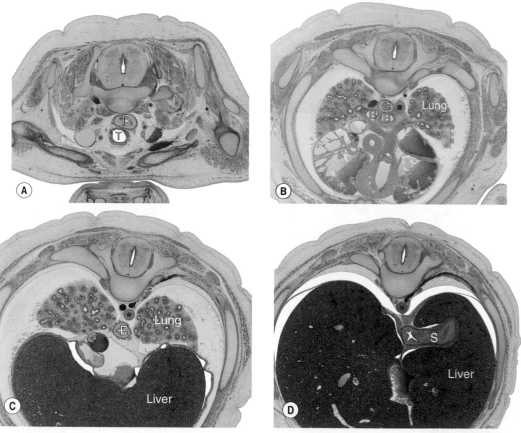

Fig. 1.8.3 A Series of Axial Plane Sections taken from Rostral to Caudal through a 56-Day-Old Embryo (Stage 23). (A) Cervical region: the trachea (T) and esophagus (E) are seen in a mass of visceral fascia bordered laterally by the dorsal aorta, anteriorly by the sternum and clavicles, and posteriorly by the cartilage of the developing vertebral body. (B&C) Thoracic region: the esophagus (E) and mainstem bronchi (B) are seen in a mass of visceral fascia that extends laterally into the root of the lungs.

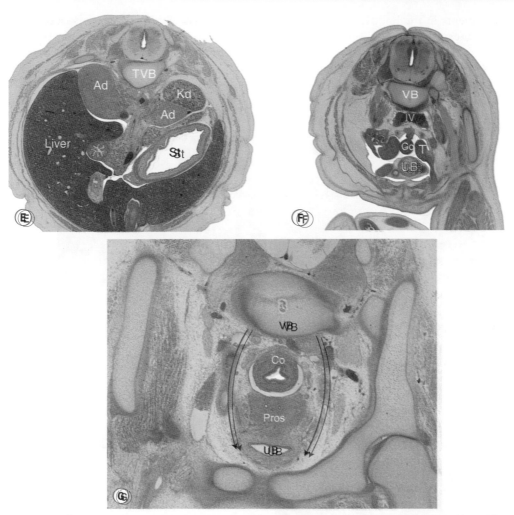

Fig. 1.8.3 Cont'd (D) Thoracoabdominal junction: the aorta is seen on the midline surrounded by a thin mass of visceral fascia and passing through the aortic hiatus of the diaphragm. (E) Abdominal region: the urogenital ridges containing the developing kidneys (Kd) and enlarged adrenal gland (Ad) are seen compressing the visceral fascia on the midline. (F) Pelvic region: the mediastinum of visceral fascia is seen anterior to the vertebral bodies (VB). (G) The mediastinal visceral fascia containing vessels and nerve is seen sweeping (arrows) around the colon (Co) to embrace the prostate (Pros) and urinary bladder (UB). The skeletal muscle bands seen on the cartilaginous precursors of the pelvic walls are embedded in parietal endopelvic fascia, an extension of the epimysium. Images modified with permission from The Virtual Human Embryo hosted by the Endowment for Human Development.

this fascial column, its posterior surface blends with the somatic prevertebral (axial) fascia that lies anterior to the anterior longitudinal ligament (Fig. 1.8.4). Most abdominopelvic organ systems develop embedded in the visceral mesoderm, near the midline, and then migrate to other locations in the body; however, they will maintain their connection with the midline through extensions of the visceral fascia in the mesenteries or mesocolons. Organs that develop with this visceral fascia but remain in the body wall are termed primary retroperitoneal organs, examples are the adrenal glands and the kidneys. Those organs that initially develop in the suspensory ligaments in the body cavity and then are compressed into the posterior body wall are referred to as secondarily retroperitoneal; examples include the duodenum and portions of the ascending and descending colon. I suggest that this medially positioned column of visceral fascia represents a continuous "mediastinum" of the body, not just in the thorax but along the entire length of the vertebral column (Fig. 1.8.4). Thus the mediastinum of the body can be described as a fascial column, arranged parallel to the vertebral

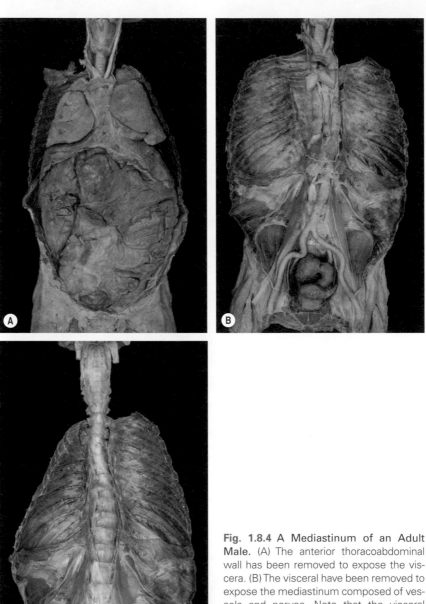

Fig. 1.8.4 A Mediastinum of an Adult Male. (A) The anterior thoracoabdominal wall has been removed to expose the viscera. (B) The visceral have been removed to expose the mediastinum composed of vessels and nerves. Note that the visceral fascia has also been removed to expose the vessels. (C) The mediastinum has been removed to expose the anterior longitudinal ligament.

column and functioning as an anchor for the visceral organs as well as a conduit through which blood vessels, nerves, and lymphatic vessels pass between the posterior body wall and the associated viscera (Anderson and Makins 1890).

KEY POINTS

- The visceral mesenchyme forms a midline column of extraperitoneal (extraserosal) fascia that extends from the cranial base to the pelvic basin, coursing parallel with the notochord and positioned directly anterior to the vertebral column.
- Most abdominopelvic organ systems develop embedded in the visceral mesoderm, near the midline, and then migrate to other locations in the body; however, they will maintain their connection with the midline through extensions of the visceral fascia in the mesenteries or mesocolons.
- This medially positioned column of visceral fascia represents a continuous "mediastinum" of the body, not just in the thorax but along the entire length of the vertebral column.

VISCERAL FASCIA

Extending from cranial base to pelvic basin and lining the body cavities, visceral fascia is by far the most complex of the four main layers of fascia. In the adult, the composition of visceral fascia is typically described as loose, irregular connective tissue containing a varying amount of adipocytes (Fig. 1.8.5).

Functionally, visceral fascia provides the packing tissue for the midline structures of the body. The midline fascia forms a column that extends from its attachments to the cranial base through the cervical region into the thorax, where it occupies the mediastinum. At the diaphragm, this column passes through the aortic and esophageal openings to enter the abdomen. Descending through the abdomen into the pelvic basin, the midline fascia forms a continuation of the mediastinum. In the pelvic basin, the visceral column of fascia surrounds the midline structures. Early studies had suggested four layers of visceral fascia are present in the walls of the body cavities: (1) muscular fascia surrounding the body wall muscles (at one time termed "parietal fascia"; see discussion in Derry 1907a, 1907b; Thompson 1901); (2) the fascia forming neurovascular sheaths; (3) fascia surrounding individual organs; and (4) fascia underlying the

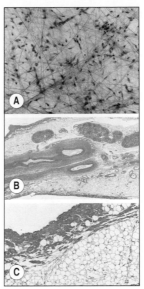

Fig. 1.8.5 Histological Views of Fascia. (A) This is a loose connective (areolar) tissue spread demonstrating a fairly random arrangement of collagenous and elastic fibers. (B) This is a cross-section taken through mesentery demonstrating a thin layer of dense, irregular collagenous fibers underlying the mesothelium with a central core of adipose tissue surrounding several vessels and lymph nodes. Note the thickened tunica adventitia of the vessels. (C) This is a magnified view of the mesentery border showing the thin layer of dense irregular collagenous fibers underlying the single cell layer of mesothelium. From the Willard/Carreiro Collection, with permission.

pleural and peritoneal linings (reviewed in Hollinshead 1956). The muscular or "parietal" fascia is essentially the axial and appendicular fascia described in Chapter 1.3. In the thorax, the fascia surrounding the costal and diaphragmatic pleura is also parietal in nature, whereas it has been proposed that visceral fascia underlies the parietal fascia surrounding the anterior and lateral aspects of the abdominopelvic cavity (Skandalakis et al. 2006). In general, the remaining fasciae, those surrounding neurovascular bundles and those surrounding organ systems, can be considered to derive from an extensive mesenchymal matrix or splanchnopleure.

Sentinel descriptions of visceral fascia can be found in the *Journal of Anatomy and Physiology* (Anderson and Makins 1890). These original descriptions emphasized the continuity of visceral fascia from the nasopharyngeal and cervical region, through the thorax and abdomen, to levator ani in the pelvic region. However, most of the anatomical research concerning visceral fascia has been done from a surgical perspective designed to solve clinical problems involving access into a specific region or excision of tissue in cases of neoplastic growth (for example, see Garcia-Armengol et al. 2008). Although the fine-grained analysis of individual fascial planes is necessary from a surgical perspective, the narrow focus of these studies tends to obscure the overall picture of this continuous fascial matrix in the body. In the remainder of the chapter, the general organization of visceral fascia in the cervical, thoracic, abdominal, and pelvic areas is presented.

 KEY POINTS

- The composition of visceral fascia is typically described as loose, irregular connective tissue containing a varying amount of adipocytes.
- On the midline, visceral fascia surrounds the vascular and lymphatic trees and provides a conduit for the fibers of the autonomic nervous system.

REGIONAL VISCERAL FASCIA

Cervical Visceral Fascia

In the cranial region, visceral fascia surrounds the pharynx and its attachment to the cranial base. Superiorly, visceral fascia includes the pharyngobasilar and pharyngobuccal fascia and, as such, fuses to the cranial base surrounding the attachments of the superior constrictor muscles (Last 1978). Cervical visceral fascia extends inferiorly into the neck, surrounding the nasopharynx, oropharynx, and remaining cervical viscera. Thus at the cranial base, cervical fascia has a flared opening surrounding the nasal passageways and the oral cavity (Fig. 1.8.6, sections 22 and 46).

In the neck, visceral fascia incorporates such regional fasciae as pretracheal, retropharyngeal, and alar (carotid sheath) fascia as well as the fascia surrounding the thyroid cartilage and thyroid gland (Fig. 1.8.6, sections 66 and 86). In this way visceral fascia can be conceived of as a continuous vertical sleeve lying internal to the hyoid muscles, anterior to the longus muscles, medial to the scalene muscles, and extending into the thorax.

Thoracic Visceral Fascia

Upon entering the thorax, the visceral fascia is forced to accommodate the two pleural cavities; this it does by compressing into the midline (Fig. 1.8.6, section 112),

forming the packing substance of the thoracic mediastinum (Fig. 1.8.6, section 112; and Fig. 1.8.7A). Here, the visceral fascia surrounds the great vessels of the heart and thickens to become the fibrous pericardium anteriorly, whereas posteriorly, the visceral fascia forms a loose matrix surrounding the aorta, esophagus, trachea, and primary bronchi, and the thoracic duct. This matrix is very loose to allow distension of the esophagus upon swallowing. Normally, no significant condensations of fascia are present in this region, otherwise they would lead to dysphagia. Finally, visceral fascia surrounds the bronchi as they pass through the root of the lung; this fascia becomes continuous with the stroma of the airways and the septa of the lung.

Abdominal Visceral Fascia

Visceral fascia also accompanies the esophagus and aorta into the abdominal cavity where it parallels the aorta and inferior vena cava in their course along the midline. Endoabdominal fascia can also be divided into parietal and visceral components. The parietal component of the endoabdominal fascia is very complex, having multiple layers (Kingsnorth et al. 2000; Skandalakis et al. 2006) that differ somewhat above and below the umbilicus due to an upward growth of a layer of mesoderm, termed secondary mesoderm, that arises out of the tissue located near the cloaca (Kingsnorth et al. 2000). This secondary mesoderm alters the layers present in the infraumbilical region of the abdominal wall as described in Wyburn (1937).

The endoabdominal visceral fascia thickens significantly along the posterior midline and forms a vertical column analogous to the visceral fascia in the mediastinum of the thoracic (Fig. 1.8.7B&C). It is along this pathway that the blood supply, innervation, and lymphatic channels reach the peritoneal organs of the abdomen. This situation is remarkably similar to that seen with the mediastinum of the thorax, where visceral fascia invests the structures in the root of the lung and accompanies these structures as they pass from the mediastinum deep into lung tissue.

On the posterior body wall the kidneys lie in a perirenal space covered by a particularly thick mass of fat and surrounded by an elastic layer of perirenal fascia, which is separate from that surrounding the peritoneal cavity (reviewed in Standring 2015). This perirenal fascia has been termed Gerota's fascia and is most likely derived from the intermediate mesoderm in the three-layered

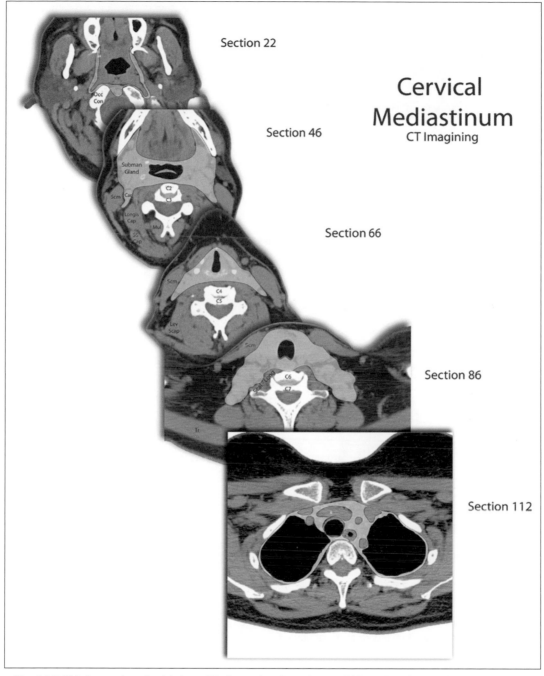

Fig. 1.8.6 This is a series of axial plane CT slices taken from the cranial base (section 22) through the cervical region to reach the cervicothoracic junction (section 86) of a 49-year-old female patient. Section 112 demonstrates the opening of the pleural sacs and the spreading of the endothoracic fascia around these sacs. From the Willard/Carreiro Collection, with permission. Abbreviations: Car, carotid sheath; Lev Scap, levator scapulae; Longus Cap, longus capitis muscle; Mul, multifidus muscle; Occ Con, occipital condyle; Scal-Long, scalene and longus muscles; SCM, sternocleidomastoid muscle; SS Cap, semispinalis capitis; Subman Gland, submandibular gland; Tr, trapezius muscle.

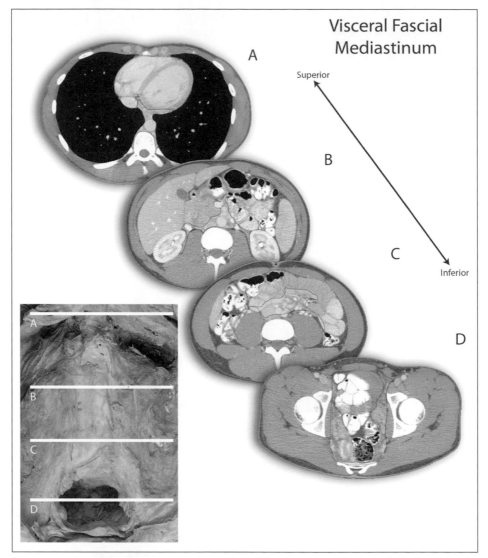

Fig. 1.8.7 A Series of Axial Plane CT Images Involving the Thorax, Abdomen, and Pelvis. The mediastinal column of visceral fascia has been shaded yellow. The inset on the lower left is a posterior body wall with all peritoneal organs removed revealing the endoabdominal fascia. The white lines indicate the levels of the corresponding CT images. The visceral fascia forms a curtain over the body wall that thickens noticeably at the midline, where it covers the major vascular and neural channels such as the abdominal aorta and the inferior vena cava. Extensions of the abdominal mediastinal fascia pass into the mesogastrium, mesentery, and mesocolon to reach the visceral organs of the abdomen. From the Willard/Carreiro Collection, with permission.

embryo. Posteriorly, the perirenal fascia blends with the parietal endoabdominal fascia covering the psoas muscle and the quadrates lumborum. Medially there is evidence that it crosses the midline to communicate with the perirenal fascia on the opposite side and inferiorly it tapers to surround and fuse to the ureters.

Pelvic Visceral Fascia

Endopelvic fascia can also be divided into parietal and visceral components. The parietal layer surrounds the internal aspect of the muscles in the pelvic region, including the iliacus, psoas, obturator internus, levator ani, and ischiococcygeus. As in the abdominal cavity, the parietal fascia is covered with a serous membrane, the parietal peritoneum. The visceral layer of endopelvic fascia is extremely complex, forming numerous condensations and planes in the area around the rectum, urinary bladder, and internal reproductive organs (Ercoli et al. 2005; Stelzner et al. 2011). Inferiorly, the visceral endopelvic fascia extends to the superior aspect of the pelvic diaphragm. The pelvic diaphragm, composed of skeletal muscle, is lined with axial or investing fascia derived from the somatic body wall. A blending of visceral fascia with the axial (investing) fascia of the pelvic diaphragm occurs on its superior (internal) surface. Inferior to the pelvic diaphragm is the ischiorectal (ischioanal) fossa; it is packed with pannicular fascia closely associated with the overlying dermis of the gluteal region (Fig. 1.8.7D and Fig. 1.8.8). The anterior and inferior border of the endopelvic visceral fascia fills the retropubic space surrounding the base of the urinary bladder (Stoney 1904).

At the level of the sacral promontory, the visceral endopelvic fascia forms a median fold surrounding the hypogastric plexus (presacral nerve) and two slightly more lateral folds surrounding the common iliac vessels and associated lymphatic channels. Inferior to the sacral promontory, the median fold divides with the hypogastric plexus to sweep laterally, joining the vessels in the lateral fold of endopelvic fascia. This allows the visceral (endopelvic) fascia to surround the midline organs—rectum, reproductive organs, and urinary bladder (Fig. 1.8.7D and Fig. 1.8.8)—and create a fascial conduit from the vasculature in the presacral region, forward to the lateral aspect of the urinary bladder (Roberts and Taylor 1970).

As in the thorax and abdomen, the visceral endopelvic fascia thickens on the midline, where it again forms a mediastinum surrounding these organs. The endopelvic fascia serves as a conduit over which the major organ systems in the pelvic basin receive their blood supply and innervation as well as their lymphatic drainage. In the female, extensions of the pelvic mediastinal component of the visceral fascia form the core of the broad ligament and condensations of visceral fascia at the base of the broad ligament form the transverse cervical ligament of the uterus. From the cervix of the uterus, posterolaterally directed bands of visceral fascia form the sacrouterine ligaments that reach back to the sacrum and underlie the prominent rectouterine folds. In both sexes, condensations of visceral fascia surround the rectum where it has been termed the mesorectum (Garcia-Armengol et al. 2008; Havenga et al. 2007).

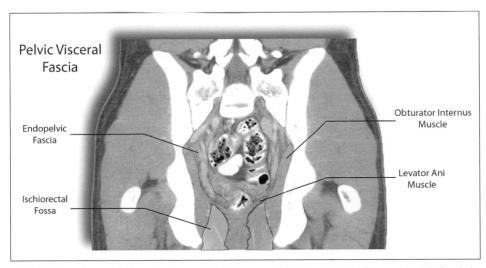

Fig. 1.8.8 This is a Coronal Plane Reformatted CT Image of the Male Pelvis. The endopelvic fascia is seen surrounding the visceral organs in the center of the pelvic basin. The levator ani separates the endopelvic fascia from the pannicular fascia located in the ischiorectal fossa. From the Willard/Carreiro Collection, with permission.

KEY POINTS

- Visceral fascia extends off from the body wall through the root of the lung, or through sheets of mesogastrium, mesentery or mesocolon to reach and surround the organs.
- At all levels, cervical, thoracic, lumbar and pelvic, of the axial body blood vessels, lymphatics and autonomic fibers course accompany the visceral fascia to reach the organ systems.

Summary

Visceral fascia can be traced from the cranial base into the pelvic cavity. It forms the packing surrounding the body cavities, where it is compressed against the somatic body wall. It also forms the packing around visceral organs, many of which it reaches by passing along the suspensory ligaments such as the mesenteries. This fascia also functions as a conduit for the neurovascular and lymphatic bundles as they radiate outward from the thoracic, abdominal, and pelvic mediastinum to reach the specific organs.

REFERENCES

Anderson, W., Makins, G.H., 1890. The planes of subperitoneal and subpleural connective tissue, with their connections. J. Anat. Physiol. 25, 78–86.

Derry, D.E., 1907a. On the real nature of the so-called "pelvic fascia." J. Anat. Physiol. 42, 97–106.

Derry, D.E., 1907b. Pelvic muscles and fasciae. J. Anat. Physiol. 42, 107–111.

Drake, R.L., Vogl, A.W., Mitchell, A.W.M., 2010. Gray's Anatomy for Students. Churchill Livingstone Elsevier, Philadelphia.

Ercoli, A., Delmas, V., Fanfani, F., et al., 2005. *Terminologia Anatomica* versus unofficial descriptions and nomenclature of the fasciae and ligaments of the female pelvis: a dissection-based comparative study. Am. J. Obstet. Gynecol. 193, 1565–1573.

Gallaudet, B.B., 1931. A Description of The Planes of Fascia of The Human Body with Special Reference to The Fascias of The Abdomen, Pelvis and Perineum. Columbia University Press, New York, p. 76.

Garcia-Armengol, J., Garcia-Botello, S., Martinez-Soriano, F., Roig, J.V., Lledo, S., 2008. Review of the anatomic concepts in relation to the retrorectal space and endopelvic fascia: Waldeyer's fascia and the rectosacral fascia. Colorectal Dis. 10, 298–302.

Havenga, K., Grossmann, I., DeRuiter, M., Wiggers, T., 2007. Definition of total mesorectal excision, including the perineal phase: technical considerations. Dig. Dis. 25, 44–50.

Hazarika, N.H., Coote, J., Downman, C.B., 1964. Gastrointestinal dorsal root viscerotomes in the cat. J. Neurophysiol. 27, 107–116.

Hollinshead, W.H., 1956. Anatomy for Surgeons: The Thorax, Abdomen and Pelvis. Hoeber-Harper, New York.

Kingsnorth, A.N., Skandalakis, P.N., Colborn, G.L., et al. 2000. Embryology, anatomy, and surgical applications of the preperitoneal space. Surg. Clin. North. Am. 80, 1–24.

Last, R.J., 1978. Anatomy: Regional and Applied. Churchill Livingstone, Edinburgh.

O'Rahilly, R., 1986. Gardner, Gray & O'Rahilly Anatomy: A Regional Study of Human Structure. W.B. Saunders Comp, Philadelphia.

O'Rahilly, R., Müller, F., 1996. Human Embryology and Teratology. Wiley-Liss, New York.

Roberts, W.H., Taylor, W.H., 1970. The presacral component of the visceral pelvic fascia and its relation to the pelvic splanchnic innervation of the bladder. Anat. Rec. 166, 207–212.

Singer, E., 1935. Fascia of the Human Body and their Relations to the Organs they Envelop. Williams and Wilkins, Philadephia.

Skandalakis, P.N., Zoras, O., Skandalakis, J.E., Mirilas, P., 2006. Transversalis, endoabdominal, endothoracic fascia: who's who? Am. Surg. 72, 16–18.

Standring, S., 2015. Gray's Anatomy, The Anatomical Basis of Clinical Practice. Elsevier Churchill Livingstone, Edinburgh.

Stelzner, S., Holm, T., Moran, B.J., et al., 2011. Deep pelvic anatomy revisited for a description of crucial steps in extralevator abdominoperineal excision for rectal cancer. Dis. Colon Rectum. 54, 947–957.

Stoney, R.A., 1904. The anatomy of the visceral pelvic fascia. J. Anat. Physiol. 38, 438–447.

Thompson, P., 1901. The arrangement of the fascia of the pelvis and their relationship to the levator ani. J. Anat. Physiol. 35, 127–141.

Wyburn, G.M., 1937. The development of the infra-umbilical portion of the abdominal wall, with remarks on the aetiology of ectopia vesicae. J. Anat. 71, 201–231.

Membranous Structures Within the Cranial Bowl and Intraspinal Space

Torsten Liem

CHAPTER CONTENTS

 KEY POINT

The intra- and extracranial dural system, in particular the fascial relationships of the spinal dura mater and the innervation and vascular supply, shows many clinically significant insights, including insights for the application of osteopathic manual treatment (OMT).

Current findings in the dural anatomy give many significant insights for the clinician as well as for the application of osteopathic manual treatment (OMT). For example, the specific innervation of the dural system and the pathophysiological significance of the myodural bridges (MDB) in cervicogenic or chronic tension-type headache or in dural pain syndrome are hypothesized. Based on these findings, specific techniques are developed (Liem et al. 2017).

EMBRYONIC GROWTH DYNAMICS OF THE DURAL MEMBRANE ACCORDING TO BLECHSCHMIDT

Understanding the dynamics of embryological development enables us to understand many structural, physiological, functional, and dysfunctional interrelationships that are important for diagnosis and therapy. In this chapter you will get an idea of the peculiar dynamic of meningeus growth and the developmental dynamics of the dura in interaction with the development of other tissue structures. With this information you can understand structural dysfunctions found during investigations. Furthermore, you can perceive, feel, understand, and treat those dysfunctions in relation to the time factor, the dynamics of pre- and postmatural dependencies, and form-building processes.

Blechschmidt (1973, 1978) explained that connective tissue forms according to the environmental forces at hand (Figs. 1.9.1–1.9.3). The well-vascularized nervous system creates different biodynamic fields that lead to tensile stress in the back of the developing embryonic spine and to compression in the front of it. In the course of that development, the base of the skull beneath the brain is flattened and compressed and is formed as cartilaginous prestructures (Fig. 1.9.4). The cranial roof is formed out of skin under tensile growth-stress, and the bony structures are created by dermal ossification of flattened and tensed membranous connective tissue. Because of that development, the outer dura mater is strongly anchored to the inside of the cranial bones. With increasing excentric growth of the cerebrum, the tensile resistance of the antibasal and

95

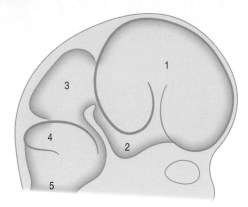

Fig. 1.9.1 Influence of the Brain on the Development of the Cranium According to Blechschmidt. Schema of brain portions of an embryo of 28 mm. 1, Cerebrum; 2, diencephalon; 3, midbrain; 4, cerebellum; 5, medulla oblongata. Modified with permission from Blechschmidt, E., 1978. Anatomie und Ontogenese des Menschen. Quelle & Meyer, Heidelberg, Wiesbaden, Germany.

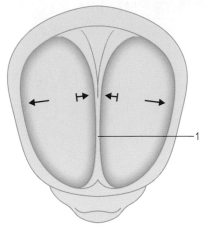

Fig. 1.9.3 View of Right and Left Dural Membranes in the Frontal Area. Left and right dural membranes are shown. Arrows: developmental push of both cerebral hemispheres. 1, Falx cerebri as very tough fascial membrane. Embryo size approx. 29 mm. Modified with permission from Blechschmidt, E., 1978. Anatomie und Ontogenese des Menschen. Quelle & Meyer, Heidelberg, Wiesbaden, Germany.

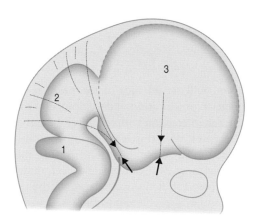

Fig. 1.9.2 Influence of the Brain on the Formation of the Cranium According to Blechschmidt. Expansion of the developing brain induces formation of a thick fascial membrane (dura) between the cerebellum and cerebrum, as well as of a smaller membrane between the frontal and temporal lobes of the cerebrum. Convergent arrows: developmental push of the brain is met by tensional resistance of dural membranes. 1, Cerebellum; 2, midbrain; 3, right cerebral hemisphere. Embryo size approx. 29 mm. Modified with permission from Blechschmidt, E., 1978. Anatomie und Ontogenese des Menschen. Quelle & Meyer, Heidelberg, Wiesbaden, Germany.

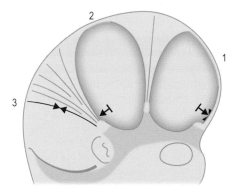

Fig. 1.9.4 Lateral View of Dural Membranes. The densation field at the basis of the dural membranes leads to later development of the cartilaginous cranial base (pointed area). Convergent arrows: dural membrane capable of resisting tension. Smaller arrows: developmental expansion of brain. Embryo size approx. 29 mm. Modified with permission from Blechschmidt, E., 1978. Anatomie und Ontogenese des Menschen. Quelle & Meyer, Heidelberg, Wiesbaden, Germany

laterodorsal cranial walls increases gradually, so that the brain regions bend away from each other. The brain fissures develop and falx and tentorium become denser. Falx cerebri and tentorium cerebellum develop by compression of mesenchymal tissue between the brain hemispheres, respectively between the cerebrum and cerebellum during embryonic brain growth.

The embryonic heart follows the diaphragm in a descending movement while the brain ascends in its growing process. The meningeal membranes envelop and support the brain and the spinal cord. They consist of three layers: the inner layer is the pia mater, then follows the arachnoidea, and the outer layer is formed of the dura mater on the inside of the skull and spine.

INTRACRANIAL MEMBRANE SYSTEM

Pia Mater (Soft Inner Layer of the Dural Membrane System)

The pia mater, which contains vessels, is the innermost layer of the three meningeal membranes. It consists of a thin layer of connective tissue with many elastic fibers and is very close to the gyri of the brain substance itself but is not fused with it. Vessels enter the brain from it. Furthermore, it creates the choroid plexus, a network of bold vessels that enter the brain ventricles and produce the cerebrospinal fluid (CSF).

Arachnoidea (Middle Layer of the Meningeal Membranes)

The arachnoidea has a gauze-like spongy structure and can be differentiated into two layers. The outward layer beyond the dura mater is separated from it by a thin cleft, the **subdural space**, which contains some veins and nerves. The inner layer consists of a trabecular framework.

Between the arachnoidea and pia mater there is the **subarachnoidal space.** Both membranes are connected by the trabecular framework in the subarachnoidal space. It is filled with CSF and forms the outer CSF spaces. It is narrow at the apex of the skull, but because the arachnoidea follows the pia mater, larger caverns are created in areas where the brain and bony cranial wall are farther apart, at the base of the cranium. These widened, CSF-filled spaces are called **cisterns** (cerebromedullar cistern, interpeduncular cistern, chiasmatic cistern, cisterna ambiens). Outgrowths of the arachnoidea, the arachnoidal villi, project into these spaces in the venous drainage of the inner skull, particularly that of the sagittal sinus. Through these villi the CSF can flow out into the venous system. The arachnoidea continues as the perineurium (nerve sheet) of the nerves passing through.

According to Ramo et al. (2018), without pia-arachnoid-complex, the spinal cord has very little inherent **stiffness** and shows significant relaxation when strained.

Dura Mater (Hard Outer Layer of the Meningeal Membranes)

The dura mater consists of dense, uneven, strong connective tissue with a lot of collagenous fibers. It is very tight and not permeable to the CSF. A special layer of flat fibroblastic cells without extracellular collagen and extracellular space can be found at the transition between the dura and arachnoidea (Haines et al. 1993). This dural borderline can be divided into **periostal dura** and **meningeal dura**. There is no epidural space like that in the spine. The dura mater continues as the **epineurium** of efferent nerves that leave the skull. The skin of the scalp and the dura are connected by emissary veins, which may be under enormous tension. In the region of the ethmoid bone cells, the tegmentum and sinus sigmoideus, the dura is very flat.

The inner layer (dura meningealis) is weaker in its structure than the outer dura layer or the arachnoidea (Haines et al. 1993). The dura of an adult can resist stronger forces than that of a newborn (Dragoi 1995). According to Arbuckle (1994), this fibrous structure enables the intracranial dura and the intraspinal dura to transmit different forces. These "pathways for transmission of forces" find their way by the fibrous structures of the dura, the so-called stress-fibers. Arbuckle defines the following groups: horizontal, vertical, transversal, and circular. The direction of fibers in the dura mater cranialis can possibly be traced back to the results of mechanical forces during embryonic development, when collagenous fibers are brought into line by stress forces (Hamann et al. 1998). Between the dura periostale and dura meningeale there are some other important structures apart from the venous blood sinuses.

- **Endolymphatic bag:** a sort of baglike tube, part of the ductus endolymphaticus, which is located at the rear wall of the petrous bone between the two dura layers.
- **Meningeal arteries:** terminal branches of the carotid arteries.
- **Sympathetic nerve fibers:** travel between the dural layers of intracranial vascular walls (coming from the superior cervical ganglion and the plexus caroticus), as do the sensitive fibers of the 5th and 10th cranial nerves and of the 1st and 2nd cervical nerves.
- **Trigeminal cave (Meckel's cavity):** a peculiar cavern of the dura for the ganglion of the 5th cranial nerve (also called trigeminal nerve ganglion, semilunar ganglion, or Gasserian ganglion), located at the front side of the apex of the petrous part of the temporal bone above the foramen lacerum.

Horizontal and Vertical Dural System

The membranes inside the cranium are connected anatomically as well as functionally and so affect each other.

Due to their different positions and orientations they can be divided into four septa: the falx cerebri, tentorium cerebella, falx cerebelli, and diaphragma sellae. Collagenous fiber bundles of the falx cerebri and falx cerebella form arcs in the anterior, intermediate, and posterior regions that cross each other perpendicularly. In the course of growth, fiber organization modulates from a 45-degree angle to a 90-degree angle (Dragoi 1995).

According to Delaire (1978), the horizontal system (tentorium cerebella and diaphragma sellae) acts as a clamp or tightener for the cranial base, whereas the vertical system (falx cerebri and falx cerebelli) tightens the cranial vault. Delaire argues that the tension in the horizontal and vertical dural system is maintained and regulated by the continuous tone of the neck muscles and the sternocleidomastoid muscle, but this is controversial. According to Ferré et al. (1990), movement of the neck muscles can be transmitted via the aponeurotic part of the scalp. However, only very weak and secondary movement can be sensed there, even though the aponeurotic structure of the scalp is clearly movable, unlike the highly immobile falx cerebri and falx cerebelli. According to Sutherland (1939), tension in every part of the membranous system can have an influence at all other parts of that system due to the structural bond. The dural membranes safeguard the integrity of the cranium, especially in early childhood, by way of their attachment to the cranial bones, in case of exposure to force. Additionally, it is thought that involuntary "jointed" movements of similar cranial bones are regulated via synchronicity with the rhythm of the primary respiratory mechanism. Every difference in tension at one side of the membrane alters the complete unit and leads to a new balance.

The falx cerebri divides each cranial hemisphere from the other. Its anterior downward border attaches at the gallic crest of the ethmoid bone, continues across the foramen caecum, the frontal crest, and the borders of the sulcus for the superior sagittal sinus of the frontal bone, then follows the parietal crest of the parietal bones and the sulcus sagittalis of the occipital bone until it gets to the internal occipital protuberance. There the falx is involved in the formation of the straight sinus, and at this structure both layers of the falx cerebri detach from each other and continue into the tentorium cerebelli. At the parietal bones it forms the sagittal sinus, and its free margin contains the inferior sagittal sinus.

The tentorium cerebelli ("Taa Tente"; Winslow, 1732) divides the cerebrum and cerebellum and stretches over the cerebellum like a tent. Above the tentorium there are, apart from the cerebral hemispheres, the subcortical nuclei and the thalamus. Like the falx cerebri and falx cerebella, the tentorium starts at the straight sinus and is attached there, too. The tentorium is attached posteriorly at the inner occipital protuberance and at both sides at the transversal groins of the internal occipital bone, where it forms the transverse sinus. Sideways, it leads along the sinus across the parietomastoideal suture and attaches for a short distance with its superior layer to the inferior back edge of the parietal bone. Meanwhile, the inferior layer can be found as an attachment to the mastoid process of the temporal bone. This is an important place, because its attachments continue from there along the mastoid process and the superior edge of the petrous part of the temporal bone, where it encloses the superior petrosal sinus. The inferior lateral layers are attached to the clinoid processes of the sphenoid bone. The free internal borders of the tentorium continue in an anterior direction, cross over the anterior inferior layers, and are attached to the anterior clinoid processes of the minor wings of the sphenoid bone. Here, where the internal branches of the tentorium cross the outer branches, the abducent nerve can be found. Obviously the abducent nerve can be disturbed by tentorium tension. A large oval opening, the tentorial incisura, is occupied anteriorly by the midbrain and the interpeduncular cistern and posteriorly by the rounded end (or splenium) of the corpus callosum.

EXTRACRANIAL MEMBRANE SYSTEM

Pia Mater Spinalis

This membrane contains vessels and nerves. From the pia mater, on both sides of the spinal cord, a connective tissue plate, the **denticulate ligament**, leads to the spinal dura mater. It fixes the spinal cord and divides the two spinal nerve roots. The pia mater follows the inner side of the spine and ends as a long, slender filament, the filum terminale, at the dorsal surface of the coccygeus bone.

Arachnoidea Spinalis

The arachnoidea has "extremely poor vascular and nerve supply" (Doppmann et al. 1969). It accompanies the dura mater to the nerve roots and allows it to be bathed in cerebrospinal fluid. The membranes follow the nerves to the intervertebral foramina, where they envelop the spinal ganglia. The arachnoidea then continues as the **perineurium** of the spinal nerve.

Spinal Dura Mater

The spinal dura mater (SDM) forms a tight tube of collagenous fiber, leading from the foramen magnum of the occipital bone, where it is fixed, to the canalis sacralis, transferring at S3 level into the filum terminale, which attaches in a fanlike manner at the periosteum of the coccygeus bone. Its course follows the curvatures of the vertebral channel. At the border between the foramen magnum and the vertebral channel there are two layers of dura mater: the outer, periosteal layer, and the interior layer, which is the true dura mater. Between the two layers there is epidural space, which enables a sliding motion between the dura and the vertebral channel. The epidural space is a fictitious cavity (Newell 1999), a "true potential space" (Breig 1960). In the upper cervical spine the epidural fat tissue is less developed (Breig 1960). There is no complete consensus concerning the structure of human dura mater, especially regarding the direction of the collagenous fibers, which are responsible for biomechanical functions. The SDM is longitudinally oriented (Patin et al. 1993), and the gills, consisting of elastin and collagen, are directed longitudinally (Patin et al. 1993; Runza et al. 1999). Longitudinal tensile strength and stiffness is much more than the transversal stress. Longitudinal stress, occurring from longitudinal spinal movements, is for the most part carried by the longitudinal collagenous fibers, and this leads farther to upwardly or downwardly situated neighboring structures.

In the upper cervical area, connective tissue follows a transverse course (von Lanz 1929). According to a study of the SDM in dogs, collagenous fibers are organized into longitudinal bundles, which are straight when stretched and curly when in a relaxed state (Tunituri 1977). Elastic fibers are oriented multidirectionally and are like a network. In the rear part of the SDM, elastin makes up 13.8% of the total, and 7.1% in the frontal part. In the thoracic region the proportion of elastin is higher than in all other regions (Nakagawa et al. 1994).

The SDM is largest at the level of the craniocervical junction and at the level of the lumbar spine (Lazorthes et al. 1953). It is only loosely attached to the spinal channel, except for its cranial and caudal fixations, enabling movement of the dura against the canal (Hogan and Toth 1999). It is supposed that the dura is able to transmit the fine movements of the CSF from the cranial bowl to the sacral bone. As a continuation of the falx cerebelli and the intracranial dura, the SDM inserts firmly into the occipital foramen. According to von Lanz (1929), the dura is fixed at the following structures in particular:

- At the basilar part of the occipital bone (leading through the membrana tectoria)
- At the ligamentum transversum atlantis
- At the ligamentum longitudinale posterius
- At the periosteum of the squama occipitalis at the arc of the atlas (C1) and axis (C2) joints
- At the atlanto-occipital and atlantoaxial joints

Furthermore, the dura is attached firmly at the third cervical vertebra (Upledger and Vredevoogd 1994), but according to our own investigations, this is not always so (Liem 2000).

Ligamenta Craniale Durae Matrae Spinalis

The attachment of the SDM to the occipital bone, supported by fibers between the arc of the atlas (C1), the arc of the axis, and the posterior rim of the atlanto-occipital joint and the foramen magnum, are called "ligamenta craniale durae matrae spinalis," according to von Lanz (1928). Rutten et al. (1997) found attachments to the ligamentum flava of C1 to C3 and the deep layer of the nuchal ligament.

Myodural Bridge

Myodural Bridge in Atlanto-Occipital Interspace

The myodural bridge (MDB), originating from the ventral part of rectus capitis posterior minor (RCPmin), travels in three directions:

1. Indirect: fibers run anteriorly and inferiorly into posterior atlantooccipital membrane (PAOM) and terminate in PAOM, which is connected to the SDM. Some fibers pass through PAOM
2. Direct: directly connects with SDM
3. Indirect: part of the fibers travel through PAOM and cross the ventral part of atlas to participate in the formation of the ventral dural ligament (VDL); indirectly connects with SDM by VDL

MDB in the Atlanto-Axial Interspace

1. Dense fibrous bundles originate from RCPmin, rectus capitis posterior major (RCPmaj), and M. obliquus inferior (OCI)
2. Converges to form atlantoaxial part of the VDL
3. Connects with SDM.

Fibrous tissues of MDB from RCPmin, RCPmaj, and OCI are composed mainly of type I collagen fibers (stained red) with strong refraction.

Function

- By means of the parallel running type I collagen fibers in the MDB, suboccipital muscle could pull the SDM strongly through effective force propagated by MDB during head movement (Zheng et al. 2018).
- Hypothesis: Right angle of myodural fibers are running to the DMS and preventing folding of the DMS in extension toward the spinal cord or proprioceptive function (McPartland and Brodeur 1999).
- Sensorimotor function
- Postural control (McPartland and Brodeur 1999)
- Maintenance of integrity of subarachnoid space and cerebellomedullary cistern (Scali et al. 2015)
- MDB, suboccipital muscle contraction may be a dynamic source of CSF circulation (Sui et al. 2013)
- Pathophysiological implications: Pathological change of MDB might cause cervicogenic or chronic tension-type headaches (Fernández-de-las-Penas et al. 2008).
- Tensed suboccipital muscles cause a transmission of tension to the DMS, which can lead to a dural pain syndrome (Palomeque-del-Cerro 2017).

Interspinal Ligaments of the SDM

The attachments from the SDM to the interior walls of the spinal canal can be divided into anteroposterior-oriented ligaments and lateral-oriented connections. As always in medicine, the borders are floating.

In the same way, attachments to the **flaval ligament** and the **posterior longitudinal ligament** transmit forces in a sagittal plane. Sometimes they are more of a protection for the soft tissues between spinal cord and spine than a real ligament. That is also true for the **trousseau fibreux de Soulié**. On the one hand they connect the dura mater with the posterior longitudinal ligament; on the other hand they connect the SDM with the periosteum. That leads on both sides to coverage of the anterior epidural venous plexus (Trolard 1888, as cited in Liem 2018).

A lateral attachment is the **ligamentum sacrodurale anterius** or **Trolard's ligament**, which is situated between the dura and vertebral bodies and arcs in the lower lumbar and sacral spine. Similarly, **Hofmann's ligaments** are situated between the SDM and the superficial layer of the posterior longitudinal ligament (Doppmann et al. 1969; Fick 1904; Schellinger et al.

1990). The **ligamentum dorsolateralia duralis** or **Hofmann's lateral ligaments** are described by Spencer et al. (1983) and form a connection between the dural coverage of the spinal nerve and the vertebral periosteum. Spencer et al. called them "lateral Hofmann's ligaments." These are supposed to prevent a posterior evasion of the spinal nerve in case of a pain-causing disc protrusion.

These attachments are also known as **meningovertebral ligaments.** At the level of every intervertebral foramen are the **opercula of Forestier**. They are a junction between the dural coverage of the outgoing spinal nerve and the periosteum of the particular vertebra (Forestier 1922, as cited in Liem 2018; Grimes et al. 2000; Lazorthes, as cited in Giradin 1996). The opercula envelop the intervertebral foramen from inside and outside, which means they are situated at the inside and outside of the vertebral canal. The **transformidal ligaments** embrace the intervertebral foramen along the outside. Giradin (1996) described them as either the greater parts of the opercula of Forestier or as the incomplete opercula or **false ligaments.** The **ligamentum denticulatum** leads from the pia mater to the dura mater and connects the spinal cord from both sides of the occipital bone to the level of L2 with the dura. This is like a supporting structure, which allows the spinal cord to be suspended in the cerebrospinal fluid. The attachment spikes of the ligament cross the subarachnoidal space laterally, penetrate the arachnoidea, and are finally fixed at the dura mater in between the dural covers of the spinal nerves (Key 1870, as cited in Rossitti 1993). The **rhomboid halter** (Key and Retzius, as cited in Lang 1981) is a diamond-shaped plate of connective tissue that embraces lower parts of the afterbrain and the upper spinal cord at its anterior side. It blends with the dura mater together with the topmost spikes of the denticulate ligament. The ventral roots of the second cervical nerve should be situated posterior of the "rhomboid halter" and the ventral roots of the first cervical nerve posterior or anterior to it. The downward-directed rhombic tip is mostly situated in the region of the fissura mediana anterior at the C4 level (Lang 1981).

All these interspinal ligaments and membranous structures are supposed to support the movement of the dural tube inside the spine and to prevent folding or other injury-causing mechanisms to the dura or the spinal cord.

VASCULARIZATION OF THE MENINGEAL MEMBRANES

Intracranial Vascularization

The dural system is vascularized arterially by, above all, the meningeal arteries—terminal branches of the inner and outer carotid arteries. They are situated between dura and bone.

Vasomotor and immunomodulatory effects are seen in cranial dura in rats (calcitonin gene-related peptide [CGRP], calcitonin receptor-like receptor [CLR], smooth muscle actin [SMA]) (Lennerz et al. 2008).

Intraspinal Vascularization

The posterior spinal arteries are found in pairs (branches of the posterior inferior cerebellum artery)—the anterior spinal artery (branch of the vertebral artery) and meningeal branches of the intercostal arteries. Anterior and posterior internal vertebral venous plexuses form in the epidural space. The internal vertebral venous plexuses are embedded in fat that is semiliquid at body temperature.

The valveless plexus veins are of special importance for physiological function and for dysfunction. Via the intervertebral canals, they communicate with the lumbar veins, the intercostal veins, the azygos and hemiazygos veins, and with venous plexuses in the nuchal region (marginal and occipital sinuses of the dura mater). These anastomoses enable multidirectional drainage of venous blood without congestion.

Meningeal, vascular irritation can lead to permanent activation of the neck and chewing muscles and has possible clinical relevance to patients with tension headaches (Hu et al. 1995). Mechanical irritation can lead to facilitation with a local hypersympathicotonus and a chemical irritation with vessel spasm.

MENINGEAL NERVE SUPPLY

Intracranial Innervations

The upper part of the dural system is innervated mainly by thin-caliber afferent axons derived from branches of the trigeminus nerve, the lower part by cervical nerves 1 to 3, and branches of the vagus nerve. Many of these afferent axons show vasomotor and immunomodulatory effects related to the CGRP receptor complex to meningeal arteries and mast cells (Lennerz et al. 2008).

All meningeal nerves contain postganglionic sympathetic fibers, which have their origin directly or indirectly in the superior cervical ganglion via the internal carotid plexus or the maxillary plexus, accompanied by branches of the medial meningeal artery.

The parasympathetic supply is achieved by the greater petrosal nerve (from the parasympathetic part of the seventh cranial nerve) and branches of the vagus nerve and glossopharyngeal nerve.

Clinically relevant in relation to dural pain syndrome and headache is also that parts of these trigeminal axons afterward penetrating the sutures between calvarial bones and project also muscles (Schueler et al. 2013).

Intraspinal Innervation

Unlike the DMC, the SDM is scarcely innervated. Meningeal branches of the spinal nerves and the nerve plexus of the posterior longitudinal ligament, as well as perivascular plexuses of the root arteries, form the intraspinal innervation. Infrequent paravascular nerves run epidurally.

As a result of the multisegmental innervation of the dura, patients can show dural pain not punctually but as regional deep pain. The nerves in the cranial area converge to the nucleus trigeminus spinalis with clinical implications. Chemical, mechanical, and thermal stimuli could cause a neurogenic inflammation reaction and dilation (without axon damage).

Transcranial collaterals of trigeminal dural afferents run to extracranial structures and could have relevance for the pathophysiology of tension headache (Messlinger 2016).

Function of the meninges:
- Protective envelope for the brain and spinal cord
- Neurocranium tensioner
- Protection against mechanical trauma
- Vibration-free absorption of mechanical loads on the skull by tension straps (together with other structures) (Drenkhahn and Zenker 1994)
- Bone growth at the suture margins is induced and controlled by an interaction of dura mater, mesenchymal cells, and cranial bones.
- DeLeon and Richtsmeier (2009) suggest that the development of cranial asymmetry is related to tension in the dura mater. However, this could not be confirmed in its entirety.
- The dura mater appears to be an important factor in preventing the sutures from ossifying (Opperman et al. 1993).
- Immune function
- Reabsorption of cerebrospinal fluid (Zenker and Kubik 1996)
- Thermoregulation of the brain (Zenker and Kubik 1996)

RECIPROCAL TENSILE MEMBRANE AND SUTHERLAND'S FULCRUM

The dura mater forms the ligamentous apparatus of the bony skull, meaning that both of the dural layers can be seen as a mechanical unit. According to Delaire (1978), the horizontal system (tentorium cerebelli, diaphragma sellae) acts as tensioner for the cranial base, whereas the vertical system (falx cerebri, falx cerebelli) acts as tensioner for the cranial roof. Tension of the vertical and horizontal systems is maintained and regulated mainly by the tone of the neck muscles and the sternocleidomastoid muscle.

From the osteopathic perspective, Sutherland (1939) calls the dural membrane system a "reciprocal tension membrane system" to show the functional unity of that membrane. The reciprocal tension membrane of the brain and spinal cord is meant to be the structural connection of the single cranial bones, with the task of guiding and limiting the range of motion of these bones. By using the structural connection of all membranes, tension in any part of the system is able to influence all other parts.

The center of this intracranial membrane system is a virtual point that is situated—according to Magoun (1976)—at the uniting point of the tentorium cerebelli, falx cerebri, and falx cerebelli in the course of the straight sinus. This point is also known as **Sutherland's fulcrum** (Magoun 1976) or the **automatic shifting suspended fulcrum**. The dynamic forces affecting the membranes are brought into balance here.

Possible Effects of Abnormal Dural Tension

- Venous drainage dysfunction of the skull via the venous sinuses
- Decreased drainage of the brain
- Vascular supply disorders of brain tissue
- Disorders in fluctuation of CSF
- Headache, intracranial, and retro-orbital pain via the sensible nerve supply of the dural membranes (CN V and X and first, second, and third cervical nerves)
- Face pain and abnormal tone of the chewing muscles via CN V and the trigeminal ganglion, which is covered with dura and is vulnerable to dural stress
- Dysfunction of any cranial nerve and nerve ganglia, for example, at the cranial openings and the intracranial dural membranes, as well as at the dural coverage of cranial nerves
- Limitation in movement and mobility of the cranial bones, the sacral bone, and the coccygeal bone
- Dysfunction of spinal nerves (at the emission points in the dura mater)
- Transmission of dural tension via fascial attachments and the epineurium of the spinal nerve
- Abnormal tension in one of the dural double layers will always affect other dural parts
- Disturbance of the pituitary gland (diaphragma sellae).

FUTURE TASKS AND OPEN QUESTIONS

There are still some remaining open questions concerning the real lines of forces within the fascial system of the cranial bowl and spine. Is there really transmission of movement? For what purpose? Where is the motor of these forces? Which effects do we obtain by using different procedures in the conservation and fixation of specimens concerning tissue characteristics (mainly concerning the transmission of tension/motion)? The surveys performed to date have mostly been with laboratory specimens.

Is it possible to transmit connective tissue tension from outside the dural system to the dura and vice versa? If yes, then by what means and for which functional and clinical meanings?

Future studies need to address these and many more inquiries, including the links between medical and engineering sciences like bionic science or the results of biomimetic robotic research and viscoelastic forces (Doschak and Zernicke 2005; Fernandez and Pandy 2006).

Based on the previously mentioned findings, specific OMT maneuvers have been developed (Liem et al. 2017).

Summary

A detailed knowledge of the functional relationships between the intra- and extracranial dural systems provides useful clinical insights for the field of osteopathic manual treatment (OMT), including the specific innervation and vascular supply of the spinal dura mater as well the anatomical structure of the myodural bridge (MBD). Dysfunctions in both areas could contribute to painful pathologies in the head/neck region and beyond.

REFERENCES

Arbuckle, B.E., 1994. The Selected Writings of Beryl E. Arbuckle. American Academy of Osteopathy, Indianapolis.

Blechschmidt, E., 1973. Die pränatalen Organsysteme des Menschen. Hippokrates, Stuttgart.

Blechschmidt, E., 1978. Anatomie und Ontogenese des Menschen. Quelle & Meyer, Heidelberg, Wiesbaden.

Breig, A., 1960. Biomechanics of the Central Nervous System: Some Basic Normal and Pathologic Phenomena. Almqvist and Wiksell, Stockholm.

Delaire, J., 1978. L'analyse architecturale et structurale cranio-faciale (de profil). Rev. Stomatol. 79, 6.

DeLeon, V.B., Richtsmeier, J.T., 2009. Fluctuating asymmetry and developmental instability in sagittal craniosynostosis. Cleft Palate Craniofac J. 46, 187–196.

Doppmann, J.L., Di Chiro, G., Ommaya, A.K., 1969. Selective Arteriography of the Spinal Cord. Warren H. Green, St. Louis.

Doschak, M.R., Zernicke, M.F., 2005. Structure, function and adaptation of bone-tendon and bone- ligament complexes. J. Musculoskelet. Neuronal Interact. 5, 35–40.

Dragoi, G., 1995. The mechanical properties of newborn dura mater. J. Leg. Med. 3, 368–374.

Drenkhahn, D., Zenker, W. (eds.), 1994. Anatomie, Bd. 1. 15. Urban & Schwarzenberg, Aufl. München, p. 489.

Fernandez, J.W., Pandy, M.G., 2006. Integrating modelling and experiments to assess dynamic musculoskeletal function in humans. Exp. Physiol. 91, 371–382.

Fernández-de-las-Penas, C., Cuadrado, M.L., Arendt-Nielsen, L., Ge, H.Y., Pareja, J.A., 2008. Association of cross-sectional area of the rectus capitis posterior minor muscle with active trigger points in chronic tension-type headache: a pilot study. Am. J. Phys. Med. Rehabil. 87, 197–203.

Ferré, J.C., Chevalier, C., Lumineau, J.P., Barbin, J.Y., 1990. L'ostéopathie cranienne, leurre ou réalité. Odontologie et Stomatologie 5. In: Corriat, R. (ed.), 1992–1993. Sutherland ou l'approche cranienne en medicine ostéopathique. Kursskript des COC an der V.U.B., 31–38.

Fick, R., 1904. Anatomie und Mechanik der Gelenke. Fischer, Jena, Germany.

Giradin, M. (Ed.), 1996. Die caudale durale Insertion und das Ligamentum sacrodurale anterius (Trolard). Naturheilpraxis 4, 528–536.

Grimes, P.F., Massie, J.B., Garfin, S.R., 2000. Anatomic and biomechanical analysis of the lower lumbar foraminal ligaments. Spine 25, 2009–2014.

Haines, D.E., Harkey, H.L., al-Mefty, O., 1993. The "subdural" space: a new look at an outdated concept. Neurosurgery 32, 111–120.

Hamann, M.C., Sacks, M.S., Malinin, T.I., 1998. Quantification of the collagen fibre architecture of human cranial dura mater. J. Anat. 192, 99–106.

Hogan, Q., Toth, J., 1999. Anatomy of soft tissues of the spinal canal. Reg. Anesth. Pain Med. 24, 303–310.

Hu, J. W., Vernon, H., Tatourian, I., 1995. Changes in neck electromyography associated with meningeal noxious stimulation. J. Manipul. Physiol. Ther. 18, 577–558.

Lang, J., 1981. Klinische Anatomie des Kopfes. Springer, Berlin, 436.

Lazorthes, G. In: Giradin, M. (Ed.), 1996. Die caudale durale Insertion und das ligamentum sac-rodurale anterius (Trolard). Naturheilpraxis 4, 528–536.

Lazorthes, G., Poulhes, J., Gaubert, J., 1953. Les variations regionales de l'epaisseur de la dure-mere. C. R. Assoc. Anat. 78, 169–172.

Lennerz, J.K., RuÄàhle, V., Ceppa, E.P., et al., 2008. Calcitonin receptor-like receptor (CLR), receptor activity modifying protein 1 (RAMP1), and calcitonin generated peptide (CGRP) immunoreactivity in the rat trigeminovascular system: differences between peripheral and central CGRP receptor distribution. J. Comp. Neurol. 7, 1277–1299.

Liem, T., 2000. Osteopathische und biomechanische Untersuchung zur Zugübertragung der Dura mater auf die bindegewebigen Strukturen der Periorbita. OSD, Hamburg.

Liem T., 2018. Kraniosakrale Osteopathie. Chapter 7: Hirn- und Rückenmarkshäute. Thieme, Stuttgart, Germany

Liem, T., Tozzi, P., Chila, A., 2017. Fascia in the Osteopathic Field. Handspring Publishing Limited, Pencaitland, Scotland.

Magoun, H.I., 1976. Osteopathy in the Cranial Field, third ed. Journal Printing Co., Kirksville, MO, p. 27.

McPartland, J.M., Brodeur, R.R., 1999. Rectus capitis posterior minor: A small but important suboccipital muscle. J. Bodyw. Mov. Ther. 3, 30–35.

Messlinger, K., 2016. Extrakraniale projektionen meningealer afferenzen und ihre bedeutung für meningeale nozizeption und kopfschmerz. Zeitschrift für Komplementärmedizin 8 14–19.

Nakagawa, H., Mikawa, Y., Watanabe, R., 1994. Elastin in the human posterior longitudinal ligament and spinal dura: A histologic and biochemical study. Spine 19, 2164–2169.

Newell, R.L., 1999. The spinal epidural space. Clin. Anat. 12, 375–379.

Opperman, L.A., Sweeney, T.M., Redmon, J., Persing, J.A., Ogle, R.C., 1993. Tissue interactions with underlying dura mater inhibit osseous obliteration of developing cranial sutures. Dev. Dyn. 198, 312–322.

Palomeque-del-Cerro, L., Arráez-Aybar, L.A., Rodríguez-Blanco, C, et al. 2017. A systematic review of the soft-tissue connections between neck muscles and dura mater: the myodural bridge. Spine 42, 49–54.

Patin, D.J., Eckstein, E.C., Hamm, K., Pallares, V.S., 1993. Anatomy and biomechanical properties of human lumbar dura mater. Anesth. Analg. 76, 535–540.

Ramo, N.L., Troyer, K.L., Puttlitz, C.M., 2018. Viscoelasticity of spinal cord and meningeal tissues. Acta Biomater. 75, 253–262.

Rossitti, S. (Ed.), 1993. Biomechanics of the pons-cord tract and its enveloping structures: an overview. Acta Neurochir. 124, 144–152.

Runza, M., Pietrabissa, R., Mantero, S., et al. 1999. Lumbar dura mater biomechanics: experimental characterization and scanning electron microscopy observations. Anesth. Analg. 88, 1317–1321.

Rutten HP, Szpak K, van Mameren H, Ten Holter J, de Jong JC, 1997. Anatomie relation between the rectus capitis posterior minor muscle and the dura mater. Spine. 22, 924–926.

Scali, F., Pontell, M. E., Nash, L. G., Enix, D.E., 2015. Investigation of meningomyovertebral structures within the upper cervical epidural space: a sheet plastination study with clinical implications. Spine J. 15, 2417–2424.

Schellinger, D., Manz, H., Vidic, B., et al., 1990. Disk fragment migration. Radiology 175, 831–836.

Schueler, M., Messlinger, K., Dux, M., Neuhuber, W.L., De Col, R., 2013. Extracranial projections of meningeal afferents and their impact on meningeal nociception and headache. Pain 154, 1622–1631.

Spencer, D., Irwin, G., Miller, J., 1983. Anatomy and significance of fixation of the lumbosacral nerve roots in sciatica. Spine 8, 672–679.

Sui, H.J., Yu S.B., Yuan, X.Y., et al., 2013. Anatomical study on the connections between the sub-occipital structures and the spinal dual mater. Chinese J. Clin. Anat. 31, 489–490.

Sutherland, W.G., 1939. The Cranial Bowl. Free Press, Mankato, MN.

Tunituri, A.R., 1977. Elasticity of the spinal cord dura in the dog. J. Neurosurg. 47, 391–396.

Upledger, J.E., Vredevoogd, J.D., 1994. Lehrbuch der Craniosacralen Therapie. 2. Aufl. Haug, Heidelberg, Germany.

von Lanz, T., 1928. Zur struktur der dura mater spinalis. Anat. Anz. 66, 78–87.

von Lanz, T., 1929. Über die rückenmarkshäute. II. Die beziehungskausale entwicklungsmechanik primitiver rückenmarkshäute, dargestellt an hypogeophis alternans und rostratus. Anat. Anz. 67, 130–139.

Winslow, J.B., 1732. Exposition Anatomique de la Structure du Corps Humain. Desprez et Desseartz, Paris.

Zenker, W., Kubik, S., 1996. Brain cooling in humans – anatomical considerations. Anat. Embryol. 193, 1–13

Zheng, N., Chi, Y.Y., Yang, X.H., et al., 2018. Orientation and property of fibers of the myodural bridge in humans. Spine J. 18, 1081–1087.

Diaphragmatic Structures

Anna Maria Vitali

CHAPTER CONTENTS

THE DIAPHRAGM AND ITS FASCIA: ANATOMICAL, EMBRYOLOGICAL, AND EVOLUTIONARY DEVELOPMENT

The diaphragm is a complex structure that is involved in multiple functions: ventilating, swallowing, vomiting, coughing, sneezing, vocalizing, controlling posture, and trunk stabilization. It is described as an "aponeurotic" dome, with an elliptical shape—a union of two domes with a central plateau.

The diaphragm has a membranous part, the phrenic center; a peripheral contractile muscular portion; a lumbar or posterior portion formed by pillars; and ligamentous arches. The trefoil-shaped phrenic center has three leaves: one anterior and two lateral, to the right and left, whose fibrous constitution on several layers helps to delimit the orifice of the vena cava.

The peripheral muscular part is subdivided into:
- sternal: two thin strips originating from the posterior aspect of the xiphoid process;
- costal: longitudinal fibers originating from the inner face and the superior margin of the last six ribs, interdigitating with the horizontal ones of the transverse muscle.

The lumbar part has an insertion on the spine forming the medial, intermediate, and lateral pillars. The right medial pillar reaches the second, third, and fourth lumbar vertebrae, whereas the left does not descend beyond the third lumbar vertebra. The intermediate pillars are small and originate from the body of the third lumbar vertebra and from the disk between the second and third lumbar vertebrae. The lateral pillars are robust fibrous structures that lead to the costiform processes of the second lumbar vertebra and are subdivided to form the medial arcuate, which surrounds the psoas muscle, and the lateral arcuate, which surrounds the quadratus lumborum muscle.

These diaphragmatic arches, often improperly defined as "ligaments," look like a thickening of the fascia of the quadratus lumborum and the psoas muscles, with which their collagen fibers mix; this fascial continuity allows for the sliding and coordination among the contractile activities of the diaphragm and both quadratus lumborum and the psoas muscles. The arches of the diaphragm, through their longitudinal insertion, connect to the fascia of the right and left transverse muscle and are arranged in a horizontal manner.

The esophageal hiatus is delimited by muscle bundles that continue in the right medial pillar, whereas the aortic hiatus is located near the body of the second lumbar vertebra and the medial pillars, slightly to the left of the midline.

The complexity of the diaphragm can be better understood if one considers the embryological and evolutionary development of the diaphragm. Starting from weeks 3 and 4, the embryo folds back on itself to form a primitive body cavity with two ends: a cephalic and a caudal one. With the descent of the cervical transverse septum in a caudal direction, a pleuropericardic cavity is formed from where the pleurae and the pericardium will originate.

The communication between the pleural and peritoneal cavities will be closed by the pleuroperitoneal membranes, by the mesenchyme associated with the anterior intestine that will give rise to the pillars, and by the migration of the muscle cells of the cervical somites.

The diaphragm is derived from the following structures:
- The septum transversum, which will form the central aponeurotic portion (phrenic center)
- The two pleuroperitoneal membranes
- The cervical somites C3–C4, which will form the muscular part
- The mesentery of the esophagus, in which the diaphragmatic pillars will develop.

From the third month onward, some dorsal bundles of the diaphragm will originate from the first lumbar vertebra. The phrenic nerve also originates from the cervical segments.

The integrity of the diaphragm and its development are essential to prevent the creation of hernias and to preserve the normal development of the lungs.

The main characteristic of the subdivision of the primitive cavity is therefore to divide but also to create a complex functional continuity of coordination, which is evident at the fascial level.

KEY POINTS

Given its embryological development, the diaphragm can be divided into:
- costal, muscular, and contractile, which are linked to respiratory function
- crural and visceral, which control the esophageal sphincter and the stability of the stomach within the abdominal cavity

To better understand the complex relationship between the sections of the trunk, neck, and diaphragm and their functions, it is useful to analyze the muscular and visceral fascia and also the diaphragm itself.

THE MUSCLE FASCIA OF THE TRUNK AND NECK AND ITS CONNECTIONS WITH THE DIAPHRAGM

The fascia of the neck and trunk have a trilaminar organization and a continuity between each of these laminae. As Carla Stecco (2015) has shown, the muscles of the trunk have the characteristics of epimysial fascia: adhering to the muscles, they contribute to forming sepiments that characterize their shape, structure, and function. Only two aponeurotic fasciae are present in the trunk: the rectus sheath anteriorly and the thoracolumbar fascia posteriorly.

The superficial plane unites muscles that functionally develop spiral/rotational movements, creating the possibility of coordinating the movements between the upper limbs, the head and neck, the contralateral pelvis, the pubic symphysis through the rectus sheath, and finally the sacrum and thoracolumbar fascia. These connections allow the hand to coordinate with the movements of the chest, pelvis, and head.

The intermediate fascial plane is formed by the clavipectoral fascia that, after having enveloped the subclavian on its lower surface, continues into the lamina medialis of the deep fascia of the neck that envelops the hyoid muscles (omohyoid, sternohyoid, and sternothyroid). This creates an ideal fascial continuity to manage mastication, swallowing, and the movements of the hand and head, such as those for picking up items or food and lifting them to the mouth.

In the thorax, below the plane formed by the intermediate lamina, we find a deep lamina that envelops the scalene muscles at the top, and then, proceeding downward, the intercostal muscles form what is called the intercostal fascia. This fascia continues into the fascia of the transverse muscle and that of the sheath of the rectus abdominis muscles, which are not in a superficial plane but a deep one.

KEY POINT

The deep lamina, receiving the scalene, the intercostal, the rectus abdominis, the pyramidalis, and the transverse muscles, achieves a fascial continuity that allows them to be coordinated, as we shall see, with the diaphragm and with the multiple functions it performs. There is also a trilaminar arrangement of the fascia in the abdomen. The broad abdomen muscles originate from a single layer of hypaxial muscle at the end of week 6.

In a first phase, three different concentric layers can be seen with a lateral disposition: an internal one corresponding to the transverse, an intermediate one corresponding to the internal oblique, and a superficial one corresponding to the external oblique extending from the fifth, sixth, and second ribs up to the level of the first lumbar vertebra. The rectus abdominis muscles can be seen at this stage as a single longitudinal muscle starting from the fifth rib that runs along the lateral edge of the three circular layers. In this phase the three lateral layers are in continuity with the intercostal muscles of the thorax, and their lower extremity is delimited by the umbilical cord in the ventral region where the precursor of the lower limb begins to appear.

In the next 3 weeks the three layers descend from their original lateral position, developing medially, while the rectus reaches the umbilical region at week 9. From week 9, the aponeurotic part relative to the lateral muscles can be seen to connect to a thick sheath that envelops the rectus abdominis muscles and is thicker on the ventral surface (Mekonen et al. 2015).

It can be seen from the embryological development of the lateral muscles of the abdomen the presence of a thin epimysial fascia with a proprioceptive function for each single layer, the presence of loose connective tissue that allows each single layer to slide to a certain degree, and the adhesions between the three different layers at the level of the lateral border of the sheath of the rectus abdominis muscle that allows the transfer of forces. In each lamina the collagen fibers have a specific orientation and each layer can slide over the other. The linea alba is formed by the decussation of the collagen fibers of the intermediate aponeuroses. The two rectus abdominis muscles are housed inside the sheath and connect the rib cage to the pelvis.

The fusion of the three distinct aponeuroses of the relative layers creates the typical structure of the aponeurotic fascia of the sheath of the rectus abdominis. The sheath of the rectus abdominis must therefore be adaptable to respond to the mechanical stresses of the trunk generated by large and complex movements that require the participation of the wide muscles of the abdomen.

The transversus abdominis muscle connects the thoracolumbar fascia to the sheath of the rectus abdominis, coordinating the elasticity and strength of the abdominal wall with the stability and motility of the spine. It is enveloped by its epimysium, which allows a relationship with, while remaining divided from, a membrane other than that of the epimysium of the transversus abdominis muscle that is called the transversal fascia and must be considered to be a visceral fascia, which is, in turn, separate from the peritoneum. This fascia contributes to the formation of the inguinal canal, relates to the bladder and to the spermatic cord, and accompanies the descent of the testicles and ovaries into the pelvis.

THE VISCERAL FASCIA OF THE TRUNK AND ITS CONNECTIONS WITH THE DIAPHRAGM

The internal fasciae can be divided into investing and insertional fasciae. The investing fasciae adhere strongly to the viscera, the glands, or the vessels; they have a greater presence of elastic fibers in order to adapt to changes in the organs' volume; they are also devoid of sensitive innervation and have autonomous innervation.

The insertional fasciae are fibrous germs rich in collagen that connect the organs with other organs and with the fascia of the trunk, creating compartments and cavities. The peritoneum and the pleura are typical insertional fasciae.

The insertional fasciae are connected in some specific points with muscle fasciae, partly to guarantee the autonomy of the internal organs during locomotion and partly to create a connection. The insertional fasciae have a dual role: to divide by creating spaces and to connect organs that have to perform their functions together (Stecco et al. 2017).

The diaphragm is covered by a thin diaphragmatic fascia of which the superior lamina merges with the pleura and the lower lamina with the peritoneum. The superior surface of the diaphragm is connected to the base of the pericardium, the bottom of the lungs, and the costodiaphramatic pleural sinuses.

KEY POINT

The parietal pleura is a visceral fascia that covers the thoracic cavity and adheres to the diaphragm below. Its inner surface adheres to the fascia of the intercostal muscles; from this unusual fusion between visceral and muscular fascia there comes endothoracic fascia, which carries out a series of complex functions connected with the contractile and visceral activity of the diaphragm—first, the expansion of the rib cage during inspiration, the control of phonation, and the ability to swallow. Proximally it contributes to forming the suprapleural membrane and securing it to the first rib and the seventh cervical vertebra, and at this level it contains some muscle fibers coming from the scalene muscles.

The endothoracic fascia distally continues in the diaphragmatic fascia, contributing to the formation of the phrenoesophageal ligament, which plays an important role in the control of the gastroesophageal sphincter during the course of each respiratory act.

The diaphragm and the base of the pericardium adhere to each other at the phrenic center's upper surface, forming the phrenicopericardial ligaments; through the pericardium an indirect connection is established with the sternum anteriorly at the level of the superior and inferior sternopericardial ligament, posteriorly with the vertebrae through the superior and inferior vertebropericardial ligament, and from above with the fascia of the thymus and with the intermediate layer of the cervical fascia. The posterior part of the pericardium contributes to the formation of the bronchopericardial membrane whose fundamental function is to make a separation between cardiac and respiratory rhythm possible (Fig. 1.10.1–Fig. 1.10.3).

The very thin fascia that covers the lower surface of the diaphragm is in direct continuity with the peritoneum, forming thickenings or ligaments that maintain a fascial connection between the diaphragm and the subdiaphragmatic organs.

In correspondence with the crural diaphragm, a thin areolar layer that is rich in elastic fibers rises along the opening between the diaphragm and the peritoneum, where it extends and continues into the transversal fascia. Part of its elastic fibers merge with the wall of the esophagus and penetrate into the submucosa. This fascial expansion forms the phrenoesophageal ligament that connects the esophagus and the diaphragm in a way that is as flexible as is necessary to allow a minimum amount of freedom of movement during acts of respiration and swallowing, and when boluses pass down the esophagus, forming a real antireflux barrier (Fig. 1.10.4).

The stomach is connected to the diaphragm via the phrenogastric ligament. The liver is connected to the lower surface of the diaphragm via the right and left triangular ligament and the coronary ligament in almost perfect correspondence with the overlying phrenopericardial ligament (Fig. 1.10.5).

Via the adrenal-diaphragmatic ligament the diaphragm connects with the adrenal gland; between the adrenal gland and the kidney there is loose connective tissue.

The kidneys, enveloped in the renal fascia, are fixed at the top of the diaphragm; the fascia retrorenalis

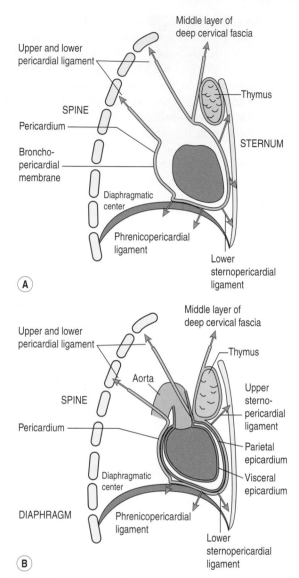

Fig. 1.10.1 Suspension ligaments of the pericardium and thymus and their connections to the diaphragm. Redrawn with permission from Stecco, L., 2012. Manipolazione Fasciale per le Disfunzioni Interne. Piccin Nuova Libraria, Padua.

merges with the fascia of the quadratus lumborum muscle and is fixed to the corpus vertebrae. The anterior fascia continues into the parietal peritoneum and joins the contralateral fascia. The fascia retrorenalis merges distally into the psoas fascia.

The phrenicocolic ligament connects the diaphragm to the spleen.

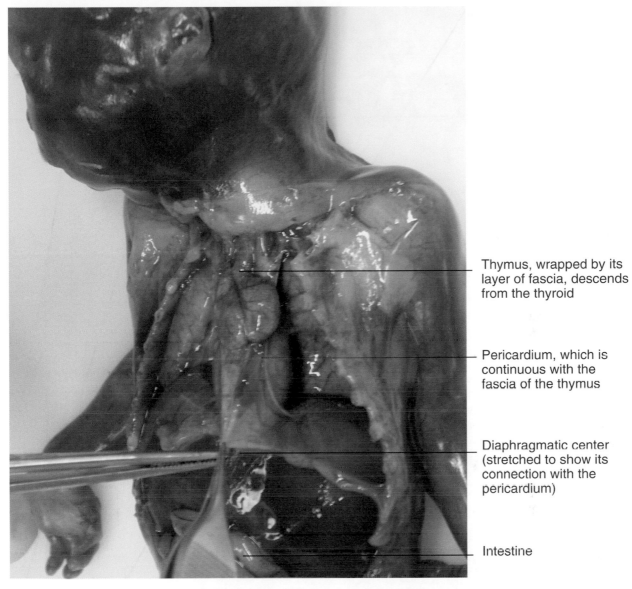

Thymus, wrapped by its layer of fascia, descends from the thyroid

Pericardium, which is continuous with the fascia of the thymus

Diaphragmatic center (stretched to show its connection with the pericardium)

Intestine

Fig. 1.10.2 Endothoracic fascia of a 22-week fetus. Image reproduced with permission from Stecco, L., 2012. Manipolazione Fasciale per le Disfunzioni Interne. Piccin Nuova Libraria, Padua.

The transversalis fascia forms an intermediate layer between the parietal peritoneum on the inside and the muscular layer of the transverse muscle covered by its epimysium. At the top it fuses with the inferior lamina of the diaphragmatic fascia. At the bottom it is fixed to the superior margin of the pelvis and fuses with the iliac fascia, which envelops the ileopsoas muscle; anteriorly it contributes to form the sheath of the rectus abdominis muscles, and posteriorly it continues to envelop the anterior surface of the quadratus lumborum muscle and the psoas major.

The transversalis fascia and the parietal peritoneum, along with the endopelvic fascia, form the fascial structures of the pelvic floor.

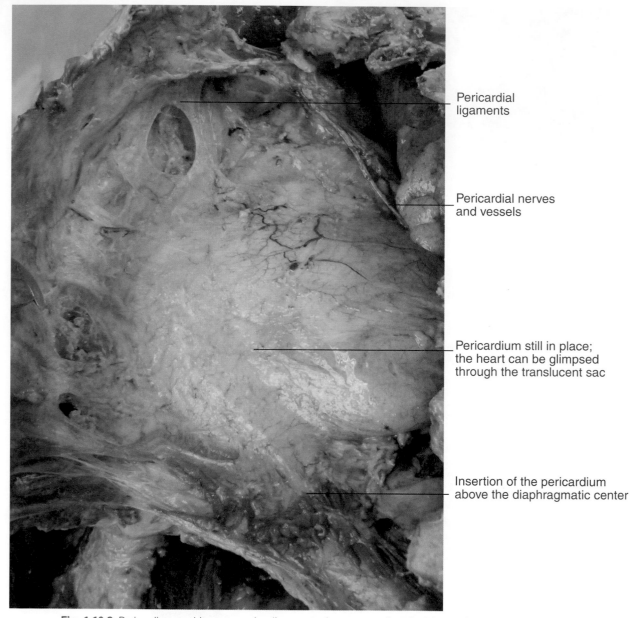

Pericardial
ligaments

Pericardial nerves
and vessels

Pericardium still in place;
the heart can be glimpsed
through the translucent sac

Insertion of the pericardium
above the diaphragmatic center

Fig. 1.10.3 Pericardium and its suspension ligaments. Image reproduced with permission from Stecco, L., 2012. Manipolazione Fasciale per le Disfunzioni Interne. Piccin Nuova Libraria, Padua.

THE FASCIA OF THE DIAPHRAGM AND ITS CONNECTIONS

The diaphragm is a respiratory muscle, but it takes part in many visceral functions; it is the main barrier between two environments that are subjected to continuous pressure changes and contributes to the expansion of the lungs, ensures that the gastric contents do not flow back into the esophagus, allows the passage of boluses, and prevents the abdominal viscera from rising into the thoracic cavity.

De Troyer et al. (1981) and Mittal (1993) have suggested differentiating between the costal and crural parts of the diaphragm. The costal diaphragm forms the contractile

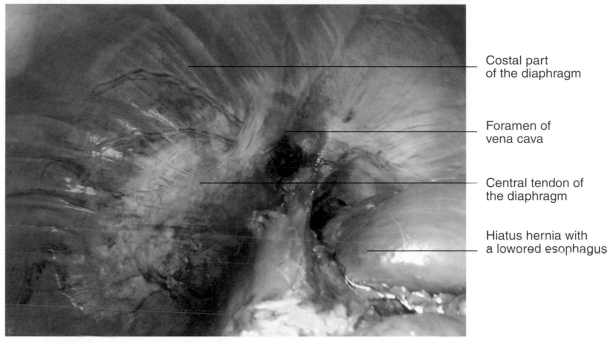

Costal part
of the diaphragm

Foramen of
vena cava

Central tendon of
the diaphragm

Hiatus hernia with
a lowered esophagus

Fig. 1.10.4 Lower view of the diaphragm. Image reproduced with permission from L. Stecco, 2012. Manipolazione Fasciale per le Disfunzioni Interne. Piccin Nuova Libraria, Padua.

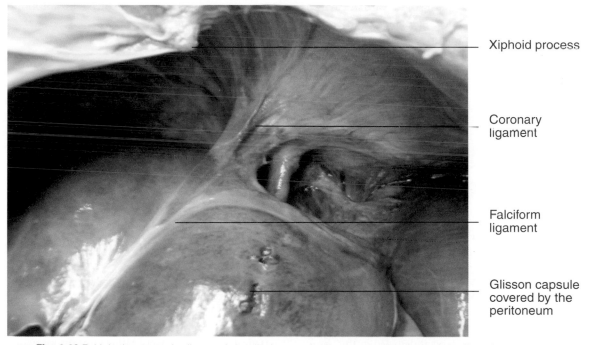

Xiphoid process

Coronary
ligament

Falciform
ligament

Glisson capsule
covered by the
peritoneum

Fig. 1.10.5 Links between the liver and the diaphragm via the coronary ligament of the liver. Image reproduced with permission from Stecco, L., 2012. Manipolazione Fasciale per le Disfunzioni Interne. Piccin Nuova Libraria, Padua.

muscular part, whose fibers converge toward the central tendon from the two hemidomes; the orientation of the muscle fascicles, which can almost be considered digastric, contribute with their contraction to lower the phrenic center. The crural diaphragm connects with the spine, and the costal and crural parts of the diaphragm act synchronously during respiration, but their activity diverges into functions such as emesis and swallowing.

The innervation of the diaphragm is also complex. The diaphragm receives sensory and motor innervation from the phrenic nerve, but the costal diaphragm is also innervated by sensory fibers, originating from six out of seven intercostal nerves (Pickering and Jones, 2002).

Young et al. have shown that the deep fibers of the crural diaphragm are not innervated by the phrenic nerve but by the vagus nerve (Young et al. 2010). This could help explain the swallowing reflex and the passage of the bolus, which requires a distension of the esophageal sphincter and relaxation of the crural fibers while the costal diaphragm contracts. During emesis, the transit takes place in reverse and the contraction of the diaphragm and the walls of the abdomen serve to increase intraabdominal pressure and facilitate ejection.

The connections with the pericardium in the cephalic direction and with the liver in the caudal direction allow better cardiac perfusion, the filling of the cardiac cavities, and the ejection of blood while maintaining cardiac and respiratory rhythm separate and favoring their integration when motor activity is increased—a hypothesis that is supported by studies that show how phrenic afferents are related to the pericardium, the hepatic parenchyma, and the inferior vena cava.

The presence of receptors in the diaphragm and their possible role in the proprioception of the diaphragm itself is debated. Recent studies on phrenic afferents (Nair et al. 2017) and on the receptors associated with them have highlighted the presence of neuromuscular spindles in the diaphragm that, in vivo, are activated during the lengthening of muscle fibers (therefore in the expiratory phase) and not during contraction. The presence of spindles has been established in the crural diaphragm but not in the costal one (Corda et al. 1965; Holt et al. 1991); this may indicate that the spindles, while being stretched in the expiratory phase, signal a potential distension of the esophageal sphincter and that they are therefore implicated in coordinating its degree of closure with the contraction of the diaphragm.

Golgi tendon organs have been detected in the tendinous portion of the diaphragm, in the central tendon, and in the myotendinous junction of the costal diaphragm; they show a low activation threshold when the diaphragm contracts in the inspiratory phase and might be involved in protecting the integrity of contractile fibers. During fatigue, the activity of the spindles increases and that of the Golgi tendon organs decreases.

Pressure-sensitive mechanoceptors have also been identified in the diaphragm in the area adjacent to the phrenic center and are considered to be Pacinian corpuscles (Corda et al. 1965).

Nair et al. (2017) showed that phrenic nerve afferents project onto the ganglion cells of the dorsal root C3–C6, to gray matter, to the cuneate fasciculus, and to the laminae V and X. It is interesting to note that the latency time is short, which might indicate that these are spinal monosynaptic projections or ones that intervene in interneuronal pathways. The study also found that the activation of spindles determines a monosynaptic excitation of the motoneurons, hence a rapid reflex pathway, while the activation of interspinal neurons seems to be connected to the reflexes connected to the costal and intercostal part.

The functional significance of the data is not yet completely clear, but cervical interneurons might transmit information coming from the diaphragm receptors directed to propriospinal neurons and/or motoneurons to the supraspinal centers involved in autonomic or respiratory control.

KEY POINT

Bearing in mind that there are receptors in the fascia and considering the different distribution of the receptors in the crural and costal diaphragm, it can be hypothesized that diaphragmatic fascia plays a fundamental role in the proprioception and coordination of the complex functions that the diaphragm integrates.

THE ROLE OF THE DIAPHRAGM IN RESPIRATORY FUNCTION AND THE CONTROL OF STATIC AND DYNAMIC POSTURE

The contraction of the diaphragm generates the following actions during inspiration:

- the diaphragm contracts and its central tendon (phrenic center) lowers; the intrapulmonary pressure decreases, increasing the vertical space in the thorax;

- the descent of the diaphragm encounters the resistance of the viscera, increasing intraabdominal pressure;
- the central tendon becomes a fixed point against the intraabdominal pressure, and as the muscle fibers of the diaphragm contract even further they pull the last six ribs vertically and laterally, increasing the transverse diameter;
- the sternum moves upward and forward, increasing the anteroposterior diameter;
- the diaphragm contraction itself increases the three diameters;
- when a larger respiratory volume is required, accessory respiratory muscles come into play.

The contraction of the diaphragm generates the following pressure changes:
- decrease in pleural pressure;
- increase in intraabdominal pressure;
- increase in the transdiaphragmatic pressure (the difference between the intrathoracic pressure and the intraabdominal).

It could be said that the diaphragm came into being in order to clearly separate the thoracic cavity from the abdominal cavity and to keep the viscera stable inside the latter, and, in the course of the evolution of mammals, it has turned into a muscularized structure.

The longitudinal, contractile costal fibers correspond to the apposition zone, in which the diaphragm is in direct contact with the deepest and lowest part of the rib cage, which is the most exposed to intrapleural pressure. When the fibers shorten just enough to eliminate the apposition zone, the descent of the phrenic center ends while the deformation of the rib cage begins more in a coronal or sagittal sense.

The contents of the viscera, predominantly fluid and incompressible, require that the intraabdominal pressure be balanced by the myofascial structures, arranged around the spine, in the abdominal wall and in the pelvic floor.

Studies conducted with paraplegic subjects show that the mere contraction of the diaphragm, without the contribution of the intercostal muscles, actually generates a decrease in intrapleural pressure, which tends to bring the upper part of the rib cage inward simultaneously with an outward displacement of the last six ribs and the abdomen. Under normal conditions, the effect, caused only by the contraction of the diaphragm, is balanced by the contraction of the scalene muscles. Their anticipatory activation might be related to the

stabilization of the rib cage in regard to the neck during the respiratory activity, thus preventing the rib cage itself from collapsing, and allowing its expansion through the stretching of the fascia.

The contraction of the diaphragm produces a displacement of the last six ribs, connected to the intercostal fascia, which merges with that of the transverse muscle and with the sheath of the rectus abdominis muscles. A partial distension of the transverse fibers is generated in the inspiratory phase, followed by a contraction in the expiratory phase that helps to stabilize the ribs with its upper part, maintain tension in the thoracolumbar fascia with its middle part, and compensate for sacroiliac movements with its lower part. The outward movement of the last six ribs also depends on the forces that resist the descent of the diaphragm so that the abdominal viscera become a fulcrum.

Experiments conducted on animals show that evisceration leads to a shortening of the fibers of the diaphragm during inspiration, which does not generate any expansion of the rib cage. The tone of the abdominal wall is therefore a factor that affects the contractile capacity of the diaphragm.

During inspiration, the descent of the phrenic center is accompanied by the sternum being pulled upward thanks to the action of the scalene muscles on the first two ribs and of the sternocleidomastoid. The rectus abdominis muscles relax, as does the transverse muscle, stretching the sheath of the rectus abdominis muscles.

The myofascial system surrounding the abdominal cylinder must adapt to the change in intraabdominal pressure by stretching, which tightens both the internal and the muscular fascia. The resulting tension in the thoracolumbar fascia has the effect of stabilizing the spine.

The orientation of the diaphragm fibers ensures that most of its contractile force is transmitted to the last six ribs; when the costal diaphragm extends them, the crural diaphragm does not participate in the deformation of the rib cage, therefore the crural diaphragm does not participate in the respiratory dynamics but has more of a role in the control of gastroesophageal functions—primarily swallowing and reflux prevention.

The mobility of the last six ribs is essential to absorb the increase in intraabdominal pressure, which would otherwise result in an increase in pressure on the pelvic floor; the myofascial system of oblique muscles, in particular the external obliques, must be particularly smooth and elastic, which also preserves pelvic continence.

The diaphragm is considered to be a key element of the abdominal cylinder (Hodges et al. 2001); together with the transverse abdominal muscle and the pelvic floor helps to maintain sufficient stability around the spine. It was demonstrated in one of experiments that the transverse abdominal muscle and the diaphragm co-contracted in a tonic way to maintain the stability of the spine before the beginning of the movements of the limbs.

Mandal, while studying the effects of laparotomy on the activation of respiratory muscles using electromyographic recordings of diaphragm and parasternal intercostal muscle activity, as well as esophageal pressure, showed that the activity of respiratory muscles increases considerably after laparotomy and that this increase persists over time. The data confirm the importance of the abdominal wall and fascial, muscular, and visceral integrity in managing and controlling the pressure differences between the two cavities and transferring the forces between abdominal wall muscles and along the fascia related to them (Mandal et al. 2016).

Wallden proposed that the viscous nature of the incompressible viscera makes them act as a fulcrum. According to his theory, the diaphragm contracts concentrically in the inspiratory phase and by pushing the viscera downward it determines a sufficient eccentric stretching of the abdominal wall and the pelvic floor to maintain the organs stable and ensure the closure of the sphincters, thanks to the coordination between the costal and crural diaphragm (Wallden 2017).

The last six ribs must be mobile and elastic to absorb the increase in intraabdominal pressure generated by the contraction of the costal diaphragm, avoiding compression of the organs and interfering with the mechanism of containment of the gastroesophageal and pelvic sphincters.

The prestretching of the pelvic and abdominal fascia allows a more effective contraction of the muscles associated with them, favoring, in the inspiratory phase, the contraction of the abdominal wall in synchrony with the myofascial structures of the pelvic floor; in this way, the viscera are pushed upward simultaneously with the lengthening of the fibers of the costal diaphragm, preventing visceroptosis. This dynamic is the result of coordinated activity between the muscles of the abdominal wall, the sheath of the rectus abdominis, the thoracolumbar fascia, the pelvic floor, and the diaphragm, which increases thoracolumbar stability in static activities.

A similar mechanism can be seen in dynamic rhythmic activities such as walking, running, and jumping and in explosive activities such as throwing and kicking. The muscles of the trunk, acting in a diagonal or spiral direction, manage the torsion of the thorax and the pelvis. Specifically, it might be useful to investigate the role played by the endothoracic fascia in the control of the emission of sounds that often accompanies the gesture of throwing or hitting.

It is necessary that these muscles maintain their elasticity and their ability to slide between the different planes in order to perceive and transmit the forces and tensions generated by the multidirectional movements that originate in the extremities, to which they are connected through the fascial system.

As already highlighted, the trunk has a trilaminar disposition of the muscles and the two aponeurotic fasciae, in turn formed by three laminae, each of which contain collagen fibers of the same orientation. Thanks to their structure, the broad muscles of the abdomen, as well as those of the respiratory and pelvic diaphragm, can almost be considered to be digastric muscles, which manage the coordination between the last six ribs, the pelvis, and the upper and lower limbs.

The correlation between breathing rhythm, heartbeat, circulatory rhythm, and rhythmic activities, the visceral and muscular fascial systems is essential to coordinate viscera stability with the contractile activity of the diaphragm.

In running, for example, the impact on the ground with the right leg, in addition to activating the fascia and muscles of the lower limb, determines the descent of the viscera. This, in turn, generates a contraction of the abdominal muscles, which pushes the viscera up toward the diaphragm, guaranteeing its stability. In this phase, it is necessary that the last six ribs open during inspiration. This action is favored by the torque generated by the external contralateral obliques. In the next step, inspiration is maintained to allow the viscera to be pushed up once more, with the same mechanism, and to facilitate the elongation of the costal diaphragm during expiration. The optimal rhythm seems to be to take two steps for each respiratory cycle.

Summary

The diaphragm has the complex role of adapting breathing and regulating intraabdominal and intrathoracic pressure to:
- avoid the dislocation of the viscera into the abdominal cavity;
- stabilize the viscera themselves;
- regulate cardiac and hepatic flux and alveolar perfusion;
- regulate the incoming and outgoing transit of boluses;
- participate in the expulsive phase of giving birth and defecation;
- allow sneezing/coughing.

The fascial system:
- intervenes to coordinate action at the peripheral level of the muscles of the thoracic wall, neck, and upper limbs, optimizing respiratory function;
- coordinates the delicate balance between the movements of the neck, trunk, and upper limbs to protect visceral functions;
- coordinates the posture of the trunk during breathing;
- coordinates rhythmic motor activities with the posture of the trunk and the movements of the limbs with the respiratory rhythm.

REFERENCES

Corda, M., Von Euler, C., Lennerstrand, G., 1965. Proprioceptive innervation of the diaphragm. J. Physiol. 178, 161–177.

De Troyer, A., Sampson, M., Sigrist, S., MacKlem, P.T., 1981. The diaphragm: two muscles Science 213, 237–238.

Hodges, P.W., Heijnen, I., Gandevia, S.C., 2001. Postural activity of the diaphragm is reduced in humans when respiratory demand increases. J. Physiol. 537, 999–1008.

Holt, G.A., Dalziel, D.J., Davenport, P.W., 1991. The transduction properties of diaphragmatic mechanoreceptors. Neurosci. Lett. 122, 117–121.

Mandal, K.C., Halder, P., Barman, S., Kumar, R., Mukhopadhyay, B., Shukla, R.M., 2016. Intragastric pressure: useful indicator in the management of congenital diaphragmatic hernia. J. Indian Assoc. Pediatr. Surg. 21, 175–177.

Mekonen, H.K., Hikspoors, J.P., Mommen, G., Köhler, S.E., Lamers, W.H., 2015. Development of the ventral body wall in the human embryo. J. Anat. 227, 673–685.

Mittal, R.K., Sivri, B., Schirmer, B.D., Heine, K.J., 1993. Effect of crural myotomy on the incidence and mechanism of gastroesophageal reflux in cats. Gastroenterology 105, 740–747.

Nair, J., Streeter, K.A., Turner, S.M.F., et al., 2017. Anatomy and physiology of phrenic afferent neurons. J Neurophysiol. 118, 2975–2990.

Pickering, M., Jones, J.F.X., 2002. The diaphragm: two physiological muscles in one. J. Anat. 201, 305–312.

Stecco, C., 2015. Functional Atlas of the Human Fascial System. Elsevier, London, 167–182.

Stecco, C., Sfriso, M.M., Porzionato, A., et al., 2017. Microscopic anatomy of the visceral fasciae. J. Anat. 231, 121–128.

Wallden, M., 2017. The diaphragm - more than an inspired design. J. Bodyw. Mov. Ther. 21, 342–349.

Young, R.L., Page, A.J., Cooper, N.J., Frisby, C.L., Blackshaw, L.A., 2010. Sensory and motor innervation of the crural diaphragm by the vagus Nerves. Gastroenterology 138, 1091–1101.e5.

Molecular Aspects of Fascia

Carla Stecco and Caterina Fede

CHAPTER CONTENTS

INTRODUCTION

It has been demonstrated that the fascia represents a complex structure composed of various kinds of cells embedded in abundant extracellular matrix and rich in nervous fibers (Kumka and Bonar 2012) (Fig. 1.11.1). It usually consists of two or three layers of parallel collagen fiber bundles, separated by thin layers of loose connective tissue (Fig. 1.11.2). The role of the cellular component is to define the metabolic properties of the tissue and enable it to adapt to and respond to varying conditions and stimuli, thanks to the receptors and cellular signaling system. Conversely, the extracellular matrix is made up of two components with differing characteristics:

- fibers: collagen fibers give support to the structure, and elastic fibers constitute the elastic part of the complex;
- the ground substance: a water-rich gelatinous substance that can transport metabolic material throughout the body.

This chapter examines the cellular components, the composition of the extracellular matrix, and the receptors expressed by the cells that regulate the fascial environment. Proper understanding of the microanatomy of the fasciae and how they respond to different stimuli is fundamental for knowledge of what alterations in them may give rise to pain.

> ### KEY POINT
>
> Fascia consists of two or three layers of parallel collagen fiber bundles, separated by thin layers of loose connective tissue. It is composed of various kinds of cells embedded in abundant extracellular matrix and rich in nervous fibers.

FASCIAL TISSUE CELLS

The main class of cells known in fascial tissue is composed of **fibroblasts** (Langevin et al. 2004); their main role is to maintain the structural integrity and organization of tissues secreting precursors of the extracellular matrix (ECM), such as collagen fibers and elastin. Fascial tissue cells are randomly distributed and not organized in flat monolayers or restricted to one side of the tissue, as is the case, for example, in epithelial tissue.

In 2018, a new class of cells was discovered in fascial tissue: the **fasciacytes** (Stecco et al. 2018). These fibroblast-like cells show some particular differences with respect to fascial fibroblasts (Fig. 1.11.3):

- morphology: whereas fibroblasts are elongated, fasciacytes are rounded—the cytoplasm being restricted to the perinuclear region—and have smaller and less elongated cellular processes;
- location: fasciacytes are not found among collagen bundles but form small clusters along the surface of

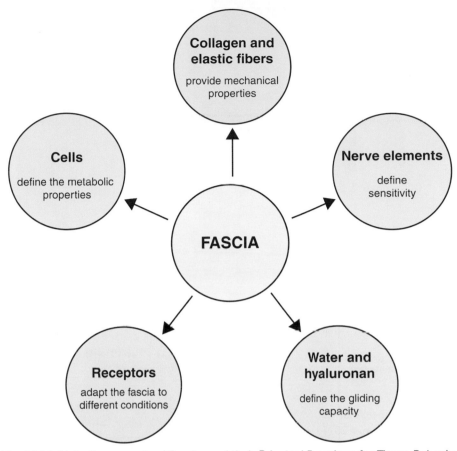

Fig. 1.11.1 Main Components of Fasciae and their Principal Functions for Tissue Behavior.

each fascial sublayer, defining the boundary between the fibrous sublayer and loose connective tissue (Fig. 1.11.2);
- function: fibroblasts produce the fibrous component, or rather collagen and elastic fibers, and play a role in regulating force transmission at a distance; fasciacytes produce hyaluronan, which allows fascial gliding among the various fascial sublayers.

Characterization of this new cell demonstrated that both cells, fasciacytes and fibroblasts, are positive to the typical markers of fibroblasts, such as vimentin, but fasciacytes also express the marker S100-A4 as a subclass of cells of chondroid metaplasia (Klein et al. 1999). This may be defined as a *reversible transformation toward a chondroid-like cell,* despite the negative reaction for the marker of the chondrocyte family, collagen II. In conclusion, this is a new type of cell, specialized for hyaluronan synthesis. In normal healthy fascia, about 30%

of the fibroblasts are fasciacytes, although this percentage may vary, according to the stimuli to which the fascial tissue is subjected.

The fascia also possesses cells with contractile activity, called **myofibroblasts** (Schleip and Klingler 2019). They show contractile activity transmitted via adherens junctions that open mechanosensitive ion channels in adjacent cells, resulting in Ca^{2+} influx (Follonier et al. 2008). Myofibroblasts can affect motor neuronal coordination, musculoskeletal dynamics, and regulation of fascial stiffness. Their contractile behavior may induce substantial contractures (~1 cm per month), and they also have significant effects on mechanical joint stability, influencing fascial tension in chronic pathological fibrotic conditions.

Lastly, fascial structures have been described as containing **telocytes**, specialized connective tissue cells provided with long thin extensions called telopodes, which

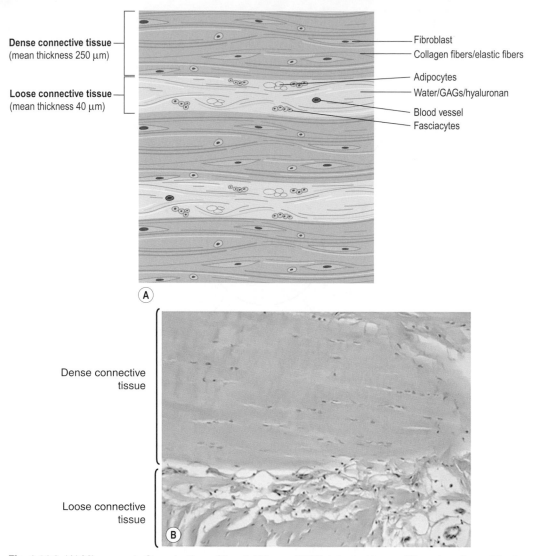

Dense connective tissue
(mean thickness 250 μm)

Loose connective tissue
(mean thickness 40 μm)

Fibroblast
Collagen fibers/elastic fibers
Adipocytes
Water/GAGs/hyaluronan
Blood vessel
Fasciacytes

(A)

Dense connective tissue

Loose connective tissue

(B)

Fig. 1.11.2 (A) Microscopic Organization of Fascial Tissue; (B) Histological Image (Hematoxylin and Eosin Staining) of Dense and Loose Connective Layers of Human Fascia Lata.

allow intercellular communication by means of cell junctions or extracellular vesicles (Chaitow 2017). Although their specific role is still under investigation, these cells are believed to be involved in cell repair, regeneration, remodeling, immune control, and cell communication, thus indicating that they also probably play an important role in regulating myofascial pain and fascial disorders. Although their morphological characteristics, distribution, and behavioral relationships are still unknown—both between each other and with other components of fascial tissue—they have been found in the tensor fascia lata, crural fascia of the leg, plantar fascia, and thoracolumbar fascia. Our research group found telocytes in the thoracolumbar fascia among tightly packed collagen bundles with various orientations (Fig. 1.11.4). Dawidowicz et al. (2016) defined the telocytes in fasciae as a "network in network" system, thanks to the complex three-dimensional communication system that they form in the interstitial extracellular matrix.

Fascial cell types also include various bundles of **nervous fibers** that follow the fasciae like a dense network, thus giving this tissue a role as a pain generator.

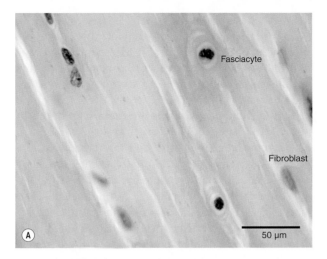

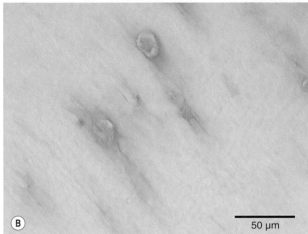

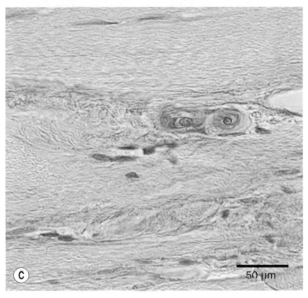

Fig. 1.11.3 (A) Hematoxylin and Eosin Stain of Human Fascial Tissue with Two Typical Cell Classes (Fasciacytes and Fibroblasts). (B, C) Fasciacytes with Hyaluronan-Rich Matrix (Pale Blue).

Table 1.11.1 lists the main types of cells in the fascia, with their morphological characteristics and main functions in tissues.

KEY POINT

Fascial fibroblasts produce the fibrous component of the extracellular matrix, or rather collagen and elastic fibers, and play a role in regulating force transmission; fasciacytes produce hyaluronan, which allows fascial gliding among the various fascial sublayers.

THE EXTRACELLULAR MATRIX: FIBROUS COMPONENT AND AQUEOUS MATRIX

The extracellular matrix is the extracellular component of the tissue. It consists of a three-dimensional and highly dynamic network composed of collagens, proteoglycans/glycosaminoglycans, elastin, fibronectin, laminins, and several other glycoproteins. All these components bind to each other, forming a complex network in which cells reside; it also permits and regulates various cellular functions, such as survival, growth, differentiation, and migration (Theocharis et al. 2016).

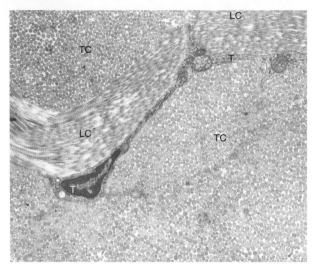

Fig. 1.11.4 Telocytes in thoracolumbar fascia of mice, visualized by transmission electron microscopy. TC, transversal collagen fibers; LC, longitudinal collagen fibers; T, telocyte. Courtesy Lucia Petrelli, Department of Neurosciences, University of Padua.

Generically, the extracellular matrix is subdivided into one fibrous and one aqueous component, with different characteristics and functions. The **fibrous component** is made up of collagen fibers and elastic fibers. Its function involves structures, connections, and containment and is fundamental in transmitting muscular force (Turrina et al. 2013; Yucesoy et al. 2003). The amount of the different types of fibers varies according to anatomical site, type of fascial tissue, and the various stimuli to which the fascia is subjected. Most collagen fibers are composed of collagen type I, which provides

the mechanical properties of tensile strength, and collagen type III, which consists of reticular fibers arranged in a mesh. The elastic fibers, made up of elastin and fibrillin, play the role of counterbalancing the amount of collagen, thus allowing tissues to cope with stretching and distension (Stecco 2015).

Elastic and collagen fibers are mainly produced by fibroblasts. These cells play a crucial role in extracellular matrix remodeling by synthesizing and organizing connective tissues, and they also modulate the production of the various fibrous components according to differing stimuli: physical, mechanical, hormonal, and pharmacological. For instance, *in vitro* and *in vivo* studies have confirmed that extracorporeal shock wave treatment enhances fibroblast proliferation and differentiation by activating gene expression for transforming growth factor β1 and collagen types I and III (Frairia and Berta 2011). In the same way, the agonists of endocannabinoid (CB1 and CB2) receptors can suppress fibroblast expression of fibrosis markers such as collagen I and fibronectin, remodeling extracellular matrix production and limiting the progress of uncontrolled fibrogenesis (Guan et al. 2017; Li et al. 2016; Garcia-Gonzalez et al. 2009). We found that *in vitro* cultured human fascial fibroblasts are able to produce **hyaluronan (HA)**-rich vesicles a few hours after treatment with the agonist of CB2 receptor, quickly released into the extracellular environment. Sex hormones can also stimulate cells of the muscular fasciae, regulating the production of some components of ECM, collagen I, collagen III, and fibrillin. At low β-estradiol hormone levels, as in postmenopausal women, the fascial tissue becomes

TABLE 1.11.1	**Fascial Cells**	
	Morphology	**Function**
Fibroblasts	Elongated, with extended cellular processes	Production of fibrous component; regulation of force transmission
Fasciacytes	Rounded, with cytoplasm restricted to perinuclear region	Synthesis of hyaluronan; gliding properties of fascia
Myofibroblasts	Large cells with undulating membranes and highly active endoplasmic reticulum	Contractile activity; effect on motor neuronal coordination, musculoskeletal dynamics, and fascial stiffness regulation
Telocytes	Long, thin extensions (longest cellular processes in the human body)	Can produce extracellular vesicles and allow intercellular communication and cell repair
Nervous fibers	Myelinated or unmyelinated fibers, or free nerve endings	Conduction of signals, nociception

enriched in collagen I and so is probably more rigid; instead, when hormone levels rise—for example, during pregnancy—fascial tissue becomes more elastic, with increased amounts of collagen III and fibrillin (Fede et al. 2019). If the fibrous component of the fasciae is altered because of hormonal imbalance, the behavior of the fascia and underlying muscle is compromised, leading to diminished elasticity and strength, modification of biomechanical properties, and increased tissue stiffness, causing myofascial disorders in many cases (Hansen 2018; Nallasamy et al. 2017).

The second component of the extracellular matrix is the **aqueous network of amorphous material**, composed of glycosaminoglycans (GAGs), most often covalently linked to proteins, forming proteoglycans. The main GAGs are heparin, heparin sulfate, chondroitin sulfate, dermatan sulfate, keratan sulfate, and HA. The increasingly important role of HA in fascial structures has been demonstrated. Initially, HA was found in the vitreous humor of the eye and considered as a molecule with only structural purposes. Subsequently, the essential role of this GAG emerged in various biological mechanisms, from cell proliferation and mobility to inflammation, angiogenesis, and its involvement in various diseases, such as cancer, diabetes, vascular alterations, and many others (Viola et al. 2015). In the human body, HA has a high turnover rate because of the simultaneous action of synthetases HAS1, HAS2, HAS3, hyaluronidases (HYAL) in their various isoforms, and other degrading molecules, such as reactive oxygen species (Tammi et al. 2002). Polymers of HA may range in size from a few kDa to 8 MDa; molecular size greatly influences the biological, physiological, and pathological functions of the molecule (Cowman et al. 2015a). In general, high molecular weight molecules have shown antiangiogenic, immunosuppressive, antiinflammatory, and tissue damage repair activity; smaller fragments show proinflammatory and proangiogenic activity. It influences all the biological activities of the ECM, including fascial tissue, in which it is particularly abundant between deep fascia and muscle, within muscle, and between the collagen layers that compose the deep fascia. The loose connective tissue between the layers of densely packed collagen fibers is rich in HA, which has a fundamental lubricating function facilitating smooth gliding between these structures (Cowman et al. 2015b).

It has also been demonstrated that, although the amount of HA in human fascia remains constant in the same anatomical site, it significantly changes according to the area and the type of fascia. The mean amount of HA is about 43 µg/g in aponeurotic fasciae, decreases drastically (about 6 µg/g) in epimysial fasciae, and increases in the retinacula (90.4 µg/g) (Fede et al. 2018). This confirms that the fasciae require a specific level of HA to allow correct gliding and the normal functions of deep fascia; in fact, variations in the amount of HA according to anatomical site correspond perfectly to the various gliding functions of the fasciae from several sites. That is, the aponeurotic fasciae are free to glide over the muscles, requiring a greater amount of HA, whereas the epimysial fasciae form a fibrous layer strongly adhering to the underlying muscles and need less HA (Stecco et al. 2009). Lastly, the retinacula represent specialized aponeurotic fasciae surrounding joints, where movements are the most intense and the highest levels of HA are found (Stecco et al. 2010).

The fascial tissue is thus able to synthesize and regulate the fibrous component of the ECM through the fibroblast cells, and the loose component by the production and regulation of HA by the fasciacytes, according to which kind of stimuli is applied to the tissues (Stecco et al. 2018). If the HA alters its density by changes in concentration, molecular weight, or temperature, or if its aggregative properties are changed by covalent or noncovalent binding of proteins, the physicochemical properties of the HA molecules also change, with consequent increases in the viscosity and elasticity of the HA-containing fluid. For example, an increase in temperature, even of only 2 degrees centigrade causes progressive break-up of the three dimensional superstructure of HA chains, with a consequent decrease in viscosity (Forgacs et al. 2003). It has been demonstrated that, although HA is stable in alkaline solution, its viscosity dramatically increases in acid solution; after intense physical exercise, muscle pH may reach a value of 6.60, with an increase of about 20% in HA viscosity (Gatej et al. 2005). Hyaluronan basically works as a lubricant. When it becomes more viscous, the thickness of loose connective tissue increases because of high concentrations of sticky hyaluronan, and the gliding of the fascial layer decreases, leading to less flexibility (Wilke et al. 2019). Thus in conclusion, if the composition of the loose connective tissue of the fasciae varies, the behavior of the whole deep fascia and the underlying muscle may be compromised, leading to stiffness and myofascial pain (Stecco et al. 2011; Cowman et al. 2015a).

KEY POINT

The ground substance of the extracellular matrix is rich in hyaluronan. Hyaluronan has a fundamental lubricating function: its amount in human fascia changes according to the anatomical site, the type of fascia, and the gliding properties of that fascia.

CELL RECEPTORS IN FASCIAL TISSUE

We demonstrated that fascial cells can modulate their environment according to various kinds of stimuli, such as sex hormones or endocannabinoids, which are retained by specific cell receptors. All cells, in fact, are constantly exposed to a variety of extracellular signals that they must first recognize, then decode according to a sequence of molecular switches (intracellular signaling pathways), and, lastly, to translate into an appropriate response (Uings and Farrow 2000). The variety of receptors on the cell plasma membrane has the role of responding specifically to the various signals, which may be soluble factors, such as hormones and growth factors, ligands on the surface of other cells, or the extracellular matrix itself, like hyaluronan molecules. According to the receptor to which it is linked, the signal molecule may make different responses. For example, hyaluronan can bind and interact with a variety of receptors, generating differing signaling pathways (Joy et al. 2018). We mention the CD44 receptor, which generally upregulates cell proliferation and migration, regulating

tumor growth and metastasis in cancer (Naor et al. 2002); RHAMM (receptor for HA-mediated mobility) promotes tissue repair and cell mobility via interactions with skeletal proteins and gap junctions between cells; and LYVE-1 (lymphatic vessel endothelial receptor 1), involved in transporting HA from tissues to lymph via lymphatic endothelial cells.

Hormones constitute other important soluble factors that can stimulate fascial cells. The documented presence of sex hormone receptors in fascial tissue represents the first step in our understanding of sex differences in the prevalence of myofascial pain: women, in fact, tend to have more myofascial problems than men. It has been demonstrated that relaxin receptor 1 (RXFP1) and estrogen receptor-alpha (ERα) are expressed in the deep fascia (crural fascia of the leg, rectus sheath of the abdomen, fascia lata of the thigh) (Fig. 1.11.5B) (Fede et al. 2016b). The expression rate is lower in postmenopausal than in premenopausal women because of decreased hormone levels. Estrogen and relaxin can stimulate fascial fibroblasts by linking with receptors on the plasma membrane, contributing to collagen and ECM remodeling, regulating fibrosis and inflammation, and consequently defining fascial stiffness. If fascial stiffness increases, the nociceptors within the fascia may be sensitized, also causing stiffness in the underlying muscle (Schleip et al. 2006). The role played by the fascia as sources and modulators of pain has been demonstrated by endocannabinoid receptor expression (Fig. 1.11.5A) (Fede et al. 2016a).

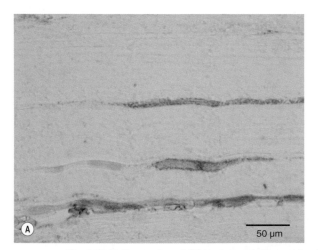

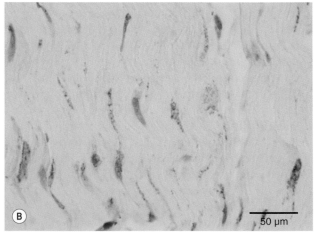

Fig. 1.11.5 Expression of CB1 receptor in human fascia lata of the thigh (A) and expression of RXFP1 in human rectus sheath of the abdomen (B). Immunohistochemical stain highlights positive cells in brown. Cell nuclei are stained in blue.

CB1 (cannabinoid receptor 1) and CB2 (cannabinoid receptor 2) are two G-protein-coupled cannabinoid receptors that allow the action of endogenous lipid mediators (endocannabinoids) and have a wide range of biological effects similar to those of marijuana. In particular, CB1 receptors are mainly distributed in the central nervous system; CB2 receptors are present in the myocardium, endothelial and smooth muscle cells, liver, and brain (Pacher and Steffens 2009). Their expression in the deep human fascia highlights their role as modulators of fascial fibrosis and inflammation: the activation of CB1 and CB2 receptors can suppress proinflammatory cytokines such as IL-1beta and TNF-alpha and increase antiinflammatory cytokines, providing antifibrotic activity (Nagarkatti et al. 2009). In this way, all the elements that can modulate CB1 and CB2 receptors are able to alter the endocannabinoid system by modifying the tissue levels of endocannabinoids themselves (in the case of manipulative treatments, exercises, stretching) or by working as agonists/antagonists of endocannabinoid receptors (if cannabis is used as a drug). These factors may trigger the release of antiinflammatory cytokines, which relieve myofascial pain.

KEY POINT

Fascial cells can modulate their environment according to various kinds of stimuli: hormones, endocannabinoids, and physical and mechanical stimuli. The signals are recognized by receptors of fascial cells and translated into an appropriate cellular response that can change the molecular composition of fascia, thereby regulating stiffness and pain.

Summary

The fasciae are not merely connective tissues with the function of supporting, joining, and protecting other tissues. The more we deepen our studies, the more we understand their organization. The fasciae represent a complex structure that includes a fibrous component, a loose connective component rich in hyaluronan, and a cellular component. All of these structures play specific roles, can respond to various kinds of stimuli, and can be modulated. All factors influencing cells or ECM behavior may result in changes in the composition of the entire fascial tissue, influencing its properties. Only clear-cut and deep understanding of fascial anatomy and of each component of the fascial tissue will allow us to understand their role and behavior in normal and pathological situations, making it possible to provide a healthy lifestyle, physical exercise, and more rational treatments.

REFERENCES

Chaitow, L., 2017. Telocytes: connective tissue repair and communication cells. J. Bodyw. Mov. Ther. 21, 231–233.

Cowman, M.K., Lee, H.G., Schwertfeger, K.L., McCarthy, J.B., Turley, E.A., 2015a. The content and size of hyaluronan in biological fluids and tissues. Front. Immunol. 6, 261.

Cowman, M.K., Schmidt, T.A., Raghavan, P., Stecco, A., 2015b. Viscoelastic properties of hyaluronan in physiological conditions. F1000Res. 4, 622.

Dawidowicz, J., Matysiak, N., Szotek, S., Maksymowicz K., 2016. Telocytes of fascial structures. Adv. Exp. Med. Biol. 913, 403–424.

Fede, C., Albertin, G., Petrelli, L., et al. 2016a. Expression of the endocannabinoid receptors in human fascial tissue. Eur. J. Histochem. 60, 2643.

Fede, C., Albertin, G., Petrelli, L., et al. 2016b. Hormone receptor expression in human fascial tissue. Eur. J. Histochem. 60, 2710.

Fede, C., Angelini, A., Stern, R., et al. 2018. Quantification of hyaluronan in human fasciae: variations with function and anatomical site. J. Anat. 233, 552–556.

Fede, C., Pirri, C., Fan, C., et al., 2019. Sensitivity of the fasciae to sex hormone levels: modulation of collagen-I, collagen-III and fibrillin production. PLoS One 14, e0223195.

Follonier, L., Schaub, S., Meister, J.J., Hinz, B., 2008. Myofibroblast communication is controlled by intercellular mechanical coupling. J. Cell Sci. 121, 3305–3316.

Forgacs, G., Newman, S. A., Hinner, B., Maier, C.W., Sackmann, E., 2003. Assembly of collagen matrices as a phase transition revealed by structural and rheologic studies. Biophys. J. 84, 1272–1280.

Frairia, R., Berta, L., 2011. Biological effects of extracorporeal shock waves on fibroblasts. A review. Muscles Ligaments Tendons J. 1, 138–147.

Garcia-Gonzalez, E., Selvi, E., Balistreri, E., et al. 2009. Cannabinoids inhibit fibrogenesis in diffuse systemic sclerosis fibroblasts. Rheumatology 48, 1050–1056.

Gatej, I., Popa, M., Rinaudo, M., 2005. Role of the pH on hyaluronan behavior in aqueous solution. Biomacromolecules, 6, 61–67.

Guan, T., Zhao, G., Duan, H., Liu, Y., Zhao, F., 2017. Activation of type 2 cannabinoid receptor (CB2R) by selective agonists regulates the deposition and remodeling of the extracellular matrix. Biomed. Pharmacother. 95, 1704–1709.

Hansen, M., 2018. Female hormones: do they influence muscle and tendon protein metabolism? Proc. Nutr. Soc. 77, 32–41.

Joy, R.A., Vikkath, N., Ariyannur, P.S., 2018. Metabolism and mechanisms of action of hyaluronan in human biology. Drug Metab. Pers. Ther. 33, 15–32.

Klein, D.M., Katzman, B.M., Mesa, J.A., Lipton, J.F., Caligiuri, D.A., 1999. Histology of the extensor retinaculum of the wrist and the ankle. J. Hand Surg. Am. 24, 799–802.

Kumka, M., Bonar, J., 2012. Fascia: a morphological description and classification system based on a literature review. J. Can. Chiropr. Assoc. 56, 179–191.

Langevin, H.M., Cornbrooks, C.J., Taatjes, D.J., 2004. Fibroblasts form a body-wide cellular network. Histochem. Cell. Biol. 122, 7–15.

Li, X., Han, D., Tian, Z., et al., 2016. Activation of cannabinoid receptor type II by AM1241 ameliorates myocardial fibrosis via Nrf2-mediated inhibition of TGF-β1/Smad3 pathway in myocardial infarction mice. Cell. Physiol. Biochem. 39, 1521–1536.

Nagarkatti, P., Pandey, R., Rieder, S.A., Hegde, V.L., Nagarkatti, M., 2009. Cannabinoids as novel anti-inflammatory drugs. Future Med. Chem. 1, 1333–1349.

Nallasamy, S., Yoshida, K., Akins, M., Myers, K., Iozzo, R., Mahendroo, M., 2017. Steroid hormones are key modulators of tissue mechanical function via regulation of collagen and elastic fibers. Endocrinology 158, 950–962.

Naor, D., Nedvetzki, S., Golan I, Melnik, L., Faitelson, Y., 2002. CD44 in cancer. Crit. Rev. Clin. Lab. Sci. 39, 527–579.

Pacher, P., Steffens, S., 2009. The emerging role of the endocannabinoid system in cardiovascular disease. Semin. Immunopathol. 31, 63–77.

Schleip, R., Naylor, I. L., Ursu, D., et al., 2006. Passive muscle stiffness may be influenced by active contractility of intramuscular connective tissue. Med. Hypotheses 66, 66–71.

Schleip, R., Klingler, W., 2019. Active contractile properties of fascia. Clin. Anat. 32, 891–895.

Stecco, A., Macchi, V., Masiero, S., et al., 2009. Pectoral and femoral fasciae: common aspects and regional specializations. Surg. Radiol. Anat. 31, 35–42.

Stecco, C., 2015. Functional Atlas of the Human Fascial System, first ed. Elsevier, Edinburgh, p. 4.

Stecco, C., Fede, C., Macchi, V., et al., 2018. The fasciacytes: a new cell devoted to fascial gliding regulation. Clin. Anat. 31, 667–676.

Stecco, C., Macchi, V., Porzionato, A., et al., 2010. The ankle retinacula: morphological evidence of the proprioceptive role of the fascial system. Cells Tissues Organs 192, 200–210.

Stecco, C., Stern, R., Porzionato, A., et al., 2011. Hyaluronan within fascia in the etiology of myofascial pain. Surg. Radiol. Anat. 33, 891–896.

Tammi, M. I., Day, A.J., Turley, E.A., 2002. Hyaluronan and homeostasis: a balancing act. J. Biol. Chem. 277, 4581–4584.

Theocharis, A.D., Skandalis, S.S., Gialeli, C., Karamanos, N.K., 2016. Extracellular matrix structure. Adv. Drug Deliv. Rev. 97, 4–27.

Turrina, A., Martínez-González, M.A., Stecco, C., 2013. The muscular force transmission system: role of the intramuscular connective tissue. J. Bodyw. Mov. Ther. 17, 95–102.

Uings, I.J., Farrow, S.N., 2000. Cell receptors and cell signaling. Mol. Pathol. 53, 295–299.

Viola, M., Vigetti, D., Karousou, E., et al., 2015. Biology and biotechnology of hyaluronan. Glycoconj. J. 32, 93–103.

Wilke, J., Macchi, V., De Caro, R., Stecco, C., 2019. Fascia thickness, aging and flexibility: is there an association? J. Anat. 234, 43–49.

Yucesoy, C. A., Koopman, B. H., Baan, G.C., Grootenboer, H.J., Huijing, P.A., 2003. Extramuscular myofascial force transmission: experiments and finite element modeling. Arch. Physiol. Biochem. 111, 377–388.

Fascia of the Pelvic Floor

Marek Jantos and Carla Stecco

CHAPTER CONTENTS

INTRODUCTION

The pelvis is a well-defined but complex anatomical region. It is commonly referred to as the *bony pelvis* or *pelvic girdle* and is likened to a basin-shaped bowel consisting of bones overlaid by layers of muscles and fasciae. Its bony structure provides protection to the organs and strength and stability to the body's framework.

KEY POINTS

The central location makes the pelvis an area of *tensional convergence* between the upper trunk and axial spine and the lower limbs (see Fig. 1.12.1).

Connecting the upper torso to the pelvis are the abdominal and lower back muscles, and connecting the pelvis to the lower limbs are the anterior hip muscles and posterior glutei. The coordination of any postural adjustment is achieved via multiple layers of muscles and the fascial system that interconnects the pelvis with all other anatomical regions. These varied and important functions rely on multiple layers of fascia; the superficial fascia that maintains form, the deep fascia that invests pelvic muscles and neurovascular bundles, and the visceral fascia that holds the pelvic organs in place.

Structurally, when the body is in a standing position, the gravitational center is located just medial to the pubis synthesis and centered between the two hip joints. The fascial and muscular systems maintain the body's balance with intricate precision through the efficient relaying of mechanical information between the upper and lower body regions. Minor postural changes shift the center of gravity and alter the body's tensional lines and the position of the body's organs, altering the pressure on fascia and ligaments that hold the organs in place (Petros 2010). The suspensory tone of fascial tissue exerts a significant influence on organ function. In a hypertonic tone it can restrict organ motility; if too lax, it can lead to pelvic organ prolapse. With ageing, as posture changes and the quality of fascial support declines, the relative positioning of organs in relation to the pelvic hiatus changes and women become predisposed to problems of prolapse and incontinence.

Fascia and muscles play a significant role in maintaining urinary and fecal continence, enabling parturition, and facilitating sexual activity. With these varied functions, the soft tissue within the bony pelvis is characterized by maximum elasticity and versatility. Elasticity can be restricted by obesity, pregnancy, nonrelaxing muscles, adhesions, and scar tissue. Obesity and pregnancy increase intraabdominal pressure; persistent muscle tension gives

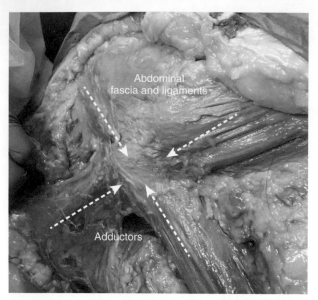

Fig. 1.12.1 The pubis as an area of tensional convergence. The abdominal fascia and ligaments converge from the upper torso and adductors from the lower limbs.

rise to functional contractures, whereas scar tissue and adhesions reduce mobility. In addition, trauma, overwork, and persistent straining also weaken ligamental support and lead to structural deficiencies and prolapse. Pelvic organ prolapse repair, where surgical procedures use mesh and synthetic tapes for organ support, is not compatible with the elasticity of native tissue and can create problems of erosion, infection, and limited mobility and can lead to chronic pain (Pike 2019).

KEY POINTS

With the reproductive, urinary, and digestive systems sharing the same immediate environment, the role of pelvic soft tissue takes on special significance, providing important insight into why so many chronic pelvic syndromes not only share the same comorbidities but are comorbid to each other.

The fascial system is a dynamic body-wide system. This is well-illustrated by the effect of breathing, which creates a resonance that reverberates in every anatomical region. With each breath the pelvic hiatus dilates during inhalation and narrows with each exhalation. Prior to every sneeze or cough, there is a reflex-mediated preemptive tightening of pelvic muscles. During birthing, the respiratory muscles maximize intraabdominal pressure, while minimizing the intrathoracic pressure, to facilitate the expulsive efforts during labor (McConnell 2013). During excursions of the respiratory diaphragm, organs in the abdominopelvic cavity—the liver, spleen, pancreas, adrenals, small intestine, and the bladder—that attach directly to the inferior aspect of the diaphragm move in synchrony with the rhythm of breath (Stecco and Stecco 2016). Each of these organs respond to movement and gravitational forces by moving around their normal axes. Adhesions, scar tissue, and loss of fascial elasticity undermine the dynamics associated with natural rhythms. Posture and malalignment of the pelvis affect not only the organs within but contribute to disorders in the upper body, shoulders, chest, neck, and jaw.

BODY-WIDE CONTINUITY OF PELVIC FASCIA

The anatomical structure of the pelvic floor consists of four principle layers: the *endopelvic fascia*, the muscular *pelvic diaphragm* made up of the *levator ani* muscle group, the *perineal membrane* known as the *urogenital diaphragm*, and the *superficial transverse perineii* (Stoker 2009). These four layers are further delineated by three fascial layers. The original work of identifying the continuity of the pelvic fascia has been the focus of extensive study by the second author (Stecco 2015; Ramin et al. 2015). The fascial layers that form this continuum, extend from the lower abdominal area, incorporate the pelvic muscles and organs, and traverse up to the lumbar area, as shown in Fig. 1.12.2. This continuity also extends laterally to the groin and the lower limbs.

In an anteroposterior direction, the innermost fascial layer begins with the *internal oblique* and *transverse aponeurosis* then invests the pubis synthesis, continues on as the deep transverse muscle of the perineum (that extends between the pubic arch and ischiopubic rami), surrounds the levator ani muscle, and attaches to the perineal body. It then goes on to form part of the deeper anococcygeal ligament and extends to the presacral and iliopsoas fascia. Below the levator ani muscles and the urogenital diaphragm there is a second fascial layer, which begins as the investing fascia of the abdominal wall muscles (*external oblique* muscles) and continues in the form of *Gallaudet's fascia*, which surrounds the superficial transverse perineal muscles and forms the superficial part of the *anococcygeal ligament* (a fibrous but elastic collagen mesh) that extends up to the posterior layer of the *thoracolumbar fascia*. This layer links with the coccyx and sacral bone and the origins of the gluteus maximus fascia. The third layer is located well below the urogenital diaphragm and consists of several segments of superficial fascia. It starts anteriorly with *Scarpa's*, *dartos*, and *Colles' fascia*; surrounds the *bulbospongiosus* and *ischiocavernosus* muscles; connects with the *superficial anal sphincter* (*corrugator cutis ani*); and continues on to the superficial fascia of the back. These form the superficial fascia, located in the middle of the hypodermis. Medially, the fibers ease into the submucous tissue and laterally blend with the true skin.

> ### KEY POINTS
>
> With fascial continuity it is possible to see how back, groin, and limb pain are linked to pelvic pain. Compensation patterns can arise anywhere within a tensional sequence.

Trauma and scar tissue disrupts tensional flow in fascia and leads to compensatory mechanism and pain, which can occur above or below scar tissue. Abdominal incisions frequently lead to pubic and urogenital pain, whereas lumbar injuries and chronic lower back pain can be associated with urinary symptoms of urge and frequency or with small bowel obstruction.

INNER STRUCTURE OF THE PELVIC CAVITY

The pelvic cavity is the inferior portion of the abdominal cavity—the largest of the body's cavities. The fibrous fascia that defines each cavity gives rise to the peritoneum, which forms the oblique roof of the pelvic cavity; the lower boundary is formed by the pelvic floor muscles, as shown in Fig. 1.12.2.

The peritoneum consists of a double layer that extends from the respiratory diaphragm down to the pelvic peritoneal space and covers the fundus of the urinary bladder, the front of the rectum, the anterior and posterior surface of the uterus, and the upper posterior vagina. The outer layer of the peritoneum is known as the *insertional fascia*, a thicker layer by which the organs attach to the walls of the cavity. The inner and thinner layer is the *investing fascia* (sometimes referred to as the *visceral fascia*), which envelopes individual organs and forms part of the internal structure of

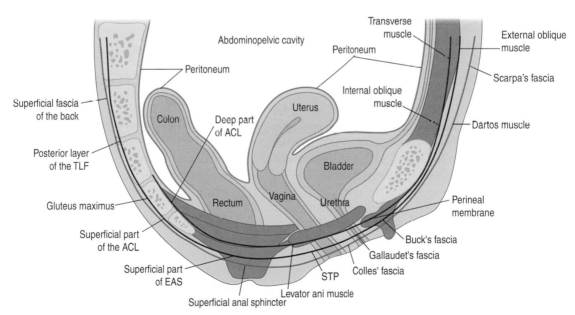

Fig. 1.12.2 Continuity of fascia linking the abdominal, pelvic, and lumbar region. ACL, anococcygeal ligament; EAS, external anal sphincter; STP, superficial transverse perineal muscle; TLF, thoracolumbar fascia.

the organ. The space between the insertional and investing fascia is referred to as the peritoneal cavity and contains peritoneal fluid that lubricates and enables smooth movement of organs—the *omentum* and *mesenteries*. The peritoneum covering the anterior and posterior section of the uterus meets and extends laterally to the side walls of the pelvis, forming fascial condensations that make up the broad ligaments that invest the fallopian tubes and hold the organ in place.

The pelvic floor is made up of the *levator ani muscle group*, also known as the *pelvic diaphragm*, as shown in Fig. 1.12.2. Bilaterally, the two walls of the pelvic cavity are formed by the *obturator internus muscle.* The front wall is formed by the pubic bones, and the posterior wall consists of the *piriformis* and *coccygeus* muscles, which provide closure to the pelvis. The levator ani muscle is held in place by laterally attaching along the white line known as the *arcus tendinous levator ani*, which consists of a strong fibrous condensation within the *obturator internus* fascia. All of the weight-bearing of the pelvic diaphragm (the levator ani muscles) is dependent on the integrity of this fascial attachment.

The center of the pelvic floor features the *pelvic outlet*, which is divided into two clearly defined components. Anteriorly, it is made up of the *urogenital hiatus*, spanned by a sheet of fascia known as the *pubocervical fascia*. The urogenital hiatus provides an opening for the *urethra*, which forms the outlet for the bladder, and the *vagina*, which forms the outlet for the uterus. Posteriorly, the *rectal hiatus* provides an opening for the anal canal and is spanned by the *rectovaginal fascia*.

The pelvic organs, which include the bladder, urethra, vagina, uterus, and rectum, all rest directly over the central hiatus and are held in place by the endopelvic fascia. Pelvic organs have no inherent strength of their own and are totally dependent on the suspensory ligaments, fascial attachments, and muscles to hold them in their correct position and ensure full and proper function (Petros 2010).

Some anatomists see the pelvic floor as a muscle hammock on which the pelvic organs rest; others see the pelvic floor as all-inclusive of muscle—pelvic viscera—held in place by ligaments and membranous structures (Herschorn 2004; Delancey and Shobeiri 2010). From this perspective, muscles, ligaments, and organs are not separate entities but are part of one unified structure held together by the endopelvic fascia.

The endopelvic fascia consists of tissue made up of elastin (distensible tissue), collagen (less distensible soft tissue), and smooth muscle. The vagina is a central organ that is suspended across the middle of the pelvis, directly over the pelvic outlet. It is held in place by connective tissue at three different levels (Stoker 2009). At the apex it is supported by attachment to the cervix and on either side by the *cardinal* and *uterosacral* ligaments (Level 1). In the midline it is held by connective tissue originating from the side walls, known as the *arcus tendinous fasciae pelvis* (Level II), and the distal portion is attached laterally to the puborectalis muscle and perineal body (Level III). The empty bladder and the urethra rest back on the vagina, with the vagina acting as a trampoline-like structure. Vaginal support of these structures is one of the key components in the urinary continence mechanism. Defects in vaginal support can lead to a descent of the urethra and bladder into the vaginal introitus and the formation of a cystocele. In the posterior section of the pelvis, laxity of the uterosacral ligaments and the rectovaginal fascia, and loss of support from the perineal body, can give rise to uterine prolapse, as well as high or low rectocele. The central outlet, spanned by muscles and fascia, is a point of weakness in the pelvic floor. If as a result of trauma, injury, or ageing, the muscles and connective tissue supporting the pelvic organs are compromised, the weakness will affect the filling, storage, and elimination of waste and impact optimal sexual function. The connective tissue is most vulnerable to damage during lifting, straining, and birthing and is affected by obesity, ageing, and hormonal status.

FASCIAL TONICITY AND ORGAN FUNCTION

The endopelvic fascia and pelvic muscles constitute the immediate environment of the pelvic organs. Pelvic muscles are the primary generators of tension, which is transmitted by the fascia that houses the ganglia that regulate peristalsis and organ function (Stecco and Stecco 2014).

Peristalsis of an organ is a local phenomenon, mediated by the microscopic ganglia within fascia (Stecco and Stecco 2016). The extramural and intramural ganglia of the autonomic nervous system act as a peripheral brain in regulating the function of organs and glands. These ganglia are highly reactive to alterations in fascial tension (Stecco and Stecco 2016; Ramin et al. 2015). Micromotions in the bladder serve as an interesting example of the relationship between nonrelaxing pelvic muscles, increased fascial tension, and peristalsis of the organ (Vahabi and Drake 2015). The term "micromotions" refers to localized contractions and stretches in the bladder wall that result in periodic slow movements, similar to those of gastrointestinal peristalsis. These peristaltic movements, first proposed by Van Duyl in 1985 (Vahabi and Drake 2015), are modulated by intramural myenteric plexuses that regulate contracting segments, consisting of bundles of smooth muscles working as interlinked functional units. An increase in micromotions results in exaggerated sensations from the bladder, even in the absence of any detected changes in bladder pressure, giving rise to a pathological sensory urge. In the absence of micromotions, there is a decrease in sensation and increased post-void residual urine. When comparing asymptomatic women with those experiencing increased bladder sensations (as in overactive bladder), the latter showed significantly higher micromotions and increased urge. Given that intravesicular pressure changes were not the main determinant, it is likely that altered myogenic properties within the smooth muscle cells influenced their excitability (Vahabi and Drake 2015). The dysregulation of bladder pacemaker action is a sign in 70% of bladder pain syndrome (BPS) patients (Bouchelouche and Bouchelouche 2013).

KEY POINTS

With evidence linking nonrelaxing muscles to overactive bladder, it seems likely that increased fascial tension may be a contributor, if not the mediator, of bladder dysfunction.

Case studies of overactive bladder responded positively to fascial manipulation and pelvic muscle relaxation, with reduction or complete resolution of bladder pain and detrusor overactivity (Pasini et al. 2015; Jantos et al. 2015b).

EXTERNAL ANATOMY OF THE PELVIS

One external structure that is often overlooked in the study of pelvic anatomy is the *bulbo-clitoral organ*, which plays no role in reproduction but has a key role in sexual pleasure. The integrity of this organ is compromised by abdominal and pelvic surgery, which modifies the tensional balance and leads to pain, sexual dysfunction, and loss of sexual desire.

Studies of the bulbo-clitoral organ have resulted in the first anatomical text, which forms the basis of this discussion (Di Marino and Lepidi 2014). The clitoris, urethra, and vagina are anatomically interconnected and held in place by fascial layers descending from the abdomen. The superior and inferior fascia links the bulbo-clitoral organ to the distal vagina and urethra in the urogenital diaphragm. Because of the organ's three-dimensional structure, its morphology is mostly studied from dissected samples ex situ.

The *glans clitoris* is the visible part of the larger bulbo-clitoral organ. It is embedded in the perineum and forms part of the vulva. It is attached to the anterior pubis by the suspensory ligament and the *retro-crural fascia*. The body of the glans clitoris is made up of two cavernous structures, also known as the roots or pillars of the clitoris. These are attached via the *ischiocavernosus muscle* to the inside surface of the ischio-pubic ramus, just below the insertion point of the urogenital diaphragm. The two crura merge to form the body of the clitoris.

The dimensions of the crura are significantly larger by comparison to those of the body of the clitoris, averaging 37 mm in length and 9 mm in diameter, compared with the glans clitoris that averages 5.1 mm in length and 3.4 mm in diameter. Within the body of the clitoris, the cavernous cylinders are surrounded by a large number of nerves and blood vessels, and these are enveloped by the *clitoral fascia* (analog to Buck's fascia in the male penis).

Immediately below the body of the clitoris are spongy structures commonly known as *vestibular bulbs*, variously referred to as "genital bulbs," "clitoral bulbs," "urethral bulbs," "vaginal bulbs," and "urethra-vaginal bulbs," reflecting the fact that these surround the urethra and vagina. The top surfaces of the bulbs insert into the perineal membrane of the urogenital diaphragm and then insert into the lateral edges of the distal portion of the urethra and vagina, whereas their lowermost part forms a cap over the top of the *greater vestibular glands* (or *Bartholin's glands*).

Anatomically, the vestibular bulbs are overlaid by fatty tissue of the *labia*, *Colles' fascia*, and the *bulbospongiosus muscle*. During different phases of the sexual cycle the bulbo-clitoral organ undergoes significant transformation (engorgement and swelling), which requires maximum elasticity of tissue that envelops the organ. Any adhesions or scarring, which is common postbirth, may restrict the elasticity and mobility of the fascial tissue, potentially giving rise to pain and a range of sexual disorders, including persistent arousal disorder (Waldinger and Schweitzer 2009).

FASCIAL TENSION AND CHRONIC PELVIC PAIN

The prevalence of chronic pelvic pain is relatively high, affecting over 30% of women. Chronic urogenital pain (CUP) forms a subcategory of pelvic disorders and affects around 10% of women, with symptoms affecting the urinary and reproductive system in the form of bladder pain syndrome (BPS) and vulvodynia (Vd).

The dilemma that confronts clinicians dealing with urogenital pain disorders is the challenge of identifying the cause, source, and mechanisms of pain. The role of the fascial system in these pain disorders has never been explored. As a result, many of the current treatments are experimental and ineffective, being focused on pharmaceutical and surgical management (i.e., cystectomies, vestibulectomies, hysterectomies), often based on the misguided belief that pain originates in the organ (Baskin 1992; Brookoff 2009).

The first author and his associates have been investigating the origins and mechanisms of pain in BPS and Vd by means of pain mapping. The term "pain mapping" refers to the process of systematic examination of pelvic soft tissue in an effort to objectively localize pain and establish a relationship between the pain source and reported symptoms (Jantos 2015a). The importance of pain mapping is that it authenticates the sufferers' report of *their* pain and symptoms and highlights the role of peripheral mechanisms of pain (Jantos et al. 2015a).

For research purposes, three pain maps were used to examine pelvic points considered relevant to CUP (Jantos 2020; Johns et al. 2017). The three maps are shown in Fig. 1.12.3A–C. Map A consists of 27 palpation points of the external urogenital area; Map B consists of 15 palpation points of pelvic muscles; and Map C consists of 12 palpation points focused on the paraurethral and bladder area, an area generally unrecognized and previously not mapped. The details of the pain-mapping procedure are outlined in several articles (Jantos et al. 2015b).

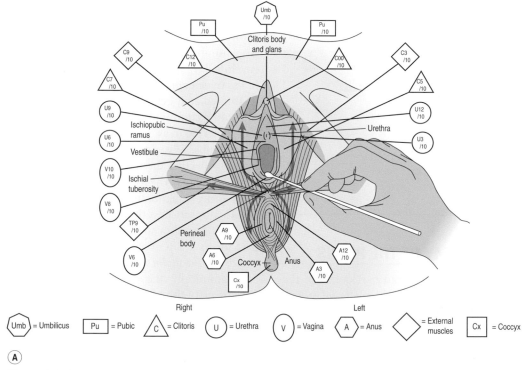

Fig. 1.12.3 (A) Urogenital pain map, identifying external assessment points. TP, transverse perineal muscle.

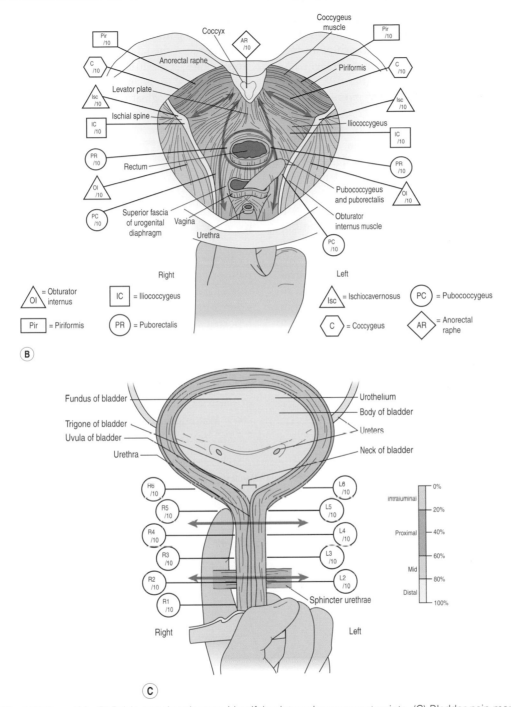

Fig. 1.12.3 cont'd (B) Pelvic muscle pain map, identifying internal assessment points. (C) Bladder pain map, identifying paraurethral assessment points. L = left; R = right. Redrawn with permission from Jantos, M., 2021. A myofascial perspective on chronic urogenital pain in women. In: Santoro, G.A., Wieczorek, P., Bartram, C., (Eds). Pelvic Floor Disorders: Imaging and a Multidisciplinary Approach to Management. Springer Press, New York.

In a study of 320 cases, CUP pain profiles were compared with those of asymptomatic controls (Jantos 2020). A summary of the pain mean scores for each point from Maps A, B, and C (see Fig. 1.12.3) are shown in Fig. 1.12.4.

Analysis showed that on Map A, the BPS and Vd cases reported high pain scores mainly in the vestibular area and urethral meatus (see Fig. 1.12.3A). Anatomically this appears to be a sensitive area for both the pain groups and even asymptomatic women. Given that these points involve the superficial perineal fascial, pain is experienced locally and was not referred to distant regions. In contrast, points on Maps B and C were consistently more painful in both of the diagnostic groups (BPS and Vd), with no pain reported in the asymptomatic control group. Points from Map B referred pain to the hips, lower back, abdomen, and groin and radiated to the anal sphincter, often reproducing fecal urge. Points from Map C produced the most severe pain; reproduced urethral and bladder pain, urge, and sensation of suprapubic pressure; and produced referred pain to the umbilicus, pubic area, inguinal quadrants, lower lumbar region, gluteal area, groin, and in some cases the soles of the feet, as shown in Fig. 1.12.5. The most extensive referred pain patterns were seen on Maps B and C and occur on account of the involvement of deep fascia as shown in Fig. 1.12.5 B and C.

Diagnostically, of all of the points tested, it was the paraurethral points on Map C that most reliably differentiated between the CUP groups and asymptomatic controls (Jantos et al. 2017; Jantos 2020). The explanation may be related to the innervation density and vascularity in the anterior vaginal wall and urethral lumen and the effect of tensional convergence in the posterior pubis area.

KEY POINTS

The evidence indicates that the paraurethral area may be the primary generator of chronic urogenital and pelvic pain symptoms, yet it is rarely palpated during diagnostic assessments.

Women with a diagnosis of Vd or BPS rarely speak of pain originating from the paraurethral area, yet palpation of these points reproduced not only what they considered to be "their pain" but also the most commonly reported symptoms, such as suprapubic pressure; burning, sharp, stabbing pain; and urge, which is commonly associated with frequency.

In the symptomatic group, a subgroup of women reported clitoral pain (a localized form of Vd) or symptoms of persistent genital arousal (Waldinger and Schweitzer 2009; Waldinger et al. 2010). Both of these symptoms

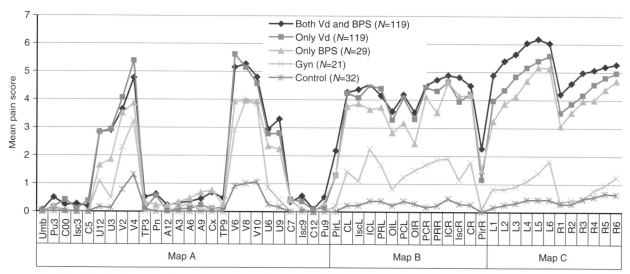

Fig. 1.12.4 Summary of pain mean score from each map and a comparison of scores for Vd, Vd and BPS, and BPS groups only, compared with a general gynecology group and an asymptomatic control group. BPS, bladder pain syndrome; Gyn, general gynecology; Pn, perineal body; Vd, vulvodynia; L = left; R = right; see Fig. 1.12.3 for the keys to the other abbreviations in this figure.

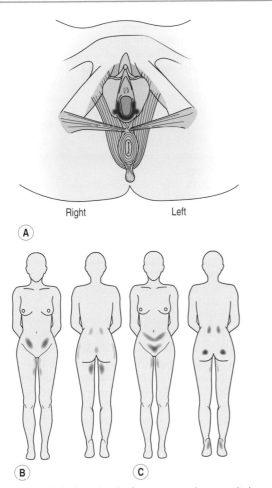

Right   Left

(A)

(B)   (C)

Fig. 1.12.5 (A) Referred pain from external urogenital area. (B) Referred pain from pelvic muscle points. (C) Referred pain from paraurethral points.

were reproduced by palpation of paraurethral points. In none of the clitorodynia cases was clitoral pain ever reproduced by Q-tip testing of the clitoral glans itself. On the basis of pain mapping, clitoral pain and persistent genital arousal form part of the CUP continuum but originate in the paraurethral area.

Pain-mapping studies highlight several important points. In order to reproduce symptoms and make an accurate diagnosis it is necessary to conduct a far more comprehensive physical exam than just a Q-tip test of the external points. Failing to do so may wrongly attribute pain to presumed diseased organs, such as the bladder, urethra, vulva, or bowel—organs that appear to

be innocent bystanders in most pelvic pain syndromes (Peters 2008). Some points on Map B and C produce pain that is passive and imperceptible to the sufferers unless it is palpated.

Studies examining the relationship between pain and endometriosis found no correlation between severity of pain and level of disease and recommend that pain of myofascial origin be explored (Orr et al. 2018; Stratton et al. 2015; Aredo et al. 2017). Another observation from pain mapping showed that the pain profiles of BPS and Vd cases are almost identical, suggesting that BPS and Vd may be one and the same disorder but diagnosed by two different specialties—urology and gynecology, respectively. Furthermore, given that one of the most common comorbidities of both BPS and Vd is irritable bowel syndrome, all of these disorders may share a common mechanism mediated by fascial dysfunction (Jantos 2020).

From the three maps used, specific points were identified that reliably differentiated between symptomatic and asymptomatic women. Using logistic regression analysis, six points from the three maps were identified that provide a 94% reliable diagnosis of BPS and Vd. These include a vestibular and urethral point on Map A, two pelvic muscle points on Map B, and two paraurethral points from Map C (Johns 2017; Jantos 2020).

Summary

The body-wide fascial system connects the pelvic area and other anatomical regions. Fascia communicates mechanical information; maintains the necessary tensional balance; and regulates the function of muscles, organs, and biological systems. Injury, surgical trauma, medications, scars, adhesions, infections, recurrent inflammation, hormonal variations, hydration, inactivity, muscle overactivation, and emotional stress affect the tensional balance and thixotropic behavior of interstitial fluids. Unfortunately, the pelvic region is subject to some of the most invasive medical procedures and laparoscopies, commonly used to investigate suspected endometriosis and organ diseases. All of these procedures affect the continuity and dynamics of the fascial system, creating a high risk of scarring, adhesions, and secondary complications of pain, small bowel obstruction, and infertility. The dynamic properties of fascia, its malleability and plasticity, should be of primary interest and focus in therapy. To this end the study of pelvic fascial anatomy is most relevant and promising.

REFERENCES

Aredo, B.S., Heyrana, K.J., Karp, B.I., Shah, J.P., Stratton, P., 2017. Relating chronic pelvic pain and endometriosis to signs of sensitization and myofascial pain and dysfunction. Semin. Reprod. Med. 35, 88–97.

Baskin, L.S., Tanagho, E.A., 1992. Pelvic pain without pelvic organs. J Urol. 147, 683–686.

Bouchelouche, K., Bouchelouche, P., 2013. Mast cell and bladder pain syndrome. In: Nordling, J., Wyndaele J.J., van de Merwe, J.P., Boucheloche, P., Cervigni, M., Fall, M. (Eds.), Bladder Pain Syndrome: A Guide for Clinicians. Springer, Boston, pp. 71–86.

Brookoff, D., 2009. Genitourinary pain syndromes: Interstitial cystitis, chronic prostatitis, pelvic floor dysfunction, and related disorders. In: Smith, H. (Ed). Current Therapy in Pain. Saunders Elsevier, Philadelphia, pp. 205–215.

Delancey, J., Shobeiri, S.A., 2010. State of the art pelvic floor anatomy. In: Santoro, G.A., Wieczorek, A.P., Bartram, C.I. (Eds.), Pelvic Floor Disorders: Imaging and Multidisciplinary Approach to Management, Springer Verlag Italia, Milano, pp. 3–15.

Di Marino, V., Lepidi, H., 2014. Anatomical Study of the Clitoris and the Bulbo-Clitoral Organ. Springer (eBook).

Herschorn, S., 2004. Female pelvic floor anatomy: The pelvic floor, supporting structures and pelvic organs. Rev. Urol. 6 (Suppl. 5), S2–S10.

Jantos, M., 2021. A myofascial perspective on chronic urogenital pain in women. In: Santoro, G.A., Wieczorek, P., Bartram, C. (Eds.), Pelvic Floor Disorders: Imaging and a Multidisciplinary Approach to Management. Springer Press, New York.

Jantos, M., Johns, S., Baszak-Radomańska, E., 2017. Testing reliability of Q-tip criteria in the diagnosis of vulvodynia. J. Low. Genit. Tract Dis. 21, (Suppl. 4), S31.

Jantos, M., Johns, S., Torres, A., Baszak-Radomańska, E., 2015a. Mapping chronic urogenital pain in women: rationale for a muscle assessment protocol - the IMAP, Part 1. Pelviperineology, 34, 21–27.

Jantos, M., Johns, S., Torres, A., Baszak-Radomańska, E., 2015b. Mapping chronic urogenital pain in women: insights into mechanisms and management of pain based on the IMAP, Part 2. Pelviperineology, 34, 28–36.

Johns, S., Jantos, M., Baszak-Radomańska, E., 2017. Refining a pain mapping tool. J. Low. Genit. Tract Dis. 21, S10.

McConnell, A., 2013. Respiratory Muscle Training. Churchill Livingstone, Edinburgh.

Orr, N.L., Noga, H., Williams, C., et al., 2018. Deep dyspareunia in endometriosis: role of the bladder and pelvic floor. J. Sex. Med., 15, 1158–1166.

Pasini, A., Sfriso, M.M., Stecco, C., 2015. Treatment of chronic pelvic pain with fascial manipulation. Pelviperineology, 35, 13–16.

Peters, K. M., 2008. Reply to letter-to-the-editor: Prevalence of pelvic floor dysfunction in patients with interstitial cystitis. Urology 71, 1232.

Petros, P.E.P., 2010. The Female Pelvic Floor: Function, Dysfunction and Management According to the Integral Theory, third ed. Springer, Heidelberg, p. 16.

Pike, H., 2019. NICE guidance overlooks serious risks of mesh surgery. BMJ. 2, 1537.

Ramin, A., Macchi, V., Parzionato, A., De Caro, R., Stecco, C., 2015. Fascial continuity of the pelvic floor with the abdominal and lumbar region. Pelviperineology 35, 3–6.

Stecco, C., 2015. Functional Atlas of the Human Fascial System. Churchill Livingstone Elsevier, Edinburgh.

Stecco, L., Stecco, A., 2016. Fascial Manipulation for Internal Dysfunctions: Practical Part. Piccini, Padua.

Stecco, L., Stecco, C., 2014. Fascial Manipulation for Internal Dysfunctions: Practical Part. Piccini, Padua, p. 19.

Stoker, J., 2009. Anorectal and pelvic floor anatomy. Best Pract. Res. Clin. Gastroenterol. 23, 463–475.

Stratton, P., Khachikyan, I., Sinaii, N., Ortiz, R., Shah, J., 2015. Association of chronic pelvic pain and endometriosis with signs of sensitization and myofascial pain. Obstet. Gynecol. 125, 719–728.

Vahabi, B., Drake, M.J., 2015. Physiological and pathophysiological implications of micromotion activity in urinary bladder function. Acta. Physiol. 213, 360–370.

Waldinger, M.D., Schweitzer, D.H., 2009. Persistent genital arousal disorder in 18 Dutch women: part II—A syndrome clustered with restless legs and overactive bladder. J. Sex. Med. 6, 482–497.

Waldinger, M.D., Venema, P.L., Van Gils, A.P.G., Schutter, E.M., Schweitzer, D.H., 2010. Restless genital syndrome before and after clitoridectomy for spontaneous orgasms: a case report. J. Sex. Med. 7, 1029–1034.

Embryology of the Fascial System

Fabiana Silva, Leonardo Sette Vieira and Jaap van der Wal

CHAPTER CONTENTS

INTRODUCTION

In humans, the period of development from conception to the 8th week of life is considered to be the embryonic period (Sadler 2019). There exist two mainstream lines of thought regarding embryonic development—one mainly genetic, the other morphological (or metabolic). The genetic theory credits development from DNA programming. The metabolic morphological theory interprets development as resulting from the relationship of cell and tissue metabolism with the environment. In the latter concept, differentiation is considered to be organized "from outside to inside": morphogenesis and organogenesis are not strictly predetermined by the genetic code but occur in morphogenetic fields (Blechschmidt 2004). Ingber (1998) showed that the state of activity of DNA in cells is greatly influenced by the interactions of cells with the extracellular environment. The intracellular environment and DNA is influenced and orchestrated by its external environment via the extracellular matrix (ECM) by means of substances like epigenetic factors and messenger globulins while internal cellular metabolism attempts to balance the new demands from the environment. The concept of reciprocal interaction between DNA and organism integrates the two theories: the genetic code is influenced via the ECM by the embryo, that is, the organism, and genetic code functions as a constraint of possibilities. The

reciprocal relationship between DNA activity and environment might also be exerted in the adult organism (Lipton 2005). The purpose of this chapter is to present the formation of the so-called fascial system regarding both of the morphogenic theories and referring to the neurofasciogenic model of Tozzi (2015).

Typically, human embryonic development of the first 8 weeks is subdivided in 23 so-called Carnegie stages (Table 1.13.1). At stages 7 and 8, around the third postconceptional week of development, the so-called gastrulation marks the beginning of morphogenesis (Moore and Persaud 2016). The totipotent cells of the epiblast differentiate into three primordial germ "layers"—the ectoderm or ectoblast, mesoderm or mesoblast, and endoderm or endoblast. The epithelial epiblast cells lose their epithelial organization, migrate, and proliferate, resulting in mesenchymal cells. Mesenchymal cells appear as primordial connective tissue, and under specific genetic and metabolic signaling conditions, the mesenchyme differentiates in various connective tissue types (Blechschmidt and Gasser 2012) (Fig. 1.13.1). The mesoderm (or "inner tissue," according to Blechschmidt) gives rise to all of the fascial tissue and derivatives. The head and neck mesenchyme are derived from the neural ectoderm (neural crest) (Douarin et al. 2007; Bordoni and Lagana 2019). The fascia in principle originates from the

TABLE 1.13.1	**Carnegie Stages (O'Rahilly and Müller 1990).**							
	Week 1	**Week 2**	**Week 3**	**Week 4**	**Week 5**	**Week 6**	**Week 7**	**Week 8**
Carnegie stages	1, 2, 3, 4	5, 6	7, 8, 9	10, 11, 12, 13	14, 15	16, 17	18, 19	20, 21, 22, 23

Modified from Hill, M.A., 2019. Embryology timeline human development. https://embryology.med.unsw.edu.au/embryology/index.php/Timeline_human_development.

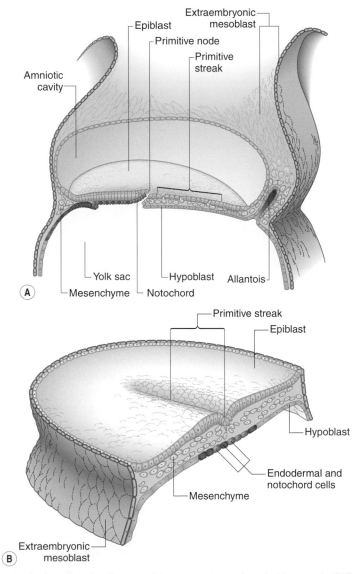

Fig. 1.13.1 (A) Longitudinal section showing mesoblast ingression at the primitive streak. (B) Transverse section through the embryonic plate at the level of the primitive streak to show the early movement of mesoblast between the epiblast and underlying hypoblast. Reproduced with permission from Standring, S., Ed., 2016. *Gray's Anatomy: The Anatomical Basis of Clinical Practice*, 41st ed. Elsevier, London, 181, Figs. 10.1 and 10.2.

mesenchyme (mainly derived from the mesoderm) in all kinds of forms and compositions. The mesenchyme also provides the metabolic conditions for the development of the ectodermal and endodermal structures.

KEY POINT

The formation of the fascial system is influenced by both genetic and environmental factors. Fascial tissue is mainly derived from mesenchyme, which in turn originates mainly from the so-called mesoderm. The body's fascial tissue develops from mesenchymal tissue, originating from mesoderm cells and in the face and neck region of mesenchymal cells from the cranial neural crest. All of these cells are related to metabolic support for the development of cells in the border tissue, endoderm and ectoderm.

NEURAL (MENINGEAL) FASCIA

Neurogenesis is the process of formation of the nervous system and begins in the differentiation of the ectodermal neural plate, which folds to form the neural groove (day 18). Next the groove merges to form the neural tube. The most dorsal part of the neural groove forms the neural crest (Hill 2019). The neural tube gives rise to the central nervous system (CNS), and the neural crest gives rise to the peripheral nervous system (PNS). The rapid growth of the neural tube needs large metabolic support, which comes from the mesenchyme (mesoderm) surrounding the neural tube that simultaneously assists in the shaping of the nervous system. The mesenchymal sheaths begin forming in Carnegie stage 10. The outer part of the neural tube is enveloped in the primitive meninges (primitive pia mater), providing nutrients for development. Because of the thin and delicate structure of the pia mater and arachnoid, they are called leptomeninges; they are derivatives from the mesoderm.

The outermost meningeal membrane, the dura mater, is constituted by a dense layer of collagenous connective tissue and is divided into two parts, an osseous or endosteal layer, which shapes the growth of the calvaria bones, and a meningeal layer that will contribute to the formation of the brain compartments, giving rise to falx cerebri, tentorium cerebelli, falx cerebelli, and diaphragm of the sella turcica. As neural cells emerge in the wall of the neural tube, they push older cells to the periphery in the direction of the primitive meninges.

This generates a mechanical stretching of the cells, influencing the shape of future neurons. Later development of the neural tube is faster because of lower tissue resistance. The anterior structures form a restrictive mechanism against this growth and cause the tube to flex forward in the region of the most cranial part of the notochord, where its bifurcation occurs, forming a transverse structure named submesencephalic septum, the future area of the midbrain. In this area the forces of the mesodermal connective tissue converge, which resists the accelerated rate of cerebral growth. These converging force vectors determine the structural and histological pattern of cranial dura mater stress (Liem 2002) (Fig. 1.13.2). Here the base of the skull is formed. The primitive dura mater grows slower than the brain, forming a restrictive mechanism that drives brain growth and is, together with the embryo's blood vessels, responsible for the formation of the brain grooves and the forebrain folds.

Spinal cord neural fasciae are constituted similarly to the cranial ones, providing nutritional support on the one hand and directing neural development on the other hand. From the primitive pia mater, the denticulated ligaments are formed that connect the spinal cord to the dura mater, providing support (Tubbs et al. 2001). The dura mater develops several ligaments responsible for maintaining a harmonious relationship between the neural tissue and the vertebral canal and spinal foramen. Spinal skeletal bone growth is faster than spinal cord growth. The meninges form important ligaments by attaching the terminal part of the medulla (in the adult at the level of vertebra L1, L2) to the coccyx. This is the terminal ligament and forms a junction of the dura mater with the pia mater (Standring 2016) (Fig. 1.13.3).

The fascial coverings in the PNS are derived from the mesenchyme that surrounds neurons of the neural crest. The neurites are enveloped by endoneurium. Sets of neurites are organized into fascicles and covered by perineurium. The nerves at the end are enveloped by the epineurium. In areas where there might be some kind of compression of the nerve a mesoneurium appears. This is a loose connective tissue sheath, formed by connective tissue, which protects the nerve and enables the nerve to glide freely (it also contains the vasa nervorum, the blood vessels of the nerve). An important feature in this respect are the (mesodermal) Schwann cells, which form the myelin sheath around the neurites and dendrites,

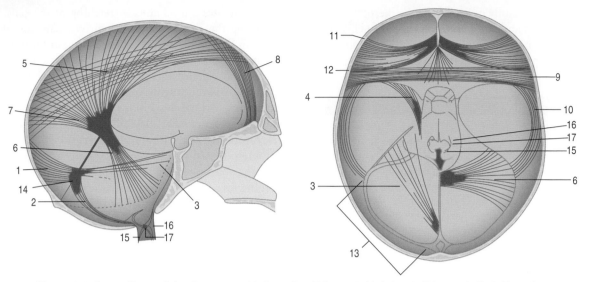

Fig. 1.13.2 Stress fibers of the dura mater. Horizontal: 1. Falx cerebri inferior. 2. Falx cerebelli. 3. Tentorium cerebelli. 4. Sphenoidal. 5. Falx cerebri superior. Vertical: 6. Tentorium. 7. Falx cerebri posterior. 8. Falx cerebri anterior. 9. Transverse. Circular: 10. Squamosal. 11. Cranial vault anterior. 12. Cranial vault medial. 13. Cranial vault posterior. 14. Cranial fossa posterior. 15–17. Spinal dura. Redrawn with permission from Arbuckle, B.E. 1994.The selected writings of Beryl E. Arbuckle, DO, FACOP. Indianapolis: American Academy of Osteopathy.

among others responsible for increasing the conduction velocity of the neural stimulus.

About 50% of the CNS is made up of neurons derived from the neural tube. The other 50% are glial cells, which are also cells of neurodermal origin and which provide physical and metabolic support for the functioning and development of the neurons. The glial cells mostly constitute the matrix and supportive and connective tissue component of the nervous tissue (without glia the neurons could not live or function). They represent a kind of "neurodermal mesenchyme" (Brodal 2010) (Fig. 1.13.4).

VASCULAR FASCIA

In the first two weeks, diffusion of nutrients is sufficient to meet the metabolic needs of the embryo. From the middle of the 3rd week on, this general diffusion mechanism is replaced by a more organized vascular system in order to meet the extremely high metabolic needs in the developing embryo (Sadler 2019). A dorsal vascular aortic system and a specialized venous network, the cardinal veins, arise. These vessels differentiate from the mesoderm because of the constant flow of liquids, ions, and glycoproteins present in the embryonic ECM. Vessels have an adventitious outer layer forming a protective fascial envelope, similar to visceral investing fasciae (Stecco and Stecco 2014).

The vascular network supports the nutrition of the neural tube, but at the same time capillaries in strands of mesenchymal connective tissue provide a restrictive mechanism. In the embryo's spine, for example, blood vessels are responsible for the somatic segmentation. In the cranial part they are, together with the primitive dura mater, responsible for the creation of folds and shapes in the developing brain (Fig. 1.13.5). In a similar way the dorsal aorta is paramount for the formation of the pharyngeal arches and consequently the formation of the face and cervical structures. From the folding of the embryo in relation to the ascending brain emerges the first pharyngeal arch around stage 12 (approximately the 4th week).

The organization of a vascular endothelial network (capillaries) is a relatively rapid process that occurs first in the cranial region of the embryo. In the early stages, when the embryo reaches 6.0 mm in length, two-thirds of the embryo body is taken up by the head and one-third by the trunk. Vascular development occurs parallel to the notochord, directing and nourishing the neural and digestive tract.

From cells in the lateral area of the mesoderm, the so-called splanchnopleure, the cardiac progenitor cells arise. The primitive heart develops in the cranial area of the embryo, surrounded by mesenchymal tissue, which will develop into the pericardium. The heart is mainly

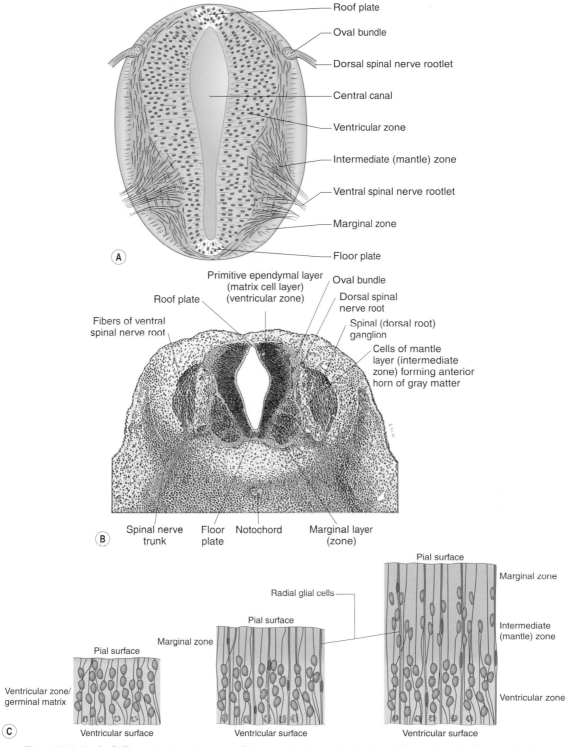

Fig. 1.13.3 (A, B, C) The early development of the neural tube and spinal cord. Reproduced with permission from Standring, S., Ed., 2016. *Gray's Anatomy: The Anatomical Basis of Clinical Practice*, 41st ed. Elsevier, London, 241, Figs. 17.4, Fig. 17.5, and Fig. 17.6.

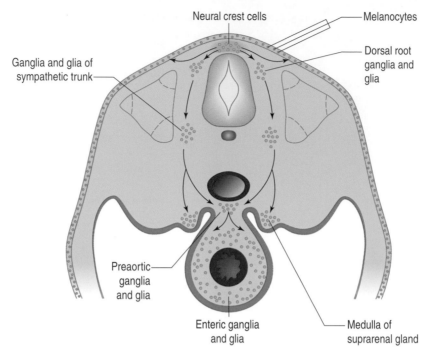

Fig. 1.13.4 The migration routes of the neural crest in the trunk. Reproduced with permission from Standring, S., Ed., 2016. *Gray's Anatomy: The Anatomical Basis of Clinical Practice*, 41st ed. Elsevier, London, 243, Fig. 17.11.

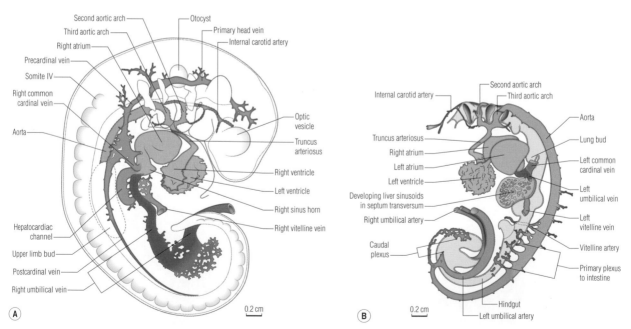

Fig. 1.13.5 Vascular network formation at the embryos. Reproduced with permission from Standring, S., Ed. 2016. *Gray's Anatomy: The Anatomical Basis of Clinical Practice*, 41st ed. Elsevier, London, 201, Fig. 13.2.

formed by two clusters of splanchnic mesodermal cells that migrate to the primary cardiogenic area in the cephalic region of the embryo (days 16–18). This area will develop the left ventricle and atrium and a part of the right ventricle. The remainder of the heart (including the arterial cone and arterial trunk) develops from a secondary cardiogenic area derived from the part of the splanchnic mesoderm that is ventral to the posterior pharynx (day 20 and 21). From mesothelial cells of the transverse septum, which is the mesodermal structure that separates the heart from the primitive liver, most of the visceral pericardium (so-called lining fascia) and coronary arteries are derived. The insertional pericardium is also derived from the lateral part of the mesoderm, this time from the somatopleure (see next section), which surrounds the pericardial cavity. With the descent of the heart from the cervical region to the mediastinal area, the insertional pericardium maintains continuity with the deep fasciae surrounding the infrahyoid and thyroid muscles. In the thoracic region

this continuity forms thickenings that help maintain the positioning of the pleura and pericardium, forming the suspensory ligaments (pericard and pleura).

VISCERAL FASCIA

The digestive tract begins its formation around the 18th day after fertilization and is subdivided into: foregut, midgut, and hindgut. Foregut and midgut exhibit a craniocaudal development gradient, the hindgut a caudocranial one (Fig. 1.13.6).

By day 20 the lateral part of the mesoderm splits into somatopleure and splanchnopleure. Somatopleure is a mesodermal layer that is directly related to the ectoderm. It will give rise to the intravisceral ligaments and plicae, the omenta of the viscera, and the "ligaments" with the abdominal wall. They provide adherence (with gliding possibility) between the various organs and to the body wall and protection and visceral adaptation to

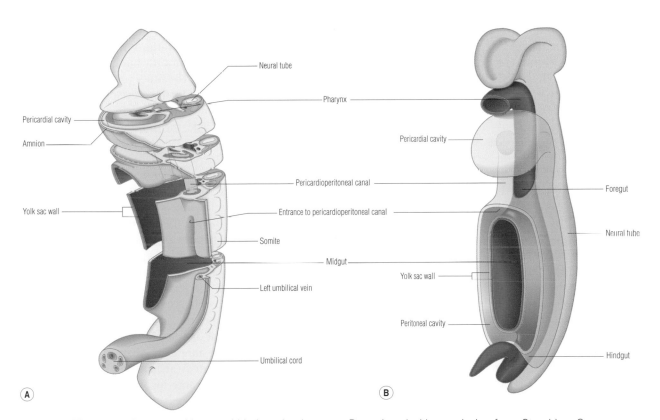

Fig. 1.13.6 Foregut, midgut, and hindgut development. Reproduced with permission from Standring, S., ed., 2016. *Gray's Anatomy: The Anatomical Basis of Clinical Practice*. 41st ed. Elsevier, London, 194, Fig. 12.1 A and B.

external movements of the trunk or to deep breathing. The somatopleure plays a fundamental role in the organization of the great vascular branches and, thus, is mainly innervated by (ortho)sympathetic nerves. This vascularization is generated to support the large metabolic activity caused by the accelerated cell growth of the digestive tract. At the same time, this vascular organization interferes with the shape and development of the entire digestive tract and surrounding fasciae.

The splanchnopleure is a mesodermal structure that is directly related to the endodermal tube and will form the investing fasciae of the gut tube. Histologically the lining fascia acquires a more elastic characteristic than the parietal fascia, allowing volume changes in the digestive and respiratory tract. The splanchnopleure provides metabolic support for the development of the digestive tract, and in adulthood the investing fasciae of the gut and abdominal organs are fundamental to the direct function of the organs and are associated with the enteric nervous system (ENS) (Sasselli et al. 2012).

At the beginning of the 4th week of development, the massive production of interstitial fluids related to the embryo's high metabolic rate form a kind of intraembryonic cavity called intraembryonic coelom. This coelom forms a single cavity that divides the lateral mesoderm of the body into two layers. The intraembryonic coelom provides room for organs to develop. At the end of the 4th week, the celiac cavity is divided into three well-defined cavities: one pericardial cavity, two pericardioperitoneal canals, and one peritoneal cavity. During the folding (flexion) of the cranial part of the embryo (the so-called cephalic fold) the heart and peripheral cavity are relocated anteriorly. With the descent of the heart, liver, and transverse septum, the pericardioperitoneal channels need to subdivide into the pericardial, pleural, and peritoneal cavities. The pleura cavity arises from the posterior space of the mediastinum, created by the anteriorization of the heart and liver. In these pleural cavities develop the endodermal cells that will form the lungs and the mesenchyme, which will form the pleural membranes. The outermost layer of the pleural mesenchyme forms the parietal pleura that unites with the somatic mesoderm that will form the deep fasciae of the trunk. In this way, the fascia endothoracica is shaped.

The three portions of the gut tube—the foregut, midgut, and hindgut—develop in a different way. The foregut is the first to develop. The foregut will be supported by an anterior (ventral) mesogastrium and a posterior (dorsal) layer. Midgut and hindgut are connected to the body wall by a dorsal mesogastrium. Foregut and midgut develop in the craniocaudal direction. The accompanying mesoderm, nourishing and directing the endodermal tube, guides vagal cranial nerve fibers into these two portions of the tube. The hindgut, developing caudacranially as discussed previously, "drags" nerve fibers from the sacral portion of the spinal cord with it. This occurs around the 8th stage of development (the end of the 3rd week).

At stage 10 of embryonic development (about the 4th week), an oropharyngeal membrane is formed. The pharyngeal (or branchial) arches are formed by the embryo's cranial folding in relation to the formation of the aortic arches of the primitive dorsal aorta. Pharyngeal arches consist of endodermal, mesodermal, and ectodermal tissue. Various structures of the face and neck are derived from them. The first pharyngeal arch will give rise to the lower jaw and part of the tongue, "carrying" the trigeminal nerve. Because they are formed in front of the foregut, the branchial arches establish a direct connection with the anterior mesogastrium, which explains the continuity of the buccopharyngeal and pharyngobasilar fasciae into the buccal cavity, digestive tract, and cranial base. The other pharyngeal arches II, III, and IV appear with further development of the digestive tract. The second arch is the innervation domain of the facial nerve (VII), the third of the glossopharyngeal nerve (IX), and the fourth of the vagus nerve (X). The fifth arch degenerates, and the existence of the sixth one is controversial in the literature.

The tongue is formed from the four pharyngeal arches, thus exhibiting innervation by the V, VII, IX, and X cranial nerves. Besides those nerves, the major innervating nerve is the hypoglossal nerve responsible for the innervation of all muscles, except for the palatoglossus muscle (which receives vagal innervation). The tongue is continuous with the pharyngeal and esophagesl fasciae called the buccopharyngeal fascia which forms the fascia of the organs of the digestive tract and enters the region of the basilar apophysis of the bone where it is continuous with the dura mater that covers all the holes in the base of the skull (Warshafsky et al. 2012).

At the midgut, the anterior (ventral) mesogastrium degenerates. Because there is no anterior fixation of the gut tube to the abdominal wall there, the mesentery allows great mobility of this intestinal region. The mesentery is a bilaminated layer derived from the posterior mesogastrium that surrounds the midgut (jejunum and ileum) and runs from the duodenojejunal flexure to the ileocecal valve. Innervation occurs by the (ortho)sympathetic minor thoracic splenic nerve, which originates from the superior mesenteric ganglion, and by branches of the vagus nerve.

The hindgut begins to develop in Carnegie stage 10 (approximately the 4th week) (Hill 2019). It develops in the sacral region of the embryo. This might explain that the distal third of the transverse colon, descending colon, sigmoid, and rectum are innervated by the parasympathetic nerve, originating from sacral spinal segments. This hindgut possesses only a posterior (dorsal) mesogastrium connection.

The intermediate mesoderm is involved in the formation of the kidney and ureter. The kidney is shaped first in the pelvis and then "ascends" to the upper lumbar region as the embryo develops (Fig. 1.13.7). The renal ascending explains the appearance and length of the ureter. The renal fasciae attach the organ to the diaphragm and extend through the ureter to the bladder where they are continuous with the insertional fascia that runs from the bladder to the sacrum. Also, the renal fascia is indirectly related to the ventral part of the thoracolumbar fascia, which also contains the psoas and quadratus lumborum muscle. Tozzi and colleagues, in 2012, demonstrated in some individuals a relationship of decreased mobility between psoas fascia and renal fascia in relation to nonspecific chronic low back pain. Around the kidney the capsula adiposa develops. It is a fascial fat layer like the subcutis, protecting the kidney against too much mobility. It is noteworthy that the

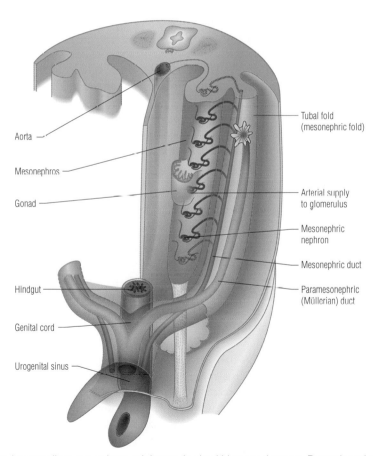

Fig. 1.13.7 The intermediate mesoderm originates in the kidney and ureter. Reproduced with permission from Standring, S. Ed., 2016. *Gray's Anatomy: The Anatomical Basis of Clinical Practice*, 41st ed. Elsevier, London, 1201, Fig. 72.3.

kidney has only an indirect relationship with the (parietal) peritoneum and is considered an extraperitoneal organ. The pelvic fasciae are situated outside the peritoneal cavity (extraperitoneal). They present an insertional fascia, a sacro-genito-vesicopubic lamina, derived from the somatopleure. This lamina is derived from mesenchymal cells that support the growth of the bladder, originating from the hindgut, endoderm, and the genitourinary system that develops from the intermediate mesoderm.

The developmental processes, as described previously, are related to the development of the dorsal (posterior) and ventral (anterior) mesogastrium that will give rise to all ligaments of the liver with the diaphragm, duodenum, and stomach. During their development the digestive tract, heart, and liver tend to "descend". In this way the primitive digestive and respiratory tubular structures, trachea and esophagus. The heart is formed in the posterior wall of the intraembryonic coelom in the thoracic region, and the liver and heart have an anterior (ventral) location. This anterior entrainment generates a space behind these organs, the pericardial cavity. The mesodermal tissue that follows the heart will give rise to the investing pericardium whereas the other layer, in contact with the skeleton, will give rise to the insertional pericardium, the sternal, and phrenicopericardial ligaments. This space formed between the heart, liver, and spine is called the heart-liver angle, and it creates a kind of "tissue vacuum" (Blechschmidt 2004). In this way space is opened for the development of a part of the foregut endoderm into the lungs. The growth of the endoderm brings with it a part of the intraembryonic coelom that will form the visceral pleura. The outermost layer of the coelom, formed by somatopleure, will give rise to the parietal pleura or insertional fascia of the lung. The inferior and lateral part of the coelom between the two mesodermal layers will give rise to the pleural recess. Part of this mesodermal pleura formation will contribute to the formation of the diaphragm.

Between the heart and the primitive liver (at first in the cervical region), the origin of a mesodermal structure called the transverse septum takes place. This structure is extremely important in the shaping of the thoracic and abdominal viscera. The "descending" of the heart, transverse septum, and liver from the cervical to the abdominal region takes place as the digestive system develops. The transverse septum is formed at the level of the fourth somite. This shows that the innervation of the diaphragm

and visceral fascial structures of the upper thoracic and abdominal region (phrenic nerve) originates from the cervical medulla spinalis (Allan and Greer 1997). The transverse septum will give rise to the tendinous center of the diaphragm. The main part of the (muscular) diaphragm is constituted by the pleuroperitoneal membrane, the mesentery of the esophagus and the ingrowing mesoderm of the sixth intercostal body wall segment. Because of this great embryonic diversity in formation, the diaphragm presents several innervations: the crura (lateral and medial) and the esophageal hiatus are innervated by the vagus nerve; the sternocostal part is sensitively innervated by the intercostal nerves T7 to T12; as to motor supply the diaphragm is innervated by the phrenic nerve (Wallden 2017). Alterations in the diaphragm can generate sensitization at several spinal level.

DEEP FASCIA OF THE MUSCULOSKELETAL SYSTEM

The musculoskeletal system, including the deep fasciae, originates mainly from the paraxial mesoderm (except for the viscerocranial bones [skull and face] that derive from the cranial neural crest mesenchyme). The paraxial mesoderm is organized in somites. Somite formation has to do with the metamerization of the trunk in which mesenchymal cell aggregates surround the neural tube and the notochord in a rhythmic way. Before the formation of those somites the nonsegmented mesoderm is located dorsolaterally, between the neural epithelium and the extraembryonic coelom. Somites first appear on the 23rd day as thick-walled vesicles. About 38 pairs of somites form during human development (days 20–30).

The dorsal part of the somite vesicle wall is close to the ectoderm. This part will eventually develop to the dermatomes that will form the subcutaneous skin of the back, neck, and trunk together with somatopleure (Schoenwolf et al. 2015). The metamerie of the skin is reflected in the innervation patterns of the cutaneous nerves that innervate the skin, epidermis, and dermis and contribute to the innervation of the superficial fascia, generating so-called (neurological) dermatomes.

The myotome develops in the intermediate zone of the somite, giving rise to the muscles, deep fasciae, and internal muscle fasciae (epimysium, perimysium, and endomysium). The innervation comes from the migration of neural crest cells to their somites and on its turn is organized in neurological myotomes. The formation of myotomes probably defines the innervation of the entire deep fascia. This nervous relationship seems to be necessary for the synchronization of motion components (Stecco et al. 2019). As the deep fascia is closely related to sympathetic innervation related to ECM vascular innervation, spinal cord segments corresponding with the (ortho)sympathetic nervous system may influence the deep fasciae (Schleip et al. 2019). Soon after the formation of somites, the myotome is divided into dorsal epimere and ventral hypomere. The epimere develops into the epaxial, deep back muscles and their respective fasciae, which are innervated by the dorsal branch of the spinal nerve. The hypomere gives rise to the hypaxial muscles and fasciae of the lateral and ventral walls of the thorax and the abdomen, which are innervated by the ventral branch of the spinal nerve.

The ventral part of the wall, which is close to the endoderm and dorsal aorta, will give rise to the sclerotomes.

The sclerotomes differentiate into vertebrae and ribs and most trunk bones.

At the end of the 1st month of life, the four limbs appear in the angular area between the neural tube and the mesothelial lining of the coelom. They form through the ventral and dorsal walls. The ventral wall gives rise to the axillary and inguinal fossae. The limb bones and sternum are formed from somatopleure and originate from the lateral mesoderm, unlike the muscles and bones of the trunk that originate from the paraxial mesoderm, that contributes to somitic formation. The different embryonic origin generates a difference (or shift) in the innervation of the dermatomes and myotomes in the limbs, a fact that does not occur in the trunk. Stecco et al. (2019) suggest that superficial fascia and skin are related to dermatome innervation whereas the deep fasciae and their respective limb compartments are related to myotome innervation. (Fig. 1.13.8)

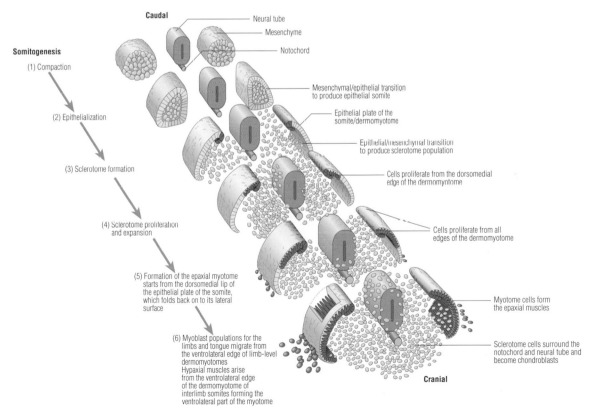

Fig. 1.13.8 Somitogenesis. Reproduced with permission from Standring, S., Ed., 2016. *Gray's Anatomy: The Anatomical Basis of Clinical Practice*, 41st ed. Elsevier, London, 752, Fig. 44.3.

Bones and periosteum are somitic derivatives of the paraxial mesoderm except for viscerocranium bones (Bordoni and Lagana 2019). The bones of the face present cranial peripheral innervation by the fifth (V) cranial nerve. Part of the trigeminal afferences synapse in the trigeminal spinal nucleus, which is found in the four cervical first levels, generating a potential for spinal cord sensitization at these levels.

CONCLUSION

The processes of embryological development are complex and fascinating. Understanding the origin of fasciae and of the "fascial system" can influence the choice of therapeutic approaches and may help understand the complex relationships of the human body.

Summary

The fascial system is complex, and this complexity begins immediately in its development in the human embryo. As environmental influences, metabolic responses integrated with genetics are relevant to fascial tissue and its neural interfaces, providing clinical associations between these systems.

REFERENCES

Allan, D.W., Greer, J.J., 1997. Embryogenesis of the phrenic nerve and diaphragm in the fetal rat. J. Comp. Neurol. 382, 459–468.

Arbuckle, B.E., 1994.The selected writings of Beryl E. Arbuckle, DO, FACOP. Indianapolis: American Academy of Osteopathy.

Bordoni, B., Lagana, M., 2019. Bone tissue is an integral part of the fascial system. Cureus 11, e3824.

Blechschmidt, E., 2004. The ontogenetic basis of human anatomy. Edited and translated by Brian Freeman. North Atlantic Books, Berkley, California, first ed.

Blechschmidt, E., Gasser, R., 2012. Biokinetics and Biodynamics of Human Differentiation. North Atlantic Books, Berkley, CA.

Brodal, P., 2010. The Central Nervous System: Structure and Function, fourth ed. Oxford University Press, Oxford, p. 19.

Douarin, N., Brito, J., Creuzet, S., 2007. Role of neural crest in the face and brain development. Brain Res. Rev. 55, 237–247.

Hill, M.A., 2019. Embryology Timeline human development. https://embryology.med.unsw.edu.au/embryology/index.php/Timeline_human_development.

Ingber, D., 1998. The architecture of life. Sci. Am. 278, 48–57.

Liem, T., 2002. La Osteopatia craneosacra, first ed. Editorial Paidotribo, Barcelona, Spain.

Lipton, B., 2005. The Biology of Belief: The Power of Consciousness Matter and Miracles. Elite Books, Santa Rosa, CA.

Moore, K. L., Persaud, T. V., N 2016. The Developing Human – Clinically Oriented Embryology. W.B. Saunders, Philadelphia.

O'Rahilly, R., Müller, F., 1990. Ventricular system and choroid plexuses of the human brain during the embryonic period proper. Am. J Anat.189, 285–302.

Sadler, T. W., 2019. Langman's Medical Embryology. Wolters Kluwer, Philadelphia, fourteenth ed.

Sasselli, V., Pachnis, V., Burns, A., 2012. The enteric nervous system. Dev. Biol. 366, 64–73.

Schleip, R., Gabbiani, G., Wilke, J., et al., 2019. Fascia can actively contract and may thereby influence musculoskeletal dynamics: a histochemical and mechanographic investigation. Front. Physiol. 10, 336.

Schoenwolf, G., Bleyl, S., Brauer, P., Francis-West, P., 2015. Larsen's human embryology. Elsevier Saunders, Philadelphia, PA, 5th ed.

Standring, S. (Ed.) 2016. Gray's Anatomy: The Anatomical Basis of Clinical Practice. Elsevier, UK, forty-first ed.

Stecco, C., Pirri, C., Fede, C., et al., 2019. Dermatome and fasciatome. Clin. Anat. 32, 896–902.

Stecco, L., Stecco, C., 2014. Fascial Manipulation for Internal Disfunctions. Piccin Nuova Libraria, Padova, Italy.

Tozzi, P., 2015. A unifying neuro-fasciogenic model of somatic dysfunction- Underlying mechanisms and treatment - Part 1. J. Bodyw. Mov. Ther. 19, 310–326.

Tozzi, P., Bongiorno, D., Vitturini, C., 2012. Low back pain and kidney mobility: local osteopathic fascial manipulation decreases pain perception and improves renal mobility. J. Bodyw. Mov. Ther. 16, 381–391.

Tubbs, R.S., Salter, G., Grabb, P.A., Oakes, W.J., 2001. The denticulate ligament: anatomy and functional significance. J. Neurosurg. 94 (Suppl. 2), 271–275.

Wallden, M., 2017. The diaphragm - more than an inspired design. J. Bodyw. Mov. Ther. 21, 342–349.

Warshafsky, D., Goldenberg, D., Kanekar, S., 2012. Imaging anatomy of deep neck spaces. Otolaryngol. Clin. N. Am. 45, 1203–1221.

BIBLIOGRAPHY

Hinrichsen, K. V., 1990. Human Embryologie. Springer-Verlag, Berlin.

Moore, K., Persaud, T. V. N, Torchia, M., 2016. Before we are born: Essentials of embryology and birth defects. Elsevier UK, ninth ed.

On the Origin of Fascia: A Phenomenological Embryology of Fascia as the "Fabric" of the Body

Jaap van der Wal

CHAPTER CONTENTS

ABOUT SO-CALLED GERM LAYERS

"Each being can only be understood from its becoming." In this way, the German biologist Ernst Haeckel (1866) summarized the importance of the embryological approach. If one wants to know more about the functional and anatomical significance of an organ, a tissue, it seems useful to examine its embryonic development. Knowing how a certain shape or structure came about simply tells more about what it is (Lesondak 2017). From the phenomenological stance the (functional) meaning of forms is more important than their causal explanation. The question as to the origin of fascia quickly can become a more morphological question: Where in the body do the relevant connective tissue structures arise? Here, however, the question of the origin of fascia has been addressed as a more philosophical item: How is fascia as the body matrix shaped and what does that mean?

With such questions, one usually ends up with the three so-called germ layers[a] (Sadler 2019). A germ layer may be defined as "a collection of cells that have the same

origin in embryogenesis and that will develop into specific body tissues" (Moore and Persaud 2016). The three germ layers in human development are formed during the so-called *gastrulation*, approximately in the third week after conception. In common embryology a germ layer is regarded as a morphological organ-forming unit from which the various tissues and organs develop, resulting in a functional organism. Embryology textbooks usually summarize which germ layer gives rise to which tissue types and to which organs (so-called derivatives).

Nowadays it is not possible to trace every organ or tissue one-to-one to a certain germ layer. Almost every organ is at least a "mixture" of several germ layer derivatives. For example, the intestine may be functionally described as a tube derived from endoderm, but it has a muscle wall derived from the so-called mesoderm. The eye is usually described as a derivative or bulge of the penultimate cerebral vesicle (diencephalon) and is therefore considered a derivative of the neuroderm (which was derived from the ectoderm). The element in the eye however that can be thought as derived from neuroderm is the retina; the eyeball itself with its sclera and extrinsic eye muscles for example are "mesoderm derivatives." Special feature of the mesenchyme of the head is that it

---

[a]Here the notion "layer" is preferred over the term "leaf."

is not a derivative of the "primary" mesenchyme that comes up during the formation of the three germ layers in the third week of development, but that it originates from a second "wave" of mesenchymal formation that appears to emerge from the neural crest of the neural tube (Le Douarin et al. 2012). Despite the nuances explained previously, in general the germinal layers are regarded as constituting elements of the body. This seems to support the idea that the body is "built up" from these three components and that various organs and tissues are derived from these three components (Table 1.14.1).

With their modern "anatomical mind" many people tend to think that organisms, that bodies are "made up of". For example of cells, of organs, of different germinal layers, which elements then are considered as "building blocks". They believe that, for example, we start as a cell, a so-called fertilized egg cell, and the body is the result—the product of cell multiplication and growth. In a phenomenological or organicistic view on development, however, we do not start as a cell but as a zygote, and a zygote is a (unicellular) body—an organism that from that moment on constantly (sub)organizes itself into cells via those cells differentiating into organs and tissues. The embryo itself demonstrates this by the phenomenon of so-called morphogenetic fields.[b] Blechschmidt (2011) refers to them as "kinetic metabolic fields." This means that, in the embryo, metabolic fields are constantly emerging, which is where

the cells, controlled by and in response to changing environment, differentiate into new types of cells. One can therefore just as well argue that embryonic existence (and therefore the entire existence of an organism) comes down to the preservation of its unity throughout all those different fields and differentiations. In this view the body, the organism, is not the product of the parts but is a self-organizing, emerging entity (unity).

WHERE DOES THE FASCIAL TISSUE COME FROM?

If one searches for anything like the "primeval fascia" or the "primary fascia," then one almost inevitably ends up with the so-called *mesenchyme*. The primary appearance of the mesoderm is mesenchyme (Blechschmidt 2012, 58–67). In the third week of human development a bilaminar disc consisting of *epiblast* (upper layer) and *hypoblast* (lower layer) is transformed with *gastrulation* in a trilaminar disc consisting of ectoderm, mesoderm, and endoderm. This tripartite or threefold organization is a necessary biological condition for the development of an animal or human body. Human beings that only consist of two germ layers are never born; a mesoderm is an absolutely necessary condition.

[b]In the developmental biology of the early twentieth century, a morphogenetic field is a group of cells able to respond to discrete, localized biochemical signals leading to the development of specific morphological structures or organs. This definition should not be confused with an extended view on this embryological notion as propagated by Sheldrake (2009).

> ### KEY POINT
>
> Three or Third? If the three germ layers are three of a kind, then the three germ layers could be considered as three equivalent or similar 'building block' elements of which the body is built up. However, a trilaminar germ disc actually already represents the animal body organization, i.e. two walls/limiting tissues with a different third dimension in between i.e. the 'meso' representing the inner or interior body.

TABLE 1.14.1	Germ layers
The endoderm forms	pharynx, esophagus, stomach, small intestine, colon, liver, pancreas, bladder, epithelial parts of the trachea and bronchi, lungs, thyroid, and parathyroid.
The mesoderm forms	muscle (smooth and striated), bone, cartilage, connective tissue, adipose tissue, circulatory system, lymphatic system, dermis, genitourinary system, serous membranes, and notochord.
The ectoderm forms	the surface ectoderm: epidermis, hair, nails, lens of the eye, sebaceous glands, cornea, tooth enamel, the epithelium of the mouth and nose; the neural crest of the ectoderm develops into: peripheral nervous system, adrenal medulla, melanocytes, facial cartilage, dentin of teeth; the neural tube of the ectoderm develops into: brain, spinal cord, posterior pituitary, motor neurons, retina.

Source: Wikipedia Germ Layer, https://creativecommons.org/licenses/by-sa/3.0/.

Mesoderm is semantically almost an impossible word. What should it mean: three skins with one skin in the middle? A middle skin? *Gray's Anatomy* (Standring 2016) indicates that it is not correct to consider the trilaminar disc as being constituted by three **epithelial** layers. The usual notions are ectoderm, mesoderm, and endoderm (sometimes referred as ectoblast, mesoblast, and endoblast). By applying the same epitheton (whether -derm or -blast) for all three components, the concept that it concerns three more-or-less equivalent constituent elements of the human body is implied. If, however, one looks at the situation histologically, this does not appear to be the case. The mesoderm initially manifests itself as a connective tissue, whereas the other two layers clearly have the character of an epithelium. The German embryologist Erich Blechschmidt (Blechschmidt 2004, 2011) urgently pointed out that here the primordial principle of a human (and also animal) body is emerging. This means a body (body organization) is characterized by two boundary layers (the term *limiting tissue* was suggested) and an intermediate "layer" of tissue in between that can be referred to as an *inner tissue*. So, the trilaminar disc is about an animal organization plan: the adult animal (including the human being) is characterized by an existence in an anatomical and psychosomatic "inner space" between two body walls. An outer (parietal) body wall (from which later limbs and head also develop) and an inner (visceral) body wall (from which later, in broad outlines, the gut and derivatives develop).

In such a vision the terms ectoderm and entoderm can be maintained as indeed the substrate or primordium of the later skins (derm = skin) or body walls or boundaries. But for the mesoderm, the epitheton "derm" no longer holds true because mesenchyme is quite a different quality of tissue: a connective tissue. Here one can speak of "inner tissue" (in German, *innegewebe*). Therefore, the term "meso" is used to emphasize that it is not a matter of three layers but of a three-part ("triune") body with an inner dimension (Fig. 1.14.1).

So "meso" (and mesenchyme) comes from a completely different perspective that can also provide a special dimension to the understanding of fascia. In Blechschmidt's view, in every tissue all cells are always kinetic or metabolically linked to each other through the transport of substances. "There are cells that absorb nutrients from the environment or from neighboring cells and mutually attract each other through this physical absorption of substances. On the other hand, they

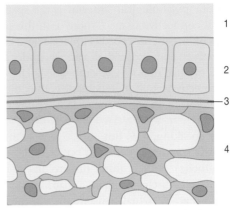

Fig. 1.14.1 Schematic diagram of the two basic tissues: limiting tissue and inner tissue. 1, Fluid; 2, cells of limiting tissue; pink: glycocalyx. 3, Basement membrane. 4, Inner tissue; light pink: intercellular material of inner tissue. Redrawn with permission from Blechschmidt E., 2012, Ontogenese des Menschen: Kinetische Anatomie, Kiener Verlag, Munchen, p. 58.

also exert mutual rejection by producing and shedding metabolic by-products. This constant interaction between uptake and excretion, between attraction and repulsion is a condition for cells to organize themselves in relation to each other and thereby to bring about certain forms. Limiting tissue forms the boundary between fluid on the one hand and the inner tissue on the other, while the inner tissues is surrounded on all sides by boundary tissues and therefore permanently 'on the inside', that is: IN the body. Inner tissue can therefore also be described as undifferentiated connective tissue (mesenchyme)" (Blechschmidt 2012).

This idea or model as applied to the adult (human) body may give a different perspective on the dimension "inner." The organs that are usually described as viscera can therefore be considered as a body wall that limits us to the outside world and enables mainly metabolic and material interaction with that outer environment. The designation "inside" is therefore meant literally; it is an inside body wall. The viscera therefore do not represent our (psychosomatic) "inner" or "innerness." Another body wall (which could therefore by analogy be called "outside-wall") forms our parietal boundary to the world. This body wall also allows us to relate to the outside world and allows (a different kind of) interaction with it—namely, perception and action. As the substrate of our so-called (psychosomatic) inner, the "meso" remains the "in between." One could argue that our "anatomical" (but also our psychological) interior is the spatiality of the original connective tissue ("meso"). In this inner, all organs (including the so-called ectodermal and endodermal derivatives and those that can be understood as derivatives of the "meso") are embedded. The original primal connective tissue mesenchyme is thus the matrix tissue, the "fabrica" in which the organs are embroidered (Levin 2012).[c]

Broadly speaking, it is not 1, 2, 3 times "the same" (three "blasts" or three "derms"), but it is (1 + 1) two limits (epithelia) with a third dimension in between them. Whereas epithelia are characterized by the fact that intercellular space is virtually absent, the absolute characteristic of mesenchyme or inner tissue is the existence of (interstitial) space between the cells. This extracellular matrix (ECM) or *interstitium* can be "filled" or formed by all kinds of substances (from interstitial organic "water" to cartilage substance or calcified bone matrix) and also always contains a third dimension—namely, *fibers* of all possible nature and quality. In this way, concepts such as fascia, connective tissue, matrix, and inner space are aligned, and it is very well possible to conceive that meso and thus fascia represents the matrix, the "fabric" of our body organization.

MESENCHYME, "TISSUE OF INNERNESS"? FASCIA, "ORGAN OF INNERNESS"?

In the previously mentioned quote from Blechschmidt, reference is made to uptake and excretion and attraction and rejection as principles of interaction between cells. These principles of relationship can also be attributed to fascia, mesenchyme, and connective tissue. Mechanically, histologically, and embryologically, one can think of two different types of interactions in the mesenchyme—namely, connecting and creating space (separation). These two dimensions have all kinds of histological and physiological appearances.

> ### KEY POINT
>
> Connecting and shaping space: Connective tissue (supporting tissue) is not only about "connection." Creating space and enabling body cavities (joint cavities) are (morphogenetic) functions of connective tissue. "Dis-connecting" enables movement. This also concerns muscle, not purely contractile tissue, which is able to connect (shortening) and shape space lengthening.

It is possible that the cell component of the mesenchyme becomes dominant. Then the cells and thereby the mesenchyme condense into (almost) purely cellular agglomerations. This is the case, for example, in fat or muscle tissue. The cells form a parenchyma embedded in a fibrous matrix. Stephen Levin (2021) said, "Think away the parenchyma of muscle cells from the muscle tissue and you get a band or ligament." The opposite (shedding of the cells, in Blechschmidt's jargon) could then be recognized in the ability of the mesenchyme to create body cavities. Consider the pleural cavities or peritoneal cavity.[d] They are not cavities, but rather "joint fissures," where two organs or a body wall and organs encounter each other but can still move against each other (contiguity). One could rightly call this the principle of creating space that makes movement possible. The mesenchyme in this case is almost "cell and fiber empty." This is how joint fissures and body cavities become movement organs.

Apply the concept of connecting and creating space to the "fascia in a broader sense." The fascia in a broader sense is that often-discussed network or system that is present everywhere in the body and that forms the "tensional network" (Schleip 2012) of our body in which all organs and structures are interwoven and embedded. In short, it is the mature representation of our "mesodermal inner" and the primary mesenchymal framework of

---

[c]Remarkably, the Latin term *fabrica* (the first book by Andreas Vesalius was entitled *De Humani Corporis Fabrica*) initially reminds us of a factory or construction, in other words, a space or building. However, the Latin word *fabrica* also means something like fabric or texture. So, mesenchyme represents the matrix in which parts are embedded, which connects the various parts with each other and creates the space between them.

[d]Pleural membranes and peritoneal membranes are often histologically described as a "mesothelium." This is an epithelium formed by mesenchyme (connective tissue). The essential difference is that the mesothelium defines an interstitial space (in fact, actively creates it) and that an epithelium usually defines an outside wall or a lumen of a tube. A mesothelium also tends to stick and adhere if the (sliding) movement that is enabled is no longer practiced. With a body cavity such as the oral cavity, covered with epithelium, that tendency will not be as pronounced.

the body, with possibly a regulatory role on multiple function levels. The fascia in the narrower sense is then the subcutaneous collection of anatomically recognizable connective tissue structures that connect, support, and enclose muscles, bones, nerves and blood vessels, and other internal organs in the form of layers, membranes, fasciae, and envelopes (Stecco 2015).

Give the two previously mentioned tendencies vectors, then the picture quickly emerges that "meso" (mesenchyme) can concentrate (densify, connect, contract) on the one hand and on the other hand may decentralize (open, create space, stretch). The two polar tendencies in the inner tissue (connective tissue) can of course also be seen in the different qualities of interstitial substance or in different relationships between fibers, cells, and interstitium. It's not for nothing that most anatomy textbooks speak of supportive and connective tissue.

So, it is proposed here to also consider body cavities and joint clefts as functions of fascia. The subcutaneous connective tissue, for example, is a loose connective tissue with a lot of interstitial space between the fibers. The functional principle focuses on separating, creating space, and enabling motion (Guimberteau and Armstrong 2015) like in tendon and muscle sheaths. In bursae the fibers are absent, a kind of "body cavity." Intermuscular septa—the classical fasciae like epimysia, fascia ante brachii, fascia lata, and many more—are meant to connect and guide tensile forces. In such case, the appearance of fascia is quite different. The fibers are dense, tight, and dominant, so that there is hardly any room for interstitium or cells (the so-called regular dense collagenous connective tissue, or RDCCT). This concerns the typical fascial layers dominating in the posture and locomotion system (PLS),[e] as described by Schleip et al. (2012), Van der Wal (2009), and Stecco (2015).

---

[e]Here the notion PLS (posture and locomotion system) is preferred for reasons that will be clear in the text. "System" is used instead of "apparatus" because the anatomical "locomotion apparatus" (consisting of bones, joints, ligaments, and muscles) is a too narrow-minded concept; at least the nervous system should be partly incorporated in order to function as a PLS. Posture and locomotion because "locomotion" is too poor a notion: in humans standing in equilibrium (posture) is typical and essential, keeping one's upright position is an integral part of our bipedal locomotion. The notion of musculoskeletal system will be shown in this text as a poor and reductionistic concept that should be abandoned.

It may also be the interstitial substance of mesenchyme or fascia that forms the mechanically connecting (or separating!) dimension. Consider in this context cartilage or bone tissue. Cartilage is known to be equipped with collagen fibers (fibrous cartilage), with elastic fibers (elastic cartilage), or with a much lower fiber content (hyaline cartilage). Often cartilage serves a relatively flexible connecting dimension or creates forms (ear). Cartilage can also serve mobility by the space-creating principle, as is the case in the fissures of the synovial joints, and sometimes also becomes visible in the formation of fissures in symphyses and the intervertebral discs.

The interstitium is the third dimension of fascia and mesenchyme. It forms in principle a hugely extensive space that can be found everywhere between organs, structures, and tissue elements. It therefore can be regarded as one large continuous "interanatomical" body cavity along which communication, coordination, and organization are also possible by means of substances (Benias et al. 2018; Oschman 2015). It is known from embryology inducing signal proteins are organized and distributed via the mesenchyme. The demonstrated gradients of epigenetic control molecules could also be established via diffusion through the interstitial space. During human embryonic development the meso provides the metabolic conditions for the development of the ectodermal structures and plays a role in their differentiation (Blechschmidt and Gasser 2012).

> ### KEY POINT
> Innerness and matrix: The mesenchyme forms—together with the blood and tissue—the matrix in which all organs are embedded and embroidered. It creates the necessary inner space and at the same time the equally necessary relationships, continuity, and coherence—what keeps us together.

Mesenchyme is always associated in the embryo with the formation of blood and blood vessels. Blood is not a fluid but a tissue and is categorized in many histology textbooks as supportive or connective tissue. The primary manifestation of blood is mesenchyme, in which (via the formation of blood islands and blood strands) capillary vessels are formed that then transport "liquid tissue"—that is, blood cells. The vast network of capillaries (estimates vary from 60,000–90,000 km!) performs what is typical for connective tissue—connecting and creating space in a dynamic way. Organs are connected by means of blood, but during evolution in animals the (perhaps also psychological) inner space for the organism can become larger as blood allows it. Mesenchymal structures may connect the organs and body parts during development in a more mechanical way; the accompanying blood ensures exchange and intermediary contact. Blood vessels (often as neurovascular bundles) can play a role in shaping the body. A strand of connective tissue surrounding a vascular structure may function as a restraining structure providing resistance and biomechanical constraint to growth, with flexion growth as consequence (for example, in developing limbs or of the pharyngeal arches) (Blechschmidt 2004).

The widespread presence of capillaries throughout the body also makes it possible to visualize the image of the fascia in a broader sense as the matrix tissue in which all organs are woven and embedded. With the corrosion technique, one can make casts of the capillary network. It is interesting that in the spatial form of such a cast one can immediately see the overall shape of the organism or organ from which the cast is made. The "anatomy" of the blood therefor makes the spatial organization of the body visible: blood and fascia "take the shape of the body" and literally create the web in which everything is embedded (Fig. 1.14.2).

IN FASCIA IT IS ABOUT TWO—BIOTENSEGRITY

A theoretical and philosophical view of fascia in a broader sense is put into words by Stephen Levin when he claims that "fascia forms the fabric of our body and that in this fabric all organs are somehow woven or embroidered" (Levin and Martin 2012). Mechanically one can think of two forces in the fascial connective tissue system: pressure and pull. The entire PLS can therefore in a certain sense be considered a biotensegrity system with compacted elements (skeletal elements) on the one hand and pull transmitting elements (ligaments, fasciae, muscles, and "dynaments") on the other. Therefore, it is no longer considered as a skeleton that is held together by means of connective tissue capsules and ligaments, which function as hinges and joints, and then is set in motion by a separate muscle apparatus. To understand a tensegrity system, one needs the tension as well as the compression (the stiff element), as "Islands of compression floatingly suspended

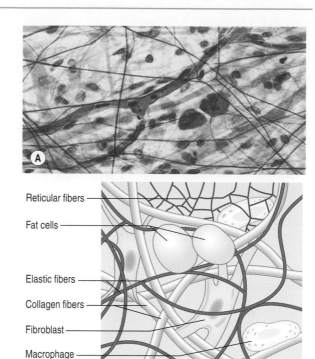

Reticular fibers

Fat cells

Elastic fibers

Collagen fibers

Fibroblast

Macrophage

Fig. 1.14.2 Histological image (A) and a schematic diagram (B) of primeval connective tissue (areolar connective tissue). Image (A) shows the three essential components of inner tissue (cells, fibers, and interstitium or ECM) and the blood component of inner tissue as the tracery of capillaries. (A) Reproduced with permission from Patton, K.T., Thibodeau, G.A., 2020, *Structure & Function of the Body*, 16th ed., Elsevier, St Louis, MO. (B) Redrawn from Anatomy and Physiology, Connexions website, OpenStax College, June 19, 2013, Creative Commons. Accessed online at https://openstax.org/books/anatomy-and-physiology/pages/1-introduction.

in a balanced sea of tension" (Myers 2020). With fascia, it is always associated with TWO functions: push and pull. So, apparatus components like muscles, ligaments, fasciae, and bones can also be interpreted as specializations of a body-wide connective tissue matrix or system (fascia in a broader sense). Bone is fascia (Sharkey 2019), muscle is fascia (Levin and Martin 2012), and dynaments are fascia (Van der Wal 2009). In this context, it has been suggested by Pauwels (1960) that the differentiation of primitive mesenchyme to the various derivatives might also be governed and influenced by mechanical stimuli like deformation (pulling) and compression stimulating to collagenous connective tissue, respectively cartilage and ossification. Blechschmidt also proposed the existence of kinetic metabolic morphogenetic fields like contusion, dilation, retention, and so on (Blechschmidt 2004, 2012).

All this is a logical consequence of the idea that fascia in a broader sense coincides with the mesoderm or, rather, "meso." Even more specifically: the concept of mesenchyme as "inner tissue" may also give an opening to the "nonscientific" concept of A.T. Still that the fascia in a broader sense could possibly be regarded as the "space of the soul": "The soul of man, with all the streams of pure living water, seems to dwell in the fascia of his body" (A.T. Still, as quoted in Lee 2005). The further elaboration of this possible psychosomatic body concept is not a subject of this chapter. Here an attempt has been made to show that fascia in a broader sense may represent "in a broader sense" our inner being.

Summary

The method par excellence for understanding the organization of the body and its systems and organs is the study of "becoming," i.e. the embryology of fascia. The primordial fascia is the mesenchyme that, in turn, is the primary appearance of the so-called mesoderm. This "meso" can also be understood as the matrix of "fabric" of the body.

REFERENCES

Benias, P.C., Wells, R.G., Sackey-Aboagye, B., et al., 2018. Structure and distribution of an unrecognized interstitium in human tissues, Sci. Rep. 8: 4947.

Blechschmidt, E., 2004. The Ontogenetic Basis of Human Anatomy, first ed. (B. Freeman, trans.). North Atlantic Books, Berkley, California.

Blechschmidt, E., 2011. Die Frühentwicklung des Menschen – Eine Einführung. Kiener Verlag, Munich.

Blechschmidt, E., 2012. Ontogenese des Menschen – Kinetische Anatomie. Kiener Verlag, Munich.

Blechschmidt, E., Gasser, R., 2012. Biokinetics and Biodynamics of Human Differentiation. North Atlantic Books, Berkley, CA.

Guimberteau, J.C., Armstrong, C. 2015. Architecture of Human Living Fascia: Cells and Extracellular Matrix Revealed through Endoscopy (book and DVD). Handspring Publishing, Pencaitland, East Lothian, Scotland.

Haeckel, Ernst, 1866. Allgemeine Anatomie der Organismen, Drittes Kapitel, Seite 23, Verlag Georg Reimer, Berlin.

Le Douarin, N.M., Couly, G., Creuzet, S.E., 2012. The neural crest is a powerful regulator of preotic brain development. Dev. Biol. 366, 74–82.

Lee, Paul, R., 2005. Interface, Mechanisms of Spirit in Osteopathy. Stillness Press, Portland OR, 61. From Still, AT, 1892, The Philosophy and Mechanical Principles of Osteopathy.

Lesondak, 2017. Fascia: What It Is and Why It Matters. Handspring Publishing, Pencaitland, Scotland.

Levin, S.M., 2021. In: Susan C Lowell de Solórzano, Everything Moves, p. 35–39.

Levin, S.M, Martin, D.C., 2012. Biotensegrity: The Mechanics of Fascia. In: R. Schleip, T. Findley, L. Chaitow, P.A. Huijing (eds.), Fascia: The Tensional Network of the Human Body. Churchill Livingstone, Edinburgh., 137–142.

Moore, K.L., Persaud, T.V.N., 2016. The Developing Human – Clinically Oriented Embryology. W.B. Saunders Company, Philadelphia.

Myers, T.W., 2020. Tension-dependent structures in a stretch-activated system. J Bodyw Mov Ther. 24, 131-133.

Oschman, J., 2015. Energy Medicine - E-Book: The Scientific Basis. Churchill Livingstone; London.

Pauwels, F., 1960. Eine neue Theorie über den Einfluß mechanischer Reize auf die Differenzierung der Stützgewebe. 10. Beitrag z. funktionellen Anatomie und kausalen Morphogenese des Stützapparates. Zeitschrift für Anatomie und Entwicklungsgeschichte. 121, 478.

Sadler, T.W., 2019. Langman's Medical Embryology, fourteenth ed. Wolters Kluwer, Philadelphia.

Schleip, R., Findley, T.W., Chaitow, L., Huijing. P.A. (eds.), 2012. Fascia - The tensional network of the human body. Churchill Livingstone Elsevier, Edinburgh.

Sharkey, J., 2019. Regarding: Update on fascial nomenclature-an additional proposal by John Sharkey. J. Bodyw Mov. Ther. 23, 6–8.

Sheldrake, R., 2009. Morphic Resonance - The Nature of Formative Causation, 4th edition, Inner Traditions Bear and Company.

Standring, S., 2016. Gray's Anatomy: The Anatomical Basis of Clinical Practice, forty-first ed. Elsevier, UK.

Stecco, C., 2015. Functional Atlas of the Human Fascial System. Churchill Livingstone Elsevier, Edinburgh

van der Wal, J., 2009. The architecture of the connective tissue in the musculoskeletal system - an often overlooked functional parameter as to proprioception in the locomotor apparatus. Int. J. Ther. Massage Bodywork 2, 9–23.

Communication

Fascia as an Organ of Communication

Robert Schleip

The previous part of this textbook demonstrated the topographical continuity and the specialized local adaptations of the global fascial network. Agreed, it is possible to dissect this continuous network into hundreds of different sheets and bundles, provided one is sufficiently talented in working with a surgical scalpel and given one has a clearly depicted guideline on where to place the cuts. However, when left without a dissection manual and looking at the tissue alone, it becomes apparent that all of those whitish collagenous membranes and envelopes seem to act together as one interconnected fibrous network. Nevertheless, for decades, ligaments, joint capsules, and other dense fascial tissues have been regarded as mostly inert tissues and have primarily been considered for their biomechanical properties.

Already during the 1990s advances were being made in recognizing the proprioceptive nature of ligaments, which subsequently influenced the guidelines for knee and other joint injury surgeries (Johansson et al. 1991). Similarly, the plantar fascia has been shown to contribute to the sensorimotor regulation of postural control in standing (Erdemir and Piazza 2004).

This chapter explores the potential of the fascial network as one of our richest sensory organs. Given the right stature, the overall mass and volume of our muscle fibers may be bigger than that of the fascial body. However, the surface area of the many million endomysial sacs and other membranous pockets endows this network with a total surface area that by far surpasses that of the skin or any other body tissue. Interestingly, compared with muscular tissue's innervation with muscle spindles, the fascial network possesses a higher quantity of sensory nerve receptors than its red muscular counterpart.

When it comes to the relative quantity of innervating nerves some of the most detailed data can be found from the respective numbers of axons in cat calf muscle tissues (Mitchell and Schmidt 1983). Fig. 2.1.1 shows the respective proportions for both efferent and afferent nerve fibers. A detailed quantitative analysis of the sensory innervation of cat calf muscles reveals that the proportion of nonspindle afferents found in these tissues is about six times larger compared with those neurons innervating the muscle spindles. This includes many different types of sensory receptors, including the usually myelinated proprioceptive endings (Golgi, Pacini, and Ruffini endings), but also a myriad of tiny unmyelinated "free" nerve endings, the latter of which are found almost everywhere in fascial tissues, but particularly in periosteum, in endomysial and perimysial layers, and in visceral connective tissues.

But how does our body-wide fascial net compare in terms of sensory nerve supply with other tissues in the human body? A detailed calculation by Martin Grunwald estimated the quantity of nerve endings in the body-wide fascial net as 100 million (Grunwald 2017). However, this calculation related to the total mass of dense fibrous connective tissues only, which based on Tanaka and Kawamura (1992) was estimated at 5 kg for an average male body. Nevertheless, there are good reasons for including the loose connective tissues into the calculation: not only because these tissues are part of the modern functional definition of "the fascial net" (Adstrum et al. 2017), but also because of the reported tendency for an even higher innervation density in the loose subcutaneous connective tissue compared with the denser fascial layers underneath (Tesarz et al. 2011). When taking these looser connective tissues into account, combined with the average human body data from Tanaka and Kawamura (1992), the mass of fibrous connective tissues

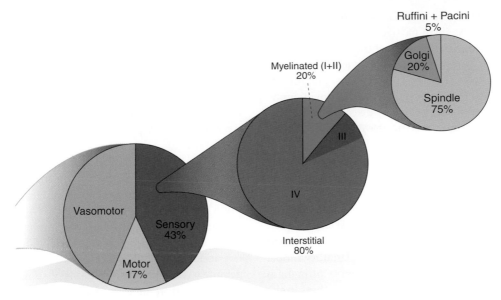

Fig. 2.1.1 Composition of Neurons Supplying a Musculoskeletal Tissue Region. The quantities of respective axons shown here are derived from detailed analysis of the combined nerve supplying the lateral gastrocnemius and soleus muscle in a cat (Mitchell and Schmidt 1983). While a small portion of the interstitial neurons may terminate inside bone, the remaining neurons can all be considered to terminate in fascial tissues. Even the sensory devices called muscle spindles are nestled within fibrous collagenous intramuscular tissues (usually within the perimysium), and their specific sensitivity is therefore greatly influenced by the compliance or stiffness of their fascial environment. Interstitial neurons terminate as free nerve endings. Some of them clearly seem to have a proprioceptive, an interoceptive, or a nociceptive main function. Investigations, however, suggest that the majority of interstitial neurons in fascia serve a polymodal function, meaning that they are open for function as a signaling device for more than one of these sensorial categories. Illustration courtesy fascialnet.com.

in the human body increases to 12.5 kg (representing 17% of the total body weight).

With this more realistic mass of the complete fascial system in mind, the total quantity of nerve endings in the fascial net can then be estimated to be approximately 2.5 times larger than the 100 million endings suggested by Grunwald, thus we arrive at the impressive number of 250 million nerve endings in the fascial net. Compared with an estimated quantity of 200 million nerve endings in the skin (Grunwald 2017) or with the estimated 126 million endings for vision in our eyes, this new calculation suggests that the body-wide fascial network may possibly constitute our richest sensory organ.

While the richness of innervation in the fascial net is certainly impressive, it could also be argued that fascia may also constitute our most important perceptual organ for perceiving our own body—whether it consists of pure proprioception, nociception, or the more visceral interoception (Schleip 2003). These three areas of

somatic self-perception will therefore be examined in detail in the following pages.

Many years ago, the author was involved in a dispute between instructors of the Feldenkrais Method of somatic education (Buchanan and Ulrich 2001) and teachers of the Rolfing Method of Structural Integration (Jacobson 2011). Advocates of the second group had claimed that many postural restrictions are due to pure mechanical adhesions and restrictions within the fascial network, whereas the leading figures of the first group suggested that "it's all in the brain,"—that is, that most restrictions are due to dysfunctions in sensorimotor regulation. In support of the sensorial hypothesis they cited the vividly published report of Trager (Trager et al. 1987; Juhan 2003), who had observed the disappearance of many muscular restrictions during general anesthesia in many of his patients. Subsequently, a small experiment was set up involving several representatives of those two schools, in which three patients undergoing orthopedic surgery gave their consent for having their range of motion tested (in passive arm elevation as well as foot dorsiflexion) in the surgical theater immediately before and after commencement of general anesthesia. Given the limited scientific rigor of this preliminary investigation, the result nevertheless was convincing to all involved: Most of the previously detected restrictions appeared to be significantly improved (if not absent) during the conditions of anesthesia. It seemed that what had been perceived as mechanical tissue fixation may at least be partially due to neuromuscular regulation (Fujishiro et al. 2013; Hollmann et al. 2018). The ongoing interdisciplinary dispute after this event led to a re-thinking of traditional concepts of myofascial therapies, and several years later a first neurologically oriented model was published as a proposed explanatory model for the effects of myofascial manipulation (Cottingham 1985), later copied and expanded by many others in the field (Chaitow and DeLany 2000; Schleip 2003).

While fascial stretch therapies and manual fascial therapies often seem to have positive effects on palpatory tissue stiffness and passive joint mobility, it is still unclear which exact physiological processes may be underlying these responses. Some of the potential mechanisms will be addressed in the clinical section of this book (Chapters 7.1–7.29); they may be due to dynamic changes in water content of the ground substance, altered link proteins in the matrix, and a different molecular expression of hyaluronan, as well as other factors. However, today an increasing number of practitioners are basing their concepts to some extent on the mechanosensory nature of the fascial net and its assumed ability to respond to skillful stimulation of its various sensory receptors.

The questions then are: What do we really know about the sensory capacity of fascia? And what specific physiological responses can we expect to elicit in response to stimulation of various fascial receptors?

This second part of our textbook will explore some of these intriguing questions. The first chapter in this part will be of particular interest, as it gives a solid overview on what is currently known of the importance of fascial tissues for our sense of proprioception. While, in the past, much emphasis was placed on joint receptors (being located in joint capsules and associated ligaments), current investigations indicate that more superficially placed mechanoreceptors, particularly in the transitional area between the fascia profunda and the fascia superficialis, seem to be endowed with an exceptionally rich density of proprioceptive nerve endings (Stecco et al. 2008). Although this may be relevant for the practice (and often profound beneficial effects) of skin taping in sports medicine—as well as for other therapeutic fields—further research is necessary to confirm whether the innervation of this superficial fascial layer does indeed play a leading role in proprioceptive regulation.

The sensory nature of fascia also includes its potential for nociception. The chapter on this concept is written by leading experts in that field, all from Heidelberg University. They summarize their many years of research about the nociceptive potential of the lumbar fascia. Their choice of the lumbar fascia as field of inquiry is, of course, not accidental. While some cases of low back pain are definitely caused by deformations of spinal discs, several large magnetic resonance imaging studies clearly revealed that for the majority of low back pain cases the origin may have to be searched for elsewhere in the body, as the discal alterations are often purely incidental (Jensen et al. 1994; Sheehan 2010). Based on this background, a new hypothetical explanation model for low back pain was proposed by Panjabi (2006) and subsequently elaborated on by others (Langevin and Sherman 2007; Schleip et al. 2007). According to these authors, microinjuries in lumbar connective tissues may lead to nociceptive signaling and further downstream effects associated with low back pain. The new findings from the Heidelberg group—reported in the next chapters—concerning the nociceptive potential of the lumbar fascia therefore promise to have potentially huge implications for the diagnosis and treatment of low back pain. As this is a newly emerging field, their research will definitely trigger further research investigations into this important (and very costly) field within modern health care.

Two other chapters will complete this part. One will cover the newly rediscovered field of fascial interoception, which relates to mostly subconscious signaling from free nerve endings in the body's viscera—as well as other tissues—informing the brain about the physiological state of the body. Although sensations from proprioceptive receptors are usually projected via the somatomotor cortex, signaling from interoceptive endings is processed via the insula region in the brain and is often associated with an emotional or motivational component. This field also promises interesting implications for the understanding and treatment of disorders with a somatoemotional component, such as irritable bowel syndrome, fibromyalgia, or posttraumatic stress disorder.

Finally, this part includes inspiring perspectives on non-neural communication dynamics within the fascial network. We invite the reader to read these pages with a healthy attitude of skeptical curiosity, because some of the potential mechanisms presented appear to be of a hypothetical nature. However, it would certainly not be the first time within the fascinating field of fascia research that a hypothesis previously considered daring might lead to new and substantial insights with clear clinical applications.

REFERENCES

Adstrum, S., Hedley, G., Schleip, R., Stecco, C., Yukesoy, C.A., 2017. Defining the fascial system. J. Bodyw. Mov. Ther. 21, 173–177.

Buchanan, P.A., Ulrich, B.D., 2001. The Feldenkrais Method: a dynamic approach to changing motor behavior. Res. Q. Exerc. Sport 72, 315–323.

Chaitow, L., DeLany, J.W., 2000. Clinical Application of Neuromuscular Techniques, vol. 1. Churchill Livingstone, Edinburgh.

Cottingham, J.T., 1985. Healing Through Touch – A History and Review of the Physiological Evidence. Rolf Institute Publications, Boulder, Colorado.

Erdemir, A., Piazza, S.J., 2004. Changes in foot loading following plantar fasciotomy: a computer modeling study. J. Biomech. Eng. 126, 237–243.

Fujishiro, T., Hayashi, S., Kanzaki, N., et al., 2013. Evaluation of preoperative hip range of motion under general anaesthesia. Hip Int. 23, 298–302.

Grunwald, M., 2017. Homo Hapticus. Droemer Verlag, Munich.

Hollmann, L., Halaki, M., Kamper, S.J., Haber, M., Ginn, K.A., 2018. Does muscle guarding play a role in range of motion loss in patients with frozen shoulder? Musculoskelet Sci. Pract. 37, 64–68.

Jacobson, E., 2011. Structural integration, an alternative method of manual therapy and sensorimotor education. J. Altern. Complement. Med. 17, 891–899.

Jensen, M.C., Brant-Zawadzki, M.N., Obuchowski, N., et al. 1994. Magnetic resonance imaging of the lumbar spine in people without back pain. N. Engl. J. Med. 331, 69–73.

Johansson, H., Sjölander, P., Sojka, P., 1991. A sensory role for the cruciate ligaments. Clin. Orthop. Relat. Res. 268, 161–178.

Juhan, D., 2003. Job's Body: A Handbook for Bodywork. Station Hill Press, Barrytown, New York.

Langevin, H.M., Sherman, K.J., 2007. Pathophysiological model for chronic low back pain integrating connective tissue and nervous system mechanisms. Med. Hypotheses 68, 74–80.

Mitchell, J.H., Schmidt, R.F., 1983. Cardiovascular reflex control by afferent fibers from skeletal muscle receptors. In: Shepherd, J.T., Abboud, F.M., (eds.), Handbook of Physiology, Section 2, The cardiovascular system, vol. III, Part 2. American Physiological Society, Bethesda, MA, pp. 623–658.

Panjabi, M.M., 2006. A hypothesis of chronic back pain: ligament subfailure injuries lead to muscle control dysfunction. Eur. Spine J. 15, 668–767.

Schleip, R., 2003. Fascial plasticity—a new neurobiological explanation. Part 1 2003 J. Bodyw. Mov. Ther. 7, 11–19.

Schleip, R., Vleeming, A., Lehmann-Horn, F., Klingler, W., 2007. Letter to the Editor concerning "A hypothesis of chronic back pain: ligament subfailure injuries lead to muscle control dysfunction" (M. Panjabi). Eur. Spine J. 16, 1733–1735.

Sheehan, N.J., 2010. Magnetic resonance imaging for low back pain: indications and limitations. Ann. Rheum. Dis. 69, 7–11.

Stecco, C., Porzionato, A., Lancerotto, L., et al., 2008. Histological study of the deep fasciae of the limbs. J. Bodyw. Mov. Ther. 12, 225–230.

Tanaka, G., Kawamura, H., 1992. Reference Man Models Based on Normal Data from Human Populations. Report of the Task Group on Reference Man, The International Commission on Radiological Protection, Nr. 23. Available from: http://www.irpa.net/irpa10/cdrom/00602.pdf.

Tesarz, J., Hoheisel, U., WiedenhoÄàfer, B., Mense, S. 2011. Sensory innervation of the thoracolumbar fascia in rats and humans. Neuroscience 194: 302–308.

Trager, M., Guadagno-Hammond, C., Turnley Walker, T., 1987. Trager mentastics: movement as a way to agelessness. Station Hill Press, Barrytown, NY.

Proprioception

Jaap van der Wal

PROPRIOCEPTION, MECHANORECEPTION, AND THE ANATOMY OF FASCIA

It may be assumed without doubt that the connective tissue continuum of fasciae and fascial tissue also serves as a body-wide mechanosensitive signaling system with an integrating function analogous to that of the nervous system and therefore also plays a substantial role in the process of proprioception (Langevin 2006; Stecco et al. 2007b; Benjamin 2009; Van der Wal 2009). Fascial structures like epi- and perimysia, membranes, septa, or superficial fascia are an intricate and integrated part of the organization of the so-called position and locomotion system (Wood Jones 1944; Standring 2005). To play its functional role in proprioception, a fascial structure should be equipped with adequate neurophysiological substrate (mainly mechanoreceptors). For the quality of the centripetal information from such substrate, however, it is of great importance **how** the mechanical architecture of the connective tissue structure at stake relates to its "mechanical environment," as there is the skeletal and muscular tissue in a given area (Benjamin 2009; Van

der Wal 2009). Only if a given fascial structure has a mechanical architectural relationship with, for example, muscular or skeletal elements is it able to provide the mechanoreceptive information needed for proprioception. This means that the aptitude of a fascial structure to provide centripetal mechanoreceptive information depends on its architecture and its structural relationship with its environment of muscular and skeletal tissue and not simply on its anatomy or topography. It is therefore the functional architecture of fascia and not its anatomical topography that defines its role in the transmission of forces (stretching, squeezing, compressing, and so on) and therefore in proprioception (and mechanoreception) (Van der Wal 2009).

In this chapter the notion proprioception is defined from the neurophysiological perspective—as the ability to sense the relative position and orientation of one's own parts of the body as well as the movement of the body and its parts and the strength of effort being employed in that movement (Anderson et al. 1994). In a stricter sense, proprioception could be defined as the process of conscious and subconscious sensing of joint position and/or motion in particular and of the body in general: **statesthesia** and **kinesthesia** (Skoglund 1973; Fix 2002). Here the term "proprioception" is not meant in the more explicit psychological definition of "proprioception" as sometimes applied (i.e., as the notion "body image sense" or "body awareness"). Proprioception, in this context, has to be differentiated from **exteroception** (relating us with the outer world) and from **interoception** (informing us about visceral and metabolic processes and the movement of internal organs), as treated elsewhere in this book.

The morphological substrate of proprioception—encapsulated or unencapsulated mechanosensitive sensory nerve endings (mechanoreceptors) and related afferent neurons (Fig. 2.2.1)—is considered to provide the centripetal information needed for the control of locomotion or for the maintenance of posture (Barker 1974). At the brain level this information is integrated with information originating from other sources, such as skin receptors and more specific "proprioceptive" sense organs like the labyrinth, to the overall conscious and subconscious awareness of body position, movement, and acceleration (kinesthesia and statesthesia).

In this context, mechanoreception therefore is not synonymous with proprioception. Proprioception relates to mechanoreception as seeing relates to the retina. The mechanoreceptive information needed for the process of proprioception originates not only from fasciae and other connective tissue structures but also from mechanoreceptive or even tactile information from muscles, joints, bones, and even skin. Mechanoreceptors are defined as receptors that are triggered by mechanical deformation like squeezing, stretching, or compressing. In order to understand their contribution to the overall proprioceptive information, it is not only important to know their topography (*where* and in which elements or tissues of the body, e.g., of the locomotor system, they are located) but also *how* they are spatially and, in particular, mechanically related to the various (tissue) components of the body or system. Proprioception in the fascia is not only provided by the mechanoreceptors that are located within or are immediately attached to the fascial structures but also the architecture of the fascia *itself* plays an instrumental role in the process of proprioception (Van der Wal 2009). It can do so by mediating forces that cause deformation of the receptors that, in fact, represents the main stimulus for mechanoreceptors. For that, the receptor does not have to be directly attached to the fascia itself. Some authors (Benjamin 2009) capture the idea that fascia could serve as a significant site of muscle attachment, constituting a kind of "soft tissue skeleton." For example, mechanoreceptors situated within muscles as anatomical units may orient as to their distribution and spatial organization to the fascial or connective tissue structures (tendons, septa, and so on) to which the muscle fascicles insert or between which muscular tissue is interposed in the process of force transmission (Fig. 2.2.2). In such cases, the fascial architecture plays an instrumental role in the process of proprioception without the necessity for the connective tissue structures themselves being

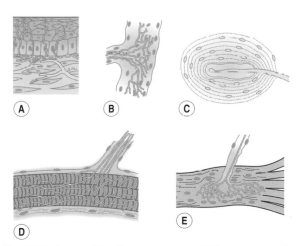

Fig. 2.2.1 Types of Mechanoreceptors. (A) Free nerve ending (FNE); (B) Ruffini corpuscle (RC) or spray-like endings; (C) lamellated corpuscle (LC) or paciniform ending; (D) muscle spindle (MS); (E) Golgi tendon organ (GTO).

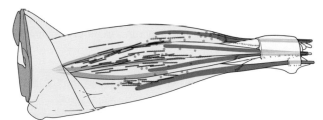

Fig. 2.2.2 The spatial distribution of muscle spindles in the superficial lateral forearm muscle in the rat. The distribution is clearly more related to the architecture of the proximal epicondylar connective tissue apparatus than to the topography of the muscles. The projections of the proximal intermuscular septa are indicated with blue, the projections of the distal tendons in red. The black lines indicate muscle spindles; the gray dots are Golgi tendon organs (GTO).

directly equipped with mechanoreceptive substrate (Van der Wal 2009).

To evaluate the significance of fascial structures as to the proprioceptive input from a certain body region, it is not only important to know the anatomy of the given fascia ("where") but also its architecture, that is, its functional relationship ("how"). Many fascial structures play a direct or indirect role in force transmission (Huijing 1999, 2007). Most anatomy textbooks, however, describe the so-called musculoskeletal system as a system built up from discrete elements involved in positioning, motion, and force transmission, like muscles (with tendons and aponeuroses) and ligaments. In this outdated concept, muscles represent the main composing elements in the system and therefore are often presented in anatomical atlases as discrete anatomical structures with the surrounding and "enveloping" connective tissue layers removed. When a connective tissue structure is recognized as a layer, a membrane or a fascia that covers a body part (e.g., an organ) of a body region, it is usually given a name derived from the anatomical component that the layer covers. Fasciae therefore are most often defined as a suborganization of the "primary" anatomy of organs (e.g., muscles). This is all related to the "dissectional mind" that still prevails in the anatomy atlases and textbooks and considers the locomotor apparatus as being "built up" from anatomical elements. If one considers the fascia as "the dense irregular connective tissue that surrounds and connects every muscle, even the tiniest myofibril, and every single organ of the body forming continuity throughout the body" (Schleip 2012) or as the "organ of form" (Varela and Frenk 1987), the fascia actually is presented as an important integrative element in human posture and organization of movement. Therefore an analytical and "dissectional" approach of the "anatomy" of the fascia cannot do justice to the role of fascial tissue and structures in proprioception.

> ### KEY POINT
>
> Architecture of connective tissue (fascia) in the so-called locomotor apparatus is complementary to the anatomy of the so-called musculoskeletal system. Understanding the function of fascial and connective tissue structures in posture and movement well, as in the process of proprioception, requires insight into not only *where* the structure is situated but also into *how* the connective tissue at stake is mechanically related to the neighboring structure or tissue.

CONNECTIVITY AND CONTINUITY

The primary connective tissue of the body is derived from the embryonic so-called "mesodermal" germ layer. It represents the matrix and environment within which the organs and structures of the body are differentiated. In fact, all the organs, including the specialized derivates from the "mesoderm" itself (like, e.g., muscles and bones) are "embedded" in a matrix of "meso" or mesenchyme. Blechschmidt (2004) distinguished the so-called "mesoderm" as an "inner tissue" and therefore discriminates it from ectoderm and endoderm, which present themselves primarily as "limiting tissues" (in fact, epithelium-like layers). He proposed not to call mesoderm a "derm" anymore but to call it "inner tissue." The primary "inner tissue" is the undifferentiated connective tissue **mesenchyme**, which in principle is organized in three components: cells, intercellular (or better, interstitial) space (the "interstitium" with interstitial fluid or substances), and fibers.

In the functional development and differentiation of the mesenchyme as primary connective tissue, there are two patterns of "connectivity." The first pattern is the development of "interstitial space(s) or cavities," mostly presented as a fissure functioning as a (sliding and slipping) space. This tendency is seen in the formation of coelom (body cavities), joint cavities, and also in bursa-like gliding spaces between adjacent tendons or muscle bellies as well as in the arachnoidian space. Such a pattern ensures spatial separation, which enables movement and mobility. The second pattern is the formation of a binding medium. That can be done by the fiber component (so it is, for example, in regular dense connective tissue structures like the **desmal** sutures in the skull, interosseous membranes, ligaments, septa, and aponeuroses) or by interstitial substrate and matrix (for example, in cartilaginous joints like intervertebral discs). In osteopathic circles, the continuum and continuity of the "connective tissue apparatus" in the human is emphasized. Such a view is in harmony with the idea that the principal function of mesoderm as "inner tissue" is "mediating" in the sense of "connecting" (binding) *and* "disconnecting" (shaping space and enabling movement), in this way creating innerness or inner space (Blechschmidt 2004).

This view of two patterns of connectivity is also applicable to the anatomy of fasciae in strict sense.

In general, the fasciae in the musculoskeletal system exhibit two different mechanical and functional aspects:

- Fasciae of muscles adjacent to spaces that are filled with loose, areolar connective tissue ("sliding tissue") and sometimes with adipose tissue. They enable the sliding and gliding of muscles (and tendons) against each other or against other structures. In such splits, spaces or sheaths, globular or oval mechanoreceptors triggered by compression and squeezing (as discussed later) could "inform the brain" about the displacement and movement of fascial tissue and related structures.

- Intermuscular and epimysial fasciae that serve as areas of force transmission and of insertion for muscle fibers that in this way can mechanically reach (the periosteum of) a skeletal element without necessarily being attached directly to the bone. Such fascia structures may appear as aponeuroses, intermuscular septa, but also as so-called superficial fasciae (like fascia cruris and fascia antebrachii), providing a broad insertion area for muscle fibers or forming stress-"containing" envelops like the fascia lata. If provided with more stretch-susceptible receptors, such fascial layers could inform about stresses of the fascial tissue in relation to the transmission of forces.

This indicates that fasciae exhibit a variety of mechanical relationships with neighboring tissue and therefore may play quite different functional roles as to proprioception as well. The fasciae of the organs and of muscles often represent the "gliding fascia" type; in this context, coelomic cavities function as "joint spaces," enabling motion of the organs. Many epimysial muscle fasciae function in a similar way, providing mobility between a muscle and its neighborhood. However, fasciae like the fascia cruris (tibial fascia) or the retinaculum patellae also may function as epimysial and epimuscular ("fascial") aponeuroses.

ARCHITECTURE IS DIFFERENT FROM AND COMPLEMENTARY TO ANATOMY

To understand the mechanical and functional circumstances of the fascial role in connecting and separating, in conveying stresses and forces, and in proprioception, it is therefore more important to know the **architecture** of the connective and muscle tissue than the regular anatomical order or topography. This applies to every fascial layer in the human body. One must know both where they are situated (anatomy) and how they are connecting and connected (architecture). Depending on the architectural relationship of the fascial connective tissue with the neighboring tissue, not only juxta-articular connective tissue (like interosseous ligaments) can provide proprioceptive information about joint movement or joint position but epimysial, intermuscular, aponeurotic, fascial layers can also play a functional role in this process (directly or indirectly).

In this context, two views on the organization of connective and muscular tissue may be described. On the one hand, there is the well-known view that muscular and connective tissue structures have to be considered as discrete anatomical elements. In this concept, muscles function as dynamic force-transmitting structures that are organized in parallel to ligamentous structures as the more passive force-transmitting elements. The nonligamentous (fascial) connective tissue is considered as auxiliary to the muscle units in the form of tendons and aponeuroses. Areolar fascial connective tissue shapes, space in between the anatomical elements, providing the opportunity for sliding and mobility. Such architecture is exhibited dominantly and clearly in the distal regions of the limbs, where separate muscle entities (bellies with tendons) function **in parallel** to underlying joint capsules with or without capsular reinforcing ligaments. Here, mechanoreceptive substrate in the fascia serves the (unconscious) perception of this sliding and movement.

On the other hand, a pattern can be described where connective tissue and muscular tissue are organized mainly **in series** with each other in a more "transmuscular" organization. Huijing et al. (2003) point out that often muscles, which from an anatomical perspective are considered as morphologically discrete elements, can no longer be considered as isolated units controlling forces and movements: there is clear evidence of transmuscular force transmitting. Detailed studies of the lateral cubital region of man and rat showed such architecture quite clearly (Van der Wal 2009). Here nearly all the deep and superficial **regular dense collagenous connective tissue** (RDCCT) layers are organized in series with muscle fascicles (presented as muscle compartment walls). Collagenous fibers that run from bone to bone—so-called ligaments thought to be stressed passively by displacement of the articulating bones—hardly occur. Instead, there occur broad aponeurotic layers of RDCCT to which relatively short muscle fascicles insert, which, on the opposite side, are directly

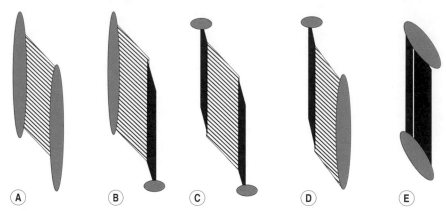

Fig. 2.2.3 The Dynament Principle. Panels A to E represent various possible appearances of a "dynament" with, on the one hand, the extreme situation A in which the muscle fibers in question immediately adhere to the periost of both bones involved, and, on the other hand, the extreme situation E without intermediating muscle tissue between the connective tissue layers or structures. (In this case the dynament acts as a "classical" ligament). Panel C represents the more-or-less "ideal dynament": one connective tissue structure/layer (fascia, aponeurosis, septum) adheres to one ("proximal") bone (top); another connective tissue structure/layer (tendon or aponeurosis) adheres to the other ("distal") bone (down). In between two RDCCT structures is a zone of muscle tissue (muscle fibers). RCDDT, regular dense collagenous connective tissue.

attached to skeletal elements. Such configurations of muscle fascicles attached to the periosteum of one articulating bone, and via a layer of RDCCT indirectly attached to another articulating bone, could be considered "dynamic ligaments." Such "dynaments" are not necessarily situated directly beside the joint cavity or in the deep part of the joint region (Van der Wal 2009) (Fig. 2.2.3).

KEY POINT

From a morphological point of view, most anatomy books have described the skeletal muscles of the human body as being discrete activators with clear origins and insertions (Standring 2015). The "muscle man" as presented in many anatomy models and atlases could therefore be considered as reduced and an "artifact."

THE SUBSTRATE OF MECHANORECEPTION

Connective tissue and fasciae are richly innervated (Stilwell 1957; Schleip 2003; Stecco et al. 2007a; Benjamin 2009). Considerations such as "architecture versus anatomy" mutatis mutandis may also apply for the spatial organization of mechanoreceptors, which represent the morphological substrate for proprioception. To interpret the role and function of mechanoreceptors in the

process of proprioception, it is not only important to know *where* they actually are located in such regions but also *how* they are or are not connected with the relating tissue elements. In general, however, textbooks report mechanoreceptors either as "muscle receptors" or as "joint receptors." Muscle receptors are thought to be mechanoreceptors present in the muscles, including their auxiliary structures such as tendons, aponeuroses, and epimysia (a more-or-less typical anatomical definition). Muscle spindles and Golgi tendon organs (GTOs) are the best-known types of such receptors (Barker 1974). Joint receptors are considered to be situated in joint capsules and related structures, including reinforcing ligaments. These receptor types are usually ordered according to the (ultra)structure of the receptor itself, physiological features, type of afferent nerve fiber, and other parameters (Freeman and Wyke 1967a, b).

Mechanoreceptors are in fact free nerve endings (FNEs), whether or not equipped with specialized end organs. The main stimulus for such receptors is deformation. Variation exists as to the microarchitecture of the ending. On the one hand, there exists the principle of lamellae around a relatively simple nerve ending. This represents the principle of the ball- or bean-shaped Vater Pacini, or paciniform corpuscles (PC), often called lamellated corpuscles (LC). On the other hand, there is the more spray-like organization of the nerve ending wrapping around and in between the deformable substrate, such as connective tissue fibers. Those are the spindle-shaped Ruffini corpuscles (RC) and GTOs. These two types of microarchitecture roughly relate to the type of mechanical deformation that is at stake: in general, compression for the lamellated bodies and traction (and torsion) for the spray-like type. Other varying parameters are threshold, adaptivity, and adjustability. In this general classification, the muscle spindle is a spindle-shaped, spray-like ending organized around specialized muscle fibers equipped with the extra possibility of adjustable length (Strasmann et al. 1990).

As stated previously, mechanoreceptors are in general reported to occur as either "muscle receptors" or "joint receptors." In this concept, muscle receptors are mechanoreceptors present in the muscles, and joint receptors are mechanoreceptors situated in joint capsules and so-called joint-related structures, such as ligaments. In this context, the concept often prevails that joint receptors play the leading role in the process of monitoring joint position or movement for the purpose of statesthesia and kinesthesia, while muscle receptors are relegated to motor functions that operate at a subconscious or reflex level (Barker 1974).

Mechanoreceptors associated with muscles, including the muscle auxiliary structures such as tendons, are usually classified as follows (see Fig. 2.2.1):
- FNEs (unencapsulated)
- muscle spindles (MS; sensory endings with encapsulated intrafusal muscle fibers)
- GTOs (type III endings, relatively large spray-like endings, i.e., 100–600 µm diameter with high threshold and very slow adapting)

The mechanoreceptors typically associated with joints are (Fig. 2.2.1):
- FNEs (unencapsulated)
- LCs (type II ending with a two- to five-layered capsule, less than 100 µm length, with low threshold and rapidly adapting). *Here, this term is preferred over the notion of "paciniform corpuscle."*
- RCs (type I ending, relatively small spray-like ending, up to 100 µm, with low threshold and slow adapting).

THE FUNCTIONAL ROLE OF ARCHITECTURE OF THE CONNECTIVE AND MUSCULAR TISSUE IN MECHANORECEPTION

In an extensive study of the spatial organization of the morphological substrate of proprioception in the proximal lateral cubital region of the rat (Van der Wal 2009),

an inventory has been made of mechanoreceptors that may occur in direct or indirect relationships with the connective tissue layers and structures in the joint region.

A spectrum of mechanosensitive substrate occurs at the transitional areas between the RDCCT layers (organized as epimysial or intermuscular layers and septa) and the muscle fascicles organized in series with them. This substrate exhibits features of the mechanosensitive nerve terminals that usually are characteristic for joint receptors *and* for muscle receptors. At the so-called superficial antebrachial fascia, as well as at the intermuscular fascial layers, RC and LC were present between the fascial layer and inserting muscle fibers. Sometimes, even, one pole of a muscle spindle was attached to those layers.

Based upon the architecture of the connective tissue and upon the spatial distribution of the substrate of mechanoreception, it is assumed that the joint receptors here are also influenced by the activity of the muscle organized **in series** with the collagenous connective tissue near those receptors. This supports the idea that the stresses during joint positioning are conveyed mainly via those collagenous layers and are involved in triggering the related mechanoreceptors. In the region studied, there exists no basis in morphology for so-called joint receptors that are deformed exclusively by passive strain in (joint-near or para-articular) collagenous connective tissue structures induced by displacement of the articulating bones. The substrate of proprioception that was found in and near the RDCCT apparatus in the lateral cubital region has features of mechanoreceptors that are usually linked with "joint receptor" substrate as well as of mechanoreceptors usually present in muscles and related tendons. It is obvious that, in cases like this, the fascial layers together with the *in-series* inserting muscular tissue function as a kind of "dynamic ligament" or "dynament."

Very often myofascial areas are richly innervated and covered by nerve plexuses. In the previously mentioned study on rats (Van der Wal 2009), it was shown that over the proximal (epimysial) antebrachial fascia, as well as over the fascia "covering" the supinator muscle (in fact a supinator aponeurosis), extensive plexuses were present. Plexiform arrangements of peripheral nerves sprouting over tendons and ligaments are a consistent feature in the innervation pattern in the periarticular aponeuroses of the knee and elbow joint (Wilson and Lee 1986). Stilwell (1957) states that such networks terminate in small "paciniform corpuscles" and in "freely ending axons" on the surface connective tissue of tendons, aponeuroses, and muscles, and in periosteal connective tissue, nearly always in the vicinity of other mechanoreceptors. The type of axons present in the nerve fascicles of the plexuses studied here (Van der Wal 2009), as well as the demonstrated (or putative) origin of those axons from the substrate of mechanoreception in the studied material, support the notion that such peri- or juxta-articular nerve plexuses are not exclusively involved in nociceptive processes, as stated by Freeman and Wyke (1967a, b). This also means that the substrate of proprioception does not necessarily have to be situated *within* the fascial fibers to play a functional role in proprioception. Regarded mechanically, the intermediate zones between fascial dense connective tissue and adjacent muscle fibers and/or adjacent loose areolar connective tissue might be of interest as a source of mechanoreceptive information. In areas where the fascial connective tissue is so dense that it allows little dislocation or deformation, as is the case in most ligamentous structures, it seems logical that the innervation is more involved in nociception or sympathetic vascular regulation. In the latter respect, it is worth mentioning that there exist ligaments that are mechanically important yet poorly innervated, and ligaments with a key role in sensory perception that are richly innervated (Hagert et al. 2007; Benjamin 2009). It all relates to the degree to which deformation is allowed (since it is deformation that forms the major stimulus for mechanoreceptive triggering), as well as to the microscopic level (the kind of mechanoreceptor) and to the macroscopic level (the architecture of the fascia and related tissue).

 KEY POINT

> The morphological substrate of proprioception in a given region is organized according to the occurrence of mechanical forces and events (pull, tension and compression, rolling and gliding) and therefore to the architecture of muscular and connective tissue rather than according to the anatomy of discrete anatomical structures like muscles and ligaments.

DYNAMENTS: MORE THAN LIGAMENTS OR MUSCLES

The findings in the studies described previously regarding spatial distribution and the organization of so-called "muscle receptors" were even more relevant to the concept

that is brought forward here. Those receptors appeared not to be organized according to principles of anatomy and topography but to cope with the functional architecture of the connective tissue complex of the epi-, inter-, and submuscular RDCCT layers in relation to muscular architecture. In all the antebrachial extensor muscles studied, the distribution of muscle spindles per muscle area is uneven. If the spatial distribution of muscle spindles is considered per muscle, it is difficult to detect a common distribution pattern in all muscles (see Fig. 2.2.2). The spatial distribution of those receptors, however, becomes understandable from the regional functional architecture of the connective tissue and fascia (i.e., the RDCCT structures). The muscular zones that are dense in muscle spindles and GTOs are the stress- and force-conveying zones of the muscle, which are in series with the connective tissue complex proximally and in series with the peripheral tendons distally**.** This arrangement provides a common principle that may explain many kinds of distribution patterns. Of course, sometimes architectural units coincide with specific topographical entities, as is the case in this study with the supinator muscle that with its aponeurosis nearly represents the anatomy of a "dynament" (see Fig. 2.2.3).

As Huijing et al. (2003) pointed out, based upon mechanical arguments that the muscles are not isolated units controlling forces and movements as often thought, apparently also on the level of spinal sensorimotor control the muscles should no longer be considered the functional entity in the position and locomotion system (English and Letbetter 1982; English and Weeks 1984; Van der Wal 2009). Such considerations again match task-dependent models of brain control well: motor units are not necessarily organized with respect to individual motor nuclei but are organized according to behavioral tasks. The concept of the locomotor apparatus being built up by architectural units of muscular tissue *in series* with collagenous connective tissue is more consistent with such trans- or supramuscular models than is the concept in which muscles function as the entities that maintain joint integrity parallel to ligamentous structures.

CLASSIFICATION OF MECHANORECEPTORS IN PROPRIOCEPTION

In consequence of the identification in the so-called locomotor apparatus of an in-series organization of muscular tissue and regular dense connective tissue structures (mainly tendons distally and muscle compartment walls proximally), three configuration types of mechanoreceptors were identified in the mentioned study (Van der Wal 2009). *Mutatis mutandis* this spectrum could also be considered to represent the substrate of proprioception of the fascia:

- Muscle spindles, GTO (RC), FNE, and LC are found in areas between muscular tissue and RDCCT layers. This configuration coincides with the conventional muscle–tendon spectrum of sensory nerve endings (Barker 1974; Von Düring et al. 1984).
- LC and FNE are found in areas in which RDCCT adjoins reticular connective tissue, gliding spaces. This configuration coincides mainly with the spectrum of sensory nerve endings usually indicated as articular receptors (Freeman and Wyke 1967a, b; Halata et al. 1985).
- Only FNE are present in the transition to the skeletal attachment (periosteum). This configuration coincides with the endotenonial spectrum of sensory nerve endings, with mainly (mechanoreceptive) FNE from group III and IV fibers (Von Düring et al. 1984).

Most plexuses in or near the regular dense connective tissue of fascial layers contain nerve fibers of types III and IV. Nerve fibers of group III (or A delta type) are afferent from mechanoreceptors; nerve fibers of group IV (or C-type) are afferents from FNE that are either nociceptive or mechanosensitive (strain).

In the previously mentioned configurations, RCs are not considered to be a separate category, but GTO and RC are considered to be the same receptor type, presenting gradual differences depending on the texture of the surrounding tissue. The quartet MS-GTO/RC-LC-FNE represents the complete spectrum of mechanoreceptors in the locomotor apparatus. In this way, the three main types of so-called muscle receptors (MS, GTO, and LC) are combined with the three types of so-called capsular (or joint) receptors (RC, LC, and FNE). Depending on the local situation, this quartet therefore represents the spectrum of mechanoreceptors involved in the proprioceptive function of fasciae and fascial structures. Therefore the role of a mechanoreceptor in proprioception is defined not only by its functional properties but also by its architectural environment. It is the architecture of the fascial connective tissue in relation to the muscular tissue components and skeletal elements that plays a major role in the coding of the proprioceptive information that is provided.

Summary

The one-liner "The brain knows nothing about the muscles" means that "above" (and actually already at) the level of the medullar ventral horn the central nervous system is organized in movements, tasks, and actions and therefore not in muscles. Because most anatomy books (still) describe the skeletal muscles of the human body as being discrete activators with clear origins and insertions, the notion "musculo-skeletal system" should be considered as functionally obsolete or at least as "poor" or "reduced." In the so-called posture and locomotion system the fascial system serves as a kind of "connective tissue skeleton" providing continuity and connectivity that is organized according to an architecture of force transmission and complementary to the anatomical components of skeletal and muscle tissue. This principle is valid also for the organization of the morphological substrate of proprioception; it is organized according to the architecture of mechanical forces not to the anatomy of discrete structures like muscles and ligaments: the fascia is instrumental in the organization of (the morphological substrate) of proprioception

REFERENCES

Anderson, K.N., Anderson, L.E., Glanze, W.D. (Eds.), 1994. Mosby's Medical, Nursing, & Allied Health Dictionary, fourth ed. Mosby-Year Book, 1285.

Barker, D., 1974. The morphology of muscle receptors. In: Barker, D., Hunt, C.C., McIntyre, A.K. (Eds.), Handbook of Sensory Physiology. Muscle Receptors, vol. II. Springer Verlag, Berlin.

Benjamin, M., 2009. The fascia of the limbs and back – a review. J. Anat. 214, 1–18.

Blechschmidt, E., 2004. The Ontogenetic Basis of Human Anatomy. North Atlantic Books, Berkeley, CA.

English, A.W., Letbetter, W.D., 1982. Anatomy and innervation patterns of cat lateral gastrocnemius and plantaris muscles. Am. J. Anat. 164, 67–77.

English, A.W., Weeks, O.I., 1984. Compartmentalization of single muscle units in cat lateral gastrocnemius. Exp. Brain Res. 56, 361–368.

Fix, J.D., 2002. Neuroanatomy. Lippincott Williams & Wilkins, Hagerstown, MD.

Freeman, M.A.R., Wyke, B.D., 1967a. The innervation of the ankle joint. An anatomical and histological study in the cat. Acta Anat. (Basel) 68, 321–333.

Freeman, M.A.R., Wyke, B.D., 1967b. The innervation of the knee joint. An anatomical and histological study in the cat. J. Anat. 101, 505–532.

Hagert, E., Garcia-Elias, M., Forsgren, S., Ljung, B.O., 2007. Immunohistochemical analysis of wrist ligament innervation in relation to their structural composition. J. Hand Surg. Am. 32, 30–36.

Halata, Z., Rettig, T., Schulze, W., 1985. The ultrastructure of sensory nerve endings in the human knee joint capsule. Anat. Embryol. (Berl) 172, 265–275.

Huijing, P., 1999. Muscular force transmission: a unified, dual or multiple system? A review and some explorative experimental results. Arch. Physiol. Biochem. 107, 292–311.

Huijing, P., 2007. Epimuscular myofascial force transmission between antagonistic and synergistic muscles can explain movement limitation in spastic paresis. J. Electromyogr. Kinesol. 17, 708–724.

Huijing, P., Maas, H., Baan, G.C., 2003. Compartmental fasciotomy and isolating a muscle from neighboring muscles interfere with myofascial force transmission within the rat anterior crural compartment. J. Morphol. 256, 306–321.

Langevin, H.M., 2006. Connective tissue: a body-wide signaling network? Med. Hypotheses 66, 1074–1077.

Schleip, R., 2003. Fascial plasticity – a new neurobiological explanation part 2. J. Bodyw. Mov. Ther. 7, 104–116.

Schleip, R., 2012. What is fascia? A review of different nomenclatures. J. Bodyw. Mov. Ther. 16, 496–502.

Skoglund, S., 1973. Joint receptors and kinaesthesis. In: Iggo, A. (Ed.), Handbook of Sensory Physiology, vol. 2. Springer Verlag, Berlin, Heidelberg, New York, 111–136.

Standring, S., 2005. Gray's Anatomy, thirty-ninth ed. Elsevier, New York.

Standring, S., 2015. Gray's anatomy, forty-first ed. Elsevier, New York.

Stecco, C., Gagey, O., Macchi, V., et al., 2007a. Tendinous muscular insertions onto the deep fascia of the upper limb. First part: anatomical study. Morphologie 91, 29–37.

Stecco, C., Gagey, O., Belloni, A., et al., 2007b. Anatomy of the deep fascia of the upper limb. Second part: study of innervation. Morphologie 91, 38–43.

Stilwell, D.L., 1957. Regional variations in the innervation of deep fasciae and aponeuroses. Anat. Rec. 127, 635–653.

Strasmann, T.H., Van der Wal, J.C., Halata, Z., Drukker, J., 1990. Functional topography and ultrastructure of periarticular mechanoreceptors in the lateral elbow region of the rat. Acta Anat. (Basel) 138, 1–14.

Van der Wal, J.C., 2009. The architecture of connective tissue as parameter for proprioception-an often overlooked functional parameter as to proprioception in the locomotor apparatus. Int. J. Ther. Massage Bodywork 2, 9–23.

Varela, F.J., Frenk, S., 1987. The organ of form: towards a theory of biological shape. J. Soc. Biol. Struct. 10, 73–83.

Von Düring, M., Andres, K.H., Schmidt, R.F., 1984. Ultrastructure of fine afferent terminations in muscle and tendon of the cat. In: Hamann, W., Iggo, A. (Eds.), Sensory Receptor Mechanisms. World Scientific Publishing, Singapore.

Wilson, A.S., Lee, H.B., 1986. Hypothesis relevant to defective position sense in a damaged knee. J. Neurol. Neurosurg. Psychiatry 49, 1462–1464.

Wood Jones, F., 1944. Structure and Function as seen in the Foot. Baillière, Tindall and Cox, London.

Interoception: A New Correlate for Intricate Connections Between Fascial Receptors, Emotion, and Self-Awareness

Robert Schleip, Joeri Calsius, and Heike Jäger

CHAPTER CONTENTS

INTRODUCTION

While the sense of proprioception and exteroception is fairly well-known to therapists working with fascia, interoception has received far less attention for quite some time. However, since the beginning of this century interoception has gained increasingly more interest in research and translational applications, such as fascial therapies. Besides being coined as a key concept for manual therapies (D'Alessandro et al. 2016), interoception seems fundamental in understanding emotional processing (Barrett 2017) and psychosomatics (Calsius et al. 2016; Cameron 2001) and has shown to be pivotal in body psychotherapies (Geuter 2015; Fogel 2009). In turn, disturbed or atypical interoceptive sensitivity seems to be associated with diabetes and obesity and may represent a general susceptibility to psychopathology (Murphy et al. 2017). Although the concept of interoception is not new—evolving from what in the nineteenth century was called coenesthesia or *Gemeingefuehl* by early German physiologists—it has been conceptually refined and adjusted based on growing research ever since (Ceunen et al. 2016; Craig 2009, 2003; Critchley et al. 2004). In this chapter we take a closer look at this evolution; describe intricate connections with fascia, emotion, and self-awareness; and briefly dwell on possible opportunities for (manual) therapy.

WHAT IS INTEROCEPTION?

At first, concepts of interoception often focused on visceral sensations only, so-called visceroception (Damasio 1994). More current concepts describe interoception as a sense of the physiological condition of the body, which includes a much wider range of physiological sensations, such as, for example, muscular effort, tickling, vasomotor sensations, sensual touch, and even taste (Box 2.3.1). These sensations share the way they are triggered by stimulation of unmyelinated, free nerve endings that project to the insular cortex rather than to the primary somatosensory cortex, which is usually considered as the main target of proprioception and exteroception (Berlucchi and Aglioti 2010; Critchley et al. 2004). In short, interoception is about how we experience what is going on with and in our body.

However, more current findings improved our understanding of interoception thoroughly. Firstly, interoception

---

BOX 2.3.1   Interoceptive Sensations

- Warmth, coolness
- Muscular activity
- Pain, tickle, itch
- Hunger, thirst
- Air hunger
- Sexual arousal
- Wine tasting (in sommeliers)
- Heartbeat
- Vasomotor activity
- Distension of bladder
- Distension of stomach, rectum, or esophagus
- Taste
- Sensual touch

---

is now more understood as *an umbrella term for the phe-nomenological experience of the body state, an experience which is ultimately a product of the central nervous system (CNS), regardless of what information the brain uses and does not use to construct this experience* (Ceunen et al. 2016, p. 1). Secondly, although we would intuitively assume that how we perceive our bodily state (body awareness) is a di-rect and (chrono-)logical consequence of what our body senses (interoception), this seems not to be the case. On the contrary, interoceptive perception is *largely a construction of beliefs that are kept in check by the actual state of the body. What you experience is in large part a reflection of what your brain predicts is going on inside your body, based on past ex-perience* (Barrett and Simmons 2015, p. 424). Thirdly, sensorimotor as well as interoceptive states are building blocks of what we call emotions (Oosterwijk and Barrett 2014) and therefore closely linked to concepts as body- and self-awareness (Mehling et al. 2011; Fogel 2009).

 KEY POINT

Interoception is an umbrella term for the phenomeno-logical experience of what is going on in the body. This experience is constructed by the central nervous sys-tem based on all available information and influenced by past experiences as well as predictive guesses about possible future scenarios.

As a consequence, body- and self-awareness are on one hand clearly interoceptive-based and "embodied" processes but at the same time also biased and con-structed "mental" phenomena. Here one can imagine

possible implications on diagnostic as well as a thera-peutic levels. But for now we conclude on interoception as a *multimodal integration not restricted to any sensory channel or mere sensations, but also relying on learned associations, memories, and emotions and integrating these in the total experience which is the subjective repre-sentation of the body state* (Ceunen et al. 2016, p. 13).

KEY POINT

Body- and self-awareness are at one hand clearly intero-ceptive-based and "embodied" processes but at the same time also biased and constructed "mental" phenomena

---

SENSUAL TOUCH

An interesting addition to the above list of interoceptive sensations is the sense of sensual or pleasant touch. In a unique case, a patient who lacked myelinated afferents reported a faint and obscure sensation of pleasant touch and general well-being while receiving slow, soft-brush-like stroking of the skin. Surprisingly, functional magnetic imaging revealed a clear activation of the insular cortex, with no activation of the primary somatosensory cortex (Olausson et al. 2010). Contrary to the idea that touch is always processed via exteroceptive pathways, this and other research led to distinguish an interoceptive pathway for specific tactile information, based on the innervation of primate skin. It was concluded that the affected sensory receptors are unmyelinated C-fiber afferents—typically with low mechanical threshold and slow conduction velocity—which are connected to the interoceptive-insular brain network (Björnsdotter et al. 2010). The affected re-ceptors are often referred to as C-tactile afferents, human tactile C-fibers, or C-tactile system.

Because these C-tactile afferents are not found in the palm of the hand, it is assumed that they are present in hairy skin only and absent in glabrous skin, capacitating the human skin with particular touch receptors (Abraira and Ginti 2013). In turn this enables a discriminative system for social touch, which underlies emotional, hor-monal (for example, oxytocin), and affiliative responses to caress-like, skin-to-skin contact between individuals and which enhances sensual salience of tactile interac-tion (Kirsch et al. 2018) (Fig. 2.3.1). Although the pro-found importance of such an affiliative touch system for human health and well-being (see also Montague 1971; Fisher et al. 1976) has been indicated since the classical

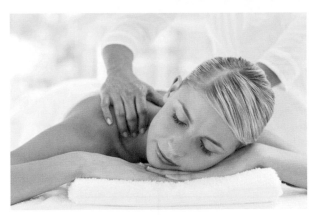

Fig. 2.3.1 The Discovery of Interoceptive Receptors in Human Skin. Besides proprioceptive nerve endings, human skin contains interoceptive C-fiber endings, which trigger a general sense of well-being. The connections of these slowly conducting receptors do not follow the usual pathway of the pyramidal tract toward the proprioceptive areas in the brain. Rather, they project to the insular cortex, a key player in the regulation of interoception. ©iStockphoto.com/Neustockimages.

study of Harlow (1958), it was not until recently that the epigenetic implications of touch were brought to light. In a prospective study (up till 4 to 5 years of life) researchers mapped the effects of early postnatal touch contact and were able to localize negative impact on DNA-methylation and lasting associations with child biology (More et al. 2017).

INTEROCEPTIVE PATHWAYS

In addition to Craig (2011, 2009, 2003), who described the afferent neurons related to interoception terminating in lamina I of the dorsal horn, Ceunen and colleagues (2016) offer further details. First they indicate that aside from the spinal homeostatic pathway (including also the second and fifth lamina), at least two other routes are into play, namely the cranial and humoral homeostatic pathways. The first concerns cranial nerve input, for example, from the vagus and glossopharyngeal nerve, while the latter reaches up to the brain by means of circulating substances. Another innovatory insight is that although these three homeostatic pathways are central to interoceptive processing, interoceptive awareness in the end is *a construction of the CNS relying on all available information* (Ceunen et al. 2016) (Fig. 2.3.2).

Zooming in on the spinal and the cranial pathways, both project via sympathetic and parasympathetic efferent routes, respectively, arriving at the main homeostatic integration sites in the brainstem, such as the nucleus tractus solitarii, the parabrachial nucleus, and the periaqueductal gray (Fig. 2.3.3). From there it goes to the thalamic region and the dorsal posterior insula where a primary homeostatic and precortical *representation* is made. Subsequently, this information moves on to the mid and anterior insula. The mid insula is known to be densely connected with the amygdala and hypothalamus and thereby central in emotional memory and ongoing metabolic processing. In fact, the mid insula is pivotal for what is called the *re-representation* of the actual body state and in that sense is at the core of interoception (Craig 2009, 2003). A further integrative level is expressed in the anterior insula whereby the left anterior insula is thought to be activated predominantly by homeostatic afferents associated with parasympathetic functions (e.g., taste), and the right one is activated predominantly by homeostatic afferents associated with sympathetic functions (e.g., pain) (Craig 2005, p. 567). The anterior insula also has intimate connections with the anterior cingulate cortex. Together they form an emotional network in which the limbic insular component is involved in sensory reception and conscious feelings, and the cingulate cortex serves as the motivational and motor component for the behavioral expression of the feelings. With the right anterior insula coming into play (relaying to the orbitofrontal cortex), the re-representational image shifts toward self-conscious perception and contributes to what is called *body awareness* (Mehling 2011; Fogel 2009).

Developments in research on body and self-awareness argue how all this starts with one of the central tasks of the brain, which is to construe *an internal model* that helps regulating the body in the midst of its environment: *"The skeletomotor prediction signals prepare the body for movement, the interoceptive prediction signals initiate a change in affect, and the extrapersonal sensory prediction signals prepare upcoming perceptions"* (Barrett 2017, p. 9). With interoception as a fundamental part, brain research shows how this internal model, in turn, depends heavily on what is identified as the default mode network (DMN) (Rebello et al. 2018; Oosterwijk and Barrett 2014; Andrews-Hanna 2012). This DMN seems to be at the core of human capacities, such as mind wandering, daydreaming, or zoning out, and offers an interesting context to explore how basic bodily processes, such as interoception, contribute to unique phylogenetic achievements, such as self-reflection and creativity.

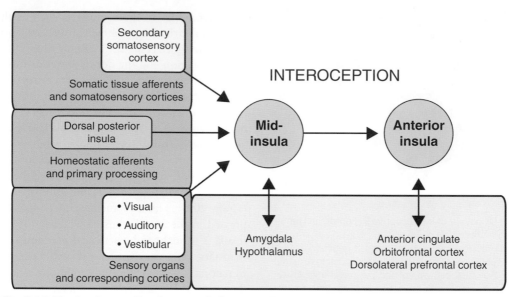

Fig. 2.3.2 The Insula as a Key Structure in Interoception. Adapted from Craig, A. D., 2008. Interoception and emotion: a neuroanatomical perspective. In Lewis, M., Haviland-Jones, J.M., Barrett, L.F. (Eds.), *Handbook of Emotions* (pp. 272–292). Guilford Press, New York; and redrawn from Ceunen, E., Vlaeyen J.W.S., Van Diest, I., 2016. On the origin of interoception. Front. Psychol. 7, 743. Open access: https://creativecommons.org/licenses/by/4.0/.

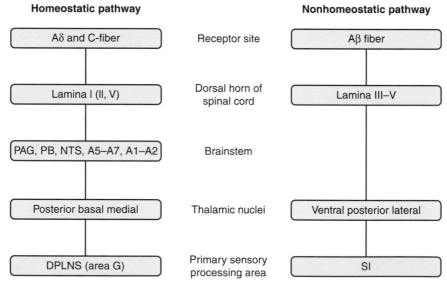

Fig. 2.3.3 Homeostatic and Nonhomeostatic Pathways in Interoception. DPLNS, dorsal posterior insula; NTS, nucleus tractus solitarii (nucleus of the solitary tract); PAG, periaqueductal gray; PB, parabrachial nucleus; SI, primary somatosensory cortex. Redrawn from Ceunen E., Vlaeyen, J.W.S., Van Diest, I., 2016. On the origin of interoception. Front. Psychol. 7, 743, which was partly based on Craig A. D., 2010. How do you feel? Lecture by Bud Craig. With the collaboration of Linköping University and Linköping University Hospital. (Video) Available at: https://vimeo.com/8170544. Open access: https://creativecommons.org/licenses/by/4.0/.

INTEROCEPTION AND SOMATOEMOTIONAL DISORDERS

At the same time, all this body-brain intertwining sheds more light on how interoception possibly relates to psychosomatic and somatoemotional disorders, such as anxiety, depression, irritable bowel syndrome, or functional somatic syndromes in general. Apparently, many complex disorders with a somatoemotional component are associated with clear differences in interoception. While this is currently a new and growing field of research in psychobiological medicine, many of the studies published reveal associations of such pathologies with interoceptive processing. However, the precise system dynamics of these associations (including the differentiation between primary causative and secondary effects) still need to be elucidated for most of the interoceptive disorders. To this end, Murphy et al. (2017) propose a model that sees atypical interoceptive sensitivity as a general susceptibility to several psychopathological conditions due to its fundamental role in the personality trait alexithymia.

For example, anxiety and depression have been shown to coincide with significant alterations in interoceptive processing. They are connected with increased and noisy interoceptive input, the processing of which is amplified by self-referential belief states via an enhanced top-down modulation in response to the poorly predictable interoceptive states (Paulus and Stein 2010). Both of these somatoemotional disorders seem not to be dysfunctions of the afferent interoceptive signaling but can be understood as altered interoceptive states as a consequence of noisy, amplified, self-referential belief states concerning the interoceptive sensations. The same relationship goes for the influence of distorted symptom perception in patients with medically unexplainable symptoms (Bogaerts et al. 2010) or the influence of alexithymia as a personality trait (Herbert et al. 2011). Here again we refer to the aforementioned research showing how the interoceptive re-representation in the CNS is influenced by *predictive guesses of the brain* and by *previous experiences* (Barrett and Simmons 2015). So with the experience of bodily stress being a central element in the development of functional somatic syndromes (Henningsen et al. 2007) interoceptive interference from "organic disease" or "dysfunctional peripheral stimuli" is more than plausible (Fig. 2.3.4).

Similarly, brain imaging studies of patients with irritable bowel syndrome revealed a disrupted modulation of insular cortex responses to visceral stimuli (such as in response to experimentally induced painful rectal distension as well as to the subsequent relaxation). It is suspected that these dysfunctional regulations may provide the neural basis for altered visceral interoception by stress and negative emotions in these patients (Elsenbruch et al. 2010).

Drug addictions, as well as other addictions, have also been proposed to be seen, at least in part, as interoceptive disorders. Apparently, the primary goal here is that the addicted individual aims to obtain the effects of the drug use ritual upon their internal body perception. The representations of the achievement of this goal in interoceptive terms by the insula contribute to how addicted individuals feel, remember, and decide about performing the related rituals. Similar interoception-related insular dynamics have been suggested for other addictions and cravings, such as excessive sex, gambling, smoking, or eating (Naqvi and Bechara 2010).

In essential hypertension an increased interoceptive awareness has been observed, even in the early stages of this disorder, and its contribution to the prospective development of this common cardiovascular syndrome has been discussed (Koroboki et al. 2010). Finally, aging and posttraumatic stress disorders have been shown to be associated with a significant decline in interoceptive awareness. Mindfulness-based therapies and so-called contemplative practices, focusing on subtle somatic sensations, are therefore suggested as helpful therapeutic approaches (Farb et al. 2015).

FASCIA AS AN INTEROCEPTIVE ORGAN

In musculoskeletal tissues only a minority of the sensory nerve endings are myelinated mechanoreceptors concerned with proprioception, such as muscle spindles, Golgi receptors, Paccini corpuscles, or Ruffini endings. The vast majority—80% of afferent nerves—terminate in free nerve endings (Schleip 2003). Termed "interstitial muscle receptors," they are located in fascial tissues such as the endomysium or perimysium and are connected with either unmyelinated afferent neurons (then called type IV or C-fibers) or myelinated axons (type III or Aδ fibers). Indeed, 90% of these free nerve endings belong to the first group, to the slowly conducting C-fiber neurons (Abraira and Ginti 2013). Functional magnetic imaging studies by Olausson et al. (2008) revealed that stimulation of these C-fiber neurons results in activation of the insular cortex (which indicates a clear interoceptive role

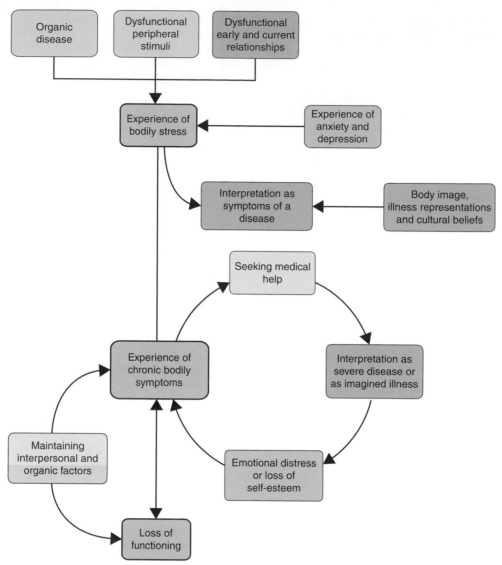

Fig. 2.3.4 Hypothetical Model for the Cause of Functional Somatic Syndromes. Redrawn with permission from Henningsen, P., Zipfel, S., Herzog, W. 2007. Management of functional somatic syndromes. Lancet 369, 946–955.

of these receptors) and not of the primary somatosensory cortex, which is usually activated by proprioceptive input.

A surprising conclusion from this is that the number of interoceptive receptors in muscular tissues by far outnumbers the amount of proprioceptive endings with a 7-to-1 ratio. Whereas some of these free nerve endings are thermoreceptors, chemoreceptors, or have multimodal functions, the majority of them do in fact function

as mechanoreceptors, which means they are responsive to mechanical tension, pressure, or shear deformation. Although some are high threshold receptors, it has been shown that a significant portion (approximately 40%) can be classified as low threshold receptors, which are responsive to touch as light as with a painter's brush (Ackerley et al. 2014). Most likely they are therefore also responsive to the tissue manipulation of myofascial therapists.

MANUAL THERAPY AND INTEROCEPTION

When treating muscular tissues, myofascial therapists are usually concerned with direct biomechanical effects on nonneural tissues or with the stimulation of specific proprioceptive nerve endings, such as muscle spindles, Golgi receptors, etc. However, interoceptive research learns that manual therapists target the interoceptive receptors and their related upstream effects to a much larger degree than is usually taught or practiced. For example, some of the interoceptive nerve endings in muscle tissues inform the insula about the work load of local muscle portions. Their mechanical stimulation has been shown to lead to changes in sympathetic output, which increases the local blood flow. Stimulation of other interoceptive nerve endings has been shown to result in an increased matrix hydration via the extrusion of plasma from tiny blood vessels into the interstitial matrix (Schleip 2003). Other effects of myofascial therapy can lie in optimizing gliding function via stimulation of hyaluronic acid and, more broadly, in the draining effect on the neuroendocrine matrix (Stecco 2015; Stecco et al. 2011). Perhaps an even more interesting role of fascial bodywork could be its contribution to regulatory processes of a vegetative nature, which comes down to the damping role of the sympathetic nervous system by facilitating the parasympathetic system. Working with a so-called slow melting pressure, "light sensual" or "haptic" touch appears to be most effective in this regard (Calsius 2020; Turvey and Fonseca 2014).

 KEY POINT

Working with a "slow melting pressure," "light sensual," or "haptic touch" appears to be most effective from an interoceptive point of view.

In this regard it is very useful to pay ongoing attention to the autonomic and the limbic–emotional (or insular) response of the client while monitoring the direction, speed, and magnitude of the applied touch during bodywork. Subsequently, it is advisable to enhance perceptual refinement and invite the client to share verbal feedback regarding the experienced interoceptive perceptions. Research indeed argues in favor of integrating room to express what one experiences during myofascial bodywork or, if possible, coworking with a psychologist (Bordoni and Marelli 2017). While proprioceptive sensations may be in the foreground during the actual stroke application, those finer interoceptive sensations are usually easier to perceive in periods of at least several seconds of rest between different manipulative strokes. Subjective sensations of warmth, lightness/heaviness, spaciousness, density/fluidity, nausea, streaming, pulsation, spontaneous affection, or a general sense of well-being may be such interoceptive sensations that can be triggered by myofascial tissue manipulation, especially when using a "light, listening" touch or working with "deep melting pressure." From the therapist's perspective, subtle changes in the client—such as an increased local tissue hydration; changes in temperature, in skin color, in breathing; micromovements of the limbs; pupil dilation; and facial expression—can serve as valuable signals for physiological effects related to interoceptive processes, with possible impact on his/her body- and self-awareness.

Therapists who apply mechanical stimulation to visceral tissues, such as visceral osteopaths, should also profit from a larger recognition of interoception and related physiological and psychoemotional effects. After all, the enteric nervous system or "belly brain" contains more than 100 million neurons (Gershon 1999), most of which are located either in the connective tissue zone between the inner and outer layers of the muscularis externa (Auerbach's plexus) or in the dense connective tissue layer of the submucosa (Meissner's plexus). Many of these visceral nerve endings are directly concerned with interoception and are connected via the spinal, cranial, and humoral homeostatic pathways with the cortical insula, as described previously. Considering that several complex disorders, such as irritable bowel syndrome, are associated with a disrupted modulation of insular responses to visceral stimuli (Van Oudenhove et al. 2016), it is conceivable that slow and careful manual work on visceral tissues could be a useful, if not ideal, approach for enhancing more healthy, interoceptive self-regulation. Myofascial and visceral therapists should also not be surprised when encountering psychoemotional responses that may include changes in internal body perception, in self-awareness, or in affiliative emotions (Fogel 2009). These may be triggered by their stimulation of interoceptive free nerve endings in the skin, in visceral connective tissues, and in muscular tissues.

MOVEMENT THERAPIES AND INTEROCEPTION

In competitive sports, the attention is often focused on external goal achievements. Frequently, it is also focused on the task of overriding internal sensations of discomfort, tiredness, etc. In contrast, contemplative practices—like Yoga, Tai Chi, Chi Gong, Feldenkrais, Pilates, Body Mind Centering, or Continuum Movement—encourage a more refined "embodied" perception of one's own body (Farb et al. 2015), which often implies skilled fine-tuning of the student's perception for interoceptive sensations. Here one can think of emphasizing sensations such as a subtle tingling under the skin, a general or localized warming, a subjective sense of internal spaciousness, a feeling of aliveness, an inner silence, an emotional "homecoming," or a meditation-like change in overall self-awareness. For example, gravity-oriented changes in body positions—such as some upside-down postures in yoga practices—could easily trigger new and interesting (and hopefully unthreatening) sensations in visceral ligaments, which can foster interoceptive refinement. Given the research indications for a close correlation of many psychoemotional disorders—such as irritable bowel syndrome, anxiety, or posttraumatic stress disorder—with a disrupted interoception, it is conceivable that some of these movement practices may have a strong therapeutic potential for these disorders. As a consequence, the integration of hands-on bodywork and hands-off movement strategies with psychotherapeutic techniques is increasingly gaining interest, especially regarding patients suffering from trauma, functional "unexplainable" symptoms, or stress-related disorders (Calsius 2020; Calsius et al. 2016).

KEY POINT

Given the importance of interoception, the integration of hands-on bodywork and hands-off movement strategies with psychotherapeutic techniques is increasingly gaining interest, especially regarding patients suffering from trauma, functional "unexplainable" symptoms, or stress-related disorders.

Typically, these therapeutic practices foster an attitude of inner mindfulness, of refining "internal listening skills," and they frequently alternate brief periods of active motor attention with subsequent periods of rest where the students pay attention to small interoceptive sensations within their body. Not surprisingly, some studies already indicate a positive health-enhancing effect of such "mindfulness-based therapies" for a large number of common clinical conditions (Astin et al. 2003)

Summary

In this chapter we tried to clarify several aspects of interoception and current insights on possible translational applications. Central to all this is how the fascial system as a dynamic and sensitive substrate for interoception can offer a unique entry point to the clients' "somatic" body and "psychological" inner world and thereby open up possibilities in therapy for structural dysfunctions and somatoemotional disorders. Also in contemplative movement practices interoception seems to be pivotal in improving general well-being and self-awareness. Regardless if we are perceiving, emoting, feeling, thinking, dreaming, moving, or touching, somewhere in the midst of all these intriguing but complex processes is always a vast share of interoception.

REFERENCES

Abraira, V.E., Ginty, D.D., 2013. The sensory neurons of touch. Neuron 79, 618–639.

Ackerley, R., Backlund Wasling, H., et al., 2014. Human C-tactile afferents are tuned to the temperature of a skin-stroking caress. J. Neurosci. 34, 2879–2883.

Andrews-Hanna, J.R., 2012. The brain's default network and its adaptive role in internal mentation. Neuroscientist 18, 251–270.

Astin, J.A., Shapiro, S.L., Eisenberg, D.M., Forys, K.L., 2003. Mind-body medicine: state of the science, implications for practice. J. Am. Board Fam. Pract. 16, 131–147.

Barrett, L.F., 2017. The theory of constructed emotion: an active inference account of interoception and categorization. Soc. Cogn. Affect. Neurosci. 12, 1–23.

Barrett, L.F., Simmons, W.K., 2015. Interoceptive predictions in the brain. Nat. Rev. Neurosci. 16, 419–429.

Berlucchi, G., Aglioti, S.M., 2010. The body in the brain revisited. Exp. Brain Res. 200, 25–35.

Björnsdotter, M., Morrison, I., Olausson, H., 2010. Feeling good: on the role of C fiber mediated touch in interoception. Exp. Brain Res. 207, 149–155.

Bogaerts, K., Van Eylen, L., Li, W., et al., 2010. Distorted symptom perception in patients with medically unexplained symptoms. J. Abnorm. Psychol. 119, 226–234.

Bordoni, B., Marelli, F., 2017. Emotions in motion. Myofascial interoception. Complement. Med. Res. 24, 110–113.

Calsius, J., 2020. Treating psychosomatic patients. In search of a transdisciplinary framework for the integration of bodywork in psychotherapy. Routledge, London.

Calsius, J., De Bie, J., Hertogen, R., Meesen, R., 2016. Touching the lived body in patients with medically unexplained symptoms: how an integration of hands-on bodywork and body awareness in psychotherapy may help people with alexithymia. Front. Psychol. 7, 253.

Cameron, O. G., 2001. Interoception: the inside story-a model for psychosomatic processes. Psychosom. Med. 63, 697–710.

Ceunen, E., Vlaeyen, J.W.S., Van Diest, I., 2016. On the origin of interoception. Front. Psychol. 7, 743.

Craig, A.D., 2003. Interoception: the sense of the physiological condition of the body. Curr. Opin. Neurobiol. 13, 500–505.

Craig, A.D., 2005. Forebrain emotional asymmetry: a neuroanatomical basis? Trends Cogn. Sci. 9, 566–571.

Craig, A.D., 2009. How do you feel now? The anterior insula and human awareness. Nat. Rev. Neurosci. 10, 59–70.

Craig, A. D., 2011. Significance of the insula for the evolution of human awareness of feelings from the body. Ann. N. Y. Acad. Sci. 1225, 72–82.

Critchley, H.D., Wiens, S., Rotshtein, P., Ohman, A., Dolan, R.J., 2004. Neural systems supporting interoceptive awareness. Nat. Neurosci. 7, 189–195.

D'Alessandro, G., Ceritelli, F., Cortelli, P., 2016. Sensitization and interoception as key neurological concepts in osteopathy and manual medicine. Front. Neurosci. doi:10.3389/fnins.2016.00100.

Damasio, A.R., 1994. Descartes' Error: Emotion, Reason, and the Human Brain. Grosset/Putnam, New York.

Elsenbruch, S., Rosenberger, C., Bingel, U., Forsting, M., Schedlowski, M., Gizewski, E.R., 2010. Patients with irritable bowel syndrome have altered emotional modulation of neural responses to visceral stimuli. Gastroenterology 139, 1310–1319.

Farb, N., Daubenmier, J., Price, C.J., et al., 2015. Interoception, contemplative practice, and health. Front. Psychol. 6, 763.

Fisher, J.D., Heslin, R., Rytting, M., 1976. Hands touching hands. Affective and evaluating effects of interpersonal touch. Sociometry 39, 416–421.

Fogel, A. (2009). The psychophysiology of self-awareness: rediscovering the lost art of body sense. W.W. Norton: New York.

Gershon, M.D., 1999. The Second Brain. Harper Perennial, New York.

Geuter, U., 2015. Körperpsychotherapie: grundriss einer theorie für die klinische praxis. Springer, Berlin.

Harlow, H.F., 1958. The nature of love. Am. Psychol. 13, 673–689.

Henningsen, P., Zipfel, S., Herzog, W., 2007. Management of functional somatic syndromes. Lancet 369, 946–955.

Herbert, B.M., Herbert, C., Pollatos, O., 2011. On the relationship between interoceptive awareness and alexithymia: is interoceptive awareness related to emotional awareness? J Pers. 79, 1149–1175

Kirsch, L.P., Krahé, C., Blom, N., et al., 2018. Reading the mind in the touch: neurophysiological specificity in the communication of emotions by touch. Neuropsychologia 116, 136–149.

Koroboki, E., Zakopoulos, N., Manios, E., et al. 2010. Interoceptive awareness in essential hypertension. Int. J. Psychophysiol. 78, 158–162.

Mehling, W.E., Wrubel, J., Daubenmier, et al., 2011. Body awareness: a phenomenological inquiry into the common ground of mind-body therapies. Philos. Ethics Humanit. Med. 6, 6.

Montague, A., 1971. Touch: The Human Significance of the Skin. Harper & Row, New York.

More, S.R., Mc Ewen, L.M., Quirt J., et al., 2017. Epigenetic correlates of neonatal contact in humans. Dev. Psychopathol. 29, 1517–1538.

Murphy, J., Brewer R., Catmur, C., Bird, G., 2017. Interoception and psychopathology: a developmental neuroscience perspective. Dev. Cogn. Neurosci. 23, 45–56.

Naqvi, N.H., Bechara, A., 2010. The insula and drug addiction: an interoceptive view of pleasure, urges, and decision-making. Brain Struct. Funct. 214, 435–450.

Olausson, H.W., Cole, J., Vallbo, A., et al., 2008. Unmyelinated tactile afferents have opposite effects on insular and somatosensory cortical processing. Neurosci. Lett. 436, 128–132.

Olausson, H., Wessberg, J., Morrison, I., McGlone, F., Vallbo, A., 2010. The neurophysiology of unmyelinated tactile afferents. Neurosci. Biobehav. Rev. 34, 185–191.

Oosterwijck, S, Barrett, L.F., 2014. Embodiment in the construction of emotion experience and emotion understanding. In: Shapiro, L. (Ed.), Routledge Handbook of Embodied Cognition. Routledge, New York, pp. 250–260.

Paulus, M.P., Stein, M.B., 2010. Interoception in anxiety and depression. Brain Struct. Funct. 214, 451–463.

Rebello, K., Moura, L.M., Pinaya, W.H.L., Rohde, L.A., Sato, J.R., 2018. Default mode network maturation and environmental adversities during childhood. Chronic Stress 2, 1–10.

Schleip, R., 2003. Fascial plasticity – a new neurobiological explanation. Part 1. J. Bodyw. Mov. Ther. 7, 11–19.

Stecco, C., 2015. Functional Atlas of the Human Fascial System. Churchill Livingstone Elsevier, London.

Stecco, C., Stern, R., Porzionato, R., et al., 2011. Hyaluron within fascia in the etiology of myofascial pain. Surg. Radiol. Anat. 33, 891–896.

Turvey, M.T., Fonseca, S.T., 2014. The medium of haptic perception: a tensegrity hypothesis. J. Mot. Behav. 46, 143–187.

Van Oudenhove, L., Levy, R.L., Crowell, M.D., et al., 2016. Biopsychosocial aspects of functional gastrointestinal disorders: how central and environmental processes contribute to the development and expression of functional gastrointestinal disorders. Gastroenterology 150, 1355–1367.

Nociception: The Thoracolumbar and Crural Fascia as Sensory Organs

Ulrich Hoheisel, Toru Taguchi, and Siegfried Mense

CHAPTER CONTENTS

INTRODUCTION

In the literature, the thoracolumbar fascia (TLF) is usually assumed to have a mechanical function connecting the latissimus dorsi muscle to the gluteal muscles, thus functionally linking the arm with the leg. Other functions are: (1) forming a sheath around muscles that reduces friction during movements, (2) facilitating the return of venous blood to the heart, (3) providing an ectoskeleton for the attachment of muscles, and (4) protecting blood vessels and muscles from mechanical damage (e.g., the lacertus fibrosus of the biceps brachii muscle or the aponeuroses of the palm or soles) (Benjamin 2009).

Recent data indicate that fascia in general is not just a passive structure but is contractile. The basis of the contractility are myofibroblasts that appear to be present in many fascia and perform very slow "contractions," lasting many minutes, when the tissue is stimulated chemically in vitro (Schleip et al. 2007). A clinical manifestation of the contractility of fascia tissue is the Dupuytren's syndrome. Data show that genetic causes contribute to the high contractility of palmar fascia tissue in Dupuytren's syndrome (Staats et al. 2016).

Finally, the fascia has been discussed as a possible source of pain in patients with nonspecific low back pain (Yahia et al. 1992). This type of back pain does not originate in bony structures of the spine or the facet joints but in the soft tissues of the low back (muscles, ligaments, fasciae). Nonspecific low back pain is one of the most common pain complaints in industrialized countries; therefore, the clarification of a possible contribution of fascia receptors to this pain would be of importance not only for our understanding but also for the management of this type of pain.

To fulfil the role of a pain source in nonspecific low back pain, the fascia should have a dense innervation with sensory fibers. However, the innervation of the TLF was largely ignored as a subject of scientific studies and, therefore, little information is available on the innervation of the fasciae and hence on the possible sensory role of the fascia. Panjabi (2006) published a comprehensive report of mechanisms of pain generation in nonspecific low back pain but did not mention the TLF as a potential source. On the other hand, there can be no doubt that most fasciae are innervated. For instance, Stecco and colleagues (2007) found abundant nerve fibers in the fasciae of the upper limb, including retinacula and the lacertus fibrosus.

Likewise, the results of a histological study on human specimens by Yahia and colleagues (1992) showed that the TLF is innervated and possesses free and encapsulated nerve endings. For the present article, the free nerve endings are particularly interesting because many of them are nociceptive and mediate pain. For the tibial anterior fascia, an important role for the pain of delayed onset muscle soreness (DOMS) has been suggested in a study on human subjects (Gibson et al. 2009). In this investigation, hypertonic saline was injected as a pain-producing agent into the muscle and the overlying structures after induction of DOMS in that muscle. The main result was that the injection directly underneath the fascia caused more pain than into the muscle itself. Schilder and colleagues arrived at the same conclusion when testing the thoracolumbar fascia (Schilder et al. 2014).

The aims of the present report were twofold: (1) find out what types of nerve fibers are present in the TLF and crural fascia (CF); (2) obtain electrophysiological data on the responses of sensory neurons in the spinal dorsal horn to stimulation of TLF and CF. The underlying question of the second aim was where in the spinal cord the information from fascia receptors was processed and how neurons with input from the fascia behave in general.

PART 1: INNERVATION OF THE THORACOLUMBAR FASCIA

Regarding the fascia's possible function as a source of pain in patients with low back pain, the afferent (sensory) fibers are expected to include nociceptive ones. In our group, we studied the innervation of the thoracolumbar fascia in rats in whole mount preparations and coronal sections, both taken from the lumbar level. Close to the spinous processes of the spine the fascia had three layers: (1) a thin outer layer consisting of parallel collagen fibers oriented transversely (in the coronal plane), (2) a thick middle layer composed of massive collagen fiber bundles running obliquely to the long axis of the body, and (3) a thin inner layer consisting of loose connective tissue covering the underlying multifidus muscle (Fig. 2.4.1A). Since many nerve fibers coursed from the connective tissue into the outer layer of the fascia proper (or vice versa), the connective tissue can be viewed as the fourth layer of the fascia. All fibers were visualized with immunohistochemical techniques. As a universal marker for all nerve fibers, antibodies to protein gene product 9.5 (PGP 9.5) were used. The coronal section in Fig. 2.4.1(A) shows PGP 9.5-immunoreactive (ir) neuronal structures mainly in the subcutaneous and outer layer as well as in the inner layer. The nerve fibers included truncated fibers of passage

(black arrows) and nerve endings (open arrows). Nerve endings are characterized by a granular structure at a low magnification that is due to the axonal expansions (varicosities) close to the nerve terminal (as discussed later). The fibers of passage did not necessarily belong to the innervation of the fascia; theoretically they may supply tissues other than the fascia.

Fig. 2.4.1(D,a) is a quantitative evaluation of the PGP 9.5-ir fibers. In a 5-mm-long part of the fascia in coronal sections, the length of all fibers and nerve endings in the various layers of the fascia were measured and the mean fiber length was calculated. The various parts of each bar graph show the mean fiber length in a given layer. The evaluation showed clearly that the great majority of all fibers were situated in the subcutaneous tissue and outer layer of the fascia. In the middle and inner layer only a small fraction of all fibers were found.

The peptidergic sensory nerve endings were identified with antibodies to the neuropeptide calcitonin gene-related peptide (CGRP) and substance P (SP; Danielson et al. 2006). CGRP is present in a high percentage of sensory fibers and serves as a general marker for these fibers (Danielson et al. 2006). The SP-containing fibers are a subpopulation of the CGRP fibers, as all SP-positive fibers also contain CGRP. Fibers containing SP are of particular interest, because they are assumed to have a nociceptive function (Lawson et al. 1997). Both SP and CGRP-ir fibers are involved in pain processes in that they induce neurogenic inflammation (i.e. vasodilation) and increase the permeability of blood vessels caused by action potentials that release CGRP and SP from free nerve endings of sensory fibers (Mense et al. 1996). These action potentials originate in the dorsal roots or peripheral nerve and invade the nerve endings antidromically (against the normal direction of propagation).

One aim of the present study was to perform a quantitative evaluation of CGRP-ir and SP-ir nerve fibers and sensory endings. Such an evaluation is important because the density of neuropeptide-ir fibers (such as SP and CGRP) had been shown to vary greatly from one tissue to the other (McMahon et al. 1984). Figure 2.4.1(D,b and c) shows a quantitative evaluation of CGRP-ir and SP-ir nerve fibers. Compared with all (PGP 9.5-ir) fibers, the CGRP fibers were much less numerous: approximately 16%. As in other tissues, the SP-ir fibers were just a small fraction of the CGRP fibers. Figure 2.4.1(B, C) shows examples of free nerve endings that were ir for these neuropeptides. A typical feature of these sensory nerve

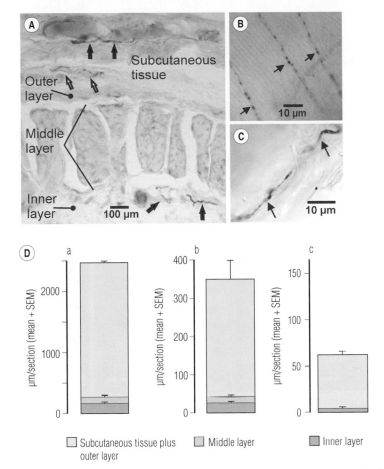

Fig. 2.4.1 Innervation of the Thoracolumbar Fascia. (A) Coronal section of the thoracolumbar fascia close to the spinous process L5 (thickness 40 μm). Outer layer: collagen fibers oriented transversely; middle layer: collagen fiber bundles orientated diagonally to the long axis of the body; inner layer: loose connective tissue covering the multifidus muscle. Black arrows mark PGP 9.5-immunoreactive (ir) nerve fibers of passage, open arrows PGP 9.5-ir nerve endings. (B) Three CGRP-ir terminal axons (arrows) with chains of varicosities in a whole mount preparation of the inner layer (dorsal view). The cross striation of the underlying multifidus muscle is visible. (C) SP-ir terminal axon (arrows) located in the subcutaneous tissue close to the outer layer (coronal section, thickness 40 μm). (D) Quantitative evaluation of the mean fiber length in the fascia layers as indicated in (A). (D,a) PGP 9.5- ir nerve fibers (PGP 9.5 is a universal marker for all nerve fibers), (D,b) CGRP-ir nerve fibers, (D,c) SP-ir nerve fibers. CGRP and SP are markers of peptidergic sensory nerve fibers. White part of the bar: subcutaneous tissue plus outer layer of the fascia; black: middle layer; gray: inner layer. Note that the middle layer of the fascia is free from SP-ir nerve fibers (D,c).

endings were the widenings of the axon (the so-called varicosities, Fig. 2.4.1B) that look like a string of beads or pearls (Fig. 2.4.2A). The varicosities are the sites where stimuli are thought to act.

In the context of this chapter the SP-ir nerve endings are particularly interesting, because they are assumed to be nociceptive. Therefore the ending shown in Fig. 2.4.1C probably represented a nociceptor. In this case it was situated in the subcutaneous tissue overlying the fascia proper. An interesting finding was that in the middle layer of the fascia no SP-ir fibers or endings were found (Fig. 2.4.1D,c). Teleologically this makes sense, because the middle layer has to transmit the forces that accompany all body movements. If nociceptive endings existed between the collagen fiber bundles of the middle layer they

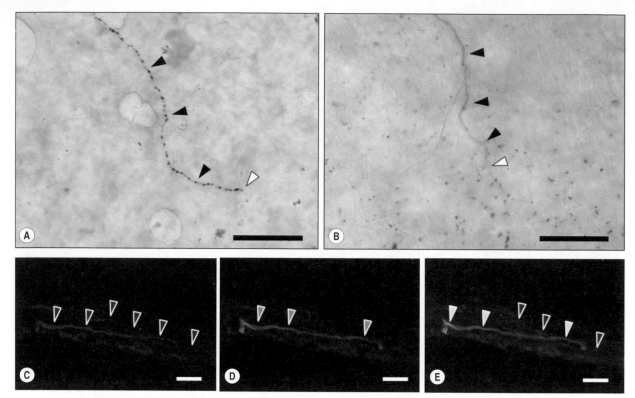

Fig. 2.4.2 **CGRP- and Peripherin-Immunoreactive (-ir) Nerve Fibers in the Crural Fascia (CF).** (A–B) Bright field images of nerve fibers from whole mount preparations of the CF. (A) A peptidergic CGRP-ir axon with a long chain of varicosities and its nerve terminal. (B) A nonpeptidergic peripherin-ir axon and its nerve terminal. Filled arrowheads: axon of immunoreactive nerve. Open arrowheads: peripheral nerve terminal. Scale bars: 50 μm. (C–E) Fluorescent images of a CGRP-ir nerve fiber (red, C), peripherin-ir (green, D), and superimposed (yellow, E) in a transverse section of the CF. Scale bars: 50 μm. (A and B) Reproduced with permission from Taguchi, T., Yasui, M., Kubo, A., et al., 2013. Nociception originating from the crural fascia in rats. Pain 154, 1103–14. (C–E) Courtesy Dr. M. Yasui, Department of Functional Anatomy and Neuroscience, Nagoya University Graduate School of Medicine.

would be excited by trunk movements. The result would be movement-induced pain even in subjects with otherwise intact lower back. The paucity of fibers in the middle layer of the fascia is in line with the statements of Hagert and colleagues (2007) who distinguished between ligaments that are mechanically important yet poorly innervated (e.g., the ligaments of the wrist) and ligaments whose main role appears to be sensory. The latter structures consist largely of loose connective tissue, and nerve fibers are predominantly located in this tissue.

Regarding the extent of sensory innervation of the TLF, the following coarse calculation can be made: the peptidergic CGRP- and SP-ir fibers are not the only sensory fibers, because there are also nonpeptidergic/lectin-positive thin sensory fibers. Even if the same number of nonpeptidergic sensory fibers are added to the peptidergic ones—which is probably too high a number, because both groups overlap (Hwang et al. 2005)—all sensory fibers would make up approximately 1/3 of all fibers. This means that about 2/3 of the innervation of the fascia is nonpeptidergic or efferent. The efferent fibers probably consist of sympathetic postganglionic fibers. Indeed, data from our group indicate that with a specific marker for sympathetic fibers (tyrosine hydroxylase, an enzyme necessary for the synthesis of [nor-]epinephrine) a large fraction of the fibers in the TLF can be labeled. This finding may explain the great influence psychological stressors have on the pain of patients with nonspecific low back pain.

KEY POINT

The thoracolumbar fascia (TLF) is densely innervated with sensory and sympathetic fibers.

PART 2: ELECTROPHYSIOLOGY

So far, just a few electrophysiological studies have addressed primary afferent fibers and dorsal horn neurons (second-order neurons) that have receptive fields (RFs) in lumbar soft tissues. The first description of mechanosensitive afferent units in lumbar intervertebral discs and adjacent muscles was made by Yamashita and colleagues (1993) in rabbits. They identified 13 mechanosensitive units. The RFs of 10 units were located in the psoas muscle, three in the intervertebral disc area. The mechanical thresholds of the afferent units from muscle were low to high. The receptors having a high mechanical threshold were considered to be nociceptive.

In the literature, there is little information about the response behavior of afferent fibers from the TLF. In 1995 unmyelinated nociceptors ($n = 57$) in paraspinal tissues of rats were described (Bove and Light 1995). Some of these receptors responded to stimulation of the fascia. The centers of the RFs were located in the tail or base of the tail in most cases when the recordings were made from the dorsal roots L6 and S1. This finding indicates that there is a caudal shift of the RFs in the deep tissues of the low back relative to the segmental level of the dorsal roots through which the afferent fibers enter the CNS.

PART 3: INNERVATION OF THE CRURAL FASCIA

1. Immunohistochemistry

Similar to the TLF, the CF is densely innervated. Figure 2.4.2(A) shows a peptidergic CGRP-ir nerve fiber in whole mount preparations of the CF. The CF exhibited also nerve fibers immunoreactive to peripherin, a neural marker for nonpeptidergic thin-fiber receptors (Fig. 2.4.2B). The distribution patterns of CGRP- and peripherin-ir nerve fibers were similar, and the two markers coexisted in the same fibers (Fig. 2.4.2C–E).

2. Response Behavior of Thin-Fiber Receptors

The response behavior of thin myelinated (Aδ-) and unmyelinated (C-) fiber afferents from the CF were systematically characterized using a single-fiber electrophysiological recording technique in vivo (Taguchi et al. 2013). After removal of the skin, receptors in the CF could be stimulated without affecting those in the tibialis anterior muscle, because the fascia has sufficient thickness to be pulled up with a forceps. Moreover, it is connected to the muscle by loose connective tissue only. This makes it possible to identify the exact location of the RF in the CF.

The electrophysiological data revealed that Aδ- and C-fibers in the CF had different characteristics in many ways:

- Rate of resting discharge. In Aδ-fibers, only 1 out of 16 (6%) had ongoing activity, and the mean discharge rate was 0.01 impulses/s. In contrast, 67% of the group C-fibers (16 of 24) showed resting activity, and the discharge rate was 0.21 impulses/s.
- Size and location of the RFs. The RFs of Aδ-fibers were distributed over the entire CF except the area medial to the edge of the tibial bone (Fig. 2.4.3A). The RFs of C-fibers were exclusively located in the distal third of the CF. Moreover, the RF size of Aδ-fibers was much larger than that of C-fibers. The reason for the different location and size of RFs between the Aδ- and the C-fibers that were recorded from the same nerve branch (i.e., peroneal nerve) is unknown.
- Responsiveness to mechanical stimulation. As shown in Fig. 2.4.3(B), both Aδ- and C-fibers exhibited increased firing rates in response to a ramp shaped mechanical stimulus (pressure of 0–392 mN in 40 s) in a roughly intensity-dependent manner up to the maximum force. The mean response magnitude in action potentials per the stimulus period was seven times higher in Aδ-fibers than in C-fibers (Fig. 2.4.3C). From the response behavior of the two fiber types, it is difficult to decide if they were mechanoreceptors or nociceptors. The higher stimulation threshold and smaller response magnitude of C-fiber receptors suggest that they may represent nociceptors. In contrast, the low stimulation threshold and high response magnitude of Aδ- receptors speaks more for a mechanoreceptive function.
- Responsiveness to chemical stimuli (Taguchi et al. 2013). Thirteen of 23 C-fibers tested (57%) were responsive to the algesic substance bradykinin (10 μM). The proportion of bradykinin-responsive C-fibers lay between the proportions found in muscle (74%; Taguchi et al. 2005)

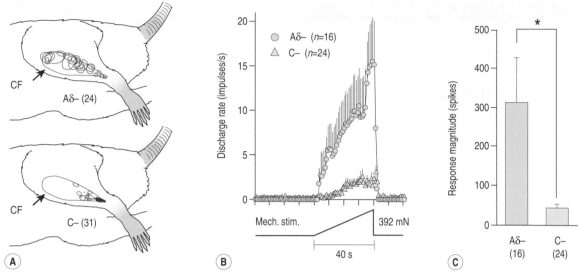

Fig. 2.4.3 Mechanical Responses of Thin-Fiber Receptors in the Crural Fascia (CF). (A) Distribution of receptive fields of fascial Aδ- (n = 24, upper panel) and C-fibers (n = 31, lower panel). (B) Mechanical response patterns of fascial Aδ- (n = 16) and C-fibers (n = 24) to a ramp-shaped mechanical stimulus (0–392 mN in 40 s). The y-axis shows mean discharge rate +SEM of all the fibers recorded (bin width: 1 s). (C) Quantitative analysis of the magnitude of the mechanical response given by net-evoked discharges during the stimulus period for 40 s in (B). Note the significantly larger mechanical response in Aδ-fibers than in C-fibers. Modified with permission from Taguchi, T., Yasui, M., Kubo, A., et al., 2013. Nociception originating from the crural fascia in rats. Pain 154, 1103–14.

and skin (33%; Taguchi et al. 2010). In the CF, only 1 out of 16 Aδ-fibers was responsive to bradykinin.

- Responsiveness to heat stimuli (Taguchi et al. 2013). Eleven out of 21 C-fibers (52%) responded to heat (from 32°C to 50°C during 30 s), whereas none of the Aδ-fibers did. The relatively high susceptibility of C-fiber receptors to heat could mean that they were equipped with TRPV1 receptor molecules. This interpretation would fit in the assumption that the C-fibers were nociceptive.

In addition, 43% of the C-fiber receptors in the CF were polymodal nociceptors responding to mechanical, chemical, and heat stimuli, while none of the Aδ-fibers were of the polymodal type.

3. Projection of Cf Afferents to the Spinal Cord

Irrespective of the function of the CF receptors (nociception or mechanoreception), the sensory information has to be transmitted to the central nervous system. The spinal projection pattern of sensory input from the CF has been demonstrated by using the neuronal activation

marker c-Fos (Taguchi et al. 2013). The c-Fos expression in response to repetitive noxious pinching of the CF with watchmaker's forceps was increased in the middle to medial part of the superficial dorsal horn (laminae I–II) of the ipsilateral side. The craniocaudal distribution extended from the spinal segments L2 to L4, peaking at segment L3. No obvious c-Fos-ir nuclei were found in ipsilateral deeper laminae (laminae III–VI) or on the side contralateral to the pinching stimuli.

PART 4: EFFECTS OF AN EXPERIMENTAL FASCIA INFLAMMATION

1. Primary Afferent Fibers

An experimental fasciitis was induced by injection of Freund complete adjuvant into the fascia. Twelve days later the density of innervation for each fiber type was determined. The histological picture of the experimentally induced fasciitis resembled an eosinophilic inflammation.

TABLE 2.4.1   Quantitative Evaluation of the Fiber Length in the Three Layers of the Rat Thoracolumbar Fascia By Immunohistochemistry (Serial Cryostat Cross-Sections at a Thickness of 40 μm)

| | FIBER LENGTH PER 1000 μm^2 | | | | | | | |
| | PGP 9.5 | | CGRP | | Substance P | | Tyrosine hydroxylase | |
Fascia:	Intact	Inflamed (CFA)	Intact	Inflamed (CFA)	Intact	Inflamed (CFA)	Intact	Inflamed (CFA)
Outer layer	3.13 μm	1.10 μm ↓	046 μm	0.24 μm	0.002 μm	0.06 μm ↑	0.24 μm	0.02 μm ↓
Middle layer	0.07 μm	0.22 μm	0.01 μm	1.02 μm	—	—	0.003 μm	0.004 μm
Inner layer	3.74 μm	5.28 μm	0.30 μm	1.01 μm ↑	—	0.05 μm ↑	0.11 μm	0.09 μm
All layers	2.31 μm	2.14 μm	0.25 μm	0.41 μm	0.001 μm	0.03 μm ↑	0.12 μm	0.07 μm ↓

Intact: data from intact fascia; inflamed: inflamed fascia 12 days after injection of Complete Freund's Adjuvant. PGP 9.5 (protein gene product 9.5): universal marker for all nervous structures. CGRP and substance P: markers for sensory peptidergic nerve fibers. Tyrosine hydroxylase: marker for postganglionic sympathetic nerve fibers. ↑ Significant increase in density in the inflamed fascia ($p < 0.05$). ↓ Significant decrease in density in the inflamed fascia ($p < 0.05$).
PGP, protein gene product 9.5; CGRP, calcitonin gene-related peptide.

The inflamed fascia exhibited a higher density of CGRP-ir and SP-ir units (Table 2.4.1). However, the density of PGP 9.5-positive units, which represented all afferent and efferent fibers in the fascia, was reduced. This result occurs because the many sympathetic units had a much lower density in the inflamed fascia. The reason for this decrease in sympathetic fiber density is not known.

The changes in innervation density of the inflamed fascia occurred in the subcutaneous tissue and the inner layer; they were almost absent in the middle layer. Moreover, we never found a SP-ir fiber in this layer, and this was valid for the intact and inflamed fascia.

The mechanism for the increased fiber length in inflamed tissue is obscure. The most likely mechanism appears to be sprouting and not increased branching of the fibers (Reinert et al. 1998).

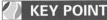
KEY POINT

In inflamed fascia the innervation density with CGRP- and SP-ir fibers was increased.

2. Dorsal Horn Neurons

KEY POINT

Dorsal horn neurons receiving input from the TLF and CF do exist.

Electrophysiological (microelectrode) recordings of dorsal horn neurons receiving input from lumbar tissues in cats were made for the first time by Gillette and colleagues (1993). They recorded the neurons extracellularly in the dorsal horn of the spinal cord. Gillette and colleagues found that most neurons (72%) received excitatory convergent input from skin and deep tissues. Some neurons (23%) had RFs restricted to the skin, and very few cells (5%) had RFs in deep somatic tissues. The deep-tissue RFs were located in facet joint capsules, periosteum, ligaments, intervertebral disc, spinal dura, low back/hip/proximal leg muscles, and tendons. Most RFs in the deep tissues of the cat's lower back were located at the vertebral level L6-L7 whereas the recordings were made in the spinal segments L4-L5.

Experiments of our group revealed the existence of nociceptive input from the TLF to dorsal horn neurons, suggesting that the TLF is a possible source of low back pain (Fig. 2.4.4). In these experiments, systematic extracellular recordings from dorsal horn neurons were made in the spinal segments Th13-L5 in rats (Taguchi et al. 2008). The fascial RFs were searched by pinching (noxious mechanical stimulation) of the TLF with a sharpened watchmaker's forceps. A sample recording of the discharges of a single neuron in the segment Th13 is shown in Fig. 2.4.4(C). The neuron showed afterdischarge following the short noxious

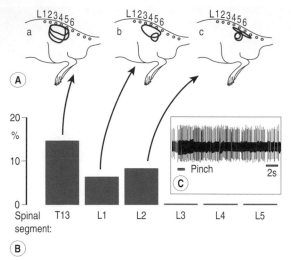

Fig. 2.4.4 Dorsal Horn Neurons Processing Input from Thoracolumbar Fascia. (A) Fascial receptive fields of dorsal horn neurons recorded in thoracic spinal segment T 13 (a) and lumbar spinal segments L1 (b) and L2 (c). Numbers indicate spinous processes of lumbar vertebrae. Note that the receptive fields were shifted caudad relative to the spinal segments in which the neurons were recorded. (B) Proportion of dorsal horn neurons with input from thoracolumbar fascia (TLF) in spinal segments T13-L5. The spinal segments Th13-L2 received TLF input, while in the segments L3-L5 it is missing. (C) Original registration of action potentials from a single dorsal horn neuron during and after pinching the fascia for approximately 1.5 s (black bar underneath the registration).

stimulus, which is seen mainly in nociceptive neurons. Many dorsal horn neurons with fascial RFs also responded to stimulation with a small cotton ball soaked with 5% hypertonic saline and put on the surface of the fascia. The responses to this stimulus often occurred at a very short latency. This finding is in line with the neuroanatomical results showing that the SP-positive nerve fibers were mainly found in the subcutaneous tissue and outer layer of the fascia (Fig. 2.4.1D,c).

Neurons with RFs in the TLF were found in the spinal segments Th13-L2, but not in L3-L5 (Fig. 2.4.4B). Approximately 6% to 14% percent of the dorsal horn neurons in the spinal segments Th13-L2 had input from the TLF. The approximate centers of RFs in the TLF were located at the vertebral levels L3-L4, L4-L5, and L5-L6 when the recordings were made in the

spinal segments Th13, L1, and L2, respectively. The location of the fascial RFs was consistently shifted three to four segments caudally relative to their recording site (Fig. 2.4.4A; Taguchi et al. 2008). Usually, all RFs in the TLF were located on the side ipsilateral to the recording site. Most of the neurons with RFs in the TLF had convergent input from the skin and other deep tissues or regions in the low back, abdominal wall, hip, and proximal/distal leg. This finding may explain the diffuse nature of nonspecific low back pain patients.

In experiments employing recordings from dorsal horn neurons with input from the gastrocnemius-soleus muscle and low back muscles, both low- and high-threshold mechanosensitive cells were found (Hoheisel et al. 2000; Taguchi et al. 2008). So far, such a classification based on the mechanical threshold of dorsal horn neurons has not been undertaken for neurons with input from the TLF. However, our results indicate that most of the neurons with fascial input behaved like wide-dynamic-range (WDR) neurons, most of which are assumed to be nociceptive.

In experiments with inflammatory lesions of muscle and fascia, the excitability of dorsal horn neurons was increased. In animals in which a tonic-chronic (6 days duration) myositis of the multifidus muscle had been induced, the proportion of neurons with fascial RFs in the thoracolumbar region rose significantly. In addition, in the spinal segment L3 that does not normally receive input from the TLF, more than 10% of the cells responded to input from the TLF in myositis animals. These electrophysiological recordings from dorsal horn neurons of rats revealed that the TLF is an important source of nociception originating from the low back and could contribute to the pain of patients with chronic low back pain.

Interestingly, after induction of the myositis the increase in the proportion of neurons responding to input from the TLF was higher than that of cells responding to input from the inflamed muscle itself. Additionally, in human subjects who had been induced with delayed onset muscle soreness (DOMS), the fascia covering the overused muscle became more sensitive to painful stimulation than the muscle itself (Gibson et al. 2009). Collectively, these findings suggest that, in patients with nonspecific low back pain, fascia tissue may be a more important pain source than the low back muscles or other soft tissues.

Summary

- The TLF is densely innervated with sensory and sympathetic fibers.
- In inflamed fascia the innervation density with CGRP- and SP-ir fibers was increased.
- Dorsal horn neurons receiving input from the TLF and CF do exist.
- The input from the TLF is processed in spinal segments cranial to L2 in animals with intact soft tissues.
- The approximate center of the RF in the TLF was always shifted several segments caudad relative to the spinal segment recorded from.
- In animals with a tonic-chronic myositis and fasciitis, the size of the RFs in the TLF expanded, the proportion of neurons with RFs in the TLF increased, and the segment L3 acquired TLF input.
- These neurophysiological findings, together with the neuroanatomical data, are relevant for a better understanding of the mechanisms of nonspecific low back pain. Under chronic pathological conditions, an enhanced nociceptive input from the TLF could contribute to low back pain in patients.

REFERENCES

Benjamin, M., 2009. The fascia of the limbs and back - a review. J. Anat. 214, 1–18.

Bove, G.M., Light, A.R., 1995. Unmyelinated nociceptors of rat paraspinal tissues. J. Neurophysiol. 73, 1752–1762.

Danielson, P., Alfredson, H., Forsgren, S., 2006. Distribution of general (PGP 9.5) and sensory (substance P/CGRP) innervations in the human patellar tendon. Arthrosc. Knee Surg. Sports Traumatol. 14, 125–132.

Gibson, W., Arendt-Nielsen, L., Taguchi, T., Mizumura, K., Graven-Nielsen, T., 2009. Increased pain from muscle fascia following eccentric exercise: animal and human findings. Exp. Brain Res. 194, 299–308.

Gillette, R.G., Kramis, R.C., Roberts, W.J., 1993. Characterization of spinal somatosensory neurons having receptive fields in lumbar tissues of cats. Pain 54, 85–98.

Hagert, E., Garcia-Elias, M., Forsgren, S., Ljung, B.O., 2007. Immunohistochemical analysis of wrist ligament innervation in relation to their structural composition. J. Hand Surg. Am. 32, 30–36.

Hoheisel, U., Unger, T., Mense, S., 2000. A block of spinal nitric oxide synthesis leads to increased background activity predominantly in nociceptive dorsal horn neurones in the rat. Pain 88, 249–257.

Hwang, S.J., Oh, J.M., Valtschanoff, J.G., 2005. The majority of bladder sensory afferents to the rat lumbosacral spinal cord are both IB4- and CGRP-positive. Brain Res. 1062, 86–91.

Lawson, S.N., Crepps, B.A., Perl, E.R., 1997. Relationship of substance P to afferent characteristics of dorsal root ganglion neurones in guinea-pig. J. Physiol. 505, 177–191.

McMahon, S.B., Sykova, E., Wall, P.D., Woolf, C.J., Gibson, S.J., 1984. Neurogenic extravasation and substance P levels are low in muscle as compared to skin the rat hindlimb. Neurosci. Lett. 52, 235–240.

Mense, S., Hoheisel, U., Reinert, A., 1996. The possible role of substance P in eliciting and modulating deep somatic pain. Prog. Brain Res. 110, 125–135.

Panjabi, M.M., 2006. A hypothesis of chronic back pain: ligament subfailure injuries lead to muscle control dysfunction. Eur. Spine J. 15, 668–676.

Reinert, A., Kaske, A., Mense, S., 1998. Inflammation-induced increase in the density of neuropeptide-immunoreactive nerve endings in rat skeletal muscle. Exp. Brain Res. 121, 174–180.

Schilder, A., Hoheisel, U., Magerl, W., et al., 2014. Sensory findings after stimulation of the thoracolumbar fascia with hypertonic saline suggest its contribution to low back pain. Pain 155, 222–231.

Schleip, R., Kingler, W., Lehmann-Horn, F., 2007. Fascia is able to contract in a smooth muscle-like manner and thereby influence musculoskeletal mechanics. In: Fascia research. Basic science and implications for conventional and complementary health care. Urban and Fischer, Munich, pp. 76–77.

Staats, K.A., Wu, T., Gan, B.S., O'Gorman, D.B., Ophoff, R.A., 2016. Dupuytren's disease susceptibility gene, EPDR1, is involved in myofibroblast contractility. J. Dermatol. Sci. 83, 131–137.

Stecco, C., Gagey, O., Belloni, A., et al., 2007. Anatomy of the deep fascia of the upper limb. Second part: study of innervation. Morphologie 91, 38–43.

Taguchi, T., Hoheisel, U., Mense, S., 2008. Dorsal horn neurons having input from low back structures in rats. Pain 138, 119–129.

Taguchi, T., Ota, H., Matsuda, T., Murase, S., Mizumura, K., 2010. Cutaneous C-fiber nociceptor responses and nociceptive behaviors in aged Sprague-Dawley rats. Pain 151, 771–782.

Taguchi, T., Sato, J., Mizumura, K., 2005. Augmented mechanical response of muscle thin-fiber sensory receptors recorded from rat muscle-nerve preparations in vitro after eccentric contraction. J. Neurophysiol. 94, 2822–2831.

Taguchi, T., Yasui, M., Kubo, A., et al. 2013. Nociception originating from the crural fascia in rats. Pain 154, 1103–1114.

Yahia, L., Rhalmi, S., Newman, N., Isler, M., 1992. Sensory innervation of human thoracolumbar fascia. An immunohistochemical study. Acta Orthop. Scand. 63, 195–197.

Yamashita, T., Minaki, Y., Oota, I., Yokogushi, K., Ishii, S., 1993. Mechanosensitive afferent units in the lumbar intervertebral disc and adjacent muscle. Spine 18, 2252–2256.

2.5

Fascia as a Body-Wide Communication System

James L. Oschman

CHAPTER CONTENTS

"A single-celled paramecium swims gracefully, avoids predators, finds food, mates, and has sex, all without a single synapse. "Of nerve there is no trace. But the cell framework, the cytoskeleton might serve."
                                      —*Sherrington (1951)*

INTRODUCTION

The opening quotation, from an eminent neuroscientist, reminds us of the existence of evolutionarily ancient communication systems present in single-celled organisms that are entirely lacking in nerves or synapses. How does a single-celled creature, such as a paramecium, lead such a sophisticated life without a nervous system? Many cell biologists are recognizing that the cytoskeleton is the "nervous system" of the cell. The extracellular coats of the "primitive" microorganisms are thought to have evolved into the mammalian extracellular matrix. Specifically, the extracellular sugar polymer coatings of individual bacteria, viruses, and protozoa extended the "reach" of these ancient organisms into their environment and formed the oldest and most pervasive information and defense system in nature. The connective tissue and fascia are thought to be the modern expressions of these ancient cell coats.

In 1858, Virchow pointed out that each of the 50 billion cells in the human body is an "elementary organism." These ancient organisms evolved into the modern mammalian cell (Puck 1972). Mammalian cells contain miniature "musculoskeletal systems" composed of microtubules (the "bones" of the cell), microfilaments (the "muscles" of the cell), and other filamentous molecules that can act as a sort of "connective tissue" within the cell. These cellular components enable cells to change shape and to migrate from place to place as they carry out their functions of tissue maintenance and repair.

In early colonial organisms such as volvox, individual cell coats combined to form a continuous inner matrix supporting the cells. Later evolutionary steps led to the first nerves and muscles, as in the coelenterates. Most biologists accept the Darwinian principle of gradual refinements during the long evolutionary process. Hence the interconnected cellular and extracellular matrices have had a much longer period of evolutionary refinement than the nervous system. We need to study the relationships between the fascia and the cells that maintain and repair injuries. Highly relevant clues come from the experiences of body therapists, body psychotherapists, and energy psychologists who have come to recognize that memory and traumatic memory are intertwined and have significant somatic components (for example, see Hansmann 2013; Schleip 2003; Grassman and Pohlenz-Michel 2007; Redpath 1995; Oschman 2006; Feinstein 2012).

COMMUNICATION AND INFORMATION PROCESSING

In his book *Wetware: A Computer in Every Living Cell*, Bray (2009) proposed that cells are built of molecular circuits that perform logical operations, as electronic devices do. He also suggested that the computational properties of cells may provide the basis for all the distinctive properties of living systems, including the ability to embody in their internal structures images of the world around them. These concepts account for the adaptability, responsiveness, and intelligence of cells and organisms.

Because of its obvious importance, the brain has been studied with a vast array of analytical tools, and we know enough about it to fill many books and journals. However, many unanswered questions remain. For example, the discovery that the connective tissue cells in the brain also form a communication system has returned the whole of neuroscience to the drawing boards. In mammals, connective tissue cells called glia (the Greek word γλια means "glue") constitute some 50% or more of the volume of the brain. Decades of research have required revision of the traditional view that glial cells function purely for mechanical and nutritional support. We now know that glial cells interact morphologically, biochemically, and physiologically with neurons throughout the brain, modulate neuronal activity, and influence behavior (Koob 2009). A new cutting-edge branch of both neuroscience and fascial research has been born based on the relationship between connective tissue cells and neuronal processes.

This chapter explores the concept that these ancient communication systems persist throughout the modern mammalian organism and that their existence helps account for several phenomena that may be difficult to explain by neural mechanisms alone.

DEFINING THE FASCIA

Findley and Schleip (2007) have defined fascia broadly to include all of the soft fibrous connective tissues that permeate the human body. Their definition has the important feature of blurring the arbitrary demarcation lines between various components of the connective tissue so that we can view the fascia as "one interconnected tensional network that adapts its fiber arrangement and density according to local tensional demands."

Pischinger (2007) described the fascial system as the largest system in the body, as it is the only system that touches all of the other known systems. Finando and Finando (2011) summarized evidence that the ancient acupuncture meridian system shares many structural, functional, and clinical characteristics with the fascial system. Like the acupuncture meridian system, the fascia may be viewed as a single organ, a unified whole, the environment in which all body systems function.

There are a number of correspondences between therapeutic approaches to the fascia and methods used in acupuncture. For example, Pischinger (2007) stated that needle puncture produces a reaction in the entire intercellular–extracellular matrix. The involvement of the fascia in dysfunction and disease is pervasive. It is believed that, to some extent, the fascia is involved in every type of human pathology (Paoletti 2006; Pischinger 2007). The fascia is the one system that connects to every aspect of human physiology. Langevin (2006) and Langevin and Yandow (2002) suggest that the fascia is a metasystem, connecting and influencing all other systems, a concept with the potential to change our core understanding of human physiology.

These perspectives help address the increasing interest in whole-systems phenomena that distinguish holistic manual therapies from methods that focus on parts rather than wholes. Experience often shows that formerly intractable health issues are sometimes resolved by taking a broader view of a patient's condition.

Along with these holistic perspectives come questions such as:

How do we account for the unitary nature of a living organism: the way it responds as a whole to any stimulus—as if every part of it knew what every other part is doing?

—*Ho (1994)*

and:

How is it that an organism behaves as a whole, and not just a collection of parts?

—*Packard (2006)*

These issues are related to the theme of this book, because much of the success of modern manual therapies stems from a willingness on the part of practitioners to unwind a patient's entire traumatic history, including all of the resulting compensations, which can be very different from treating a current complaint.

 KEY POINT

The quality of functioning and continuity of the living matrix is of obvious importance to athletes, dancers, musicians, martial arts practitioners, and others for whom skilled and integrated movement is a goal and a way of life.

The existence of a system that is all pervasive and that connects every part of the organism with every other part stands out as a possible integrator of diverse physiological processes at all levels of scale. Study of regulatory communications opens many new and unique perspectives about the fascia that are being explored by body therapists and body psychotherapists. Minor or major disruptions in such global regulatory systems can have significant health consequences, possibly relating to some of the intractable or difficult-to-treat health issues that might be successfully approached by considering the quality of functioning and continuity of the living matrix. This is of obvious importance to athletes, dancers, musicians, martial arts practitioners, and others for whom skilled and integrated movement is a goal and a way of life.

Many of the hypotheses introduced here are highly speculative, but they are made with the confidence that emerging technologies will eventually validate or refute them. Modern noninvasive research tools can be used to probe regulatory functioning at the cell and molecular levels in health and disease. For example, Pienta and Coffey (1991) discussed harmonic information transfer through a tissue tensegrity-matrix system: "Cells and intracellular elements are capable of vibrating in a dynamic manner with complex harmonics, the frequency of which can now be measured and analyzed in a quantitative manner by Fourier analysis." In the decades since that statement was made, other technologies have been developed that can characterize activities in the molecular fabric of the body. One valuable resource is a series of symposia on ultrafast phenomena in semiconductors and nanostructure materials, including living

tissues. For example, the development of powerful ultrafast laser pulsing technologies has led to the use of terahertz scanning near-field infrared microscopy of biological materials (Schade et al. 2005).

A second application of terahertz technologies involves spectroscopic methods for measuring the interactions between water and proteins at very small time scales (Havenith 2010). Atomic force microscopy can provide topographical information and measurements of mechanical stiffness, electrical conductance, resistivity, and magnetic properties at micro- and nanoscales in living material (Darling and Desai 2012).

The fascinating ideas of Bray (2009)—that is, a biochemical basis for "a computer in every cell"—may be testable using the revolutionary femtosecond spectroscopic methods introduced by Ahmed Zewail, for which he received the Nobel Prize in 1999. Zewail showed that it is possible, with the world's fastest camera, to see how atoms in a molecule move during chemical reactions on the time scale in which the reactions occur (Zewail 2001). During chemical reactions atoms move at a velocity that compares with that of a rifle bullet (about 2500 feet per second, or 1700 miles per hour). Raman and infrared spectroscopic techniques are now enabling rapid and sensitive chemical characterization of samples based strictly on the vibrational signatures of the molecules present in a sampling volume. When applied to biological systems, the techniques provide highly complex spectra that document changes taking place in the entire genome, proteome, and metabolome; real-time noninvasive in-vivo applications are possible. A whole issue of the *Journal of Biophotonics* was devoted to developments in this field (Krafft and Bird 2013).

THE LIVING MATRIX

The concept of a systemic living matrix emerged from the following sequence of discoveries:

1. Bretscher (1971) discovered that the polypeptide part of the principal glycoprotein on the surface of human erythrocytes extends through the membrane barrier to the interior surface of the cell membrane (Fig. 2.5.1B). Using novel chemical methods on human erythrocytes, he was the first to demonstrate the existence of oriented transmembrane proteins. His research led him to propose new principles of biological membrane structure, which are widely accepted.

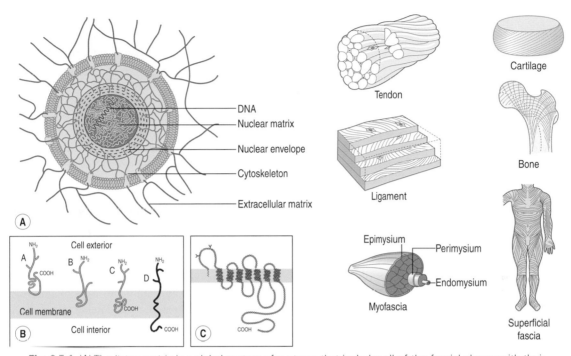

Fig. 2.5.1 (A) The living matrix is a global system of systems that includes all of the fascial planes with their connections to muscles, nerves, bones, organs, and vascular tissues, as well as connections to the cytoskeletons and nuclear matrices of cells throughout the body. (B) The key discovery leading to the living matrix concept was published by Bretscher (1971), who asked if the polypeptide part of the principle glycoprotein (glycophorin) on the surface of human erythrocytes sticks to the outer surface of the membrane, A; extends into the membrane, B; extends deeply into the membrane, C; or, perhaps, extends all the way through the membrane barrier to the inner surface, D. He demonstrated that the protein traverses the membrane. He was the first to demonstrate the existence of oriented transmembrane proteins. (C) Most if not all of the receptors on cell surfaces are composed of long helical proteins that snake back and forth across the membrane from 7 to 24 times. Seven-transmembrane-helix (7TM) receptors such as this one are responsible for transducing information initiated by signals as diverse as photons, odorants, tastants, hormones, and neurotransmitters. Several thousand such receptors are now known, and the list continues to grow. These are sometimes referred to as serpentine receptors because the single polypeptide chain "snakes" back and forth across the membrane.

2. By 1981, it was realized that Bretscher's discovery could enable an important revision of our understanding of cell structure in relation to the connective tissue and fascia (Oschman 1981).

3. The idea of transmembrane links between extracellular matrix and actin microfilaments and other structures within cells was well-established by the mid-1970s, but it took nearly a decade before the links were definitively identified (Hynes and Yamada 1982).

4. By 1997 a summary by Horwitz entitled "Integrins and Health" was published in *Scientific American* with the subtitle "Discovered only recently, these adhesive cell-surface molecules have quickly revealed themselves to be critical to proper functioning of the body and to life itself." Apparently, Horwitz was unaware of Bretscher's seminal discoveries some 26 years earlier. As major adhesion receptors, integrins signal across the plasma membrane in both directions (Hynes 2002).

KEY POINT

The integrin concept was a turning point in comprehending the significance of the term *holistic*. From a structural and functional perspective, the integrins link the connective tissues, fascia, and myofascial systems with the cellular and genetic domains throughout the body.

5. Further research confirmed that this arrangement exists in many cells and that it is pivotal for various physiological processes. Integrins are not individual molecules but are complex molecular assemblies that are responsible for adhesion of cells to each other. They are also receptors for various kinds of signal molecules that trigger cascades of reactions within cells (Fig. 2.5.2). The integrin concept was a turning point in comprehending the significance of the term *holistic*. From a structural and functional perspective, the integrins link the connective tissues, fascia, and myofascial systems with the cellular and genetic domains throughout the body. From a biological perspective, the integrins provide a physical and energetic connection between the realms of physiology, cell biology, membrane biology, and molecular genetics.

KEY POINT

The living matrix is well-defined from a molecular perspective because most of its major components have been extracted and characterized individually.

From the perspective of complementary and alternative medicine, the integrins have enabled us to complete the picture of the body as a whole system. Moreover, this system is thoroughly definable from a molecular perspective, because most of the major components of the living matrix have been extracted and characterized individually. Here, then, is a valuable connection between reductionism, the study of isolated parts, and holism, the study of how those parts go together to make a functioning organism. In 1993 we coined the term **living matrix** to describe this interconnected system (Oschman and Oschman 1993). Holistic therapists readily relate to the living matrix concept because it helps understand some of the remarkable therapeutic successes that come from therapies based on the concept of the body as an interconnected system.

6. Connections with the nuclear envelope (Berezney et al. 1982) suggested that the nuclear matrix may be a continuation of an overall cell matrix distributed throughout the cell, from the plasma membrane to the nuclear interior.
7. Links across the nuclear envelope are shown in Fig. 2.5.3. A spectacular example of a relationship between the nuclear envelope and the cytoskeleton known as the cellular geodome structure (Lazarides and Revel 1979) is shown in Fig. 2.5.3A. This structure is composed of actin, tropomyosin, and alpha-actinin. Fig. 2.5.3B shows the KASH, SUN, and related proteins that connect the cytoskeleton with the nuclear matrix.

SIGNALING PATHWAYS AND HUMAN PERFORMANCE—THE ZONE: NEUROLOGY OR BIOPHYSICS?

Albert Szent-Györgyi often mentioned his insight that life is too rapid and subtle to be explained by slow-moving chemical reactions and nerve impulses. A search for examples of such phenomena eventually led to a phenomenon that is often discussed by athletes and performers of all kinds, an altered state of consciousness called "the zone." A close look at these phenomena, inspired by remarkable performances of an Olympic figure skater, Midori Ito, led to a book entitled *Energy Medicine in Therapeutics and Human Performance* (Oschman, 2003) and a summary article by Oschman and Pressman (2014). One conclusion of that inquiry was the concept of **systemic cooperation**, a state of consciousness in which all parts of the organism function together to produce well-coordinated actions. It is of interest to determine the nature of the communications that might give rise to these phenomena. There are several possible perspectives and approaches to study regarding this issue, which is fundamental to our understanding of fascia and its roles in regulatory biology. It must be emphasized that we do not know the answer to this puzzle, but it is worthwhile to consider the possibilities to lay the groundwork for future investigations.

BIOPHYSICS

Biophotons

A pioneering German biophysicist, Fritz-Albert Popp, used the term *Gestaltbildung* to reference a condition in

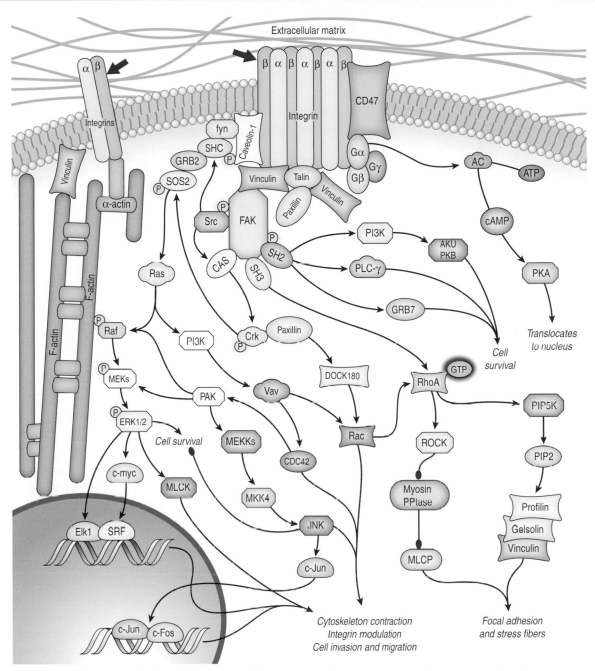

Fig. 2.5.2 Integrins (red arrows) are not individual molecules but are complex molecular assemblies that are responsible for adhesion of cells to each other and are implicated in important biological functions of the cell, such as virus binding, cell-surface antigenicity, cell–cell recognition, cell–cell communication, cellular transformation, transport, energy transduction, etc. They are also receptors for various kinds of signal molecules that trigger cascades of reactions within the cell. Redrawn with permission from an SABiosciences illustration.

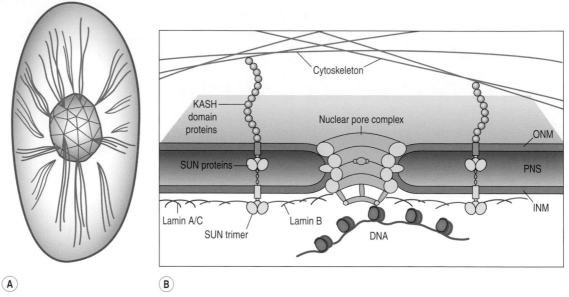

Fig. 2.5.3 (A) A spectacular example of a relationship between the nuclear envelope and the cytoskeleton known as the cellular geodome structure described by Lazarides and Revel (1979). This structure is composed of actin, tropomyosin, and alpha-actinin. Panel (B) details the nuclear envelope, showing SUN, KASH, and related components of the system connecting the cytoskeleton with the interior of the nucleus. INM, inner nuclear membrane; KASH, Klarsicht, ANC-1, Syne homology; lamin A/C, a protein that in humans is encoded by the LMNA gene; lamin B, a protein that in humans is encoded by the LMNB1 gene; ONM, outer nuclear membrane; PNS, perinuclear space; SUN, SUN proteins (for Sad1 and UNC-84). From Preston, C.C., Faustino, R.S., 2018. Nuclear envelope regulation of oncogenic processes: roles in pancreatic cancer. Epigenomes 2, 15, Sept. issue. Open access: https://creativecommons.org/licenses/by/4.0/.

which every cell "knows" what every other cell is doing. The research of Popp and his colleagues, beginning in 1974, focused on light or biophotonic communications (Popp 2003).

Electrons and Other Subatomic Particles

In the late 1950s, Szent-Györgyi developed a research interest in cancer and began to apply the theories of quantum mechanics to the biochemistry (quantum biology) of cancer. Meeting Szent-Györgyi and his colleagues in the early 1980s led to discussions of the idea that proteins are semiconductors (Gascoyne et al. 1981). An important conclusion of that article was that a small change in the degree of hydration of collagen led to an enormous increase in its conductivity. The concept of semiconduction in the fascia and living matrix was supported by the images of living fascia obtained by Guimberteau and Armstrong (2015). The images show that living fascia is highly reflective or shiny. This property is characteristic of materials such

as metals and semiconductors that have free or mobile electrons. Szent-Györgyi was convinced that regulatory information was carried by electrons and protons. Other mobile energetic phenomena can also be considered: excitons, holes, phonons, and solitons (Oschman 1996).

It must be emphasized that at the present time we have little direct information about these hypotheses.

NEUROLOGY

Current textbooks in the extensive field of motor control explain high-speed precision performances via feedforward calculations in the cerebellum (which in humans is equipped with far more neurons than the forebrain) and related adjustments. Cerebellar computation provides an example of feedforward processing of signals in order to improve movement accuracy. Feedforward control combines sensory inputs via mossy fibers (the fastest neurons owing to their high frequencies; Delvendahl and Hallermann 2016) and previous experience to predict the appropriate output. This allows quick reactions because errors are anticipated rather than detected (reviewed by Ohyama et al. 2003). In this way faulty motor commands are altered to prevent errant movements.

There are good reasons to look at the living matrix as a proteinaceous semiconductor system—essentially an electronic circuit (Fig. 2.5.4). A presentation of these concepts at the New England School of Acupuncture attracted the interest of two scholars who were exploring the possible scientific basis of the acupuncture meridian system (Matsumoto and Birch 1988). They became fascinated with the possibility that the collagenous living matrix and semiconduction of electrons and protons (as suggested by Szent-Györgyi) might provide a scientific basis for some forms of the Ch'i or circulating life energy that are thought to be inherent in all things, as described in Chinese philosophy.

These ideas gained virtually no traction in the biomedical research community. The paradox is that Szent-Györgyi's insights, which continue to be ignored by academics, actually provided the foundation for one of the largest and most rapidly growing industries in the world, the field of molecular electronics. A distinguished contributor to this field acknowledged Albert Szent-Györgyi and Robert Milliken for the key foundational insights that enabled this field to flourish (Hush 2006). The key concepts were semiconduction in proteins (Szent-Györgyi) and molecular orbital theory (Milliken).

An aspect of fascia strongly supports Szent-Györgyi's concepts of what he called electronic biology. One of the major functions of the fascial ground substance is the storage of electrons essential to the immune response (Oschman et al. 2015). The study of Earthing or grounding of the human body has demonstrated that connecting our bodies with the surface of the Earth can lead to a very rapid and well-documented resolution of inflammation anywhere in the body. Figure 2.5.5 is an example of rapid antiinflammatory effects of connecting the body with the earth and its abundant supply of electrons, which are probably nature's first and most effective antioxidants. The most parsimonious explanation for the rapid resolution of inflammation is rapid semiconduction of electrons from the Earth through the living matrix/meridian system (for reference, see Oschman et al. 2015).

Much of the confusion that prevents physicians and other allopathic therapists from understanding complementary and alternative medicine arises because energy therapists have learned to work with vital communication and control systems that are not yet recognized by the prevailing medical paradigm, with its primary focus on nerves, biochemistry, and chemical messengers. As the story of energetics unfolds, we are acquiring valuable new information and concepts that cannot help but improve everyone's understanding of physiology and medicine and enhance the effectiveness and appreciation of all clinical approaches. There is much to learn from the experiences of wholistic therapists and from the study of peak performances of elite athletes, musicians, dancers, and others. Study of these phenomena led to a search for physiological communications that might be faster than nerve impulses. The following are some of these very fast processes that have been identified:

- Semiconduction in the living matrix
- Wetware as described by Dennis Bray
- Metabolons
- Bioelectric and biomagnetic fields
- Biophotons
- Quantum coherence (see Hansmann 2013)
- Superconduction (see Geesink and Meijer 2019)

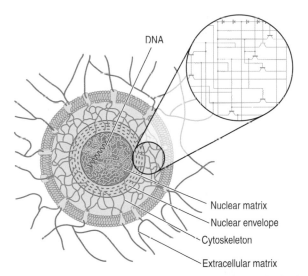

DNA

Nuclear matrix
Nuclear envelope
Cytoskeleton
Extracellular matrix

Fig. 2.5.4 The living matrix is compared with an electronic circuit containing resistors, diodes, transistors, and related solid-state electronic components. Although this may seem like a fantasy, it is actually the basis for the burgeoning modern molecular electronics industry based on molecular circuits.

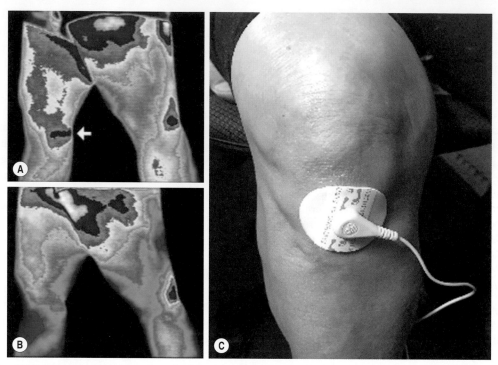

Fig. 2.5.5 Medical infrared imaging of a 33-year-old woman who had a gymnastics injury at the age of 15. She had an 18-year history of chronic right knee pain, swelling, and instability. (A) Arrow points to the exact location of patient's pain and shows significant inflammation. (B) Lower image was taken after 30 minutes of exposure to clinical Earthing using patch system shown in the inset (C). Note significant reduction of inflammation in the knee area. Rapid reduction in response to clinical Earthing provides strong support for Albert Szent-Györgyi's suggestion that proteins such as collagen are electronic semiconductors.

CONCLUSION

The existence of a living matrix underlying all parts of the body gives rise to the question of whether or not meaningful signals are propagated through this network, and whether or not these signals are integrating the activities of cells and tissues and organs throughout the body. A universal teaching is that the nervous system is the master control and communication system in the body. Another class of widely studied regulatory mechanisms involves molecular messages: hormones, neurohormones, neurotransmitters, antigens, growth factors, cytokines, and intracellular messengers such as cyclic AMP and calcium. Since publication of the first edition of this book, the field of nitric oxide research has made vast progress and become popular (relating to very fast gaseous signaling dynamics). There may be additional communication and control systems that are just as

important and vital as the nervous, hormonal, and second messenger systems. For example, a close look reveals that the nervous system actually plays only a small role in regulating the repair of an injury or in the body's response to a disease. The fascia and living matrix represent an exciting frontier for investigation. In the introduction it was mentioned that memory and traumatic memory are intertwined and have significant somatic components. A variety of body therapists recognize that physical or emotional trauma can become recorded in tissue structure and/or body shape. This is revealed when appropriate interventions nudge an individual into letting go of the tensions or body shapes they are holding and release a flow of information that brings into awareness memories that have long been held in the subconscious. Remarkable as these events appear, they confirm Dr. Candace Pert's assertion that, "your body is your subconscious mind" (Pert 2004). This is a reminder that the experiences of body therapists can provide important clues about how the fascia functions in relation to trauma. We look forward to the time when the modern research tools listed here can reveal more detail about how physical and emotional traumas affect the living matrix.

Summary

Evolutionary origins of fascia and extracellular matrix—the extracellular coats of the "primitive" single-celled microorganisms—evolved into the mammalian extracellular matrix. The connective tissue and fascia are thought to be the modern expression of these ancient cell coats. Discovery of the integrins—vital links between fascial and cellular matrices—gave rise to the living matrix concept. Cell biologists have suggested that the cytoskeleton is the "nervous system" of the cell. Some researchers are convinced that the acupuncture meridian system resides within the fascia. The quality of functioning and continuity of the living matrix is essential to athletes, dancers, musicians, martial arts practitioners, and others for whom skilled and integrated movement is a goal and a way of life. We know much about the language of the nervous system, but little about the kinds of messages that might be conducted through the living matrix. New methods will enable us to learn about this language. Albert Szent-Györgyi and his colleagues focused on protons and electrons as high-speed messengers, and this is supported by the reflectivity of living fascia and by the fast resolution of inflammation by Earthing or grounding the body.

DEDICATION

This chapter is dedicated to the memory of Dr. Mae-Wan Ho (1941–2016), an inspiring biophysicist, artist, humanitarian, and fearless advocate for life and sanity in science. Her *Science in Society* website is a rich and artistic archive of scientific reports, journalism, and audiovisual material representing two decades of work by the Institute for Science in Society (https://www.i-sis.org.uk/index.php). The magazine she created with her physicist husband Dr. Peter Saunders, *Science in Society*, was labeled, "The only radical science magazine on earth." The magazine has been widely circulated to the public, politicians, and policy makers worldwide.

ACKNOWLEDGMENT

The author is very grateful to the editor, Robert Schleip, for valuable suggestions.

REFERENCES

Bray, D., 2009. Wetware: A Computer in Every Living Cell. Yale University Press, New Haven, CT.

Berezney, R., Basler, J., Bucholtz, L.A., Smith, H.C., Siegel, A.J., 1982. Nuclear matrix and DNA replication. In: Maul, G.G., (Ed.), The Nuclear Envelope and the Nuclear Matrix. Alan R. Liss, New York, pp. 183–197.

Bretscher, M.S., 1971. A major protein which spans the human erythrocyte membrane. J. Mol. Biol. 59, 351–357.

Darling, E.M., Desai, H.V., 2012. Force scanning for simultaneous collection of topographical and mechanical properties. Microsc. Anal. 26, 7–10.

Delvendahl, I., Hallermann, S., 2016. The Cerebellar Mossy Fiber Synapse as a model for high frequency transmission in the mammalian CNS. Trends Neurosci. 39, 722–737.

Feinstein, D., 2012. What does energy have to do with energy psychology? Energy Psychol. 4, 59–78.

Finando, S., Finando, D., 2011. Fascia and the mechanism of acupuncture. J. Bodyw. Mov. Ther. 15, 68–176.

Findley, T.W., Schleip, R., 2007. Fascia Research: Basic Science and Implications for Conventional and Complementary Healthcare. Elsevier Urban & Fischer, Munich.

Gascoyne, P.R.C., Pethig, R., Szent-Gyorgyi, A., 1981. Water structure-dependent charge transport in proteins. Proc. Natl. Acad. Sci. 78, 261–265.

Geesink, H.J.H., Meijer, D.K.F., 2019. Superconductive properties in animate and inanimate systems are predicted by a novel biophysical quantum algorithm. Available from: https://www.researchgate.net/publication/330652340_Superconductive_properties_in_animate_and_inanimate_systems_are_predicted_by_a_novel_biophysical_quantum_algorithm.

Grassman, H., Pohlenz-Michel, C., 2007. Access to the Present Moment: Trauma Somatics® The Reorganization of the Somatic Memory System. IASI Yearbook, 1–10.

Guimberteau, J.C., Armstrong, C., 2015. Architecture of Human Living Fascia: Cells and Extracellular Matrix as Revealed by Endoscopy. Handspring, Edinburgh.

Hansmann, B., 2013. Working with beliefs reflected in liquid crystal. In the body water reflects not only what is but also what was. IASI Yearbook of Structural Integration, pp. 44–54.

Havenith, M., 2010. THz spectroscopy as a new tool to probe hydration dynamics. In: Song, J.J., Tsen, K.T., Betz, M., Elezzabia, A.Y.K. (Eds.), Ultrafast Phenomena in Semiconductors and Nanostructure Materials XVI. SPIE Press, Bellingham, WA, pp. 1–5.

Ho, M.W., 1994. The Rainbow and the Worm. World Scientific, Singapore.

Horwitz, A.F., 1997. Integrins and health. Discovered only recently, these adhesive cell-surface molecules have quickly revealed themselves to be critical to proper functioning of the body and to life itself. Sci. Am. 276, 68–75.

Hush, N.S., 2006. An overview of the first half-century of molecular electronics. Ann. N. Y. Acad. Sci. 1006, 1–20.

Hynes, R.O., 2002. Integrins: bidirectional, allosteric signaling machines. Cell. 110, 673–687.

Hynes, R.O., Yamada, K.M., 1982. Fibronectins: multifunctional modular glycoproteins. J. Cell Biol. 95, 369–377.

Koob, A., 2009. MIND. The Root of thought: What do glial cells do? Nearly 90% of the brain is composed of glial cells, not neurons. Sci. Am. October 27, 2009. Available https://www.scientificamerican.com/article/the-root-of-thought-what/.

Krafft, C., Bird, B., (Eds.), 2013. Biomedical vibrational spectroscopy (editorial). J. Biophotonics 6, 5–6.

Langevin, H., 2006. Connective tissue: a body-wide signaling network? Med. Hypotheses 66, 1074–1077.

Langevin, H., Yandow, J., 2002. Relationship of acupuncture points and meridians to connective tissue planes. Anat. Rec. 269, 257–265.

Lazarides, E., Revel, J.P., 1979. The molecular basis of cell movement. Sci. Am. 240, 100–113.

Matsumoto, K., Birch, S., 1988. Hara Diagnosis – Reflections on the Sea. Paradigm, Brookline MA.

Ohyama, T., Nores, W.L., Murphy, M., Mauk, M.D., 2003. What the cerebellum computes. Trends Neurosci. 26; 222–227.

Oschman, J.L., 1981. Structure and properties of ground substances. Am. Zool. 24, 199–215.

Oschman, J.L., 1996. The nuclear, cytoskeletal, and extracellular matrixes: a continuous communication network. In: The Cytoskeleton: Mechanical, Physical and Biological Interactions, November 15–17, 1996, sponsored by The Center for Advanced Studies in the Space Life Sciences, Marine Biological Laboratory, Woods Hole, Massachusetts, supported by the National Aeronautics and Space Administration.

Oschman, J.L., 2003. Energy Medicine in Therapeutics and Human Performance. Butterworth Heinemann, London.

Oschman, J.L., 2006. Trauma energetics. J. Bodyw. Mov. Ther. 10, 21–34.

Oschman, J.L., Chevalier, G., Brown, R., 2015. The effects of grounding (earthing) on inflammation, the immune response, wound healing, and prevention and treatment of chronic inflammatory and autoimmune diseases. J. Inflamm. Res. 8, 83–96.

Oschman, J.L., Oschman, N.H., 1993. Matter, energy, and the living matrix. October 1993 issue of Rolf Lines, the news magazine for the Rolf Institute, Boulder, Colorado, 21, pp. 55–64.

Oschman, J.L., Pressman, M.D., 2014. An anatomical, biochemical, biophysical and quantum basis for the unconscious mind. Int. J. Transpers. Stud. 33, 77–96.

Packard, A., 2006. Contribution to the whole (H). Can squids show us anything that we did not know already? Biol. Philos. 21, 189–211.

Paoletti, S., 2006. The Fasciae: Dysfunction and Treatment. Eastland Press, Seattle.

Pert, C., 2004. Your Body is your Unconscious Mind. [Audio CD] Sounds True, Louisville, CO.

Pienta, K.J., Coffee, D.S., 1991. Cellular harmonic information transfer through a tissue tensegrity-matrix system. Med. Hypotheses 34, 88–95 see p. 88.

Pischinger, A., 2007. The Extracellular Matrix and Ground Regulation. North Atlantic Books, Berkeley.

Popp, F.A., 2003. Properties of biophotons and their theoretical implications. Indian J. Exp. Biol. 41, 391–402.

Preston, C.C., Faustino, R.S., 2018. Nuclear Envelope Regulation of Oncogenic Processes: Roles in Pancreatic Cancer. Epigenomes 2, 15.

Puck, T.T., 1972. The Mammalian Cell as a Microorganism. Holden Day, San Francisco, CA.

Redpath, W., 1995. Trauma Energetics: A Study of Held-Energy Systems. Barberry Press, London.

Schade U, Holldack K, Martin MC, Fried D. 2005. THz near-field imaging of biological tissues employing synchrotron radiation. In: Ultrafast Phenomena in Semiconductors and Nanostructure Materials IX. Proceedings of SPIE 5725:46–52 (Kong-Thon Tsen; Jin-Joo Song; Hongxing Jiang, Eds).

Schleip, R., 2003. Fascial plasticity – a new neurobiological explanation: Part 1. J. Bodyw. Mov. Ther. 7, 11–19.

Sherrington, C.S., 1951. Man on his Nature. Doubleday Anchor, New York, p. 265.

Virchow, R., 1858. Die Cellularpathologie in ihrer Begründung und in ihrer Auswirkung auf die physiologische und pathologische Gewebelehre. Verlag A. Hirschwald, Berlin.

Zewail, A.H., 2001. Femtochemistry: Atomic-Scale Dynamics of the Chemical Bond Using Ultrafast Lasers (Nobel Lecture). In: De Schryver, F.C., De Feyter, S., Schweitzer, G. (Eds.), Femtochemistry: With the Noble Lecture of A. Zwail. Wiley-VCH Verlag GmbH, Weinheim, FRG (chap. 1).

PART 3

Force Transmission

Force Transmission and Muscle Mechanics: General Principles

Peter A. Huijing

CHAPTER CONTENTS

INTRODUCTION

Muscle force is generated within sarcomeres within myofibers (i.e., muscle fibers). The sarcomere forces (summed according to the rules for serial and parallel arrangement) need to be exerted outside myofibers to be able to cause movement of body parts.

 KEY POINT

Rules for addition of forces and displacement govern all force transmission.

In short, the rules for summation of sarcomere effects indicate that forces are added for sarcomeres arranged in parallel, and shortening velocities are added for sarcomeres arranged in series. This can be understood intuitively by realizing the following: for serial arrangements of sarcomeres, the force generated within one sarcomere needs to be exerted at the next one, and this can only happen if this next sarcomere can bear that force. The typical expression is that a chain (i.e., serial arrangement of chain elements) is as strong as its weakest link. Both serial sarcomeres can change length and these length changes, as well as shortening velocities, will be added. For this reason many sarcomeres are

arranged in series in human muscles (e.g., the myofibers of medial head of gastrocnemius contains more than 20,000 serial sarcomeres) to bring shortening from the microlevel of one sarcomere to the macrolevel of moving muscles.

For parallel arrangement of sarcomeres (i.e., within adjacent myofibrils) each of these sarcomeres will transmit force onto the next (serial) one, and as a consequence forces will be added, but not length change and velocity of shortening. In this case the change from the micro to macro level is made by having many myofibrils, as well as myofibers, arranged in series.

There are two fundamental ways to look at force transmission.

1. The direct (mechanics) way: considers a force transmitted from the sarcomeres of a muscle onto, for example, the tendon and from there to bone, to cause movement of a body segment.
2. The inverse mechanics way deals with questions: which structures are the sources of so-called reaction forces that allow the muscle to exert force? An active or stretched passive muscle will shorten unless opposed by a load (an opposing force) that will prevent shortening to a length at which no force can be generated (slack length). This opposing force is a reaction force that is equal to the force exerted by the muscle (action = reaction) but has an opposite direction.

It may be exerted by the tendon or by other structures arranged in series with the sarcomeres.

It is clear that the two approaches should yield the same answers. Even though the concept of inverse mechanics seems more complex initially, we will use this approach because it is easier to avoid mistakes.

As there are two types of structures arranged in series with sarcomeres—tendons or tendon plates (aponeuroses) and fascia—two types of force transmission are distinguished.

MYOTENDINOUS FORCE TRANSMISSION

Each myofiber (muscle fiber) is equipped (at least at one end) with a myotendinous junction (Fig. 3.1.1A). The thin filaments of the last sarcomere of myofibrils within myofibers are attached sideways through the sarcolemma to collagen fibers of the aponeurosis (tendon plate) that invade the invaginations of the myofibers but remain

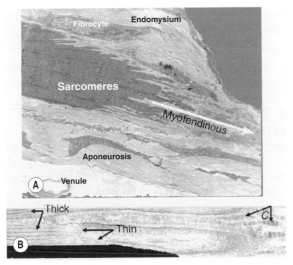

Fig. 3.1.1 The Myotendinous Junction. (A) Low power electron micrograph showing this junction of one myofiber. The intracellular parts (e.g., sarcomeres) are dark, and light areas are extracellular materials. A considerable area of contact between the two exists because of many invaginations of the myofiber. The aponeurosis is made up from many little tendons belonging to single myofibers. (B) High power electron micrograph showing one invagination containing collagen fibrils C that will form the myofiber's small tendon (further to the right). Within the intracellular part, thick and thin filaments of the last sarcomere are indicated. Across the sarcolemma and basal lamina (dark line border of the invagination and myofiber) the thin filaments are connected to the collagen fibrils.

outside of the cell. The supramolecular structures involved in such connections are shown schematically in Fig. 3.1.2A–C. The myotendinous loads exerted on the last sarcomeres are transmitted to the next sarcomeres in series within each myofibril. If this should be the only type of force transmission, forces in all sarcomeres in series within a myofibril need to be equal. If this is the exclusive reaction force available, and if all sarcomeres have identical properties, such sarcomeres will shorten to a length until their identical force is in equilibrium with the reaction force. In static final conditions, this will yield identical sarcomere lengths within the myofiber, unless more paths are available force transmission from the initial sarcomere than just the sarcomere to serial pathway. The biological dangers in case of such a unique system are clear: even if only one sarcomere in such a series breaks down (for example, out of 20,000 found to be arranged in series within myofibers of human medial gastrocnemius muscle), the whole myofibril becomes unable to exert force. It should also be realized that the number of serial sarcomeres readily adapts to altered conditions, even as the muscle is active; and that this should be a considerable problem.

MYOFASCIAL FORCE TRANSMISSION

Via the intracellular cytoskeleton and transsarcolemmal molecules, connections between sarcomeres and surrounding collagenous fibers do not exist only at the ends of myofibers but are present along their full periphery. Therefore, multiple reaction forces are exerted onto sarcomeres within a myofiber. If these sideways connections supply a notable part of the reaction forces (which can also best be considered as a load on the sarcomere additional to the myotendinous one), we have force transmission onto the endomysium. We refer to such transmission as *myofascial force transmission*. As a consequence, not all sarcomeres in series need to be at identical lengths and forces: forces of subsequent sarcomeres need not be identical because myofascial and myotendinous reaction forces can prevent some of them from shortening more than others exposed exclusively to myotendinous loads (Fig. 3.1.1B).

It should be noted that some authors consider intramuscular myofascial force transmission as limited to transmission solely between adjacent muscle fibers (e.g., Chapter 1.2). In contrast, we will argue that the muscular connective tissue stroma itself is a pathway of force

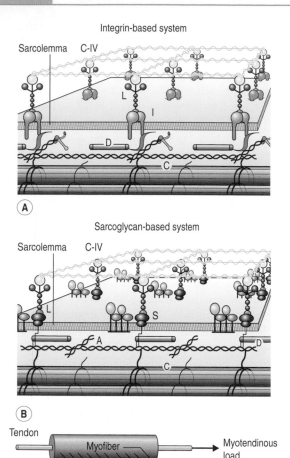

Fig. 3.1.2 Connections of Sarcomeres to Extracellular Structures. Schematic examples of two systems of transsarcolemmal connections via the basal lamina to the endomysium (not shown). The two molecular systems are named by the molecules that connect across the sarcolemma (myofiber cell membrane). (A) The integrin-based system. (B) The sarcoglycan-based system. The abbreviations indicate the following molecules or structures: C = cytoskeleton within the myofiber to which sarcomeres are attached at Z-disks (at double lines) and at M-lines. A = strings of actin on the inside of the sarcolemma. D = dystrophin molecule connecting actin and sarcoglycans (S, in part B) and connecting the two systems. Absence of this molecule causes very serious disease. Talin connects subsarcolemmal actin strings to integrin molecules (I, in part A). For both systems, the connections to a network of collagen IV molecules (C-IV) are made by laminin (L). (C) The mechanical effect of such myofascial connections (thin black line) is a loading of the myofiber in addition to myotendinous loading.

transmission leading to force transmission beyond the fascicle and even further beyond the borders of muscle (Chapter 3.2).

DISTRIBUTION OF FORCES IN A MULTIPATH SYSTEM

The fact that connections exist between different structures potentially involved in force transmission is no guarantee that substantial forces are transmitted via them.

> ## KEY POINT
>
> If multiple paths for force transmission are available, the ratios of the stiffness of each of these pathways determine the division of forces.

The connections have to be stiff enough to be able to transmit force. In fact the forces will be divided over the different pathways according to the ratio of the stiffness of each of these pathways. So stiffness is the determining factor and not the strength of the connections; nevertheless, the pathways need to be strong enough (i.e., not to break down) under repeated loading to have any functional significance.

INTRAMUSCULAR SUBSTRATES OF MYOFASCIAL FORCE TRANSMISSION

Endomysia constitute tubes for each myofiber. Note, however, that endomysial walls are shared between adjacent tubes (and myofibers). This causes a continuous honeycomb type of structure of muscular connective tissues until the fascicle borders are reached (see also Chapter 1.2).

The collections of fascicles are made up in a similar way, having the perimysium as borders delimiting fascicles, so that within a muscle a stroma of continuous tubes is present that is delimited by the epimysium, surrounding the whole muscle. Note that the word stroma (of Greek origin) actually refers to a supporting function.

Myofascial force transmission limited to the intramuscular domain is called *intramuscular myofascial force* transmission. This term is used also in the case of force transmission of a single myofiber or fascicle operating within its endomysial or perimysial tunnel (Chapter 8.3). In those cases, and that of a fully dissected muscle, reaction forces have to be exerted via tendons as these are then the only effective connections to the outside world (Huijing et al. 1998).

Experimental evidence, proving the feasibility of intramuscular myofascial force transmission, comes from animal experiments involving cutting tendons or aponeuroses. For example, when four of the five heads of a maximally dissected rat EDL were removed by tenotomy of their distal tendons, the force transmission of 55% of the muscle bulk was prevented, but the muscle still exerted 85% of the force (Huijing et al. 1998).

REFERENCES

Huijing, P.A., Baan, G.C., Rebel, G., 1998. Non myo-tendinous force transmission in rat extensor digitorum longus muscle. J.Exp. Biol. 201, 682–691.

Epimuscular Myofascial Force Transmission: An Introduction

Peter A. Huijing

CHAPTER CONTENTS

INTRODUCTION: EPIMUSCULAR MYOFASCIAL FORCE TRANSMISSION AND ITS SUBSTRATE

If *myofascial* loads (i.e., reaction forces from fascial structures) are exerted onto the muscle stroma (Huijing and Baan 2001), force is via the epimysium. Therefore such transmission is called *epimuscular myofascial force transmission*.

Two pathways are available for such transmission:

- Directly between two adjacent muscles (by definition occurring exclusively within a muscle group: synergistic muscles). We call this specific case intermuscular myofascial force transmission.
- Between a muscle and some extramuscular structures, such as the neurovascular tract (i.e., the collagen-reinforced structure in which blood vessels, lymphatics, and nerves are embedded), intermuscular septa between muscle groups, interosseal membrane, periosteum, general (or deep) fascia, etc. We call this extramuscular myofascial force transmission to emphasize the role of extramuscular tissues. Forces exerted this way may play a role

in stabilizing joints or be exerted on bones and other extramuscular structures, but may also be exerted on other muscles.

All of the tissues discussed (with the exception of the aponeuroses and tendons) are part of a continuous fascial system. By itself, the fact that they are connected will not warrant force transmission; if the connections are very compliant (i.e., not stiff), force will only be transmitted after very high length changes that will stiffen connections. Note that some research groups entertain the idea that, for healthy people, this is the normal condition within the physiological length range and relative positions. Such ideas will be discussed in detail in Chapter 8.5.

However, experiments indicate that after more moderate length changes sizable fractions of muscular force may be transmitted. This means that fascial structures, even those that are not dense depositions of collagen fibers as in tendons and aponeuroses, also may transmit some of the muscular force; therefore, it has been argued that the term "loose connective tissue" for such structures is inadequate (Huijing and Langevin 2009) and the term "areolar" is preferred for such tissues.

EFFECTS OF EPIMUSCULAR MYOFASCIAL FORCE TRANSMISSION

Proximodistal Force Differences

> ### KEY POINT
>
> The presence of proximodistal force differences of a muscle constitutes absolute proof of myofascial force transmission.

Because of additional myofascial loading, forces exerted at the origin and insertion of muscle are not equal (e.g., Huijing and Baan 2001). The net myofascial load (i.e., the vector sum of all such loads, involving size and direction) will keep sarcomeres at one end of myofibers within muscle longer than at other locations within the same myofibers—that is, different active forces are exerted locally (Fig. 3.2.1A). A force equal to the additional load is integrated into the force exerted at the opposite end of the muscle. Active force of several muscles may appear also at the insertion of another muscle, as long as myofascial connections to the extratendinous tissues are intact and stiff (e.g., Rijkelijkhuizen et al. 2005, 2009).

Distributions of Sarcomere Lengths Within Muscle and its Myofibers

Myofascial loading will cause a distribution of lengths of sarcomeres arranged in series within myofibers (serial distribution). Most of such additional force is borne by active sarcomeres (because they are very stiff)

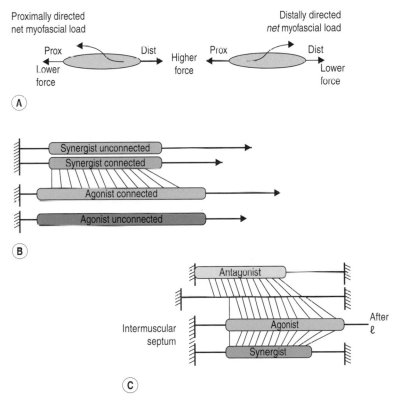

Fig. 3.2.1 Myofascial Force Transmission and Some of its Consequences. (A) Proximodistal force differences. The net myofascial load on the muscle is integrated into either the proximal force (left panel) or the distal force (right panel) depending on the loading direction. (B) Comparison of distal forces of unconnected and myofascially connected muscles after distal lengthening. As the agonistic muscle is lengthened the force in the synergistic muscle drops. (C) Connections and myofascial loading of antagonistic muscles across the intermuscular septum. In these conditions part of the antagonistic muscle force will be exerted at the distal tendon (right) of the agonistic muscle.

but may also be borne by the connective tissue stroma of muscle and will be added to the active force exerted.

If the point of application of myofascial loads on myofibers and their size and direction were identical, sarcomere length distributions would be limited to serial ones.

KEY POINT
Serial distribution of sarcomere length is serious evidence for myofascial force transmission.

However, a simple test illustrates that the situation is more complex. If one suspends equal masses from the tendon of a (horizontal) muscle, the muscle is pulled down, exposing the extramuscular neurovascular tract (Fig. 3.2.1A), but this tract is pulled down more at the distal tendon than at the proximal tendon. This indicates that the tract is stiffer at the proximal than at the distal end of the muscle. As a consequence, myofibers located proximally within muscle will, on average, be longer than more distal ones. Therefore in addition to the serial distribution of sarcomere lengths within myofibers, a parallel distribution of mean myofiber sarcomere lengths will be present as well. The nature of both types of distributions will vary with the specific conditions of myofascial loading. It is hard to measure such distributions, but finite element modeling (also discussed in Chapter 8.5) allows the study of such principles even in quite complex conditions of loading.

Myofascial Interaction Between Muscles

Dissection experiments (Maas et al. 2005) indicate that intermuscular transmission plays a role, but extramuscular myofascial force transmission is the more important mechanism for muscular mechanical interaction. Indirect intermuscular mechanical effects are present through two coupled events of extramuscular myofascial force transmission (muscle to extramuscular tissues to another muscle). Myofascial interaction was shown for synergistic muscles involving both intermuscular and extramuscular transmission (Huijing and Baan 2001; Huijing 2003). During experiments this is apparent as follows: after the agonist muscle is lengthened at its distal tendon while its synergistic muscle is kept at constant length (Fig. 3.2.1B), distal force of the isometric synergistic muscle is decreased (compared with the unconnected case) with increasing lengths of its adjacent muscle. The lengthened muscle creates, or enhances, a distally directed myofascial load on the

isometric synergistic muscle. At its proximal tendon, this load is integrated into force exerted by the muscle (as in Fig. 3.2.1A). In contrast, distally exerted force is decreased because of such loading conditions.

Myofascial force transmission between antagonistic muscles is (by definition) only possible via extramuscular pathways, as such muscles are separated by compartment walls. Stiff connections are made between compartments by neurovascular tracts (i.e., the collagen fiber reinforced collection of nerves, blood vessels, and lymphatics), but also other extramuscular fascial structures are expected to play a role. The effects and explanation of myofascial interaction between two muscle groups located at opposite sides of an intermuscular septum or interosseal membrane (Fig. 3.2.1B) are similar to those described for synergistic muscles (Huijing 2007; Huijing et al. 2007; Meijer et al. 2007; Rijkelijkhuizen et al. 2007). In a series of experiments in rats, we have shown that such mechanisms and effects are active between all muscles of the lower leg (for an overview of results, see Rijkelijkhuizen et al. 2009). So, even antagonistic muscles located at opposite sides of the leg interact (e.g., m. tibialis anterior and triceps surae muscles; see Chapter 5.8 for similar physiological results in mice) and cannot be considered as fully independent entities. It should be realized that this means that part of the force exerted by active sarcomeres within a muscle may be exerted at the tendon of its antagonistic muscle. In fact, the proximal sarcomeres of myofibers may be in series not only with more distal sarcomeres of the same myofiber, but via myofascial loading also with distal sarcomeres (and their adjacent endomysia) in the lengthened antagonistic muscle(s).

Muscular Relative Position also Affects Muscular Force Exertion

Several experiments (Huijing 2002; Maas et al. 2004), as well as finite element modeling (Maas et al. 2003a and b; Yucesoy et al. 2006), indicate that a muscle kept at constant length and moved through its natural fascial context exerts tendon forces in proximal or distal direction that will vary according to the myofascial loading conditions that are altered with changes in relative position (Figs 3.2.2 and 3.2.3).

KEY POINT
Relative to the position of muscle with respect to other muscles, fascial structures of bone are a codeterminant of force exerted at origin and insertion of the target muscle.

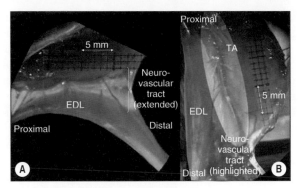

Fig. 3.2.2 The Neurovascular Tract. (A) Rat m. extensor digi-torum longus (EDL) while loaded vertically with equal weights (not shown) at proximal and distal tendons exposing the neuro-vascular tract. (B) The neurovascular tract (highlighted area) in its original position. This tract is exposed by laterally cutting and medially deflecting m. tibialis anterior (TA).

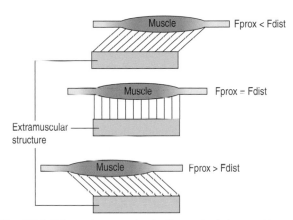

Fig. 3.2.3 Schematic example of effects of relative position on myofascial connections and loading. As the muscle of constant length is moved its relative position is changed with respect to other structures (e.g., other muscles or extramuscular struc-tures). The effects for myofascial connections and the direction of loading on the muscle are indicated with the consequences for muscle force exerted at proximal (left) and distal (right) tendons.

The artificial conditions in these studies were neces-sary to prove the principle of relative movement and its effects. It should be realized that muscular movement relative to bones or neuromuscular tracts also plays a role in this phenomenon.

In vivo, relative movements between synergistic muscles occur because of differences in the moment arms of the joints crossed, and for bi- or polyarticular muscles because of movement in a joint not crossed by its adjacent monoarticular synergistic muscle. Relative

movement of antagonistic muscles is the order of the day, because movement of a joint will have opposite ef-fects on muscular length—for example, joint flexion will lengthen its extensor muscles and shorten its flexor muscles.

COMPLEXITY OF MYOFASCIAL LOADING OF MUSCLE

We have provided the simplest examples of myofascial loading to clarify its principles. In reality, within the integrated myofascial system, loading of muscles will be very complex.

Multiple and opposite loads on a muscle are consid-ered common (for example, a proximally directed load by the neurovascular tract and a distally directed load by compartmental fascia). The latter is particularly evident for shorter muscles but also present at higher lengths. If one cuts a tendon (as is done as an experimental interven-tion, but also seen in some surgery, as in Chapter 5.3), its passive muscle retracts somewhat, indicating being under tension before tenotomy. If such tenotomized muscle is activated, it will shorten only a little more, indicating a distal myofascial load keeping the muscle at length.

By changing the length and position of muscles, the direction of net loading may change because of (1) rotating a fascial component with respect to mus-cle or (2) making the mechanical effects of another fascial structure dominant.

If simultaneously exerted proximal and distal myofas-cial loads on a muscle are equal, the proximodistal force difference will be zero. Therefore the presence of such a difference constitutes absolute proof of epimuscular myofascial force transmission, but its absence does not necessarily mean that such force transmission is absent!

Because myofascial loading of a muscle under con-sideration may originate from all muscles with the body segment, it is clear that a lot needs to be known before the conditions determining the target muscle's force are specified in detail.

In addition, myofascial force transmission between muscles in adjacent segments is likely, because of the stiff-ness of the neurovascular tract coursing through the tis-sues of the body segments. There are some indications that intersegmental myofascial transmission occurs (Vleeming et al. 1995; Huijing et al. 2009; and from the Wilke group, e.g., 2016, 2019), but this needs further confirmation, par-ticularly for living and active muscles (Huijing 2009).

Proving the feasibility of epimuscular myofascial force transmission and its basic effects and principles were the goal of the first 10 years of our experimental and modeling work on myofascial force transmission. It is good to realize that the control needed for solid experimental proof precludes getting close to in-vivo conditions, and conditions were chosen accordingly. Since that time, more attention has been given to some aspects of the in-vivo conditions (see Chapter 5.3). In any case, it is clear that we have only scratched the surface of this intricate and complex system of force transmission, and a lot more scientific and clinical work is needed to reveal the principles and effects of its complexity.

ADDITIONAL FACTORS TO CONSIDER

As indicated, experimental work discussed previously has many limitations that need to be considered in a more generalized view (see also Chapter. 5.3). On the other hand, if one performs experiments in vivo in human or animal studies, it is often impossible to attain sufficient control of the conditions, and it is wise also to keep such limitations clearly in mind.

Joint Movement

Joint movement to new positions (rather than direct muscle lengthening) affects actual stiffness of fascial components; for example, the length and, particularly, tension within neurovascular tracts are very dependent on joint positions (Huijing 2009). Therefore a study by Maas and Sandercock (2008) extended experiments (to cats) and manipulated actual joint movement. Evidence of epimuscular myofascial force transmission between synergistic muscles of the calf was reported only if the soleus muscle was at a length deviating from that imposed by the specific ankle angle. These authors concluded that epimuscular myofascial force transmission does not occur for in-vivo physiological conditions but may play a role when conditions deviate from normal. There is no doubt of the validity of their finding. However, in its generality, their conclusion about myofascial force transmission occurring exclusively in nonphysiological conditions is premature (see also discussion in Chapter 8.5).

Contrasting evidence has been emerging, with similar experiments using magnetic resonance imaging work in humans (Huijing et al. 2011; Yaman et al. 2013; Pamuka et al. 2016; Karakuzu et al. 2017): changing the knee angle caused local changes of strain, not only in gastrocnemius muscle but also in synergistic soleus muscle kept at constant length due to a fixed ankle angle. The same was found for the full remainder of antagonistic muscles of the lower leg that also do not cross the knee.

Previously, some other studies indicated evidence of in-vivo epimuscular myofascial force transmission (Yu et al. 2007). One could argue, as was done by Herbert and co-authors (2008), that if only a small percentage of muscle force is transmitted myofascially, we could afford to neglect the whole process. However, having epimuscular myofascial force transmission as a fundamental mechanism of intact tissues does change completely the view of functioning of those tissues, even if the size of the related phenomena may be small in specific conditions.

Levels of Muscular Activation

One important aspect of the work discussed is that even though different levels of activation have been studied by varying firing rates of muscles (Meijer et al. 2006; 2008), such changes were always imposed uniformly on all muscle studied. In vivo, different muscles or muscle groups are active at varying levels of activation. By stimulating different nerves or their branches (Maas and Huijing 2009), this may be mimicked. These results do not affect the principles as described previously in a major way.

EFFECTS ON FUNCTIONING OF THE SENSORY APPARATUS

As our view of in-series and parallel arrangements of structures is renewed, it is clear that our views on neural sensors need to be adapted as well: many more receptors outside of muscle (e.g., in periosteum, intermuscular septa, compartment) will receive information about muscular conditions. Also intramuscularly, conditions for receptors may be different than thought previously. Classically, muscle spindles are considered as arranged in parallel to myofibers, and Golgi tendon organs as arranged in series with them. However, if a part of the stroma that contains muscle spindles is in series with sarcomeres, this receptor will also operate in series. Preliminary results indicate that this may be the case (Arikan et al. 2009). In any case, in accordance with results on epimuscular myofascial force transmission, receptors in muscle kept at constant muscle-tendon complex length increase their firing rates, as other muscles within the same segment are lengthened.

Summary

The most important basic principles of epimuscular myofascial force transmission have been discussed. On the basis of that, the conclusion is warranted that if we do not take such force transmission into account we will never fully understand muscular function. Similarly, it is likely that at least acute effects of manual therapy will involve some of these mechanisms.

REFERENCES

Arikan, Ö.E., Huijing, P.A., Güçlü, B., Yucesoy, C.A., 2009. Altered afferent response of restrained antagonistic muscles after passive stretching of gastrocnemius indicates a remarkable role of epimuscular myofascial force transmission in the sensory level. In: Society for Neuroscience's Meeting. Society of Neuroscience. Washington D.C.

Herbert, R.D., Hoang, D., Gandevia, S.C., 2008. Are muscles mechanically independent? J. Appl. Physiol. 104, 1549–1550.

Huijing, P.A., 2002. Intra-, extra- and intermuscular myofascial force transmission of synergists and antagonists: effects of muscle length as well as relative position. J. Mech. Med. Biol. 2, 1–15.

Huijing, P.A., 2003. Muscular force transmission necessitates a multilevel integrative approach to the analysis of function of skeletal muscle. Exerc. Sport Sci. Rev. 31, 167–175.

Huijing, P.A., 2007. Epimuscular myofascial force transmission between antagonistic and synergistic muscles can explain movement limitation in spastic paresis. J. Electromyogr. Kinesiol. 17, 708–724.

Huijing, P.A., 2009. ISB Muybridge Award lecture 2007: Epimuscular myofascial force transmission, its ubiquitous presence across species and some of its history, effects and functional consequences. J. Biomech. 42, 9–21.

Huijing, P.A., Baan, G.C., 2001. Extramuscular myofascial force transmission within the rat anterior tibial compartment: Proximo-distal differences in muscle force. Acta Physiol. Scand. 173, 1–15.

Huijing, P.A., Langevin, H.M., 2009. Communicating about fascia: history, pitfalls and recommendations. In: Huijing, P.A., Hollander, P., Findley, T.W., Schleip, R. (Eds.), Fascia Research II. Basic Science and Implications for Conventional and Complementary Health Care. Elsevier, München.

Huijing, P.A., Langenberg, R.W., van de Meesters, J.J., Baan, G.C., 2007. Extramuscular myofascial force transmission also occurs between synergistic muscles and antagonistic muscles. J. Electromyogr. Kinesiol. 17, 680–689.

Huijing, P.A., Yaman, A., Ozturk, C.O., Yucesoy, C., 2011. Effects of knee joint angle on global and local strains within human triceps surae muscle: MRI analysis indicating in vivo myofascial force transmission between synergistic muscles. Surg. Radiol. Anat. 33, 869–879.

Karakuzu, A., Pamuk, U., Ozturk, C., Acar, B., Yucesoy, C.A., 2017. Magnetic resonance and diffusion tensor imaging analyses indicate heterogeneous strains along human medial gastrocnemius fascicles caused by submaximal plantar-flexion activity. J. Biomech. 57, 69–78.

Maas, H., Baan, G.C., Huijing, P.A., 2004. Muscle force is determined also by muscle relative position: isolated effects. J. Biomech. 37, 99–110.

Maas, H., Baan, G.C., Huijing, P.A., Yucesoy, C.A., Koopman, B.H., Grootenboer, H.J., 2003a. The relative position of EDL muscle affects the length of sarcomeres within muscle fibers: experimental results and finite-element modeling. J. Biomech. Eng. 125, 745–753.

Maas, H., Huijing, P.A., 2009. Synergistic and antagonistic interactions in the rat forelimb: acute effects of coactivation. J. Appl. Physiol. 107, 1453–1462.

Maas, H., Meijer, H.J.M., Huijing, P.A., 2005. Intermuscular interaction between synergists in rat originates from both intermuscular and extramuscular myofascial force transmission. Cells Tissues Organs 181, 38–50.

Maas, H., Sandercock, T.G., 2008. Are skeletal muscles independent actuators? Force transmission from soleus muscle in the cat. J. Appl. Physiol. 104, 1557–1567.

Maas, H., Yucesoy, C.A., Baan, G.C., Huijing, P.A., 2003b. Implications of muscle relative position as a co-determinant of isometric muscle force: a review and some experimental results. J. Mech. Med. Biol. 3, 145–168.

Meijer, H.J.M., Baan, G.C., Huijing, P.A., 2006. Myofascial force transmission is increasingly important at lower forces: firing frequency-related length-force characteristics. Acta Physiol. (Oxf.) 186, 185–195.

Meijer, H.J.M., Baan, G.C., Huijing, P.A., 2007. Myofascial force transmission between antagonistic rat lower limb muscles: effects of single muscle or muscle group lengthening. J. Electromyogr. Kinesiol. 17, 698–707.

Meijer, H.J., Rijkelijkhuizen, J.M., Huijing, P.A., 2008. Effects of firing frequency on length-dependent myofascial force transmission between antagonistic and synergistic muscle groups. Eur. J. Appl. Physiol. 104, 501–513.

Pamuka, U., Karakuzu, A., Ozturka, C., Acar, B., Yucesoy, C.A., 2016, Combined magnetic resonance and diffusion tensor imaging analyses provide a powerful tool for in vivo assessment of deformation along human muscle fibers. J. Mech. Behav. Biomed Mater. 63, 207–219.

Rijkelijkhuizen, J.M., Baan, G.C., de Haan, A., de Ruiter, C.J., Huijing, P.A., 2005. Extramuscular myofascial force transmission for in situ rat medial gastrocnemius and plantaris muscles in progressive stages of dissection. J. Exp. Biol. 208, 129–140.

Rijkelijkhuizen, J.M., Baan, G.C., de Haan, A., de Ruiter C.J., Huijing, P.A., 2009. Extramuscular myofascial force transmission for in situ rat medial gastrocnemius and plantaris muscles in progressive stages of dissection. J. Exp. Biol. 208, 129–140.

Rijkelijkhuizen, J.M., Meijer, H.J.M., Baan, G.C., Huijing, P.A., 2007. Myofascial force transmission also occurs between antagonistic muscles located in opposite compartments of the rat hindlimb. J. Electromyogr. Kinesiol. 17, 690–697.

Vleeming, A., Pool-Goudzwaard, A.L., Stoeckart, R., van Wingerden, J.P., Snijders, C.J., 1995. The posterior layer of the thoracolumbar fascia. Its function in load transfer from spine to legs. Spine 20, 753–758.

Wilke, J., Engeroff, T., Nürnberger, F., Vogt, L., Banzer, W., 2016. Anatomical study of the morphological continuity between iliotibial tract and the fibularis longus fascia. Surg. Radiol. Anat. 38, 349–352.

Wilke, J., Krause, F., 2019. Myofascial chains of the upper limb: A systematic review of Anatomical Studies Clinical Anatomy. Clin. Anat. 32, 934–940.

Yaman, A., Ozturk, C., Huijing, P.A., Yucesoy, C.A., 2013. Magnetic resonance imaging assessment of mechanical interactions between human lower leg muscles in vivo. J. Biomech. Eng. 135, 91003.

Yu, W.S., Kilbreath, S.L., Fitzpatrick, R.C., Gandevia, S.C., 2007. Thumb and finger forces produced by motor units in the long flexor of the human thumb. J. Physiol. 583, 1145–1154.

Yucesoy, C.A., Maas, H., Koopman, B.H., Grootenboer, H.J., Huijing, P.A., 2006. Mechanisms causing effects of muscle position on proximo-distal muscle force differences in extra-muscular myofascial force transmission. Med. Eng. Phys. 28, 214–226.

Myofascial Chains: A Review of Different Models

David Lesondak

CHAPTER CONTENTS

INTRODUCTION

The spiritual notion that "it's all connected" may not be so true anywhere as it is in the world of fascial anatomy. However, if so true, that knowledge is clinically meaningless without coherent, plausible maps of this anatomical connectivity. While the myofascial meridians of Thomas Myers—*Anatomy Trains* (Myers 2014)—are well-known (and are covered in Chapter 3.4), Myers himself readily admits that there are more connections and fascial continuities to be explored and mapped.

What follows is an overview of some of the other acknowledged whole-body continuities. There are often similarities within and between the various models. What follows is not meant to be a literature review of all the models but instead to highlight some the diversity among them. For reasons of space, what follows must be cursory, but it is my hope that these overviews will stimulate the clinician, trainer, and researcher to study further these other models in order to improve their fundamental understanding and practical outcomes.

KURT TITTEL

Professor Emeritus of the Functional Anatomy Department of the University of Halle, Germany, and author of over 500 papers, Dr. Tittel did not rely on the musculoskeletal topography of cadavers when developing his models. Instead he preferred to study active function, believing that the best way to understand the parts was to understand their relationship to the whole organism, and that this relationship exists all the way down to the cellular level.

His book *Muscle Slings in Sports,* which has been in print for more than 60 years, presents his muscle slings in painstaking detail. It includes over 100 illustrations (Fig. 3.3.1) outlining his concepts (Tittel 2015). They are categorized into:

1. Flexor slings of the lower extremity
2. Extensor slings of the lower extremity
3. Extensor slings in whole body movement
4. Flexor and extensor slings in whole body movement
5. Muscle slings in lateral inclination and rotation
6. Muscle slings in static sequences
7. Other sling combinations.

The slings are additionally organized by more than two dozen basic sports or functional movements. For example, lower leg flexor slings are shown for both ballistic movements and ballet; static sequences include bracing scenarios (i.e., a gymnast on parallel bars, or on the rings, and so on).

While Tittel is much more functional-anatomy focused in the presentation of his slings (and this is a strength), he

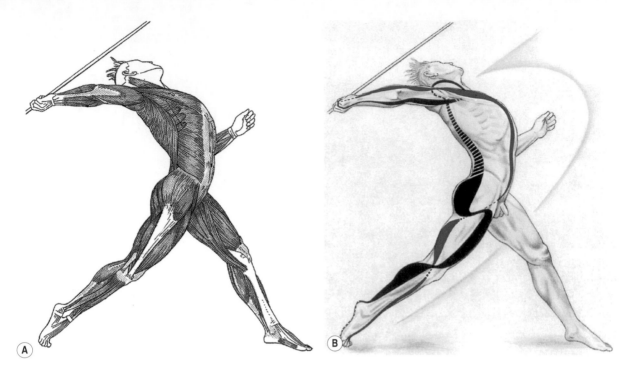

Fig. 3.3.1 Tittel's Diagram of a Javelin Thrower in the Last Moment of "Drawing The Bow" Before Throwing The Javelin. The figure on the right shows the relationship between the extensor sling in red and the flexor sling in black at this exact phase of movement. The schematic on the left gives a thorough breakdown of all the myofascial units (muscles) involved. This level of dynamics and detail is inherent in all of Tittel's models. Reproduced with kind permission from Tittel, K., 2015. Muscle Slings in Sport. Kiener Press, Munich.

does single out the thoracolumbar fascia (TLF), long before the research of Vleeming et al. (see Willard et al. 2012). Recognizing the importance of TLF in both regulating and stabilizing posture, he also highlights its superficial layer serving as an origin for the lattisimus dorsi and the serratus posterior inferior, as well as the important relationship between the deep layer of the TLF with the transverses abdominis.

> ### 🌱 KEY POINT
>
> Tittel's models were the result of painstaking analysis of the human body in motion. With a strong focus on sports, his models may be best suited for those in sports medicine or who work with athletes.

GODELIEVE DENYS-STRUYF

Godelieve Denys-Struyf was a Belgian physiotherapist with osteopathic training and a background in art. She made use of her art skills by drawing postural profiles of her patients, rendering these in anterior, posterior, and lateral aspects. As she began to amass these profiles (sources indicate in the thousands across two decades) she began grouping them into similar patterns. She also cross-referenced the physical patterns with accumulated anecdotal observations of behavior and personality patterns. Even something like the simple observation of the postural differences between feeling happy or depressed led her to believe that the body often expresses what language cannot. Or, as she simply states, "The body is language." As such, her work may be of heightened interest to the more trauma-oriented somatic practitioner. Her work is currently being republished in multiple volumes (Campignon 2018a, 2018b).

Her path to decoding and translating this language was the development of six common myofascial chains, with tension being transmitted from one muscle to the next via both aponeurosis and myotatic (stretch) reflexes. Biomechanically, Denys-Struyf held that asymmetrical distortions and poor posture are not caused by the pull of gravity but by excessive muscle actions struggling against this pull.

Considering the fascia to be the "liaison" between the superficial and the deep, the muscles and the skeleton, the skeleton and the viscera, and the viscera and the muscles, she also considered these intersystem interfaces to be areas of information exchange because of the high number of nerves and blood vessels within the fascia.

She typified six common myofascial chains, with tension transmitted from one muscle to the next via aponeurosis and myotatic (stretch) reflexes, these further interact with a system of levers and pivots (i.e., joints), which can perform in functional ways deemed to be primary, acting, adjusting, or adaptive, depending on use. She further associated the chain with different developmental movements. Also of import in that all of these chains, save one, connect the torso to the extremities.

  KEY POINT

Denys-Struyf based her models on six commonalities discovered in detailed postural analysis of over 2000 patients across two decades. She also made correlations between the models and behavioral/emotional states.

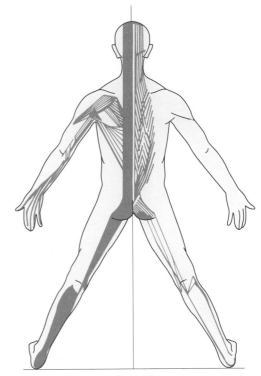

Fig. 3.3.2 The Postero-Median Chain comprises connections along the posterior aspect of the body. Similar to other posterior chains it links the soleus posterior up the soleus through the medial hamstrings but continues into the glutes and erector spinae. It branches out to include the latissimus, trapezius, and the medial posterior arm muscles. Redrawn with kind permission from Godelieve Denys-Struyf, *Les Chaînes Musculaires et Articulaires*. First ed.: SBO-RTM 1979. Edition and copyright: ICTGDS 1987.

1. The Postero-Median Chain (Fig. 3.3.2) begins at the toe flexors and rises up the soleus to the semimembranosus and semitendinosus, continuing up the back and neck via the erector spinae. It branches out along the latissimus to the shoulder via the middle trapezius, infraspinatus, teres minor, posterior deltoid, and down into the fingers via the triceps and flexor group.

2. The Antero-Median Chain (Fig. 3.3.3) starts at the anterior neck with the sternocleidomastoid and scalene, branching out to the upper limb via the subclavius, anterior deltoid, and brachialis; down the supinators; and into the thumb via the adductor pollicis. Back in the trunk it continues down from the sternal head of the sternocleidomastoid (SCM) to include the transversus thoracis, sternalis (when present) intercostals, and rectus abdominis to the muscles of the pelvic floor. It translates to the lower limb via relationship to the pyramidalis, adductor group, and medial aspect of the gastrocnemius to the adductor hallucis.

3. The Postero-Lateral Chain (Fig. 3.3.4) starts with the upper portion of the trapezius, along the supraspinatus to the middle deltoid, continuing down the lateral aspect of the triceps to the anconeus, flexor, and extensor carpi to the muscles of the palm. The leg portion comprises the gluteus medius, connecting to both the biceps femoris and vastus lateralis down the peroneals and gatrocnemius, including the plantaris to the lateral foot.

4. The Antero-Lateral (AL) Chain's (Fig. 3.3.5) upper portion goes from the clavicular head of the SCM to the pectoralis minor and continues along the deltoid where it forms additional connections with the latissimus, teres major, and subscapularis. It also continues down the arm through the biceps, supinator, brachioradialis, and extensor muscles of the fingers to the palmaris longus, thenars, and lumbricals. The lower

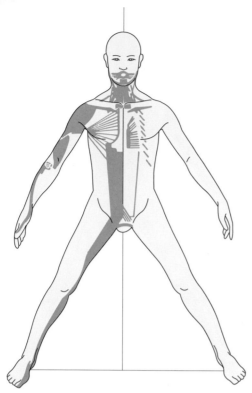

Fig. 3.3.3 The Antero-Median Chain connects the anterior medial aspect of the lower leg to the rectus abdominus, the pectorals, scalene group, and subclavius to the deltoid and supinators into the thumb. Redrawn with kind permission from Godelieve Denys-Struyf, *Les Chaînes Musculaires et Articulaires*. First ed.: SBO-RTM 1979. Edition and copyright: ICTGDS 1987.

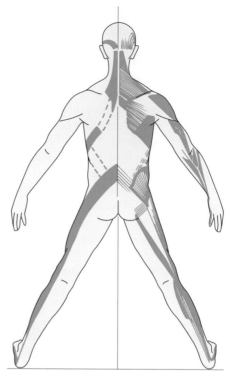

Fig. 3.3.4 The Postero-Lateral Chain comprises the upper trapezius through the middle deltoid to the flexors via the anconeus, while the lower aspect links the lateral foot to the gluteus medius by way of the peroneals, biceps femoris, and vastus lateralis. Redrawn with kind permission from Godelieve Denys-Struyf, *Les Chaînes Musculaires et Articulaires*. First ed.: SBO-RTM 1979. Edition and copyright: ICTGDS 1987.

portion of the AL comprises the gluteus medius, tensor fascia lata, tibialis anterior and posterior, planters, interosseous membrane, and lumbricals of the foot.

5. The Postero-Anterior (PA) Chain (Fig. 3.3.6) includes the scalene longus colli and capitis, intercostals, and paraspinals, including the transverse and rectus abdominis and diaphragm. There are no extremities involved here, but the PA activates during inhalation to provide fixed points for respiration, as such it alternates in reciprocal relationship with the Postereo-Lateral Chain.

6. The Antero-Posterior Chain (Fig. 3.3.7) includes the pectorals minor and coracobrachialis down the biceps to the finger extensors. In the lower portion, it includes the iliacus, quadriceps, and the toe extensors.

A study published in *Physical Therapy* (Díaz-Arribas et al. 2015) looked at the efficacy of Godelieve Denys-Struyf method (GDS) for low back pain in a cluster randomized controlled trial. GDS was measured against typical PT protocols with data collected in 2-, 6-, and 12-month intervals for changes in both LBP and leg radiculopathy. While there was no change in pain level between the two groups, there was an overall disability difference of 0.8 to the positive in the GDS group compared with the control group. It was hypothesized that the GDS group performed better because they exercised more, as the interventional nature of GDS is more exercise-based.

JOSEPH SCHWARTZ

Schwartz is a licensed massage therapist who has been studying the intricacies of the somatic world for over three decades. A devoted rock climber with a passion for sheer verticals and challenging crevasses, his injury of a broken talus in December 1985 became a case study at

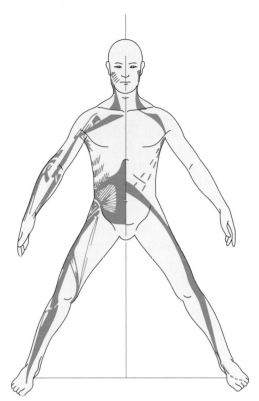

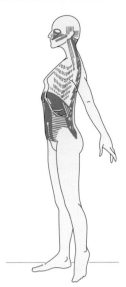

Fig. 3.3.6 The Postero-Anterior Chain Connects the Diaphragm to Both the Rectus and Transversus Abdominis Anteriorly and via the Intercostals to the Paraspinals and from there to the Scalenes, Longus Colli, and Capitis. Redrawn with kind permission from Godelieve Denys-Struyf, *Les Chaînes Musculaires et Articulaires*. First ed.: SBO-RTM 1979. Edition and copyright: ICTGDS 1987.

Fig. 3.3.5 The Antero-Lateral Chain. The complexity of the Antero-Lateral Chain links the clavicular of the sternocleidomastoid to the pectoralis minor, deltoid, and aspects of the rotator cuff through the biceps and other linkages to the extensors. The lower aspect connects the gluteus medius, tensor fascia lata, tibialis posterior, and anterior to the lumbricals. Redrawn with kind permission from Godelieve Denys-Struyf, *Les Chaînes Musculaires et Articulaires*. First ed.: SBO-RTM 1979. Edition and copyright: ICTGDS 1987.

Stanford; it also started him on his somatic studies, which include certifications in physical education, Iyengar, and Anusara yoga. He published a sports-specific manual for muscle testing in 2015.

Schwartz's *The 5 Primary Kinetic Chains* (Schwartz, 2016, 2017) serves as a template for human locomotion. The chains operate interdependently, with each requiring the other in order to move with smooth efficiency. Each chain is a complex interrelation of parts and includes the additional classifications of subsystems (influenced by Vleeming), prime movers, synergist, and fascial springs.

While the concept involves reciprocal muscle actions operating simultaneously in concert across the human frame, it is hypothesized that the fourth and fifth chains

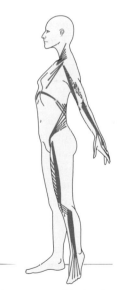

Fig. 3.3.7 Working in concert with the Postero-Lateral Chain, the Postero-Anterior Chain includes the extremities in both the arms via pectoralis minor and coracobrachialis, and the iliacus to the quadriceps to the toe extensors. Redrawn with kind permission from Godelieve Denys-Struyf, *Les Chaînes Musculaires et Articulaires*. First ed.: SBO-RTM 1979. Edition and copyright: ICTGDS 1987.

use and release the elastic storage capacity inherent in the fascial system via the Fascial Springs. The system begins as follows:

1. The Intrinsic Kinetic Chain's (IKC) principal action is breathing and facilitating the relationship between breathing and the nervous system. The IKC begins at the cranial sutures and connects with the temporalis, and deeper to the pterygoids and masseter. It continues to encompass the entire hyoid group, all three scalenes, sternocleidomastoid, and suboccipitals. It continues posteriorly to include the erector spinae group and multifidus all the way to the thoracolumbar fascia, psoas, and quadratus lumborum, wrapping around the obliques, transversus abdominis, and up the rectus abdominis. Laterally it expands along the internal intercostals, pectoralis minor, and serratus posterior superior.

2. The Deep Longitudinal Kinetic Chain (DLKC) is about shock absorption—the ability of kinetic energy to travel through the body joint by joint and buffer appropriately. It then transfers that energy engaged by heel strike into the swing phase via the Anterior Spiral Kinetic Chain (ASKC). Starting at the foot at the extensor digitorum longus and brevis, it passes through the lower subsystem (tibialis anterior, peroneus longus, and biceps femoris) continuing up the leg on both sides at the rectus femoris, adductor magnus, iliotibial band, and gluteus medius. The subsystem continues via the connection to the sacrotuberous ligament across the SI joint through the TLF to the erector spinae of the opposite side. There it translates to the shoulder girdle via the upper trapezius, serratus anterior, pectoralis, middle deltoid, and down the brachialis to the extensor muscles, forming a complement to the opposite leg and hip.

3. The Lateral Kinetic Chain's (LKC) principal action is axial stabilization. It translates ground engagement into ground-force reaction, stabilizing contralateral weight transition during gait and movement. The LKC starts at the flexor hallucis longus. The plantar aponeurosis and Achilles tendon, arising with the peroneus longus, soleus, tibialis posterior deep to that, and the vastus lateralis and iliotibial band to the thoracolumbar fascia and quadratus lumborum, then proceeds up the latissimus dorsi to the middle and upper trapezius, where it continues down the extensors into the lumbricals of the hand. The LKC is ipsilateral.

4. The Posterior Spiral Kinetic Chain's (Fig. 3.3.8) primary function is to store elastic energy and features four fascial springs: the plantar aponeurosis, Achilles tendon, iliotibial band, and the thoracolumbar fascia (referenced as the "master spring"). They work synergistically and ease the energy usage of the associated muscles. They also work contralaterally through the oblique subsystem, which includes the gluteals, TLF, and latissimus, and can transmit force to the opposite shoulder and down the arm extensors girdle via the deltoid and up into the head via the splenius capitis and SCM.

5. The Anterior Spiral Kinetic Chain is the complementary compartment to PSKC, redirecting the elastic energy of the PSKC into the swing phase of gait. This becomes the forward motion that becomes the next

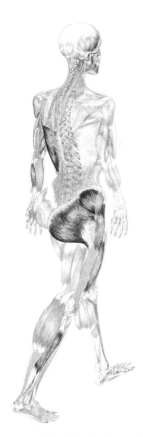

Fig. 3.3.8 The Posterior Spiral Kinetic Chain functions to store elastic energy during gait via the fascial "springs" of the plantar aponeurosis, Achilles tendon, iliotibial band, and the thoracolumbar fascia. With kind permission from Schwartz, J., 2016. The 5 Primary Kinetic Chains Dynamic Neuromuscular Assesment Lyons, Colorado.

shock absorption of the DLKC, and so on, throughout the cycle. It also contains a subsystem that includes the adductor longus, rectus abdominis, and both abdominal obliques, allowing for translation of movement through the trunk and again supporting and assisting synergistic movement into the shoulder girdle and arm.

> ### KEY POINT
> The five Kinetic Chains serve as a template for human locomotion. Four fascial springs form a primary feature of the Posterior Spiral Kinetic Chain, which serves in an elastic storage capacity for the swing phase of gait.

SERGE PAOLETTI

Osteopath Serge Paoletti graduated from the European School of Osteopathy. He would go on to teach there, as well as in Vienna, Hamburg, and several schools in France. Paoletti postulates that fascial chains exist everywhere in the body, given the ubiquity of fascia and its role in force transmission. Therefore it is possible for any given myofascial unit to act as a "transmission belt" for another unit and so on. Furthermore, the most important fascial chains are also the most extensive, topographically speaking, linking one end of the body to the other. In his view this is somewhat clinically unwieldy, given all the different types of collagen as well as fiber thickness and direction. Potential cross-linking via fiber direction is also very important to these models.

In trying to establish common fascial chains based on common human movements, Paoletti postulates a total of nine chains—three external chains, three internal chains, one meningeal chain, and one chain each for the medial and lateral aspects of the upper limb. His chains contain numerous transfer points (TPs) that are often, but not exclusively, centered around bony landmarks and joints (Paoletti 2006).

Paoletti thought it vital to understand that force transmission through these chains was omnidirectional, passing not just upward and downward but also from the outside of the body toward the inside and vice versa. While examined separately, these chains always exist in relationship to each other. They often make sudden changes in direction, as well as from superficial to deep (which then presents a challenge in evocative renderings). Of particular note in the Paoletti model is his keenness to explore the anatomical connections between the myofascial, neurofascial, and visceral fascia, and their potential to influence one another.

Another unique feature of the Paoletti models are the introduction of horizontal chains. Though not as detailed, they feature prominently in the meningeal chain and at transfer points involving the pelvis. They will be designated as HC.

It should also be noted that some of Paoletti's chains are less anatomically specific, for example, citing the "lateral fascia of the leg" without naming specific muscle units (IT band, peroneals, one assumes). Likewise, when he refers to "superficial fascia" he is referring to the overall layer. We will keep our nomenclature consistent with his.

The External Chains

1. The External Lateral Chain (ELC)

    The ELC begins at the peroneals to transfer points (TP) at the fibular head and patella, where it continues up the iliotibial tract and tensor fascia lata to TPs at the hip and pelvis. From here it ascends both anteriorly and posteriorly and to the perineum via an HC comprising the obturators and piriformis.

    Anteriorly the ELC travels to the rectus abdominis and thoracic fascia to a TP at the clavicle, where it continues up the superficial fascia of the lateral aspect of the neck to the lateral cranial fascia.

    Posteriorly the ELC goes from the hip TP along the thoracolumbar fascia to a TP at the posterior part of the scapula. Continuing along the external rotators of the shoulder, posterior deltoid, infraspinatus, and teres minor, it arrives at the posterior base of the skull via the trapezius, splenius, and longissimus capitis.

2. The External Anterior Chain (EAC) starts at the foot and follows the anteromedial fascia to a TP at the knee. From there Paoletti states that via oblique fascial fibers any forces from the anterolateral part of the thigh can be transmitted to adductors, therefore it follows the adductors to a TP at the pubis and inguinal ligaments before mimicking the LEC by rising up the rectus abdominis. At the pelvis it also encounters two internal chains via the iliacus and perineal chain via the superficial perineal fascia.

3. The External Posterior Chain (EPC) begins at the calf fascia continuing through a TP at the posterior knee, along the biceps femoris to an elaborate TP comprised of the ischium, coccyx, sacrum, and the sacrotuberous ligament. It continues up the erector

spinae. The EPC can crossover to the opposite side via oblique fibers of the thoracolumbar fascia. The EPC can also influence the perineal HC through the coccyx, sacrotuberous, and sacrospinous ligaments. Through those same structures there is also a connection to dura mater and the vertically oriented Meningeal Chain.

Internal Chains

4. The Internal Peripheral Chain (IPC) begins at the perineum continuing upward via either the transversalis fascia and/or the peritoneum, forming a TP at the diaphragm. From there it follows the endothoracic fasciae to a TP at the scapula, following the path to the other external chains to the occipital ridge. Paoletti declaims that the force transmission can also pass laterally via the pleura to the shoulder TP and once again up the neck to the base of the skull.

5. The Internal Central Chain (ICC) starts at the diaphragm/pericardium interface along the pharyngeal aponeurosis to the thoracic outlet forming a connection to the middle and deep cervical fascia, as well as a TP at the hyoid (and therefore could influence the superficial fascia of the neck). The ICC continues along the pterygotemporomaxillary and interpterygoid fasciae from where it continues to the dura mater.

6. The Internal Mixed Chain (IMC) also starts at the perineum and follows the umbilico-prevesical fascia (as such, this should include the retropubic space of Retzius and encompass the bladder) to a TP at the umbilicus where it meets the transversalis and follows both the round and falciform ligaments of the liver, forming a transfer point at the diaphragm, and follows the same path as either the IPC or ICC.

Meningeal Chain

7. The Meningeal Chain begins at the coccyx and can be influenced by any of the other chains and vice versa. From the coccyx it arises and comprises the entire vertebral column where the potential exists to make contact with a myriad of potential TPs. Given this plethora of possibilities, Paoletti chooses to highlight the following:

   - Anterior TPs travel along the common posterior ligament (which spans the entire column), the strongest of these TPs being the lower aspect of the coccygeal ligament and the upper attachments of C2 and C3.

   - Lateral meningeal extensions travel with the nerve as far as the intervertebral foramen. These extensions are continuous with the dura mater. These extensions strongly attach to the bone and also serve to prevent overstretching of the nerve roots and spinal cord.

   - From here the spinal cord enters the cranium via the foramen magnum, spreading spherically throughout the cranial cavity with pronounced articulations at the base of the skull. This continuity also forms the large septa of the tentorium, and the faux cerebelli and faux cerebri, providing horizontal and sagittal anchoring, respectively, for the brain.

8. The External Medial Arm Chain (EMAC) starts at the hand and flows the anteromedial edge of the forearm muscle to the medial epicondyle of the humerus to form a TP at the elbow, continuing along the medial intermuscular septum and coracobrachialis fascia to a TP at both the clavicle and acromion, arriving at the anterolateral cranium via the scalene and superficial cervical fascia.

9. The External Lateral Arm Chain (ELAC) starts at the wrist and can follow both the anterolateral and posterolateral edge of the fascia along the radius to a TP at the lateral aspect of the elbow. The ELAC then follows the lateral intermuscular septum to the deltoid where it can then split into two different directions:

   - along the medial and anterior portion of the deltoid fascia to the pectoral fascia where it can interact with the Internal Chains in a cephalad direction.

   - along the lateral and posterior edge of the deltoid to a TP at the spine of the scapula. Here Paoletti writes of the ELAC meeting a "posterior oblique chain" (that he does not elsewhere describe), which comprises the latissimus and lateral shoulder rotators and arrives at the base of the skull via the EPC.

It should also be noted that Paoletti clinically observed that the ELAC required the most consistent osteopathic treatment due to the heavy workload engendered by this structure.

 KEY POINT

The Paoletti models represent some of the most elaborate models yet postulated with, unlike other models, frequent changes in direction and depth. Paoletti was keen to explore the various possible connections between muscular, visceral, and meningeal fascia.

DISCUSSION

Since the fascia connects "everything" within the body, many anatomical connections can and will be made. Although these connections have local aspects, what should be prima facie in all models is that they serve to plausibly map the terrain of whole-body movements and compensations to better inform the clinician, physiotherapist, trainer, et.al. in making decisions for intervention beyond the typical local focus of other models.

It is also curious to note that all of the previously discussed models, save Denys-Struyf, are explicit about the importance of the lumbodorsal fascia.

In practicum and for use with patients when confronted with conflicting models (along with the unique and idiosyncratic nature of human beings), this author recommends applying Occam's razor as much as possible.

Summary

Different models for myofascial chains can exist because of the inherent nature of fascia as a connecting tissue and system. These models have a global perspective, focusing on whole-body patterns, movements, and restrictions. Different models should subscribe to their own internal logic and be consistent within themselves, or at least acknowledge where they are not. Different models can both contradict as well as support each other. A working knowledge of various myofascial chain models may lead the curious clinician or researcher to different questions or hypotheses for treatment.

REFERENCES

Campignon, P., 2018a. Muscle and Articulation Chains, GDS Method, Biomechanical Aspects. Kindle edition.

Campignon, P., 2018b. Muscle and Articulation Chains, GDS Concept, Relational Chains Book 1. Kindle edition.

Díaz-Arribas, M.J.D., Kovacs, F.M., Royuela, A., et al., 2015. Effectiveness of the Godelieve Denys-Struyf (GDS) method in people with low back pain: cluster randomized controlled trial. Phys. Ther. 95, 319–336.

Myers, T., 2014. The Anatomy Trains. Churchill Livingstone Elsevier, Edinburgh.

Paoletti, S., 2006. The Fasciae: Anatomy, Dysfunction and Treatment. Eastland Press, Seattle.

Schwartz, J., 2016. The 5 Primary Kinetic Chains. Dynamic Neuromuscular Assessment™ [posters], Dynamic Neuromuscular Assesment Lyons, Colorado.

Schwartz, J., 2017. The 5 Primary Kinetic Chains. Desktop edition. Dynamic Neuromuscular Assesment Lyons, Colorado.

Tittel, K., 2015. Muscle Slings in Sport. Kiener Press, Munich.

Willard, F.H., Vleeming, A., Schuenke, M.D., Danneels L, Schleip R., 2012. The thoracolumbar fascia: Anatomy, functions and clinical considerations. J. Anat. 221, 507–536.

Anatomy Trains: Myofascial Force Transmission in Postural Patterns

Thomas W. Myers

CHAPTER CONTENTS

INTRODUCTION—FASCIA AS METAMEMBRANE

We humans have a biblical and Aristotelian penchant for naming parts. Anatomists must admit, nevertheless: no matter how many of the bottomless barrel of terms they know, every human being is grown organically from a single egg, not assembled like a car from parts. The familiar industrial images that pervade our thinking about the body—the heart is a pump, the lungs are bellows, the brain is a computer, etc.—subtly promote the idea of isolated action of quasi-independent machines. We know in our heart of hearts, however, and should remember in our everyday clinical thinking, that the scientific truth is that our body always does and always has worked together in an unbroken concert from the exuberance of our conception to the mystery of finally becoming truly still.

Starting at about 14 days in embryological development, as cells proliferate and specialize they create an extracellular matrix (ECM) between them (Moore and Persaud 1999). This delicate weblike intercellular gel provides the immediate environment of most cells, mixing varying proportions of fiber, gluey proteoaminoglycans, and water with diverse and circulating metabolites, cytokines, and ionized mineral salts (Williams 1995).

It is this ECM that provides most of the "tissue" bulk in many connective tissues, as the cells alter the ECM to form bone, cartilage, ligaments, aponeuroses, areolar webs, interstitial conduits, and the rest (Snyder 1975). The ECM grows along with the cells themselves and together they form a single "exosymbiosis" for the cellular community. All 70 trillion of your cells are connected, joined, and held together or allowed to glide separately by the ECM.

KEY POINT

The extracellular matrix is an organismic "metamembrane" and forms the living environment for every cell, especially muscle. One may question whether the nervous system "thinks" in terms of individual muscles, or whether the muscle, a convenient division for the dissector, is even a distinct physiological unit. Neuromotor units or fascicles within muscles may be a more useful division. Global patterns may also tell us something useful that an individual muscle analysis misses.

More than just a container, the ECM is intimately connected to cell membranes and through them to the cytoskeleton via hundreds or thousands of binding transmembranous proteins like integrins on the cell surface (Ingber 1998). Forces from outside the cell are transmitted via these adhesive connections to the inner workings of the cell (Ingber 2006b). We have known for a long time that each cell is "tasting" its chemical milieu. Now, we know that each cell is additionally "feeling" and responding to its mechanical environment—leading to the relatively new field of "mechanobiology" (Ingber 2006a). Forces also move in the other direction—from the cell to the ECM, for example, from striated or smooth muscle or (myo) fibroblast contraction that is conveyed through the membrane to the surrounding ECM (Tomasek et al. 2002), lending stability or causing contracture.

Fibroblast cells and their cousins are particularly adept at promulgating and maintaining this system of the ECM, which operates under the following design constraints.

To allow trillions of cells to stand up and walk around in an organismic fashion, the ECM must:

- Invest every tissue without exception—muscle, nerve, epithelia, and of course all the connective tissues themselves, from blood to bone. Only the open lumens of the lungs and digestive system are free of it.
- Be permeable enough to allow all local cells to be in the flow of metabolism yet tough enough to protect those cells from endogenous and exogenous forces (Benias 2018).
- Vary widely, both across the body from tough bone and resilient cartilage to the delicate lymphatic network of the breast and the aqueous humor of the eye.
- Transmit forces from one tissue to another with maximum precision and maximal adaptability to sudden changes in load while sustaining minimal cellular tissue damage.
- Be able to remodel itself over time to meet altered biomechanical conditions in growth, performance, healing, and repair (or pathologically in disease or degeneration—for instance, the steady loss of elasticity in the bands of connective tissue that hold our lens, leading to increased focal length, and reading glasses, as we age).

Injury and disease mark its limits, but the ECM is a highly adaptable "metamembrane" for the organism, creating an organismic boundary, restraining and directing movement, protecting delicate tissues, and maintaining the recognizable shape most of us function in from day to day (Juhan 1987; Varela and Frenk 1987).

DIVIDING THE INDIVISIBLE

Although the ECM is manifestly one single whole, it is convenient to divide it into three sections:

- The tissues of the dorsal cavity—the numerous glia within the nervous system itself and the pia, arachnoid, and dural meninges around the brain and spinal cord—with the perineural extensions out the peripheral nerves into the rest of the body (Upledger and Vredevoogd 1983).
- The tissues of the ventral cavity—the strings, sheets, and sacs that separate the organs; allow glide between them; and hold them to the body wall, including the mesentery, mediastinum, plaura, and peritoneum (Barral and Mercier 1988).
- The tissues of the locomotor system, such as the bones, joints, capsules, ligaments, fasciae, aponeuroses, and all the tissues surrounding and investing the skeletal muscles—endomysium, perimysium, epimysium, and their tendinous and intermuscular extensions (Chaitow 1980).

This last section, which because of the necessity for transmission of strong forces accounts for a significant percentage of the total protein of the body, can again be divided functionally into:

- An "outer" myofascial layer consisting of 600 or so muscles embedded in the fascia necessary to hold them together, organize their movement, and deliver their force effectively to the bones and other tissues.
- An "inner" layer of joint capsules, ligaments, and periostea that surrounds the skeleton and organizes its growth, protects it from dismemberment, and limits movement, thus providing efficient force transmission from one joint to the next (Myers 2020).

All of the divisions mentioned are imprecise. Because of the integrated nature of the ECM, it is sometimes impossible to tell where one section stops and the other begins, and functionally they are all in league with each other. This last division between the outer and inner "bags" within the musculoskeletal system is particularly porous, because these structures have been shown to work more often in series than in parallel (Van der Wal 2009).

ISOLATING A MUSCLE

After this preamble to holism, the remainder of this chapter will focus on some patterns within this "outer bag" of myofasciae. Our traditional view of anatomy on the one hand has broadened our knowledge considerably. On the other, it has been a limited reductionistic parsing of the body, largely with a scalpel. The result is "the muscle" as the predominant label for making named units within the unified soft tissue of this layer. Once a muscle is dissected from its neurovascular fascia, from its overlying areolar and profundis layer, and from its neighbors right and left, and the ligaments below, the muscle is then analyzed solely in terms of what would happen if the two end points north and south (the so-called proximal and distal attachments) were pulled together in a concentric, isometric, or (with an opposing outside force) eccentric contraction (Williams 1995; Biel 2005; Muscolino 2010).

This isolationist muscle analysis separates *one* function out of the many and raises it to the level of *the* function. *All* of the fasciae discussed previously are also attachments of that muscle, and all contribute to an integrated cybernetic response. Most analyses of posture and movement proceed from the idea that individual muscles move bones whereas individual ligaments stabilize them (Kendall and McCreary 1983). Despite the couple of centuries of kinesiology since Borelli that have taken this model to its limits, one may now question whether the nervous system "thinks" in terms of individual muscles, or whether the muscle, a convenient division for the dissector, is even a distinct physiological unit. Neuromotor units or fascicles within muscles may be a more useful division (Van der Wal 2009), and global patterns—our focus for the rest of this chapter—may also tell us something useful about human movement and stability functioning.

More current thinking, much of which is described in the previous chapter, has focused on functional wholes and interconnected patterns within this outer layer, rather than looking for the muscle or particular fascial structure as the culprit for systemic failure such as injury (or more pointedly, lack of injury repair). The Anatomy Trains myofascial meridians map is yet another of these maps, owing much to the work that has come before, from Raymond Dart through Tittel, Mezières, Hoepke, Vleeming, and others, yet at the same time this system has some unique features (Hoepke 1936; Dart 1950; Tittel 2015; Vleeming et al. 1995).

THE ANATOMY TRAINS

The Anatomy Trains, then, is an attempt to describe common pathways of functional force transmission

through the outer layer of myofascia (Fig. 3.4.1, Myers 2020). They differ from the previously mentioned iterations of kinetic chains in that the Anatomy Trains trace connections directly through the fascial fabric whereas the others trace more functional connections. The quadriceps often work with the soleus—they are functionally connected in any squat and leap—but they are not connected fascially in the same strap of biological fabric. By mapping the sinewy "guy-wires" of the outer myofascia (especially important in our high center of gravity, small base of support structure, and unique gait), Anatomy Trains has more to do with the postural "set" that underlies functional coordination.

> ### KEY POINT
> Anatomy Trains myofascial meridians trace connections through the fascial fabric, whereas earlier similar systems often trace functional connections. The quadriceps often work with the soleus and gastrocnemius—they are functionally connected in any squat and leap—but they are not connected fascially in the same strap of biological fabric. Thus the Anatomy Trains map of fascial connections is more implicated in how posture sets the underlying conditions for functional coordination.

Although they share some common ground with the meridians of acupuncture, Anatomy Trains' meridian mapping is based entirely on classical Western fascial anatomy. Any resemblance to the acupuncture meridians is purely coincidental—or perhaps an indication that "chi" travels along the planes of fascia (Fig. 3.4.2).

Not all myofascial connections are created equal. To qualify as a myofascial meridian, it must conform to the following rules:

• *Follow the grain of the (myo)fascial fabric* from structure to structure. Unless there are demonstrable myofascial or collagen fibers running in the same direction to connect any two adjacent structures, they cannot be linked in this scheme (except through the skeleton as in normal biomechanics). These fibers are easy to find from the hamstrings over the ischial tuberosity to the sacrotuberous ligament, for example, whereas finding significant fibers to justify a pull from, say, the rectus femoris to the quadratus lumborum is conceivable but unlikely.

• *Go more or less in a straight line.* Meridians are lines of pretensed tissue, and pulls cannot go around corners

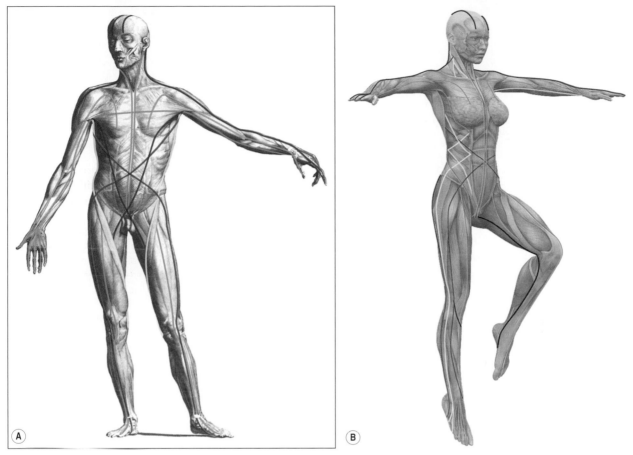

Fig. 3.4.1 (A) The Anatomy Trains mapped onto a familiar figure from Albinus. (B) The current Anatomy Trains logo. (C) The structures of the four arm lines diagrammed. From Myers, T.W., 2020. *Anatomy Trains*, 4th ed. Elsevier, with permission.

except via "pulleys"—for example, tendons under the retinaculae in the ankles and wrists. The more pull in the tissues in the meridian, the straighter the meridian tends to become. Hamstrings to sacrotuberous ligament tracks a meridian; hamstrings to the adjacent quadratus femoris involves a sharp turn and is therefore disallowed.

- *Do not pass through intervening walls of fascia or hard tissues* that would block the force transmission. Myofascial meridians are therefore continuous lines of fabric running outside, not through, the bones.

Parsing the body in this way reveals 12 sets of connections through the parietal myofascia, which are more fully described elsewhere (Myers 2020; www.Anatomy-Trains.com). Generally, there are distinct and coherent lines of dissectable myofascial connection along the

front of the body, along its back, lining the sides, running around the trunk and under the arches, along the arms, connecting contralateral girdles, and through the core of the legs and trunk to the cranial base.

We have dissected these 12 meridians, most in both embalmed and untreated cadavers. The dissection method for exposing these lines involves turning the scalpel sideways and lifting the myofascia off in a continuous layer, as in Fig. 3.4.3. Dissected from an untreated cadaver, the plantar fascia was cut from the bases of the toes, but the integrity of the fascia around the calcaneus to the Achilles tendon was maintained. The soleus was detached from the tibia and fibula, but the gastrocnemii connections to the hamstrings were maintained—and so on up the sacrotuberous ligament and sacral fascia into the erector spinae, which clearly

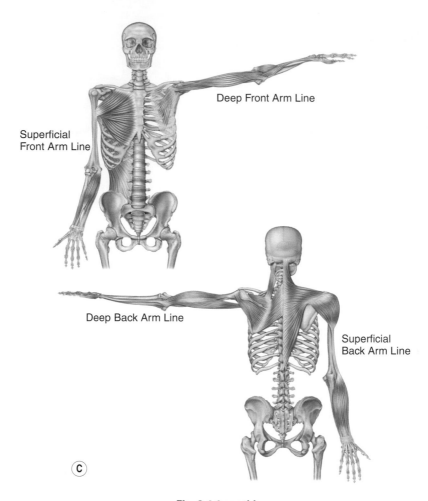

Fig. 3.4.1 cont'd

interface with the galea aponeurotica of the scalp. The Superficial Back Line runs from the bottom of the toes to the bridge of the nose in one band of myofascial fabric along the dorsal surface.

Here follows the fascial and myofascial soft-tissue structures involved in each line. The attachments of the individual muscles within the lines are known as "stations" within the Anatomy Trains schema, to denote that even though the line is connected to the "inner bag" of periosteum and ligaments at these junctures, the force transmission carries on via the fascia beyond the muscle attachment (Wilke 2016). The degree, timing, and precise mechanism of such force transmission has yet to be measured and confirmed, but early evidence suggests that it is worth our

consideration to think that muscles are connected to muscles via the fascia (Huijing 2009). This idea might usefully be added to the more accepted convention: muscles attach to bones. Of course, no muscle attaches to any bone anywhere in the body; it is always via the intervening connective tissue structures (Van der Wal 2009).

- Superficial Front Line: Toe extensors, anterior crural compartment, quadriceps, rectus abdominis and abdominal fasciae, sternalis and sternal fascia, sternocleidomastoid.
- Superficial Back Line: Short toe flexors and plantar aponeurosis, triceps surae, hamstrings, sacrotuberous ligament, sacrolumbar fascia, erector spinae, epicranial fascia.

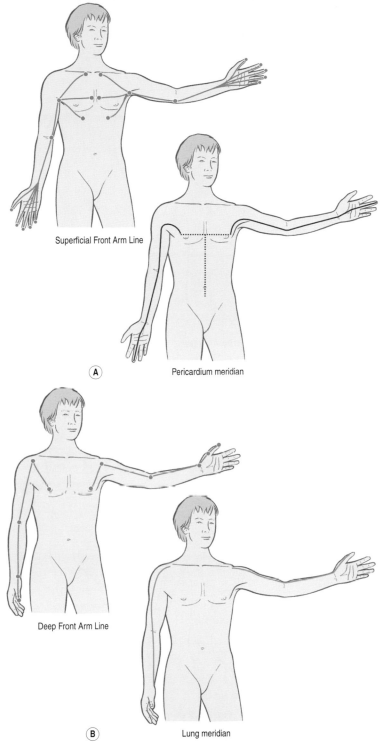

Fig. 3.4.2 A comparison of the myofascial meridians and the acupuncture meridians in the arms, by Dr. Peter Dorsher. From Myers, T.W., 2020. *Anatomy Trains*, 4th ed. Elsevier, Appendix 4, with permission.

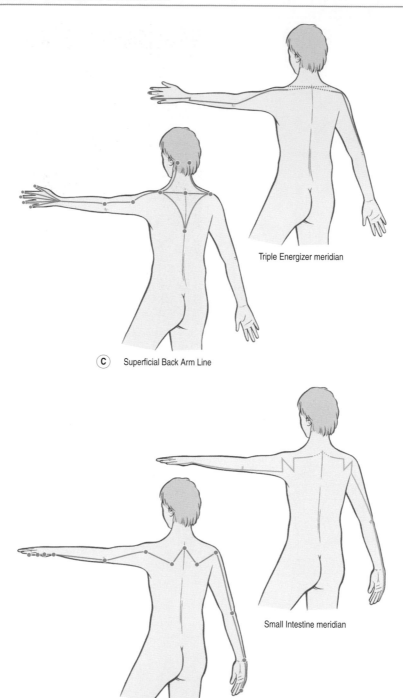

Triple Energizer meridian

(C)   Superficial Back Arm Line

Small Intestine meridian

(D)   Deep Back Arm Line

Fig. 3.4.2 cont'd

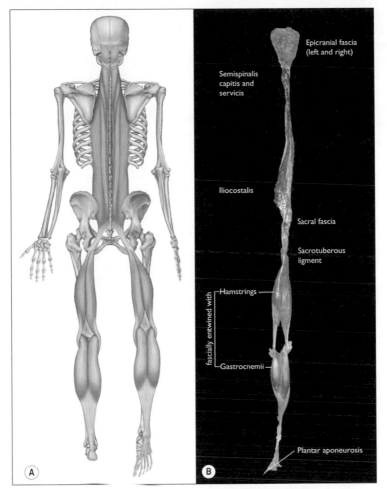

Fig. 3.4.3 (A) The Superficial Back Line in diagram, and (B) dissected as one continuous band of myofascia up the back of the body from toes to nose. By using the scalpel to separate myofascial layers, fascial fabric continuity can be maintained along a given fascial plane. Each of the myofascial meridians described has been dissected in this way. From Myers, T.W., 2020. *Anatomy Trains*, 4th ed. Elsevier, with permission.

- Lateral Line: Fibularis muscles, lateral crural compartment, iliotibial tract, hip abductors, lateral abdominal obliques, internal and external intercostals, sternocleidomastoid, and splenii.
- Spiral Line: Splenii (contralateral) rhomboids, serratus anterior, external oblique, (contralateral) internal oblique, tensor fasciae latae, anterior iliotibial tract, tibialis anterior, fibularis longus, biceps femoris, sacrotuberous ligament, (contralateral) long dorsal sacroiliac ligament, erector spinae.
- Superficial Back Arm Line: Trapezius, deltoid, lateral intermuscular septum, extensor group.

- Deep Back Arm Line: Rhomboids, levator scapulae, rotator cuff, triceps, fascia along ulna, ulnar collateral ligaments, hypothenar muscles.
- Superficial Front Arm Line: Pectoralis major, latissimus dorsi, medial intermuscular septum, flexor group, carpal tunnel.
- Deep Front Arm Line: Pectoralis minor, clavipectoral fascia, biceps, radial fascia, radial collateral ligaments, thenar muscles.
- Front Functional Line: Pectoralis major (lower edge), semilunar line, pyramidalis, (contralateral) anterior adductors (longus, brevis, and pectineus).

- Back Functional Line: Latissimus, lumbosacral fascia, (contralateral) gluteus maximus, vastus lateralis.
- Ipsilateral Functional Line: Latissimus (outer edge), external abdominal oblique, sartorius.
- Deep Front Line: Tibialis posterior, long toe flexors, deep posterior compartment, popliteus, posterior knee capsule, adductor group, pelvic floor, anterior longitudinal ligament, psoas, iliacus, quadratus lumborum, diaphragm, mediastinum, longus muscles, hyoid complex, floor of mouth, jaw muscles.

It is important to note at this point that Anatomy Trains is only a scheme, a map. It is supported by clinical observation, common sense, and initial dissection work, but the degree of sustained force transmission across these lines has yet to be quantified let alone reproduced at a scientifically verifiable level (Wilke 2015). It is also important to note that Anatomy Trains is not a treatment method but a way of seeing that has been shown to be supportive of a number of approaches in physiotherapy and rehabilitation, personal and performance training, and manual therapies of all types (Avison 2015; Larkam 2017; Fredrick 2014; Gabler 2017; Earls 2014; Killens 2018).

Each myofascial meridian can be seen to have a function beyond the function of each individual muscle within it, and some of these meridians lend themselves to a "meaning" within human experience. These subjective but compelling elements can be observed in the clinic, suggesting global treatment plans that support the restoration that the therapist applies to locally strained or damaged tissues.

Running through the system briefly in this way, we can see that the Superficial Front Line, which runs up the body from the top of the toes to the mastoid process, is often shortened in patterns of chronic fear (as seen across the mammalian spectrum in the startle response). Though not yet scientifically verified, this pattern has been observed so often as to make it a truism: strong or chronic emotions of fear often leave a discernible mark in the postural and movement patterning of the body that manifests as muscular (and eventually fascial) shortening of the structures of the Superficial Front Line (see Fig. 3.4.4).

If this pattern is observed in a client, then opening, lengthening, and lifting the tissues of the Superficial Front Line will tend to support the longevity and efficacy of whatever treatment mode is chosen. Expressed in the negative, failing to include such global considerations in

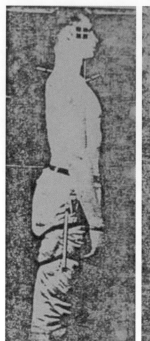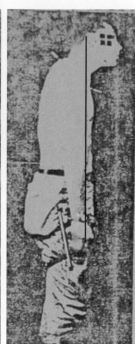

Fig. 3.4.4 A subject just before and just after an unexpected loud noise. The "startle response" (a common cross-species and cross-cultural reaction) can be seen as a reflexive attempt to protect the vulnerable parts of the body through a strong contraction of the Superficial Front Line. Courtesy Frank Jones.

local treatment will leave the tendency for the patient to return to the patterns that led to the segmental failure in the first place.

The Superficial Back Line (see Fig. 3.4.3) must shorten and strengthen to bring us from the primary fetal curve into adult standing, which involves a balance among the spinal curves. Disturbance in this developmental process can result in imbalances among the primary and secondary curves. These imbalances in turn tend to guide the body toward chronically held muscular compensation. Chronically held muscle leads over time to fascial contracture, densification, and adhesion, but the hypothesis based on observation is that this force can be transmitted (or more accurately "distributed"—see the next section on Tensegrity) to other spots in the body (Pavan et al. 2014).

These meridians of myofascial fibers in continuous connection are offered as common (but not exclusive) pathways of myofascial transmission from one segment to another. The result is a common and recognizable pattern of posture that is held neurologically, muscularly, and (ultimately) fascially. It is the aim of many fascially based therapies to free these patterns so that the muscles and habit patterns have a chance to be changed for the better. In the absence of freeing these fascial adhesions, techniques designed to change muscle tone or neurological habit will be fighting an "uphill battle."

To apply this logic to the client illustrated (see Fig. 3.4.5), the neck pain suffered by this preteen is directly related to the position of her knees. In bringing the knees into hyperextension, thus turning a "secondary" curve into a primary (convex dorsally, concave ventrally), she forces her body to compensate in the other two secondary curves, which could have resulted in low back pain or (as in this case) neck pain.

(This pattern may have been established in reverse order—we do not know simply by looking at a photograph. The order of layered compensations within a pattern is a matter of interest, but not of necessity: it is enough that the knee position and neck position are "related" and must be dealt with as a whole, regardless of the historical order in which they are acquired.)

Whatever locally has broken down or strained in her neck, the best and most lasting work will supplement whatever local treatment was applied with "fascial reeducation" (many methods could be employed) of her chronic plantarflexion at the ankle, and hyperextension at the knee and lumbar spine. The posttreatment picture on the right shows how such patterns can (and need to be) considered as a whole. Notice how the Superficial Back Line presents itself as a series of balanced curves in the posttreatment picture. This tends to reinforce the new pattern and promote longevity in results.

> ### KEY POINT
>
> Analyzing posture and function via the Anatomy Trains will assist any practitioner in making manual therapy and training work more efficient by delineating what needs to be lengthened or freed and by showing what other parts of the body are linked to the pattern in question.

TENSEGRITY

The unique properties of tensegrity engineering are well-explored elsewhere in this volume. Whether a human being's locomotor structure can accurately be described as a formal tensegrity as it is defined mathematically is open to question, but the fact that humans are "tension-dependent structures" is not. A bunch of human bones cannot be stacked on each other to recreate the skeleton. Even with the ligaments in place, our structure is hardly self-sufficient or sturdy. Only when these outer layers of "myofascialature" span evenly around the skeleton does the creature stand, adjust, and stabilize in a functional way (see Fig. 3.4.6).

It is worth considering that these myofascial meridians act as the global, geodesic tension complexes that simultaneously stabilize and allow adjustments within the skeletal frame. In other words, the body is not (unless injured or misused) the "strain-focusing machine" described in biomechanical texts but is rather a tensegral "strain-distribution machine." The myofascial meridians provide common (again, not exclusive) pathways for force transmission in the "neuromyofascial web" to:

- Add prestress for stiffening via muscular or myofibroblast contraction.

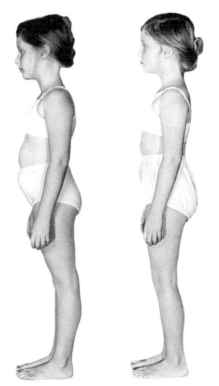

Fig. 3.4.5 Though problems always manifest locally, this girl clearly has a global imbalance in the Superficial Back Line pretreatment (left) and is more coherent and balanced posttreatment (right), which will support the durability of the local results. Courtesy Robert Toporek.

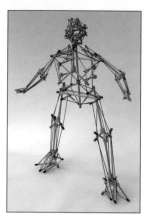

Fig. 3.4.6 If the body works in a manner similar to this intriguing tensegrity model by the late Tom Flemons, then the Anatomy Trains can be seen as the long "elastics" that create the sea of tension in which the isolated compression struts of the bones float. © T.E. Flemons, www.intensiondesigns.com.

- Relax prestress for adjustability via the muscles, myofibroblasts, or treatment.
- Relieve strain in one area of the body by exporting some of it to other parts up or down the "line."

CONCLUSION

Anatomy Trains myofascial meridians is an "argument from design" rather than an established scientific fact. This author understands that further research will modify the specifics of the lines, or expand the scope, or replace it with a better map. No map matches the territory, and new imaging methods will produce new maps.

Whatever new research brings to evidence-based practice of soft-tissue manipulation and training, "practice-based evidence" and increasing clinical anecdotes demonstrate what can be gained in terms of efficacy and duration of results by including global considerations and "whole fascial net" connections in assessment and treatment.

Summary

Within the body-wide extracellular matrix surrounding parietal myofasciae, 12 identifiable myofascial meridians, termed the Anatomy Trains, can be identified and dissected intact from the body. The Anatomy Trains can be used in a wide variety of treatment and assessment methods to specify areas of treatment and related compensation.

REFERENCES

Avison, J., 2015. Yoga-Fascia, Anatomy, and Movement. Handspring Publishers, Edinburgh.

Barral, J.P., Mercier, P., 1988. Visceral Manipulation. Eastland Press, Seattle.

Benias, P., Wells, R.G., Sackey-Aboagye, B., et al. 2018. Structure and distribution of an unrecognized interstitium in human tissues. Sci. Rep. 8, 4947.

Biel, A., 2005. Trail Guide to the Body, third ed. Books of Discovery, Boulder, CO.

Chaitow, L., 1980. Soft Tissue Manipulation. Thorson's, Wellingborough, UK.

Dart, R., 1950. Voluntary musculature in the human body: the double spiral arrangement. Br. J. Phys. Med. 13, 265–268.

Earls, J., 2014. Born to Walk. Lotus Publishing, Chichester.

Fredrick, A.C., 2014. Fascial Stretch Therapy. Handspring, Edinburgh.

Gabler, K., 2017. Your Body's Brilliant Design. Skyhorse Publishing, New York.

Hoepke H., 1936. Das Muskelspiel des Manschen. Stuttgart: G Fischer Verlag.

Huijing, P.A., 2009. Epimuscular myofascial force transmission between antagonistic and synergistic muscles can explain movement limitation in spastic paresis. In: Huijing P.A, Hollander P., Findley T.W., Schleip R., (Eds.) Fascia Research II: Basic Science and Implications for Conventional and Complementary Health Care. Elsevier GmbH, Munich.

Ingber, D., 1998. The architecture of life. Sci. Am. 98, 48–57.

Ingber, D., 2006a. Cellular mechanotransduction: Putting all the pieces together again. FASEB J. 20, 811–827.

Ingber, D., 2006b. Mechanical control of tissue morphogenesis during embryological development. Int. J. Dev. Biol. 50, 255–266.

Juhan, D., 1987. Job's Body. Station Hill Press, Barrytown, NY.

Kendall, F., McCreary, E., 1983. Muscles: Testing and Function, third ed. Williams & Wilkins, Baltimore.

Killens, D., 2018. Mobilizing the Myofascial System. Handspring Publishing, Edinburgh.

Larkam, E., 2017. Fascia in Motion. Handspring Publishers, Edinburgh.

Moore, K., Persaud, T., 1999. The Developing Human, sixth ed. W.B. Saunders, London.

Muscolino, J., 2010. The Muscular System Manual. Mosby Elsevier, Maryland Heights, MO.

Myers, T.W., 2020. Anatomy Trains: Myofascial Meridians for Manual Therapists and Movement Professionals, fourth ed. Elsevier, Edinburgh.

Pavan, P.G., Stecco, A., Stern, R., Stecco, C., 2014. Painful connections: densification versus fibrosis of fascia. Curr. Pain Headache Rep. 18, 441.

Snyder, G., 1975. Fasciae: Applied Anatomy & Physiology. Kirksville College of Osteopathy, Kirksville, MO.

Tittel, K., 2015. Muscle Slings in Sport. Kiener, Munchen.

Tomasek, J., Gabbiani, G., Hinz, B., Chaponnier, C., Brown, R.A., 2002. Myofibroblasts and mechanoregulation of connective tissue modeling. Nat. Rev. Mol. Cell Biol. 3, 349–363.

Upledger, J., Vredevoogd, J., 1983. Craniosacral Therapy. Eastland Press, Chicago.

Van der Wal, J., 2009. The architecture of the connective tissue in the musculoskeletal system – an often overlooked functional parameter as to proprioception in the locomotor apparatus. In: Huijing P.A, Hollander P.,

Findley T.W., Schleip R., (Eds.) Fascia Research II. Elsevier GmbH, Munich.

Vleeming, A., Pool-Goudzwaard, A.L., Stoeckart, R., van Wingerden, J.P., Snijders, C.J., 1995. The posterior layer of the thoracolumbar fascia. Its function in load transfer from spine to legs. SPINE. 20, 753–758.

Varela, F., Frenk, S., 1987. The organ of form. J. Soc. Biol. Struct. 10, 73–83.

Wilke, J., Krause, F., Vogt, L., Banzer, W., 2016. What is evidence-based about myofascial chains? A systematic review, Arch. Phys. Med. Rehabil. 97, 454–461.

Williams, P., 1995. Gray's Anatomy, thirty-eighth ed. Churchill Livingstone, Edinburgh.

Biotensegrity and the Mechanics of Fascia

Stephen M. Levin and Graham Scarr

CHAPTER CONTENTS

INTRODUCTION

Fascia is the fabric of the body; not the vestments covering the corpus but the material that gives it form: the warp and the weft. Muscle and bone, liver and lung, gut and urinary, brain and endocrine are all embroidered into the fascial web. It is a continuum, a tissue that emerges from the simple-celled embryo and evolves into a complex structural heterarchy that pervades the entire organism (Simon 1962), from the interstitium that surrounds virtually every cell in the body to the extracellular matrix and fascial network with all their specialized variations (see Chapter 3.6). In fact, all the "connective tissues" developed out of the embryonic mesenchyme, which means that the structures we label as muscles, bones, tendons, ligaments, and fascia, etc., are all derived from what is essentially the same tissue. As a result, it is likely that they share some similarities in their behavior, with biotensegrity currently representing the most comprehensive approach to explaining this: the mechanics of fascia.

BIOTENSEGRITY

The biotensegrity concept recognizes that all living structures result from interactions between some basic principles of self-organization, or rules of physics, and that that these apply to everything from the smallest of molecules to the complete organism (Levin 2015; Martin 2016; Scarr 2018). At the most basic level, atoms interact with each other in different ways that can be categorized as those that attract and those that repel (van der Waal's forces, covalency, hydrogen bonding, and steric repulsion, etc.), and they spontaneously organize themselves into the most stable and energy-efficient configurations to form crystals and flexible molecules. Each one develops as a distinct structural entity and effectively becomes a physical representation of the invisible forces that hold it together.

KEY POINT

Biological structures emerge from interactions between some basic principles of self-organization.

These structures form as they do because they are constrained by some basic principles of self-organization—geodesic geometry, close packing, and minimal energy—and as attraction and repulsion always operate in conjunction with each other, they enable dynamic systems to automatically move toward a lower and more stable state of energy. The same principles also apply at higher size scales where we now refer to these invisible forces as tension and compression and are able to physically model their interactions (Connelly and Back 1998).

THE TENSEGRITY MODEL

Figure 3.5.1(A) shows a tensegrity structure consisting of six compression struts suspended within a tensioned network of cables, where the reciprocal action of these forces balances and maintains its particular shape. Each structural element is either under tension *or* compression, which means that tensegrity models are also displays of the invisible forces that hold them together: a three-dimensional "diagram of forces" in mechanical terms (Fuller 1975; Heartney 2009) (Fig. 3.5.1B). They are geodesics because their structural elements transfer these forces over the shortest distance; they are close-packed because their component parts automatically get as close as they can to each other; and they naturally balance in the simplest state of minimal energy. Such models are strong, light in weight, flexible, and resilient. They can change shape with the minimum of effort and always return to the same position of stable equilibrium (dynamic stability), and their physical properties are very similar to living tissues. Each part is mechanically integrated with all the others so that when one part moves, everything is involved, thus enabling forces, power, and information to be transferred from one part of the system to another in a controlled way.

To add to this, each cable and strut could itself be constructed from a modular chain of smaller, similar tensegrities, with each individual part maintaining its own structural role within the global heterarchy (Fig. 3.5.2). Such close-packed configurations are intrinsically stable; they optimize the load-bearing ability and provide a mechanism for distributing potentially damaging stresses throughout the structure (Connelly and Back 1998). They are also ubiquitous in biology where each "part" is made from smaller parts, smaller parts, smaller parts . . . with each one nested and integrated within all those surrounding it to form a complete structural and functional unit (Reilly and Ingber 2018). So, although living organisms appear to be highly complicated, both the simple tensegrity model and complex anatomy are formed through the same principles of self-organization and the combined actions of these physical forces, as outlined by Thompson (1917), but there is a problem.

Orthodox Biomechanics

Current biomechanical theory is based on the laws of classical mechanics as formulated by Galilei, Newton, and Hooke, etc., and applied to the behavior of manmade machines from the seventeenth century (Borelli 1680),

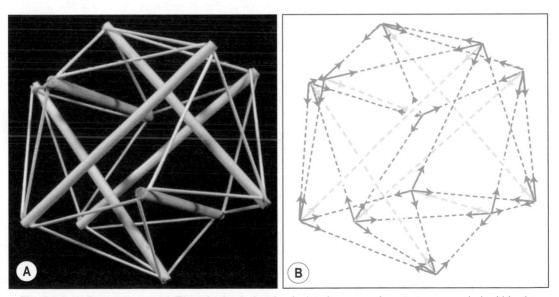

Fig. 3.5.1 (A) Tensegrity model (T-icosahedron) showing isolated compression struts suspended within the global tension network of cables. ©Rory James. Reproduced from Scarr, G., 2018. Biotensegrity: The Structural Basis of Life, second ed. Handspring Publishing, Pencaitland, East Lothian, Scotland, Fig. 3.3B (B) The vectored diagram of forces.

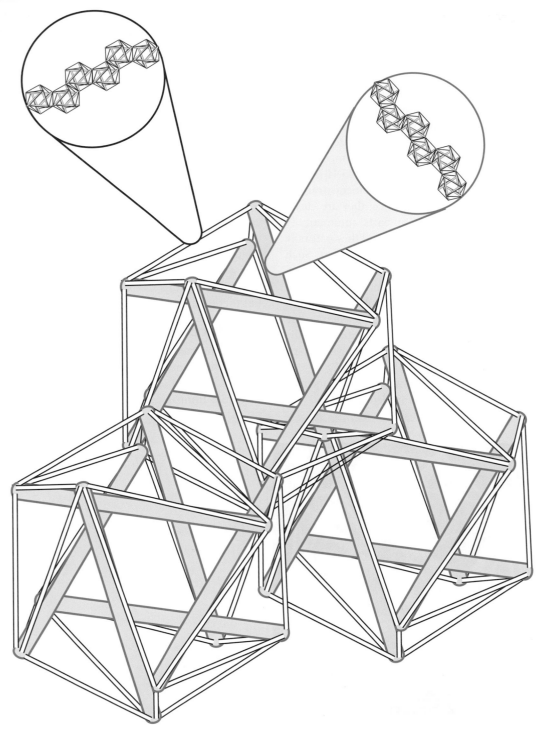

Fig. 3.5.2 Modular tensegrities showing how the same configuration can repeat itself at multiple levels within the global heterarchy.

and it has remained largely unchanged ever since. The problem is that these rules were discovered on inanimate objects and they do not necessarily apply to the nonlinear dynamics of living tissues (Fig. 3.5.3).

For example, biomechanics has taken the more "vertical" part of the stress/strain curve to be a straight line purely because this simplifies the analysis, but it is a fudge! "True linearity does not exist in biology—not even as an approximation. Such a living system that is so profoundly complex at all its different levels and size-scales (10^{-9}–10^1) cannot behave in a linear way—it is fundamentally impossible" (Blyum 2020). In addition, the nonlinear curve never reaches zero stress because of the intrinsic tension contained within the system (Schleip and Klingler 2019). From a biotensegrity perspective, it is much more likely that biological structures operate within the more "horizontal" low-stress/strain region where they will be more responsive, consume less energy, and operate more efficiently (Levin 2015).

The lever theory of joint motion (Borelli 1680) also presents a problem because such mechanisms inherently generate bending moments, shear stresses, and potentially damaging stress concentrations (this is not the case in tensegrity configurations), and it is most unlikely that

developing tissues would be able to withstand the disastrous consequences of these (Levin 2015). In addition, bones do not revolve around the fixed fulcrum of a lever; the mechanical behavior of cadavers is not the same as in living tissues, and the role of connective tissues is frequently ignored in the analysis. The nervous system is also incapable of controlling the huge complexity of joint movements on its own, all of which suggests that something else must be going on (Cabe 2019).

These problems have persisted simply because there has been nothing else to explain them, but they have led biomechanics down a blind alley from which it is only just starting to recover. There is nothing wrong with classical mechanics, but it should be recognized that its value in a biological context is questionable because of the kinematic indeterminacy inherent within the latter, and biotensegrity now offers a more comprehensive perspective that resolves all these issues (Table 3.5.1).

THE MECHANICS OF FASCIA

A popular misconception about the structure of the human body, and biotensegrity, is that it is simply a system of compressed bones suspended within a tensioned

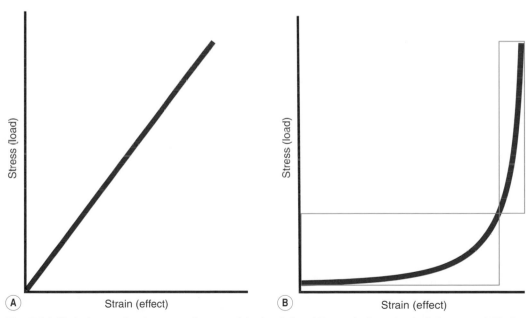

Fig. 3.5.3 Typical stress/strain curves for materials that follow (A) standard mechanical theory and (B) the nonlinear dynamics of tensegrity and living tissues—note that the curve origin does not start from zero stress. Reproduced with permission from Scarr, G., 2020. Biotensegrity: What is the big deal? J. Bodyw. Mov. Ther. 24, 134–137.

TABLE 3.5.1 **Comparison of Properties of Biological Systems, Lever Mechanics, and Tensegrity Icosahedron**

Biological Systems	Lever Systems	Tensegrity Icosahedron
Nonlinear	Linear	Nonlinear
Global	Local	Global
Structurally continuous	Discontinuous	Structurally continuous
Gravity independent	Gravity dependent	Gravity independent
Omnidirectional	Unidirectional	Omnidirectional
Low energy	High energy	Low energy
Flexible joints	Rigid joints	Flexible joints

network of muscles and fascia, but this view is far too simplistic. Anatomy is NOT a collection of isolated bits that operate in a local piecemeal-like way but a complex, fully integrated, nested modular arrangement where the function of each part is dependent on all those surrounding it (Fig. 3.5.2).

Fascia is a continuous body-wide architectural system containing multilevel subsystems, or compartments, that ultimately surround individual cells. Within the higher-level compartments are bones, muscles, lungs, heart, liver, bladder, etc. Smaller fascial compartments enclose glands, blood vessels, nerves, and other tissues, while individual muscle cells are encapsulated within tubular endomysial, perimysial, and epimysial compartments.

 KEY POINT

Fascia is a tensioned network encapsulating a heterarchical system of tissue compartments under compression.

All these different compartments are regional specializations of what is essentially the same tissue with each one playing a subtly different role. The parenchymal cells within them provide the "power" (myofiber, cardiac, hepatic, nerve, adipose, etc.) while the fascia contains the cells and supports their functions. From an embryological, biotensegrity, and logical perspective, bones must then also be considered as compartmental specializations of fascia (mineralized but still flexible) with their own parenchymal cells (osteocytes, osteoblasts, and osteoclasts) (Bordoni and Lagana 2019; Levin 2018).

The fascia is also continuous, with tendons, ligaments, aponeuroses, membranes, etc., as it is *within* every bone

and organ in the body, so that at the microscopic level there is no clear distinction between where one ends and the other begins (see Chapter 3.6). It is intrinsically tensioned (Schleip and Klingler 2019) but cannot operate without a compressional component, which is neatly provided by the cells, fluid-bound proteoglycans, and other structures within each compartment. Muscles are then not so much "organs of movement" but rather dynamic tensioners of the system. The "mechanics of fascia" is thus something of a misnomer because the same principles that led to its formation also express themselves through a unified mechanical system that includes *every* part of the body.

Closed-Chain Kinematics

Closed kinematic chains (CKCs) have been used in mechanical engineering for hundreds of years, because they provide a simple and efficient mechanism with multiple applications and are also well-described in biology (Levin et al. 2017). Closed-chain kinematics couple multiple parts into continuous mechanical loops, with each one influencing the position, motion, and stability of all the others in the system and enabling the controlled transfer and amplification (or attenuation) of force, speed, and kinetic energy. They also describe the basic mechanics of tensegrity (Fig. 3.5.4).

 KEY POINT

The mechanics of fascia are based on a body-wide system of closed-chain kinematics operating within a tensegrity configuration.

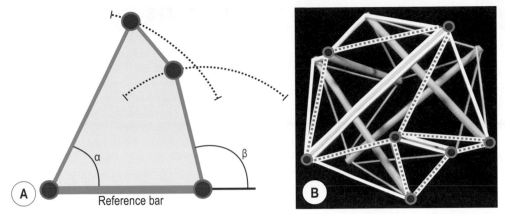

Fig. 3.5.4 (A) Planar four-bar closed kinematic chain (CKC) system showing the trajectories and limits of three moving bars in relation to a fixed reference bar, and how the motion of each bar is controlled by the relative positions of all the others. Modified with permission from Levin, S.M., Lowell de Solórzano, S., Scarr, G., 2017. The significance of closed kinematic chains to biological movement and dynamic stability. J. Bodyw. Mov. Ther. 21, 664–672, Fig. 1A. (B) Tensegrity model highlighting some of the stable three-bar "tension triangles" (white, 2-D) that allow the nonplanar four-bar CKCs (blue dotted, 3-D) to change shape in a controlled way. ©Rory James. Reproduced from Scarr, G., 2018. Biotensegrity: The Structural Basis of Life, second ed. Handspring Publishing, Pencaitland, East Lothian, Scotland, Fig. 4.8B.

Kinematics is all about the "geometry of motion," and the simplest arrangement that enables the structure itself to control this is the planar four-bar, where the length and position of each linkage bar (linkage) determines the mechanical behavior of all the others in the system, and the changing angular relationships between them (α and β) define their characteristic nonlinear properties. In comparison, three-bar triangular shapes can be relatively rigid and are important because of their stability, whereas those with five or more bars can be uncontrollable on their own but are crucial to more complicated systems. Note that this mechanical system is not synonymous with exercise regimes that take a similar name.

At first sight, these closed-chain linkages might appear to be just complex lever systems, but this is not the case in a biological context where every bar and connection between them ("pin-joint") consists of multiple structures acting within their own CKC subsystems (Fig. 3.5.2). Each one will be active in either tension *or* compression (at that particular size scale) and evolutionarily developed in response to the forces flowing through it. There is thus no true fulcrum or bending moment around which a lever can act, and "automatic shifting-suspension mechanism" might be a better description.

The mechanics of CKCs in a biotensegrity context apply equally well to the omnidirectional interactions within and between different molecules, cells, tissues (e.g., fascia), joints, and the whole body, with their nonlinear responses intrinsically related to the heterarchical geometry (Fig. 3.5.3B). Like a pantograph, they enable such systems to amplify (or attenuate) force, speed, and kinetic energy, and thus operate much faster than muscles can contract, with the structure itself guiding motion. As the positional status of each "joint" is dependent on the interactions between a vast number of different fascia-linked tissues, the effect of every muscle contraction can then become distributed over a wide anatomical field. Conversely, multiple muscles can transfer and concentrate their power through the CKC system and cause movement patterns that might otherwise seem impossible.

Such configurations allow the body to respond instantly to rapidly changing conditions and regulate complex movements in ways that are beyond the sole capability of the nervous system (Cabe 2019), where control and the processing of information (force and direction) are embedded within the structure itself and allow the system to perform its own logic computations in synergy with the neurology. CKCs arrangements also have distinct evolutionary advantages, as they enable multiple mechanical functions to become optimized throughout the entire system, during embryological development, and provide a mechanism for increasing diversity (Levin et al. 2017; Scarr 2018).

Biotensegrity recognizes that living organisms are physical representations of a complex balance of invisible force vectors, and that it is the efficient separation of tension and compression into different structural modules (bars) that enables them to change shape with minimal effort and remain completely stable throughout (dynamic stability). CKC mechanics enable the structural system to efficiently distribute forces over a wide variety of different pathways and compensate for any deficits that arise within the system. As a degenerate system, it would also enable the cooperation of fundamentally different components to produce consistently reliable outputs under diversely fluctuating conditions (Wilson and Kiely 2016).

Whenever nature uses the same strategy in a variety of different situations there is probably an underlying energetic advantage to its appearance, and embryological development and evolution consistently favor those patterns and shapes that are the most efficient in terms of stability, materials, and mass. Biology is not dependent on those contrived laws that govern the behavior of manmade machines (e.g., lever theory) but conforms more to the newly emerging physics of soft matter—the characteristics and behavior of bubbles, foams, colloids, polymers, and liquid crystals (Hirst 2013). Biotensegrity now reverses the centuries-old concept of the skeleton as the "frame upon which the soft tissue is draped" and replaces it with an integrated, dynamic, and multilevel fascial heterarchy fit for 21st-century biomechanics.

Summary

Biotensegrity recognizes that complex living structures result from interactions between some basic principles of self-organization and that these apply to everything from the smallest of molecules to the complete organism. Each one is a physical representation of the invisible forces that led to its formation and continue to flow through it. It thus appreciates the fascia as a continuous, heterarchical tension system containing multilevel sub-systems (compartments) under compression, with the mechanics described through a complex system of closed-chain kinematics operating within the global tensegrity configuration at every level. An appreciation of biotensegrity increases our understanding of what is taking place within the body and thus has the potential to improve therapeutic protocols and movement training.

REFERENCES

Blyum, L., 2020. The unreasonable effectiveness of light touch. In: Trewartha, J.E., Wheeler, S.L. (Eds.), Scars, Adhesions and the Biotensegral Body: Science, Assessment and Treatment. Handspring Publishing, Pencaitland, East Lothian, Scotland.

Bordoni, B., Lagana, M.M., 2019. Bone tissue is an integral part of the fascial system. Cureus 11, e3824.

Borelli, G.A., 1680. De Motu Animalium. Petrum Vander As, Lugduni Batavorum.

Cabe, P.A., 2019. All perception engages the tensegrity-based haptic medium. Ecol. Psychol. 31, 1–13.

Connelly, R., Back, A., 1998. Mathematics and tensegrity. Am. Scient. 86, 142–151.

Fuller, R.B., 1975. Synergetics: Explorations in the Geometry of Thinking. Collier Macmillan, London.

Heartney, E., 2009. Kenneth Snelson: Forces Made Visible. Hard Press Editions, MA.

Hirst, L.S., 2013. Fundamentals of Soft Matter Science. CRC Press, Taylor & Francis Group, Boca Raton, FL.

Levin, S.M., 2015. Tensegrity: The new biomechanics. In: Hutson, M., Ward, A., (Eds.), Textbook of Musculoskeletal Medicine, second ed., Oxford University Press, Oxford, pp. 69–80.

Levin, S.M., 2018. Bone is fascia. Available at https://www.researchgate.net/publication/327142198_Bone_is_fascia.

Levin, S.M., Lowell de Solórzano, S., Scarr, G., 2017. The significance of closed kinematic chains to biological movement and dynamic stability. J. Bodyw. Mov. Ther. 21, 664–672.

Martin, D.C., 2016. Living biotensegrity: Interplay of Tension and Compression in the Body. Keiner, Munich.

Reilly, C.B., Ingber, D.E., 2018. Multi-scale modeling reveals use of hierarchical tensegrity principles at the molecular, multi-molecular, and cellular levels. Extreme Mech. Lett. 20, 21–28.

Scarr, G., 2018. Biotensegrity: The Structural Basis of Life, second ed. Handspring Publishing, Pencaitland, East Lothian, Scotland.

Schleip, R., Klingler, W., 2019. Active contractile properties of fascia. Clin. Anat. 32, 891–895.

Simon, H.A., 1962. The architecture of complexity. Proc. Am. Philos. Soc. 106, 467–482.

Thompson, D., 1917. On Growth and Form. Cambridge University Press, Cambridge.

Wilson, J., Kiely, J., 2016. The multi-functional foot in athletic movement: extraordinary feats by our extraordinary feet. Hum. Mov. 17, 15–20.

Human Living Microanatomy

Jean-Claude Guimberteau

CHAPTER CONTENTS

INTRODUCTION

This re-edit of the previous version of this chapter proposes to introduce the actors behind the scene in an attempt to look at the subject matter from a different perspective, to try to give a sense to all these explorations and observations and offer new hypotheses for thought (Guimberteau and Armstrong 2015).

In the past we tried to understand what we had seen under the skin, not only at the level of the tendon or muscle but in all the zones of the body. The major conclusion is that it is the same structural organization everywhere. The organization of living matter appears to be global.

Actually, in some particular areas, mostly when there is tissue friction, we find seemingly free spaces, which could be disconcerting for the global theory, but in fact not only do these areas belong to the global system, they reinforce the basic concept.

The observation of living matter by intratissular endoscopy and the study of our microanatomy with high magnification offer a way of thinking that is unique from traditional anatomical research, from cadaver dissection, and from laboratory observations (Fig. 3.6.1).

 KEY POINT

Dead fragments cannot reveal the reality of what is live.

THE PHYSICAL FACTORS

They reside within us but are often forgotten because they are deemed to be trivial. They cannot be ignored. The permanent, powerful endogenous force exerted by blood pressure is a good example. When we observe the edges of skin draw away from an incision, or the separation of the incised edges of an aponeurosis, the permanent tension

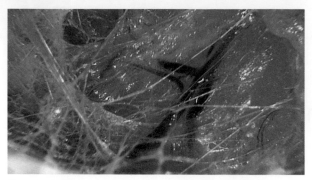

Fig. 3.6.1 Perimuscular and subcutaneous fibrillar network during intratissular surgical endoscopy of a living patient.

within the prestressed tissues is obvious. Less visible forces include osmotic pressure, Van Der Waals forces, and pH gradients. They all determine a set of specifications necessary for biological life. These basic, essential forces were underlined by D'Arcy Thomson, an 18th-century Scottish biologist and mathematician, but his work was submerged by the wave of evolutionary thinking (Thompson 1917).

Back then, the main conclusion suggested through observations is that from the skin to the muscle, from the tendon to the periosteum, at all the different zones, and at all the tissular levels, the body is one and has the same multifibrillar architecture possessing constant intra- and interfibrillar movements with different cellular and morphological specifications.

From now on, we can account for the anatomical structures differently.

TISSUE CONTINUITY—NO LAYERS, NO EMPTY SPACES

 KEY POINT

The first major observation is the continuity of structures. The fibrillar architecture forms a continuous framework that *structures* the entire body from the surface of the skin to the cell interior, from macroscopic to microscopic down to the molecular level and atomic structures.

Simple, contiguous physical spatial relationships can be defined within living matter. They determine a structured, continuous form that can be represented, drawn, and schematized. This ties in with the concept of a bodywide matrix. There is total physical continuity within living tissue, and this renders the concepts

of virtual spaces, separate planes, and other artificial divisions within living tissue obsolete.

We are looking at a continuum of living matter.

This fibrillar irregular network is our interior architecture.

We believe that it is a fibrillar *constitutive*, and *continuous* architecture.

The role of connective tissue is not simply to connect and separate organs and specific anatomical structures, it is *constitutive*, providing a global, three-dimensional architecture in which different types of cells can perform their specific roles.

This represents a fundamental paradigm shift. Anatomy manuals still describe highly stratified layers of tissue, a model first described by Vesalius in the 16th century (Vesalius 1543). This model must now be reconsidered in the light of current scientific thinking that integrates life sciences with modern physics and new mathematics.

DISPERSED PATTERNS WITH NO REGULARITY

What is also really disturbing is that this framework of *constitutive* fibers, with its wide variety of shapes and forms, displays **no symmetry or regularity**. We cannot find any known Euclidean forms. There are no vertical, horizontal, or parallel fibers, no lozenges or circles. Instead, we find a tangled mesh of fibers, a mishmash of complete chaos (Fig. 3.6.2).

There is no discernible beginning or end to this irregular, global network. However, this continuity is accompanied by the uniqueness of all its elements,

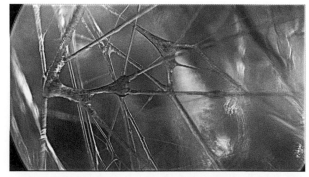

Fig. 3.6.2 Perinervous fibrillar mesh in which the fibers are arranged in a complete disorderly appearance.

such as the polyhedrons of the skin, the fatty lobules, and the structures of the fibrillar network, as well as the cells. Everything seems similar but not identical.

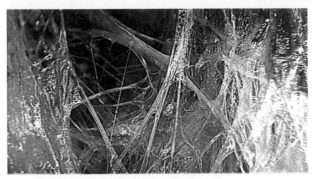

Fig. 3.6.3 Intersection: intertwining of fibrils in three dimensions that form an irregular polyhedral unit of volume

First of all, this brings us to the notion of *rupture of symmetry* developed by Nobel Prize winners Kobayashi and Maskawa in 2008 (Kobayashi and Maskawa 1970). They explained that at the moment of the Big Bang, the universe was symmetrical and without structure. As it cools, the universe ruptures one symmetry after another, thus allowing the appearance of an increasingly differentiated structure by separation of matter and antimatter and producing the germ of the wide variety of structures currently present in the universe. Life, like all biological processes, is also a rupture of symmetry.

To accept that the architecture of the sliding system, to which we owe the harmonious movement of the body, is apparently completely irregular and chaotic questions the basic principles of linear causality. Traditional anatomical teaching prepares us to discover a well-oiled, organized, rational human machine governed by the principles of classical Newtonian physics. Actually, this apparent chaotic and dispersed pattern has structural movements, and these fibrillar movements within the multifibrillar network clearly have a functional finality, which is mobility. But how?

MAINTAINING TISSUE CONTINUITY DURING MOBILITY: MOVEMENTS OF FIBERS, MECHANICAL BEHAVIOR

We have observed that during movements, fibers can stretch, slide, divide, and behave coherently in three dimensions (Fig. 3.6.3).

We realize that the fibrillar mechanism is full of surprises on a purely mechanical level. We have seen that the fibrillar system is able to absorb an applied force by diffusing it across the network, thus permitting both interdependence of separate anatomical structures and optimal transmission of the force (Guimberteau et al. 2005).

Let us look more closely at this set of movements.

REVERSING THE PROCESS OF ENTROPY

Could this be an example of an irreversible dissipative structure, as described by Ilya Prigogine, who was awarded the Nobel Prize for chemistry in 1977 (Prigogine and Stengers 1979)? That is to say, it is a structure that functions contrary to the second principle of thermodynamics, which states that in an isolated system, loss of energy is inexorable and increases over time. This is called entropy, and in traditional physics entropy is associated with disorder and the loss of information.

But Prigogine goes further. He suggests that an open system that is not in a state of equilibrium does not necessarily evolve toward maximal entropy, but on the contrary is capable of transforming lost energy produced by any disturbance. This energy is "dissipated" and utilized for the creation of a newly organized project that is more complex and enables the structure to adapt to its function. He stated that the particularity of life is to reverse the process of entropy with a subsequent increase in complexity that opens up a world of possibilities.

This could be an explanation to understanding all the spatial movements made by the human body in three dimensions with minimal loss of energy and reduced entropy.

IRREVERSIBILITY OF TIME

At the same time, Prigogine expressed or developed the notion of irreversibility in the process of time—that it to say, characterized by time going only in one direction. This concept of the irreversibility of time may appeal to researchers who noticed that the fibers did not all function in the same way and at the same time. Some were fixed, stable, and therefore determined to behave in a predictable way. But for others, the behavior is unpredictable, prepared to deal instantly with all internal or external mechanical constraint. These comportments are clear examples of unpredictability of the movement and trajectory of the fibers, but also of nondeterminism and nonreversibility within this chaos of fibers (Fig. 3.6.4).

This amazing behavior at the molecular level is mind boggling!

How can all these collagen molecules peel away from each other and then stick back together again in an instant, smoothly and without rupture? If we think about it, the combination of these movements at a specific time and place will never be repeated.

 KEY POINT

Deterministic, nonlinear, chaotic behavior is one of nature's potential dynamic capabilities. It broadens the field of possible solutions and allows them to be explored more efficiently.

The association of all these individual movements represents incalculable combinations that cannot be resolved mathematically and ensures that each movement we make is not reproducible in space and time. Each movement is therefore unique, in a creative nondeterministic universe that allows for the possibility of multiple solutions. But finally at the end of the movement the tissular memory may make possible the perfect return to the initial rest position.

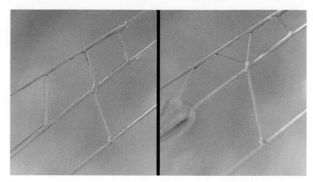

Fig. 3.6.4 Fibers: fibrils have the capacity to lengthen, slide, and divide, facilitating the dispersion of energy in 3D.

The observation of all this uncertainty inevitably may lead one to quantum physics, especially since we are talking about microscopic scales of about a micron that can be influenced either by Newtonian or quantum physics, or both. Confronted with the observation of apparent disorder resulting in efficiency, and the mixture of quantum and Newtonian physics with a dose of thermodynamic physics, it is obvious that we need to change our way of thinking.

QUANTUM PHYSICS AND CHAOS THEORY

Chaotic Systems—Their Appearance and Underlying Order

The term chaos is not a wise choice, because it is misunderstood and often discredits the value of the subject.

In fact, it is the study of the forms and patterns of life and nature. We, humans, are living products of nature.

Chaos theory refers to chaos as described by modern physics.

Many disciplines, such as sociology, cosmology, computer science, engineering, economics, philosophy, and of course biology, have already sought to find solutions to this problem.

The study of complex nonlinear systems such as ecosystems allows us to address complex natural phenomena that are unstable and cannot be accounted for by classical mathematics and physics. Ecosystems do not express themselves with the forms of classical geometry, such as straight lines, planes, circles, spheres, triangles, and cones.

Euclidian measurements, such as length, width, and height, cannot account for irregular forms like clouds, waves, turbulence in a torrent of water, or the distribution of the branches in a tree (Fig. 3.6.5). Clouds are not spheres, mountains are not cone-shaped, and lightning does not move in straight lines. Natural geometry is interlaced, entangled, and twisted.

The classical linear model of Platonic harmony turns out to be inadequate, and it cannot help us understand complexity, because it favors order and stability.

CHAOS THEORY IS A MODERN DISCOVERY

In 1795, Laplace, the master of determinism, declared in his book *A Philosophical Essay on Probability* that order is the result of random events. This in turn leads to unpredictability and instability (Laplace 1825).

Henri Poincaré, a mathematician, physicist, and philosopher of the late 19th century, was the precursor of chaos theory. He asserted that the laws of nature do not deal with certainties, but possibilities. The future is not given; it is in the making (Poincaré 1912).

The meteorologist and mathematician Edward Lorenz, who won the Crafoord Prize in 1983, established the legitimacy of chaos theory through the discovery of the notion of strange attractors (Lorenz 1963). In 1963, he succeeded in reducing meteorology to its simplest expression by modeling the movements of air and water using simple computer-assisted equations based on fluid mechanics.

To his great surprise, he discovered that two meteorological models calculated from almost identical initial conditions give rise to two divergent curves as time passes. Lorenz thus highlights the chaotic nature of meteorology. It was he who famously declared that a butterfly flapping its wings in the Amazon forest could cause a hurricane in Washington. In other words, the effect is not proportional to the cause. This is nonlinearity.

KEY POINT

Deterministic chaotic behavior broadens the scope of possible solutions, allows for more efficient exploration of these solutions, and permits greater complexity. It is one of the potential dynamic capabilities of nature. This apparent disorder is governed by an underlying dynamic order. This provides an explanation for previously incomprehensible natural phenomena and the behavior of ecosystems.

FLUIDS

It was also necessary to explore fluids and volumes in the body. Fluids such as blood, bile, urine, cerebrospinal fluid, and intra-articular fluid are omnipresent during surgery. All tissues are humidified at all times.

But when the surgeon makes an incision in the skin, water doesn't flow freely from the incision. We notice a little liquid known as lymph along the edges of the incision, but that is all. So the fluids that represent 85% of our body weight do not escape through the incision. Their distribution appears to be organized, but how?

In the first part of this chapter written in 2012, we noted, thanks to intratissular endoscopy, areas that resemble bright mirrors. They reflect the light of the endoscope, and they are the result of the intercrossing of fibers in three dimensions. This irregurity is not the result of chance or accident. These forms are not

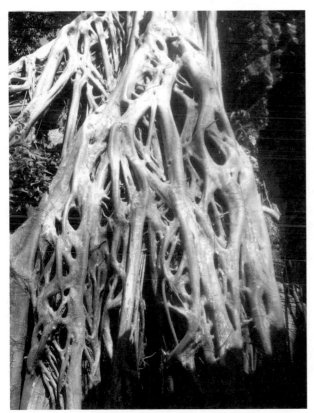

Fig. 3.6.5 Euclidian measurements cannot account for irregular forms like the distribution of the roots of a tree.

imperfections. They are irregular, and this irregularity enables the occupation of space more efficiently compared with Euclidian forms. All the surgeons of the universe can see them during surgery.

INTERCROSSING FIBERS IN 3D CREATE IRREGULAR POLYHEDRAL MICROVOLUMES

These microvolumes are irregular polyhedral forms that are all different—the same forms we find at the surface of the skin. Their seemingly chaotic disposition, their variable forms, and their nonsystematized contiguity nevertheless reveal an underlying order. These microvolumes are known as microvacuoles (Fig. 3.6.6). It took scientists a while to understand that the colloidal gels they contain are in a state of emulsion induced by atmospheric pressure that enters the body through the incision made by the surgeon's scalpel. They appear a few minutes after incision and eventually evaporate.

This observation provides us with essential information. The subdivision of living matter into microvolumes allows us to tackle the thorny problem of the distribution of fluids within living matter, and the adaptability of this living matter to external physical forces. When skin is compressed, the internal pressure of the microvolumes varies simply because the fibers, consisting mainly of collagen, move and then return to their original spatial configuration caused by the preexisting stress of the fibers. This is also possible because the microvacuoles are not hermetic, thanks to the tensioactive properties of their membranes. However, the overall volume of the microvacuoles remains constant. Their form is thus maintained.

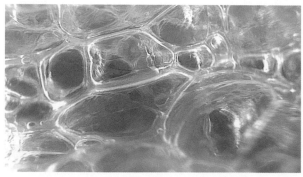

Fig. 3.6.6 Microvolume, resulting from the intercrossing of fibers, is a real morphological entity.

Inside the constantly changing polyhedral framework of the microvacuoles are fluids, but there are no rivers or underground lakes. Living matter is soaked in fluid, rather like the juice inside the pulp of an orange.

Colloidal states are an "ultradivided" state of matter consisting of various proteins, mineral salts, water, and various other contents. Their presence is permanent but in varying concentrations.

They have a capacity to disperse that generates an excellent exchange surface, which increases considerably at the interface. For example, the surface area of foam is much greater than the surface area of a bubble. Their ultralight masses are animated by Brownian movement, and so they seem to escape the force of gravity, as well as the van der Waals forces.

Minute modifications in these systems can lead to significant changes in their overall behavior, on all scales.

TURBULENCE AND PHASE TRANSITION

This is called turbulence, and the final result is "phase transition," which in the terminology of the physics of complex chaotic systems is the capacity of a dynamic state to rapidly swing in one direction or another.

These phase transitions that occur across all scales obey nonlinear mathematics, and so predictions of their future state are said to be random.

ADAPTATION AND TRANSFORMATION: MEGAVACUOLE

Phylogenesis

In old hematomas, and olecranon bursitis, we first observe an edematous reaction with enlarged microvacuoles and fibers.

The microvolumes are drawn or pushed apart, and the fibers separate, forming a space filled with glycosaminoglycans and free of fibers. We also note the presence of numerous bubbles within the fibers.

In these cases, a transition phase is a functional adaptation with a change in physical and metabolic behavior. The multifibrillar, microvacuolar system is progressively transformed into a megavacuole (Fig. 3.6.7).

On the other hand, this notion of changes in state that is observed in living human beings is very useful when attempting to interpret anatomical situations hitherto poorly explained. For example, the carpal tunnel in

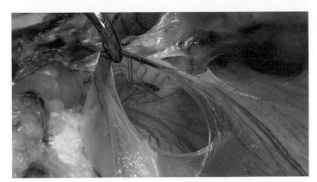

Fig. 3.6.7 Megavacuolar transformation at the level of carpal tunnel under the repetitive longitudinal and lateral forces.

the wrist is the primary area of external mechanical constraint during flexion. The flexor tendons are subjected to this constraint as they pass below the annular ligament and pulleys. The multifibrillar sliding system adapts to repetitive mechanical pressure during flexion of the wrist and fingers by forming what appear to be carpal and digital canals but are actually megavacuolar morphological variations.

> **KEY POINT**
>
> This observation is very important because it also provides an explanation for certain anatomical spaces in the body, such as the spaces surrounding the heart—the pericardium, around the lungs—the pleura, and even the peritoneum.
>
> These spaces all have one thing in common. Inside these spaces, there is permanent, repetitive movement.

A Strong Impression of Total Coherence Emerges From These Observations

All these changes are structurally coherent with the multifibrillar architectural organization of the entire human body. The same fibrillar system is found everywhere.

It is this structural coherence that is fundamental, because it is then possible for us to describe a body that is structured by the same architectural framework, with two essential components:

First, there is a **mobile component,** either with or without functional adaptations, brought about by phase transition. These are the sliding areas, composed essentially of fibers and fluids and containing few cells. These areas play a *shock absorbing role.* They deal with endogenous or external constraint by absorbing and spreading the load.

Second, there is an **operative/productive component** of the same multifibrillar system but essentially filled with cells and few fluids. Examples are fatty lobules, the thyroid gland, the kidneys, and the adrenal glands, each with specific functional roles.

Moreover, there is another observation that is unavoidable in endoscopic exploration. This is the observation of fractalization. We now know that some fibers in the multifibrillar network are able to divide into subfibrils. In this way, force is dispersed throughout the structure right down to the molecular level. The force of gravity is also diminished in this way, at all scales, from macroscopic to microscopic.

FRACTALIZATION ADDS ANOTHER DIMENSION TO THE CHAOTIC ASPECT OF LIVING MATTER

> **KEY POINT**
>
> Fractal structures lack regularity, but this irregularity is neither random nor arbitrary. There is regularity in the irregularity.

From the outset we observed this phenomenon of fractalization at the surface of the skin. But we now know that it also occurs in the fibers and subfibrils and down to the molecular level (Fig. 3.6.8).

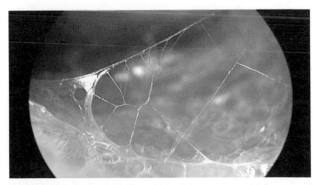

Fig. 3.6.8 Fractalized fibrillar network is an essential feature of the living human body. This process can occur during mechanical behavior.

Fractalization, or scale invariance theory, was first described by Benoit Mandelbrot, mathematician. He coined the word "fractal" and is recognized for his contribution to the field of fractal geometry. A fractal structure looks similar no matter what distance we view it from. Whatever the scale under which it is examined, each part possesses the same structure as the whole. This property is called self-similarity. Fractal structures display regularity within their irregularity, and this adds another dimension to the chaotic aspect of living matter (Mandelbrot 1982).

Fractalization is a widespread phenomenon in anatomy. In this way, a large surface can be contained within a small volume, thus providing a larger surface area for exchange. This is the case with the alveoli in the lungs but also the intestinal villi. This solution has been retained by nature because it increases metabolic efficiency and maximizes the exploitation of space. Unlike Mandelbrot's drawings, nature offers us irregular fractalization, which is not inert; it is dynamic.

This dynamic, instantaneous fractalization helps us understand the resistance of living matter to gravity and gives an answer to this trivial question: How is this volume of colloidal living matter, containing at least 75% of fluids, able to overcome gravity, the strongest fundamental force in our universe? How can we grow?

BIOTENSEGRITY

A tensegrity structure provides a global response to a local mechanical stress. The result is a degree of independence from the force of gravity.

Stephen Levin coined the term *biotensegrity* when he applied the concept of tensegrity to living organisms. Although debated, it represents a major advance in our understanding of the organization of anatomical structures and helps us to understand how the multifibrillar network is able to grow and withstand the force of gravity (Levin 1982).

 KEY POINT

This capacity to resist gravity is fundamental, because it throws new light on the processes of morphogenesis and organogenesis.

Of course, the discovery of homeobox genes that regulate the expression of other genes provides essential answers regarding the localization of the blueprint, but provides no explanation of spatial organization and contiguity. Yet again, this continuous fibrillar organization may provide answers.

UNDERSTANDING GROWTH AND MORPHOGENESIS

Self-assembly is made possible by the fractalization of fibers in the multifibrillar network, and this enables the transition from one stable form to another when sufficient energy is available. Under the influence of growth hormones, the network multiplies, develops, and grows without rupture. Cells develop within this fibrillar framework. The fundamentals of mechanical behavior are respected at all times.

The ability of the fibrils to reproduce the basic polyhedral forms, combined with the phenomenon of dynamic fractalization, helps us to better understand how all the forms we observe in the human body can be created. Standard 3D design software is a very efficient tool to illustrate this. For example, if we take a set of lines with irregular intersections as previously described, all we need to do is impose a longitudinal force to obtain cylindrical structures. Tendons are examples of longitudinal structures. The intermuscular septa and some articular ligaments are also longitudinal structures, but the spatial arrangement of their fibers is different. The formation of hollow tubular structures like blood vessels, the bronchial tree, the intestines, and excretory ducts occurs spontaneously. The formation of a canal is simply the continuation of an imposed constraint in the same structure.

Bone is simply a reinforcement of the fibrillar system with hydroxyapatite. The respiratory system can be considered to be the result of the penetration of air into the fibrillar system. It is the same process for joints. The thyroid is the result of that area of the fibrillar system being inhabited by cells that group together to perform specific physiological functions. The vascular, nervous, lymphatic, and muscular systems are completely integrated into this network.

There is a global coherence at all levels of organization within the fibrillar network. Moreover, two avenues of reflexion can be considered. One is of a more general nature.

THE STRUCTURAL SIMILARITY OF LIFE

This organizational model is comparable to that of a tree, which is a perfect example of the fractalization of life. This occurs across all scales, from the trunk to the main and secondary branches and stems and the framework of the leaf down to the plant cells themselves.

Confronted with this polyhedral human architectural framework, it is difficult to ignore the fact that it is found in all other living species—animal, vegetable, and even mineral. From the skin to the pulp of an orange and volcanic rock, the list is long. This encourages us to think, or even affirm, that all biological systems employ the same universal mechanisms for evolution and complexification.

The use of the irregular polyhedron as the fundamental unit of form seems to be a necessary consequence of the basic physical forces acting on living organisms.

After the first physiological and scientific aspect, the second touches on our work as therapists. It is now possible to explain and define pathologies such as edema—swelling of the microvacuoles without lasting alterations to the multifibrillar, microvacuolar system. Inflammation is a dilatation of the microvacuoles and the vessels, and an alteration of fluids.

We now better understand why a scar can have multiple consequences because of the loss of fibrillar harmony that is replaced by stiffness. We have clear mental images of obesity, an overloading of the microvacuoles by adipocytes. The microvacuoles become so heavy that they can no longer resist gravity. Finally, we understand the programmed aging of all the components that is the revenge of gravity and leads inexorably to the sagging of our contours. There is so much more left to discover about the human body.

CONCLUSION

It may no longer be possible to consider human anatomy as it has been taught since Vesalius. New technological advances have allowed us to lift a corner of nature's veil, and we have been able to observe the ocean of apparent disorder that generates the order of life. Life can no longer be defined solely from the perspective of the cell. It is now necessary to take into account the cell's external environment, the fibrillar architecture.

KEY POINT

From now on, it will be difficult to ignore this extracellular "interior architecture" that forms a symbiosis with the cytoskeleton.

Its organization is a continuous, irregular, mobile, adaptive, fractal, chaotic, and nonlinear vector, from the surface of the skin to the smallest constituents of our structure, of that most beautiful of optimal efficiencies—life.

Could this bodywide, fibrillar network be defined as "fascia"?

Summary

The anatomical model described by Vesalius and our elders must now be reconsidered in the light of current scientific thinking that integrates life sciences with modern physics and new mathematics.

The classical linear model of Platonic harmony turns out to be inadequate, and it cannot help us to understand complexity, because it favors order and stability.

The study of our microanatomy and fibrillar architectural network through the observation of living matter by intratissular endoscopy has encouraged me to leave my traditional academic world to study the science of complexity and of chaotic, nonlinear systems.

The study of complex nonlinear systems such as ecosystems allow us to address complex natural phenomena that are unstable and cannot be accounted for by classical mathematics and physics.

The physical factors and actors behind the scene are introduced in an attempt to look at things from a different perspective and offer new ground for thought, in particular concerning the chaotic and irregular of the fibrillar architecture inside the body.

There is still much to discover about human anatomy, but new technological advances and theories in the fields of physics and mathematics have allowed us to lift a corner of nature's veil. The multifibrillar, microvacuolar network appears to be an ocean of apparent disorder that generates the order of life. This architectural fibrillar network, previously known as "connective tissue" but is in fact constitutive, can no longer be neglected.

Its globality and continuity give meaning and definition to the term "fascia."

REFERENCES

Guimberteau, J.C., Armstrong, C., 2015. Architecture of Human Living Fascia. The Extracellular Matrix and Cells Revealed Through Endoscopy. Handspring Publishing, Edinburgh.

Guimberteau, J.C., Sentucq-Rigall, J., Panconi, B., Mouton, P., Bakhach, J., 2005. Introduction to the knowledge of subcutaneous sliding system in humans. Ann. Chir. Plast. Esthet. 50, 19–34.

Kobayashi, M., Maskawa, T., 1970. Chiral symmetry and eta-x mixing. Progr. Theor. Phys. 44, 1422–1444.

Laplace, P.S., 1825. Essai philosophique sur les probabilités, fifth ed. Bachelier, Paris.

Levin, S.M., 1982. Continuous tension, discontinuous compression: a model for biomechanical support of the body. Bull. Struct. Integration 8, 31–33.

Lorenz, E.D., 1963. Deterministic nonperiodic flow. J. Atmos. Sci. 20, 130–141.

Mandelbrot, B.B., 1982. The Fractal Geometry of Nature. WH Freeman, New York.

Poincaré, H., 1912. Calcul des probabilités, second ed. Gauthier-Villars, Paris.

Prigogine, I., Stengers, I., 1979. La Nouvelle alliance. Gallimard, Paris.

Thompson, D.W., 1917. On Growth and Form, vol. 1. Cambridge University Press, Cambridge.

Vesalius, A., 1543. De humani corporis fabrica libri septem. Ex Officina Joannis Oporini, Basel.

The Fascial Net: Resonance Frequency With Links to Thermodynamics

L'Hocine Yahia and Nathan Nyamsi Hendji

CHAPTER CONTENTS

INTRODUCTION

In biomechanics, the human spine is often defined as a complex structure whose principal functions are to protect the spinal cord and transfer loads from the head and trunk to the pelvis. However, the function of the spine remains controversial, and some researchers believe that it plays an important role in locomotion (Gracovetsky 1985). If we do not understand the function of the spine and its components, we cannot model it or clarify the disorders that affect it. It is known that in nature, organs and tissues do not have a single function. As such, fully understanding the different functions of the spine and its components is essential for the clinicians and other spine researchers.

This process of trying to better understand the spine function led to a novel study that was initiated with the collaboration of the Laboratory of Innovation and Analysis of Bio Performance at Prof. L'Hocine Yahia's lab at École Polytechnique de Montréal, Canada, and Prof. Mark Driscoll's Musculoskeletal Biomechanics Research Lab at McGill University in Montreal, Canada. This study focuses on the thoracolumbar fascia (TLF)

and its potential role in the locomotive function of the spine (Nyamsi Hendji 2019). A few studies in spine and fascia research had already focused on this, so the aim of this work was to explore new potential research paths. More precisely, the goal of the study was to assess how the TLF could affect spine resonant frequencies. Research work based on locomotion as the spine's primary function encourages the study of its biomechanics from a different perspective and could bring riveting insight into both spine and fascia research.

LOCOMOTION THEORIES

Role of Spine in Locomotion

In mammals, few studies have been devoted to the role of the trunk in walking. To our knowledge, no study is precisely interested in the activity of the trunk during the initiation of locomotion. Gracovetsky was among the first to challenge the classical thinking regarding the role of the human spine and to assume that it is the engine of locomotion (Gracovetsky 1985).

KEY POINTS

According to spinal engine theory, animals must travel from one point to another consuming minimum energy in a constant gravitational field and minimizing the stress experienced by the various anatomical structures. Anatomy therefore emerges as the solution and not the given parameter of the evolutionary problem. Thus if the primary function of the spine is locomotion, its anatomy is the result of that particular function.

The spine is considered the "primary" engine, in the etymological sense of the word. This primary engine, so obvious in our ancestors, the fish, has not traveled toward the lower limbs over time. In bipedal locomotion the pelvis, linked to the lumbar spine, initiates the motion by rotating and is then followed by the legs. The rotation occurs because of the coupled motion of the lumbar spine. The natural curvature of the lumbar spine (lordosis) combined with the lateral flexion moment generated by the firing of the trunk muscles (deep back muscles and obliques) results in the rotation of the pelvis. This is the coupled motion of the lumbar spine (Gracovetsky 1985).

In summary, locomotion was first achieved by the motion of the spine. The limbs came after, as an improvement, not as a substitute; and yet, analysis of bipedal gait concentrates almost exclusively on the motion of the limbs. Indeed, some studies consider only the legs for locomotion and the spine as a passive element (Andriacchi and Alexander 2000; Raibert 1986). On the contrary, not only does the spine play a stabilizing role but it also helps maintain good posture during locomotion (Schilling and Carrier 2010; Zhao et al. 2014). This theory has been successfully applied in the robotics field (Karakasiliotis 2013; Zhao et al. 2012; Zhao et al. 2014). Development of fixed-leg quadruped robots with flexible spines has shown that activation of the spine alone allows locomotion, proving its key role (Zhao et al. 2012; Zhao et al. 2014). Flexible spine not only allows the robot's locomotion, but it also helps in controlling and adjusting the posture, making the locomotion more efficient (Schilling and Carrier 2010; Zhao et al. 2014).

One of the basic goals of any design—both animate and inanimate—is to get maximum output for minimum energy. Locomotion can be represented as a flow of mass from one location to another (Bejan and Marden 2006).

Animals move on the surface of Earth in the same way as rivers, winds, and oceanic currents. They seek and find paths and rhythms that allow them to move their mass the greatest distance per expenditure of useful energy while minimizing thermodynamic imperfections such as friction. Animals move in different ways for different purposes, but effective use of energy is the common factor because it is important over a lifetime. Therefore the basic design of most animals should evolve toward locomotion systems that optimize distance per energy cost subject to minimum stress requirements. Bejan (2006) proposed that animal and human locomotion is "guided locomotion." It is movement with design—efficient, economical, safe, fast, dynamic, and purposefully straight. This is the constructal design of animal and human locomotion.

Resonance in Locomotion

One way this energy optimization can be achieved is with resonance. Nearly all objects and structures are characterized by a set of natural (or resonant) frequencies. When solicited at one of those frequencies, the structure stores energy and therefore experiences high displacements. This is known as resonance. When it occurs, a minimal force input produces a maximum motion output.

In engineering, the goal of any design is usually to avoid resonance. The large amplitudes that may be created are unwanted in the static structures built by man. Indeed, the strain of large amplitude oscillations can lead to spectacular catastrophic failure, as in the collapse of the Tacoma Narrows Bridge, for example (Yahia et al. 2019a). Mechanical properties and geometries are therefore selected so that the lowest resonant frequency of the structure is well above the expected frequencies that it will experience.

In biology, however, large amplitude oscillations obtained with a minimum of power input are often desirable (e.g., locomotion). In the absence of wheels, oscillatory periodic motion is the basis of all locomotion. For periodic motions of fins, wings, and legs, fluid and/or solid mass components are made to swing, and the organs that power this have elastic components so that resonance can occur (Yahia et al. 2019a).

Locomotion often involves resonance. This phenomenon helps in obtaining maximum amplitudes for a minimum input energy.

Any body part held by elastic forces can perform oscillatory motion at a characteristic resonance frequency f0. Mechanical energy is always saved if f0 is tuned to other body frequencies, such as the leg or the wing beat frequency. If the driving force frequency f is tuned to the member frequency so that f = f0, a small periodic force can maintain a large amplitude oscillation. This amplification process is of great technological and biological significance. Animals make use of it in walking, running, swimming, and flying (Ahlborn et al. 2006).

Animals that locomote at their resonance frequency achieve the best possible energy efficiency, because twice in each stride cycle they convert the necessarily expended gravitational (or elastic) potential energy into kinetic energy. Thereby large deflection amplitudes can be achieved with a minimum of muscle force (Yahia et al. 2019a).

Locomotion benefiting from resonance has been successfully applied on a smaller scale to the design of a one-legged hopper robot, showing an improved hopping impact efficiency (Wanders et al. 2015).

The drawback of operating at the resonance frequency is that large amplitudes are only obtained in a narrow frequency range near the resonant frequency. This does not mean that animals can only move at fixed speeds. As shown by Ahlborn et al. (2006), the resonant frequencies can be tuned by changing the mass distribution relative to a rotation axis, the relevant vertical acceleration, the oscillating mass, and the effective spring constants. Using these principles, animals can vary their resonant frequencies and move with high energy efficiency at various speeds.

From a neuromotor point of view, the control of locomotion is achieved by intrinsically active neural networks called central pattern generators (CPGs) that produce the rhythmic patterns of muscle activation necessary for the rhythmic movements of locomotion (MacKay-Lyons 2002). Experimental studies suggest that resonance tuning also occurs at the level of those CPGs that synchronize to the mechanical resonant frequency of the oscillating limbs for which they control muscle activation (Abe and Yamada 2003; Holt et al. 1990; Jeng et al. 1997).

LINKING THE LOCOMOTION THEORIES WITH THE THORACOLUMBAR FASCIA: A NOVEL APPROACH

The locomotion theories briefly presented here suggest the important, yet underestimated, role of the spine in locomotion. Research in the 2010s has proved that the

TLF is a central piece in the spine's structure and plays an important role, in many different ways, in the spine's function, biomechanics, and mechano-pathobiology (Avila Gonzalez et al. 2018).

By simple deduction, the involvement of the TLF in the locomotion mechanics then seems inevitable. But a question remains: what exactly is the function of the TLF in locomotion?

To put all the elements presented previously in a nutshell: we first have the spinal engine theory, which states that locomotion is initiated by the rotation of the lumbar spine, and we have the theory of locomotion benefiting from resonance, which says that the frequency of the moving limbs is naturally tuned to their resonant frequency during locomotion, which results in minimum force requirements.

With all those elements in mind, the following reasoning resulted:

- Resonance in locomotion is tunable so that it can be maintained for various speeds (Ahlborn and Blake 2002; Ahlborn et al. 2006). Sadly, similarly to the locomotion studies in general, the spine is also overlooked in those resonance studies, the focus being mainly on the resonance of the swinging limbs. However, though Ahlborn and Blake (2002) only considered limbs resonance in their work, they concluded that other body parts such as the spine could also resonate, thus contributing to making the locomotion even more efficient.
- Previous resonance tuning studies have shown that sensory feedback is essential to adjust the frequency of the CPGs to the mechanical resonant frequency (Hatsopoulos 1996; Williamson 1998). Biological systems have evolved with several strategies to synchronize the mechanical and neural dynamics using sensory feedback.
- Two of the main features of the TLF are: its dense innervation (Yahia et al. 1992; Wilke et al. 2017), which allows feedback to the central neural system, and its musclelike properties, with the presence of myofibroblasts (Yahia et al. 1993; Schleip et al. 2005) potentially allowing it to modulate its tension.
- It was proposed that the TLF innervation allows sensory feedback to regulate muscle tension in order to optimize spine mobility and stability (Yahia et al. 2019a).

Based on these elements, researchers supposed that the sensory feedback provided by the TLF, along with its muscle-like properties, could also allow for modulating its own tension in order to optimize the spine's resonant frequency and adapt to different locomotion speeds.

KEY POINTS

The hypothesis of the project was that during locomotion the spine resonates along with the limbs, and this allows for energy-efficient locomotion. To maintain that at different speeds, the spine's resonance frequency is tuned by the TLF, which modulates its tension accordingly (Fig. 3.7.1).

A SIMPLIFIED LUMBAR SPINE FINITE ELEMENT MODEL WITH MIDDLE AND POSTERIOR LAYERS OF THE THORACOLUMBAR FASCIA

The objective of this research project was to determine whether the influence of the TLF on the spine resonant frequencies is significant by means of a finite-element (FE) model of the lumbar spine.

METHODS

In order to achieve the objective, the first step was to develop the finite-element model. A previously validated, simplified finite-element model of the lumbar spine (L1-S1) was first reproduced from Sadouk (1998; Fig. 3.7.2), and the middle and posterior layers of the TLF were then added according to the information found in the literature. The software used was the Mechanical APDL module of ANSYS (18.1). Vertebrae were modeled as rigid and linked by nonlinear beams defined to take into account the combined properties and behavior of the intervertebral discs, facet joints, and

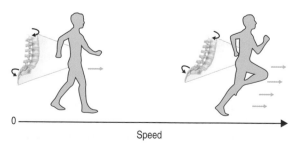

Fig. 3.7.1 Spine's resonance maintained at different speeds.

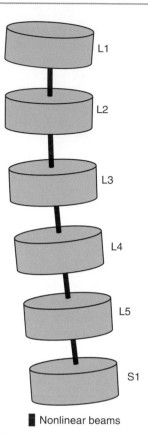

■ Nonlinear beams

Fig. 3.7.2 Simplified model of lumbar spine (after Sadouk 1998).

the different ligaments. The middle and posterior layers of the TLF were modeled by individual fibers with elastic isotropic properties ($E = 100$ MPa; $\nu = 0.3$) inserting on the back and side of the vertebrae at the different lumbar levels and merging laterally in the lateral raphe. Tensioning of the TLF was achieved by applying a lateral tensile force on the lateral raphe modeling the action of the transverse abdominal muscles (Fig. 3.7.3).

The second step consisted of a partial validation of the developed model by means of static loading tests to make sure that the model was behaving consistently. Moments in the sagittal and frontal planes up to 10 N.m were applied on L1 while keeping the sacrum fixed. The impact of the tension in the TLF on the displacements at L1 was then assessed.

In the end, a modal analysis of the lumbar spine finite-element model was run to study, in this locomotion context, the influence of the TLF on the spine's resonant frequencies. For this part of the study the boundary conditions were changed to better represent

Lateral raphe

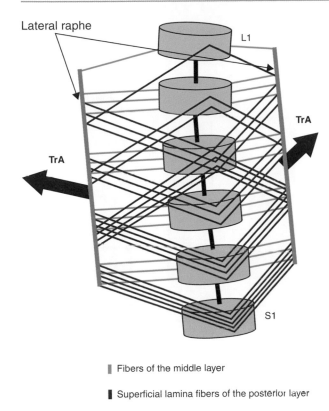

L1

TrA

TrA

S1

▌ Fibers of the middle layer

▌ Superficial lamina fibers of the posterior layer

▌ Deep lamina fibers of the posterior layer

Fig. 3.7.3 Final model with middle and posterior layers of TLF merging in the lateral raphe and tension applied by forces representing the transverse abdominal muscles (Nyamsi Hendji 2019).

locomotion conditions (L1 fixed and S1 free), and material properties (E = 10 GPa ; ν = 0.3) were assigned to the rigid vertebrae. Rigid bodies have null resonant frequencies, which could have affected the results. Additionally, masses and inertias were assigned to each vertebra according to what was done in a previous dynamic study using this same simplified model (Bazrgari 2007). The mass and inertia assigned to S1 were those of a full pelvis to better represent reality. First, a sensitivity analysis was achieved to assess the influence of the model's parameters on its resonant frequencies. Then a more detailed study of the calculated resonant frequencies and the impact of the TLF's properties was carried out to assess for a potential link to locomotion. Two different sets of parameters were defined for the material properties of the vertebrae and intervertebral discs (values of mass, inertia, and elastic moduli changed by plus or minus 10%), which corresponded to

two different morphological and anatomical configurations. For each of them a modal analysis was run. These two different sets of parameters were meant to verify if the same results were obtained for different morphologies, which would be equivalent to different individuals.

RESULTS

The results of the static study first showed that the passive lumbar spine model was successfully reproduced and that, after implementation of the TLF, its behavior was in agreement with results obtained from previous studies on either numerical or experimental models. For the first test of flexion in the sagittal plane, a 50 N tension force applied bilaterally on the lateral raphe caused a translation restriction of 1.78% at L1 level for a 10 N.m flexion moment and 9.81% for a 2 N.m flexion moment (Fig. 3.7.4). For the second test of lateral flexion, a 20 N tension force applied unilaterally on the lateral raphe on the opposite side of the motion caused a translation restriction of 8.51% at L1 level for a 10 N.m flexion moment and 37.74% for a 2 N.m flexion moment (Fig. 3.7.5).

Sensitivity coefficients that quantify the effects of a given parameter on the model response were calculated for each parameter of the model. The results showed that the impact of the mass and inertia of the vertebrae on the model's resonant frequencies is not significant, with relative sensitivity coefficients of 0.003 and 0, respectively. The Young's modulus of the vertebrae has a medium impact (0.08). The shear modulus of the nonlinear beams modeling the intervertebral discs has a medium impact as well (0.12). Finally, the Young's modulus of the TLF had a high impact (0.45).

The modal analysis showed for the first morphological configuration a resonant frequency of 1.16 Hz corresponding to a torsion mode. For the second morphological configuration, the same torsion mode was found for a slightly different frequency: 1.28 Hz. For both configurations a 10% variation of the TLF's Young's modulus was enough to produce a variation of that frequency in a range of equal size as that of the locomotion range of frequencies, 1.4 to 2.8 Hz.

As explained in the spinal engine theory, it is by a rotation movement that the spine initiates locomotion (Gracovetsky 1985). Therefore having a resonant frequency corresponding to a torsion mode close to the locomotion range of frequencies brings an element in favor of that theory. Furthermore, the results obtained

Sagittal flexion

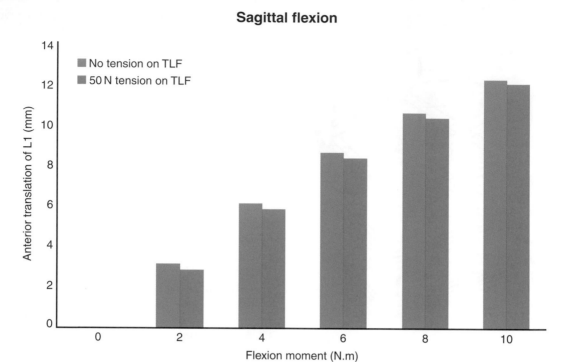

Fig. 3.7.4 Results of the sagittal flexion test (Nyamsi Hendji 2019).

Lateral flexion

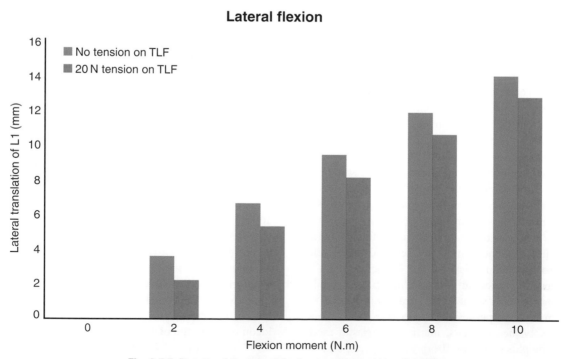

Fig. 3.7.5 Results of the lateral flexion test (Nyamsi Hendji 2019).

also indicate that the TLF could have the most significant effect on the spine's resonant frequencies and that it has the potential to easily modulate those frequencies by changing its properties. This means that the frequency of the torsion mode mentioned previously could be tuned by the TLF to the locomotion frequency.

CONCLUSION

The model presented here has several limitations that were all discussed in depth in the master's thesis in which it was presented (Nyamsi Hendji 2019). Even though it cannot be completely validated, this model was able to reproduce results from the literature for static cases in terms of movement restriction in both lateral and sagittal flexion. Regarding the dynamic part of the study, the results of the modal analysis were not validated whatsoever, simply because such a study has not been done before. Several studies performing modal analysis on lumbar spine models exist, but none of them include the TLF. Achieving such studies in vivo seems difficult at the moment, as no technology allows for making such measurements. We can only rely on developing better numerical models to try and validate those results. Therefore this preliminary study can be seen as an exploration research project aiming at opening new research paths and providing ideas on how we can challenge and rethink the actual approaches in spine biomechanics and change the perspective from which it has been studied.

To take this work further, complete modeling of all the muscle groups involved in the spine's function will be necessary (back muscles and gluteus maximus), especially integrating the hydrostatic effect of the erector spinae muscles (Vleeming et al. 2014; Creze et al. 2019). Modeling of the full pelvis and real vertebrae rather than discs will also be necessary to better reproduce the anatomy and the insertion of the TLF and all the muscles involved. Elements such as the viscoelastic behavior of the TLF and its potential auxetic properties (negative Poisson's ratio) should also be considered.

Human movement is a complex system. For scientists and engineers, dynamics and evolution of complex systems are not easy to predict. A fundamental approach to studying complex systems is far from equilibrium thermodynamics. From that point of view, complex systems are self-organized systems extending over multiple hierarchical levels at different scales and behaving in a nonlinear fashion (Yahia et al. 2019b). Such systems are characterized by emergent properties.

KEY POINTS

Emergence is a consequence of complexity at multiple scales of organization. A particular system behavior is considered emergent if it cannot be predicted by studying the component parts at the finer scales of system organization. In other words, interactions of components in the finer scales lead to structural or functional properties in the higher scales of the system that are absent in the components themselves (Yahia et al. 2019b).

Complexity endows the system with the capacity to adapt when the environment changes so that the system can continue to exist and function. Modeling such complex systems can appear as a difficult task in biomechanical studies. A solution to that would be to incorporate multiscale modeling approaches coupled with artificial intelligence algorithms. This would allow the development of realistic models able to interact with their environment and adapt to it through feedback loops allowing constant reconfiguration without user input.

Summary

Two theories on locomotion have been introduced in this chapter: the spinal engine theory (locomotion is initiated by the spine) and locomotion benefitting from resonance (body parts resonant frequency is tuned to locomotion rhythm to minimize force and energy requirements). Both these theories have been successfully applied in robotics applications. A research project aiming to link these theories and the TLF's function was then presented. In this project a finite-element model of the lumbar spine, including the middle and posterior layers of the TLF, was developed. The work presented is the first to ever investigate the effect of the TLF on the spine's resonant frequencies. This preliminary study shows that the lumbar spine has a torsional resonant mode for a frequency value near the range of the locomotion frequencies, suggesting that locomotion benefitting from the resonance phenomenon could be possible. Furthermore, small changes in the TLF properties can easily modulate this frequency, which could help in maintaining resonance for various speeds. Overall, the results indicate that the TLF could play a role in locomotion. Further studies integrating thermodynamics approaches and detailed models using evolved techniques and tools will be necessary to continue this work and confirm the results obtained.

REFERENCES

Abe, M.O., Yamada, N., 2003. Modulation of elbow joint stiffness in a vertical plane during cyclic movement at lower or higher frequencies than natural frequency. Exp. Brain Res. 15, 394–399.

Ahlborn, B.K., Blake, R.W., 2002. Walking and running at resonance. Zoology 105, 165–174.

Ahlborn, B.K., Blake, R.W., Megill, W.M., 2006. Frequency tuning in animal locomotion. Zoology 109, 43–53.

Andriacchi, T.P., Alexander, E.J., 2000. Studies of human locomotion: Past, present and future. J. Biomech. 33, 1217–1224.

Avila Gonzalez, C.A., Driscoll, M., Schleip, R., et al., 2018. Frontiers in fascia research. J. Bodyw. Mov. Ther. 22, 873–880.

Bazrgari, B., 2007. Biodynamic of the Human Spine. (Unpublished doctoral dissertation). École Polytechnique de Montréal, Montréal (QC), Canada.

Bejan, A., Marden, J.H., 2006. Constructing animal locomotion from new thermodynamics theory: Although running, flying and swimming appear to be distinctly different types of movement, they may have underlying physics in common. Am. Sci. 94, 342–349.

Creze, M., Soubeyrand, M., Gagey, O., 2019. The paraspinal muscle-tendon system: Its paradoxical anatomy. PLoS One 14, e0214812.

Gracovetsky, S., 1985. An hypothesis for the role of the spine in human locomotion: A challenge to current thinking. J. Biomed. Eng. 7, 205–216.

Hatsopoulos, N.G., 1996. Coupling the neural and physical dynamics in rhythmic movements. Neural Comput. 8, 567–581.

Holt, K.G., Hamill, J., Andres, R.O., 1990. The force-driven harmonic oscillator as a model for human locomotion. Hum. Mov. Sci. 9, 55–56.

Jeng, S.F., Liao, H.F., Lai, J.S., Hou, J.W., 1997. Optimization of walking in children. Med. Sci. Sports Exerc. 29, 370–376.

Karakasiliotis, K., 2013. Legged locomotion with spinal undulations. (Unpublished doctoral dissertation). Swiss Federal Institute of Technology, Lausanne, Switzerland.

MacKay-Lyons, M. 2002. Central pattern generation of locomotion: a review of the evidence. Phys. Ther. 82, 69–83.

Nyamsi Hendji, N., 2019. Fascia thoracolombaire : vers une meilleure compréhension de la biomécanique de la colonne vertébrale et de la locomotion humaine. (Unpublished master's thesis). École Polytechnique de Montréal, Montréal (QC), Canada.

Raibert, M.H., 1986. Legged Robots that Balance. Cambridge, MA: MIT Press, p. 233.

Sadouk, S., 1998. Analyse mécanique par éléments finis du système actif-passif de la colonne lombaire humaine. (Unpublished master's thesis). École Polytechnique de Montréal, Montréal (QC), Canada.

Schilling, N., Carrier, D.R., 2010. Function of the epaxial muscles in walking, trotting and galloping dogs: implications for the evolution of epaxial muscle function in tetrapods. J. Exp. Biol. 213, 1490–1502.

Schleip, R., Klingler, W., Lehmann-Horn, F., 2005. Active fascial contractility: Fascia may be able to contract in a smooth muscle-like manner and thereby influence musculoskeletal dynamics. Med. Hypotheses 65, 273–277.

Vleeming, A., Schuenke, M.D., Danneels, L., Willard, F.H., 2014. The functional coupling of the deep abdominal and paraspinal muscles: the effects of simulated paraspinal muscle contraction on force transfer to the middle and posterior layer of the thoracolumbar fascia. J. Anat. 225, 447–462.

Wanders, I., Folkertsma, G.A., Stramigioli, S., 2015. Design and analysis of an optimal hopper for use in resonance-based locomotion. IEEE International Conference on Robotics and Automation (ICRA), Seattle, pp. 5197–5202.

Wilke, J., Schleip, R., Klingler, W., Stecco, C., 2017. The lumbodorsal fascia as a potential source of low back pain: A narrative review. Biomed Res. Int. 2017, 5349620.

Williamson, M., 1998. Neural control of rhythmic arm movement. Neural Netw. 11, 1379–1394.

Yahia, L.H., Klingler, W., Newnan, N., et al. 2019a. Fundamental biophysics of the human spine - Beyond the classical biomechanics [abstract]. J Theor Biol. [unpublished].

Yahia LH, Klingler W, Newnan, N., Lucia, U., Schliep, R., 2019b. Holism versus reductionism in spine biomechanics [abstract]. J Theor Biol. [unpublished]

Yahia, L.H., Pigeon, P., DesRosiers, E.A., 1993. Viscoelastic properties of the human lumbodorsal fascia. J. Biomed. Eng. 15, 425–429.

Yahia, L.H., Rhalmi, S., Newman, N., Isler, M., 1992. Sensory innervation of human thoracolumbar fascia. Acta Orthop. Scand. 63, 195–197.

Zhao, Q., Nakajima, K., Sumioka, H., Yu, X., Pfeifer, R., 2012. Embodiment enables the spinal engine in quadruped robot locomotion. IEEE/RSJ International Conference on Intelligent Robots and Systems, Vilamoura, Portugal, 2449–2456.

Zhao, Q., Sumioka, H., Nakajima, K., Yu, X., Pfeifer, R., 2014. Spine as an engine: Effect of spine morphology on spine-driven quadruped locomotion. Adv. Robotics 28, 367–378.

PART 4

Physiology

The Physiology of Fascia: An Introduction

Frans van den Berg

Manual therapists, chiropractors, physiotherapists, and osteopaths all need a thorough understanding of anatomy and physiology for the examination and treatment of a patient. Without knowledge of the anatomy of the locomotor apparatus, examination and making a diagnosis are impossible. A plausible explanation for the patient's symptoms can only be found with anatomical knowledge. This is the sense in which Cyriax (1978) regarded the examination of a patient as "applied anatomy." Anatomy shows us which structure is affected, whereas physiology teaches us which pathophysiological processes have taken place in the patient's tissue, why symptoms occur, and which therapeutic stimulus is necessary for healing and regeneration.

In the field of manual therapy we are interested predominantly in the physiology of the locomotor apparatus and the connective tissue. For effective treatment, the therapist must know the construction, function, and physiological forces that stimulate the connective tissue. This is the only way that suitable therapeutic stimuli can be applied after injury and/or degeneration.

Kaltenborn (1989) saw in manual therapy a treatment application for so-called somatic dysfunctions (disorders of the locomotor apparatus). These are manifested by pain, problems with joint mobility (hypomobility or hypermobility), and changes to other tissue (skin, subcutis, fascia, ligaments, muscles, etc.). This means that changes in the connective tissue caused by injury are not just limited to the primarily affected structure.

Our whole body physiology changes as a result of pain. The activity of the neuroendocrine system and the function of the internal organs change in this way. Muscle tone, the activity of the autonomic nervous system, the wake–sleep rhythm, and not least our behavior and conduct also change as a result of pain. All these changes are independent of the location or type of structure causing the pain.

An example will help us to understand this: if the primary pain is caused by a small tear in the annulus fibrosus (L5-S1), changes to all the structures in this area quickly appear. A "connective tissue zone" develops because of the changed tension and mobility of skin and subcutis against the body fascia. A "periosteal zone" also develops, with slight swelling and increased sensitivity to pressure, a hypertonic "muscle zone," and hypomobility of the relevant joints. Changed sensitivity to pressure and slight swelling of the ligaments also arise. All these changes are found not just locally in the area of the pain (L5-S1) but also in the autonomic area of origin—in our example, the area of about T10-L2.

Let us now accept the inverse argument that the primary pain is caused by an irritation of the uterus, the ovaries, the bladder, the kidneys, the prostate, the large intestine, etc. In this case, too, the same changes occur in the autonomic area of origin at about the level of T10 to L2 by means of a viscerosomatic reflex. For the therapist, this mutual exertion of influence on the tissue means that it is sometimes very difficult to impossible to establish in the end which structure caused the primary pain.

Correspondingly, we run the risk in manual therapy that the symptoms felt by the patient in the locomotor apparatus are attributed exclusively to the locomotor apparatus as the cause—and the examination and later treatment will be limited to the musculoskeletal system. We also have to see patients as human beings and not reduce them to their locomotor apparatus. As explained, their symptoms can also be organic or have other causes (Van den Berg 2008).

CONNECTIVE TISSUE OF THE LOCOMOTOR APPARATUS

In this chapter we restrict ourselves primarily to the connective tissue of the locomotor apparatus. The types of connective tissue relevant to manual therapy are hyaline joint cartilage and the unformed, taut, fibrous connective tissue. The latter can be found in the joint capsule, the fascia, and in the intramuscular and intraneural connective tissue. Networks are built by the collagen fibers, and these can move and unfold in different directions. These networks occur because the tissue is strained and distorted in different directions. This gives rise to the mobility, which is typical for these structures.

Additional connections (pathological crosslinks) can arise under pathophysiological circumstances between the intercrossing collagen fibers in the network. These reduce mobility in the network and lead to capsule shrinkage and muscle shortening (see also Chapter 4.3) (Akeson et al. 1973, 1977, 1987, 1991; Grodzinsky 1983; Videman 1987; Brennan 1989; Currier and Nelson 1992).

The unformed, taut, fibrous connective tissue is definitely different from formed connective tissue, which is found in tendons, ligaments, retinacula, aponeuroses, etc. As this tissue is always stressed in the same direction, the collagen fibers tend to run parallel to each other. The therapeutic options are limited here, predominantly to deep frictions (performed after injury), with the aim of promoting circulation and optimizing healing (Van den Berg 2010).

Collagen has a tensile strength of about 500 to 1000 kg/cm². This extremely high stability explains why collagen and connective tissue—whether a joint capsule or a ligament—cannot be significantly extended (Leadbetter et al. 1990; Currier and Nelson 1992; Aaron and Bolander 2005). The original joint mobility is the maximum that can be achieved by using joint mobilization and/or muscle stretching. In adults, it is virtually impossible to achieve greater mobility than was originally there. The reason lies once more in the physiology: connective tissue can only become longer by the deposit of collagen molecules strung sequentially together. This usually happens under the influence of growth hormones; the optimum influence occurs in the first 8 years of life. Think of gymnasts or ballet dancers who begin in childhood and train to achieve the required mobility. Appropriate mobility and extension stimuli are also applied far more often among top athletes than in manual therapy treatment or even in a patient's home exercise program.

After periods of longer immobilization it is usually very difficult to regain the former level of mobility. The majority of patients invest too little time in performing the necessary exercises and think that two visits a week to the manual therapist are sufficient (Van den Berg 2007).

Paoletti (2001) describes the whole connective tissue of the locomotor apparatus as fascia. It is certainly true that the fascia apparatus holds together all the structures in our body, from our head to the tips of our fingers and toes. You could say that the joint capsule is a specialized fascia and that the ligaments are functional adaptations or swellings of the fascia.

CONSTRUCTION AND FUNCTION

Connective tissue consists of cells and extracellular matrix. We differentiate between fibroblasts, chondroblasts, and osteoblasts. Sometimes we talk of fibrocytes, chondrocytes, and osteocytes. The difference lies in the synthesis activity: blasts have a higher synthesis activity than cytes, which are characterized by more mitochondria and a larger endoplasmic reticulum (Leadbetter et al. 1990; Currier and Nelson 1992; Finerman and Noyes 1992; Aaron and Bolander 2005).

In the embryo, all connective tissue cells stem from mesenchymal cells. The type of connective tissue cell into which the mesenchymal cells will develop is predominantly determined by the mechanical stress to which the cells and their cell membrane are subjected. As the cell membrane does not possess any great mechanical stability, the cell forms an extracellular matrix to protect against mechanical stress. The construction and composition of the extracellular matrix again depends on the form of the mechanical demands (Van den Berg 2010).

TRACTION OR TENSILE LOAD VERSUS PRESSURE

If the force on the tissue is predominantly traction, the fibroblasts formed as a result produce predominantly type I collagen fibers and only a few elastic fibers and a small quantity of ground substance. For example, the matrix of a tendon or a ligament is constructed of up to 97% collagen fibers. Only about 1% to 2% of the dry weight are elastic fibers and about 0.5% to 1% are ground substance. Ground substance serves here to reduce the friction during movement between the collagen fibers and allows diffusion in the tissue by deposit of water (Van den Berg 2010).

On the other hand, if pressure is the dominant force, as in hyaline cartilage and nucleus pulposus, the chondroblasts formed here produce almost entirely ground substance. The nucleus pulposus therefore consists of about 98% to 99% ground substance and up to about 1% to 2% very thin type II collagen. The collagen here has the task of mechanically protecting and stabilizing the ground substance (see also Chapter 4.2) (Buckwalter et al. 1989; Eyre et al. 1989; Currier and Nelson 1992).

The physiological construction of the connective tissue determines the required treatment, depending on the injuries: if there is an injury to the joint capsule, gradually increased extension (frequent movement without pain) should be applied to the tissue or cells, so that the original construction and stability of the joint capsule can be achieved.

However, if there is injury or degeneration of the joint cartilage, treatment should consist of the application of physiological force by compression. Accordingly, the joint should be regularly treated with gradually increased application and relief of axial force.

PHYSIOLOGICAL STIMULI

It is therefore questionable that manual therapists frequently treat patients with problems in the area of the joint cartilage with traction. It is often advised that strain (axial loading) should also be minimized. It is obvious that this cannot lead to repair of the cartilage structures—there are no physiological stimuli.

Even after injuries to the intervertebral disc—this is usually a lesion of the annulus fibrosus that lends itself to traction—physiological stress should be included in the treatment. This means that flexion and rotation movements must be made. (In reality, however, this important stimulus to regeneration is very often forbidden to patients.)

Similar considerations should be taken into account for injuries to the meniscus as well; although it repeatedly says in the literature that the meniscus has a weight-bearing function, this is very doubtful if you look at its histological construction. The meniscus consists largely of type I collagen and has only 1%–2% type II collagen and hardly any ground substance. It follows that the meniscus is primarily designed for traction. As a result, therapy should include traction exercises for the meniscus. This is achieved by gradually increasing rotation with the knee joint flexed (Van den Berg 2010).

WOUND HEALING AND MANUAL THERAPY

While the type of stimulus for a tissue can be derived from the histology and physiology, the wound healing phase tells us at what intensity we have to apply the necessary physiological forces/loading/stimuli during therapy.

Wound healing is divided into three or four phases (Fig. 4.1.1). The first "inflammatory phase" usually lasts 5 days and is divided into a vascular phase (trauma to day 2) and a cellular phase (days 3–5). Immediately after the injury, bleeding normally occurs in the tissue. This bleeding activates the cells in the vascular phase to release important substances that initiate processes such as coagulation and wound healing. In the subsequent cellular phase, mobile fibroblasts migrate from the surroundings into the injury area. These cells are then called myofibroblasts. They promote wound contraction and are responsible for stabilizing the wound

Wound healing

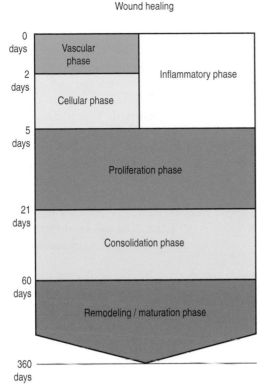

Fig. 4.1.1 Time scale for wound healing.

Note that the proliferation phase in poorly perfused tissue, such as tendon, ligament, meniscus, or intervertebral disc, can also last up to 6 weeks. However, since the therapist is basically guided by information on pain from the patient, this does not have any consequence at all for the type of treatment. In this case it is only necessary for the amount of weight bearing to be increased more slowly.

Once the wound has been closed with type III collagen after conclusion of the proliferation, it is followed by the "reconstruction phase" (days 21–28 to day 360). A type of interim "consolidation" phase is also mentioned in some of the literature (days 21–28 to day 60) (Kloth et al. 1990; Cohen et al. 1992; Currier and Nelson 1992; Finerman and Noyes 1992; Clark 1996; Aaron and Bolander 2005). As far as therapy is concerned, stress on the tissue should now be slowly increased to push ahead the reconstruction of unstable type III collagen into stable type I collagen and return the tissue to its original stability. The increase in weight bearing in the therapy is dependent on what the patient requires of weight bearing on the tissue for his work or sport. This means that if the patient has to lift a weight of 200 kg in his daily life, therapeutic training should continue until the training weight corresponds to the everyday weight.

CONDITIONS FOR WOUND HEALING

Drugs

The starting point of physiological wound healing is inflammation. Logically, drugs that inhibit or even eliminate inflammation are counterproductive for wound healing. This disastrous effect is most obviously seen in tissue such as tendons, ligaments, and insertions. As these structures bleed very little when injured, due to the small amount of vascularization, only a small amount of inflammation is generated. The poorer the inflammatory reaction, however, the worse the prognosis for wound healing. The negative influence of antiinflammatory drugs on wound healing has already been evidenced by many studies (Ng 1992; Billingsley and Maloney 1997; Muscará et al. 2000; Elder et al. 2001; Yugoshi et al. 2002; Marsolais et al. 2003; Sikiric et al. 2003; Bergenstock et al. 2005; Kaftan and Hoseman 2005; Murnaghan et al. 2006; Tortland 2007).

From a therapeutic point of view the standard method here is deep friction. The increased release of

(Kloth et al. 1990; Cohen et al. 1992; Currier and Nelson 1992; Finerman and Noyes 1992; Clark 1996; Aaron and Bolander 2005). In both phases, therapy with mechanical tissue stress must be very restrained. It is important to avoid further bleeding. Exercise and weight bearing are only allowed in an area of movement that is totally pain free. However, a prerequisite for this is appropriate pain perception by the patient, which is not dulled by analgesia.

In the subsequent "proliferation phase" (day 5 to days 21–28), the matrix synthesis started in the cellular phase is much intensified. Wound closure is achieved by a filigree network of type III collagen. This collagen is relatively thin and does not provide the tissue with any great mechanical stability. For this collagen network to attain an almost identical construction to the original tissue, the tissue in this phase of wound healing must be confronted with its normal physiological stress (Kloth et al. 1990; Cohen et al. 1992; Currier and Nelson 1992; Finerman and Noyes 1992; Clark 1996; Aaron and Bolander 2005).

inflammatory mediators induced by stimulation of the tissue improves perfusion and wound healing.

Even the use of analgesics can be a disruptive factor for wound healing. The great danger of analgesic drugs is that the patient is no longer informed of the current ability to withstand stress on the tissue. As the natural warning signal, which is pain, is missing, the patient or even the therapist continues to exceed the physiological stress limits and thereby causes new and permanent damage. The wound-healing process stagnates in a repetitive inflammatory phase (Bisla and Tanelian 1992; Brower and Johnson 2003; Dormus et al. 2003; Northcliffe and Buggy 2003; Scherb et al. 2009).

Nutrition

Because connective tissue consists predominantly of proteins, the take-up of protein through nutrition is very important. Protein is available in the form of plant or animal products. It is problematic that animal protein is acid-forming and can lower the interstitial pH value. If the pH value falls below 6.5, fibroblasts find it difficult to carry out their normal synthesis function. As a result, the tissue degenerates and healing can no longer take place (Geiersperger 2009; Van den Berg 2010).

As the energy from the mitochondria is predominantly made available by burning up glucose, a sufficient quantity of sugar in our diet is also important. However, if sugar is predominantly added through short-chain carbohydrates, the strain on the pancreas is increased. The result can be the development of type 2 diabetes, a disease of modern civilization. If the blood sugar level is permanently too high, regeneration and healing are also made more difficult. Refined sugar is also extremely acid forming (see previous discussion).

Finally, the consumption of fat should concentrate mostly on unsaturated fatty acids. Important here are the essential unsaturated omega 3 and omega 6 fatty acids. Prostaglandin 2, which is important after an injury, is produced from omega 6 fatty acids. Omega 3 fatty acids enable the formation of prostaglandins 1 and 3, which control inflammation as antagonists of prostaglandin 2. (In the western diet there is a predominance of omega 6 fatty acids.) An excess of saturated fatty acids, on the other hand, can cause atherosclerosis and tissue perfusion problems.

Vitamins, minerals, and trace elements are also essential for connective tissue stability. These substances allow stabilizing connective bridges in the collagen

(Geiersperger 2009; Van den Berg 2010) (see also Chapter 7.23).

Perfusion

In order to make the right nutrients for their synthesis processes available to the cells (as part of the healing process)—particularly after injury—the tissue must be sufficiently perfused. This is demonstrated not least in the classic signs of inflammation, such as heat, swelling, and redness. The most negative influences on tissue perfusion are smoking (Holm and Nschemson 1988; Battié et al. 1991; Silcox et al. 1995; Hadley and Reddy 1997, Iwahashi et al. 2002; Oda et al. 2004; Zakaria and Sina 2007), atherosclerosis (Kurunlahti et al. 1999; Dwivedi et al. 2003; Turgut et al. 2008; Kauppila 2009), and increased sympathetic reflex activity.

Stress

Psychological stress causes the release of an increased level of stress hormones, such as cortisol. Cortisol inhibits collagen synthesis and slows or even prevents healing and regeneration. Sympathetic reflex activity is also increased by stress (as discussed previously).

Internal Organs

For the macronutrients from the diet to be reconstructed into micronutrients valuable for the cells, the function capacity of the digestive tract must be known. For optimum digestion, food should be well-chewed to increase the contact surface between the food and the digestive enzymes. The smaller the portion that lands in the stomach, the easier it is for further digestion to take place. If it is too large, the gastric entrance is also mechanically stressed. Drinking during the meal thins the gastric juices and transports incompletely digested particles into the small intestine. This reduces the uptake of nutrients in the small intestine. If nonsteroidal antiinflammatory drugs are taken, the mucous membranes of the stomach and small intestine are weakened, restricting the uptake of nutrients (Van den Berg 2010).

The liver, the gall bladder, and the pancreas are among the organs responsible for the production of digestive enzymes and the conversion of glucose to fat or of fat to glucose. The liver also plays an extremely important role in detoxification and the neutralization of acids. Other detoxification organs are the large intestine, the kidneys, the skin, and the lungs. Water is required for all detoxification processes and must be added in sufficient quantity (Van den Berg 2010).

Immune System

An immune weakness can develop as a result of dietary deficiency, poor large intestine function, the frequent taking of antibiotics, or as a result of the surgical removal of important parts of the immune system, such as the appendix, the tonsils, etc. This can lead to auto-immune reactions that can then lead to chronification of inflammation and poor regeneration and healing.

REFERENCES

Aaron, R.K., Bolander, M.E., 2005. Physical Regulation of Skeletal Repair. Symposium of the American Academy of Orthopaedic Surgeons, Rosemont, IL.

Akeson, W., Amiel, D., Mechanics, G., 1977. Collagen cross-linking alterations in joint contractures: Changes in reducible cross-links in periarticular connective tissue collagen after nine weeks of immobilization. Connect. Tissue Res. 5, 15–19.

Akeson, W., Woo, S.L.Y., Amiel, D., 1973. The connective tissue response to immobility: Biochemical changes in periarticular connective tissue of the immobilized rabbit knee. Clin. Orthop. 93, 356–361.

Akeson, W.H., Amiel, D., Abel, M.F., Garfin, S.R., Woo, S.L., 1987. Effects of immobilization on joints. Clin. Orthop. Relat. Res. 219, 28–37.

Akeson, W.H., Amiel, D., Kwan, M., Abitbol, J.-J. Garfin, S.R., 1991. Stress dependence of synovial joints. In: Hall, B.K. (Ed.), Bone, Volume 5: Fracture Repair and Regeneration. CRC Press, Boca Raton, FL.

Battié, M.C., Videman, T., Gill, K., et al., 1991. Volvo Award in clinical sciences: Smoking and lumbar intervertebral disc degeneration: An MRI study of identical twins. Spine 16, 1015–1021.

Bergenstock, M., Min, W., Simon, A.M., Sabatino, C., O'Connor, J.P., 2005. A comparison between the effects of acetaminophen and celecoxib on bone fracture in rats. J. Orthop. Trauma 19, 717–723.

Billingsley, E.M., Maloney, M.E., 1997. Intraoperative and postoperative bleeding problems in patients taking warfarin, aspirin, and non-steroidal anti-inflammatory agents. A prospective study. Dermatol. Surg. 23, 381–383.

Bisla, K., Tanelian, D.L., 1992. Concentration-dependent effects of lidocaine on corneal epithelian wound healing. Invest. Ophthalmol. Vis. Sci. 33, 3029–3033.

Brennan, M., 1989. Changes in the cross-linking of collagen from rat tail tendons due to diabetes. J. Biol. Chem. 264, 20953–20960.

Brower, M., Johnson, M., 2003. Adverse effects of local anesthetic infiltration on wound healing. Reg. Anesth. Pain Med. 28, 233–240.

Buckwalter, J.A., Smith, K.C., Kazarien, L.E., et al., 1989. Articular cartilage and intervertebral disc proteoglycans differ in structure: an electron microscopic study. J. Orthop. Res. 7, 146–151.

Clark, R.A.F. (Ed.), 1996. The Molecular and Cellular Biology of Wound Repair, second ed. Plenum Press, New York.

Cohen, K.I., Diegelmann, R.F., Lindblad, W.J., 1992. Wound Healing, Biochemical and Clinical Aspects. WB Saunders Company, Philadelphia.

Currier, D., Nelson, R., 1992. Dynamics of Human Biologic Tissues. FA Davis Company, Philadelphia.

Cyriax, J., 1978. Textbook of Orthopaedic Medicine, seventh ed. Baillière Tindall, London.

Dormus, M., Karaaslan, E., Ozturk, E., et al., 2003. The effects of single-dose dexamethasone on wound healing in rats. Anesth. Analg. 97, 1377–1380.

Dwivedi, S., Kotwal, P.P., Dwivedi, G., 2003. Aortic atherosclerosis, hypertension, and spondylotic degenerative disease: A life-style phenomenon, coincidence, or continuum? JIACM 4, 134–138.

Elder, C.L., Dahners, L.E., Weinhold, P.S., 2001. A cyclooxygenase-2 inhibitor impairs ligament healing in the rat. Am. J. Sports Med. 29, 801–805.

Eyre, D.R., Benya, P., Buckwalter, J., et al., 1989. Intervertebral disc: basic science perspectives. In: Frymoyer, J.W., Gordon, S.L. (Eds.), New Perspectives on Low Back Pain. American Academy of Orthopaedic Surgeons, Park Ridge, IL.

Finerman, G.A.M., Noyes, F.R. (Eds.), 1992. Biology and Biomechanics of the Traumatized Synovial Joint: The Knee as a Model. American Academy of Orthopaedic Surgeons, Rosemont, IL.

Geiersperger, K., 2009. Wundheilung und Ernährung. Master Thesis für der Universitätslehrgang für Sports Physiotherapy. Paris Lodron Universität Salzburg – Abteilung Sportwissenschaften.

Grodzinsky, A., 1983. Electromechanical and physiochemical properties of connective tissue. Crit. Rev. Biomed. Eng. 9, 133–199.

Hadley, M.N., Reddy, S.V., 1997. Smoking and the human vertebral column: a review of the impact of cigarette use on vertebral bone metabolism and spinal fusion. Neurosurgery 41, 116–124.

Holm, S., Nachemson, A., 1988. Nutrition of the intervertebral disc: acute effects of cigarette smoking. An experimental animal study. Ups. J. Med. Sci. 93, 91–99.

Iwahashi, M., Matsuzaki, H., Tokuhashi, Y., Wakabayashi, K., Uematsu, Y., 2002. Mechanism of intervertebral disc degeneration caused by nicotine in rabbits to explicate intervertebral disc disorders caused by smoking. Spine 27, 1396–1401.

Kaftan, H., Hosemann, W., 2005. Systemic corticoid application in combination with topical mitomycin or dexamethasone. Inhibition of wound healing after tympanic membrane perforation. HNO 53, 779–783.

Kaltenborn, F.M., 1989. Manual Mobilization of the Extremity Joints. Banta, Minneapolis, MN.

Kauppila, L.I., 2009. Atherosclerosis and disc degeneration/ low-back pain – a systemic review. Eur. J. Vasc. Endovasc. Surg. 37, 661–670.

Kloth, L.C., McCulloch, J.M., Feedar, J.A. (Eds.), 1990. Wound Healing: Alternatives in Management. FA Davis Company, Philadelphia.

Kurunlahti, M., Tervonen, O., Vanharanta, H., Ilkko, E., Suramo, I., 1999. Association of atherosclerosis with low back pain and the degree of disc degeneration. Spine 24, 2080–2084.

Leadbetter, W.B., Buckwalter, J.A., Gordon, S.L. (Eds.), 1990. Sports-Induced Inflammation: Clinical and Basic Science Concepts. American Academy of Orthopaedic Surgeons, Park Ridge, IL.

Marsolais, D., Cote, C.H., Frenette, J., 2003. Nonsteroidal anti-inflammatory drug reduces neutrophil and macrophage accumulation but does not improve tendon regeneration. Lab. Invest. 83, 991–999.

Murnaghan, M., Li, G., Marsh, D.R., 2006. Nonsteroidal anti-inflammatory drug-induced fracture non- union: an inhibition of angiogenesis? J. Bone Joint Surg. Am. 88, 140–147.

Muscará, M.N., McKnight, W., Asfaha, S., Wallace, J.L., 2000. Wound collagen deposition in rats: Effect of an NO-NSAID and a selective COX-2 inhibitor. Br. J. Pharmacol. 129, 681–686.

Ng, S.C., 1992. Non-steroidal anti-inflammatory drugs: uses and complications. Singapore Med. J. 33, 510–513.

Northcliffe, S.A., Buggy, D.J., 2003. Implications of anesthesia for infection and wound healing. Int. Anesthesiol. Clin. 41, 31–64.

Oda, H., Matsuzaki, H., Tokuhashi, Y., Wakabayashi, K., Uematsu, Y., Iwahashi, M., 2004. Degeneration of intervertebral discs due to smoking: experimental assessment in a rat-smoking model. J. Orthop. Sci. 9, 135–141.

Paoletti, S., 2001. Faszien. Urban & Fischer Verlag, Munich-Jena.

Scherb, M.B., Courneya, J.P., Guyton, G.P., Schon, L.C., 2009. Effect of bupivacaine on cultured tenocytes. Orthopedics 32, 26.

Sikiric, P., Seiwerth, S., Mise, S., et al., 2003. Corticosteroid-impairment of healing and gastric pentadecapeptide BPC-157 creams in burned mice. Burns 29, 323–334.

Silcox, D.H., Daftari, T., Boden, S.D., et al. 1995. The effect of nicotine on spinal fusion. Spine 20, 1549–1553.

Tortland, P.D., 2007. Sports injuries and nonsteroidal anti-inflammatory drug (NSAID) use. Conn. Sportsmed., Winter 2007, 1–4.

Turgut, A., Sönmez, I., Cakit, B., Koşar, P., Koşar, U., 2008. Pineal gland calcification, lumbar intervertebral disc degeneration and abdominal aorta calcifying atherosclerosis correlate in low back pain subjects: A cross- sectional observational CT study. Pathophysiology 15, 31–39.

Van den Berg, F., 2007. Angewandte Physiologie – Band 3; Therapie, Training und Tests. Kapitel 1–1 (Applied Physiology, vol. 3. Treatment, training and tests. Chapter 1–1). Thieme Verlag, Stuttgart.

Van den Berg, F., 2008. Angewandte Physiologie – Band 4; Schmerzen verstehen und beeinflussen (Applied Physiology, vol. 4. Understanding and influencing pain). Thieme Verlag, Stuttgart.

Van den Berg, F., 2010. Angewandte Physiologie – Band 1; Das Bindegewebe des Bewegungsapparates; verstehen und beeinflussen (Applied Physiology, vol. 1. The connective tissue of the locomotor apparatus; understanding and influencing). Thieme Verlag, Stuttgart.

Videman, T., 1987. Connective tissue and immobilization. Clin. Orthop. 221, 26–32.

Yugoshi, L.I., Sala, M.A., Brentegani, L.G., Lamano Carvalho, T.L., 2002. Histometric study of socket healing after tooth extraction in rats treated with diclofenac. Braz. Dent. J. 13, 92–96.

Zakaria, P.M., Sina, P., 2007. Smoking and lumbar disc degeneration: a case-control study among Iranian men referring to lumbar MRI. Res. J. Biol. Sci. 2, 787–789.

Fascia is Alive: How Cells Modulate the Tonicity and Architecture of Fascial Tissues

Robert Schleip, Heike Jäger, and Werner Klingler

CHAPTER CONTENTS

CELLULAR POPULATIONS IN FASCIA

Cells constitute only a minor portion of the volumetric quantity of fascial tissues. Nevertheless, they play a major role in modulating their architecture and stiffness. Among various cell types such as the cells of the immune system, the fibroblasts and sublineages are the most prominent cell line in fascia. These cells are like nomadic construction workers, as well as cleaners and repair handymen, for the extracellular matrix (ECM). Their life span is estimated to be several months. Besides secreting precursors of most of the components of the extracellular matrix, and in secreting precursors for enzymes like collagenase and metalloproteinases that degrade ECM material again; besides building and regenerating the ECM, they also play important roles in tissue injury repair.

There are usually only a few immune cells like macrophages, a few mast cells, and some sporadic lymphocytes present in fascia. The mast cells contain granules rich in histamine and heparin, which play a key role in the inflammatory process. When activated, mast cells rapidly release these granules into the ground substance, activating blood flow and immune defense.

Macrophages are a type of white blood cell and important for the cellular immunity. As the name macrophage indicates (*makrós* means large and *phagein* means to eat) macrophages do internalize and digest all cellular debris and non-body cells in a process called phagocytosis. Further they secret TGF-β1. Macrophages are free mobile-like fibroblasts that use the fascia as space in between the cells to control for bacterial and other pathogens that infect our body.

KEY POINTS

A macroscopic widespread fluid-filled space exists within and between tissues.

In a model system for low back pain in mice, it could be shown that moderate stretching of the animals improved the healing processes. Therefore histology and macrophage expression in the connective tissue of the low back was analyzed, and it could be shown that the macrophage number in the low back area of stretched animals dropped much faster than in the no treatment individuals (Corey et al. 2012).

There are further indications that the cells in the interstitium/fascial space have a highly sophisticated way of cooperating in tissue repair. Pakshir and colleagues (2019) just found out that a coordinated interplay of fibroblasts and macrophages occurs in the areas of tissue injury. In *in vitro* experiments they show that fibroblasts create a deformation field and that macrophages are able to sense these spatial deformations of the matrix around them. It is proposed that macrophages possess highly mechano-sensitive channels or receptors to monitor velocity gradients of local displacements in their surrounding. This information is used by the macrophages to crawl toward the fibroblasts where they secrete growth factors that the fibroblasts differentiate into myofibroblasts. This is a highly efficient and synergistic behavior of two free mobile cell types in fascial tissue that depends on a certain physiological tension created by contractile fibroblasts that is sensed by macrophages over quite long distance.

KEY POINTS

Macrophage-fibroblast interactions improve tissue repair after injury.

New research data show that such a space where cells of the fascia communicate does exist.

Confocal laser endomicroscopy made real-time imaging available up to a depth of 60 to 70 μm. This offers for the first time the observation of living tissue over a distance of about 10 cell layers in height. On submucosa samples, Benias and coworkers found interstitial fluid-filled spaces stabilized by ECM material and collagen bundles that are lined partly by fibroblast-like cells. For the first time it could be shown that this macroscopic widespread fluid-filled space exists within and between tissues. Future research will show if this space is one of the "highways" that free mobile cells of the fascia use to protect and renew tissue (Benias et al. 2018).

An often-undervalued cell population within fascial tissues are univacuolar adipocytes. They are particularly abundant in areolar connective tissues, yet also in areas where fascial tissues frequently are engaged in shear and sliding motions. In addition, they are present in areas like the heel pad that are exposed to frequent pressure in addition to tensional loading. Here, the fat cells are arranged much more tightly and in smaller units than elsewhere, forming a most effective cushion. Although many people tend to regard these cells as less precious elements of their body, they fulfill important functions. This includes their endocrinal functions: adipocytes are not only important producers of estrogen, but also of several other peptides and cytokines. Through these they influence appetite regulation, insulin/glucose regulation, angiogenesis, vasoconstriction, and blood coagulation, and can even express proinflammatory conditions in the body. Besides macrophages, they are also one of the producers of the important cytokine transforming growth factor (TGF)-β1, which we will address later. The detrimental effects of severe obesity on many physiological functions of the body are largely caused by several of these peptides and cytokines. Additionally, the common cosmetic surgery of liposuction can be expected to perturb local and global physiology and should therefore be considered with a degree of caution similar to a partial removal of other endocrine organs in the body. The humoral factors are transmitted to and from the adipocytes via the bloodstream. Fat tissue is well-vascularized, especially below the superficial fascial layer. Therefore another portion of cells in fascia makes vascular, lymphatic, and neural tracts, however small those vessels may be.

A new cell type named telocyte was discovered in the interstitial/fascial space. These telocytes have an unusual, irregular shape, they are very long, and have thin cytoplasmic processes (telopodes) extending from a small cell body. Telocytes reach a length of several hundreds of micrometer. In comparison, fibroblasts have an elongated spindlelike shape and are about 10 to 15 micrometers long. Telocytes are a particular interstitial cell type and are found in dense connective tissue like the fascia lata (Davidowicz et al. 2015) and other interstitial spaces of organs, such as the heart, skeletal muscles, skin gastrointestinal tract, uterus, and urinary system.

Telocytes are able to release extracellular vesicles that are involved in paracrine signaling and are therefore considered important players in intercellular communication (Cretoiu and Popescu 2014). For this purpose, cistern-like regions with a lot of caveolae, mitochondria, and endoplasmic reticulum are present in the long processes the telopodes, which are possibly involved in calcium uptake/release. Interestingly, telopodes are able to build up a 3D network by interacting with each other by cellular junctions; this was shown for the human myometrium.

In addition, a novel type of connective tissue cell has been discovered by a team of researchers at Padova University. They suggested the name "fasciacyte" for this cell type, which seems to be primarily focused on a rapid production of hyaluronan. These cells express a rather round cell shape—in contrast to the spindle-like shape of regular fibroblasts—and are frequently found in the upper and lower portions of loose connective tissue layers, that is, at their transition to denser fascial layers adjacent to them (Stecco et al. 2018).

Usually hyaluronan is considered as lubricant, meaning it decreases friction between adjacent tissue layers. This function is supported by a recent histological study in which it was shown that the concentration of fascial tissues, which are exposed to a large degree of shearing/sliding motions, express hyaluronan concentrations up to 10 times higher compared with fascial tissues that are exposed to very little deformation (Fede et al. 2018). This suggests that providing a fascial region with regular shearing motions could induce a higher hyaluronan concentration in this region.

Based on the hydrophilic quality and other biochemical properties of hyaluronan, it can be assumed that fasciacytes are capable of influencing the water content of the ground substance, the viscoelastic tissue properties, and also the pro-/anti-inflammatory milieu in fascial tissues.

> **KEY POINTS**
>
> Cells are sparse in fascia. However, fascial cells contribute to the functional integrity and repair/regeneration mechanisms of fascial tissues and to homeostasis, water binding, viscoelastic properties, and intercellular communication.

FASCIA AND IMMUNOLOGY

Components of the immune system are the innate immunity as an evolutionary old "fast defense system" and the adaptive immune response, which is an antigen-specific strategy requiring complex interactions. Indeed, there are roughly 300 different types of proteins in the extracellular matrix. Among this plethora of substances there are humoral factors modifying the immune response. Most notably, the extracellular matrix is a reservoir of cytokines and growth factors such as TGF-ß1. TGF-ß1 is necessary for the production of specific interleukins. An animal model of a TGF-ß1 depletion leads to a lethal immunopathology (Boyd and Thomas 2017). Fascia is constantly challenged with physical stretch, changes of the biochemical milieu,

minor lesions and entry of microorganisms, or even reaction to a body-wide alertness of the immune system (Zullo et al. 2017; Tomlin and Piccinini 2018). Fasciae also form important biological barriers for infections. Additionally, a bacterial infection of the fascia itself leads to detrimental and severe disease. Because of the introduction of widely available antibiotics in the middle of the last century, treatment of these severe fascial infections was made possible. But still today, mortality is high in patients suffering from the so-called necrotizing fasciitis, a severe form of bacterial infection propagating along fascial sheaths, for example, originating from penetrating trauma.

> **KEY POINTS**
>
> - Fascia and its extracellular matrix are key elements of the immune response.
> - Macrophages have manifold functions and are involved in wound repair, muscle regeneration, and inflammation processes.

MYOFASCIAL TONICITY

In an examination of human lumbar fascia, a group of biomechanical investigators (Yahia et al. 1993) discovered its ability for tissue contraction. Three years later, the German anatomy professor Staubesand, in an examination of the human fascia profunda of the lower leg, documented the presence of smooth musclelike cells (Staubesand and Li 1996). As he also found a rich presence of sympathetic nerve fibers in their vicinity, he postulated a potential close connection between sympathetic activation and fascial tonus regulation. Indeed, many clinicians report a frequent association between long-term psychological stress and a perceived increase in palpatory myofascial stiffness. Such increase in tissue stiffness seems to be present also at rest, a condition for which most electromyography experts agree that most skeletal muscles are electrically silent (Basmajian and DeLuca 1985). It has therefore been suggested that human resting muscle tone may be significantly influenced by changes in fascial stiffness (Masi and Hannon 2008).

This was the background for the authors' research group to provide a more thorough examination of human fasciae for the presence of contractile cells. In a collection of biopsy tissues—taken from human lumbar fascia, iliotibial tract, interspinous ligament, and plantar fascia—immunohistochemical staining for the presence of α-smooth muscle actin (αSMA) stress fiber bundles was performed. Such staining is commonly used to identify the presence of cells with smooth musclelike contractile features. Subsequent microscopic analysis then revealed that some of the stained cells could be identified as smooth muscle cells, which were then involved with the formation of blood vessels. The remaining cells were myofibroblasts, a type of connective tissue cell whose presence in fascia had previously been reported only from wound healing or pathological tissue contractures (Fig. 4.2.1A). These highly contractile cells—generally considered as a special phenotype of fibroblasts—were found in all tissue samples, although with very large density variations (Schleip et al. 2019).

Unexpectedly, it was also revealed that the intramuscular perimysium seemed to express a higher density of myofibroblasts than the endomysium, perimysium, or fascia profunda (Fig. 4.2.1B). Interestingly, meat scientists report that tonic muscles tend to contain a thicker perimysium, giving them the appearance of tough meat (in contrast to the tender meat quality of phasic muscles, which have a much thinner perimysium; Borg and Caulfield 1980). It has therefore been suggested that the augmented resting stiffness of some tonic muscles could be related to an enhanced myofibroblast density in their perimysium (Schleip et al. 2006b).

In some tissue samples of the lumbar fascia, a dramatically increased density of myofibroblasts was found. The density was comparable to that reported in Dupuytren contracture or frozen lumbars. This could suggest that the lumbar fascia may sometimes express a pathological condition similar to those two common fascial tissue contractures (Fig. 4.2.1A).

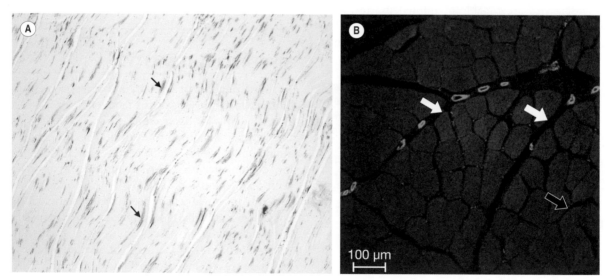

Fig. 4.2.1 (A) Indications for fascial pathology of "frozen lumbar." Section of the posterior layer of the lumbar fascia at the level of L2. Note the high density of myofibroblasts, which in this patient is comparable to their reported density in the shoulder capsule during a "frozen shoulder" pathology. This suggests that, at least in this patient, the low back region could be affected by fascial contracture and stiffening similar to that of a "frozen shoulder." Arrows indicate examples of stress fiber bundles containing α-smooth muscle actin (a differential marker for myofibroblasts), which are stained here in dark gray. Length of image 225 μm. Adapted from Schleip, R., Klingler, W., Lehmann-Horn, F., 2006a. Fascia is able to contract in a smooth muscle-like manner and thereby influence musculoskeletal mechanics. In: Liepsch, D. (Ed.), 5th World Congress of Biomechanics, Munich, July 29–August 4, 2006. Medimond International Proceedings, Bologna, pp. 51–54, with permission. (B) Immunofluorescence imaging of two representative sections of intramuscular fascia from the human lumbar region. Bright green: elements that are positively stained for the presence of αSMA. Note the apparently increased presence of myofibroblasts in the perimysial zones (white arrows) as opposed to endomysial zones (black arrows) in both sections. Illustration from Schleip et al. 2019. Front Physiol. 10, 336. Open access. https://creativecommons.org/licenses/by/4.0/.

KEY POINTS

Myofascial tone is determined by forces generated by skeletal muscle fibers in combination with fascial stiffness regulation. Both components are influenced by neuronal input and osmotic pressure.

FROM MYOFIBROBLAST CONTRACTION TO TISSUE CONTRACTURES

It is assumed that most myofibroblasts develop out of regular fibroblasts. This transition is stimulated by an increase in mechanical strain and by specific cytokines (Fig. 4.2.2). Myofibroblasts play an important role during wound healing and are also involved in many pathological fascial contractures (such as Peyronie's disease, hypertrophic scar, plantar fibromatosis, Dupuytren contracture, or frozen shoulder). Because of their possession of dense αSMA stress fiber bundles, their contractile capacity is four times stronger than regular fibroblasts.

In order to further investigate the potential contractile function of fascial myofibroblasts, the authors' group performed mechanographic in vitro examinations for active fascial tissue contractions. Using rat lumbar fascia within an organ bath environment, several substances were shown to induce measurable tissue contractions.

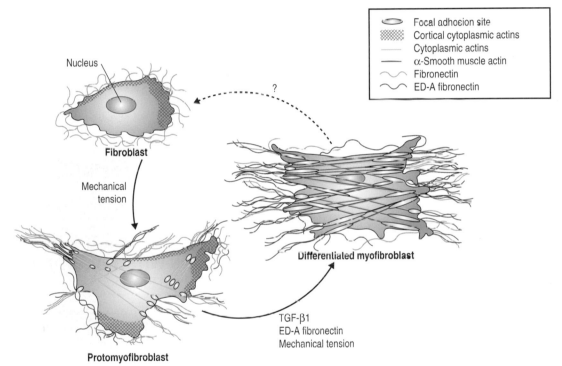

Fig. 4.2.2 Two states of myofibroblast differentiation. In vivo, fibroblasts might contain actin in their cortex but they neither show stress fibers nor do they form adhesion complexes with the extracellular matrix. Under mechanical stress, fibroblasts will differentiate into protomyofibroblasts, which form cytoplasmic actin-containing stress fibers that terminate in fibronexus adhesion complexes. Protomyofibroblasts also express and organize cellular fibronectin—including the ED-A splice variant—at the cell surface. Functionally, these cells can generate contractile force. TGF-β1 increases the expression of ED-A fibronectin. Both factors, in the presence of mechanical stress, promote the modulation of protomyofibroblasts into differentiated myofibroblasts that are characterized by the de novo expression of α-smooth muscle actin in more extensively developed stress fibers and by large fibronexus adhesion complexes (in vivo) or supermature focal adhesions (in vitro). Functionally, differentiated myofibroblasts generate greater contractile force than protomyofibroblasts, which is reflected by a higher organization of extracellular fibronectin into fibrils. Redrawn with permission from Tomasek, J.J., Gabbiani, G., Hinz, B., et al., 2002. Myofibroblasts and mechano-regulation of connective tissue remodelling. Nat. Rev. Mol. Cell Biol. 3, 349–363.

These include the cytokine TGF-β1 and thromboxane, a lipid produced by blood platelets and which is associated with blood clotting and vasoconstriction via a G-protein PLC/IP3 coupled raise in calcium in the cells. Interestingly, thromboxane has been associated with the arachidonic acid pathway characteristic of chronic silent inflammations. Tissue contractions in the organ bath could be elicited in a time frame of 5 to 30 minutes, and the measured forces were strong enough to predict a potential influence on mechanosensory regulation and motoneuronal reflex regulation. However, they were significantly lower (and slower) compared with skeletal muscle contractions with a similar cross-sectional diameter (Schleip et al. 2006a).

Although myofibroblasts are able to induce small tissue contractions only (up to 4.1 μN/cell) during a time frame of several minutes, an incremental addition of such cellular contractions over several hours and days can lead to long-term tissue contractures, which include matrix remodeling (Fig. 4.2.3). Figure 4.2.4 describes how an increased migratory and contractile activity of moving fibroblasts is able to induce such tissue contractures. It is therefore conceivable that appropriate changes in the biochemical or mechanostimulatory environment of the fascial myofibroblasts could induce profound changes in tissue stiffness.

 KEY POINTS

Myofibroblasts modify biomechanical properties of fasciae.

MODULATORS OF FASCIAL CONTRACTILITY

Let us explore which factors can influence fascial tonicity. The reported finding of the stimulatory effect of thromboxane—together with general physiological considerations on the contractile kinetics of fibroblasts and myofibroblasts—suggests that a proinflammatory biochemical milieu may tend to foster an increase in fascia stiffness. In return, an anti-inflammatory (nutritional or other) biochemical condition may go along with a tendency toward a moderate or lower fascial rigidity. For manual therapists it is therefore of interest that cell culture experiments by Meltzer and Standley (2007) showed that a treatment protocol simulating the mechanostimulatory pattern of repetitive strain injury

motions induced an increased fibroblast expression of proinflammatory cytokines, whereas the application of the mechanostimulatory pattern of an osteopathic indirect treatment protocol induced a more anti-inflammatory cytokine expression.

The surprising discovery of important signaling properties of the gaseous messenger molecule nitric oxide in the 1980s revolutionized the field of physiology; it was also subsequently honored with a Nobel Prize. This versatile messenger substance is produced by many cells in the body and has been shown to be a profound relaxant on vascular smooth muscle cells. Although systematic examinations of the effect of nitric oxide on fascial contractility have not yet been reported, the molecular dynamics involved in its effects on vascular cells suggest that it may also exert a similar relaxing effect on myofibroblastic contractile activity. If so, this would suggest that nutritional support with arginine and associated amino acids, as well as meditation founded on mindfulness-based stress reduction (Stefano and Esch 2005), could influence fascial tonicity. For a discussion of the influence of tissue pH and temperature on fascial tonicity, see Chapter 4.4.

 KEY POINTS

Tissue pH, temperature, and humoral factors such as inflammatory messengers influence fascial tonicity.

INTERACTION WITH THE AUTONOMIC NERVOUS SYSTEM

In his classic treatise on fascial tonicity, Staubesand suggested a strong influence between the autonomic nervous system (ANS) and fascial tonus (Staubesand and Li 1996). In particular, he suggested that sympathetic activation may lead to an increased cellular contraction within fascial tissues. Schleip et al. (2006a) used their in-vitro mechanographic examinations of fascial tissues to investigate whether they could elicit any measurable tissue contractions with sympathetic neurotransmitters (epinephrine [adrenaline], norepinephrine [noradrenaline], acetylcholine, or, respectively, their chemical equivalents). Nevertheless, in, spite of the great motivation and patience of all the investigators involved, no such effect could be found. It appeared that Staubesand's theory, as beautiful as it

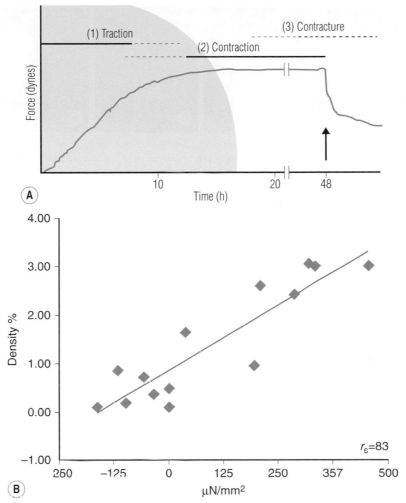

Fig. 4.2.3 (A) Active cellular contraction as a step toward chronic tissue contracture. Three phases of force generation of connective tissue cells in an in-vitro collagen lattice environment are shown. Migrating fibroblasts exert tractional forces on a compliant substratum. With sufficient stiffness of the substratum, fibroblasts transform into myofibroblasts, which express a much higher capacity for cellular contraction. Creation of new matrix components then assist in stabilizing the new collagen organization, which leads in small incremental steps via collagen-matrix remodeling to long-lasting tissue contracture. Addition of cytochalasin D, an inhibitor of filamentous actin formation in the contraction phase shortly after the force plateau is reached, results in a total loss of force (not shown). By contrast, addition of cytochalasin D much later in the putative contracture phase (arrow) results in residual tension remaining in the matrix. This residual tension is due to irreversible remodeling-shortening of the collagen network. Redrawn with permission from Tomasek, J.J., Gabbiani, G., Hinz, B., et al., 2002. Myofibroblasts and mechano-regulation of connective tissue remodelling. Nat. Rev. Mol. Cell Biol. 3, 349–363. (B) The myofibroblast density of several samples of rat lumbar fascia was assessed (via immunostaining for αSMA) subsequent to their mechanographic examination in an organ bath environment. Statistical analysis revealed a strong positive correlation between the two factors, where higher myofibroblast density was associated with more forceful contractile response ($n = 14$). Redrawn from Schleip et al. 2019. Front Physiol. 10, 336. Open access. https://creativecommons.org/licenses/by/4.0/.

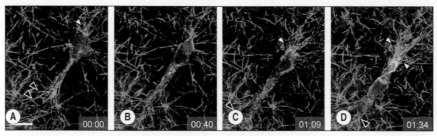

Fig. 4.2.4. Dynamic imaging of a cell migrating through a 3D collagen lattice over a total time period of 1.5 hours. Notice how the migratory movement of the cell densifies the collagen lattice (green) in the area it leaves behind (upper right area in last two images). Black arrowheads: leading edge of cell. Scale bar = 10μm. Time is indicated in h:min. Reproduced with permission from Friedl, P., 2004. Dynamic imaging of cellular interactions with extracellular matrix. Histochem. Cell Biol. 122, 183–190.

seemed, did not match with the complex physiological dynamics in real bodies. It also seemed to be in some conflict with the finding that fibroblasts, as well as myofibroblasts, often migrate through the tissue to a considerable degree, which seems to make a synaptic signaling transmission from sympathetic nerve endings difficult, if not impossible (see Fig. 4.2.4).

It therefore came as a considerable surprise when a team of researchers from the field of psychoneuroimmunology reported that they had finally found a missing link between sympathetic activation and altered T3 cell expression in the lymph nodes, and that this link is the cytokine TGF-β1, a well-known myofibroblast stimulator (Bhowmick et al. 2009). Note that, previous to this finding, it had been known for a long time that sympathetic activation, such as in psychological stress or anxiety, tends to have profound effects on the T3 cell activation of the immune system. However, it was not known through which exact pathway or cytokine transmission the communication between the ANS and this response of the immune system is accomplished. Their new clarification of this pathway now suggests that sympathetic activation has the potential of modifying TGF-β1 expression, and—because this cytokine is known as the most potent stimulator of myofibroblast contraction—that this may also lead to a modified fascial contractility.

A potent stimulatory effect of TGF-β1 on myofibroblasts has been documented in cell culture environments (Brown et al. 2002). In addition, examinations by the authors' team have confirmed that the addition of this cytokine at small physiological concentrations tends to elicit clear tissue contraction of whole bundles of rat lumbar fascia in an organ bath (Schleip et al. 2019).

This allows us to revisit—or rehabilitate—Staubesand's basic model of a close connection between fascial tonus and the ANS. The fact that the pathway via TGF-β1 expression seems not to be dependent on a local synaptic connection fits well with the slow contractile kinetics observed in fascial contractions (see Fig. 4.2.3). In addition to the effect of TGF-β1 already discussed, it is possible that sympathetic activation may exert other changes in the biochemical milieu of the extracellular matrix, which influences cellular activity in fascia. One such effect could be a sympathetically induced change in pH in the ground substance. In fact, an in-vitro study by Pipelzadeh and Naylor (1998) indicated that myofibroblast contractility can be significantly increased by a lowering of the pH. In addition, a pH-dependent myofibroblast differentiation has been shown to occur in idiopathic pulmonary fibrosis (Kottmann et al. 2012). More detailed considerations on the effect of the microenvironment on fascia will be found in Chapter 4.4.

Figure 4.2.5 illustrates a possible two-way interaction between ANS activation and fascial tonicity. Besides the influence of the ANS on cellular contractility in fascia, this graph also emphasizes the potential influence of therapeutic fascial stimulation on ANS tuning. Stimulation of nonnociceptive mechanosensory free nerve endings (belonging to either unmyelinated C-fibers or to myelinated Aδ fibers) can influence ANS tuning. In addition, stimulation of Ruffini corpuscles—which are reportedly particularly sensitive to slow shear application—tends to inhibit sympathetic activation (Terui and Koizumi 1984).

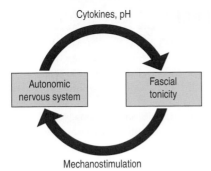

Cytokines, pH

Autonomic
nervous system

Fascial
tonicity

Mechanostimulation

Fig. 4.2.5 Proposed interaction between the autonomic nervous system and fascial tonicity. Sympathetic activation tends to activate TGF-β1 expression (and probably other cytokines) in the body, which has a stimulatory effect on myofibroblast contraction, thereby leading to an increase of fascial stiffness. In addition, shifts in the autonomic nervous system state can induce changes in pH, which affects myofibroblast contraction as well (see Chapter 4.4). On the other hand, skillful therapeutic stimulation of mechanoreceptors in fascia—particularly of Ruffini or free nerve endings—can induce changes in the autonomic nervous system. Illustration from Fascialnet.com, with permission.

 KEY POINTS

The autonomic nervous system interacts with the release of the cytokine TGF-β1, which activates myofibroblast contraction.

INDICATIONS FOR RHYTHMIC OSCILLATIONS OF FASCIAL TISSUES?

It has been known for some time that connective tissue cells—when embedded in a cell culture medium with a collagen grid—tend to express periodic oscillations. In particular, it has been shown that they express rhythmic calcium oscillations and that these oscillations are accompanied by contractions of these cells upon their immediate environment (Salbreux et al. 2007). A study by Follonier et al. (2010) specifically demonstrated that myofibroblasts tend to oscillate in such an environment in temporal synchronicity, given that they are in mechanical contact with each other (Fig. 4.2.6). This study could also demonstrate that the synchronization of the observed contractions is not mediated via the gap junctions but via their adherence junctions. (Note that gap junctions are specialized for chemical signaling between cells. Adherence junctions on the other side are thickenings in the cell membrane—a typical characteristic of myofibroblasts—through which these cells exchange mechanical signals via integrin fibers with the extracellular matrix.) The observed myofibroblastic oscillations had a period length of 99 seconds (with a standard deviation of ±32 seconds).

It is an intriguing question whether the very slow rhythm observed in these cell cultures—with one cycle

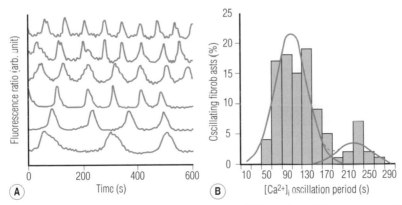

Fig. 4.2.6 Myofibroblasts express rhythmic calcium oscillations. (A) Recording of fluorescence activity of five individual cells, which were previously stained with Flura-2. (B) Fourier analysis of the dominant wavelengths of oscillating connective tissue cells in a cell culture environment. Further analysis revealed a common peak around 99 ± 32 seconds for 87% of the cells and a second maximum of 221 ± 21 seconds for 13% of the cells. Although most cells in the first group were myofibroblasts, the latter population fulfilled the morphological criteria of ASMA-negative fibroblasts. Redrawn with permission from Follonier, C.L., Buscerni, L., Godbout, C., et al., 2010. A new lock step mechanism of matrix remodeling based on subcellular contractile events. J. Cell Sci. 123, 1751–1760.

taking more than 1.5 minutes—could be related to the so-called long tide oscillations that are taught in biodynamic osteopathy (Becker 2001; Sills 2004). According to Sutherland (1990), this pulse can be felt through the listening hands of a trained practitioner who is in a deep state of mindful relaxation. Also called "breath of life," it has a reported period length of 100 seconds.

The almost exact congruence of reported period lengths between this clinical concept and the myofibroblast oscillation studies is remarkable. Whether they are indeed related to each other remains to be examined. A more than coincidental congruence between these two reported rhythms would require several preconditions. One of them is that there is indeed a sufficient interrater reliability of the palpatory perception. Another is that myofibroblasts in the real body express the same synchronization of their contractile activity as they do in the very differently composed—and more crowded—cell culture environment. Given that the integrin fibers are able to transmit mechanical cell-to-cell signaling over some distance, it cannot be excluded that this may be possible. However, further research is necessary to elucidate whether the "breath of life" perception is indeed related to an active fascial contractile rhythm, or whether it is more likely due to other processes, such as the ideomotor perceptions of the practitioner (Minasny 2009).

 KEY POINTS

- It remains speculative whether in-vitro observations of rhythmic myofibroblast contractions are clinically relevant.

Summary

Fascial tissues are populated by many different cell types, such as fibroblasts, myofibroblasts, macrophages, adipocytes, telocytes, fasciacytes, and others.

Although they make up a minor portion of the total tissue volume only, they are involved in many different and very dynamic physiological functions. These functions include tissue repair and regeneration, tissue remodeling, stiffness regulation, water binding of the ground substance, production of many different cytokines (some of which are involved in inflammation), signal transmission, and immune defense functions.

REFERENCES

Basmajian, J.V., De Luca, C.J., 1985. Muscles Alive: Their Functions Revealed by Electromyography, fifth ed. Williams & Wilkins, Baltimore, 245–248.

Becker, R., 2001. Life in Motion. Stillness Press, Portland, Oregon.

Benias, P.C., Wells, R.G., Sackey-Aboagye, B., et al., 2018. Structure and distribution of an unrecognized interstitium in human tissues. Sci. Rep. 8, 4947–4955.

Bhowmick, S., Singh, A., Flavell, R.A., et al., 2009. The sympathetic nervous system modulates CD4(þ) FoxP3(þ) regulatory T cells via a TGF-beta-dependent mechanism. J. Leukoc. Biol. 86, 1275–1283.

Borg, T.K., Caulfield, J.B., 1980. Morphology of connective tissue in skeletal muscle. Tissue Cell 12, 197–207.

Boyd, D., Thomas, P., 2017. Towards integrating extracellular matrix and immunological pathways. Cytokine 98, 79–86.

Brown, R.A., Sethi, K. K., Gwanmesia, I., et al., 2002. Enhanced fibroblast contraction of 3D collagen lattices and integrin expression by TGF-beta1 and -beta3: mechanoregulatory growth factors? Exp. Cell Res. 274, 310–322.

Corey, S.C., Vizzard, M.A., Bouffard, N.A., Badge, G.J., Langevin, H.M. 2012., Stretching of the back improves gait, mechanical sensitivity and connective tissue inflammation in a rodent model. PLoS One 7, e29831.

Cretoiu, S.M., Popescu, L.M., 2014. Telocytes revisited. Biomol. Concepts 5, 353–369.

Dawidowicz, J., Szotek, S., Matysiak, N., Mielańczyk, L., Maksymowicz, K., 2015. Electron microscopy of human fascia lata: focus on telocytes. J. Cell. Mol. Med. 19, 2500–2506.

Fede, C., Angelini, A., Stern, R., et al., 2018. Quantification of hyaluronan in human fasciae: variations with function and anatomical site. J. Anat. 233, 552–556.

Follonier, C.L., Buscerni, L., Godbout, C., Meister, J.J., Hinz, B., 2010. A new lock step mechanism of matrix remodeling based on subcellular contractile events. J. Cell Sci. 123, 1751–1760.

Friedl, P., 2004. Dynamic imaging of cellular interactions with extracellular matrix. Histochem. Cell Biol. 122, 183–190.

Kottmann, R.M., Kulkarni, A.A, Smolnycki, K.A, et al., 2012. Lactic acid is elevated in idiopathic pulmonary fibrosis and induces myofibroblast differentiation via pH-dependent activation of transforming growth factor-β. Am. J. Respir. Crit. Care Med. 186, 740–751.

Masi, A.T., Hannon, J.C., 2008. Human resting muscle tone (HRMT): Narrative introduction and modern concepts. J. Bodyw. Mov. Ther. 12, 320–332.

Meltzer, K.R., Standley, P.R., 2007. Modeled repetitive motion strain and indirect osteopathic manipulative techniques in regulation of human fibroblast proliferation and interleukin secretion. J. Am. Osteopath. Assoc. 107, 527–536.

Minasny, B., 2009. Understanding the process of fascial unwinding. Int. J. Ther. Mass. Bodyw. 2, 10–17.

Pakshir, P., Alizadehgiashi, M., Wong, B., et al., 2019. Dynamic fibroblast contractions attract remote macrophages in fibrillar collagen matrix. Nat. Commun. 10, 1850.

Pipelzadeh, M.H., Naylor, I.L., 1998. The in vitro enhancement of rat myofibroblasts contractility by alterations to the pH of the physiological solution. Eur. J. Pharmacol. 357, 257–259.

Salbreux, G., Joanny, I.F., Prost, J., Pullarkart, P., 2007. Shape oscillations of non-adhering fibroblasts. Phys. Biol. 4, 268–284.

Schleip, R., Gabbiani, G., Wilke, J., et al., 2019. Fascia is able to actively contract and may thereby influence musculoskeletal dynamics: A histochemical and mechanographic investigation. Front. Physiol. 10, 336.

Schleip, R., Klingler, W., Lehmann-Horn, F., 2006a. Fascia is able to contract in a smooth muscle-like manner and thereby influence musculoskeletal mechanics. In: Liepsch, D. (Ed.), 5th World Congress of Biomechanics, Munich (Germany) July 29–August 4, 2006. Medimond International Proceedings, Bologna, pp. 51–54.

Schleip, R., Naylor, I.L., Ursu, D., et al., 2006b. Passive muscle stiffness may be influenced by active contractility of intramuscular connective tissue. Med. Hypotheses. 66, 66–71.

Sills, F., 2004. Craniosacral Biodynamics, part 2. North Atlantic Books, Berkeley.

Staubesand, J., Li, Y., 1996. Zum Feinbau der Fascia cruris mit besonderer Berücksichtigung epi- und intrafaszialer Nerven. Manuelle Medizin 34, 196–200.

Stecco, C., Fede, C., Macchi, V., et al., 2018. The fasciacytes: A new cell devoted to fascial gliding regulation. Clin. Anat. 31, 667–676.

Stefano, G.B., Esch, T., 2005. Integrative medical therapy: examination of meditation's therapeutic and global medicinal outcomes via nitric oxide (review). Int. J. Mol. Med. 16, 621–630.

Sutherland, W.G., 1990. Teachings in the Science of Osteopathy. Sutherland Cranial Teaching Foundation, Fort Worth, Texas.

Terui, N., Koizumi, K., 1984. Responses of cardiac vagus and sympathetic nerves to excitation of somatic and visceral nerves. J. Auton. Nerv. Syst. 10, 73–91.

Tomasek, J.J., Gabbiani, G., Hinz, B., Chaponnier, C., Brown, R.A., 2002. Myofibroblasts and mechano-regulation of connective tissue remodelling. Nat. Rev. Mol. Cell Biol. 3, 349–363.

Tomlin, H., Piccinini, A., 2018. A complex interplay between the extracellular matrix and the innate immune response to microbial pathogens. Immunology 155, 186–201.

Yahia, L.H., Pigeon, P., DesRosiers, E.A., 1993. Viscoelastic properties of the human lumbodorsal fascia. J. Biomed. Eng. 15, 425–429.

Zullo, A., Mancini, M., Schleip, R., et al., 2017. The interplay between fascia, skeletal muscle, nerves, adipose tissue, inflammation and mechanical stress in musculo-fascial regeneration. J. Gerontol. Geriatr. 65, 271–283.

Extracellular Matrix

Boris Hinz

CHAPTER CONTENTS

INTRODUCTION

Extracellular matrix (ECM) is a secretion product of various cell types and is essential to organize cells into coherent tissues by performing multiple functions. ECM provides architectural structure, mechanical support, protection, and boundaries for organs (Manou et al. 2019). Historically being viewed as a mere structure-giving scaffold, ECM performs a plethora of additional functions, including cell signaling through chemical and mechanical cues, providing a "sticky" reservoir for diffusible cell-derived growth factors and microvesicles and regulating osmotic and electrolyte homeostasis. Moreover, controlled digestion (proteolysis) by specific cell enzymes can release subdomains from ECM proteins that then act as *bona fide* signaling growth factors. The functional diversity of ECM is reflected in the different forms it can assume in the body, including calcified ECM of teeth and bones, fluid-retaining cartilage, the perfectly transparent vitreous body of eyes, sheetlike basement membranes of epithelial and muscular tissues, and the highly aligned ECM in tendon and ligaments (Fig. 4.3.1).

Functionally and by location, one can discriminate between pericellular ECM (mostly basement membrane-type structures) and interstitial ECM that encompasses all other ECM structures including loose and dense connective tissues. Loose connective tissue ECM is not only loose in its definition but also in its mechanical properties; it gives shape to adipose tissue, interspaces muscle cells in the heart, makes up the outer layers of blood vessels, gives structure to delicate lung alveoli while allowing gas exchange, surrounds most internal organs, and fills the space in between. Dense connective tissue comprises the dermis of skin, ligaments, tendons, aponeuroses, and specialized cartilage and bone (Fig. 4.3.1). Depending on the definition and its location, fascia has properties of both loose and dense connective tissue that may well reflect its mediating function in the human body (Fig. 4.3.1).

THE MATRISOME

More than 300 core components compose the so-called matrisome—that is, everything that can be measured in protein mass spectroscopy analysis from tissue isolates after removing the residing cells (Naba et al. 2016). Major ECM components of connective tissue, such as fascia, are collagens, elastic fibers, and fibrous glycoproteins like fibronectin that collectively provide resilience. Fibrous ECM is infiltrated with sugar-based glycosaminoglycans (GAGs) and GAGs that are bound

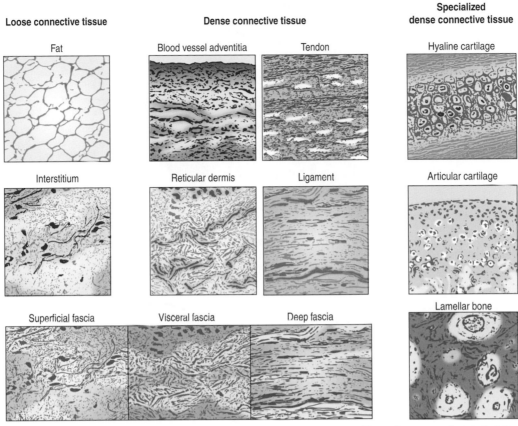

Fig. 4.3.1 Different Types of Connective Tissues. Despite being constructed from the same principle building blocks, connective tissues greatly vary in form and function. To illustrate the wide span of different morphologies at the cell level, histology sections have been graphically rendered. Images are not to scale.

to a core protein (proteoglycans) that sequester water to lubricate tissues and provide compression resistance (Fig. 4.3.2). Minor (by occurrence) constituents of connective tissue ECM include fiber-associated proteins such as fibulins and specific collagens and the so-called matricellular proteins with predominant signaling functions (Theocharis et al. 2016). All these ECM contributors—minor or major—compose multiple domains, that is, specific regions for interaction partners that can be other ECM proteins, soluble extracellular proteins (e.g., growth factors), or cell receptors. The complexity of the resulting different possible combinatorial interactions is only beginning to be understood.

Other components of the matrisome that are not typically classified as ECM proteins include proteolytic enzymes (synonymously also called proteases or peptidases) and their regulators, which process ECM molecules during maturation, maintain ECM homeostasis, generate signaling molecules by cleaving ECM (called matricryptins or matrikines), and remodel ECM in conditions of physiological repair and disease. Classical examples for ECM proteases are the matrix metalloproteases (MMPs) and proteolytic enzymes of the plasminogen/plasmin cascade (Fig. 4.3.1). Other ECM modulating enzymes have cross-linking functions and stabilize ECM proteins and networks, such as transglutaminases, lysyl oxidases, and lysyl oxidase-like enzymes. These crucial ECM "accessories" will not be further discussed in this chapter but are the subject of excellent reviews (Apte and Parks 2015; Vallet and Ricard-Blum 2019; Wells et al. 2015).

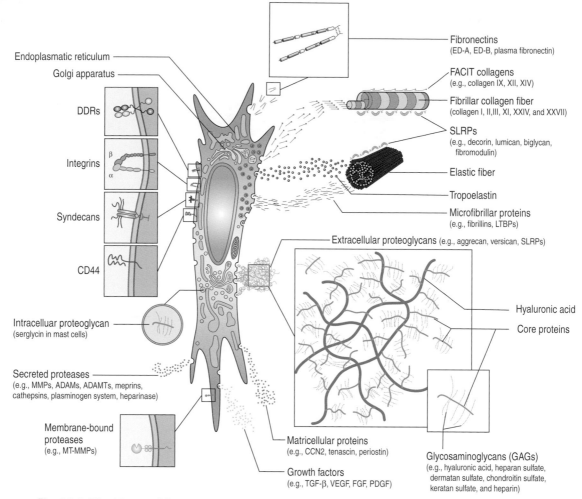

Fig. 4.3.2 Fibroblast and Components of the Extracellular Matrix. Fibroblasts are the main producers of connective tissue extracellular matrix. Note that not all displayed elements are produced by the same cell at the same time. ADAMs, A disintegrin+ and metalloproteinases; ADAMTs, a disintegrin and metalloproteinase with thrombospondin motifs; DDRs, discoidin domain receptors; ECM, extracellular matrix; FACITs, fibril associated collagen with interrupted triple helices; FGF, fibroblast growth factor; GAGs, glycosaminoglycans; HA, hyaluronic acid; LTBPs, latent TGF-β binding proteins; MMPs, matrix metalloproteases; MT-MMPs, membrane-type matrix metalloproteases; PDGF, platelet-derived growth factor; SLRPs, small leucin-rich proteoglycans.

MAIN EXTRACELLULAR MATRIX PLAYERS

Collagens

Collagen Types and Function

Collagen is the most abundant protein in the human body and makes up ~30% of the total protein mass. Collagen is predominantly produced by fibroblasts and fibroblast-like mesenchymal cells (Holmes et al. 2018). All collagens are constructed from three polypeptide chains with α-helix structure that form one coiled-coil triple-helix. Each α-helix is encoded by one distinct gene, and 46 different collagen α-helices are known that combine into 28 different collagen variants, numbered collagen I to collagen XXVIII (Bella and Hulmes 2017). The high-abundance major collagens I, II, and III and the low-abundance minor collagens XI, XXIV, and XXVII are fibrillar collagens, which provide mechanical strength, enabling tissues to tolerate and distribute high compressive and tensile forces.

This mechanical function is most obvious in fascia, tendons, and ligaments; in skin dermis; in arterial and venous vessel walls; and in cartilage, anchorage of teeth, and bone. Human tendons, for instance, support repeated cyclical loading over the course of a day (and a lifetime) that can be as high as 70 MPa—that is, one tendon with cross-section area of 1 cm² can sustain a load of 700 kg (on Earth). Collagen I is the main constituent of tendons, ligaments, fascia, and loose connective tissues. Collagen II is highly abundant in cartilage, and collagen III (together with collagen I) is the major collagen in the connective tissue layer (adventitia) of blood vessels and accumulates in healing tissue after an injury (Karsdal et al. 2017).

Collagen Structure and Fibril Formation

The triple helix molecule is stable because of the high content (30%) of the amino acid proline in the single helices and hydroxylation to 4-hydroxyproline at specific positions in the amino acid chain. The enzyme-performing proline hydroxylation is dependent on vitamin C (ascorbate); vitamin C deficiency causes scurvy with some of the main symptoms being related to collagen structure loss, such as loss of tooth anchorage. Single collagen fibrils can have a wide variety of lengths (μm to cm) and diameters (10–500 nm). To avoid intracellular fibril formation blowing up the producing cell, elaborate mechanisms evolved to promote collagen fibrillogenesis into the large fibers that are visible at the anatomical level. With the aid of collagen-specific intracellular chaperones (that support proper protein folding) and trafficking proteins (that sort proteins for secretion), fibrillar collagens are initially produced as procollagens. The propeptides at both ends of procollagens are then cleaved by ADAMTs (a disintegrin and metalloproteinase with thrombospondin motifs), bone morphogenetic protein (BMP)-1, and meprin proteinases (Apte and Parks 2015; Mead and Apte 2018; Prox et al. 2015) during or after secretion into the extracellular space. The propeptide-released ~300-nm-long single molecules are free to aggregate in a staggered fashion into larger fibrils, which is partly controlled by their C-terminal and N-terminal "telopeptides"—pieces that stand out of the triple-helix (Holmes et al. 2018). The unique staggered arrangement produces the characteristic ultrastructure of collagen fibrils with ~60 nm periodically alternating so-called D-bands (Fig. 4.3.3), but the structural basis for staggering is still a matter of debate and not all fibrillar collagen exhibit the same pattern (Holmes et al. 2018).

KEY POINTS

The collagen protein family comprises 28 known members that collectively make up ~30% of the total protein mass of our body. Fibrillar collagens provide connective tissues with high stress resistance like in ligaments, tendon, and deep fascia. In theory, one collagen fiber of 1 cm³ cross-section area can lift an adult African buffalo—I repeat, in theory.

Collagen fibrils are not exclusively composed of one single collagen but comprise complex mixtures of different collagen types and associated noncollagenous proteins and proteoglycans. In addition to combinations of different fibrillar collagens within one fibril (e.g., collagen I and II mix in skin collagen), nonfibrillar FACITs (fibril-associated collagens with interrupted triple helices), and SLRPs (small leucine-rich proteoglycans) cover the surface of collagen fibrils (Bella and Hulmes 2017; Holmes et al. 2018) (Fig. 4.3.2). They help regulating fibril formation and interaction between adjacent fibrils, for example, the gliding along each other. The next section discusses how and which proteoglycans, including SLRPs, contribute to the properties of ECM.

GAGs and Proteoglycans
GAGs

Single collagen fibrils are hydrated and thus retain some water, but most of the water in connective tissues is stored in the "ground substance," that is, the noncellular filling material that interspaces protein fibrils and fibers. Major components are nonprotein GAGs that can either exist on their own or bound to a core protein to form so-called proteoglycans (Fig. 4.3.2). GAGs are linear chains of different sugars (N-acetylglucosamine, N-acetylgalactosamine, glucuronic acid, iduronic acid, or galactose) that are in most cases sulfated. GAGs are classified into hyaluronic acid (HA), heparan sulfate, dermatan sulfate, chondroitin sulfate, keratan sulfate, and heparin, depending on the sugar types, the sequence, sulfonation, and the linkages between the sugars (Iozzo and Schaefer 2015; Theocharis et al. 2016). Because of their high negative charge, GAGs attract positive cations that exert osmotic influx of water. Together with their relative stiff character, swelling by great amounts of water makes GAGs ideal space fillers that give volume to tissues and can sustain mechanical compression. For instance, higher order structures

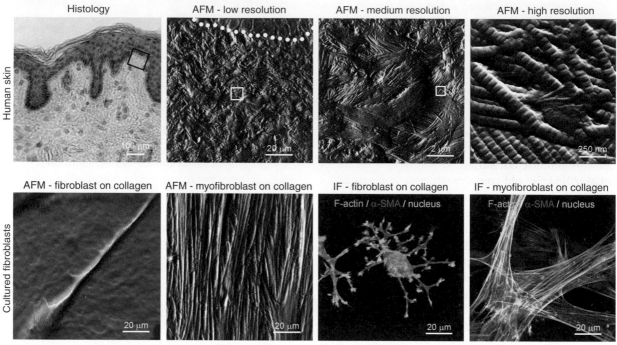

Fig. 4.3.3 Collagen D-Banding Pattern in Human Skin Dermis, and Collagen Interaction with Cultured Fibroblasts. Top row: Atomic force microscopy (AFM) micrographs show low- to high-resolution surface images from fresh cut human skin dermis of the regions indicated by boxes. Bottom row: AFM and immunofluorescence (IF) images show phenotypic conversion of fibroblasts in low-stiffness collagen gels into myofibroblasts in high-stiffness collagen gels. Courtesy Dr. Lara Buscemi, Lausanne University Hospital (CHUV), Switzerland.

where several proteoglycans bind to core chains of HA can fill the volume equivalent to one bacterium ($\sim 2 \ \mu m^3$) (Fig. 4.3.2).

The functional versatility of GAGs in connective tissues is well-illustrated by HA, also known as hyaluronan or hyaluronate (Maytin 2016). HA is a simple nonsulfated GAG and ubiquitous component of different connective tissue ECMs. The viscous and water reservoir properties of HA confer lubrication to cartilage and synovial surfaces (Knudson et al. 2019). HA also has signaling functions by binding to specific cell surface proteins of which toll-like receptors (TLR)-2/4 and CD44 are the best studied HA receptors (Theocharis et al. 2019). Through binding to these and other receptors, different-sized HA versions have different regulatory effects on the immune system, acting either pro- or antiinflammatory. As a side chain component of proteoglycans but also scaffold for multiple proteoglycans to bind, HA confers structure to skin dermis as part of versican and to cartilage as part of aggrecan proteoglycans (Maytin 2016) (Fig. 4.3.2).

> ### 🕮 KEY POINTS
>
> Glycosaminoglycans and proteoglycans have little molecular mass but high negative charges that make them ideal water retainers and space fillers in the ECM. In cartilage of joints and intervertebral disks, glycosaminoglycans provide resistance to compression but they also have important cell signaling functions.

Proteoglycans

Proteoglycans are constructed from a variety of different core proteins that covalently link to any of the GAGs or combinations thereof (Iozzo and Schaefer 2015). Proteoglycans can be secreted by cells into the interstitial ECM as huge entities, like versican and aggrecan, or contribute to the construction of basement membranes such as perlecan (Maytin 2016). They can also remain an integral part of the cell plasma membrane like syndecans and CD44 or, in the one known case of serglycin, even exist intracellularly (Gondelaud and Ricard-Blum

2019; Maytin 2016) (Fig. 4.3.2). In addition to the water retention and mechanical properties conferred by their GAG side chains, proteoglycans facilitate the assembly of ECM from its building blocks and incorporation of cell signaling growth factors into the ECM. For instance, the SLRPs decorin, biglycan, lumican, and fibromodulin assist in collagen fibril formation (Holmes et al. 2018) (Fig. 4.3.2). SLRPs are the largest class of proteoglycans and are directly regulating cell functions by binding and thereby presenting growth factors in the ECM, or by directly binding cell surface signaling receptors (Neill et al. 2015). To add complexity, cell membrane-bound proteoglycans, such as syndecans, glypicans, and CD44 can have receptor functions on their own either as core-ceptors of cell transmembrane integrins to bind glyco-proteins (e.g., fibronectin) and/or by directly binding to fibrillar ECM components (e.g., collagens) (Manou et al. 2019; Theocharis et al. 2016).

Water in the ECM

Up to 70% of the mass of the human body is water, which is not even as much as in some species of sponges with up to 90% water content or jellyfish that are 95% water. Approximately two-thirds of the human body's water is enclosed within cells and one-third is found in the extracellular space, including blood, spinal, and lymphatic fluids. Even "solid" cortical bone has a water content of 20% (Granke et al. 2015). In connective tissue ECM, water plays numerous essential roles. Ex-amples for lubricating functions are the synovial fluids existing between the surfaces of contacting joints; syno-via also cover tendons, ligaments, nerves, and fascia where they reduce friction between gliding or moving elements of the connective tissue. Because of its incom-pressibility, water further provides the HA-rich ECM of cartilage with resistance to compression, which is criti-cal for joints and vertebral disks. Nevertheless, cartilage, and to some extent bone, "squeeze out" water under compression and absorb water under relaxation of the stress. This flow transports solutes, including ions, growth factors, cellular waste products, and nutrients in and out of the cartilage structure, which is not directly connected to blood supply (McNulty and Guilak 2015). Even without the external driving forces of stress and strains, water continuously percolates with slow flow rates though the ECM of loose connective tissues—a biological process called interstitial flow. In a healthy adult, ~8 liters of interstitial fluid per day are channeled through the lymphatic drainage system, which collects plasma that continuously leaks out of the blood circula-tion at small capillaries (Maisel et al. 2017).

Elastic fibers

Elastic Fibers are Multiprotein, Multicomponent Complexes

Elastic fibers are crucial structural components of con-nective tissue ECM that must sustain mechanical forces exerted to skin, blood vessels, bladder, joints, heart, lungs, ligaments, and "energy-storing" tendons. The main constituents of this diverse group of glycoproteins are elastin and fibrillins, but also fibulins, emilins, microfibril-associated glycoprotein-1, elastin-binding protein, and latent TGF-β (transforming growth factor-β-binding proteins (LTBPs) (Thomson et al. 2019) (Fig. 4.3.2). Connective tissue fibroblasts, smooth mus-cle cells, endothelial cells, and epithelial cells (e.g., air-way epithelium) are the main producers of elastic fibers. There are important functional differences between elastic and collagen fibers. Although collagen fibers pro-vide great tensile strength but are not very stretchable at the single fiber level, elastic fibers are highly distensible and recoil after extension but provide lower resistance to strain. One good example of how these different fiber types work together are arteries: elastin in the muscular (media) layer of arteries provides resistance and restores vessel lumen diameter after normal peristaltic contrac-tions and vessel strain by blood pressure during normal systole (heart contraction). Conversely, the network of collagen fibers in the outer vessel (adventitia) layer is structured not unlike a nylon-braided sleeve used to organize household electrical cables and fully engages at the highest blood pressures to prevent the blood vessel from bursting. The functional difference of the two fiber types is a consequence of their different molecular structure; whereas collagen is highly structured, elastin has a dramatically lower degree of intrinsic order.

Elastin

Elastin is deposited and organized in the ECM during late fetal and early neonatal periods; elastin turnover rates are then reduced during adulthood in healthy tis-sues, comparable with the low "maintenance" rates of fibrillar collagens. Elastin is produced from tropoelastin building blocks that are coded by one single gene and spliced at the mRNA level into different varieties (Vindin et al. 2019). It is still debated how the three-dimensional structure of elastin confers its specific properties. It emerges that the overall elastic properties of tropoelastin cannot be reproduced experimentally in any single subdomain but depends on the interaction between subdomains in the full-length protein (Kozel and Mecham 2019). Upon secretion, tropoelastin self-organizes extracellularly at the cell plasma membrane into tropoelastin particles with ~200 nm diameter, which then fuse into larger particles (~2 µm) that coacervate into ~6 µm diameter aggregates. Association with fibrillin microfibrils and chemical crosslinking then forms the mature elastic fibers. This complex process, called elastogenesis, is dependent on multiple additional components, including GAGs, fibulin proteins, fibronectin, and microfibrillar glycoproteins (Fig. 4.3.2).

> **KEY POINTS**
>
> Elastogenesis is one example of how multiple building blocks of the extracellular matrix, such as tropoelastin, fibrillins, proteoglycans, and fibronectin, cooperate to form mature elastic fibers. Elastic fibers allow connective tissues to return to their original state after physiological strain—not unlike a rubber band.

Microfibrillar Proteins: Fibrillins and Latent TGF-β Binding Proteins

The microfibrillar proteins belong to one superfamily consisting of the three larger fibrillin isoforms fibrillin-1, -2, and -3 and the four smaller LTBP isoforms LTBP-1, -2, -3, and -4. All members are characterized by highly repetitive, disulfide-rich protein domains. Fibrillins, and possibly LTBP-1, polymerize into longer fibers after proteolytic processing and interaction of their unique carboxy- and amino-termini. Further stabilization is introduced by transglutaminase enzymes that establish covalent crosslinks at touching points within and between fibrillin molecules. The resulting fibrillar structure has a characteristic diameter of 20 nm and length of ~148 nm. Fibrillin multimerization alone is not enough to generate mature microfibrils but requires the support by other ECM components, most notably the GAG heparan sulfate and fibronectin (Godwin et al. 2019).

Microfibrils are not only a template for tropoelastin binding during elastogenesis but also provide attachment sites for specific cell receptors and growth factors such as TGF-β and BMP-1 (Rifkin et al. 2018; Sengle and Sakai 2015). In fact, the main function of LTBP-1,

-3, and -4 seems to be acting as repositories for inactive (latent) TGF-β. Binding of LTBP-1 to the ECM is essential for active TGF-β1 release by integrin-mediated cell pulling, not unlike pulling a candy (active TGF-β1) out of its wrapper (the latency-conferring complex) (Hinz 2015). All LTBPs additionally aid in microfibril formation and elastogenesis in close interaction with the glycoprotein fibronectin.

Fibronectin

Fibronectins, central ECM glycoproteins in connective tissues, are dimers of two quasi-identical subunits that are covalently linked by two disulphide bonds close to their carboxyl-termini (Zollinger and Smith 2017) (Fig. 4.3.2). Fibronectin is encoded by one single gene and comes in two major variants that are produced by alternative splicing of the mRNA. (1) Plasma fibronectin is produced by liver cells and released as a soluble protein into the blood plasma. (2) Cellular fibronectin is produced and organized into insoluble fibrillar networks by a variety of tissue-resident cell types, including fibroblasts. Fibronectin fibrils can have diameters of tens of nm to µm and lengths of several µm. Each fibronectin "leg" is built from the repeating homologous fibronectin domains type I, II, and III. Two extra domain (ED) type III repeats, ED-A and ED-B, can be independently inserted into cellular but not plasma fibronectin by alternative splicing (Zollinger and Smith 2017).

> **KEY POINTS**
>
> Fibronectin is the prototype of a multipurpose extracellular matrix glycoprotein. Its modular domain structure allows polymerization into fibrils, binding of growth factors, and cell-matrix receptors to perform signaling functions. Some of these domains are cryptic and only become functional under certain conditions—such as high tissue strain.

Fibronectin is the Swiss army knife among the ECM proteins: (1) Fibronectin plays a wide variety of different functions, including structural, signaling, and cell/ECM integrating. (2) These multiple roles are enabled by the multidomain structure and multiple docking sites within each domain. Fibronectin is a hub for a plethora of growth factors and covalently binds latent TGF-β-storing LTBPs. Likewise, different domains of fibronectin recruit multiple GAGs and the proteoglycans heparin, HA, and chondroitin sulfate and can thereby mediate between other ECM proteins that bind the same GAG partners (e.g., fibrillins, collagens, elastin). Collagen also directly binds fibronectin (Vogel 2018). Cells seem to follow a "fibronectin-first" policy and fibronectin fibrillogenesis has been shown to precede and act as a template for both collagen and elastic fiber formation. Fibronectin also provides specific recognition sites for cell transmembrane integrin receptors, including integrins $\alpha v\beta3$, $\alpha v\beta5$, and $\alpha5\beta1$ (all fibronectins), and integrins $\alpha4\beta7$, $\alpha4\beta1$, and $\alpha9\beta1$ (ED-A fibronectin). Curiously, integrin binding sites in ED-A fibronectin are not necessarily located in the ED-A domain itself but in adjacent domains that would also be present in the ED-A-lacking fibronectin molecule. This reveals—literally—another fibronectin feature shared with the Swiss army knife: (3) Cryptic domains, that is, domains that are present but not available for cell- or ECM-interactions because they are hidden in the protein structure. Such cryptic domains are made available by insertion of the ED-A and ED-B splice domains, leading to local unfolding of the full-length protein. Additional cryptic domains are pulled open by mechanical forces applied either through the ECM or by cell integrins. The domains of fibronectin required to self-assemble into fibrillar ECM are prototypical for cell-mediated mechanical unraveling, followed by the discovery of multiple other mechanosensitive cryptic sites that mediate cell signaling functions (Vogel 2018).

ECM-ASSOCIATED FACTORS AND MATRICELLULAR PROTEINS

Fibronectin is a classic case of an ECM protein that provides both structural and signaling functions. Other *bona fide* ECM constituents with cell-signaling function but no or unknown structural functions are referred to as "matricellular proteins," including thrombospondin-1, tenascin-C, periostin, osteopontin, thrombospondins (-1, -2, and -5), secreted protein acidic and rich in cysteine (SPARC), and members of the CCN protein family (Murphy-Ullrich and Sage 2014). Tenascin-C is a prototypical member of the tenascin family of ECM proteins that also include tenascins-X, -R, and -W. Tenascin-C is classically regarded as a marker for the immature ECM in the earlier phases of tissue repair, promoting population of provisional ECM with repair cells by generating a migration-supporting adhesive environment and exerting chemokinetic effects. The signaling functions of different matricellular proteins are exerted by direct binding to cell-ECM receptors like syndecans, integrins, and CD44; by binding to growth factor receptors like the vascular endothelial growth factor (VEGF) receptor and TGF-β receptors; or by binding and thereby modulating the action of growth factors like VEGF, fibroblast growth factor-2, and TGF-β (Theocharis et al. 2016).

ECM MECHANICS AND FIBROBLAST MECHANOSENSING

The essential function of structural ECM components in providing resistance to strain (e.g., tendon, ligaments, and fascia) or compression (e.g., cartilage and bone) in performing global body functions has been discussed previously. This section views from the perspective of cells residing within connective tissues. Fragile cellular residents sustain ~1000-times lower stresses than collagen fibrils and must be protected from external mechanical strain by the ECM in healthy connective tissues. Simultaneously, cells must be able to adapt ECM to changes in mechanical load and to detect and repair defects as ECM housekeepers (Lampi and Reinhart-King 2018; Walraven and Hinz 2018). ECM is continuously turned over by fibroblastic cell-mediated degradation and ECM production activities. Even in healthy tendon where core collagen fibers remain essentially unaltered during adulthood, peripheral collagen fibrils that are subject to substantial wear and tear are renewed almost daily (Yeung and Kadler 2019). Another example for physiologically connective tissue adaptation is when fibroblasts reinforce the supporting collagen architecture of our heart to sustain higher mechanical loads during prolonged exercise. Conversely, reduced ECM mechanical challenge is balanced by fibroblasts by higher ECM degradation activities—a process called "tensional homeostasis."

The real power of fibroblast mechanoresponses is witnessed during connective tissue repair after injury. When the protective architecture of the ECM is lost, residing fibroblasts start producing stabilizing scar tissue mainly composed of fibrillar collagens I and III and develop mechanoresistant intracellular stress fibers. This phenotypic and functional shift is called "myofibroblast activation" (Fig. 4.3.3). Myofibroblasts sense and modulate ECM stiffness by connecting their intracellular contractile stress fibers to extracellular fibers via transmembrane integrins and discoidin receptors.

Outside-in mechanical signaling through these receptors then triggers and maintains complex signaling cascades that drive cellular repair programs (Coelho and McCulloch 2016; Hinz et al. 2019). Examples of acute and beneficial repair are the scars forming in skin after a cut, in the heart after infarction, in the liver upon viral infection and alcohol abuse, and in lungs after injury of the outer and inner airways (Hinz et al. 2019). If the damage becomes chronic or if acute repair is insufficient, myofibroblasts persist and replace functional organ into stiff scar tissue—fibrosis ensues.

CONCLUSION

This chapter reviews ECM and its components mainly in the context of healthy tissues. However, the fundamental importance of ECM in maintaining body functions becomes evident when the genes for critical ECM components bear mutations in congenital diseases, beyond dysregulated repair in fibrosis. Depending on the ECM genes affected, such patients suffer from cardiovascular, muscular, kidney, eye, bone, and cartilage defects, or even multiple organ diseases. For instance, mutations in collagens result in severe pathologies with dramatic consequences, such as different types of epidermolysis bullosa (skin-blistering disease), types of corneal and muscular dystrophies, arterial aneurysms, chondrodysplasia, osteogenesis imperfecta, osteoporosis, osteoarthrosis, Alport syndrome (a multiorgan disease, including severe kidney disease), Knobloch syndrome (affecting vision and skull formation), and Ehlers-Danlos syndrome (mostly affecting joints and skin). Disruption of microfibrillar assembly or growth factor association with fibrillins and LTBPs due to mutations within the respective genes causes clinical relevant pathological connective tissue conditions such as Marfan's syndrome, Urban-Rifkin-Davis syndrome (autosomal recessive cutis laxa type 1C), and congenital contractual arachnodactyly (Ramirez et al. 2018; Rifkin et al. 2018; Sakai and Keene 2019).

Summary

This chapter focuses on the molecular components and mechanical properties of the connective tissue extracellular matrix that are fundamental to confer form and function to fascia. Extracellular matrix is the cell-derived but noncellular material that fills most of the space in connective tissues. Most prominent in connective tissues are structure-giving fibrous components. Collagen fibers sustain high stresses and provide strength, whereas elastic fibers support high strains and confer elasticity. Extracellular matrix glycosaminoglycans are long chains of sugars that—either alone or as proteoglycans bound to core proteins—fill space, resist compression, and lubricate connective tissue surfaces by retaining water. However, extracellular matrix components achieve so much more than structure by performing and enhancing cell signaling functions and provide cells with information on position and health state of the tissue. In fact, matricellular proteins of the extracellular matrix only have signaling functions and play no substantial structural role—like graffiti on the wall of a building.

ACKNOWLEDGMENTS

The author's research is supported by foundation grant #375597 for the Canadian Institutes of Health Research (CIHR), the Canada Foundation for Innovation (CFI), and the Ontario Research Fund (ORF) (grants #36050 and #36349). Dr. Lara Buscemi (University of Lausanne, Switzerland) is acknowledged for producing atomic force microscopy images in Fig. 4.3.3.

REFERENCES

Apte, S.S., Parks, W.C., 2015. Metalloproteinases: A parade of functions in matrix biology and an outlook for the future. Matrix Biol. 44–46, 1–6.
Bella, J., Hulmes, D.J., 2017. Fibrillar collagens. Subcell. Biochem. 82, 457–490.
Coelho, N.M., McCulloch, C.A., 2016. Contribution of collagen adhesion receptors to tissue fibrosis. Cell Tissue Res. 365, 521–538.
Godwin, A.R.F., Singh, M., Lockhart-Cairns, M.P., Alanazi, Y.F., Cain, S.A., Baldock, C., 2019. The role of fibrillin and microfibril binding proteins in elastin and elastic fibre assembly. Matrix Biol. 84, 17–30.
Gondelaud, F., Ricard-Blum, S., 2019. Structures and interactions of syndecans. FEBS J. 286, 2994–3007.
Granke, M., Does, M.D., Nyman, J.S., 2015. The role of water compartments in the material properties of cortical bone. Calcif. Tissue Int. 97, 292–307.
Hinz, B., 2015. The extracellular matrix and transforming growth factor-beta1: Tale of a strained relationship. Matrix Biol. 47, 54–65.

Hinz, B., McCulloch, C.A., Coelho, N.M., 2019. Mechanical regulation of myofibroblast phenoconversion and collagen contraction. Exp. Cell Res. 379, 119–128.

Holmes, D.F., Lu, Y., Starborg, T., Kadler, K.E., 2018. Collagen fibril assembly and function. Curr. Top. Dev. Biol. 130, 107–142.

Iozzo, R.V., Schaefer, L., 2015. Proteoglycan form and function: A comprehensive nomenclature of proteoglycans. Matrix Biol. 42, 11–55.

Karsdal, M.A., Nielsen, S.H., Leeming, D.J., et al. 2017. The good and the bad collagens of fibrosis - Their role in signaling and organ function. Adv. Drug Deliv. Rev. 121, 43–56.

Knudson, W., Ishizuka, S., Terabe, K., Askew, E.B., Knudson, C.B., 2019. The pericellular hyaluronan of articular chondrocytes. Matrix Biol. 78-79, 32–46.

Kozel, B.A., Mecham, R.P., 2019. Elastic fiber ultrastructure and assembly. Matrix Biol. 84, 31–40.

Lampi, M.C., Reinhart-King, C.A., 2018. Targeting extracellular matrix stiffness to attenuate disease: From molecular mechanisms to clinical trials. Sci. Transl. Med. 10, eaao0475.

Maisel, K., Sasso, M.S., Potin, L., Swartz MA., 2017. Exploiting lymphatic vessels for immunomodulation: Rationale, opportunities, and challenges. Adv. Drug Deliv. Rev. 114, 43–59.

Manou, D., Caon, I., Bouris, P., et al. 2019. The complex interplay between extracellular matrix and cells in tissues. Methods Mol. Biol. 1952, 1–20.

Maytin, E.V. 2016. Hyaluronan: More than just a wrinkle filler. Glycobiology 26, 553–539.

McNulty, A.L., Guilak, F., 2015. Mechanobiology of the meniscus. J. Biomech. 48, 1469–1478.

Mead, T.J., Apte, S.S., 2018. ADAMTS proteins in human disorders. Matrix Biol. 71-72, 225–239.

Murphy-Ullrich, J.E., Sage, E.H., 2014. Revisiting the matricellular concept. Matrix Biol. 37, 1–14.

Naba, A., Clauser, K.R., Ding, H., Whittaker, C.A., Carr, S.A., Hynes, R.O., 2016. The extracellular matrix: Tools and insights for the "omics" era. Matrix Biol. 49, 10–24.

Neill, T., Schaefer, L., Iozzo, R.V., 2015. Decoding the Matrix: Instructive roles of Proteoglycan receptors. Biochemistry 54, 4583–4598.

Prox, J., Arnold, P., Becker-Pauly, C., 2015. Meprin alpha and meprin beta: Procollagen proteinases in health and disease. Matrix Biol. 44-46, 7–13.

Ramirez, F., Caescu, C., Wondimu, E., Galatioto, J., 2018. Marfan syndrome; A connective tissue disease at the crossroads of mechanotransduction, TGFbeta signaling and cell stemness. Matrix Biol. 71–72, 82–89.

Rifkin, D.B., Rifkin, W.J., Zilberberg, L., 2018. LTBPs in biology and medicine: LTBP diseases. Matrix Biol. 71–72, 90–99.

Sakai, L.Y., Keene, D.R., 2019. Fibrillin protein pleiotropy: Acromelic dysplasias. Matrix Biol. 80, 6–13.

Sengle, G., Sakai, L.Y., 2015. The fibrillin microfibril scaffold: A niche for growth factors and mechanosensation? Matrix Biol. 47, 3–12.

Theocharis, A.D., Manou, D., Karamanos, N.K., 2019. The extracellular matrix as a multitasking player in disease. FEBS J. 286, 2830–2869.

Theocharis, A.D., Skandalis, S.S., Gialeli, C., Karamanos, N.K., 2016. Extracellular matrix structure. Adv. Drug Deliv. Rev. 97, 4–27.

Thomson, J., Singh, M., Eckersley, A., Cain, S.A., Sherratt, M.J., Baldock, C., 2019. Fibrillin microfibrils and elastic fibre proteins: Functional interactions and extracellular regulation of growth factors. Semin. Cell Dev. Biol. 89, 109–117.

Vallet, S.D., Ricard-Blum, S., 2019. Lysyl oxidases: from enzyme activity to extracellular matrix cross-links. Essays Biochem. 63, 349–364.

Vindin, H., Mithieux, S.M., Weiss, A.S., 2019. Elastin architecture. Matrix Biol. 84, 4–16.

Vogel, V. 2018. Unraveling the mechanobiology of extracellular matrix. Annu. Rev. Physiol. 80, 353–387.

Walraven, M., Hinz, B., 2018. Therapeutic approaches to control tissue repair and fibrosis: Extracellular matrix as a game changer. Matrix Biol. 71–72, 205–224.

Wells, J.M., Gaggar, A., Blalock, J.E., 2015. MMP generated matrikines. Matrix Biol. 44–46, 122–129.

Yeung, C.C., Kadler, K.E., 2019. Importance of the circadian clock in tendon development. Curr. Top. Dev. Biol. 133, 309–342.

Zollinger, A.J., Smith, M.L., 2017. Fibronectin, the extracellular glue. Matrix Biol. 60–61, 27–37.

The Influence of pH and other Metabolic Factors on Fascial Properties

Jörg Thomas and Werner Klingler

CHAPTER CONTENTS

pH REGULATION AND INFLUENCE ON FASCIAL TISSUE

Intra- and extracellular pH is one of the main determinants of all biochemical reactions in the body. The name relates to the Latin expression *potentia hydrogenii* and is a measure for the strength of acidity (i.e., concentration) of protons (H^+). The organs, the immune system, coagulation, and all other systems of the body need to work in a specific microenvironment with a pH-optimum. In blood, the normal range of pH is very tight and has to be between 7.36 and 7.44 for ideal conditions. Under pathophysiological conditions, with a blood pH lower than 7.0 and higher than 7.7, there is a high probability for the individual to die due to organ dysfunction.

The kidney and the lungs work together to help maintain a blood pH of 7.4 by affecting the components of the buffers in the blood. To a lesser extent, acids are egested by skin, liver, and bowels. In the body there are at least three buffer systems: first, the most important is the carbonic acid–bicarbonate buffer; second, the phosphate buffer, which plays a minor role; and third, the hemoglobin protein, which can reversibly bind either H^+ or O_2. During exercise, hemoglobin helps to control the pH of the blood by binding some of the excess protons that are generated in the muscle.

How does the most important buffer system, the carbonic acid–bicarbonate buffer work, and what are the influences of lungs and kidney on this buffer system?

Acid–base buffers in the blood keep the pH constant when hydrogen ions or hydroxide ions are added or removed. An acid–base buffer typically consists of a weak acid and its conjugate base. When protons are added to the solution, some of the base components are converted to the weak acid, and when hydroxide ions are added, protons are dissociated from the weak acid molecule. As mentioned above, the most important buffer is the carbonic acid–bicarbonate buffer in the blood. The simultaneous equilibrium reactions of interest in the blood are as follows:

$$H^+ + HCO_3^- \rightleftarrows H_2CO_3 \rightleftarrows H_2O + CO_2$$

(H^+, hydrogen ion; HCO_3^-, bicarbonate ion; H_2CO_3, carbonic acid; H_2O, water; CO_2, carbon dioxide.)

Furthermore, the Henderson–Hasselbach equation gives an idea of how this buffer system works:

$$pH = pK - \log([CO_2]/[HCO_3^-])$$

The pH of the buffer solution is dependent on the ratio of the amount of the partial pressure of CO_2 and the HCO_3^- in the blood. This ratio is relatively constant, because the concentrations of both buffer components are very large, compared with the amount of H^+ added or removed in the body during normal circumstances. Under heavy exercise or pathophysiological situation, the added H^+ protons may be too great for the buffer alone to control the blood pH. When this happens, another organ must help maintain a constant pH in the blood.

Figure 4.4.1 gives an idea how the most important organs, the kidney and lungs, influence the bicarbonate–acid buffer. Physical exercise, for example, leads to a significant increase of acidic metabolites such as lactate and CO_2 due to glycolysis and the cellular respiratory chain. An increase of the partial CO_2 pressure in the blood, measured in the brainstem and in peripheral chemoreceptors located in the aortic arch and carotid arteries, is the most dominant breathing stimulator for the breathing center located in the brainstem. Activation of the breathing center leads to deeper and faster breathing, thereby increasing ventilation. Therefore, CO_2 can be eliminated, which helps to keep the blood pH constant. Furthermore, under pathophysiological conditions—like in septic patients with a metabolic acidosis (pH < 7.3, and low buffer base)—breathing is often enormously activated to counteract the metabolic acidosis. Instead, patients with a metabolic alkalosis (pH > 7.5, and high buffer base), for example, due to excessive vomiting, may show a depression of respiration with an increase of partial CO_2 pressure in the blood to keep the pH in the physiological range. However, this compensation mechanism is limited, because hypoventilation is only tolerated in narrow ranges. The kidneys provide a mechanism of saving basic metabolites by regeneration of the bicarbonate (HCO_3^-) and secretion of H^+. Moreover, the kidney is important in respiratory diseases, like chronic obstructive pulmonary disease, where the patients suffer from a chronic high partial CO_2 in the blood, which induces a so-called respiratory acidosis (high CO_2, normal bicarbonate at the beginning). The kidney has the ability to counteract this acidosis by regeneration of more bicarbonate and an increase of acid secretion with the urine. In contrast to the lung, the counteraction of the kidney to keep the pH constant is slower.

Taken together, the carbonic acid–bicarbonate buffer is the most important buffer for maintaining acid–base balance in the blood and is mainly influenced by the kidney and lungs. This means, on the other hand, that in patients with lung and/or kidney disease it is important to control pH levels.

Chronic hyperventilation—also called "breathing pattern disorder"—tends to lead to a state of reduced CO_2 in the blood, known as hypocapnia. Hypocapnia goes along with increased alkalosis and leads to vasoconstriction and to increased nerve and muscle excitability. Hypocapnic alkalosis has been observed in

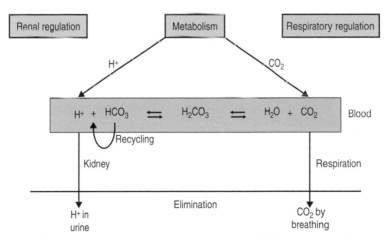

Fig. 4.4.1 Influence of lung and kidney function on the carbonic acid–bicarbonate buffer. Metabolic acidosis is counteracted in the short run by hyperventilation and thereby increases CO_2 elimination. In the longer run the kidney increased H^+ secretion and reabsorption of bicarbonate (HCO_3). Metabolic alkalosis is counteracted by hypoventilation and thereby decreased CO_2 elimination. Respiratory acidosis is reversed by an increased H^+ secretion and reabsorption of HCO_3 and vice versa in respiratory alkalosis.

anxiety as well as in other negative affective states and traits (Chaitow et al. 2002). Reversing sustained or spontaneous hyperventilation with therapeutic capnometry has proven beneficial effects in the treatment of panic disorder as well as asthma (Meuret and Ritz 2010). Interestingly, patients with psychogenic hyperventilation frequently show elevated lactate levels. Although high lactates are usually associated with acidosis, it has been shown that in patients with psychogenic hyperventilation this correlation is not valid due to adaptation processes (Ter Avest et al. 2011).

In this connection, it is very interesting that psychiatric disorders like panic disorders (PD) with chronic or acute hyperventilation may have an influence on fascial function. For example, in a meta-analysis it has been shown that patients with benign joint hypermobility syndrome (BJHS) have significantly higher incidences for fear, agoraphobia, anxiety, depression, and panic disorders than those without BJHS (Smith et al. 2014; Martín-Santos et al. 1998). In another study, patients with PD suffered significantly more often with prolapse of the mitral valve, also indicating more lax connective tissue (Tamam et al. 2000). However, there are other studies that could not detect any significant relationship between PD and joint hypermobility syndrome or mitral valve prolapse (Gulpek et al. 2004). Furthermore, the exact pathomechanism behind these findings is still unknown. Genetic studies, for example, have looked at elastin polymorphism and could not find any association with PD (Philibert et al. 2003). It is known that patients with PD often have electrolyte disturbances, like hypophosphatemia (indicator of chronic hyperventilation), elevated lactate levels in the brain, and increased CO_2 sensitivity (Sikter et al. 2007; Maddock et al. 2009). Whether these electrolyte disturbances may be explanations for the higher incidence of lax connective tissue in patients with PD has to be proven in the future.

Acid–base status is strongly linked with the electrolyte balance in the cells. Protons (H^+) and potassium (K^+) are the cations to which resting cellular membranes are permeable. This is the reason why H^+ and K^+ supersede each other in order to hold an electrochemical equilibrium across the membranes. However, the effect of acid–base status on the serum potassium is very complicated and depends on the nature of the disorder. In general, extracellular K^+ concentration rises in acidic conditions and falls in alkalosis. This is important because K^+ is stabilizing the resting membrane potential, and K^+ deviations can lead to heart arrhythmia, for example, and muscle fatigue. However, exercise can lead to a significant increase of extracellular K^+ in the muscle. Indeed, K^+ levels rise significantly after extensive physical exertion. Emergency medics need to treat cardiac arrhythmias in almost every marathon event, where of course factors other than high K^+ contribute to heart instability. The K^+ accumulation in the muscular microenvironment (i.e., within the transverse tubular system) has also been linked to muscle fatigue, which is counteracted by simultaneous elevation of muscle temperature, lactic acidosis, and the presence of endogenous catecholamine (Pedersen et al. 2003).

Not only global pH maintenance can be disturbed, but also a specific region in the body can be affected by local accumulation of acids. This is the case in inflammations, and for local acidosis it is not relevant if the cause is traumatic, infectious, or autoimmune.

KEY POINTS

- All organs as well as the immune- and coagulation system of the body work in a specific microenvironment with a pH-optimum.
- Therefore, blood pH is tightly regulated by different buffer systems, whereas the carbonic acid–bicarbonate buffer is the most important.
- Different psychiatric disorders are associated with joint hypermobility syndrome; however, the exact link between these disorders is still unknown.

WHAT IS THE IMPACT OF pH ON FASCIAL FUNCTION?

Until now there have not been sufficient studies on the influence of pH on fascial function. However, Pipelzadeh and colleagues were able to demonstrate in the superficial fascia of the lower dorsum of rats, when superperfused with lactic-acid-containing Krebs solution (pH 6.6), that the contractions of the myofibroblasts induced by adenosine or mepyramine were significantly increased (Pipelzadeh and Naylor 1998). In contrast, alkaline conditions had no influence on the agonist-induced contraction of the myofibroblasts. It should be noted that this study used a small sample size only and that their results have not yet been verified (or falsified) by additional examinations. However, the authors conclude that this pH phenomenon could be an important factor in wound contraction and healing beside other factors like growth factors, etc. One study partially confirmed this hypothesis by having demonstrated better wound healing in rats after surgical induced tympanic membrane perforations in an acidotic environmental pH (Akkoc et al. 2016). On the other side, every tissue injury induces a local acidosis by a different, mostly immunological mechanism, which may interfere with fascial function and thereby contribute to different pain syndromes, such as lower back pain (Wilke et al. 2017). In this context, a recent study demonstrated in the thoracolumbar fascia of rats an upregulation of nociceptors by inducing an inflammation, which in general goes along with a local acidification of the tissue (Mense et al. 2016) (Fig. 4.4.2). In summary, pH changes may interfere with fascial function, but most likely local pH changes in fascial tissue have a bigger impact than global pH changes in the body.

KEY POINT

Fascial function is probably influenced by pH changes, especially when local pH becomes acidotic under pathological circumstances, like inflammation.

EFFECT OF METABOLIC FACTORS AND HORMONES ON FASCIAL FUNCTION

Growth Factors

Collagen is produced in tendon fibroblasts, which are arranged in parallel along the main direction of tension. It is well-known that the tendon fibroblast is considered a key player in tendon maintenance, adaption to changes in homeostasis, and remodeling in the case of disturbances to tendon tissue. Furthermore, fibroblasts are the major mechanoresponsive cells in the tissue (Kjaer et al. 2009). Induction of collagen expression in response to increased loading has been demonstrated in many cell and tissue types and has been suggested to depend on a mechanically induced expression of collagen-inducing growth factors. These growth factors are then thought to work in an auto/paracrine manner to induce extracellular matrix protein (ECM) production (Kjaer et al. 2009). Several growth factors that stimulate collagen synthesis are expressed in response to mechanical loading. The most important ones are transforming growth factor-$\beta 1$ (TGF-$\beta 1$), connective tissue growth factor (CTGF), and insulin-like growth factor-I (IGF-I). Importantly, in human ligaments the loading-induced collagen I and III expressions appear to depend directly on TGF-$\beta 1$ activity (Nakatani et al. 2002). In conclusion,

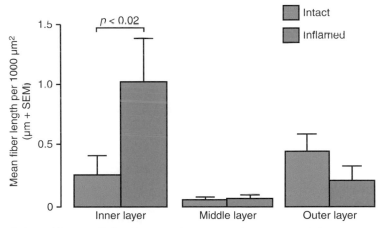

Fig. 4.4.2 Stimulation with an antiinflammatory substance tends to augment the presence of substance P-positive fibers (which are presumably nociceptive) in rat thoracolumbar fascia. Quantitative evaluation of the fiber length in the inner layer (covering the multifidus muscle), middle layer (thick layer of collagen fiber bundles oriented obliquely to the axis of the spine), and outer layer of the thoracolumbar fascia (just underneath the subcutaneous tissue). P, statistical difference between intact and inflamed; SEM, standard error of the mean. Redrawn with permission from Mense S., Hoheisel U., 2016. Evidence for the existence of nociceptors in rat thoracolumbar fascia. J. Bodyw. Mov. Ther. 20, 623–28.

the named growth factors seem to play a very important role in tendon adaption in response to mechanical loading by the induction of an increased collagen expression in fibroblasts.

It is, furthermore, interesting that hindlimb suspension (immobilization of the back legs) for 14 days in rats shows a dramatic muscle mass decrease in the soleus muscle and has almost no effect on tendon mass or expression of collagen I and III, TGF-β1, and CTGF either in tendon or muscle. This means that the general response of tendon to unloading does not appear to follow a pattern opposite to that of the loading response. This could indicate that tendon tissue is protected from rapid changes in tissue mass during unloading, while muscle, which is known to act as a protein store, is subjected to substantial and fast changes in tissue mass (Kjaer et al. 2009). Under pathological circumstances growth hormone receptors (e.g., vascular endothelial growth factor receptor) are also expressed or overexpressed in fascia tissue, which has been shown for Dupuytren's disease (DD) (Holzer et al. 2013). DD is a benign fibroproliferative connective tissue disorder characterized by contracture of the palmer fascia and shows similarities with wound healing (Kang et al. 2014).

> ### KEY POINTS
> - Different growth factors and corresponding receptors are important in tendon adaption due to mechanical loading.
> - An expression or overexpression of growth hormone receptor in the palmar fascia has been shown in Dupuytren's disease.

SEX HORMONES

An age-dependent expression (post- versus premenopausal) of sex hormone receptors (estrogen receptor [ER]; relaxin receptor I), was demonstrated in different human muscle fascia of women, especially in the deep fibroblast of the muscle fascia (Fede et al. 2016). In postmenopausal women the expression of these two receptors was lower and could be one link between hormonal factors and myofascial pain. Estrogen and relaxin (see also next subsection) seem to play a role in extracellular matrix remodelling by inhibiting fibrosis and inflammatory activities, which are important factors affecting fascial stiffness and sensitization of fascial nociceptors (Fede et al. 2016). Estrogen receptors have been also localized in synoviocytes in the synovial lining, fibroblasts in the anterior cruciate ligament (ACL), and cells in the blood vessel wall of the ligament (Liu et al. 1997). A more than 40% reduction in collagen synthesis and a reduction in fibroblast proliferation was observed in vitro in tissue samples from the ACL when estradiol was administered in physiological doses (Liu et al. 1997). The authors conclude that this may be one explanation for the greater risk of women compared with men for certain kinds of injury in, for example, cruciate ligament rupture and disease of collagen-rich tissue. In this regard, the risk of women soccer players for traumatic injuries during premenstrual and menstrual periods were higher with respect to other periods of their menstrual cycle (Möller-Nielsen and Hammar 1989). Furthermore, women with chronic intake of oral contraceptives (OC) have a higher risk of lower back pain, bone fracture, persistent pelvic pain, and pelvic joint instability. An explanation for this phenomenon was given in an in-vivo study, which demonstrated a lower exercise-induced increase in tendon collagen synthesis in women with high synthetic estradiol serum levels (HE-OC) from the intake of OC, compared with the women with no OC intake (LE-NOC) (Hansen et al. 2008). Furthermore, serum and the interstitial peritendinous tissue concentration of IGF-I and IGF-binding proteins showed reduced bioavailability in HE-OC compared with LE-NOC. Taken together, this study indicates that estradiol either directly, or indirectly via reduction of IGF-I, inhibits exercise-induced collagen synthesis (Hansen et al. 2008).

RELAXIN

Relaxin is a dimeric peptide hormone that is structurally related to the insulin family of peptides. It was discovered nearly 80 years ago and was found to be mainly produced in the ovary and placenta during pregnancy and so initially regarded as a hormone of pregnancy. Humans have three relaxin genes, H1, H2, and H3, where H2 relaxin is the major circulating and stored form of relaxin (Samuel 2005). The most consistent biological effect of relaxin is its ability to stimulate the breakdown of collagen. It acts on cells and tissue to inhibit fibrosis, the process of tissue scarring, which is primarily the result of excessive collagen deposition (Samuel 2005). Fibrosis itself is a universal response to chronic injury and inflammation of several organs and manifests as an excess accumulation of connective tissue. This results in an irreversible loss of tissue function, like in hepatic cirrhosis, pulmonary fibrosis, or renal fibrosis. The primary receptor on which relaxin influences collagen turnover is the relaxin receptor (LGR7/RXFP1) (Samuel 2005). Relaxin gene knock-out (RLX$^{-/-}$) mice demonstrated an age-related progression of interstitial fibrosis in the lung, heart, and kidneys, leading to organ damage and dysfunction (Samuel et al. 2005a). Furthermore, the RLX$^{-/-}$ mice developed a progressive scleroderma. This was shown by an age-related progression of dermal fibrosis and thickening in male and female RLX$^{-/-}$ mice associated with marked increases in types I and III collagen (Samuel et al. 2005b). These data provided the first evidence that relaxin is an essential mediator of collagen turnover and protects several organs against fibrosis (Samuel et al. 2005a, b). Furthermore, it is interesting that administration of human recombinant H2 relaxin could reverse the organ fibrosis in RLX$^{-/-}$ mice. With those data and other studies, relaxin has emerged as a potential antifibrotic agent for the future in different diseases. The future will show if relaxin could also be a potential drug for fascial contractures induced by fibrosis, for example, in chronic inflammation or in Dupuytren's disease (Kang et al. 2014).

> **KEY POINT**
>
> Female sex hormones and relaxin and corresponding receptors are important for extracellular matrix remodeling of fascia by inhibiting fibrosis and inflammatory activities and thereby affecting the fascial stiffness.

CORTICOSTEROIDS

Overload tendon injuries are frequent in recreational and elite sports. One common treatment option is the local application of corticosteroids to diminish local inflammation and to reduce pain. However, the direct effects and side effects of corticosteroid administration on the tissue are not fully understood. In rats, the injection of methylprednisolone in the tail tendon significantly reduced tensile fascicle yield strength compared with the NaCl-injected rats (control group)

(Haraldsson et al. 2009). Another group speculates that corticosteroid injection affects in some way the components of ECM and the mode by which these components contribute to the tensile strength of the fibril (Fratzl et al. 1998). Furthermore, corticosteroids should reduce decorin gene expression and inhibit the proliferation and activity of tendon tenocytes, leading to suppression of collagen production (Chen et al. 2007). Additionally, tendon cell migration, which is fundamental for tendon healing, is delayed after corticosteroid injection (Tsai et al. 2003). These corticoid-associated disturbances of tendon cell metabolism may affect the structural integrity of the tendon and weaken its mechanical properties.

However, the analgesic effects of corticosteroids in athletes with chronic pain both in the upper and lower extremities have been reported in many studies. The exact mechanism behind this pain relief effect of corticosteroids in tendinopathy remains elusive. However, the comparison of pain relief for patients with tennis elbow either receiving corticosteroid injection or physiotherapy favors the long-term outcome of physiotherapy (Bisset et al. 2006). In addition, a Cochrane analysis on plantar heel pain due to fasciitis found only poor evidence that local steroid injections compared with placebo or no treatment may slightly reduce heel pain up to 1 month but not subsequently (David et al. 2017).

Taken together, corticosteroids are still widely used and accepted drugs in tendinopathy or noninfectious fasciitis. However, inconsiderate injection of corticosteroids in tendon injuries or chronic pain in fascial structure should be avoided.

> **KEY POINT**
>
> Local corticosteroids are widely used in the treatment of tendinopathy, but long-term treatment should be avoided due to their known adverse effect on tendon function.

LACTATE

Until the early 1970s, lactate (HLa) was largely considered a dead-end waste product of glycolysis resulting from hypoxia, the primary cause of the O_2 debt following exercise, a major cause of muscle fatigue, and a key factor in acidosis-induced tissue damage (Gladden 2004). This paradigm has shifted in the last 40 years.

Lactic acid is more than 99% dissociated into La^- and H^+ at physiological pH. During exercise and muscle contractions muscle and blood La^- and H^+ can rise to very high levels. The evidence of many experimental studies indicated that elevated H^+ could depress muscle function by various mechanisms, for example, by inhibiting maximal shorting velocity and myofibrillar ATPase, inhibiting glycolytic rate, and reducing Ca^{2+} reuptake by inhibiting the sarcoplasmatic ATPase (leading to subsequent reduction of Ca^{2+} release) (Gladden 2004). However, studies have demonstrated that increased H^+ under physiological temperatures does not have such dramatic negative effects on muscle function (Bangsbo et al. 1996). Furthermore, it has been shown that lactic acidosis protected against detrimental effects of elevated external K^+ on muscle excitability and force (Nielsen et al. 2001). In the 1990s, La^- itself was considered to play some role in muscle fatigue. However, more current studies have demonstrated an effect of La^- on muscle fatigue and pain only in combination with other metabolic factors (adenosine-tri-phosphate [ATP], H^+) (Pollak et al. 2014). Furthermore, it is very interesting that La^- is considered to play an important role in wound healing by enhancing collagen deposition and angiogenesis (Trabold et al. 2003). La^- is considered to stimulate collagen synthesis by an increase of collagen promoter activity leading to an increase of procollagen messenger RNA production and collagen synthesis. In the case of La^--stimulated angiogenesis in wounds, the major pathway appears to be enhanced vascular endothelial growth factor (VEGF) production in macrophages (Trabold et al. 2003).

In summary, La^- is no longer only a "bad guy" and has important functions in wound healing, by first enhancing collagen production in fibroblasts and, second, improving angiogenesis by an increased secretion of VEGF from macrophages.

KEY POINTS

Lactate plays an important role in wound healing by promoting collagen production, but a direct effect on fascial function has not been demonstrated until now.

Summary

In the human body, strict adherence to the blood pH value in a narrow range is essential, because all organs respective of their cells only work correctly in a specific pH range. In humans and animals, therefore, different buffer systems and organs (lungs/kidneys) work together to maintain a stable pH value under different conditions. The function of cells (fibroblasts) in fascial tissue is also pH-dependent and can be increased for better wound healing under local inflammatory conditions where environmental pH becomes acidotic. On the other hand, chronic inflammation in combination with acidotic environmental pH can cause pain syndromes such as low back pain by increasing fascial stiffness and upregulation of nociceptors. In this respect female sex hormones, like estrogen or relaxin, are important for extracellular matrix remodelling of fascia/tendon and thereby coresponsible for reducing fascial/tendon stiffness. Also, growth hormones and corresponding receptors in fibroblasts are important in adaptive response to increased force (e.g., in tendons or in wound healing). However, in fascial tissue, overexpression of these growth hormone receptors may be involved fibroproliferative disorders, like Dupuytren's disease. Whether other metabolic factors like lactate have an impact on fascial function may answer further research in the future.

REFERENCES

Akkoc, A., Celik, H., Arslan, N., et al., 2016. The effects of different environmental pH on healing of tympanic membrane: an experimental study. Eur. Arch. Otorhinolaryngol. 273, 2503–2508.

Bangsbo, J., Madsen, K., Kiens, B., Richter, E.A., 1996. Effect of muscle acidity on muscle metabolism and fatigue during intense exercise in man. J. Physiol. 495 (Pt 2), 587–596.

Bisset, L., Beller, E., Jull, G., et al., 2006. Mobilisation with movement and exercise, corticosteroid injection, or wait and see for tennis elbow: Randomised trial. BMJ 333, 939.

Chaitow, L., Bradley, D., Gilbert, C., 2002. Multidisciplinary Approaches to Breathing Pattern Disorders. Churchill Livingstone, Edinburgh.

Chen, C.H., Marymont, J., Huang, M.H., et al., 2007. Mechanical strain promotes fibroblast gene expression in presence of corticosteroid. Connect. Tissue Res. 48, 65–69.

David J.A., Sankarapandian V., Christopher P.R., et al., 2017. Injected corticosteroids for treating plantar heel pain in adults. Cochrane Database Syst. Rev. 11, CD009348.

Fede, C., Albertin, G., Petrelli L., et al., 2016. Hormone receptor expression in human fascial tissue. Eur. J. Histochem. 60, 2710.

Fratzl, P., Misof, K., Zizak, I., et al., 1998. Fibrillar structure and mechanical properties of collagen. J. Struct. Biol. 122, 119–122.

Gladden, L.B., 2004. Lactate metabolism: a new paradigm for the third millennium. J. Physiol. 558 (Pt 1), 5–30.

Gulpek, D., Bayraktar, E., Akbay, S.P., et al., 2004. Joint hypermobility syndrome and mitral valve prolapse in panic disorder. Prog. Neuropsychopharmacol. Biol. Psychiatry 28, 969–973.

Hansen, M., Koskinen, S.O., Petersen, S.G., et al., 2008. Ethinyl oestradiol administration in women suppresses synthesis of collagen in tendon in response to exercise. J. Physiol. 586 (Pt 12), 3005–3016.

Haraldsson, B.T., Aagaard, P., Crafoord-Larsen, D., Kjaer, M., Magnusson, S.P., 2009. Corticosteroid administration alters the mechanical properties of isolated collagen fascicles in rat-tail tendon. Scand. J. Med. Sci. Sports 19, 621–626.

Holzer, L.A., Cör, A., Pfandlsteiner, G., Holzer, G., 2013. Expression of VEGF, its receptors, and HIF-1α in Dupuytren's disease. Acta Orthop. 84, 420–425.

Kang, Y.M., Choi, Y.R., Yun, C.O., et al., 2014. Down-regulation of collagen synthesis and matrix metalloproteinase expression in myofibroblasts from Dupuytren nodule using adenovirus-mediated relaxin gene therapy. J. Orthop. Res. 32, 515–523.

Kjaer, M., Langberg, H., Heinemeier, K., et al., 2009. From mechanical loading to collagen synthesis, structural changes and function in human tendon. Scand. J. Med. Sci. Sports 19, 500–510.

Liu, S.H., Al-Shaikh, R.A., Panossian, V., Finerman, G.A., Lane, J.M., 1997. Estrogen affects the cellular metabolism of the anterior cruciate ligament. A potential explanation for female athletic injury. Am. J. Sports Med. 25, 704–709.

Maddock, R.J., Buonocore, M.H., Copeland, L.E., Richards, A.L., 2009. Elevated brain lactate responses to neural activation in panic disorder: a dynamic 1H-MRS study. Mol. Psychiatry.14, 537–545.

Martín-Santos, R., Bulbena, A., Porta, M., et al., 1998. Association between joint hypermobility syndrome and panic disorder. Am. J. Psychiatry 155, 1578–1583.

Mense, S., Hoheisel, U., 2016. Evidence for the existence of nociceptors in rat thoracolumbar fascia. J. Bodyw. Mov. Ther. 20, 623–638.

Meuret, A.E., Ritz, T., 2010. Hyperventilation in panic disorder and asthma: Empirical evidence and clinical strategies. Int. J. Psychophysiol. 78, 68–79.

Möller-Nielsen, J., Hammar, M., 1989. Women's soccer injuries in relation to the menstrual cycle and oral contraceptive use. Med. Sci. Sports Exerc. 21, 126–129.

Nakatani, T., Marui, T., Hitora, T., et al., 2002. Mechanical stretching force promotes collagen synthesis by cultured cells from human ligamentum flavum via transforming growth factor-beta1. J. Orthop. Res. 20, 1380–1386.

Nielsen, O.B., de Paoli, F., Overgaard, K., 2001. Protective effects of lactic acid on force production in rat skeletal muscle. J. Physiol. 536 (Pt 1), 161–166.

Pedersen, T.H., Clausen, T., Nielsen, O.B., 2003. Loss of force induced by high extracellular $[K^b]$ in rat muscle: effect of temperature, lactic acid and beta2-agonist. J. Physiol. 551 (Pt 1), 277–286.

Philibert, R.A., Nelson, J.J., Bedell, B., et al., 2003. Role of elastin polymorphisms in panic disorder. Am. J. Med. Genet. B. Neuropsychiatr. Genet. 117B, 7–10.

Pipelzadeh, M.H., Naylor, I.L., 1998. The in vitro enhancement of rat myofibroblast contractility by alterations to the pH of the physiological solution. Eur. J. Pharmacol. 357, 257–259.

Pollak, K.A., Swenson, J.D., Vanhaitsma, T.A., et al., 2014. Exogenously applied muscle metabolites synergistically evoke sensations of muscle fatigue and pain in human subjects. Exp. Physiol. 99, 368–380.

Samuel, C.S., 2005. Relaxin: antifibrotic properties and effects in models of disease. Clin. Med. Res. 3, 241–249.

Samuel, C.S., Zhao, C., Bathgate, R.A., et al., 2005a. The relaxin gene-knockout mouse: a model of progressive fibrosis. Ann. N. Y. Acad. Sci. 1041, 173–181.

Samuel, C.S., Zhao, C., Yang, Q., et al., 2005b. The relaxin gene knockout mouse: a model of progressive scleroderma. J. Invest. Dermatol. 125, 692–699.

Sikter, A., Frecska, E., Braun, I.M., Gonda, X., Rihmer, Z., 2007. The role of hyperventilation: hypocapnia in the pathomechanism of panic disorder. Braz. J. Psychiatry. 29, 375–379.

Smith, T.O., Easton, V., Bacon, H., et al., 2014. The relationship between benign joint hypermobility syndrome and psychological distress: a systematic review and meta analysis. Rheumatology 53, 114–122.

Tamam, L., Ozpoyraz, N., San, M., Bozkurt, A., 2000. Association between idiopathic mitral valve prolapse and panic disorder. Croat. Med. J. 41, 410–416.

Ter Avest, E., Patist, F.M., Ter Maaten, J.C., Nijsten, M.W., 2011. Elevated lactate during psychogenic hyperventilation. Emerg. Med. J. 28, 269–273.

Trabold, O., Wagner, S., Wicke, C., et al., 2003. Lactate and oxygen constitute a fundamental regulatory mechanism in wound healing. Wound Repair Regen. 11, 504–509.

Tsai, W.C., Tang, F.T., Wong, M.K., Pang, J.H., 2003. Inhibition of tendon cell migration by dexamethasone is correlated with reduced alpha-smooth muscle actin gene expression: a potential mechanism of delayed tendon healing. J. Orthop. Res. 21, 265–271.

Wilke, J., Schleip, R., Klingler, W., Stecco, C., 2017. The lumbodorsal fascia as a potential source of low back pain: A narrative review. Biomed Res. Int. 2017, 5349620.

Fluid Dynamics in Fascial Tissues

Guido F. Meert

INTRODUCTION

It is easy to forget that the concentration quotients of salts (NaCl, KCl, CaCl$_2$) in interstitial fluid and in the water of an ocean are nearly identical. Our cells are, in a manner of speaking, swimming gel-like structures in an ocean of interstitial fluids, and we are carrying that ocean around with us.

Connective tissue consists of cells (fibroblasts and leukocytes), interstitial water, fibers (collagen and elastin), and matrix molecules (glycoproteins and proteoglycans). Interstitial fluids create a transport space for nutrients, waste materials, and messenger substances and actually facilitate homeostasis between the extracellular and the intracellular region. In addition, the lymphatic system filters his supply out of the ocean of interstitial fluids and drains it into the venous system.

Research into connective tissue has produced many interesting results. Schleip and colleagues investigated the contractility of fascial tissue, a very exciting aspect for manual myofascial therapy (Schleip et al. 2005). We also know now that all the cells of the human body are connected with one another via the connective tissue and are building an ingenious tensegrity-like construction. By mechanotransduction, mechanical signals are being transduced to the nucleus and other organelles of the cells and even open the way to genetic "adjustments" (Ingber 2006).

We should search for answers as to how the living connective tissue and cytoplasm differs from a simple nonliving mixture of the same chemical constituents in solution!

PROPERTIES OF INTERSTITIAL WATER

The structure of water is not completely understood. Formed from tiny molecules, water is very versatile. Szent-Györgyi (1957) called water the "matrix of life," and it interacts with cells and molecules in complex, subtle, and essential ways.

In the human body, and therefore also in connective tissue, we are dealing with interfacial and bulk water, and the interfacial water seems to interact with the protein function (Bellissent-Funel 2005). Water molecules seem to build "icosahedron," cubes with 20 surfaces, by their strong hydrogen bonds. But water is not static: hydrogen bonds are constantly forming and breaking in a period of some femtoseconds to picoseconds. Rearrangements of water molecules are ultrafast (Fayer et al. 2009). Simplified, the icosahedrons are presented in two states: a low-density expanded water-icosahedron and a high-density collapsed water-icosahedron. Water molecules are able to convert between the expanded and the collapsed version without breaking the hydrogen bonds (Chaplin 2004).

Water is also able to form large regions of so-called "structured water" or "liquid crystalline water." In structured water, water molecules move together, like a shoal of fish, without losing mobility. Liquid crystalline water has special features—namely, a greater molecular stability, a negative electrical charge, a greater viscosity, molecular stringing together, and the ability to absorb certain spectra of light (Pollack 2002).

Water in bulk seems to behave differently from water in confined spaces, but more research into this is needed (Ye et al. 2004). Water seems to have a fourth phase, beside gas, liquid, and solid, and that occurs at interfaces (Pollack 2002). It is surprising that the presence of an interface is more important for the dynamics of the hydrogen bonds than the chemical nature of the interface (Fenn et al. 2009). In the human body, fascial sheets, fibers, cell membranes, molecules, and so on are building bigger and smaller interfaces with a hydrophobic or hydrophilic character for the interstitial fluids. Research reveals that water inside nanotubes appears to build "water cylinders," which allow protons to jump ultrafast. Biochemical reactions take place in confined spaces with interfacial water, comparable to nanotubes, at the surface of proteins, membranes, etc.

There is a great affinity between the polymers and the water molecules of the cell, which condenses the gel into a compact structure and enables the cell to move or to open ion channels without breaking down. The extracellular matrix (ECM) builds also a gelatinous fiber network and "binds" the containing water (Fig. 4.5.1).

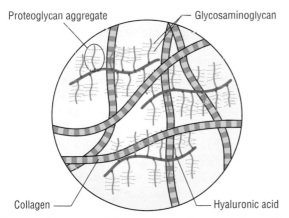

Proteoglycan aggregate — Glycosaminoglycan

Collagen — Hyaluronic acid

Fig. 4.5.1 The extracellular matrix contains a gelatinous fiber network with a high water-binding capacity. Hyaluronan (also called hyaluronic acid) often serves as a core protein for the attachment of glycosaminoglycans within the ground substance. ©Mfigueiredo, Wikimedia Commons, CC-BY-SA 3.0. For the free licensing conditions of this illustration, see https://commons.wikimedia.org/wiki/File:Glycosaminoglycans.png.

There are three "populations" of water molecules in contact with collagen fibers (Peto and Gillis 1990):

- Water, bound within the triple helix of the collagen molecules.
- Water molecules, bound on the surface of the triple helix or bound with matrix molecules (proteoglycans, glycoproteins, glycosaminoglycans).
- "Free" water in the space between the fibrils and fibers.

I would like to emphasize that the flowing of this interstitial water happens in all directions between the cell–matrix interface. I will refer to the interstitial flow later.

MORPHOLOGICAL QUALITY OF INTERSTITIAL FLUIDS

The molecules and fibers of the ECM determine the properties of the interstitial gel. Furthermore, fibroblasts, matrix molecules, enzymes, and enzyme inhibitors regulate the composition of the gelatinous ground substance of the connective tissue. This is important, as the composition of this interstitial matrix determines the transport for nutrients and waste materials between capillaries and parenchymal cells, as well as the mechanical properties of the connective tissue.

The German anatomist and embryologist Blechschmidt (2004) found that the movement of microscopic particles occurs in an ordered manner and has a kinetic aspect, which he called "metabolic movements." The flow of water, nutrients, and waste materials lead to a canalization in the inner embryological tissue and helps to form blood vessels. By slowing and condensing, catabolites build the ground substance of the inner embryological tissue. In "dilatation fields," by condensation of catabolites, water tends to flow toward this tissue and pushes cells apart. On the other hand, when water is pushed out of the embryological tissue, a "densation field" develops and the cells pack closely together. The flow of fluids develops creative morphological forces to help in forming the embryological tissues. It seems that the flow of water even plays some role in the folding of proteins, and there seems to be interaction between the shell of water surrounding the proteins and the shape and characteristics of those proteins; therefore, water "tunes" the way proteins, the building blocks of life, are functioning (Ball 2008).

Proteins have to fluctuate in order to work, and there are two types of fluctuation. The α-fluctuations proceed in the bulk of water, surrounding the protein, and β-fluctuations take place in the shell of water (two layers) around the protein (Frauenfelder et al. 2009). Biochemistry has to deal with the interactions between the molecule and its environment. The environment for molecules (cytokines, neurotransmitter, hormones, growth-factors, etc.) released by cells is made up of interstitial fluids and the ECM.

INTERSTITIAL FLUIDS AS A MEDIUM OF COMMUNICATION BETWEEN THE CELLS

Both collagens and water molecules have electric conductive and polarization properties, as do the matrix molecules. Polarization waves are possible, and protons can "jump" along the collagen fibers much faster than electrical signals can be conducted by nerves (Jaroszyk and Marzec 1993). The network of water molecules in the matrix network establishes an extraordinary, fascinating communication system.

Water molecules build dipoles and hence water flow also means the flow of energy and information. It is therefore not a total surprise that some investigators suggest that chains of water molecules along collagen fibrils are acupuncture meridians (Ho 2008).

I think that the clue to the communication of connective tissue has multiple components:
- Mechanically: the tensegrity-building of the collagenous network with the geometry of fibers, matrix molecules, and water molecules.
- Electrically and electromagnetically: the electron transport, the water bridges, and hydrogen bonds with the ion charges of dissolved substance and the hydrophobic and hydrophilic characteristics of biomolecules.
- Chemically: the interaction of the amino acids, carbohydrates, and fatty acids with their hormonal, neuronal, immunological, reparative, and growth properties and functions. The interstitial flow is an important driving force to enable the biochemical machinery.
- Energetically: liquid crystalline water is able to transmit signals and let information flow.

THE "BREATHING" OF THE TISSUES

Fibroblasts exert tensile forces on collagen fibers of the ECM via integrins and thereby squeeze the ground substance. By decreasing their tension upon the collagen fibers, the ECM is allowed to take up fluids and to swell up (Reed et al. 2010). The squeezing of the ECM by the fibroblast–collagen network is stimulated, for example, by platelet-derived growth factor (PDGF-BB) or β1-integrins, and the swelling of the ECM by relaxation of the fibroblast–collagen network is generated by proinflammatory cytokines. The major proinflammatory components seem to be prostaglandin E1 (PGE1), interleukin (IL)-1, IL-6, and tumor necrosis factor-α (TNF-α) (Martin and Resch 2009). There seem to be parallels between substances that decrease the interstitial fluid pressure (IFP) and substances that trigger the squeezing of the ECM; substances that increase the IFP cooperate with substances that release the swelling of the ECM (Reed et al. 2010).

The IFP falls during acute inflammation within minutes and acts as a driving force for the formation of edema. That occurs because of the osmotic activity of the glycosaminoglycans (hyaluronan), which leads to a swelling of the interstitial matrix. The swelling of the tissue is balanced by the collagen network. Some cytokines (IL-1, IL-6, TNF-α, etc.) are able to lower the interstitial fluid pressure; others (prostaglandin F2α, vitamin C, etc.) manage to raise it.

Dynamic mechanical stresses and pressure gradients raise small fluid flows through the ECM of all the living tissues (Fig. 4.5.2). Because of the high flow resistance of the ECM, the interstitial flow is in all directions and flows much more slowly than the blood flow in vessels (Rutkowski and Swartz, 2006). Although scientific investigation on interstitial flow is desperately needed, it is difficult to measure the interstitial flow in living persons.

It can be helpful to compare connective tissue with a sponge. By stretching or compressing the tissue, water is being extruded out of the connective tissue and makes the tissue more pliable and supple. After a while, water is resorbed and the tissue finds a new equilibrium. Manual therapies use this principle and squeeze and refill the tissue by pump and soft tissue techniques (Meert 2006). On the one hand, by pumping the connective tissue therapists try to wash out proinflammatory substances and waste products. On the other, they attempt to dissolve adherences of the collagen network to enable the supply with oxygen and nutrients.

Compression, traction, torsion, and shear stresses and also fluid shear stress exert forces on cells, receptors, and proteins. If the flow of interstitial fluids is decelerated, a contraction of the lymphatics and an increase of

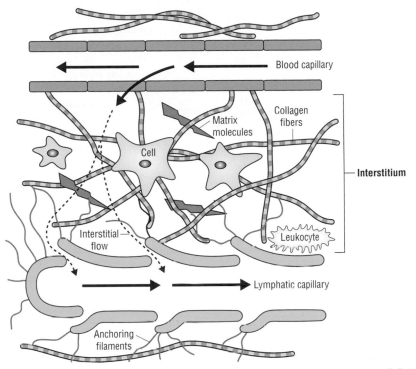

Fig. 4.5.2 Interstitial flow from a microscopic view. Adapted with permission from Meert, G.F., 2012. Veno-Lymphatische Kraniosakrale Osteopathie. Elsevier, München.

the frequency and amplitude of the active lymph pump (lymphatic vasomotion) is being induced (Gashev et al. 2002). Individual lymphangions are able to accommodate themselves independently to local changes of the flow of interstitial fluids (Venugopal et al. 2007). Endothelial cells of the vessels seem to be able to "feel out" the flow or the absence of flow of the interstitial fluids and react to it by secreting chemokines and several cytokines (Ng et al. 2004). By this interstitial flow, the cells seem to reveal the state of their environment and interact with cell migrations, cell differentiation, matrix remodeling, and secretion of proteins and cytokines. Because proteins are too large to simply diffuse, flow in the interstitial spaces is necessary for the transport of those proteins from the blood to the cells and vice versa. Investigations demonstrated that new capillary organization of endothelial cells occurred primarily in the presence of both vascular endothelial growth factor and interstitial flow (Helm et al. 2005).

It is one of the most fascinating experiences to learn to palpate, stimulate, and channel those individual and subtle waves through the tissues of a patient. After breaking up fascial adherences by myofascial techniques,

it makes sense to irrigate and purify the connective tissue. Finally, the battle between infections and the body's defenses is mostly fought in the connective tissue, leaving behind remains and fragments.

The dynamics of the interstitial fluids seem to be an important key for normal tissue function and homeostasis, and we can look hopefully to future research to decipher those mechanisms and bring some "fresh flow" in therapy and tissue engineering.

It is not for nothing that Andrew Taylor Still (1992) instructed us: "Let the lymphatics always receive and discharge naturally. If so we have no substance detained long enough to produce fermentation, fever, sickness and death."

REFERENCES

Ball, P., 2008. Water as an active constituent in cell biology. Chem. Rev. 108, 74–108.
Bellissent-Funel, M.C., 2005. Hydrophilic-hydrophobic interplay: from model systems to living systems. C. R. Geosci. 337, 173–179.

Blechschmidt, E., 2004. The Ontogenetic Basis of Human Anatomy. A Biodynamic Approach to Development from Conception to Birth. North Atlantic Books, Berkeley, California.

Chaplin, M.F., 2004. The importance of cell water. Sci. Soc. 24, 42–45.

Fayer, M.D., Moilanen, D.E., Wong, D., et al., 2009. Water dynamics in salt solutions studied with ultrafast 2D IR vibrational echo spectroscopy. Acc. Chem. Res. 42, 1210–1219.

Fenn, E.E., Wong, D.B., Fayer, M.D., 2009. Water dynamics at neutral and ionic interfaces. Proc. Natl. Acad. Sci. U. S. A. 106, 15243–15248.

Frauenfelder, H., Chen, G., Berendzen, J., et al., 2009. A unified model of protein dynamics. Proc. Natl. Acad. Sci. U. S. A. 106, 5129–5134.

Gashev, A.A., Davis, M.J., Zawieja, D.C., 2002. Inhibition of the active lymph pump by flow in rat mesenteric lymphatics and thoracic duct. J. Physiol. 540, 1023–1037.

Helm, C.E., Fleury, M.E., Zisch, A.H., Boschetti, F., Swartz, M.A., 2005. Synergy between interstitial flow and VEGF directs capillary morphogenesis in vitro through a gradient amplification mechanism. Proc. Natl. Acad. Sci. U. S. A. 102, S15779–S15784.

Ho, M.W., 2008. The Rainbow and the Worm. The Physics of Organisms. World Scientific Publishing, New Jersey.

Ingber, D.E., 2006. Cellular mechanotransduction: putting all the pieces together again. FASEB J. 20, S811–S827.

Jaroszyk, F., Marzec, E., 1993. Dielectric properties of BAT collagen in the temperature range of thermal denaturation. Ber. Bunsenges. Phys. Chem. 97, 868–872.

Martin, M., Resch, K., 2009. Immunologie. Verlag Eugen Ulmer, Stuttgart.

Meert, G.F., 2006. Das Venöse und Lymphatische System aus Osteopathischer Sicht. Elsevier, Munich.

Ng, C.P., Helm, C.L., Swartz, M.A., 2004. Interstitial flow differentially stimulates blood and lymphatic endothelial cell morphogenesis in vitro. Microvasc. Res. 68, 258–264.

Peto, S., Gillis, P., 1990. Fiber-to-field angle dependence of proton nuclear magnetic relaxation in collagen. Magn. Reson. Imaging 8, 703–712.

Pollack, G., 2002. The cell as a biomaterial. J. Mater. Sci. Mater. Med. 13, 811–821.

Reed, R.K., Liden, A., Rubin, K., 2010. Edema and fluid dynamics in connective tissue remodelling. J. Mol. Cell. Cardiol. 48, 518–523.

Rutkowski, J.M., Swartz, M.A., 2006. A driving force for change: interstitial flow as a morphoregulator. Trends Cell Biol. 17, 44–50.

Schleip, R., Klingler, W., Lehmann-Horn, F., 2005. Active fascial contractility: Fascia may be able to contract in a smooth muscle-like manner and thereby influence musculoskeletal dynamics. Med. Hypotheses 65, 273–277.

Still, A.T., 1992. Philosophy of Osteopathy. Eastland Press, Seattle.

Szent-Györgyi, A. 1957. Bioenergetics. Academic Press Inc, New York, p. 26.

Venugopal, A.M., Stewart, R.H., Laine, G.A., Dongaonkar, R.M., Quick, C.M., 2007. Lymphangion coordination minimally affects mean flow in lymphatic vessels. Am. J. Physiol. Heart Circ. Physiol. 293, H1183–H1189.

Ye, H., Naguib, N., Gogotsi, Y., 2004. TEM Study of water in carbon nanotubes. JOEL News Magazine 39, 2–7.

BIBLIOGRAPHY

Lee, R.P., 2007. The living matrix. In: Findley, T.W., Schleip, R. (Eds.), Fascia Research. Basic science and implications for conventional and complementary health care. Elsevier, Munich.

Clinical Application

Mark Driscoll and Carla Stecco

Fascia-Related Disorders

Fascia-Related Disorders: An Introduction

Mark Driscoll and Thomas W. Findley

It is often difficult to find the source of musculoskeletal disorders or the reason for performance, for that matter. Both ends of this spectrum continue to intrigue researchers. Part 5 of this book seeks to touch on disorders related to the musculoskeletal system. Many efforts to decipher this puzzle are pursued and often comprise factors such as genetics, biology, and nutrition. Part 5 approaches this subject through the mechanical lens. Provided much of our anatomy was shaped during evolution, and being subject to mechanical forces, this lens most often seems to gather most attention. Whether or not such areas may be considered fascia-related is a perception put forth in this book but not purported to be an exhaustive interpretation of all the plausible factors involved. Some chapters present local conditions, whereas others address systemic processes affecting multiple parts of the body. They are intended to stimulate thought and discussion regarding the role of fascia in manual therapies among clinical practitioners and basic and clinical scientists.

Dupuytren's disease (Chapter 5.2) illustrates the contractile power that can be generated by the fascia. In the early stages, vertical fibers that run from the palmar fascia to the skin create indentations or "pits" where they attach; later on, palmar nodules develop between the palmar fascia and the skin. Longitudinal cords develop, particularly generating deformities in the little and ring fingers. There are surgical, local, and systemic pharmacological treatments directed at the mechanical connections or the underlying processes.

Spastic paresis (Chapter 5.3) provides an example of a neurological condition affecting the ability to control and contract muscles, which may become atrophied, hypertrophied, or fibrotic. Surgical and medical interventions have been developed to reduce muscle tone.

Reviewing the muscle function, particularly during surgery to balance contraction power between wrist flexors and wrist extensors, has led to an appreciation of the role of the fascial connections between adjacent muscles, and even between muscles on opposite sides of a joint. These connections may vary a great deal from person to person. Further elucidation of these connections and how they form may lead to treatment plans more effectively tailored to the individual patient. A similar analysis may be useful in other neurological conditions, such as stroke, multiple sclerosis, and spinal cord injury, which lead to increased tone in the muscles and have anecdotal reports of changes with manual therapies.

The "diabetic foot" (Chapter 5.4) affecting over 200 million people is seen in almost 15% of persons with diabetes. Diabetes is a disease of small blood vessels in the body, affecting not only the pancreas but also the nerves (hence "diabetic neuropathy") and peripheral skin. The elevated blood glucose levels lead to glycosylation of structural proteins in connective tissue, with fascial tissues becoming thicker and stiffer. Structural changes in the plantar fascia, Achilles tendon, and joint mobility of the lower extremity result in a constellation of changes that are termed the diabetic foot.

Myofascial trigger points (Chapter 5.5) are identified by manual palpation in everyday clinical practice in a wide variety of patients. Pathophysiological changes point to localized hypoxia with connective tissue shortening and crosslink, commonly induced by direct trauma, acute or chronic strain. Taut bands develop in conjunction with trigger points, resulting in restricted motion or coordination, decreased blood flow or sensation, or compression of neural or vascular structures.

Whereas most of this part deals with conditions causing tissue shortening, Chapter 5.6 addresses the issue of tissue hypermobility seen in inherited connective tissue disorders, such as Marfan and Ehlers–Danlos syndromes. Patients have muscle weakness, pain, and fatigability, with reduction in vibratory sense. Such tissue alterations may also be caused by over-compliant tissues involved in joint stability; how they got to this point is the question. Extracellular tenascin-X acts as a bridge between collagen fibrils and enhances stiffness of connective tissues. Deficiency in this seems to be directly related to the muscle symptoms in humans, and studies of a mouse model with tenascin-X deficiency show reduced epimuscular myofascial force transmission.

Chapter 5.7 addresses the normal anatomy and biomechanical function of the plantar fascia and the clinical signs, imaging, and histopathology in plantar fasciitis. The author proposes that normal physiological loading is not sufficient to create an overuse injury in normal plantar fascia, as it may lie within the range of strain free of damage. Rather, there is an imbalance of loading with tissue threshold for remodeling, from an underlying fascial defect that reduces tissue ability to accommodate load or from a neuromuscular defect that increases loading on otherwise normal tissues. This chapter also describes in detail the composition and geometry of the plantar fascia and ends with treatment options.

Chapter 5.8 is a new addition to this book that discusses the notion of low back pain, which impacts so many lives today. The chapter discusses the current scientific literature with the symptom that is low back pain, while shining light on the implications of fascia. Lastly, Chapter 5.9 summarizes the latest notions in regard to cancer and the role of its local environment, including fascia, which is receiving growing attention.

The current state-of-the-art science leaves therapists primarily relying on their palpation skills (see Chapter 6.2), coupled with an understanding of the underlying physiological processes, to design and direct therapy. New measurement tools are however starting to offer new means by which to objectively quantify tissue behavior (Chapter 6.4). This section illustrates a number of the physiological changes associated with both decreased and increased motion of fascial tissues that may be assessed by either of these methods in clinical practice.

The noninvasive imaging techniques described in Chapter 8.2 of this book have the potential to provide much more specific guidance to direct therapy and monitor tissue changes. Particularly important will be the development of ways to quantify the visual image, similar to what is now done in tissue elastography of the breast to detect more dense cancerous tissues. As these techniques become more widely used, the role of fascia in other conditions will become better documented and therapies will become more specific.

Dupuytren's Disease and Other Fibrocontractive Disorders

Ian L. Naylor

CHAPTER CONTENTS

INTRODUCTION

The importance of the structural integrity of fascia is beautifully shown by the complexity of the many precisely controlled movements the hands can achieve. When fascial elements in the hands are altered by disease, this precision is lost. One such alteration is found in Dupuytren's disease.

Surprisingly, 188 years after Baron Dupuytren first described this condition of the hand, many fundamental details about the disease remain uncertain or unknown. What *is* known, however, is that because this disease causes the fascia to contract, it is classified as one of the fibrocontractive disorders. It is a very good example of the contractile power that fascial elements within a structure can exert when they become "diseased."

This contractile disorder has received consideration in a limited number of textbooks. Highly recommended to the reader is the text *Dupuytren's Disease*, written by Tubiana and colleagues in 2000. Despite being 21 years old, this textbook is still the most comprehensive approach to the disease and should be consulted for details that cannot be addressed in this short chapter. Rather, this chapter draws on and considers in some detail the most current findings in an attempt to shed some light on the causes, consequences, and possible treatments of this enigmatic disease.

Throughout history, the use of the hand has been fundamental to man's development, and many people have praised the hand for its "design" and complex abilities. One such person was the Englishman Thomas Traherne (c.1637–1674), who described the hands as:

The hands are a sort of feet, which serve us in our passage towards Heaven, curiously distinguished into joints and fingers, and fit to be applied to any thing which reason can imagine or desire. (Traherene 1992, Meditations on the Six Days of Creation, p. 78)

DUPUYTREN'S DISEASE

In an individual afflicted by Dupuytren's disease, there is usually a progressive decrease in their ability to carry out any tasks they could "imagine or desire." Individuals are brought to the point of severe frustration and annoyance as the disease progressively and irreversibly develops, causing a permanent deformity of the hand. Finally, with fingers firmly lodged against the palm, the hand(s) are incapable of performing their everyday, normal functions (Pratt and Byrne 2009). This, it is fully accepted, is the most extreme form of the condition, but even in those people who are suffering less severe forms of the disease, the tasks of trying to carry out *"anything which reason can imagine or desire"* become very difficult.

WHO IS AFFLICTED BY THIS DISEASE?

Dupuytren's disease is primarily a disease of Northern Europeans, especially those who come from a Celtic or Scandinavian origin. In men, who are more likely to suffer this condition than women, it usually starts during the fourth or fifth decade of life, with a peak incidence at 50 years. In contrast, for women, the peak incidence is 60 to 70 years. It does occur in other racial groups throughout the world but at a much lower incidence. Statistics suggest that there is no occurrence even within a specific Caucasian population. From all the collected evidence, there appears to be a hereditary component as the disease has a familial trait with, in some cases, autosomal dominance.

Other suggested risk factors include: type 1 diabetes, alcoholism, smoking, antiepileptic drugs, and occupations where physical forces are applied to the palm of hand. Some of these factors are more controversial than others. This is just one of the many areas of uncertainty about the disease's etiology that remains to be resolved.

A further complication that makes the disease even more complicated to understand is that not all individuals show the same rate of progression; usually, the later it starts the less aggressive it proves to be. The disease has an association with other fibrocontractive disorders such as Peyronie's and Ledderhose's disease (as discussed later).

THE BASIC PROBLEMS OF DUPUYTREN'S DISEASE

The beautiful delicacy, complexity, and dexterity of the hand is brought about by the highly coordinated interaction of nerves, muscles, tendons, and bones, which just like everywhere else in the body, are all connected together by fascial elements. In the hand these elements are arranged in a very complex way, none more so than those that are found directly under the palmar skin. These elements are somewhat unusual because they form a thickened sheet of connective tissue, which is termed the palmar aponeurosis. This thickened layer of connective tissue is thought to provide physical protection for the flexor tendons lying directly underneath it on their route to the fingers, so ensuring that despite complex stresses and loads placed upon the palm, the fingers can be manipulated. This ensures that these tendons are able to carry out their delicate and complex tasks free from constraints resulting from externally applied forces.

It is this connective tissue structure, the aponeurosis, which is considered to be central to the palmar problems of Dupuytren's disease. There is great speculation as to why the disease affects this structure and what factor(s) initiate the disease. There has also been speculation about what factors cause the condition to progress once it starts. Perhaps these factors could be the same or different. Before speculating about these factors and what they could potentially do, it may be useful to give a brief outline of the condition, with special reference to the involvement of the fascial elements in the hand.

BASIC ANATOMY OF DUPUYTREN'S DISEASE

Many studies, from the perspectives of both basic anatomy (gross and microscopic) and clinical medicine, have established that the first palmar signs of Dupuytren's disease are the development of "skin pits," especially at the position of the distal palmar crease. These pits are caused by changes in the underlying vertical fibers of the aponeurosis attached to the overlying subcutaneous fascia of the skin. They are usually slow to develop and are caused by progressive "stimulation" of the existing vertical connective tissue elements within the aponeurosis.

It should be stressed that the vertical fibers are fewer in number than the more extensive longitudinal and transverse arrangement of fibers within the structure, which provide skin anchorage when the palmar skin is subjected to shearing forces. So, the power of the vertical fibers to exert a force on the overlying skin is normally relatively low. However, once "stimulated," these fibers transmit a force causing the pits as a result of the contraction pulling against the more distensible skin rather than anchorage points in the palmar aponeurosis.

This suggests that from the very beginning of the disease, the palmar fascia has changed from a highly complex, organized, passive protective structure to one that develops the capacity to be contractile. Despite considered speculation, there is still no clear evidence as to why the vertical transmission of the contractile force that forms the pits should first occur. However, whatever the causes, the presence of such fibers as demonstrated in the microdissection studies of McGrouther in 1982 is not in any doubt. He clearly demonstrated in a series of elegant anatomical studies these vertical connections of the palmar aponeurosis to the skin at the site of the distal palmar crease.

PALMAR NODULES

After the "pits" formation, the disease can enter a highly variable period. In some people, the disease does not progress from this stage or progresses very slowly. In others, there is proliferation of cells on the surface of the palmar aponeurosis and over time, as the number of cells increases, their mass is such that they can form a distinct, palpable, and eventually, externally visible nodule full of cells (palmar nodules). It should be stressed that palmar nodules are superficial to the palmar aponeurosis and not an integral part of it. They exist between the palmar aponeurosis and the fascia of the overlying skin to which they can be adherent.

The proliferation of the cells in palmar nodules can be so pronounced that in the past, when they were examined histologically, they were sometimes diagnosed as malignant tumors (such as a sarcoma), resulting in amputation. Greater knowledge of the disease means that such radical surgery is avoided. The proliferating cells are found in a meshwork of connective tissues so dense that when they are cut using a scalpel blade the term "gritty" is used to give an indication of their density, which is unlike that of the unaffected palmar fascia.

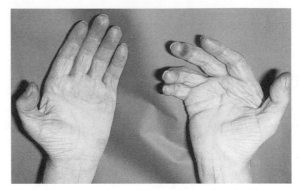

Fig. 5.2.1 Dupuytren's Contracture. Reproduced with permission from Forbes, C., Jackson, W., 2002. Color Atlas and Text of Clinical Medicine. Mosby Ltd, St. Louis, Figure 9.46.

Consequently, new connective tissue fibers and new cells occur in a location where there should be no connective tissue or additional cells.

Biochemical studies have established that the newly formed connective tissue collagen fibers are a mixture of type III and type I. The cells within the nodules have some of the functional characteristics of fibroblasts—synthesizing this new collagen—and ultrastructural similarities to some aspects of smooth muscle cells, giving rise to the contraction seen in the disease (Fig. 5.2.1).

 KEY POINT

Dupuytren's disease is still poorly understood in terms of both initiation, disease progression, and treatment. Myofibroblasts play a key role in all stages of the disease.

MYOFIBROBLASTS

These cells that develop within the palmar nodules have some rather unusual morphological characteristics when viewed using both optical and electron microscopy. They exhibit nuclear pleiomorphism using both techniques. The greater resolution of the electron microscope showed that their cytoplasm contains myofilaments and associated dense bodies. It is interesting to note that in 1972 Gabbiani et al. used these ultrastructural appearances in such palmar nodules to further develop their ideas as to the existence and possible role(s) of myofibroblasts.

As the disease develops further and more nodular cells are formed, the greater contractile force generated by the increasing number of myofibroblasts is transmitted to the rest of the aponeurosis along the longitudinal fibers. These consequently thicken and exert force on the proximal metacarpophalangeal (MP) joint. Further disease progression results in palmar "cords" being formed due to the newly produced collagen, spreading the contractile effects of the myofibroblasts to the MP joint, causing deformity.

PALMAR CORDS

The structures known as "cords" are histologically different from palmar nodules. They have fewer cells and relatively more collagen. These structures are said to cause more deformities of the fingers than palmar nodules. The cords are clearly abnormal collagenous structures formed along the preexisting fascia. One curious observation is that if the little finger is affected by the disease, resulting in a finger deformity that is seen as a flexion contracture of the proximal interphalangeal (PIP) joint, this can actually occur without any palmar nodules being present. This again demonstrates how complex this disease can be, as it would be expected that palmar nodules were essential for the progression of the condition. This is simply not always the case. Why? Nobody knows.

WHY ARE SOME FINGERS AFFECTED MORE THAN OTHERS?

The most commonly affected fingers are the little and ring finger. Why this should be so is unclear, as all flexor tendons to the fingers are potentially covered by the same aponeurosis. It would be of great interest to know whether there are regional structural variations in the palmar aponeurosis, but as yet this has not been reported. This is not a criticism but a realization that there is great difficulty in studying its normal structure, as control samples for obvious reasons are almost impossible to obtain. Sometimes in cases of trauma to the hand small samples may be available—but the damage may result in the normal architecture being deranged, resulting in false conclusions. The problem is further compounded because there is no animal model for the disease. This is indicated because no other species has a comparable hand structure.

ARE ALL MYOFIBROBLASTS THE SAME?

The lack of a suitable animal model has made understanding both the initiation and progression of the disease a very slow task. The problem is further compounded by samples of the early form of the disease not being available for laboratory study, because operative procedures to remove tissue are not usually carried out until the disease is troublesome and requires some form of surgical correction; in other words, well after the disease has started. Using samples from later in the disease process presents other problems. For example, in the more developed cases regression of the cells may also be present. Working out the types and properties of receptors present in such cells is little help in establishing the initiation factors of the disease. As in many other diseases, working out how to prevent either disease initiation or progression in the early stages would avoid later problems. To date, these problems have received little attention. Innervation of myofibroblast nodules and cords has never been established, indicating their initiation, progression, and contractile activity must be regulated by local or systemic "factors." What these are is very uncertain, but there may be underlying inflammatory causes.

INFLAMMATORY MODELS

The problem of there being no animal model for the disease has caused serious difficulty in attempting to test, in a rational way, potentially new pharmacological treatments in a rational way. Whereas it is true that myofibroblast can be "grown" in a variety of animal models, there is not one accepted method of doing this. One early technique was to use croton oil to induce the formation of a "granuloma pouch" in the back of a rat. In this technique, croton oil in maize oil is injected into an air blister made in the loose subcutaneous tissue space. The croton oil clearly provokes a major inflammatory reaction and within 14 to 21 days causes a rapid and profound induction of a myofibroblast-containing capsule—their origin being from fibroblasts present in the surrounding subcutaneous tissue space.

There is always the fundamental problem that the cells induced in the subcutaneous tissue space in rodents by this cocarcinogen, croton oil, may be different from cells induced by a fibrocontractive disease. These rapidly induced inflammatory-stimulated myofibroblasts, being formed in a matter of days rather than weeks or months in the human conditions, may have potentially different receptors than those induced by the much slower development of a pathological process such as Dupuytren's disease. Whereas it is true the croton oil–induced cells have all the ultrastructural features of myofibroblasts, whether or not they have the same receptors as those found in human conditions is a fundamental point to establish. For example, this capsular tissue responds to serotonin, whereas no human myofibroblast–containing capsular material sourced from Dupuytren's nodules, around tissue expander capsules, prosthetic devices, and breast implants, although being stimulated by documented myofibroblast agonists, have ever been stimulated by serotonin.

MYOFIBROBLAST RECEPTORS

In Vitro Studies

An alternative to animal models is to grow cells in tissue culture derived from nodules and cords of surgical specimens of Dupuytren's patients. This has been carried out on a number of occasions, but there are difficulties in this approach too. Many authors, although not all, assume that cells grown from explants represent the "transformed by disease" cells found in the nodules and cords. However, these may be the more motile cells, or in fact the structural cells from the aponeurosis in the tissues, not those involved in the disease. The cord cells differ from the nodule cells since they are clearly new structures, and this criticism may be invalid. But in the cords there are fewer cells to migrate and develop.

The final problem is that cells that are grown in tissue culture do so in a somewhat unusual environment, albeit designed to mimic "normal" conditions of growth. The presence of antibiotics, fetal calf serum, and complex mixtures of ions may induce changes in cells that are already transformed. The problem of trying to simplify conditions may, in the long run, actually complicate understanding of which receptors are actually present. The final twist is that the mere presence of a receptor does not necessarily mean that it is involved in the process of Dupuytren's disease. The complexities of this enigmatic disease continue to frustrate attempts at understanding it fully.

A further complication of extending basic research on myofibroblasts to Dupuytren's disease is that some of the more current papers have used cells in culture derived from the lung. These are perhaps best termed "structural myofibroblasts." Although they have all the structural characteristics as pathologically induced cells, whether they are directly comparable to disease-induced cells, in terms of their receptors, remains for future research to discover.

This problem needs to be thoroughly addressed if rational treatments based on receptors are to be devised.

WHAT IS THE ORIGIN OF THE CELLS THAT CAUSE THE "PITS" AT THE DISTAL PALMAR CREASE?

When we consider such a question we enter the land of speculation rather than proven science. There are two possible sources for such cells. Either they develop from existing cells in the aponeurosis, which for some reason change their resting state to become capable of a phenotypic change, or they are derived from a source outside the aponeurosis and migrate to the superficial areas of this structure, growing and bringing about a change in the function of the aponeurosis. In the latter case, the most obvious local source would be the connective tissue within the overlying palmar skin. It should be noted that the nodules never form on the ventral side of the aponeurosis.

That subcutaneous cells from the overlying skin could give rise to the source of the problem was suggested as long ago as 1963 (Hueston 1963). Hueston once told me it was compulsory for his surgical registrars to both read and understand his textbook prior to them being allowed to operate on his Dupuytren's patients. Even in 1963 it was considered to be a complex disease! Hueston's theory has been reinforced over the years by available evidence, and one piece of evidence is particularly powerful in supporting his hypothesis. If the skin that overlies the palmar nodules is removed when the palmar nodules and/or cords are excised and a skin graft is applied from a non-palmar source (using the technique known as dermofasciectomy), then the condition's recurrence is significantly less compared with those in whom the original skin is simply sutured together. This suggests that the subcutaneous fascia of the palmar skin in Dupuytren's patients may be unusual in its capacity to act as a reservoir of potentially "mobile and reactive fibroblasts" that move and are then transformed into cells that can bring about the contractile effect (the myofibroblast). But why some fingers are more prone to the effect of the overlying subcutaneous cells remains unknown.

WHAT "INSTRUCTS" THE CELLS IN THE APONEUROSIS TO CONTRACT?

When trying to develop logical strategies to treat this condition (either surgical or pharmacological), it is essential to address this question. In truth, we know very little about what instructs the cells to contract but evidence has suggested a number of possibilities.

Some of this evidence has been obtained from tissue culture experiments. The ideas presented by Hinz et al. (2007) should be read, concerning the placement of fibroblasts into conditions where they transform into myofibroblasts.

WHAT "INSTRUCTS" THE CELLS IN THE APONEUROSIS TO PROLIFERATE?

Agents that cause cell fibroblast/myofibroblast proliferation are much better understood than those agents that cause fibroblast/myofibroblast contraction. Mitogens have usually been studied in tissue culture using explants of cells growing from Dupuytren's nodules. Platelet-derived growth factor (PDGF) and basic fibroblast growth factor (bFGF) have been shown to be mitogenic for both normal fibroblasts and cells derived from Dupuytren's disease. Transforming growth factor (TGF)-beta receptors have been shown to present in cells derived from Dupuytren's disease. This growth factor exists in many forms: namely, $\beta1$, $\beta2$, and $\beta3$. The $\beta1$ and $\beta2$ forms have been shown to be mitogenic for myofibroblasts and a combination of the two is especially effective at high plating densities. Wipff et al. (2007) have also demonstrated the role of stress and TGF-$\beta1$ in converting fibroblasts into myofibroblasts, albeit in lung myofibroblasts.

CURRENT TREATMENTS

Surgical Approach

The traditional treatment of Dupuytren's disease has been surgical, using fasciotomy, fasciectomy, and more recently dermofasciectomy. The first of these techniques severs the connections of the nodule from the skin. The second removes the nodules but leaves the original overlying skin, and the third removes the nodules and replaces the overlying skin with a skin graft. No guarantees can be given for their success, and the problem of recurrence in the first two techniques is a major drawback.

The problem of recurrence necessitates surgical revision. These surgical revisions of the condition give rise to scar tissue, and the growth of this can cause problems of displacement of digital nerves, which, with the potential to damage them during further surgery, are not inconsequential. The large number of different techniques for surgical treatment of the disease suggests that this condition is far from easy to treat; in fact, some have suggested that the deformity that can follow surgery can in some cases be worse than the original disability.

A STRATEGY FOR A PHARMACOLOGICAL APPROACH

As an alternative, we may be able to use our increasing knowledge of the types of receptors possessed by myofibroblasts to design a specific and rational treatment, so avoiding the need for surgery. This will involve the use of "drugs" given either locally by injection into nodule or cord, or systemically to have an action(s) on:

1. Stopping the initiation of the transformation of the cells from superficial fascia, or another source, to grow above the palmar aponeurosis.
2. Stopping the proliferation of cells once they have been initiated.
3. Inhibiting the cellular powers of contractility so as to avoid the induction of more cells and to stop the movement of the MP or IP joint toward the palm.
4. Inhibiting the cells' capacity to produce collagen so as to inhibit nodule and/or cord formation and so delay/inhibit nodules/cord formation.
5. Selectively removing the collagen that has already been deposited.

DRUGS INJECTED INTO THE CORDS

Perhaps the most well-known use of a locally administered drug is the injection of corticosteroids, for example, triamcinolone, directly into the palmar nodules over a period of 6 weeks. However, this is a technically difficult procedure and the results have always been somewhat controversial. Beneficially, the steroids may cause an inhibition of nodular cell division and reduce collagen synthesis, resulting in softening and flattening of the nodules. But they but may have an adverse effect on existing surrounding noninvolved fibroblasts, collagenous structures in the fascia, and in the skin above the palmar nodules and cords.

A safer, more selective alternative technique was first attempted in 1973 by Hueston. This involved selective removal of the collagen in the nodules and cords using a mixture of collagenolytic enzymes and was described as "enzymic fasciectomy." Few reports have ever been published as to its success, but a more current technique with the same basic concept (Hurst et al. 2009) used a much more powerful collagenase derived from *Clostridium histolyticum*. A very high success rate has been claimed for this technique with nodules and cords involving the MP joint in the palm, and at present, it is preferred over surgery in the United States.

An alternative approach was aimed at reducing the proliferation of myofibroblasts by using the cytotoxic drug 5 fluorouracil (5FU), which is normally used for solid tumors, breast cancer, and colorectal and skin cancers. Disappointingly, the results did not fulfill the expectations of the theoretical background (Bulstrode et al. 2004).

Another approach was to use a drug that decreases the collagen release from the fibroblasts/myofibroblasts, namely, the calcium channel blocker verapamil. This has been formulated for topical use as a 15% gel, and although it was first made available in 1998, we are still awaiting comprehensive results (Rayan et al. 1996).

The oral use of tamoxifen (an antiestrogen/estrogen) has been suggested, but trials in Dupuytren's patients have not taken place. Drugs suggested for the treatment of Dupuytren's disease are shown in Table 5.2.1.

A MODERN DEVELOPMENT

The most current strategy was used by Nanchahal et al. in 2018, who injected the anti-TNF mononclonal antibody adalimumab into the cords. In a single-dose, short-term study, the injected antibody reduced the expression of alpha-smooth muscle actin and protocollagen I in the treated cords, indicating an antimyofibroblast action. Serendipitously, this drug has been used to treat rheumatoid arthritis, Crohn's disease, and ulcerative colitis and therefore has the great advantage of already having an established safety record. Multiple drug injection studies plus a more extensive follow-up period are planned. It will be very interesting to see what happens to the progression of the disease with multiple doses.

TABLE 5.2.1 **Drugs that are Being Used for the Treatment of Dupuytren's Disease**

Drug	Usual Clinical Action
Verapamil 15% gel	Calcium channel blocker
Imiquimod	Antiwart treatment
N-acetyl L-cysteine	Mucolytic agent
Sulfonate (MESA)	Used in some types of chemotherapy
Vitamin E	Nutrition, antioxidant
Neprinol–nattokinase	Proteolytic enzymes, serrapeptase
Tamoxifen	Antiestrogen
5 fluorouracil	Cytotoxic
Bromelin	Proteolytic enzyme
Collagenase from Clostridium histolyticum	Proteolytic enzyme
Humira (Adalimumab)	Anti-TNF alpha

 KEY POINT

Alleviation of Dupuytren's disease was traditionally by surgery. The use of drugs has proven limited success. Using anti-TNF monoclonal antibody therapy suggests a major improvement may be possible in the future.

Two other fibrocontractive disorders will be very briefly considered, as progress in understanding their etiology and putative treatment(s) is even more controversial than for Dupuytren's disease.

PEYRONIE'S DISEASE

This fibrocontractive disease is less understood than is Dupuytren's disease. The site of the problem is well-known to be in the Buck's fascia of the penis. The transformed fibroblast-like cells grow into thickened plaques in this fascial layer, causing irregularities to be seen when the corpus cavernosus fills with blood during the process of erection. Myofibroblasts have been identified in the plaques, but little is known about the receptors they possess.

To correct this deformity, surgical correction by excision of the plaque has been used. Some attempts at pharmacological modifications have been made using some of the same drugs used for Dupuytren's disease.

Both surgical and pharmacological approaches are problematic. This is an area for much more investigation to be carried out.

LEDDERHOSE'S DISEASE

This condition is very similar in many ways to Dupuytren's disease but occurs in the fascia of the feet, where it results in a thickened plantar aponeurosis, and in the arch of the foot. The nodules form similarly to palmar nodules but contractility is not as great a problem. The nodules can be removed surgically but with limited degrees of success. No pharmacological treatment is used.

CONCLUSION

So we finish almost where we started. Thomas Traherne suggested, *"The hands are a sort of feet,"* and little did he know all those years ago that, in terms of fibrocontractive disorders, hands and feet are remarkably similar in the diseases from which they suffer—Dupuytren's and Ledderhose's: the hands *are* a sort of feet, and vice versa!

Summary

The fascial involvement in a poorly understood condition, Dupuytren's disease, is described. The central role of the myofibroblast is considered in all stages of the disease from initiation to the deposition of disfiguring, permanent, newly formed collagen palmar cords. A list of drugs is provided, most of which have been used with very limited success. The inclusion of antitumor necrosis factor monoclonal antibodies, used as recently as 2018, suggests interest in this enigmatic fascial disease is still a challenge to the medical community. A better therapeutic strategy may at last have been found.

REFERENCES

Bulstrode, N.W., Bisson, M., Jemec, B., et al. 2004. A prospective randomised clinical trial of the intra-operative use of 5-fluorouracil on the outcome of Dupuytren's disease. J. Hand Surg. Br. 29, 18–21.

Gabbiani, G., Hirschel, B.J., Ryan, G.B., et al. 1972. Granulation tissue as a contractile organ. A study of structure and function. J. Exp. Med. 135, 719–34.

Hinz, B., Phan, S.H., Thannickal, V.J., et al. 2007. The myofibroblast – one function, multiple origins. Am. J. Pathol. 170, 1807–1816.

Hueston, J.H., 1963. Dupuytren's Contracture. Churchill Livingstone, Edinburgh.

Hurst, L.C., Badalamente, M.A., Hentz, R.A., et al., 2009. Injectable collagenase *Clostridium histolyticum* for Dupuytren's contracture. N. Engl. J. Med. 361, 968–979.

McGrouther, D. A., 1982. The microanatomy of Dupuytren's contracture. J. Hand Surgery (European Volume)14, 215–236.

Nanchahal, J., Ball, C., Davidson, D., et al., (2018) Anti-tumour necrosis factor therapy for Dupuytren's disease: A randomized dose response proof of concept Phase 2a clinical trial. EBioMedicine 33, 282–288.

Pratt, A.L., Byrne, G., 2009. The lived experience of Dupuytren's disease of the hand. J. Clin. Nurs. 18, 1793–1802.

Rayan, G.M., Parizi, M., Tomasek, J.J., 1996. Pharmacologic regulation of Dupuytren's fibroblast contraction in vitro. J Hand Surg Am. 21, 1065–1070.

Traherne, T., Guffey, G.R. [Editor] 1992. Meditations on the six days of creation, Augustan Reprint Society, Grand Rapids, USA.

Tubiana, R., Leclercq, C., Hurst, L.C., Badalamente, M., Mackin, E., (Eds.), 2000. Dupuytren's Disease. Martin Dunitz, London.

Wipff, P.J., Rifkin, D.B., Meister, J.J., Hinz, B., 2007. Myofibroblast contraction activates latent TGF-b1 from the extracellular matrix. J. Cell. Biol. 179, 1311 1323.

Spastic Paresis

Peter A. Huijing and Richard T. Jaspers

CHAPTER CONTENTS

INTRODUCTION

Spastic paresis is a common term to denominate typical presentations of the motor disorders in a specific type of cerebral palsy. By definition, spastic cerebral paresis (SCP), also called cerebral palsy, describes a group of disorders of development of movement and posture, causing activity limitation, that are attributed to nonprogressive disturbances that occurred in the developing fetal or infant brain (Bax et al. 2005). Spasticity is a neurological symptom characterized by a velocity-dependent increase in tonic stretch reflexes with exaggerated tendon jerks resulting from hyperexcitability of the stretch reflex (Smeulders and Kreulen 2007).

The term SCP suggests a mechanism, but in effect the muscles susceptible to spasticity are supposed to exert more force (due to their spasticity) and are not sufficiently opposed by antagonistic muscles (paresis). In practice the term does not mean much more than is indicated by the altered position of joint crossed by affected muscle. The patients develop characteristic positions, for example, at the wrist or ankle, toward endorotation, flexion, pronation, and adduction. Such positions at joints are not caused directly by spastic contractions, indicating that secondarily to the spastic condition some adaptation of muscles and/or fascia at the joint has occurred and may progressively become more serious.

KEY POINT

The specific positions of hand and foot seen in spastic cerebral paresis are not a direct result of spastic contractions themselves and, therefore, must be related to secondary adaptation of muscles involved and their connections.

Note that these typical positions can acutely be altered if spastic contractions are avoided (slow movement), after careful manipulation or under anesthesia. The potential role of fascia in these effects are underexposed in literature.

INTRAMUSCULAR CONNECTIVE TISSUE CHANGES IN SPASTIC PARESIS AND CONTROL HUMAN MUSCLE

To get closer to possible mechanisms it is important to know and understand how adaptation to the spastic condition secondarily changes the muscle and its myofascial connections. Usually, samples of muscle are not readily available, but in a long-lasting project (several years) our group managed to obtain small samples of flexor carpi ulnaris muscle (FCU), of what can be considered healthy muscle, and spastic muscle of patients undergoing tendon transplant surgery. These samples were analyzed for stiffness of segments of fascicles and of single myofibers and were also analyzed histologically (intramuscular connective tissues) and histochemically (myofiber type distribution) (de Bruin et al. 2014).

KEY POINT

Samples from spastic muscle are almost indistinguishable from healthy muscle.

Box 5.3.1 shows the surprisingly high number of variables analyzed for which no difference was found between spastic and healthy muscle.

The conclusion must be that spastic fascicle and myofiber segments were not stiffer, nor was there widespread fibrosis within the muscle stroma.

KEY POINT

Within the variables studied, the only difference found was the size of the intermuscular part of the neurovascular tract being enhanced in spastic muscle samples.

There was an exception to the overall consistent general results (Fig. 5.3.1)—namely, for the tertiary perimysium that does not envelop a particular fascicle but is in fact an intramuscular continuation of the extramuscular neuromuscular tract that forms the collagen fiber–reinforced pathway for nerves and blood vessels to get access to the muscle. The thickness of this structure in spastic muscle is almost threefold that of

---

> **BOX 5.3.1   What is Not Altered in Spastic Muscle?**
>
> Comparison of characteristics of small fascicle segment samples obtained from FCU muscle of SCP and control human subjects
> Physiological variables:
> - Stiffness of passive isolated fascicle segment: N.S.
> - Stiffness of passive single myofiber segments: N.S.
> - Sarcomere slack length (mean 2.5 μm): N.S.
>
> Histochemical variable (ATPase stained):
> - Myofiber type distribution: N.S.
>
> Histological variables (Sirius Red–stained cross-sections):
> - Thickness of endomysium per myofiber cross-section: N.S.
> - Area proportion (%) taken up by endomysium: N.S.
> - Thickness of primary (i.e., small fascicles envelopes) (p1): N.S.
> - Thickness of secondary perimysium (i.e., larger fascicles envelopes) (p2): N.S.
> - Myofiber cross-sectional area (after correction for mean age differences): no difference

N.S., No significant difference.

healthy muscle. As the neurovascular tract is supposed to play an important role in epimuscular myofascial force transmission, it is quite conceivable that the increased thickness is an adaptation to being exposed to enhanced myofascial loads. Such changes may be caused by the maintained altered position relative to other muscles and bony structures within the arm.

SURGICAL TREATMENT OF THE UPPER EXTREMITY IN SPASTIC PARESIS

Generally, interventions are aimed at decreasing postural effects of spasticity and improving function and cosmesis by various conservative therapy regimes, splinting regimes, pharmaceutical treatment, and/or surgery. The remainder of this chapter focuses on the surgical treatment of the upper extremity in SCP, because the role of fascia in spastic paresis of the upper extremity is best illustrated from observations during surgery. Surgical treatment is indicated only in carefully selected patients. It is paramount for the success of treatment that the desired goal of the patient is in agreement with a realistic and a surgically attainable goal. Patients with a desire for an improved manipulation of objects have to meet more

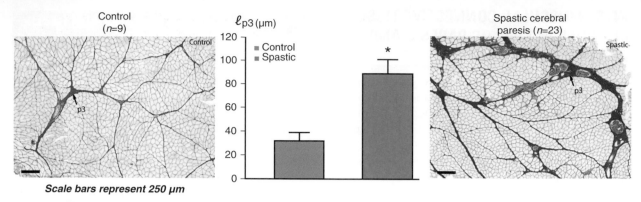

Scale bars represent 250 μm

Fig. 5.3.1 An example of the difference in thickness of the tertiary perimysium between control and spastic muscle. The central panel shows mean values and standard errors of the same variable, indicating the difference to be significant and approximately three times as thick on average. *Indicates significant difference between the control and spastic cerebral paresis group at $p < 0.01$.

strict criteria than patients with only a desire to relieve pain or an improved position for hygiene purposes. Goals of treatment can be (a) an improvement of active manual dexterity of the affected hand, (b) an improvement of bimanual dexterity by better positioning of the affected hand, (c) improved cosmetic appearance, and (d) relief of pain and/or positioning of the hand for practical purposes such as personal hygiene. Before surgery, all patients are required to have (1) realistic expectations of what can be achieved, (2) an explicit motivation to reach that goal, and (3) access to a well-organized postoperative rehabilitation regime. If the goal of treatment includes an improvement of manual dexterity, the patient is also required (4) to have voluntary muscle control over the hand and forearm, (5) to show an active prehension of the affected extremity, and (6) to have sufficient insight into the principles of treatment to actively engage in the rehabilitation regime.

The next step is to compose the optimal combination of surgical procedures in one session that will meet the goal of treatment. A surgical plan is made combining three types of procedures: (1) decreasing unwanted function by means of tenotomy, aponeurotomy, tendon lengthening, or muscle release procedures; (2) reinforcing the desired function on the paretic side by tendon transfer or tendon rerouting procedures; and (3) stabilization of joint instability by arthrodesis (definite joint fusion), capsulodesis (tightening the joint capsule), or tenodesis (limiting joint function by tendon fixation) procedures. A long clinical experience with different surgical regimes is described in the literature, but evidence

for a reliable algorithm is lacking. Surgical interventions are based on current assumptions about the nature of muscle function in spastic paresis and how they contribute to the awkward joint positions we aim to correct. The results of these interventions are not consistent in all patients and tend to be unpredictable. Therefore patient selection as described previously is very strict, and international consensus exists to plan and perform surgery only at no risk of losing any existing hand function and to set modest expectations of the clinical outcome.

A better understanding of how the interplay of the differently affected muscles in spastic paresis contributes to the disabling joint positions of the upper extremity might allow for a more reliable and predictable rationale in tailoring the surgical techniques to meet the desired functional result.

OBSERVATIONS DURING SURGERY

Obviously during tendon transplant surgery the distal tendon of FCU muscle must be cut from its insertion, which also makes it available for direct measurement of active and passive muscle force. Mechanical measurement of passive length-force characteristics of partially dissected human spastic flexor carpi ulnaris muscle (FCU) (Smeulders et al. 2004) did *not* show unusual muscular characteristics that would explain the abnormal wrist position. Note that this finding is in agreement with those described previously for muscle samples.

The two types of results combined indicate that changes occurred either within the myofibers (e.g., decrease of serial sarcomere number) or at the myofascial interaction between the muscle, or both simultaneously.

Some decreased serial sarcomere number was reported (Kinney et al. 2017). However, if this should be the only, or most important, cause creating the typical joint position, the passive length force curve should be affected by a shift to lower lengths, which may become apparent as very high forces at higher lengths.

In addition, we noticed that after tenotomy of FCU, even if the muscle was excited maximally (nerve stimulation) it did *not* result in a major retraction of the muscle to its active slack length. Instead, on tenotomy and after activation FCU shortened a little but remained relatively close to its former insertion (Fig. 5.3.2) (Kreulen et al. 2003). Even more surprisingly, as the

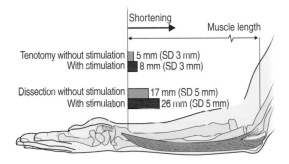

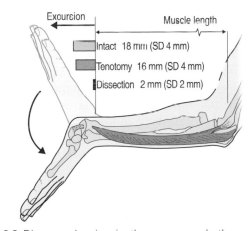

Fig. 5.3.2 Diagram showing in the upper graph the mean shortening of the flexor carpi ulnaris (FCU) muscle after tenotomy and after dissection, before and after tetanic contraction in millimeters (mm). The lower graph shows the mean passive excursion of the FCU during movement of the wrist from maximal flexion to maximal extension before tenotomy, after tenotomy, and after muscle dissection. SD, standard deviation.

wrist was moved passively from flexion to extension during surgery, *tenotomized* FCU (not spanning the wrist any longer) was lengthened almost to a similar extent as the intact FCU, indicating that the FCU is connected to structures that span the wrist via epimuscular or epitendinous connective tissues (creating a distally directed myofascial load on FCU) (see also Chapter 3.2). Even after tenotomy, such connections pull the FCU along on passive wrist extension. On wrist flexion, FCU retracted elastically so the process was repeatable during cyclic movement of the wrist. Apparently, the connective tissues involved were so stiff that they could transmit the full FCU force and strong enough so that they did not break on such force exertion. Such FCU length changes after tenotomy diminished greatly but did not fully disappear after partial dissection in distal-proximal direction (along 50%–60% of the muscle belly, necessary for subsequent fluent tendon rerouting). These results place the concept regarding the role of the fascia in spastic joint positions in a whole new perspective. Previously, the role of connective tissues as a force-transmitting matrix had hardly been considered.

We also showed length–force characteristics measured at the distal tendon of (partially dissected) FCU to vary dramatically between patients with comparable spasticity-related joint positions (Kreulen and Smeulders 2008), implying that the variables of the passive and active length–force characteristics of muscles in those conditions themselves cannot be the determining factor for developing similar abnormal joint positions.

Both active and passive length–force curves of the tenotomized FCU varied significantly when the muscles and connective tissues adjacent to the FCU were kept short (by manipulation of the wrist angle, not affecting FCU length), compared with when they were held at lengthened position (Smeulders et al. 2005). This proves that the relative length and position of adjacent structures codetermine the FCU characteristics and functional capabilities. Some patients showed differences in the length–force characteristics between flexion and extension of the wrist, particularly at low FCU lengths, and the passive force was highest in the flexed position of the wrist, whereas others showed differences at high FCU lengths, and FCU passive force was highest in the extended position of the wrist. Differences between patients were not directly related to the clinical presentation and severity of the spastic paresis (movement limitation), but these findings do prove that epimuscular fascial connections directly affect characteristics of spastic muscle and therefore its functional capabilities.

TOWARD AN EXPLANATION OF SPASTICITY-RELATED JOINT POSITIONS

The equilibrium resulting from the interplay of both muscles under spastic control and muscles under physiological neural control that yields the SCP-related joint positions induces specific conditions of the involved limbs, because muscles that are affected by spastic stretch reflexes and hypertonicity are often kept in shortened position compared with unaffected muscles. This will affect the myofascial loads on these muscles. The shortened position of one or more spastic muscles in relation to its surroundings may be more extreme than encountered in unaffected limbs. It has been shown that the distal myofascial load is high in shortened muscle (Huijing et al. 2007; Meijer et al. 2007; Rijkelijkhuizen et al. 2007), and that positional changes of the wrist did affect the force that was exerted at the distal tendon in spastic FCU, indicating a distally directed myofascial load (Huijing and Baan 2001). The fraction of force exerted by the muscle that is transmitted onto the distal tendon is affected; as with greater distal myofascial loads (yielding higher connective tissue stiffness), increasing percentages of the exerted force will be exerted via myofascial pathways. Therefore forces of spastic muscles may not be merely exerted at the distal tendons but may well be exerted mainly via epimuscular connections onto synergistic muscles that are shortened less, or onto extramuscular tissues. However, such distal myofascial force transmission alone would not explain the high moments that are required to cause the pathological and rigid joint positions of the spastic limbs, because a shortened muscle operates within a disadvantageous length range of its length–force curve and would not be able to exert high forces.

Our hypothesis (Huijing 2007) is that the extreme conditions within a spastic limb cause proximally directed epimuscular myofascial loads originating from antagonistic muscles to be exerted on spastic or synergistic muscles, through pathways similar to those that have been shown to be effective in experimental work on healthy animals (Huijing et al. 2007; Meijer et al. 2007; Rijkelijkhuizen et al. 2007). The antagonistic extensor muscles are at high length (because of the angle

of the flexed joint), as will be their adjacent connective tissues. Therefore they will be subjected to a distally directed epimuscular myofascial load creating a path for force transmission via extramuscular fascial structures. Such a path may pass through the intermuscular septa (e.g., via neurovascular tracts) and transmit force onto the spastic muscle, and thus exert a proximally directed myofascial load on its myofibers and connective tissue stroma (Fig. 5.3.2). At the location of loading, this will keep sarcomeres long. This high force could, in principle, be exerted (1) at the distal tendon of the spastic muscle or (2) via the distal myofascial pathways (distal load), and therefore create a flexion moment at the joint. This would explain the patient's rigid joint flexed position, because the more active antagonistic muscles are, the higher flexion moment would be exerted. Obviously such rigidity is enhanced by hyper-reflexivity and cocontraction of the spastic muscle. Also, because of the presence of a distally directed load on the spastic muscle (as discussed previously), the most distal sarcomeres with myofibers of the spastic muscle will be unloaded (and shorten) and the situation will be somewhat more complex: part of the force will be transmitted either on synergistic muscles and exerted at their distal tendons (exerting flexion moments as well) or on extramuscular connective tissues passing the joint at the flexor side (therefore also capable of exerting flexor moments). Therefore, in these more complex conditions, a flexed joint angle is inevitable.

CONCLUSION

Again, we feel the need to emphasize that this hypothesis for the explanation of joint positions through epimuscular force transmission is based on scientific experimental work and clinical observations that need scientific confirmation. Nevertheless, it fits the available data on spastic muscle and provides a new pathway of thinking about the nature of joint positions in spastic paresis and possible therapeutic interventions.

However, it is clear that the role of fascia in the musculoskeletal balance within the body cannot be ignored. The extent of its contribution to clinical pathology, the exact location of its mechanism, its adaptive features after therapeutic intervention, and its variability between patients are still unknown. Further scientific research unraveling mechanisms of myofascial force transmission in a functioning human extremity will affect therapeutic regimes in the future. The surgeon and therapist may be able to more objectively tailor their treatment plan to the specific needs of the patient.

REFERENCES

Bax, M., Goldstein, M., Rosenbaum, P., et al., 2005. Proposed definition and classification of cerebral palsy. Dev. Med. Child Neurol. 47, 571–576.

de Bruin, M., Smeulders, M.J., Kreulen, M., Huijing, P.A., Jaspers, R.T., 2014. Intramuscular connective tissue differences in spastic and control muscle: A mechanical and histological study. PLoS One 9, e101038.

Huijing, P.A., 2007. Epimuscular myofascial force transmission between antagonistic and synergistic muscles can explain movement limitation in spastic paresis. J. Electromyogr. Kinesiol. 17, 708–724.

Huijing, P.A., Baan, G.C., 2001. Extramuscular myofascial force transmission within the rat anterior tibial compartment: Proximo-distal differences in muscle force. Acta Physiol. Scand. 173, 297–311.

Huijing, P.A., van de Langenberg, R.W., Meesters, J.J., Baan, G.C., 2007. Extramuscular myofascial force transmission also occurs between synergistic muscles and antagonistic muscles. J. Electromyogr. Kinesiol. 17, 680–689.

Kinney, M.C., Dayanidhi, S., McCarthy, J.J., et al., 2017. Reduced skeletal muscle satellite cell number alters muscle morphology after chronic stretch but allows limited serial sarcomere addition. Muscle Nerve 55(3), 384–392.

Kreulen, M., Smeulders, M.J., 2008. Assessment of flexor carpi ulnaris function for tendon transfer surgery. J. Biomech. 41, 2130–2135.

Kreulen, M., Smeulders, M.J., Hage, J.J., Huijing, P.A., 2003. Biomechanical effects of dissecting flexor carpi ulnaris. J. Bone Joint Surg. Br. 85, 856–859.

Meijer, H.J., Rijkelijkhuizen, J.M., Huijing, P.A., 2007. Myofascial force transmission between antagonistic rat lower limb muscles: Effects of single muscle or muscle group lengthening. J. Electromyogr. Kinesiol. 17, 698–707.

Rijkelijkhuizen, J.M., Meijer, H.J., Baan, G.C., Huijing, P.A., 2007. Myofascial force transmission also occurs between antagonistic muscles located within opposite compartments of the rat lower hind limb. J. Electromyogr. Kinesiol. 17, 690–697.

Smeulders, M.J., Kreulen, M., 2007. Myofascial force transmission and tendon transfer for patients suffering from spastic paresis: A review and some new observations. J. Electromyogr. Kinesiol. 17, 644–656.

Smeulders, M.J., Kreulen, M., Hage, J.J., Huijing, P.A., van der Horst, C.M., 2004. Overstretching of sarcomeres may not cause cerebral palsy muscle contracture. J. Orthop. Res. 22, 1331–1335.

Smeulders, M.J., Kreulen, M., Hage, J.J., Huijing, P.A., van der Horst, C.M., 2005. Spastic muscle properties are affected by length changes of adjacent structures. Muscle Nerve 32, 208–215.

Diabetic Foot

Sicco A. Bus

CHAPTER CONTENTS

INTRODUCTION

Diabetes mellitus is a chronic disease affecting over 425 million people worldwide, and in one of two adults with diabetes, the disease is undiagnosed (International Diabetes Federation 2019). Diabetes may lead to several vascular and neurological complications, including ulceration, infection, or destruction of deep tissue in the foot. This "diabetic foot" affects approximately 15% of patients (Boulton et al. 2004), and it is estimated that 19% to 34% of patients will have a foot ulcer in their life (Armstrong et al. 2017). The foot ulcer is the key clinical problem in the diabetic foot that can cause infection and lead to lower-extremity amputation. Foot ulcer incidence is 7.2% per year in diabetic patients with peripheral neuropathy (Abbott et al. 1998) but is 40% in the first year after a foot ulcer has healed (Armstrong et al. 2017). Peripheral neuropathy leads to a loss of protective sensation, which makes the patient unaware of foot trauma caused by the repetitive action of elevated mechanical foot pressures (Armstrong et al. 2017). These high foot pressures are secondary to structural abnormalities, which include claw-toe and Charcot deformity, prominent metatarsal heads, and changes in subcutaneous and periarticular connective tissue (i.e., tendon, fascia, ligaments, and joint capsule). Morphological changes in the plantar fascia and Achilles tendon, and limitations in joint mobility, have been reported in diabetes. Changes in these foot structures share a common etiology related to long-standing hyperglycemia, and they may influence foot mechanics during gait and lead to foot ulcers. The goal of this chapter is to provide insight into the changes that occur as a result of diabetes in the plantar fascia, Achilles tendon, and joint mobility of the lower extremity. The underlying mechanisms of these changes are discussed, together with their biomechanical and clinical implications and available treatment options.

METHODOLOGY OF TESTING

Different methods can be used to assess changes in foot structure, joint mobility, and biomechanical function in the diabetic foot.

Assessment of Fascia, Tendon, and Ligament

Morphological changes in subcutaneous and periarticular tissues in the foot and lower leg are best assessed using in-vivo imaging techniques. With high-resolution ultrasonography the geometrical boundaries of superficial structures in the foot and lower leg can be assessed, from which tissue thickness can be measured (D'Ambrogi et al. 2003; Giacomozzi et al. 2005; Afolabi et al. 2019). More detailed qualitative and quantitative information of superficial and deep structures can be obtained using magnetic resonance imaging (MRI). MRI is superior to other imaging techniques in distinguishing soft tissue, such as muscle, tendon, ligament, fascia, and fat, and can be used to measure tissue thickness and assess the presence of rupture. The plantar fascia can be tested functionally using Jack's test, in which the hallux is passively dorsiflexed while weight-bearing (Chuter and Payne 2001). A normal response is tightening of the fascia and a raise of the foot arch. Failure may indicate fascia dysfunction or rupture.

Assessment of Joint Mobility and Stiffness

The so-called prayer sign was originally used to classify patients with limited joint mobility (LJM). This is present when the patient fails to approximate the metacarpal–phalangeal joints while opposing the palmar surfaces of the hands in a praying position. Although this method is simple in use, it is not a direct measure of LJM in the foot. Typically, a goniometer is used to assess mobility of the foot and ankle joints in a non weight-bearing position. Goniometric measurements of joint mobility are quite reliable, with reported coefficients of variation of 8.5% for the subtalar joint and 7.4% to 11.0% for the first metatarsal–phalangeal (MTP) joint (Delbridge et al. 1988; Zimny et al. 2004). Mobility and stiffness of the first MTP joint can be assessed using a mechanical testing device (Birke et al. 1995). Joint stiffness can be calculated from vertical displacement of the first metatarsal head plotted against the applied force to the metatarsal head.

Pressure Distribution Measurement

Biomechanical function of the foot is most often assessed in diabetic patients by measuring the dynamic plantar pressure distribution underneath the foot. Patients walk barefoot across a platform, which consists of a matrix of hundreds to thousands of sensors measuring the vertical (normal) pressure or stress (Fig. 5.4.1). Most often the peak pressure and the time integral of this peak pressure are calculated for multiple anatomical regions in the foot, so that conclusions on local pressure effects can be drawn. A detailed discussion of measurement of mechanical pressure in the diabetic foot is given by Lazzarini et al. (2019).

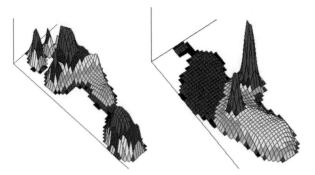

Fig. 5.4.1 Peak pressure distribution images of a healthy subject (left) and a patient with diabetic foot disease with a midfoot rocker-bottom deformity based on Charcot neuro-osteoarthropathy (Right).

NONENZYMATIC GLYCOSYLATION

Structural changes in plantar fascia, Achilles tendon, and joint mobility in diabetic patients share a common etiology—namely, nonenzymatic glycosylation of structural proteins in connective tissue secondary to the permanent hyperglycemic state in patients with diabetes mellitus (Bailey 1981; Brownlee et al. 1988). With nonenzymatic glycosylation, free glucose spontaneously attaches to structural proteins such as collagen and keratin (Schnider and Kohn 1980; Delbridge et al. 1985). Glycosylation of collagen causes an increase in intermolecular cross-linking and significant alterations in the structural stability of different collagen-rich sub cutaneous and periarticular connective tissues, such as tendon, ligament, fascia, and joint capsule (Delbridge et al. 1988). Glycosylation of keratin causes hyperkeratosis of the skin (Delbridge et al. 1985). These tissues show reduced flexibility, increased tensile strength, and other morphological adaptations (Crisp and Heathcote 1984), which are likely the cause for some of the structural abnormalities found in the diabetic foot.

PLANTAR FASCIA

The plantar fascia, or aponeurosis, is an important connective tissue structure that provides support, rigidity, and stability in the foot under dynamic conditions (Hicks 1954; Sarrafian 1983; Sharkey et al. 1998). The aponeurosis consists of longitudinally oriented collagen and elastic fibers. It originates from the posteromedial calcaneal tuberosity and divides into five bands at the midmetatarsal level, with each band inserting into the plantar plate and the skin (Bojsen-Moller and Flagstad 1976; Theodorou et al. 2000, 2002). According to the windlass mechanism described by Hicks (1954), extension of the MTP joint during the propulsion phase of gait causes the aponeurosis to tighten and to draw the calcaneus and the metatarsal heads together (Fig. 5.4.2). This results in a raised longitudinal arch and rearfoot supination, thereby making the foot a stable rigid lever in propulsion. On weight-bearing in the first half of the stance phase, the arch flattens, which increases tension in the aponeurosis. This tension unwinds the "windlass," causing flexion at the MTP joint. Failure of the plantar aponeurosis most often occurs proximally. In nondiabetic subjects, aponeurosis rupture may reduce its stabilizing action and lead to collapse of the longitudinal arch or claw-toe deformity, and may increase pressures in the forefoot (Hicks 1954; Sarrafian 1983; Sharkey et al. 1999). Fascia thickening may alter the height of the longitudinal arch (Arangio et al. 1998). The effects that diabetes has on the plantar fascia are largely unknown.

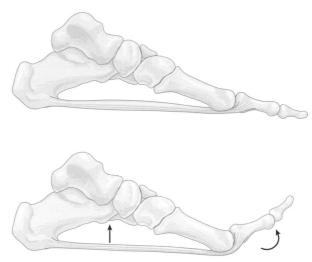

Fig. 5.4.2 The windlass mechanism. Reproduced with permission from Greisberg, J., 2007. Foot and ankle anatomy and biomechanics. In: DiGiovanni, C.W., Greisberg, J., eds. Core Knowledge in Orthopedics: Foot and Ankle. Elsevier, Philadelphia.

 KEY POINT

Structural changes in plantar fascia, Achilles tendon, and joint mobility in diabetic patients share a common etiology: nonenzymatic glycosylation of structural proteins in connective tissue secondary to the permanent hyperglycemic state in patients with diabetes mellitus.

Rupture and Fasciitis

The plantar fascia of diabetic patients with claw-toe deformity showed discontinuity, indicating rupture, in one MRI study (Taylor et al. 1998). The authors suggest that the effects of nonenzymatic glycosylation may render the aponeurosis less compliant and more prone to rupture. However, none of the patients with claw-toe deformity in another MRI study showed discontinuity of the aponeurosis (Fig. 5.4.3) (Bus 2004). Also, signal intensity increases and substantial thickening of the aponeurosis at the calcaneal insertion compatible with plantar fasciitis have been found in neuropathic diabetic patients. However, these changes did not differentiate patients with toe deformity from those without (Bus 2004). Clearly, the data on fascia rupture and the role the aponeurosis plays in causing toe deformity in diabetic patients remain inconclusive.

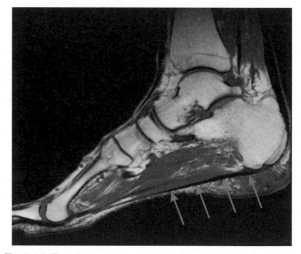

Fig. 5.4.3 The plantar aponeurosis shown as a low-signal-intensity structure on this sagittal plane magnetic resonance image of the foot of a neuropathic diabetic patient. The aponeurosis does not show discontinuity that would be indicative of fascia rupture.

Plantar Fascia Thickening

The plantar fascia may be thicker in diabetic patients than in healthy controls (D'Ambrogi et al. 2003; Bolton et al. 2005; Abate et al. 2012). High-resolution ultrasound images showed on average 2.0 mm thickness at the calcaneal insertion in healthy controls, 2.9 mm in diabetic patients, 3.0 mm in neuropathic diabetic patients, and 3.1 mm in diabetic patients with a history of foot ulceration (D'Ambrogi et al. 2003). With computed tomography, a thicker aponeurosis was found in diabetic patients than in healthy controls (mean 4.2 vs 3.6 mm) (Bolton et al. 2005). Abate et al. showed plantar fascia thickness to be significantly positively correlated with body mass index ($r = 0.749$, $p < 0.0001$). Increased fascia thickness in diabetes is likely also associated with nonenzymatic glycosylation of collagen; a reduction of 30% in collagen content in the plantar fascia has been found in diabetic patients (Andreassen et al. 1981). Apparently, with long-standing diabetes, geometrical changes of the plantar fascia shown as thickening of this connective tissue structure may occur.

KEY POINT

The plantar fascia of diabetic patients may be thicker than in healthy controls. This may cause higher plantar forefoot pressures, but the clinical implications of plantar fascia change are largely unknown.

Biomechanical Implications

Thickening of plantar fascia can influence biomechanical foot function in diabetes. Dynamic forefoot pressures were found to be significantly higher in diabetic patients with thicker plantar fascia than in diabetic and healthy control subjects with thinner plantar fascia (D'Ambrogi et al. 2003; Giacomozzi et al. 2005). Additionally, a trend in results suggests that fascia thickness and forefoot pressure in these patients were collated ($r = 0.52$). This association may be explained by the role plantar fascia plays in countering the flattening of the foot during midstance of gait. The vertical forces acting on the forefoot during arch flattening are countered by horizontal forces generated in passive structures such as the plantar fascia, which try to tie the forefoot and rearfoot together. With fascia thickening, resistance increases, meaning that larger vertical forces measured as higher pressures are required at the forefoot in order to flatten the foot during stance.

In patients with Charcot's neuroarthropathy, plantar fascia dysfunction or rupture may be indicated, based on a negative response to Jack's test (Chuter and Payne 2001). Additionally, rupture of the plantar fascia has been suggested as a potential factor in the increased forefoot-to-rearfoot pressure ratio that is found in neuropathic

diabetic patients compared with healthy controls (Caselli et al. 2002). A suggested forefoot drop as a result of fascia rupture (Sharkey et al. 1999) may cause increased loading in the forefoot and explain these results. More research is required to improve our understanding of the role that the plantar fascia plays in altering biomechanical function of the foot in diabetes.

Clinical Implications and Treatment

The clinical implications of structural changes in the plantar fascia in diabetic patients are not known. This may be the reason for the paucity of data on treatment options. Alterations in foot function associated with plantar fascia dysfunction may be indicative of its contributing role in foot ulceration in diabetic patients (Caselli et al. 2002; D'Ambrogi et al. 2003). In that sense, the release of plantar fascia may have an effect on ulcer healing and has been proposed as an alternative procedure to Achilles tendon lengthening (see next subsection) for the management of diabetic foot ulcers (Dallimore and Kaminski 2015). One study assessed the effect of plantar fascia release on the healing of originally non-healing plantar foot ulcers and found that 36 of 60 ulcers healed in 6 weeks (Kim et al. 2012) However, more direct assessments of this relationship are needed.

ACHILLES TENDON

The Achilles tendon is a fibrous structure that originates at the midcalf position and inserts into the middle part of the posterior surface of the calcaneus. It is the thickest and strongest tendon in the body. Contraction of the calf muscles pulls the Achilles tendon, resulting in plantar flexion at the talocrural joint. Injuries or abnormalities of the Achilles tendon include tendinosis, rupture, and shortening (equinus deformity). In diabetes, the Achilles tendon has been studied mainly for morphological adaptations (length and thickness) and for lengthening of the tendon as treatment option in foot ulcer patients.

Achilles Tendon Shortening/Equinus Deformity

Using electron microscopic evaluations, reductions in the collagen content of the Achilles tendon in diabetic patients have been found and are likely related to the effects of nonenzymatic glycosylation (Grant et al. 1997). These changes cause a loss of resilience and a functionally shorter tendon, which increases joint stiffness and reduces the amount of dorsiflexion. The prevalence of equinus deformity (dorsiflexion <0°) in diabetic patients may be as high as 10.3% (Lavery et al. 2002), which shows that limitations in ankle joint mobility are prevalent and require serious attention in diagnosis and treatment.

Achilles Tendon Thickening

Just like the plantar fascia, the Achilles tendon may be thicker in diabetic patients (D'Ambrogi et al. 2003; Giacomozzi et al. 2005; Evranos et al. 2015; Afolabi et al. 2019). Tendon thickness at the calcaneal insertion was found to be 4.0 mm in healthy subjects, 4.6 mm in diabetic subjects, 4.9 mm in neuropathic diabetic patients, and 5.2 mm in patients with a history of ulceration (D'Ambrogi et al. 2003; Giacomozzi et al. 2005). Again, the likely cause of tendon thickening is nonenzymatic glycosylation. Alternatively, different walking strategies adopted by diabetic patients as a result of muscle weakness and/or neuropathy may lead to abnormal cumulative stresses in the tendon and cause the tendon to thicken (Maluf and Mueller 2003). Thickening of the Achilles tendon and plantar fascia is inversely correlated above a threshold of 3.0 mm fascia thickness (r^2 = 61%–79%) (Giacomozzi et al. 2005). As explanation, the dynamics of the foot during gait with a more flat-footed initial contact caused by plantar fascia thickening may lead to less mechanical stress in the tendon and, therefore, a lower rate of tendon thickening (Giacomozzi et al. 2005). This contrasts with the above-mentioned "walking strategy hypothesis" for tendon thickening and points to the need for prospective analyses to understand these relationships.

> ### 🔑 KEY POINT
>
> Reductions in the collagen content of the Achilles tendon in diabetic patients cause a loss of resilience and a functionally shorter tendon, increasing joint stiffness and reduced dorsiflexion. Additionally, the Achilles tendon may be thicker in diabetic patients. This causes an increase in peak plantar forefoot pressure. Achilles tendon lengthening significantly reduces this forefoot pressure and can be effective in healing and secondary prevention of plantar diabetic foot ulcers.

Biomechanical and Clinical Implications

Achilles tendon shortening or thickening has both biomechanical and clinical implications. Patients with

equinus deformity show higher dynamic forefoot pressures, likely because limited dorsiflexion causes an earlier heel rise during stance, which reduces the effective area to distribute pressures underneath the foot (Lavery et al. 2002; Orendurff et al. 2006; Searle et al. 2017). Patients with equinus have nearly three times greater risk for high foot pressure (>850 kPa) (Lavery et al. 2002). Furthermore, dorsiflexion range of motion (ROM) is significantly inversely correlated ($r = -0.39$) with forefoot pressure (Orendurff et al. 2006). Univariate analysis shows patients with equinus deformity to be at greater risk of having a foot ulcer (odds ratio 2.3) (Lavery et al. 1998). In multivariate models, inclusion of other factors such as hallux rigidus, claw-toe deformity, and elevated foot pressure removes the significance of equinus deformity.

Achilles tendon thickness has only been associated with foot pressure in multivariate models that also include plantar fascia thickness and first MTP joint mobility as factors (Giacomozzi et al. 2005). There is, overall, a low correlation ($r = 0.41$) between these structural parameters and foot pressure, but this increases substantially ($r = 0.83$) above a threshold of vertical forefoot loading (94% body weight), suggesting an important role for connective tissue changes in high foot pressures measured in diabetic patients. The Achilles tendon of diabetes patients has a reduced energy-saving capacity during walking and this is an important factor contributing to the increased metabolic cost of walking in these patients (Petrovic et al. 2018). Furthermore, nondiabetic tendons exhibit a superior biomechanical profile over diabetic tendons with regard to elasticity, maximum load, stiffness, toughness, load, energy, strain and elongation at break point, tenacity, and strain at automatic load drop ($p < 0.05$ for all comparisons) (Guney et al. 2015). The clinical implications of tendon thickening in the diabetic foot are not known. Overall, these data demonstrate the multicomponent pathogenesis of high foot pressures and ulceration in diabetes in which Achilles tendon changes may have a contributing role without being the most dominant explanatory factor.

Treatment: Achilles Tendon Lengthening

Lengthening of the Achilles tendon (ATL) has been used to overcome limited ankle dorsiflexion and to treat forefoot ulcers in equinus feet. In the immediate period after ATL treatment, forefoot pressures may reduce by as much as 27% (Armstrong et al. 1999; Maluf et al. 2004).

Additionally, dorsiflexion ROM may increase 15°, and plantar flexor power during gait may decrease 65% (Maluf et al. 2004). However, these biomechanical effects are not sustained over longer periods of time (8 months). The close association between forefoot pressures and plantar flexor muscle strength ($r = 0.60$) suggests that the return of pressure levels to baseline values over time may be due to a restrengthening of the plantar flexor muscles after ATL (Maluf et al. 2004).

Lengthening of the Achilles tendon can also be effective in healing and secondary prevention of plantar diabetic foot ulcers (Dallimore and Kaminski 2015; Colen et al. 2013). Between 93% and 100% of patients may heal successfully in about 40 days after ATL treatment, compared with 88% of patients healing in 58 days after total contact casting (Lin et al. 1996; Mueller et al. 2003). Furthermore, ulcer recurrence rates between 0% and 38% after 7 to 24 months have been found in patients treated with ATL compared with rates between 59% and 81% in patients treated with casting alone (Lin et al. 1996; Mueller et al. 2003). Colen et al. (2013) found that 25% of patients who received wound closure surgery alone developed recurrent ulceration requiring reoperation, compared with only 2% of patients who additionally underwent ATL, which represents a 94% relative risk reduction ($p < 0.001$). Despite these positive clinical results, several concerns have risen with using ATL treatment in diabetic patients (Mueller et al. 2004; Salsich et al. 2005; Dallimore and Kaminski 2015). Heel pressures can increase substantially, and as a result patients may develop plantar heel ulcers (Mueller et al. 2004). Self-perceived physical functioning may be reduced compared with pre-ATL levels and compared with conservative treatment (Mueller et al. 2004). This may require rehabilitative treatment aimed at improving gait performance and physical functioning in these patients. These complications have reduced the popularity of ATL in the treatment of plantar foot ulcers and has led to the discussion if there is still place for ATL in treatment of the diabetic foot (Tagoe et al. 2016). Thus, even though ATL seems a biomechanically and clinically effective treatment for foot ulcer patients, caution is required with this procedure because complications can arise and the effects may not persist over time.

LIMITED JOINT MOBILITY

Adequate mobility in the joints of the foot and ankle is an important prerequisite for normal gait. Motion at the talocrural, subtalar, and MTP joints allows for adaptation to the surface and shock-absorption in initial stance, progression of the foot and tibia in midstance, foot rigidity for leverage in propulsion, effective push-off in terminal stance, and foot clearance in swing. Joint mobility limitations can disturb normal foot progression and lead to biomechanical changes that may be of clinical importance. LJM affects 30% to 50% of diabetic patients (Frost and Beischer 2001).

Limited Joint Mobility in the Foot and Ankle

The results from several studies on joint mobility in the talocrural, subtalar, and MTP joints are summarized in Table 5.4.1. Joint ROM is significantly reduced in diabetic patients with a history of ulceration compared with diabetic and nondiabetic control subjects (Delbridge et al. 1988; Mueller et al. 1989; Fernando et al. 1991; Birke et al. 1995; Viswanathan et al. 2003; Zimny et al. 2004). Furthermore, subtalar joint ROM is significantly associated with first MTP joint ROM ($r = 0.53–0.59$) and was found to be smaller in patients who have been diagnosed with LJM in the hands, based on the "prayer sign." LJM affects the joints of the upper extremity and lower extremity to a more or less similar extent (Delbridge et al. 1988; Fernando et al. 1991). In Caucasian patients, LJM seems to be more prevalent than in Black or Hispanic patients (Veves et al. 1995; Frykberg et al. 1998).

Joint stiffness tends to follow the same pattern as joint mobility: stiffer joints in cases with more severe foot disease (Birke et al. 1995). Whereas nonenzymatic glycosylation is probably causative of LJM seen in diabetic patients, this does not fully explain the different findings with different states of foot disease. The role of peripheral neuropathy in joint mobility in diabetic patients is not clear (Viswanathan et al. 2003; Zimny et al. 2004). Analysis of disease progression in conjunction with the development of LJM is necessary and will require prospective studies.

 KEY POINT

Joint range of motion is significantly reduced in diabetic patients, which causes an increase in forefoot plantar pressure and higher risk of developing foot ulcers. Mobilization training may improve joint range of motion but has only a small effect of peak pressure.

TABLE 5.4.1   Joint Range of Motion (ROM) and Stiffness Data for the Foot and Ankle in Different Groups of Diabetic Patients and Healthy Controls

	Diabetes and Previous Ulcer	Diabetes and Neuropathy	Diabetes Control	Healthy Control
Subtalar joint ROM (°)				
Delbridge et al. (1988)	17.9		31.1	35.2
Mueller et al. (1989)	26		31	35
Fernando et al. (1991)		29, 18[a]	29, 20[a]	30
Birke et al. (1995)	24.7,[b] 25.7[c]		32.3	31.7
Viswanathan et al. (2003)	28.8	34.3	48.0	55.3
Zimny et al. (2004)		17.9	28.4	31
Talocrural Joint Dorsiflexion (°)				
Birke et al. (1995)	2.2,[b] 3.6[c]		5.9	5.9
First MTP Joint ROM (°)				
Birke et al. (1995)	34.7,[b] 31.6[c]		46.8	47.2
Viswanathan et al. (2003)	44.5	53.3	73.0	91.3
Zimny et al. (2004)		35.3	62.0	59.4
First MTP Joint Stiffness (kg/cm)				
Birke et al. (1995)	12.1,[b] 10.3[c]		8.9	9.7

[a]Patients with diagnosed LJM based on the "prayer sign."
[b]Patients with previous ulcer at the first metatarsal head.
[c]Patients with previous ulcer at other locations.
Abbreviations: LJM, limited joint mobility (LJM); MTP, metatarsal–phalangeal joint.

Biomechanical Implications

Foot pressures can be substantially higher in diabetic patients with LJM than in patients without LJM. In one study, average peak pressures were 1425 kPa in neuropathic diabetic patients with LJM, 1250 kPa in diabetic patients with LJM, 1010 kPa in neuropathic patients without LJM, 565 kPa in diabetic controls, and 550 kPa in healthy controls (Fernando et al. 1991). Furthermore, joint ROM is strongly associated with measured dynamic forefoot pressures (Fig. 5.4.4) (Fernando et al. 1991; Birke et al. 1995; Zimny et al. 2004). Correlation coefficients were −0.67 to −0.70 for subtalar joint mobility (Fernando et al. 1991; Zimny et al. 2004) and −0.62 to −0.71 for first MTP joint ROM (Birke et al. 1995; Zimny et al. 2004). In the presence of LJM, the foot and ankle seem to lose their capacity to absorb shock and progress the foot effectively through stance, resulting in a reduced efficacy to maintain normal foot pressures. Finally, LJM measured at the first MTP and subtalar joints was found to be 80% sensitive and 90% specific to differentiate between high- and low-risk patients (Zimny et al. 2004). For these reasons, joint mobility assessment may accurately identify patients with high plantar foot pressures who are at risk for plantar ulceration and may therefore be useful for foot screening purposes.

Clinical Implications

As was discussed in a previous paragraph, diabetic patients with a history of foot ulceration have smaller joint ROM and stiffer joints (Delbridge et al. 1988; Birke et al. 1988). In these patients, subtalar joint ROM seems smaller in the affected foot (with ulcer) than in the non-affected foot. The foot site showing the most significant LJM matched the site of prior foot ulceration in 79% of cases (Mueller et al. 1989). Additionally, patients with LJM show a much higher prevalence of prior foot ulcers (65%) than patients without LJM (5%) (Fernando et al. 1991). Although these findings support the hypothesis of a link between LJM and foot ulceration in diabetic patients, in which elevated plantar foot pressure is probably the mediating factor (Fernando et al. 1991), cause-and-effect relationships cannot yet be established.

Joint mobility has been assessed as part of a multicomponent analysis of foot ulceration in several prospective

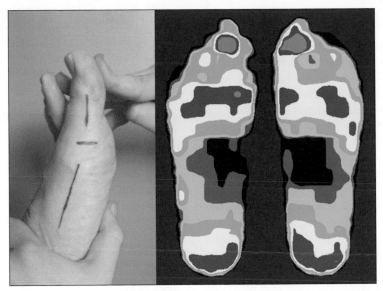

Fig. 5.4.4 The association between limited joint mobility (LJM) in the first metatarsal–phalangeal (MTP) joint and the elevated dynamic plantar foot pressures measured at the great toe in both feet shown as warm pink and red colors.

studies. These show that LJM in the foot and ankle may be a risk factor in foot ulceration (univariate model odds ratio 2.1:4.6) (Lavery et al. 1998; Boyko et al. 1999). However, in multivariate analysis only LJM at the MTP joint (hallux rigidus), albeit in combination with the presence of claw-toe deformity, remained a significant factor (Lavery et al. 1998). Joint mobility was significantly reduced by 2 degrees in the subtalar joint and by 14 degrees in the first MTP joint in patients who developed an ulcer. However, odds ratios were small (0.97) and not significant in multivariate analysis (Pham et al. 2000). These data suggest that although LJM is a contributing factor in diabetic foot ulceration, other factors such as neuropathy and some foot deformities have more prominent roles. Although joint mobility assessment may be used for foot-screening purposes, simple measures of neuropathy and foot deformity may be more important to determine risk for foot ulceration.

Treatment: Joint Mobilization

In clinical practice, generally only the consequences of LJM are treated; for example, by prescribing therapeutic footwear to patients with LJM. Joint mobilization through physical therapy is applied on only a small scale, even though it has been suggested that this may potentially benefit these patients (Mueller et al. 1989). The effects of mobility-related exercises on outcomes of joint mobility, plantar pressure, and neuropathy symptoms has been extensively reviewed and shows that

neuropathy symptoms and joint mobility may improve and that effects on plantar pressure are variable and small (van Netten et al. 2020b). These studies do show that patients may require lifelong treatment in order to achieve lasting improvements. Such foot-related mobility exercises do not appear to help prevent a diabetic foot ulcer (van Netten et al. 2020a). More well-designed prospective studies are required on these topics.

CONCLUSIONS

The diabetic foot is a complex and serious complication of diabetes, with many negative outcomes requiring medical treatment. This chapter emphasized changes occurring in the subcutaneous and periarticular structures of the foot that may have implications for foot biomechanics and diabetic foot ulcer risk. Consistent findings are the presence of thicker plantar fascia, thicker and shorter Achilles tendon, and limitations in the mobility of the foot and ankle joints, all leading to increased plantar foot pressures in diabetic patients. Data on the presence of plantar fascia rupture in diabetes are inconclusive. Nonenzymatic glycosylation of connective tissue is regarded as the mechanism for these changes, even though a direct association has never been established. Although data are lacking for plantar fascia, patients with the other structural abnormalities are at greater risk for foot ulceration, but the contribution of other patient-related and biomechanical factors in ulcer development may be more significant. There is little research on the management of these structural abnormalities. Only lengthening of the Achilles tendon in diabetic patients has been shown to be effective in healing and secondary prevention of foot ulcers; although, complications may arise that caution the application of this procedure in the diabetic foot and may require adequate rehabilitative treatment to improve physical functioning. Foot-related exercises may improve joint mobility in order to treat LJM in the foot and ankle but has no significant effect on peak pressure. No treatment options are known for changes in plantar fascia and thickening of the Achilles tendon. Clearly, more research is needed to improve our understanding of the treatment of plantar fascia, Achilles tendon, and joint mobility abnormalities in patients with a diabetic foot.

Summary

The diabetic foot is a complex and serious complication of diabetes, with many negative outcomes requiring medical treatment. Changes in the subcutaneous and periarticular structures of the foot may have implications for foot biomechanics and diabetic foot ulcer risk. Consistent findings are the presence of thicker plantar fascia, thicker and shorter Achilles tendon, and limitations in the mobility of the foot and ankle joints, all leading to increased plantar foot pressures in diabetic patients. Nonenzymatic glycosylation of connective tissue is regarded as the mechanism for these changes, even though a direct association has never been established. Although data are lacking for plantar fascia, patients with the other structural abnormalities are at greater risk for foot ulceration, but the contribution of other patient-related and biomechanical factors in ulcer development may be more significant. There is little research on the management of these structural abnormalities. Only lengthening of the Achilles tendon in diabetic patients has been shown to be effective in healing and secondary prevention of foot ulcers; although, complications may arise that caution the application of this procedure. Foot-related exercises may improve joint mobility in the foot and ankle but has no significant effect on peak pressure. No treatment options are known for changes in plantar fascia and thickening of the Achilles tendon. Clearly, more research is needed to improve our understanding of the treatment of plantar fascia, Achilles tendon, and joint mobility abnormalities in patients with diabetic foot disease.

REFERENCES

Abate, M., Schiavone, C., Di Carlo, L., Salini, V., 2012. Achilles tendon and plantar fascia in recently diagnosed type II diabetes: Role of body mass index. Clin. Rheumatol. 31, 1109–1113.

Abbott, C.A., Vileikyte, L., Williamson, S., Carrington, A.L., Boulton, A.J., 1998. Multicenter study of the incidence of and predictive risk factors for diabetic neuropathic foot ulceration. Diabetes Care 21, 1071–1075.

Afolabi, B.I., Ayoola, O.O., Idowu, B.M., Kolawole, B.A., Omisore, A.D., 2019. Sonographic evaluation of the Achilles tendon and plantar fascia of type 2 diabetics in Nigeria. J. Med. Ultrasound 27, 86–91.

Andreassen, T.T., Seyer-Hansen, K., Oxlund, H., 1981. Biomechanical changes in connective tissues induced by experimental diabetes. Acta Endocrinol. (Copenh.) 98, 432–436.

Arangio, G.A., Chen, C., Salathe, E.P., 1998. Effect of varying arch height with and without the plantar fascia on the mechanical properties of the foot. Foot Ankle Int. 19, 705–709.

Armstrong, D.G., Boulton, A.J.M., Bus, S.A., 2017. Diabetic foot ulcers and their recurrence. N. Engl. J. Med. 376, 2367–2375.

Armstrong, D.G., Stacpoole-Shea, S., Nguyen, H., Harkless, L.B., 1999. Lengthening of the Achilles tendon in diabetic patients who are at high risk for ulceration of the foot. J. Bone Joint Surg. Am. 81, 535–538.

Bailey, A.J., 1981. The nonenzymatic glycosylation of proteins. Horm. Metab. Res. Suppl. 11, 90–94.

Birke, J.A., Cornwall, M.W., Jackson, M., 1988. Relationship between hallux limitus and ulceration of the great toe. J. Orthop. Sports Phys. Ther. 10, 172–176.

Birke, J.A., Franks, B.D., Foto, J.G., 1995. First ray joint limitation, pressure, and ulceration of the first metatarsal head in diabetes mellitus. Foot Ankle Int. 16, 277–284.

Bojsen-Moller, F., Flagstad, K.E., 1976. Plantar aponeurosis and internal architecture of the ball of the foot. J. Anat. 121, 599–611.

Bolton, N.R., Smith, K.E., Pilgram, T.K., Mueller, M.J., Bae, K.T., 2005. Computed tomography to visualize and quantify the plantar aponeurosis and flexor hallucis longus tendon in the diabetic foot. Clin. Biomech. (Bristol, Avon) 20, 540–546.

Boulton, A.J., Kirsner, R.S., Vileikyte, L., 2004. Clinical practice. Neuropathic diabetic foot ulcers. N. Engl. J. Med. 351, 48–55.

Boyko, E.J., Ahroni, J.H., Stensel, V., et al. 1999. A prospective study of risk factors for diabetic foot ulcer. The Seattle Diabetic Foot Study. Diabetes Care 22, 1036–1042.

Brownlee, M., Cerami, A., Vlassara, H., 1988. Advanced glycosylation end products in tissue and the biochemical basis of diabetic complications. N. Engl. J. Med. 318, 1315–1321.

Bus, S.A., 2004. Foot Deformity in Diabetic Neuropathy: A Radiological and Biomechanical Analysis. Doctoral dissertation. University of Amsterdam, Amsterdam, The Netherlands.

Caselli, A., Pham, H., Giurini, J.M., Armstrong, D.G., Veves, A., 2002. The forefoot-to-rearfoot plantar pressure ratio is increased in severe diabetic neuropathy and can predict foot ulceration. Diabetes Care 25, 1066–1071.

Chuter, V., Payne, C., 2001. Limited joint mobility and plantar fascia function in Charcot's neuroarthropathy. Diabet. Med. 18, 558–561.

Colen, L.B., Kim, C.J., Grant, W.P., Yeh, J.T., Hind, B., 2013. Achilles tendon lengthening: friend or foe in the diabetic foot? Plast. Reconstr. Surg. 131, 37e–43e.

Crisp, A.J., Heathcote, J.G., 1984. Connective tissue abnormalities in diabetes mellitus. J. R. Coll. Physicians Lond. 18, 132–141.

Dallimore, S.M., Kaminski, M.R., 2015. Tendon lengthening and fascia release for healing and preventing diabetic foot ulcers: a systematic review and meta-analysis. J. Foot Ankle Res. 8, 33.

D'Ambrogi, E., Giurato, L., D'Agostino, M.A., et al., 2003. Contribution of plantar fascia to the increased forefoot pressures in diabetic patients. Diabetes Care 26, 1525–1529.

Delbridge, L., Ellis, C.S., Robertson, K., Lequesne, L.P., 1985. Non-enzymatic glycosylation of keratin from the stratum corneum of the diabetic foot. Br. J. Dermatol. 112, 547–554.

Delbridge, L., Perry, P., Marr, S., et al., 1988. Limited joint mobility in the diabetic foot: relationship to neuropathic ulceration. Diabet. Med. 5, 333–337.

Evranos, B., Idilman, I., Ipek, A., Polat, S.B., Cakir, B., Ersoy, R., 2015. Real-time sonoelastography and ultrasound evaluation of the Achilles tendon in patients with diabetes with or without foot ulcers: a cross sectional study. J. Diabetes Complications 29, 1124–1129.

Fernando, D.J., Masson, E.A., Veves, A., Boulton, A.J., 1991. Relationship of limited joint mobility to abnormal foot pressures and diabetic foot ulceration. Diabetes Care 14, 8–11.

Frost, D., Beischer, W., 2001. Limited joint mobility in type 1 diabetic patients: associations with microangiopathy and subclinical macroangiopathy are different in men and women. Diabetes Care 24, 95–99.

Frykberg, R.G., Lavery, L.A., Pham, H., et al. 1998. Role of neuropathy and high foot pressures in diabetic foot ulceration. Diabetes Care 21, 1714–1719.

Giacomozzi, C., D'Ambrogi, E., Uccioli, L., Macellari, V., 2005. Does the thickening of Achilles tendon and plantar fascia contribute to the alteration of diabetic foot loading? Clin. Biomech. (Bristol, Avon) 20, 532–539.

Grant, W.P., Sullivan, R., Sonenshine, D.E., et al., 1997. Electron microscopic investigation of the effects of diabetes mellitus on the Achilles tendon. J. Foot Ankle Surg. 36, 272–278.

Guney, A., Vatansever, F., Karaman, I., et al., 2015. Biomechanical properties of Achilles tendon in diabetic vs. non-diabetic patients. Exp. Clin. Endocrinol Diabetes. 123, 428–432.

Hicks, J.H., 1954. The mechanics of the foot. II. The plantar aponeurosis and the arch. J. Anat. 88, 25–30.

International Diabetes Foundation, 2019. IDF Diabetes Atlas, ninth ed. Available from: https://diabetesatlas.org.

Kim, J.Y., Hwang, S., Lee, Y., 2012. Selective plantar fascia release for nonhealing diabetic plantar ulcerations. J. Bone Joint Surg. Am. 94. 1297–1302.

Lavery, L.A., Armstrong, D.G., Boulton, A.J., 2002. Ankle equinus deformity and its relationship to high plantar pressure in a large population with diabetes mellitus. J. Am. Podiatr. Med. Assoc 92, 479–482.

Lavery, L.A., Armstrong, D.G., Vela, S.A., Quebedeaux, T.L., Fleischli, J.G., 1998. Practical criteria for screening patients at high risk for diabetic foot ulceration. Arch. Intern. Med. 158, 157–162.

Lazzarini, P.A., Crews, R.T., van Netten, J.J., et al., 2019. Measuring plantar tissue stress in people with diabetic peripheral neuropathy: A critical concept in diabetic foot management. J. Diabetes Sci. Technol. 13, 869–880.

Lin, S.S., Lee, T.H., Wapner, K.L., 1996. Plantar forefoot ulceration with equinus deformity of the ankle in diabetic patients: The effect of tendo-Achilles lengthening and total contact casting. Orthopedics 19, 465–475.

Maluf, K.S., Mueller, M.J., 2003. Novel Award 2002. Comparison of physical activity and cumulative plantar tissue stress among subjects with and without diabetes mellitus and a history of recurrent plantar ulcers. Clin. Biomech. (Bristol, Avon) 18, 567–575.

Maluf, K.S., Mueller, M.J., Strube, M.J., Engsberg, J.R., Johnson, J.E., 2004. Tendon Achilles lengthening for the treatment of neuropathic ulcers causes a temporary reduction in forefoot pressure associated with changes in plantar flexor power rather than ankle motion during gait. J. Biomech. 37, 897–906.

Mueller, M.J., Diamond, J.E., Delitto, A., Sinacore, D.R., 1989. Insensitivity, limited joint mobility, and plantar ulcers in patients with diabetes mellitus. Phys. Ther. 69, 453–459.

Mueller, M.J., Sinacore, D.R., Hastings, M.K., et al. 2004. Impact of achilles tendon lengthening on functional limitations and perceived disability in people with a neuropathic plantar ulcer. Diabetes Care 27, 1559–1564.

Mueller, M.J., Sinacore, D.R., Hastings, M.K., Strube, M.J., Johnson, J.E., 2003. Effect of Achilles tendon lengthening on neuropathic plantar ulcers. A randomized clinical trial. J. Bone Joint Surg. Am. 85-A, 1436–1445.

Orendurff, M.S., Rohr, E.S., Sangeorzan, B.J., Weaver, K., Czerniecki, J.M., 2006. An equinus deformity of the ankle accounts for only a small amount of the increased forefoot plantar pressure in patients with diabetes. J. Bone Joint Surg. Br. 88, 65–68.

Petrovic, M., Maganaris, C.N., Deschamps, K., et al., 2018. Altered Achilles tendon function during walking in people with diabetic neuropathy: Implications for metabolic energy saving. J. Appl. Physiol. (1985) 124, 1333–1340.

Pham, H., Armstrong, D.A., Harvey, C., et al. 2000. Screening techniques to identify people at high risk for diabetic foot ulceration. Diabetes Care 23, 606–611.

Salsich, G.B., Mueller, M.J., Hastings, M.K., et al. 2005. Effect of Achilles tendon lengthening on ankle muscle performance in people with diabetes mellitus and a neuropathic plantar ulcer. Phys. Ther. 85, 34–43.

Sarrafian, S.K., 1983. Anatomy of the Foot and Ankle. JB Lippincott Co, Philadelphia, PA.

Schnider, S.L., Kohn, R.R., 1980. Glucosylation of human collagen in aging and diabetes mellitus. J. Clin. Invest. 66, 1179–1181.

Searle, A., Spink, M.J., Ho, A., Chuter, V.H., 2017. Association between ankle equinus and plantar pressures in people with diabetes. A systematic review and meta-analysis. Clin. Biomech. 43, 8–14.

Sharkey, N.A., Donahue, S.W., Ferris, L., 1999. Biomechanical consequences of plantar fascial release or rupture during gait. Part II: alterations in forefoot loading. Foot Ankle Int. 20, 86–96.

Sharkey, N.A., Ferris, L., Donahue, S.W., 1998. Biomechanical consequences of plantar fascial release or rupture during gait. Part I: disruptions in longitudinal arch conformation. Foot Ankle Int. 19, 812–820.

Tagoe, M.T., Reeves, N.D., Bowling, F.L., 2016. Is there still a place for Achilles tendon lengthening? Diabetes Metab. Res. Rev. 32 (Suppl. 1), 227–231.

Taylor, R., Stainsby, G.D., Richardson, D.L., 1998. Rupture of the plantar fascia in the diabetic foot leads to toe dorsiflexion deformity. Diabetologia 41, A277.

Theodorou, D.J., Theodorou, S.J., Kakitsubata, Y., et al., 2000. Plantar fasciitis and fascial rupture: MR imaging findings in 26 patients supplemented with anatomic data in cadavers. Radiographics 20, Spec No, 181–197.

Theodorou, D.J., Theodorou, S.J., Resnick, D., 2002. MR imaging of abnormalities of the plantar fascia. Semin. Musculoskelet. Radiol. 6, 105–118.

Van Netten, J.J., Raspovic, A., Lavery, L.A., et al., on behalf of the International Working Group on the Diabetic Foot (IWGDF), 2020a. Prevention of foot ulcers in the at-risk patient with diabetes: a systematic review (update). Diabetes Metab. Res. Reviews, 36 (Suppl. 1), e3270. doi:10.1002/dmrr.3270

Van Netten, J.J., Sacco, I.C.N., Lavery, L.A., et al., on behalf of the International Working Group on the Diabetic Foot (IWGDF), 2020b. Treatment of modifiable risk factors for foot ulceration in persons with diabetes: a systematic review. Diabetes Metab. Res. Reviews, 36 (Suppl. 1), e3271. doi:10.1002/dmrr.3271.

Veves, A., Sarnow, M.R., Giurini, J.M., et al., 1995. Differences in joint mobility and foot pressures between black and white diabetic patients. Diabet. Med. 12, 585–589.

Viswanathan, V., Snehalatha, C., Sivagami, M., Seena, R., Ramachandran, A., 2003. Association of limited joint mobility and high plantar pressure in diabetic foot ulceration in Asian Indians. Diabetes Res. Clin. Pract. 60, 57–61.

Zimny, S., Schatz, H., Pfohl, M., 2004. The role of limited joint mobility in diabetic patients with an at-risk foot. Diabetes Care 27, 942–946.

Trigger Points as a Fascia-Related Disorder

Roland U. Gautschi

CHAPTER CONTENTS

TRIGGER POINTS

Myofascial trigger points (mTrPs) very commonly play a role in patients with problems in the musculoskeletal system, including tension-type headaches, migraine, neck pain, nonspecific back pain, shoulder pain, shoulder pain associated with subacromial impingement, lateral elbow pain, forearm and hand pain, posture and stress-related pains associated with computer use, hip and groin pain, knee pain, foot pain, temporomandibular joint disease, and pains in the bladder and urogenital region (Gautschi 2019).

 KEY POINTS

TrPs are widespread and are a very common cause of pain and/or dysfunction.

In the original sense of the word, a trigger point (TrP) is a point from which symptoms known to the patient, mostly in the form of referred pain, are caused (or triggered). Various types of TrPs have been distinguished (Travell and Simons 1999; Gautschi 2019):
- *Active or latent TrPs.* Active TrPs already demonstrate their characteristic pain pattern during physiological strain or movement, and sometimes even at rest. Provoking an active TrP by using pressure or stretching (or needling), this mechanical stimulation reproduces the pain (localized or referred) familiar to the patient. In contrast to this, latent TrPs are not spontaneously painful at rest or during physiological strain/exercise; latent TrPs are clinically silent. Not until the latent trigger point is provoked by strong pressure, a pain—mostly referred pain—can be triggered; but the patient is not familiar with this pain from his/her everyday experiences. Latent TrPs can demonstrate all the clinical characteristics of active TrPs—with one exception: it is not possible to reproduce the current symptoms from latent TrPs.
- Depending on the manner and time of occurrence of a TrP, primary TrPs are differentiated from secondary TrPs (into synergists and antagonists) and satellite TrPs (arising in the referred pain zone of a primary TrP).
- If a TrP is in the muscle tissue, it is described as a myofascial trigger point. If a TrP lies in a tendon, a ligament, or in the periosteum, etc., it is known, respectively, as a tendinous, ligamentary, or periosteal TrP.

 KEY POINTS

There are different types of mTrPs:
- active or latent mTrPs
- primary, secondary, or satellite TrPs
- myofascial, tendinous, ligamentary, or periosteal TrPs

Pathophysiology

Myofascial trigger points (mTrPs) are nowadays a scientifically thoroughly researched phenomenon in the field of neuromusculoskeletal medicine.

There is pathophysiological evidence of localized hypoxia in the center of an mTrP (Brückle et al. 1990), a changed EMG potential, which can be interpreted as a sign of the malfunction of motor endplates (Travell and Simons 1999), and characteristic changes in the biochemistry. In the immediate surroundings of an mTrP, the concentration of substance P and CGRP; bradykinin; serotonin; norepinephrine (noradrenaline); tumor necrosis factor-α (TNF-α); and interleukin (IL)-1β, IL-6, and IL-8 are markedly elevated, whereas the pH value is definitely reduced (Shah et al. 2005, 2008). The low pH value (5.4 instead of 6.6) and the two to four times increased concentration of pain and inflammatory mediators (compared with the reference tissue without active mTrPs) lead to a change in nociceptor activity in the sense of peripheral sensitization.

> ### KEY POINTS
>
> The biochemical milieu of muscle at the site of mTrPs is altered:
> - Increased concentration of mediators for pain and inflammation (substance P, CGRP, bradykinin, and others)
> - Lower pH value (acid environment)

Rigor complexes have been histomorphologically documented in the core zone of mTrPs (myosin and actin filaments persisted in maximally close position) with reactive overextension of the bordering sarcomeres (Simons and Stolov 1976) and intramuscular connective tissue changes (Feigl-Reitinger et al. 1998).

The pathophysiological changes are like individual mosaic stones that fit together to form a picture. The factors that combine in the formation of mTrPs are summarized in the "energy crisis model" (Fig. 5.5.1) (Travell and Simons 1999; Mense et al. 2001).

Dysfunctional motor endplates (characterized by low-threshold distribution of acetylcholine; Fig. 5.5.1, arrow A) or traumatic damage to the sarcoplasmic reticulum (by strain, traumatic overextension, or direct injury of a muscle with partial rupture of the sarcoplasmic reticulum; Fig. 5.5.1, arrow B) cause a permanent contraction of locally restricted muscle fiber sections (contraction knot). Contraction knots compress the local blood vessels, and the reduced perfusion (local ischemia) causes a local oxygen deficit (hypoxia). The permanent contraction in the contraction knot is associated with an increased energy requirement (ATP). The combination of increased metabolic requirements (from continuous activity of the contractile elements) and the reduced perfusion with diminished oxygen supply causes a pronounced, locally circumscribed energy crisis (ATP deficiency) with an area of local hypoxia at its center.

Local ischemia, which leads to local hypoxia, prevents the synthesis of sufficient adenosine triphosphate (ATP) in the muscle tissue. As a result of the ATP deficiency, the calcium ion pump fails (so that the contraction process in the muscle continues constantly—which also exhausts the available ATP) and the "softening effect" of the ATP, which is necessary to lose the actin-myosin bond, cannot function. Myosin and actin filaments therefore remain interconnected (rigor complex). Persistent rigor complexes in locally circumscribed areas of muscle fibers are the pathophysiological substrate of a myofascial trigger point. The muscle fiber sections bordering the shortened sarcomeres are overextended and lengthened as compensation. The affected muscle fibers are overall shortened and palpable as taut bands.

> ### KEY POINTS
>
> The center of an mTrP is characterized by severe hypoxia (Brückle et al. 1990).

The local ischemia within the mTrP can produce local tissue necrosis and thus cause local inflammatory processes. Freshly formed connective tissue begins to contract under the influence of myofibroblasts (van Wingerden 1995) and results in the formation of a connective tissue scar. The shortened connective tissue prevents the decontraction of the shortened sarcomeres in the TrP-region, thus fixating them structurally (Dejung 2009). Connective tissue shortening and changes (pathological crosslinks) gather both intramuscular collagenic tissue (endomysium, perimysium) and muscle fascia and intermuscular collagenic tissue over time (i.e., with chronic myofascial pain syndromes).

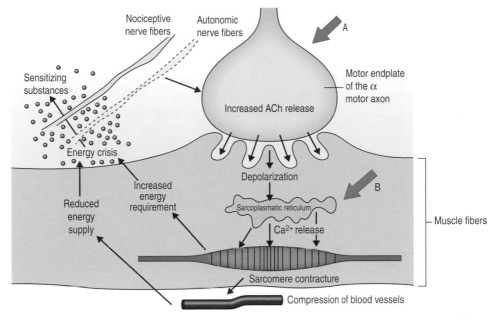

Fig. 5.5.1 Model of energy crisis for the developing of mTrPs. From Travell, J.G., Simons, D.G., 1999. Myofascial Pain and Dysfunction. The Trigger Point Manual. vol. 1, second ed. Williams & Wilkins, Baltimore, with permission.

Histomorphological examination shows that in muscle tissues with mTrPs, the endomysial spaces between the individual muscle fibers are always narrower than in controls without mTrPs (Feigl-Reitinger et al. 1998; Fig. 5.5.2). This can be interpreted as a sign of the previously described shrinking process.

Local ischemia acts as a nociceptive stimulus and leads to the release of sensitizing substances; myofascial pain is thus ischemic pain (Dejung 2009).

> **KEY POINTS**
>
> Local hypoxia is the core of the energy crisis model. Local hypoxia has been proven experimentally (Brückle et al. 1990). Hypoxia results in the insufficient production of ATP and leads thus to rigor complexes (lack of softening effect of ATP). Local hypoxia provokes local tissue necrosis and thus local inflammatory process. This causes connective tissue alterations (shrinking, pathological crosslinks).

Clinical Symptoms

Disturbances directly induced by mTrPs are manifest in the form of:

- *Pain (local and referred)* with manifold qualities (dragging, stabbing, burning, or dull; definitely delimited or diffuse; superficial or "deep in the joint", etc.). The trigger point activity is sometimes expressed in the form of paresthesia, dysesthesia, or hypoesthesia (tingling, burning, feeling "as if restricted by a tight cuff" or feeling "something is swollen," numbness, etc.).
- *Motor dysfunction:* Muscle weakness without atrophy, induced reflexively or by pain, and intramuscular and intermuscular coordination disorders are directly caused by mTrPs (Travell and Simons 1999; Lucas et al. 2004, 2010; Ivanichev 2007; Arendt-Nielsen and Graven-Nielsen 2008; Ibarra et al. 2011; Ge et al. 2012, 2014).
- *Autonomic symptoms:* TrPs frequently cause autonomic phenomena (Travell and Simons 1999). They can manifest themselves in many ways, both in the area of the trigger point itself and in the

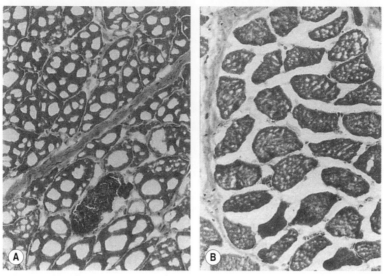

Fig. 5.5.2 In muscle tissue with mTrPs, the endomysial spaces are always narrower than in controls without mTrPs. Electron microscope image, enlarged 300 times. (A) Muscle tissue with mTrPs: shrunken endomysium. (B) Control without mTrPs: endomysium normal. From Feigl-Reitinger, A., Radner, H., Tilscher, H., et al., 1998. Der chronische Rückenschmerz: Histomorphologische Veränderungen der Muskulatur entlang der Wirbelsäule als Substrat der Myogelose. In: Feigl-Reitinger, A., Bergsmann, O., Tischer, H. (Eds.), Myogelose und Triggerpunkte. Facultas, Wien, with permission.

referred pain area: increase of skin temperature in the area of the mTrP, changes to the skin temperature and metabolism in the area of the referred pain, increased sweat secretion, nausea or dizziness, sleep disturbances, etc. They are interpreted as reflex responses of the sympathetic nervous system (Dejung 2009).

MTrPs cause taut bands and connective tissue changes, which themselves can cause a series of problems. Such **disturbances indirectly induced by mTrPs** include, for example:

- *Impaired intramuscular and intermuscular coordination:* Economy of movement is prevented by taut bands and connective tissue changes. As a result, this leads to poor posture and strain of the muscles and joints as well as poor muscle-fascia interaction (e.g., reduced catapult effect; details in Gautschi 2019).
- *Restricted range of motion:* Taut bands induce muscle shortening, which in turn leads to reduced range of motion and articular dysfunction (Lewit 2007). Fascia adhesions between neighboring muscles often cause drastically restricted mobility.

- *Perfusion disorders:* If the taut bands compress the blood vessels, this leads to perfusion disorders (formation of edema) and trophic/metabolic disorders.
- *Neuromuscular entrapment:* Neural structures perforate the muscles at many sites. If at these sites there are fascial changes or tensed muscle fibers as a result of mTrPs, they exert pressure on the nerve structure. The nerve tissue is less well perfused, and symptoms such as dysesthesia, weakness, and metabolic disorder/trophism develop in the area supplied by the nerve.
- *Irritation of deep sensitivity, proprioception, and nociception:* Connective tissue disorders alter the flow of impulses coming from the receptors that lie in the connective tissue of the muscle.
- *Peripheral chronification:* Connective tissue shortening overlie and fix the rigor complex, which means peripheral chronification of myofascial pain.

The sum of all the direct and indirect disturbances induced by mTrPs and fascial disorders is known as **myofascial syndrome** (MFS).

> ### KEY POINT
>
> The term "myofascial syndrome" (MFS) refers to all the symptoms that are triggered directly or indirectly by mTrPs and fascial disorders.

Diagnosis

Manual palpation is the most commonly used method to identify mTrPs in everyday clinical practice. Diagnosis by palpation is based on three main criteria (Fernandez-de-Las-Penas and Dommerholt 2018; Gautschi 2019; Travell and Simons 1999):

- Identification of the taut band belonging to the mTrP.
- Finding the most tender spot along the taut band.
- Reproduction of the pain pattern and/or other symptoms recognized by the patient on mechanical provocation of the mTrP (pressure, stretching, needling).

Other characteristics occur with many, but not all, mTrPs and help confirm the diagnosis. These may include palpable knots at the site of the mTrP, referred pain, or a local twitch response to mechanical stimulation of the mTrP.

The reliability of the clinical diagnosis of mTrPs has been tested in various studies. It was revealed that the intertest reliability of the identification of mTrPs varies a great deal and indeed depends on the knowledge and experience of the therapist. The kappa values differ a great deal depending on the study, and they range from poor reproducibility ($k = 0.35$) for nontrained and/or inexperienced therapists (Nice et al. 1992; Wolfe et al. 1992) to moderate (Njoo and van der Does 1994; Hsieh et al. 2000) and excellent reproducibility ($k = 0.8$) for specifically trained therapists and those experienced in palpation (Gerwin et al. 1997; Sciotti et al. 2001; Al-Shenqiti and Oldham 2005; Bron et al. 2007; Licht et al. 2007; Myburgh et al. 2011; Mayoral Del Moral et al. 2018; Barbero et al. 2019; Dommerholt et al. 2019).

Etiology

At the center of trigger point pathology there is a locally pronounced hypoxia (in particular an energy crisis; Fig. 5.5.1). Various causes can lead to a lack of oxygen and reduced energy (ATP deficiency) in the muscle tissue and, as a result, to persistent rigor complexes and thus to contraction knots. The most common

etiological factors can be summarized as developing mechanisms in the following categories:

- Direct trauma (e.g., muscle injury as a result of direct forceful impact in sports activities, accidents, etc.).
- Acute overstretch injury of the muscles (e.g., caused by sports activities or accident).
- Acute overload (e.g., caused by sports activities or accident).
- Chronic overload of the muscles (e.g., caused by poor posture, repetitive motion sequences at work or in training, long-term muscle activity in shortened or stretched position, eccentric muscle activity, stress-induced strain, etc.).
- Trigger point activity in other muscles (functional chains with secondary TrPs in synergists and antagonists, trigger point chains with satellite TrPs).

The indicated etiological factors frequently lead initially to the formation of latent TrPs, which are clinically silent. Latent TrPs can be activated by the further effect of developing mechanisms but also by contributory factors such as cold, wet, draught, stress, etc. which do not have a damaging effect in healthy muscle tissue (so-called activating mechanisms; Fig. 5.5.3). Active TrPs for their part can be retransformed by deactivation processes (such as rest, the body's own regeneration processes, therapy) to latent TrPs or healthy muscle tissue (Fig. 5.5.3).

Chronic myofascial pain is largely caused by a combination of various factors, when predisposing (e.g., poor level of fitness with reduced stamina), causative (e.g., acute overload or overstretch), and perpetuating

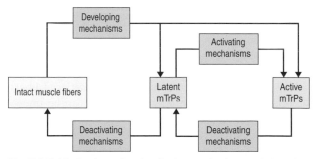

Fig. 5.5.3 Mechanisms for developing, activation, and deactivation of mTrPs. Relationship between latent and active myofascial trigger points. From Gautschi, R., 2019. Manual Trigger Point Therapy. Recognizing, Understanding, and Treating Myofascial Pain and Dysfunction. Thieme, Stuttgart, with permission.

factors (e.g., poor posture at work, trigger point activity in synergists or antagonists, reduced endogenous deactivation mechanisms) frequently work together (details in Gautschi 2019).

KEY POINTS

From the clinician's viewpoint, mTrPs are most commonly caused by:

- **Acute factors**
  - Direct trauma
  - Acute muscle overstretch injury
  - Acute overload (e.g., caused by sports or injury)
- **Chronic muscle overload**
  - Long-lasting contraction in an approximated position (postural, work, or sport related)
  - Repetitive strain injury
  - Eccentric muscle activity
  - Stress-induced overload
  - Nonmuscular primary factors (arthrogenic, neurogenic, viscerogenic, fascial, or psychogenic factors) can cause reflexive muscle tension and overload (secondary myofascial syndrome [MFS]).
- **Trigger point activity in other muscles**: Trigger point chains with secondary TrPs in synergistic/antagonistic muscles or satellite TrPs).

Various factors frequently work together in the development of mTrPs.

FASCIA AND MYOFASCIAL TRIGGER POINTS

Fascial tissue—in the widest sense—includes all the collagen-containing fibrous tissue formations (see Part 1: Topograhical Anatomy). Fascial structures thus form a network that surrounds and perforates the whole body and all the organs and is organized in many different ways into pockets and chambers and connects everything with everything else. The different developments in the form of diversified septa, surrounding interlaced fibers, ligamental and capsular thickening, etc., can be understood as local adjustments of a coherent network to specific localized tension (Schleip 2009). Not only the outer muscle fascia (epimysium) but also the thin intramuscular connective tissue structures (such as the endomysium that surrounds each individual muscle fiber and the perimysium that surrounds the whole muscle fiber bundle) belong to this fascial network (Trotter and Purslow 1992).

The muscle is structurally thus inseparably linked with the fascia organ, or to put it more specifically: it *is* a part of the fascia organ. In the myofascial system, the contractile elements of the muscles dynamize the fascial network and thus affect both the optimal pretension of the tension elements of the hypothesized tensegrity structure (see Chapter 3.5) and the movement of the whole system. The muscle cells, therefore, move around in the fascial network, so to speak, like fish in a fishing net. Their movement induces traction on the fascial structures that transfer into the periosteum, whereby the tensile force is transferred to the bones. Looked at from this angle, there is only one muscle, which "loafs around" in 600 or more fascial pockets (Myers 2020).

The fascia and the muscles are, therefore, in immediate and inseparable interrelation. They mutually induce each other to share a common fate—in both good times and bad.

Dysfunctional fascia structures can in this manner provoke or maintain dysfunctions of the muscles (mTrPs), just as muscular pathology in the form of mTrPs always has a fascial component as well and can be the cause of fascia dysfunction (as discussed later) (Fig. 5.5.4).

Fascia-Induced Muscle Dysfunction

Pathological changes to the fascial structures can be caused by a number of factors: for example, inflammatory processes, mechanical strain, metabolic dysfunction, injury, etc. (Fig. 5.5.4, arrow 1; see also Part 4: Physiology). Once fascia dysfunction has occurred, it can lead to muscular problems in particular mTrPs (Fig. 5.5.4, arrow 2).

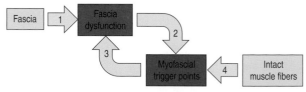

Fig. 5.5.4 Interrelation between fascia dysfunction and myofascial trigger points.
1. Factors that lead to fascia dysfunction.
2. Fascia dysfunction as possible cause of the formation/perpetuation of mTrPs.
3. MTrPs as possible cause of the formation/perpetuation of fascia dysfunction.
4. Factors that lead to the formation of mTrPs.

Fascia Dysfunction in its Role in the Formation and Activation of mTrPs

Dysfunctional fascia can contribute in different ways to the developing and perpetuation of mTrPs.

Chronic Muscle Strain as a Result of a Disorder of Fascial Mechanics. Intramuscular and extramuscular connective tissue changes cause alterations to the pattern of movement: pathological crosslinks reduce the elasticity of the muscle connective tissue (Fig. 5.5.5); intramuscular shortening, narrowing, and adhesion of fascial structures (endomysial and perimysial structures, see Peripheral Chronification) affect the intramuscular coordination and local metabolic supply; extramuscular fascia shortening and intermuscular fascia adhesions lead to restricted range of motion and disorders of intermuscular interaction. Localized stress or strain does not remain locally restricted but spreads

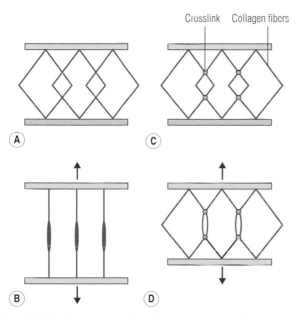

Fig. 5.5.5 Deformation of the collagen network of the muscle connective tissue by pathological crosslinks.
(A) Normal situation relaxed.
(B) Normal situation stretched.
(C) Situation with pathological crosslink relaxed.
(D) Situation with pathological crosslink stretched.
From Gautschi, R., 2019. Manual Trigger Point Therapy. Recognizing, Understanding, and Treating Myofascial Pain and Dysfunction. Thieme, Stuttgart; adapted from van den Berg, F., 2011. Angewandte Physiologie: Das Bindegewebe des Bewegungsapparates verstehen und beeinflussen. 3. Aufl. Thieme, Stuttgart, with permission.

globally in the myofascial network—following the dynamics of tensegrity architecture (see Chapter 3.5).

Fascia changes—whatever the reason they arise—regularly lead to changed posture and altered movement patterns. The resulting deviations from economic weight-bearing patterns create uneven strain on the musculoskeletal system so that myofascial (and also articular) structures are very probably in a chronically incorrect posture or chronically strained. Chronic overload is one of the most common etiological factors for the developing and activation of mTrPs.

Myofascial dysfunction frequently leads, not only locally, to the formation of mTrPs in individual muscles. As a result of persistent incorrect tension, tendinous TrPs often form in the muscle tendon transition zones and periosteal TrPs in the area of the insertion zone of the muscle. This is how multiple mTrPs develop along structural or functionally kinetic chains (see Part 3: Force Transmission) in synergistically active muscle groups.

Changes in Sensory Input. Fasciae have an important task as a receptor organ (see Part 2: Communication), and fascia dysfunctions always lead to a changed flow of impulses from the fascial mechanoreceptors as well. Fascia disorders therefore change sensory function (interoception, proprioception).

The control of motor function is an integrative sensorimotor task and the sensory input that comes from the myofascial unit is important in the generation of motor function output. A changed sensory impulse flow therefore changes muscle activation and movement control, which leads to muscular strain and can favor the formation and the activation of mTrPs.

There is evidence that a changed muscle activation pattern can be a result of trigger point activity (Lucas et al. 2004). Whether and to what extent this could stand in connection with a changed sensory provision of fascial receptors has not yet been investigated.

It is likewise obvious that autonomic regulation in the muscle is also modified by a change in sensory information. Changes in perfusion and metabolism are possible consequences.

Autonomic Disorders. Local perfusion and metabolism of muscle tissue can be permanently disturbed by fascia dysfunction. Changes in sensory input can be just as much the cause as direct mechanical influences.

The superficial fascia of the muscle must ensure access for the nerve and vascular structures that supply the

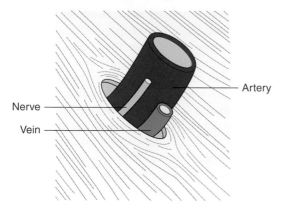

Fig. 5.5.6 Perforating triad as it passes through the surface fascia of a muscle. Diagram of a hole in the fascia with "perforating triad." In each case a vein (perforating vein), an artery (perforating artery), and a nerve (perforating nerve) penetrate the surface of the fascia of a muscle. From Staubesand, J., 1994. Die Perforanten-Trias: Ein funktionelles System. Vasomed. 6, 447–450, with permission.

muscle (to enable optimum muscle function). Nerves, arterial, and venous blood vessels all pass through the muscle fascia (perimysium) as "perforators" (Staubesand 1994; Staubesand and Li 1996; see Fig. 5.5.6). If the resistance of the superficial fascia of a muscle is increased, the neural and vascular structures at these perforator sites can be compressed.

Such entrapment of the most distal nerve sections by the superficial fascia of a muscle restricts the optimum function of the nerve—and thereby the muscle. Motor, sensory, and autonomic nerve fibers may be affected. On the one hand, strength, coordination, and mobility of the muscles are reduced; at the same time, the irritation of vasomotor fibers can change the perfusion of the muscle and with it reduces its capacity for regeneration.

As arterial and venous blood vessels usually perforate the superficial fascia of the muscle together with the nerve, the muscles' perfusion and regeneration potential can be directly affected in this way too.

Such distal entrapment of autonomic nerve fibers or blood vessels can permanently reduce the regeneration capacity of the muscles. The strain limit of the muscles is thus reached earlier, which favors the formation of mTrPs. As long as these entrapments remain, they can frustrate or weaken the positive effect of any treatment—both passive and active rehabilitation.

With the release of such minientrapments in the site of the perforation by using targeted therapy (discussed later), one of the possible perpetuating factors for a neuromusculoskeletal problem can be eliminated: motor, sensory and autonomic nerve fibers are no longer irritated. This is the optimal prerequisite for the best possible innervation (motor, sensory, and also vasomotor) and for the perfusion of the muscle, making it fully functional again.

Peripheral Chronification

Intramuscular and extramuscular fascia changes play an eminently important (and until now underestimated) role as chronification factors in the periphery. On the one hand, they can work continually as mechanisms for the formation and activation of musculoskeletal problems (see previous discussion and Fig. 5.5.3). On the other hand, fascial disorders frequently prevent the spontaneous remission of mTrPs: the endogenous, autonomic deactivation mechanisms (Fig. 5.5.3) are prevented by fascia dysfunctions. Pathological crosslinks, connective tissue shortening, and adhesions mechanically affect the recovery of myofascial structures, whereas the irritation of the fascial receptor system changes the sensory input (and with it causes a faulty motor function output). Furthermore, as a result of minientrapments in the area of dysfunctional superficial fascia of the muscles, the local metabolism is restricted—and with it the regeneration potential of the muscle tissue.

It should be particularly emphasized that intramuscular connective tissue changes probably play a crucial role in the chronification of myofascial problems. Myofascial pain usually occurs interrelated with ischemic damage stimuli in the muscle. Pronounced ischemia in the area of the mTrP is verified (Brückle et al. 1990) and can cause localized tissue necrosis. This ischemically caused necrosis generates reparations with localized inflammatory processes and collagen fibers deposited in the course of wound healing. Freshly formed connective tissue begins to contract under the influence of myofibroblasts (van Wingerden 1995). The connective tissue thereby goes through a shrinking phase, whereby inflammatory mediators strengthen the activity of the myofibroblasts and a low pH value (acid milieu) increases the contractility of the myofibroblasts (Pipelzadeh and Naylor 1998); the whole process ends with the formation of a scar. Dejung (2009) postulates that endomysial and perimysial connective tissue shortening in the TrP region thus formed overlays the contracted sarcomeres and fixes their structure. The connective tissue shrinks and prevents the decontraction of the sarcomeres of the rigor complex. This is the first stage of myofascial chronification; a chronification that represents a peripheral - not a central - chronification.

KEY POINTS

Fascia disturbances induce muscle dysfunction through:
- chronic muscle strain as a result of a disorder of fascial mechanics (pathological crosslinks, connective tissue shortening);
- changes in sensory input;
- autonomic disorder (neurovascular entrapments); and
- peripheral chronification: endomysial and perimysial connective tissue shortening overlies and fixes the rigor complexes (mTrPs).

Trigger Point–Induced Fascia Dysfunction

On the one hand, fascia dysfunction can cause the formation and persistence of mTrPs (Fig. 5.5.4, arrow 2). On the other hand, mTrPs cause fascia dysfunction (Fig. 5.5.4, arrow 3).

Mechanically Induced Fascia Dysfunction

MTrPs always occur in association with taut bands. Taut bands induce adjustment and often disorders of the fascia architecture and function.
- Taut bands put fascial structures under permanent tension (especially in the area of the transition from muscle to tendon and the muscle insertion sites) so that at these sites tendinous or periosteal TrPs often result ("insertion tendinopathies").
- Taut bands can lead to muscle shortening. Restricted range of motion, and altered movement and posture patterns occur and this can generate adaptation processes and the decompensation of fascial structures.

Biochemically Induced Fascia Dysfunction

There are marked localized changes in the biochemical milieu in the site of mTrPs. There is evidence of:
- Pronounced hypoxia (Brückle et al. 1990)
- A definite increase in inflammatory mediators such as bradykinin, substance P, and CGRP (Shah et al. 2005, 2008).

- A significantly lower pH value; that is, the tissue milieu is predominantly acidic (Shah et al. 2005, 2008).

These changes in the biochemical milieu favor the formation and perpetuation of fascia dysfunction. The disposition to fascial shortening is strengthened in an acid tissue milieu and by messenger substances associated with inflammation in the body (Pipelzadeh and Naylor 1998). The special significance of the inflammatory process has already been pointed out, because the inflammatory process itself is a reaction to ischemic tissue necrosis leading to fascia dysfunction in general and to peripheral chronification of myofascial problems in particular.

KEY POINTS

Trigger points induce fascia disturbances through:
- mechanical factors (taut bands, rigor complexes, restricted ROM) and
- biochemical factors (hypoxia, increases inflammatory mediators, low pH value).

KEY POINTS

The development of mTrPs and of fascial changes run parallel to each other, and they mutually influence and strengthen each other.

THERAPEUTIC CONSEQUENCES

The causal therapy of (myo)fascial dysfunction is carried out based on the underlying (patho)physiology. In short, localized ischemia leads to localized hypoxia, which is at the center of the pathogenesis of myofascial pain and function disorders. The consequences of hypoxia are:
- ATP deficiency (energy crisis), which leads to the rigor complex (lack of the "softening effect" of ATP).
- Localized inflammatory processes, which cause connective tissue reactions (adhesions, shrinkage) (see previous discussion).

Myofascial (trigger point) pathology that has become chronic is characterized by two factors: rigor complexes and connective tissue changes (adhesions, shortening), the latter being largely responsible for the chronification of a myofascial problem. Treatment that will be effective in a sustained manner must take both factors into account—rigor complexes and connective tissue changes.

Muscle release techniques that work exclusively by means of reflexes or therapy techniques that are mainly directed to treat the rigor complexes (dry needling, shock wave therapy) insufficiently affect the fascial aspect. Consistent and thorough treatment of the rigor complexes *and* the changed fascial structures, using manual techniques targeted on the connective tissue, is necessary. It is a sole characteristic of the myofascial trigger point therapy IMTT, founded by Dejung (1988, 2009), that the rigor complex and the connective tissue changes are equally at the center of the therapeutic intervention (Swiss approach). Four manual techniques are used to target treatment on both the rigor complex itself and the reactive changes to fascia structures (Table 5.5.1). Manual techniques are supplemented in the concept of myofascial trigger point therapy by stretching (technique V), functional strengthening of the muscles, and ergonomic measures (technique VI). Exercises at home to stretch/relax interrupt monotonous work postures and promote the regeneration capacity of the muscle fibers and the remodeling of fascial structures. Functional training supports the healing process thanks to physiological weight-bearing and exercise and makes the myofascial unit able to bear more weight, whereas ergonomic interventions reduce incorrect loading. For sustained treatment success of chronic myofascial pain, additional to local therapy of the myofascial structures, the perpetuating factors also have to be recognized and included in the treatment. Myofascial trigger point therapy IMTT is a

TABLE 5.5.1   Trigger Point Therapy (Swiss Approach): Treatment Techniques and their Local Effects

Technique	Measures	Local Tissue-Specific Therapeutic Effects
I	Manual compression of the mTrP	Squeezing out the "inflammatory soup" and the local edema Ischemia, followed by reactive hyperemia → improved metabolism Reflexive relaxing of the taut band associated with the mTrP
II	Manual stretching of the TrP region	Squeezing out the "inflammatory soup" and the local edema Ischemia, followed by reactive hyperemia → improved metabolism Reflexive relaxing of the taut band associated with the mTrP Destruction of the local rigor complex Stretching out the reactively developing connective tissue adhesions (pathological crosslinks) and connective tissue shortening: → improved intramuscular elasticity and intramuscular supply
III	Fascia stretching technique (manual stretching of the superficial and intramuscular fascia)	Loosening reactively developing connective tissue adhesions (pathological crosslinks) and shortening: → improved intramuscular mobility and supply → improved muscle elasticity Stimulation of fascial mechanoreceptors → reflexive relaxing of the taut band associated with the trigger point → Decreased sympathetic nerve activity, decreased global resting muscle tone
IV	Fascial separation technique (manual release of intermuscular fascial adhesions)	Release of adhesions between fasciae of adjacent muscles → Improved intermuscular mobility
V	Stretching, relaxing	Relaxing/improved muscle flexibility
VI	Functional training, ergonomics	Physiological loading and movement supports the regeneration process and makes the muscles more resilient Ergonomic measures reduce inappropriate muscle loading

Gautschi, R., 2008. Myofasziale Triggerpunkt-Therapie. In: van den Berg, F. (Ed.), Angewandte Physiologie, Bd. 4: Schmerzen verstehen und beeinflussen. 2. Erweiterte Auflage. Stuttgart, Thieme, pp. 310–366.

differentiated method being performed by specially trained physiotherapists and physicians.

Summary

Sustained treatment success of chronic myofascial pain requires
- treatment of the rigor complexes (mTrPs) and
- treatment of the fascial changes through hands-on (manual myofascial trigger point therapy) and hands-off (functional training) strategies
- consideration of perpetuating factors.

REFERENCES

Al-Shenqiti, A.M., Oldham, J.A., 2005. Test-retest reliability of myofascial trigger point detection in patients with rotator cuff tendonitis. Clin. Rehabil. 19, 482–487.

Arendt-Nielsen, L., Graven-Nielsen, T., 2008. Muscle pain: sensory implications and interaction with motor control. Clin J. Pain. 24, 291–298.

Barbero, M., Schneebeli, A., Koctsier, E., Maino, P., 2019. Myofascial pain syndrome and trigger points: evaluation and treatment in patients with musculoskeletal pain. Curr. Opin. Support. Palliat. Care. 13, 270–276.

Bron, C., Franssen, J., Wensing, M., Oostendorp, R.A., 2007. Interrater reliability of palpation of myofascial trigger points in three shoulder muscles. J. Man. Manip. Ther. 15, 203–215.

Brückle, W., Sückfull, M., Fleckenstein, W., Weiss, C., Müller, W., 1990. Gewebe-Po₂-Messung in der verspannten Rückenmuskulatur. Z. Rheumatol. 49, 208–216.

Dejung, B., 1988. Triggerpunkt- und Bindegewebsbehandlung – neue Wege in Physiotherapie und Rehabilitationsmedizin. Physiotherpeut 6, 3.

Dejung, B., 2009. Triggerpunkt-Therapie: Die Behandlung akuter und chronischer Schmerzen im Bewegungsapparat mit manueller Triggerpunkt-Therapie und Dry Needling. 3., überarbeitete und erweiterte Auflage (Erstauflage 2003). Hans Huber, Bern.

Dommerholt, J., Gerwin, R.D., Courtney, C.A., 2019. Pain sciences and myofascial pain. In: Donnelly, J.M. (Ed.), Travell, Simons & Simons' Myofascial Pain and Dysfunction: The Trigger Point Manual, third ed. Wolters Kluwer, Baltimore.

Feigl-Reitinger, A., Radner, H., Tilscher, H., et al., 1998. Der chronische Rückenschmerz: Histomorphologische Veränderungen der Muskulatur entlang der Wirbelsäule als Substrat der Myogelose. In: Feigl-Reitinger, A., Bergsmann, O., Tischer, H. (Eds.), Myogelose und Triggerpunkte. Facultas, Wien.

Fernandez-de-Las-Penas, C., Dommerholt, J., 2018. International consensus on diagnostic criteria and clinical considerations of myofascial trigger points: A Delphi study. Pain Med. 19: 142–150.

Gautschi, R., 2008. Myofasziale Triggerpunkt-Therapie. In: van den Berg, F. (Ed.) Angewandte Physiologie, Bd. 4: Schmerzen verstehen und beeinflussen. 2. erweiterte Auflage. Stuttgart, Thieme, pp. 310–366.

Gautschi, R., 2019. Manual Trigger Point Therapy. Recognizing, Understanding, and Treating Myofascial Pain and Dysfunction. Thieme, Stuttgart.

Ge, H.Y., Arendt-Nielsen, L., Madeleine, P., 2012. Accelerated muscle fatigability of latent myofascial trigger points in humans. Pain Med. 13, 957–964.

Ge, H.Y., Monterde, S., Graven-Nielsen, T., Arendt-Nielsen, L., 2014. Latent myofascial trigger points are associated with an increased intramuscular electromyographic activity during synergistic muscle activation. J. Pain. 15, 181–187.

Gerwin, R.D., Shannon, S., Hong, C.Z., Hubbard, D., Gevirtz, R., 1997. Interrater reliability in myofascial triggerpoint examination. Pain 69, 65–73.

Hsieh, C.Y., Hong, C.Z., Adams, et al., 2000. Interexaminer reliability of the palpation of trigger points in the trunk and lower limb muscles. Arch. Phys. Med. Rehabil. 81, 258–264.

Ibarra J.M., Ge, H.Y., Wang, C., Martínez Vizcaino, V., Graven-Nielsen, T., Arendt-Nielsen, L., 2011. Latent myofascial trigger points are associated with an increased antagonistic muscle activity during agonist muscle contraction. J. Pain. 12, 1282–1288.

Ivanichev, G.A., 2007. Myofaszialer Schmerz. Russian Kazan University Press, Russisch Kazan.

Lewit, K., 2007. Das wissenschaftliche Konzept der manuellen Therapie. Punkt für Punkt. Manuelle Medizin 45, 309–313.

Licht, G., Müller-Ehrenberg, H., Mathis, J., Berg, G., Greitemann, G., 2007. Untersuchung myofaszialer Triggerpunkte ist zuverlässig. Intertester-Reliabilität an insgesamt 304 Muskeln überprüft. Manuelle Medizin 45, 402–408.

Lucas, K., Karen, R., Polus, B., Rich, P., 2004. Latent myofascial trigger points: Their effects on muscle activation and movement efficiency. J. Bodyw. Mov. Ther. 8, 160–166.

Lucas K.R., Rich P.A., Polus B.I., 2010. Muscle activation patterns in the scapular positioning muscles during loaded scapular plane elevation: the effects of latent myofascial trigger points. Clin. Biomech. 25, 765–770.

Mayoral Del Moral, O., Torres Lacomba, M., Russell, I.J., Sánchez Méndez, Ó., Sánchez Sánchez, B. 2018. Validity and reliability of clinical examination in the diagnosis of myofascial pain syndrome and myofascial trigger points in upper quarter muscles. Pain Med. 19, 2039–2050.

Mense, S., Simons, D.G., Russel, I.J., 2001. Muscle Pain: Understanding its Nature, Diagnosis and Treatment. Williams & Wilkins, Philadelphia.

Myburgh, C., Lauridsen, H.H., Larsen, A.H., Hartvigsen, J., 2011. Standardized manual palpation of myofascial trigger points in relation to neck/shoulder pain; the influence of clinical experience on interexaminer reproducibility. Man. Ther. 16, 136–140.

Myers, T.W., 2020. Anatomy Trains. Myofascial Meridians for Manual and Movement Therapists. Elsevier, Amsterdam.

Nice, D., Riddle, D., Lamb, R., Mayhew, T.P., Rucker, K.,1992. Intertester reliability of judgments of the presence of trigger points in patients with low back pain. Arch. Phys. Med. Rehabil. 73, 893–898.

Njoo, K., van der Does, E., 1994. The occurrence and inter-rater reliability of myofascial trigger points in the quadratus lumborum and gluteus medius: A prospective study in non-specific low back pain patients and controls in general practice. Pain 58, 317–323.

Pipelzadeh, M.H., Naylor, I.L., 1998. The in vitro enhancement of rat myofibroblast contractility by alterations to the pH of the physiological solution. Eur. J. Pharmacol. 357, 257–259.

Schleip, R., 2009. Myofasziale Triggerpunkte und Faszien. In: Irnich, D. (Ed.), Leitfaden Triggerpunkte. Elsevier Urban & Fischer, München.

Sciotti, V.M., Mittak, V.L., DiMarco, L., et al., 2001. Clinical precision of myofascial trigger point localisation in the trapezius muscle. Pain. 93, 259–266.

Shah, J.P., Phillips, T.M., Danoff, J.V., Gerber, L.H., 2005. An in vivo microanalytical technique for measuring the local biochemical milieu of human skeletal muscle. J. Appl. Physiol. 99, 1977–1984.

Shah, J.P., Danoff, J.V., Deshai, M.J., et al., 2008. Biochemicals associated with pain and inflammation are elevated in sites near to, and remote from active myofascial trigger points. Arch. Phys. Med. Rehabil. 89, 16–23.

Simons, D.G., Stolov, W.C., 1976. Microscopic features and transient contraction of palpable bands in canine muscle. Am. J. Phys. Med. 55, 65–88.

Staubesand, J., 1994. Die Perforanten-Trias: Ein funktionelles System. Vasomed. 6, 447–450.

Staubesand, J., Li, Y., 1996. Zum Feinbau der Fascia cruris mit besonderer Berücksichtigung epi- und intrafaszialer Nerven. Manuelle Medizin 34, 196–200.

Travell, J.G., Simons, D.G., 1999. Myofascial pain and dysfunction. The trigger point manual. vol. 1, second ed. Williams & Wilkins, Baltimore.

Trotter, J.A., Purslow, P.P., 1992. Functional morphology of the endomysium in series fibered muscles. J. Morphol. 212, 109–122.

van den Berg, F., 2011. Angewandte Physiologie: Das Bindegewebe des Bewegungsapparates verstehen und beeinflussen. 3. Aufl. Thieme, Stuttgart.

van Wingerden, B.A.M., 1995. Connective tissue in rehabilitation. Scipro, Vaduz.

Wolfe, F., Simons, D., Fricton, J., et al., 1992. The fibromyalgia and myofascial pain syndromes: a preliminary study of tender points and trigger points in persons with fibromyalgia, myofascial pain syndrome and no disease. J. Rheumatol. 19, 944–951.

Joint Hypermobility Due to Pathologically Increased Compliance of Extra- and Intramuscular Connective Tissues

Peter A. Huijing

CHAPTER CONTENTS

INTRODUCTION

Joint hypermobility has been known clinically for more than 2500 years: the already famous physician of Cos, Hippocrates (460–377 BCE), was aware that hypermobile joints could be a problem, as they can lead to luxation of the joint (see his treatises "Airs, Waters and Places" [referred to by Parapia and Jackson 2008] and "On Joints," which have been available in translations in several languages since the 16th century [Hippocrates 1840; 1923]). The incidence of luxation at that time seemed to have been much higher than in our present times.

At times, spectacular external effects of overcompliant connective tissues drew medical attention and were described in the literature. For example, in the 17th century a Spanish patient with some medical problems who ended up in St. Pieters Gasthuis of Amsterdam was described in some detail, and not uncommon at that time, even his name was published by Job van Meek'ren (1611–1666).

The author was Amsterdam's municipal surgeon at that hospital and fulfilled other respectful functions in the city (Meek'ren 1668, 1675, 1682). An image of this 23-year-old patient ended up on the frontispiece of the books and as an illustration in the dedicated chapter (Fig. 5.6.1).

Such fascia-related disorders are defined as disorders resulting from decreased stiffness or increased compliance of the fascia. (Stiffness is defined as the actual change in force for a given change in length [i.e., $\Delta F/\Delta l$]. Compliance is the inverse of stiffness [i.e., $\Delta l/\Delta F$].) Increased compliance of fascia yielding hypermobility occurs in various inherited connective tissue disorders (e.g., Ehlers–Danlos syndrome (EDS), Marfan syndrome, cutis laxa, and osteogenesis imperfecta). Such multiorgan disorders are characterized by varying involvement of vessels, skin, joints, bones, internal organs, eyes, heart, skeletal muscle, and the peripheral and central nervous system.

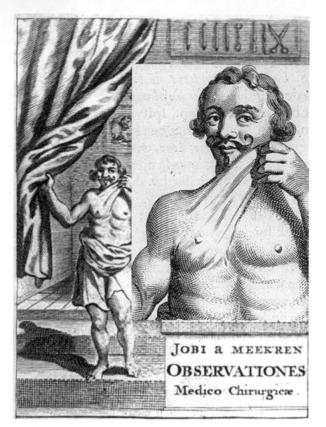

Fig. 5.6.1 Image of the "compliant Spaniard." Superimposed images of 23-year-old patient from the frontispiece and 29th chapter of one of the Dutch versions of Job van Meek'ren's book on medicosurgical observations. It illustrates the extremely compliant skin of this Spanish patient (public domain).

PHYSICAL OR MANUAL THERAPY IN EHLERS–DANLOS SYNDROME

Physical or manual therapy in Ehlers–Danlos syndrome (EDS) and Marfan syndrome focuses on reduction of musculoskeletal pain, maintenance of muscle force, increase of joint stability, reduction of scoliosis, and functional improvement (Braverman 1998). A case study on a patient with back muscle pain reported that treatment of trigger point injections combined with stretching exercises under analgesic cover for the first week may play a role in treating myofascial pain syndrome in patients suffering from EDS (Tewari et al. 2017). For those patients with respiratory muscles affected (Reychler

et al. 2019), strength training of those muscles is reported to be helpful to improve inspiratory muscle strength, lung function, functional exercise performance, anxiety, and depression. In any case, the abnormal ECM composition in these disorders may affect muscle physiology (i.e., as a result of increased compliance) or biochemistry (i.e., altered signaling by ECM molecules).

The remainder of this chapter focuses on potential changes in muscle characteristics related to increased fascia compliance, particularly in EDS. The syndrome is named after Edvard Ehlers (1863–1937) and Henri-Alexandre Danlos (1844–1912), Danish and French dermatologists, respectively ((Ehlers 1901; Danlos 1908). In 1936 an English physician, Frederick Parkes-Weber, suggested that the disorder be named Ehlers-Danlos syndrome (Enerson 2004). Since then it has become clear that the first complete description of this condition was given by A. N. Chernogubow in 1892, but this remained unknown or unrecognized outside of Russia.

It should be noted that EDS, regarding its symptoms and genetics, is a heterogeneous group of inherited connective tissue disorders characterized by joint hypermobility, skin hyperextensibility, and tissue fragility. A classification of EDS into six major types based on clinical and biochemical features was suggested (Beighton et al. 1998). These types are: the classical, hypermobility, vascular, kyphoscoliotic, arthrochalasia, and dermatosparaxis types. The hypermobility type is the most common in EDS, followed by the classical type. Together, they account for approximately 90% of all cases (Steinmann et al. 2002). The vascular type is far less common but is associated with the occurrence of arterial dissections (i.e., tears within the wall of blood vessels, which allow blood to separate wall layers) and aneurysms (i.e., localized, blood-filled dilation: balloon-like bulge of a blood vessel caused by disease or weakening of the wall) that may cause severe neurological complications. The kyphoscoliotic, arthrochalasia, and dermatosparaxis types are rare. In a review study, Theocharis and colleagues (2019) examined the common features and differences among these subtypes and also their relation to other diseases with disturbed—that is, abnormal—ECM assembly in tissues and the multitasking roles for ECM in diseases such as osteoarthritis, fibrosis, cancer, and genetic diseases.

NEUROMUSCULAR INVOLVEMENT OF EDS

 KEY POINT

Muscular involvement in Ehlers-Danlos syndrome has long been overlooked. But the principles of myofascial force transmission makes the involvement likely.

Overlooked for a long time, neuromuscular involvement in EDS is expected based on mechanical interactions between muscle fibers and their extracellular matrix (ECM) molecules (Voermans et al. 2008). Muscle hypotonia, muscle rupture, fatigue, and musculoskeletal pain are included in the diagnostic criteria of EDS (Beighton et al. 1998), and some muscle weakness was reported in EDS patients (Voermans et al. 2009).

Neuromuscular involvement was defined as consistent abnormal findings on questionnaires and/or physical examination, supported by abnormal results of appropriate investigations. Muscle weakness, myalgia, and rapid fatigability are often reported by the majority of patients. Nerve conduction studies revealed axonal polyneuropathy in five patients (13%; predominantly occurring in the TNX-deficient type). Needle electromyography showed mainly myopathic features in nine patients (26%) and a mixed neurogenic–myopathic pattern in most (60%). Muscle ultrasound images revealed increased echo intensity (48%) and atrophy (50%). Mild myopathic features (i.e., increased variation of fiber diameter, sporadic isolated atrophic fibers, and a mild increase of internal nuclei) were seen on muscle biopsy of five patients (28%). Creatine kinase was mildly elevated in four patients. Furthermore, patients with complete absence of TNX (i.e., TNX-deficient-type EDS) are associated with more severe neuromuscular symptoms than those with reduced TNX serum levels and with reduced staining of TNX within muscle (i.e., hypermobility-type EDS caused by TNXB haploinsufficiency). An inverse relation between residual TNX quantity in serum and muscle and degree of neuromuscular involvement is suggested by these results (Voermans et al. 2009.) They also confirm the findings of previous case reports on neuromuscular symptoms in EDS (Bilkey et al. 1981; Banerjee et al. 1988; Bertin et al. 1989; Takaluoma et al. 2007; Voermans et al. 2007.)

The results regarding inherited connective tissue disorders raise the question whether relatively mild myopathic changes in muscle biopsies in the minority of patients suffice to explain the mild-to-moderate neuromuscular involvement in the majority of EDS patients. Nonneuromuscular features of EDS syndrome may contribute to various neuromuscular symptoms: for example, musculoskeletal pain, increased fatigability, and mild impairment may be caused by articular and skeletal problems in EDS (Voermans et al. 2009). The finding of a close relationship between residual TNX levels and degree of neuromuscular involvement in EDS suggest other pathophysiological mechanisms may take part.

There has been criticism voiced at the inherited nature of the hypermobility EDS (for a review, see Martin 2019): the sole focus on isolating mendelian patterns, without exploring the impact of environmental influences on how hypermobile EDS manifests, may deter useful results in deciphering its multifactorial condition. Therefore according to Ann Martin, the task for future research is to explore environmental influences and control for anatomical variations.

In 2001, a new autosomal recessive type of EDS was identified as caused by deficiency of TNX (Schalkwijk et al. 2001). Subsequently, TNXB gene haploinsufficiency was found to be associated with the hypermobility type of EDS in a minority of patients (Zweers et al. 2003).

EFFECTS OF TNX-DEFICIENCY ON MUSCLE CHARACTERISTICS IN A MOUSE MODEL OF EDS

The widespread effects of this deficiency may be illustrated by modern studies. Abnormalities in muscle ECM composition may affect aspects of myofascial force transmission and may contribute to muscle weakness (for details on myofascial force transmission, see Chapter 3.2 and Huijing 2007). Knowing such effects of altered myofascial force transmission may help understand why muscle force is mildly to moderately reduced in the majority of EDS patients, whereas conventional histological analysis of muscle shows only mild abnormalities in a minority of patients.

TNX is an ECM glycoprotein abundantly expressed in various tissues during embryonic development (e.g., tendons and perimysium of skeletal muscle [Matsumoto et al. 1994; Burch et al. 1995]). In adults, TNX is predominantly expressed in connective tissues of skeletal and cardiac muscle (Matsumoto et al. 1994) and is involved in collagen deposition and maturation (Schalkwijk et al. 2001; Egging et al. 2006). Several studies suggest that TNX acts as a bridge between collagen fibrils that are organized in bundles (Lethias et al. 1996) and may be important for nonpathological stiffness of connective tissues (Lethias et al. 2006). The chemical structure of the TNX molecule (disulfide-linked trimer structure) is important for such bridging functions. TNX interacts with types I, III, and V fibrillar collagen molecules and with decorin and binds to the fibril-associated types XII and XIV collagens (Lethias et al. 2006). Finally, the FNIII domains of the TNX molecule may be important for elastic properties of the molecule itself (Lethias et al. 2006). For more chemical details, see Sawle and Pope (2019).

THE ULTRASTRUCTURE OF MUSCLE EXTRACELLULAR MATRIX IN TNX KNOCKOUT MICE IS DISTORTED

TNX knockout mice have so far been used for detailed dermatological phenotyping and dermatological features of TNX-deficient-type EDS (Mao et al. 2002; Bristow et al. 2005; Egging et al. 2007a and b).

To investigate the effects of TNX-deficiency on muscle characteristics we used such male mice to study aspects of myofascial force transmission and compare results to that of comparable but healthy mice.

ISOMETRIC CONTRACTIONS

During an isometric contraction the muscle–tendon complex length is set at a constant value. However, actual length of active myofibers is dependent on the properties of the series elastic component (SEC). Note that because of the effects of myofascial force transmission, SEC is not only determined by aponeuroses and tendons but also by the *intra*muscular network of endo-, peri-, and epimysium in the case of a fully dissected muscle and by the *inter*muscular connective tissues in the case of a muscle working within its full natural connective tissue context. In fact, sarcomeres within myofibers are linked to these

types of SEC elements (tendinous and fascial connective tissues), which themselves are arranged mechanically in parallel to each other. Total compliance of SEC affects the rate of length change of the myofibers during the initial phase of isometric force exertion and hence affects the rate of force build-up in time. The ratio of compliance of myofascial and myotendinous pathways will determine what percentage of the force exerted is transmitted in each pathway. In any case, the least compliant (i.e., stiffer) pathway will transmit most force. Vice versa, increased fascia compliance occurring in inherited connective tissue disorders is hypothesized to yield reduced myofascial interaction between muscles.

We tested this hypothesis in a study focused on both *intra*muscular aspects (force–time characteristics of *maximally dissected* medial gastrocnemius muscle [GM]) and *epi*muscular aspects (length–force characteristics of tricep**s** surae muscle [TS] and anterior crural muscles [TA + EHL and EDL]) *without major dissection* to detect changes in mechanical interaction between muscle groups of both TNX knockout and wild-type mice.

 KEY POINT

In standardized conditions, mechanical interaction, presumably due to epimuscular myofascial force transmission, between antagonistic triceps surae and anterior crural muscles is still present but is very much reduced in TNX-deficient compared with wild-type mice.

The results show that altered properties of the SEC of muscle due to TNX deficiency affect characteristics of muscle function. More specifically, study of the *intra*muscular aspects points to changes in the SEC within the (maximally dissected) muscle-tendon complex. Results of the study of *inter*muscular mechanical interaction show a reduction of myofascial interaction between muscles active within the full context of their surrounding connective tissues. An example is shown in Fig. 5.6.2A. Note that myofascial force transmission is also present for TNX-deficiency but to a much lower degree.

 KEY POINT

In standardized conditions, the magnitude of the proximo-distal force difference for EDL muscle (not shown) is reduced in TNX-deficient compared with the wild-type mice.

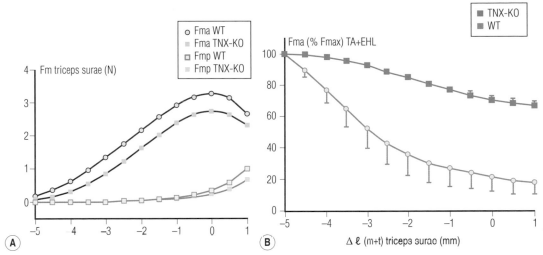

Fig. 5.6.2 TNX-deficiency diminishes myofascial interaction between antagonistic muscles. (A) Active and passive length–force characteristics of the triceps surae muscle complex (TS) of healthy (WT) and TNX-deficient rats (TNX-KO). The muscles are operating within their regular connective tissue context. (B) Summed force exerted by the tibialis anterior and extensor hallucis longus muscles (TA+EHL) kept at constant length. In both healthy rats (WT) and TNX-deficient mice (TNX-KO), TA+EHL force is lowered after TS muscle–tendon complex is lengthened [$\Delta l/(m+t)$] progressively. However, this decrease in force is much lower (<25%) for diseased rats. Active force is expressed as percent of initial force (at low triceps surae length). *Fm*, muscle force; *Fma*, active muscle force; *Fpa*, passive muscle force.

Affected intra- and epimuscular myofascial force transmission may drastically alter the required muscular coordination in physiological movements and interfere with mechanical interaction between antagonistic muscles (Matsumoto et al. 1994; Huijing 2007; Voermans et al. 2007; Huijing and Bann 2008).

INTRAMUSCULAR CHANGES: INCREASED MUSCLE COMPLIANCE

At optimum length (λ_o) several properties of dissected GM are unchanged in TNX knockout mice compared with wild-type mice: (1) maximal isometric force and maximal power production; (2) stimulation frequency–force relationship; and (3) fatigability during a series of repeated isometric contractions. In contrast, at low lengths (λ_o −4, λ_o −3.5, and λ_o −3) some GM properties were affected significantly in TNX knockout mice: (4) active force exerted at lower lengths was lower; (5) the maximal rate of relaxation was lower; and (6) the time delay between first stimulation pulse and the time of attainment of 2% of maximal active force was longer in TNX knockout mice.

This last finding is consistent with the hypothesis that relatively more slack must be taken up at lower lengths in TNX knockout mice. The other findings are related to the increased SEC compliance present in the disease, which causes more shortening to be imposed on the myofibers in TNX-deficient mice at the onset of contraction at low lengths. Vice versa, more lengthening is imposed on the myofiber at the onset of relaxation at low lengths.

INTERMUSCULAR CHANGES: REDUCED EPIMUSCULAR MYOFASCIAL FORCE TRANSMISSION

The most important result is that TNX deficiency strongly affects myofascial force transmission within the lower mouse limb (Huijing et al. 2010).

The EDL proximo-distal force difference that constitutes absolute proof of epimuscular myofascial force transmission is lower in TNX-deficient than in healthy mice. The deficiency significantly affects net epimuscular myofascial force transmission, not only in the magnitude of the net myofascial load on EDL but also in direction of loading. Whereas in wild-type mice the direction changes rapidly with increasing TS length from proximal to distal loading of EDL, this change of direction does not occur in TNX knockout mice.

Mechanical interaction between muscles was decreased in a major way: normalized distal active force of agonistic muscle (TA+EHL with triceps surae lengthening, as in Fig. 5.6.2B, and vice versa, not shown) with increasing length of the antagonistic muscle.

CONCLUSIONS

It is concluded that TNX knockout muscles act more independently than healthy muscles. It seems inevitable that such altered function will require altered patterns of muscular coordination to allow effective movement. Taken together, these findings indicate that the SEC of the muscle–tendon complex located within and between muscles is changed in TNX knockout mice. Therefore these findings support the hypothesis that TNX deficiency reduces the stiffness of myofascial pathways and thus causes a pathological reduction of the force transmitted this way (Voermans et al. 2007). This study and previous animal experiments have shown that myofascial force transmission occurs between antagonistic muscles, which points to interdependence of muscles and their role in higher levels of motor organization (Huijing 2007). Whether and to what extent altered myofascial force transmission affects muscular coordination and interferes with mechanical interaction between antagonist muscles in TNX-deficient EDS patients needs to be studied in detail. If neuromuscular control is not optimized for this situation, altered myofascial force transmission may explain symptoms of enhanced fatigability in patients suffering from EDS.

Summary

In conclusion, altered muscular function in TNX knockout mice is explained at least in part by changes of myofascial series elastic component of the muscle–tendon complex, resulting in reduced intermuscular myofascial interaction between antagonistic muscles.

REFERENCES

Banerjee, G., Agarwal, R.K., Shembesh, N.M., el Mauhoub, M., 1988. Ehlers Danlos syndrome – masquerading as primary muscle disease. Postgrad. Med. J. 64, 126–127.

Beighton, P., De Paepe, A., Steinmann, B., Tsipouras, P., Wenstrup, R.J., 1998. Ehlers–Danlos syndromes: revised nosology, Villefranche, 1997. Ehlers–Danlos National Foundation (USA) and Ehlers-Danlos Support Group (UK). Am. J. Med. Genet. 77, 31–37.

Bertin, P., Treves, R., Julia, A., Gaillard, S., Desproges-Gotteron, R., 1989. Ehlers–Danlos syndrome, clotting disorders and muscular dystrophy. Ann. Rheum. Dis. 48, 953–956.

Bilkey, W.J., Baxter, T.L., Kottke, F.J., Mundale, M.O., 1981. Muscle formation in Ehlers–Danlos syndrome. Arch. Phys. Med. Rehabil. 62, 444–448.

Braverman, A.C., 1998. Exercise and the Marfan syndrome. Med. Sci. Sports Exerc. 30, S387–S395.

Bristow, J., Carey, W., Egging, D., Schalkwijk, J., 2005. Tenascin-X, collagen, elastin, and the Ehlers– Danlos syndrome. Am. J. Med. Genet. C Semin. Med. Genet. 139, 24–30.

Burch, G.H., Bedolli, M.A., McDonough, S., Rosenthal, S.M., Bristow, J., 1995. Embryonic expression of tenascin-X suggests a role in limb, muscle, and heart development. Dev. Dyn. 203, 491–504.

Chernogubow, N.A., 1892. Über einen Fall von Cutis laxa. (Presentation at the first meeting of Moscow Dermatologic and Venerologic Society, Nov 13, 1891.) Monatshefte für praktische Dermatologie, Hamburg, 14, 76.

Danlos, H., 1908. Un cas de cutis laxa avec tumeurs par contusion chronique des coudes et des genoux (xanthome juvénile pseudo-diabetique de MM Hallopeau et Macé de Lépinay). Bull. Soc. Franc. Dermatol. Syphiligr. (Paris), 19, 70–72

Egging, D., van den Berkmortel, F., Taylor, G., Bristow, J., Schalkwijk, J., 2007a. Interactions of human tenascin-X domains with dermal extracellular matrix molecules. Arch. Dermatol. Res. 298, 389–396.

Egging, D., van Vlijmen-Willems, I., van Tongeren, T., Schalkwijk, J., Peeters, A., 2007b. Wound healing in tenascin-X deficient mice suggests that tenascin-X is involved in matrix maturation rather than matrix deposition. Connect. Tissue Res. 48, 93–98.

Egging, D.F., van Vlijmen, I., Starcher, B., et al., 2006. Dermal connective tissue development in mice: an essential role for tenascin-X. Cell Tissue Res. 323, 465–474.

Ehlers, E.L. 1901, Cutis laxa. Neigung zu Haemorrhagien in der Haut, Lockerung mehrerer Artikulationen. Dermatologische Zeitschr. (Berlin) 8, 173–174.

Enerson, O.D., 2004. Ehlers-Danlos syndrome. who named it? -A dictionary of medical eponyms. Available from: http://www.whonamedit.com/synd.cfm/2017.html.

Hippocrates, 1840. Oeuvres Complètes d'Hippocrate. Tome second [vol. 2]. Translated by E. Littré. J.B. Bailliere, Paris, pp. 75–88 [in Greek and French].

Hippocrates, 1923. On joints. In: Hippocrates. Volume III. Loeb Classical Library No. 149. Translated by E. T. Withington. Heinemann, Putnam, London; New York, pp. 201–397 [in Greek and English].

Huijing, P.A., 2007. Epimuscular myofascial force transmission between antagonistic and synergistic muscles can explain movement limitation in spastic paresis. J. Electromyogr. Kinesiol. 17, 708–724.

Huijing, P.A., Baan, G.C., 2008. Myofascial force transmission via extramuscular pathways occurs between antagonistic muscles. Cells Tissues Organs 188, 400–414.

Huijing, P.A., Voermans, N.C., Baan, G.C., Busé, T.E., van Engelen, B.G., de Haan, A., 2010. Muscle characteristics and altered myofascial force transmission in tenascin-X deficient mice, a mouse model of Ehlers–Danlos syndrome. J. Appl. Physiol. 109, 986–995.

Lethias, C., Carisey, A., Comte, J., Cluzel, C., Exposito, J.Y., 2006. A model of tenascin-X integration within the collagenous network. FEBS Lett. 580, 6281–6285.

Lethias, C., Descollonges, Y., Boutillon, M.M., Garrone, R., 1996. Flexilin: a new extracellular matrix glycoprotein localized on collagen fibrils. Matrix Biol. 15, 11–19.

Mao, J.R., Taylor, G., Dean, W.B., et al., 2002. Tenascin-X deficiency mimics Ehlers-Danlos syndrome in mice through alteration of collagen deposition. Nat. Genet. 30, 421–425.

Martin, A., 2019. An acquired or heritable connective tissue disorder? A review of hypermobile Ehlers Danlos Syndrome. Eur. J. Med. Genet. 62, 103672.

Matsumoto, K., Saga, Y., Ikemura, T., Sakakura, T., Chiquet-Ehrismann, R., 1994. The distribution of tenascin-X is distinct and often reciprocal to that of tenascin-C. J. Cell Biol. 125, 483–493.

Meek'ren. Job Janszoon van, 1668. Heelkundige aanmerkingen. t'Amsterdam by Casparus Commelijn.; Chapter XXIX. Een rekkelyke Spanjaerd. 170–171(in Dutch).

Meek'ren. Job Janszoon van, 1675. Rare und wunderbare chyrurgisch- und geneesskünstige Anmerckungen. XXIX. Von einem weichlichen Spanier in Verlegung Paul Fürstens. pp. 186–188 (in German).

Meek'ren. Job Janszoon van, 1682. Observationes Medico-Chirurgicae / ex Belgico in Latinem translate. Amstelodami ex officina Henrici & viduae Theodori Boom, Cap. XXXII. De dilatabilitate extraordinaria Cutu; viro qaedam Hispano. pp.134–136 (in Latin).

Parapia, L.A., Jackson, C., 2008. Ehlers-Danlos syndrome – a historical review. Br. J. Haematol. 141, 32–35.

Reychler, G., Liistro, G., Piérard, G.E., Hermanns-Lê. T., Manicourt, D., 2019. Inspiratory muscle strength training improves lung function in patients with the hypermobile Ehlers–Danlos syndrome: A randomized controlled trial. Am. J. Med. Genet. 179A, 356–364.

Sawle, P.J., Pope, F.M., 2019. Chapter 13: Connective tissue disorders ED syndrome. In: Whitehouse, D., Rapley, R., (Eds.), Genomics and Clinical Diagnostics. Royal Society of Chemistry, London, pp. 376–404.

Schalkwijk, J., Zweers, M.C., Steijlen, P.M., et al., 2001. A recessive form of the Ehlers-Danlos syndrome caused by tenascin-X deficiency. N. Engl. J. Med. 345, 1167–1175.

Steinmann, B., Royce, P.M., Superti-Furga, A., 2002. The Ehlers–Danlos syndromes. In: Steinmann, B., Royce, P.M. (Eds.), Connective Tissue and its Heritable Disorders. John Wiley & Sons Inc, New York, pp. 431–523.

Takaluoma, K., Hyry, M., Lantto, J., et al., 2007. Tissue-specific changes in the hydroxylysine content and cross-links of collagens and alterations in fibril morphology in lysyl hydroxylase 1 knock-out mice. J. Biol. Chem. 282, 6588–6596.

Tewari, S., Madabushi, R., Agarwal, A., Gautam, S.K., Khuba, S., 2017. Chronic pain in a patient with Ehlers-Danlos syndrome (hypermobility type): The role of myofascial trigger point injections. J. Bodyw. Mov. Ther. 21, 194–196.

Theocharis, A.D. Manou, D., Karamanos, N.K., 2019. The extracellular matrix as a multitasking player in disease. FEBS J. 286, 2830–2869.

Voermans, N.C., Altenburg, T.M., Hamel, B.C., de Haan, A., van Engelen, B.G., 2007. Reduced quantitative muscle function in tenascin-X deficient Ehlers–Danlos patients. Neuromuscul. Disord. 17, 597–602.

Voermans, N.C., Bonnemann, C.G., Huijing, P.A., et al., 2008. Clinical and molecular overlap between myopathies and inherited connective tissue diseases. Neuromuscul. Disord. 18, 843–856.

Voermans, N.C., van Alfen, N., Pillen, S., et al., 2009b. Neuromuscular involvement in various types of Ehlers–Danlos syndrome. Ann. Neurol. 65, 687–697.

Zweers, M.C., Bristow, J., Steijlen, P.M., et al., 2003. Haploinsufficiency of TNXB is associated with hypermobility type of Ehlers–Danlos syndrome. Am. J. Hum. Genet. 73, 214–217.

Anatomy of the Plantar Fascia

Carlo Biz and Chenglei Fan

CHAPTER CONTENTS

INTRODUCTION

The plantar fascia (or plantar aponeurosis) is one of the most important connective tissue structures, having a fundamental biomechanical role in supporting and maintaining the medial longitudinal arch of the foot, intervening in the mechanisms of propulsion during walking, jumping, running, and other dynamic conditions (Sarrafian 1993). The plantar fascia (PF) originates in the plantar tuberosity of the calcaneus and courses along the plantar foot, dividing into five slips that insert in the base of the proximal phalanges of the toes by the plantar plate and in the plantar skin by superficial extensions (Stecco et al. 2013). Because of its material properties and mechanical behavior, the plantar fascia (PF) can be considered a unique anatomical structure in the sole of the foot, playing an important role in foot stability by being a major contributor of three-plane stability of different tarsal joints (Pavan et al. 2011; Tweed et al. 2009). It is also capable of storing strain energy and converting it into propulsive force, behaving as a quasielastic tissue (Boukerrou et al. 2007). In the *Terminologia Anatomica* (FCAT 1998), only the term plantar aponeurosis is used to indicate this structure, whereas the terms "plantar fascia" and "plantar aponeurosis" are used interchangeably in the various anatomical textbooks. The term "aponeurosis" is generally used to indicate a tissue with a unidirectional arrangement of collagen fibers, whereas a fascia is a structure with a multidirectional arrangement of the fibers (Langevin and Huijing 2009). One microscopic study confirmed that the collagen fibers of this structure were found arranged mainly in a proximal-to-distal longitudinal direction, but there were also various fibers lying in vertical, transverse, and oblique directions. This multilayer configuration of the collagen fibers is a typical feature of fasciae rather than aponeurosis, so the authors suggest that the term "plantar fascia" would be a more appropriate name for this tissue (Stecco et al. 2013). Therefore the term "plantar fascia" is used to indicate this structure in this chapter.

MACROSCOPIC AND MICROSCOPIC CHARACTERISTICS

The PF is a tissue firmly joined to plantar muscles, the digital flexor tendons, and skin. There are numerous fat pads located on the bottom of the foot (Fig. 5.7.1A). The calcaneal fat pad is the largest fat pad and located in the heel directly below the calcaneus. This fat pad is a complex structure of adipose and connective tissue. There are strong vertical, fibrous septa that connect the heel and PF with the skin and divide the subcutaneous fat tissue into isolated compartments. This three-dimensional network of fibroelastic tissue and fat provides a strong anchoring of the skin to the underlying planes while optimizing its response to load. These fat pads act as cushions or shock absorbers; they mitigate shock generated during the gait or running cycle and make it possible to achieve a smooth distribution of pressure (Stecco 2014).

The PF has two fibrous layers: superficial and deep layer. The superficial layer is formed by longitudinal fibers, making up three distinct bands (medial, central, and lateral) that originate posteriorly from the medial process of the tuberosity of calcaneus (heel bone) into the forefoot. Among these, the central band is the thickest, largest, and most prominent (Fig. 5.7.1B). Distally, the central band of the PF divides unequally into five separate components that continue into the fascial sheets of the five toes, including onto the plantar plate and sesamoids. The deep layer is thinner and is not present throughout all of the PF. Further, fibers from the PF blend into the fascia of the intrinsic muscles of the

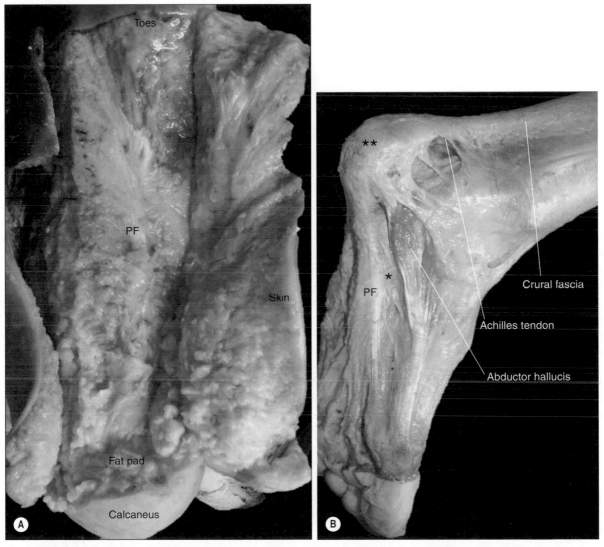

Fig. 5.7.1 (A) A calcaneal fat pad. (B) The plantar fascia is in continuity with the crural fascia (**) and the deep fasciae enveloping the abductor hallucis (*). PF, plantar fascia. Modified with permission from Stecco, C., Corradin, M., Macchi, V., et al., 2013. Plantar fascia anatomy and its relationship with Achilles tendon and paratenon. J. Anat. 223, 665–676.

feet and attach to the skin of the sole of the foot (Kho et al. 2019; Stecco et al. 2013). The PF extends medially, continuing with the deep fasciae enveloping the abductor hallucis and extending laterally, continuing with the deep fascia of digiti minimi muscles (Fig. 5.7.1B). From the superficial aspect of the PF, many vertical fibrous septa (retinaculum cutis superficialis) originate, strongly connecting the PF with the skin. The PF is also attached to the Achilles tendon, which is the tendinous extension of the lower leg muscles, the calf muscles (Benjamin 2009). In one MRI radiological study, the authors showed that the PF's origin does not change with respect to age or sex, but the continuity between the PF and Achilles tendon decreases during aging (Pękala et al. 2019). However, one study showed that the PF is more closely connected to the paratenon of the Achilles tendon than to the Achilles tendon itself through the periosteum of the heel. Stecco et al. (2013) has demonstrated that a connection between PF and the paratenon of the Achilles tendon, via a fascial sheet over the calcaneous bone, is present at all ages. In fact, the crural fascia is in continuity with the paratenon and splits around the tendon to form the paratenon of the Achilles tendon. The posterior portion of the crural fascia is stretched distally due to the continuity between it and the PF. The PF gives insertions to many intrinsic muscles, and traction occurs between the heel and the posterior region of the crural fascia. The fascia lata, "crural fascia" in the leg, and the "PF" and "dorsal fascia of the foot" are just topographical nomenclature according to location. All of them belong to the deep fasciae in the inferior limb, and defined boundaries of the deep fasciae cannot be clearly identified because of fascial continuity. According to the "theory of a whole-body fascial linkage," the PF is also connected to the trunk, the neck, the head, and the internal region, guaranteed by musculoskeletal fasciae and visceral fasciae (Myers 2013; Stecco 2004; Stecco and Stecco 2013). From the anatomical point of view, all the muscles related to the PF are connected to each other and work with exceptional synergy.

Almost all the tissue of PF is formed of type I collagen, whereas only in the loose connective tissue where the large fibrous bundles change directions is there also type III collagen, as seen with immunohistochemical stains. Few elastic fibers could be revealed in the loose connective tissue (Stecco et al. 2013). Under pathological circumstances, due to changes in the density of ground substance, the collagen fibers get closer to each other and may form pathological crosslinks. This may prevent the ability of a normal collagen network to develop the PF and further influence the normal function of the PF (Pawlina and Ross 2018; Stecco 2014).

The PF is also composed of an extracellular matrix (ECM), which is a complex and intricate structural network that surrounds and supports cells within the PF. One study found that the ECM in PF is highly rich in hyaluronan/hyaluronic acid (HA), probably produced by fibroblastic-like cells described as "fasciacytes" (Fede et al. 2018a; Stecco et al. 2013). HA molecules are very large (100–10,000 kDa) and can hold a large volume of water. The pressure, or turgor, that occurs in these giant hydrophilic proteoglycan aggregates accounts for the ability of PF to resist compression without inhibiting flexibility, making them excellent shock absorbers. In addition, HA provides a lubricant for PF as it glides over the skin and superficial fascia or under the plantar muscles. It is likely that these gliding interactions are influenced by the composition and efficacy of the HA-rich ECM. This HA-rich layer also is particularly plentiful during embryogenesis and in tissues undergoing rapid growth and is present wherever repair and regeneration occur (Pawlina and Ross 2018; Stecco 2014). If the HA amount, molecular size, and metabolism change, it could affect the functions of the PF as an excellent lubricant, shock absorber, immobilizer, efficient insulator, and wound healer.

Nerve endings and Pacini and Ruffini corpuscles are present in the PF, particularly in the medial and lateral portions where it joins with the fasciae of the abductor hallucis and abductor digiti minimi muscles, and where the sole muscles are inserted. Pacinian corpuscles, which are also found in the skin, joint capsules, and periosteum, adapt rapidly to stimuli. Ruffini corpuscles are found in the skin and joint capsules as well and adapt slowly to stimuli (Abraira and Ginty 2013). Hence, stretching, twisting, or pressure affecting a joint can activate Pacinian or Ruffini afferent corpuscles and affect efferent activity of relevant muscles of the PF (as described previously). Interestingly, Adams et al. report that free nerve endings, although categorized as nonspecialized, can function as mechanoreceptors, nociceptors, and thermoreceptors or in a polymodal manner (Adams et al. 1997). If the relevant muscles of PF contract excessively, the PF and the nerve endings it contains might be overstretched. These findings suggest that the PF has a role not only in supporting the longitudinal arch of the foot but also in its proprioception and peripheral motor coordination. Its relationship with the crural fascia and the paratenon of the Achilles tendon is consistent with the idea of triceps surae structures being involved in PF pathology, so their rehabilitation can be considered appropriate. These properties of the PF shed new light on this complex tissue. The fascia could be seen as a coachman guiding the muscles in the sole of the foot and helping to coordinate all of these structures during movement (Stecco et al. 2013).

> ### KEY POINT
>
> The plantar fascia gives insertions to many intrinsic muscles, and traction occurs between the heel and the posterior region of the crural fascia. The plantar fascia and the dorsal fascia of the foot and the fascia lata and the crural fascia in the leg belong to the deep fasciae, and defined boundaries of the deep fasciae cannot be clearly identified because of fascial continuity. The plantar fascia has a role not only in supporting the longitudinal arch of the foot but also in its proprioception and peripheral motor coordination because nerve endings and Pacini and Ruffini corpuscles are present in the PF. The PF is also composed of an extracellular matrix and is highly rich in hyaluronan.

BIOMECHANICAL IMPLICATIONS

> ### KEY POINT
>
> The stress–strain curve of PF, similar to other connective tissues with high elastin content such as ligaments, shows a nonlinear response: a "toe" region, a linear region, and a failure region.

The toe region is typically from small strains in the undeformed state. In this region the tissue has low stiffness, a mechanical characteristic that is related to the crimping conformation of the collagen fibers and the large compliance of elastin fibers. In experimental tests carried out on samples of PF, the toe region was found to extend up to 4% of strain. Over this value (linear region), the tissue shows greater stiffness and an almost linear response. In this region, the stress increment is proportional to the strain increment. In some samples of PF, a progressive failure was found at higher than 12% strain. This failure is caused by damage in the collagen fibers and results in progressive reduction of the stiffness. The maximum strength of the tissue is expressed by the maximum value of the stress shown by the stress–strain curve. This maximum strength of the tissue occurs in a region where damage phenomena occur. The physiological range of strain is limited to a region free from damage phenomena. This means that the PF generally works with a safety factor based on its strength (Fig. 5.7.2) (Pavan et al. 2011; Stecco 2014).

Carano and Siciliani (1996) demonstrated that stretching fibroblasts could increase turnover by increasing the secretion of collagenase, an enzyme that plays an important role in the degradation of collagen fibers. These authors demonstrated that cyclical stretching is more effective than a continuous stretch. Stretching or compressing delivers an immediate and proportional deformation of the fibroblasts, but after 10 to 15 minutes the cell morphology begins to readapt to the new mechanical environment, causing a loss of the biological activation. This suggests that a new mechanical stimulus is necessary to induce a new biological reaction. In relaxation tests using cadavers without specific foot pathologies, the stress was reduced 35% to 40% in 120 seconds, which was found independent of the level of the applied strain (Pavan et al. 2011). The mechanical characteristics of the PF is helpful to understand its response to overuse and clinical results of different manual and physical therapies that use heat, pressure, or stretch to modify the PF.

High tension in the PF could also cause a periosteal lifting at its insertion on the calcaneus, and bone healing could cause growth of a spur that might be seen at the calcaneus. The direction and amount of pull from the fascia on the calcaneus form the bone spur, because mechanical stress influences and modulates bone growth. Onwuanyi (2000) found that plantar heel pain in combination with heel-spur formation occurs in about 50% of patients, although other researchers doubt the contribution of the heel spur to the condition. Tountas and Fornasier (1996) found that the intrinsic changes within the PF rather than the heel spur itself resulted in the condition. The plantar heel pain occurs not from the bone spur but from the excessive tension applied to the PF (Bolgla and Malone 2004).

PLANTAR FASCIA THICKNESS AND STIFFNESS

The thickness and stiffness of the PF could vary with the site, gender, body mass index (BMI), and different

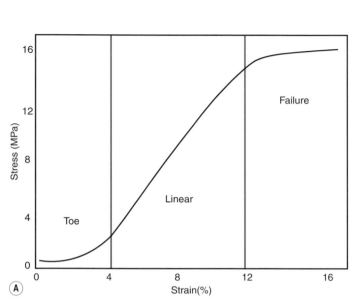

Fig. 5.7.2 (A) Biomechanical characteristics of the healthy plantar fascia, described as stress vs strain. The "toe" region receives 0% to 4% of the strain, the linear region responds to 4% to 12% of the strain, and the failure region occurs over 12% of strain in the tissue. (B) Tissue characteristics corresponding to the biomechanical behavior. The toe region is related to the crimping conformation of the collagen fibers. The linear region corresponds to the linear conformation of the collagen fibers. The failure region is caused by damage in the collagen fibers. Modified with permission from Stecco, C., 2014. Functional Atlas of the Human Fascial System. E-Book. Churchill Livingstone Elsevier, Oxford, UK.

pathologies (plantar fasciitis, diabetes, etc.), but it seems to remain constant with age. The mean thickness values reported ranges from 3.0 to 4.0 mm on the long axis using ultrasound, depending on the study (135 healthy participants, with a mean age range of 23–45 years, 50 men and 62 women) (Fig. 5.7.3A) (Fede et al. 2018b); However, the thickness of the PF could vary with sites of PF. According to Huerta et al. (2008), the mean PF thickness evaluated with ultrasound was 1.99 ± 0.65 mm, 3.33 ± 0.69 mm at the insertion, 2.70 ± 0.69 mm at 1 cm distal from the insertion, and 2.64 ± 0.69 mm at 2 cm distal from the insertion. According to Moraes do

Carmo et al. (2008), the PF, evaluated by dissection, presented a mean thickness of 4.4 mm in its central part and 2.7 mm in its lateral part, whereas its medial portion was thin. Shiotani et al. (2019) demonstrated that the PF thickness varies according to site and gender. The proximal sites of PF around the calcaneal attachment were significantly thicker and stiffer than the middle and distal sites. In addition, females had significantly thinner PF in proximal and middle sites than males while being significantly stiffer regardless of the sites compared with males. One study, in vitro, demonstrated that fascial cells can modulate the production of some

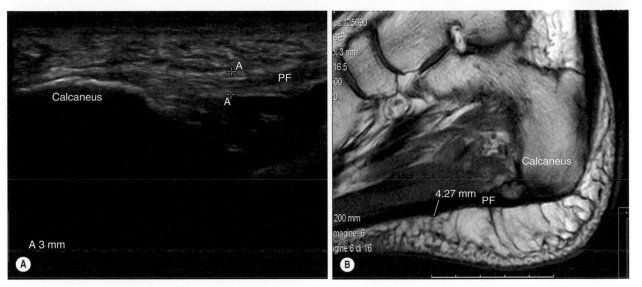

Fig. 5.7.3 (A) Ultrasound image showing plantar fascia thickness (3 mm) in a healthy subject. (B) MRI image showing plantar fascia is thicker (4.27 mm) in patients with Achilles tendon inflammation. PF, plantar fascia. A in the image (A) indicates the thickness of the plantar fascia.

components of the extracellular matrix according to hormone levels (Fede et al. 2019). The PF elasticity change during the menstrual cycle might have effects on posture sway and tremor, which could cause a potential risk of falling (Petrofsky and Lee 2015). Another study also found that females had a lower PF and heel fat pad thickness compared with males. In addition, correlation analysis results suggest that higher PF and heel fat pad thickness in males may be related to higher body mass and height (Taş 2018). Increased BMI causes a decrease in the stiffness of the PF and an increase in the thickness of the PF, as well as the thickness and stiffness of the heal pad. Increased BMI could cause changes in the mechanical properties of the heal pad and the PF (Taş et al. 2017). Taş and Bek (2018) demonstrated that the morphological and mechanical properties of the PF and the heel fat pad play an important role in balance performance (Taş and Bek 2018). Higher PF and heel fat pad stiffness and thickness are related to higher postural sway in anterior-posterior and medial-lateral directions based on single-leg balance tests.

In plantar fasciitis, different studies have found an increased thickness of the PF, varying from 2.9 to 6.2 mm, depending on the study and the points evaluated. Fabrikant and Park (2011) performed ultrasound tests on patients affected by plantar fasciitis, highlighting a thickening of the PF during the disease while a

decrease was observed if the patient underwent clinical treatment, suggesting that the PF thickening is related to inflammation episodes. Wu et al. (2011) used sonoelastography to demonstrate that PF softens with age in subjects with plantar fasciitis. In one MRI radiological study, Stecco et al. (2013) showed that the PF was thicker (3.43 ± 0.48 mm) in 27/52 patients with Achilles tendon inflammation and/or degeneration (Fig. 5.7.3B) as opposed to 2.09 ± 0.24 mm in patients with no Achilles tendon diseases. In the group of 27/52 patients with tendinopathies, the PF was more than 4.5 mm thick in five patients (they exceeded the threshold for a diagnosis of plantar fasciitis). None of the other patients (25/52) had a PF of more than 4 mm thick. There was a statistically significant correlation between the thicknesses of the PF and the paratenon.

The PF may be thicker in diabetic patients than in healthy controls. High-resolution ultrasound images showed an average 2.0 mm thickness at the calcaneal insertion in healthy controls, 2.9 mm in diabetic patients, 3.0 mm in neuropathic diabetic patients, and 3.1 mm in diabetic patients with a history of foot ulceration (D'Ambrogi et al. 2003). The thickness of the PF and of the Achilles tendon was measured by ultrasound tests and highlighted a thickening of both these structures in patients affected by diabetes, especially in those who were affected also by neuropathy (Giacomozzi et al. 2005). The thickening of the PF was associated with a more rigid foot, leading to alterations of the gait cycle and of the plantar pressure distribution. With computed tomography, a thicker PF was found in diabetic patients than in healthy controls (mean 4.2 vs 3.6 mm) (Bolton et al. 2005). Increased fascia thickness in diabetes is probably also associated with nonenzymatic glycosylation of collagen; a reduction of 30% in collagen content in the PF has been found in diabetic patients (Andreassen et al. 1981). Apparently, with longstanding diabetes, geometrical changes of the PF, shown as thickening of this connective tissue structure, may occur.

 KEY POINT

The thickness and stiffness of the PF can vary with site, gender, body mass index (BMI), and different pathologies (plantar fasciitis, diabetes, etc.), but it seems to remain constant with age.

CLINICAL IMPLICATIONS AND TREATMENT

The PF is a major arch support structure of the feet, being a fibrous tendon that maintains the longitudinal arch of the foot and starts at the calcaneal tubercle and ends at the metatarsals. During walking, the load on the PF exceeds its capacity, which results in a degenerative change or PF injury that causes inflammatory pain. Plantar heel pain can be due to local causes, but plantar fasciitis is the most common cause of heel pain (Wu et al. 2019). The etiology of plantar fasciitis is believed to be multifactorial. The highest incidence is seen between the ages of 40 and 60 years. Increased body weight and presence of calcaneal spur are main risk factors along with increased age, reduced ankle dorsiflexion, decreased first metatarsophalangeal joint extension, and prolonged standing (Mao et al. 2019). According to biomechanical studies, PF abnormalities, based on the windlass mechanism, describe overpronation and underpronation to help formulate possible relationships between conditions and treatments. Clinicians or physical therapists can reproduce the heel pain at the medial calcaneal tubercle in a weight-bearing position using the windlass test, which is useful in determining PF irritation. Use of this approach may improve clinical

outcomes, because rehabilitation intervention does not merely treat physical symptoms but actively addresses the influences that resulted in the condition (Bolgla and Malone 2004).

Plantar heel pain can also be due to referred causes, S1 radiculopathy, or systemic illness (Allam and Chang 2019). Weakness in the gluteus medius, gluteus minimus, tensor fascia latae, or quadriceps muscles inhibits their ability to assist with the lower extremity load response and further contribute to PF abnormalities, which can accelerate lower extremity pronation as well. Therefore proximal muscle weaknesses can lead to poor shock absorption and decreased pronation control (Bolgla and Malone 2004). Local pain in the prostate can also radiate referred pain to the abdomen region, lower back region, and leg and the plantar region (Purves et al. 2004). According to the "theory of a whole-body fascial linkage," PF abnormalities could lead to a dysfunction of the PF itself; the symptoms can arise directly from the area or from a distance, as a result of fascial continuity. In a similar manner, dysfunctions in the musculoskeletal and visceral system far from the PF could be capable of producing referred pain in the PF. Understanding referred pain can lead to an accurate diagnosis that might otherwise be missed. Therefore every physical examination of a patient with heel pain should include an evaluation of the PF, the fasciae, and the corresponding muscles in the inferior limb, the trunk, the neck, the head, and the internal system, based on the medical history, for tissue tightness and fascial restrictions related to fascial continuity (Stecco et al. 2013). After careful review of the patient's medical history, physical evaluation and appropriate radiology (ultrasound, MRI, and sonoelastography or radiological instruments) are necessary to discern important local causes (alterations of the PF to assess its status) and/or referred causes (proximal muscle weaknesses, fascial densification, internal disfunction). Some authors believe that the ultrasound-based diagnosis of plantar fasciitis is an effective, objective, economical, and noninvasive method (Wu et al. 2019). Certainly the practitioner needs to take into account all of the possibilities that could influence the thickness or stiffness as well, such as gender, age, BMI, and different pathologies.

Treatment is clearly directed toward the causes (local or referred causes) according to accurate diagnostic testing. Initial treatment for heel pain may include physical therapy

(Renan-Ordine et al. 2011), padding and strapping of the foot, therapeutic orthotic insoles, oral antiinflammatories, and interventional injection therapy (corticosteroid injection and high molecular-weight HA) (Kumai et al. 2018). Patient-directed treatment is also important in resolving symptoms, including regular stretching of the Achilles tendon and the PF, avoidance of flat shoes and barefoot walking, cryotherapy applied directly to the affected part, over-the-counter arch supports and heel cups, and limitation of extended (high-impact) physical activities. Referred causes must be considered, especially for patients with little or no improvement after local treatment and/or history of trauma, concomitant pain, or internal dysfunction. Patients usually have a clinical response within 6 weeks of initiation of treatment. If improvement is noted, the initial therapy program is continued until symptoms are resolved. If little or no improvement is noted and the diagnosis is accurate for local causes, the patient should be referred to a foot and ankle surgeon. Surgical management is indicated for persistent pain despite all efforts with nonoperative intervention. Endoscopic plantar fasciotomy is an alternative to traditional open proximal partial fasciotomy, but concerns with endoscopic release are poor visualization and the possibility of unintended complete release. Complete surgical release of the PF will alter the foot biomechanics, as the windlass effect may be lost after surgery. However, a prospective case series by De Prado revealed that percutaneous total fascia release did not produce a significant drop in arch height on radiographs (De Prado et al. 2019). In cadaveric studies, it has been shown that PF tension is directly proportional to Achilles tendon tension (Mao et al. 2019). Many surgical techniques aimed at dividing the gastrocnemius at different anatomical levels have been proposed for the operative treatment of isolated gastrocnemius tightness (Hamilton et al. 2009).

KEY POINT

Plantar heel pain can be due to local causes, such as plantar fasciitis, and referred causes, such as S1 radiculopathy or systemic illness. Understanding referred pain can lead to an accurate diagnosis that might otherwise be missed. Treatment is clearly directed toward the causes (local or referred causes) according to accurate diagnostic testing.

Summary

The plantar fascia has typical features of fasciae, as opposed to aponeuroses, because the collagen fibers are arranged in a multilayer configuration. The plantar fascia gives insertions to many intrinsic muscles and has continuity with the deep fasciae in the inferior limb, the trunk, the neck, the head, and the internal region, guaranteed by musculoskeletal fasciae and visceral fasciae according to the "theory of a whole-body fascial linkage." Therefore all of the muscles related to the PF are connected to each other and work with exceptional synergy. The plantar fascia has a role in proprioception and peripheral motor coordination because nerve endings and Pacini and Ruffini corpuscles are present in the PF. The PF is also composed of an extracellular matrix and is highly rich in hyaluronan.

The stress–strain curve of the PF, similar to other connective tissues, shows a nonlinear response: a "toe" region, a linear region, and a failure region. The thickness and stiffness of the PF can vary with site, gender, body mass index (BMI), and different pathologies (plantar fasciitis, diabetes, etc.), but it seems to remain constant with age. Plantar heel pain can be due to local causes, such as plantar fasciitis, and referred causes, such as S1 radiculopathy or systemic illness. Understanding referred pain can lead to an accurate diagnosis that might otherwise be missed. Treatment is clearly directed toward the causes (local or referred causes) according to accurate diagnostic testing.

REFERENCES

Abraira, V.E., Ginty, D.D., 2013. The sensory neurons of touch. Neuron 79, 618–639.

Adams, R.D., Victor, M., Ropper, A.H., 1997. Principles of Neurology, sixth ed. McGraw-Hill, New York.

Allam, A.E., Chang, K.V., 2019. Plantar Heel Pain. In: StatPearls [Internet]. StatPearls Publishing, Treasure Island, FL. Available from: https://www.ncbi.nlm.nih.gov/books/NBK499868/.

Andreassen, T., Seyer-Hansen, K., Oxlund, H., 1981. Biomechanical changes in connective tissues induced by experimental diabetes. Acta Endocrinol. 98, 432–436.

Benjamin, M., 2009. The fascia of the limbs and back—a review. J. Anat. 214, 1–18.

Bolgla, L.A., Malone, T.R., 2004. Plantar fasciitis and the windlass mechanism: a biomechanical link to clinical practice. J. Athl. Train. 39, 77.

Bolton, N.R.M., Smith, K.E., Pilgram, T.K., Mueller, M.J., Bae, K.T., 2005. Computed tomography to visualize and quantify the plantar aponeurosis and flexor hallucis longus tendon in the diabetic foot. Clin. Biomech. 20, 540–546.

Boukerrou, M., Boulanger, L., Rubod, C., et al., 2007. Study of the biomechanical properties of synthetic mesh implanted in vivo. Eur. J. Obstet. Gynecol. Reprod. Biol. 134, 262–267.

Carano, A., Siciliani, G., 1996. Effects of continuous and intermittent forces on human fibroblasts in vitro. Eur. J. Orthod. 18, 19–26.

D'Ambrogi, E., Giurato, L., D'Agostino, M.A., et al., 2003. Contribution of plantar fascia to the increased forefoot pressures in diabetic patients. Diabetes Care 26, 1525–1529.

De Prado, M., Cuervas-Mons, M., De Prado, V., Golanó, P., Vaquero, J., 2019. Does the minimally invasive complete plantar fasciotomy result in deformity of the Plantar arch? A prospective study. Foot and Ankle Surg. 26, 347–353.

Do Carmo, C. C. M., de Almeida Melão, L. I. F., de Lemos Weber, M. F. V., Trudell, D., & Resnick, D. 2008. Anatomical features of plantar aponeurosis: cadaveric study using ultrasonography and magnetic resonance imaging. Skeletal Radiol. 37, 929–935.

Fabrikant, J.M., Park, T.S., 2011. Plantar fasciitis (fasciosis) treatment outcome study: plantar fascia thickness measured by ultrasound and correlated with patient self-reported improvement. Foot 21, 79–83.

FCAT (Federative Committee on Anatomical Terminology), 1998. Terminologia Anatomica: International Anatomical Terminology. Georg Thieme Verlag, New York.

Fede, C., Angelini, A., Stern, R., et al., 2018a. Quantification of hyaluronan in human fasciae: variations with function and anatomical site. J. Anat. 233, 552–556.

Fede, C., Gaudreault, N., Fan, C., et al., 2018b. Morphometric and dynamic measurements of muscular fascia in healthy individuals using ultrasound imaging: a summary of the discrepancies and gaps in the current literature. Surg. Radiol. Anat. 40, 1329–1341.

Fede, C., Pirri, C., Fan, C., et al., 2019. Sensitivity of the fasciae to sex hormone levels: Modulation of collagen-I, collagen-III and fibrillin production. PloS One 14, e0223195.

Giacomozzi, C., D'ambrogi, E., Uccioli, L., Macellari, V., 2005. Does the thickening of Achilles tendon and plantar fascia contribute to the alteration of diabetic foot loading? Clin. Biomech. 20, 532–539.

Hamilton, P.D., Brown, M., Ferguson, N., et al. 2009. Surgical anatomy of the proximal release of the gastrocnemius: a cadaveric study. Foot Ankle Int. 30, 1202–1206.

Huerta, J.P., Garcia, J.M.A., Matamoros, E.C., Matamoros, J.C., Martínez, T.D., 2008. Relationship of body mass index, ankle dorsiflexion, and foot pronation on plantar fascia thickness in healthy, asymptomatic subjects. J. Am. Podiatr. Med. Assoc. 98, 379–385.

Kho, J.S., Almeer, G., McGarry, S., James, S.L., Botchu, R., 2019. Technical report: dynamic assessment of plantar fasciitis and plantar fascia tears utilising dorsiflexion of the great toe. J. Ultrasound 1-4.

Kumai, T., Samoto, N., Hasegawa, A., et al., 2018. Short-term efficacy and safety of hyaluronic acid injection for plantar fasciopathy. Knee Surg. Sports Traumatol. Arthrosc. 26, 903–911.

Langevin, H.M., Huijing, P.A., 2009. Communicating about fascia: history, pitfalls, and recommendations. Int. J. Ther. Massage Bodywork 2, 3.

Mao, D.W., Chandrakumara, D., Zheng, Q., Kam, C., King, C.K.K., 2019. Endoscopic plantar fasciotomy for plantar fasciitis: A systematic review and network meta-analysis of the English Literature. Foot 41, 63–73.

Myers, T.W., 2013. Anatomy Trains: Myofascial Meridians for Manual and Movement Therapists, third ed. [E-book]. Churchill Livingstone Elsevier, Edinburgh, UK.

Onwuanyi, O., 2000. Calcaneal spurs and plantar heel pad pain. Foot 10, 182–185.

Pavan, P., Stecco, C., Darwish, S., Natali, A., De Caro, R., 2011. Investigation of the mechanical properties of the plantar aponeurosis. Surg. Radiol. Anat. 33, 905–911.

Pawlina, W., Ross, M.H., 2018. Histology: A Text and Atlas: With Correlated Cell and Molecular Biology, eighth ed. Wolters Kluwer, Philadelphia, PA.

Pękala, P.A., Kaythampillai, L., Skinningsrud, B., et al., 2019. Anatomical variations of the plantar fascia's origin with respect to age and sex—an MRI based study. Clin. Anat. 32, 597–602.

Petrofsky, J., Lee, H., 2015. Greater reduction of balance as a result of increased plantar fascia elasticity at ovulation during the menstrual cycle. Tohoku J. Exp. Med. 237, 219–226.

Purves, D., Augustine, G.J., Fitzpatrick, D., et al., 2004. Neuroscience. Sinauer Associates. Inc, Sunderland, MA.

Renan-Ordine, R., Alburquerque-Sendĺn, F., Rodrigues De Souza, D.P., Cleland, J.A., Fernández-de-las-Peñas, C., 2011. Effectiveness of myofascial trigger point manual therapy combined with a self-stretching protocol for the management of plantar heel pain: a randomized controlled trial. J. Orthop. Sports Phys. Ther. 41, 43–50.

Sarrafian, S.K., 1993. Anatomy of the Foot and Ankle: Descriptive, Topographic, Functional, second ed. Lippincott Williams & Wilkins, Philadelphia, PA.

Shiotani, H., Yamashita, R., Mizokuchi, T., Naito, M., Kawakami, Y., 2019. Site-and sex-differences in morphological and mechanical properties of the plantar fascia: A supersonic shear imaging study. J. Biomec. 85, 198–203.

Stecco, C., 2014. Functional Atlas of the Human Fascial System. E-Book. Churchill Livingstone Elsevier, Oxford, UK.

Stecco, C., Corradin, M., Macchi, V., et al., 2013. Plantar fascia anatomy and its relationship with Achilles tendon and paratenon. J. Anat. 223, 665–676.

Stecco, L. 2004. Fascial Manipulation for Musculoskeletal Pain. Piccin, Padua, Italy.

Stecco, L., Stecco, C., 2013. Fascial Manipulation for Internal Dysfunctions. Piccin, Padua, Italy.

Taş, S., 2018. Effect of gender on mechanical properties of the plantar fascia and heel fat pad. Foot Ankle Spec. 11, 403–409.

Taş, S., Bek, N., 2018. Effects of morphological and mechanical properties of plantar fascia and heel pad on balance performance in asymptomatic females. Foot 36, 30–34.

Taş, S., Bek, N., Ruhi Onur, M., Korkusuz, F., 2017. Effects of body mass index on mechanical properties of the plantar fascia and heel pad in asymptomatic participants. Foot Ankle Int. 38, 779–784.

Tountas, A., Fornasier, V., 1996. Operative treatment of subcalcaneal pain. Clin. Orthop. Relat. Res. 332, 170–178.

Tweed, J.L., Barnes, M.R., Allen, M.J., Campbell, J.A., 2009. Biomechanical consequences of total plantar fasciotomy: a review of the literature. J Am. Podiatr. Med. Assoc. 99, 422–430.

Wu, C.H., Chang, K.V., Mio, S., Chen, W.S., Wang, T.G., 2011. Sonoelastography of the plantar fascia. Radiology 259, 502–507.

Wu, J., Zhang, Y.Z., Gao, Y., Luo, T.Y., 2019. Assessment the reliability of ultrasonography in the imaging of the plantar fascia: A comparative study. BMC Med. Imaging 19, 1–7.

Fascia and Low Back Pain

Mark Driscoll and Khaled El-Monajjed

CHAPTER CONTENTS

THE EPIDEMIC OF LOW BACK PAIN

What is Low Back Pain?

The distinction between *pain* and *disability* is clearly identified in the medical field. Although disability is the inability of one to perform a certain activity considered to be normal to human beings, pain, as defined by the International Association for the Study of Pain, is an unpleasant emotional or sensory experience associated with actual or potential tissue damage. This incorporates both a psychological and physiological foundation attesting to its subjective nature, which presents an inherent complexity in clinical assessments.

Consequently, it comes as no surprise that there is little consensus on the definition of *low back pain* in the medical field. The Danish Institute for Health Technology Assessment (1999) defines Low Back Pain (LBP) as "a tiredness, discomfort or pain in the low back region, with or without radiating symptoms to the leg or legs." Although some researchers define LBP as a common musculoskeletal disease that must be addressed as a complex disease (Allegri et al. 2016), the World Health Organization (WHO) disproves LBP as a disease or diagnostic entity of any sort. In fact, WHO defines LBP

as "a term attributed to pain in an area of the anatomy that it has become a paradigm of responses to external and internal stimuli – for example, 'Oh, my aching back' is an expression to mean that a person is troubled." Other researchers identify pain as a warning and settle on the definition that LBP is a whole symptom regardless of the cause and condition (Waddell 2004).

Types of LBP are usually classified according to their duration. Although the exact values vary, an accepted estimate for LBP is as follows:

- Acute LBP (ALBP): less than 6 weeks
- Subacute LBP (SLBP): between 6 to 12 weeks
- Chronic LBP (CLBP): more than 12 weeks
- Recurrent LBP (RLBP): LBP returns at some time in the future after recovering from episode.

A GLIMPSE INTO LOW BACK PAIN HISTORY

The earliest surviving writings of LBP in historiography date back to 7th century BCE, noted in a compilation of Edwin Smith Papyrus. In this, 6 of 48 published reports deal with spinal injuries to great accuracy in the clinical descriptions presented. Ironically, the last and only case written in the script (i.e., case 48) illustrating acute LBP cuts off abruptly midway when describing the treatment adopted. The next record on workings of low back pain adhere to Corpus Hippocrates (circa 400 BCE) from his collected writings of the Greek Library at Cos and Cnidus (Allan and Waddell 1989). The writings were investigated and built upon by Galen of Pergamon (circa CE 150) and his disciples who basically ruled LBP medicine for the next 1200 years. The literature described the acknowledgment of LBP as a symptom associated with various disorders related to joint and muscle. The overall attitude conformed toward a rather relaxing solution, including spas and soothing exercises. After the fall of the Greco-Roman Empire, medical practice was adopted by exiled Christians in Persia. Following the rise of the Islamic Empire, two well-known treatments adopted during that era were massaging with olive oil and Hijama (Farhadi et al. 2009).

It was not until medicine took its toll in the European Renaissance that LBP was reinvestigated. In fact, Paracelsus (1493–1541) opposed the early clinical writings to practice diagnosis and treatment solely. Indeed, this later allowed practitioners to observe and provide personal conclusions. Notably, Sydenham (1624–1689), later within the same era, simplified low back pain (also called lumbago) to rheumatism, a disorder of the musculoskeletal system. Alternatively, physicians of the 19th century were directed to finding the causes behind LBP. Conclusively, two main postulates of the 19th century, which are also considered as a conceptual basis from which medical diagnostics were built on today, are: LBP originates from the spine and LBP is a result of trauma. It is worthy to note that Brown was the first to realize LBP, in 1828, was sourced from what he called "spinal irritation" to describe the "vertebral tenderness" and the nervous system (Waddell 2004). Until that era, doctors, medical practitioners, and patients gave little attention to the fact that low back pain could be the result of injury up until the Industrial Revolution. Erichsen (1866) diagnosed what he called the "railway spine" (or what is known today as Erichsen's disease) when he observed survivors of railway crashes enduring pain with no apparent injuries to explain it. This progression then leads to the modern medicine of the present time.

KEY POINTS

Low back pain awareness and historical treatment logs suggest this syndrome has long plagued humanity.

EFFECT OF LOW BACK PAIN ON HUMANS AND ECONOMIES

Although LBP has been constantly coupled in context with other spinal disorders, including degenerative spines, it has been given very little attention. The obvious question becomes then, why have we regarded LBP as a serious medical concern? LBP resulting from injury became popular after the beginning of the industrial revolution (Benzel 2005). LBP is the leading cause of activity limitation and work productivity inhibition around the world, causing an economic burden on families, companies, and governments (Hoy et al. 2010). Today, LBP has become the fifth most common reason for all physician visits (Mafi et al. 2013), but around 10 years ago, LBP was considered to be a Western issue only. It was not until studies of LBP were popularized in other parts of the world that we have seen it widespread in mid- and low-income countries (Hoy et al. 2010). Yet still most epidemiological studies and data collection surveys are most widely conducted in North America. Even then, the epidemiology of this condition is not yet clear, with a substantial difference in previously reported prevalence and incidence data (Hartvigsen et al. 2018). Low back pain is common, with a peak onset at an average age of 35 years and a lifetime incidence of 85%. An increase in chronic LBP cases of 23.5% occurred between 1990 and 2016. It is estimated that the number of years lived with disability as a result of LBP has increased by 23.4% from 6.2 million in 1990 to 7.7 million in 2016 in China alone (Wu et al. 2019).

Low back pain has a direct effect on human's physiological and emotional well-being. Studies have shown that people with chronic low back pain have twice the risk of suicide compared with healthy individuals (Tang and Crane 2006). Nevertheless, prior studies have reached a consensus that LBP indeed affects the performance of activities of daily living. Additionally, reduced sexual functionality has been previously reported to be associated with LBP (Grabovac and Dorner 2019).

Even though chronic LBP is 5% to 20% of LBP cases, the costs associated with chronic LBP consume more than 85% of the total LBP costs. Direct medical costs in the United States alone have been estimated at approximately $560 to $635 billion, annually affecting 100 million people with chronic and acute LBP. The annual cost of LBP in Australia was estimated to be AU$9 billion (i.e., US$350 to

$400 per resident) (Institute of Medicine 2011). In addition to incurred medical costs and disability compensation, the cost of pain includes lost school days, lost productivity and employment, reduced incomes, and a lower quality of life.

CURRENT TREATMENTS OF LOW BACK PAIN

In 2018, the *Lancet* Low Back Pain Series Working Group established the existence of a global problem in the mismanagement of LBP (Traeger et al. 2019). Treatments for LBP are perceived as more of diagnostics conducted on the patient to specify as accurately as possible a conceivable "interventional management" of pain. Clinicians agree that the goals of treatment for ALBP are to relieve the patient from the displeasing sensation of pain, improve the ability to refunction normally, reduce time spent off work, and educate the patient on proper practices.

The issue is that prevalence studies show that cases of LBP are mostly nonspecific and, thus, cannot be attributed to one cause directly. Therefore clinicians depend on a diagnostic method that can carefully narrow down treatment requirements. Moreover, it allows clinicians to rule out "Red Flags" that usually require a promptly aggressive diagnosis, including trauma due to injury causing fracture, major progressive neural deficiency, urinary retention, etc. (Casazza 2012). A number of guidelines exist for the diagnosis of LBP, such as those published by the Royal College of General Practitioners (1998) or the Institute for Clinical System Improvement (2012). Most guidelines have similar recommendations for the diagnosis of LBP, and a review of most guidelines has shown that they do not contemplate specific recommendations for treatments with only a few showing acceptable results (Arnau et al. 2006). Initially, the diagnostic is a series of structured questions posed to help understand the patient's history, environment, habits, lifestyle, and working conditions (Nasser 2005). The clinician then conducts a physical examination in various positions in an attempt to localize the pain. The clinician should then specify a certain treatment within these guidelines for the patient after the first or second visit depending on the diagnosis (Nasser 2005). Treatments can initially begin with drug therapy, which includes nonsteroidal antiinflammatory drugs (NSAIDs), opioids, muscle sedatives/relaxants, and analgesics (i.e., tramadol). If the clinician is able to specify the exact

pain region, therapeutic injections could be used with minimal effects, which includes trigger-point injections, selective joint injections, and epidural injections with steroids. In other cases, when LBP is not complicated, physical modalities including therapeutic heat, cryotherapy, electrotherapy, and traction could be used given that the patient is showing progress. Should the patients show no signs of improvement over a prolonged period of time, the clinician refers him to a specialist who would later recommend invasive surgery. The specific causes of low back pain for most cases remain inaccurate enough for prescriptions of proper treatment (Nasser 2005).

 KEY POINTS

In measuring pain in LBP, current methods reside on clinicians' experience and/or the use of questionnaires for patients, such as the Oswestry scale or Roland-Morris scores, whereas an array of treatment options are practiced.

POTENTIAL SOURCES OF LOW BACK PAIN

Studies have shown that 85% of patients who visit clinics for LBP are cases in which no specific cause can be attributed—that is, nonspecific low back pain. Recently, however, with a better attribution to different pain generators, researchers have come to believe that the notion of 80% to 90% of cases of LBP being unknown to be less likely (Allegri et al. 2016). Clinicians are usually advised to consider that causes of LBP could be attributed to psychological factors, such as stress or depression and anxiety (Deyo et al. 2015). Kuslich et al. specified intervertebral discs, facet joints, sacroiliac joints, ligaments, fascia, muscles and nerve root dura as tissues that are capable of transmitting pain in the lumbar region (Kuslich et al. 1991).

In many cases, acute low back pain (ALBP) is the leading cause of chronic low back pain (CLBP). While most patients who suffer from acute low back pain (ALBP) are eventually relieved, others may progress to onset CLBP. Nevertheless, CLBP may also originate from injury, disease, or stresses on different structures of the body (Rizk et al. 2012). After a series of diagnoses, causes of CLBP may be the result of a malignancy, vertebral infection, cauda equina syndrome, vertebral compression fracture, ankylosing spondylitis, progressive/ neurological deficits, herniated discs, and spinal stenosis (Chou et al. 2007). Most cases of ALBP are unknown and cannot be attributed with a specific cause, but there are possible causes that should be considered (Casazza, 2012). They are essentially divided into three categories:

1. Intrinsic spine: Compression fracture resulting from trauma, herniated nucleus pulposus, lumbar strains, spinal stenosis, spondylolisthesis, spondylolysis
2. Systematic: Connective tissue disease, inflammatory spondyloarthropathy, malignancy, vertebral diskitis/osteomyelitis
3. Referred: Abdominal aortic aneurysm, gastrointestinal conditions, herpes zoster, pelvic conditions, retroperitoneal conditions.

Pain is the result of nociceptors (i.e., specialized peripheral sensory neurons) transducing signals to the central nervous system as a result of stimuli. CLBP occurs when the noxious stimulus persists, resulting with processes in the central and peripheral sensitization, which converts ALBP to CLBP. Central and peripheral sensitization is the increase in the excitability of neurons, which transforms normal inputs into abnormal responses (Tominaga et al. 2003). This occurs in several chronic pain disorders, including LBP, osteoarthritis, fibromyalgia, headaches, etc. Anatomically, joints, discs, and bones are richly innervated by A-delta fibers that have a strong contribution to the central sensitization upon continuous stimulation (Allegri et al. 2016). Studies identify that the most common cases of LBP are the result of either muscle tension or spasm, whereas in the other cases it is attributed to different pain generators that have specific characteristics that include radicular, facet joint, sacroiliac, and discogenic pain, including spinal stenosis. It is thought that pain could be generated by ligamentous or capsular tension, extraneous compression or shear forces, hypermobility, and altered joint mechanics. In addition to muscle, ligaments and tendons function as load bearing and fascial tissues act as elastic springs with load-bearing functions during oscillatory movements and are densely innervated by myelinated nerve endings. Thus microtearing and/or inflammation of fascia could be a direct source of musculoskeletal pain causing LBP indirectly (Schleip et al. 2010).

FASCIA: FOE OR ALLY?

The Fascial Network

The efficiency of human locomotion is the culmination of harmonized active and passive systems fortified around the foundational support of the thoracolumbar spine (Fig. 5.8.1). This stability is complemented by a structure exhibiting springlike behavior of fascial substance engulfing the torso and penetrating through the different muscular layers assisting, in particular, with load transfer—the *thoracolumbar fascia* (TLF). Composed of a complex network of interweaved aponeurotic and fascial layers, the TLF distinctly cleaves the paraspinal muscles from the posterolaterally located muscles of the abdominal wall (i.e., transversus abdominis, internal oblique, external oblique). In the thoracic region, the TLF spans the entire thoracic vertebrae around the extensor muscles to make its way laterally, attaching onto the ribs. In the lumbar region, the TLF also connects to the lumbar vertebrae but envelops within the surrounding paraspinal layers to connect laterally with the abdominal wall muscles through the *common tendon of transverse abdominis* (cTrA). Vertebra-wise, the TLF is attached to the capsule of facet joints and the supraspinous and interspinous ligaments (Willard et al. 2012).

Medially, the TLF branches out into three main layers, posterior (PLF), medial (MLF), and anterior (ALF). Researchers have identified two models to use when dealing with the TLF—two-layered and three-layered TLF. The two-layered TLF model defines the ALF as an extension of the transversalis fascia, whereby the posterior layer surrounds the back of the paraspinal muscles and the anterior deep layer is embedded between the paraspinal muscles' quadratus lumborum (QL) in the lumbar region. In the three-layered TLF model, this anterior deep layer defines the MLF, whereas the ALF is a thin sheath that passes along the anterior section of the QL to make its way posteriorly between the QL and the psoas major muscles. Furthermore, the posterior layer is further composed of two layers, the deep lamina and the innervated superficial layer that joins the deep lamina in the lumbar region. In both models, the paraspinal muscles are embedded within fascial layers (Vleeming et al. 2014).

In general, the TLF renders as an encapsulation of various paraspinal muscle compartments engulfing the torso as it connects to the abdomen. This unique anatomy raises questions as to its involvement in general pathologies related to LBP.

KEY POINTS

The TLF is a very involved tissue in the human body that highlights its inherent importance in spine biomechanics and thus may serve to add clarity or, conversely, complicate one's mechanical or clinical interpretation of LBP.

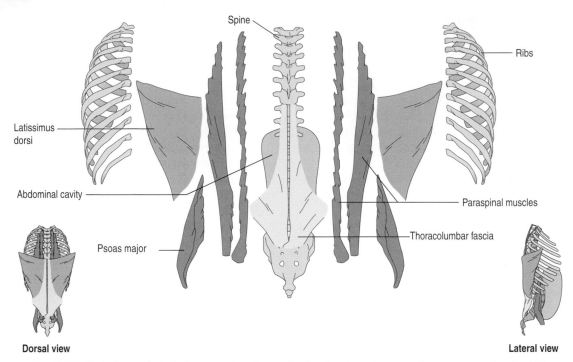

Fig. 5.8.1 Posterior exploded view showing thoracolumbar fascia and surrounding components of a 3D model created for finite-element analysis studies. Courtesy Ibrahim El-Bojairami of the McGill Musculoskeletal Biomechanics Research Lab, Montreal, QC.

WHY FASCIA?

In the past, the TLF structure was mostly ignored in studies, with a focus solely on spinal structures (vertebra, intervertebral discs, facet joints and spinal ligaments). However, positioned as a key structure covering the majority of the human back area, the TLF has become a center of interest when discussing LBP. TLF attachment to various vertebral protrusions and anatomical adhesion to contacting soft tissue, for example, skin or underlying paraspinal muscles, has encouraged researchers to investigate its innervation capacity as a source of pain. Anatomical investigations on rats and humans have shown that nociceptive nerve endings, in fact, do exist within the fascia (Tesarz et al. 2011). These have been conducted using both immunohistochemical techniques (i.e., immunoreactivity for substance P) and neurophysiological techniques (i.e., nerve excitation). Schilder et al. observed reports of higher degrees of pain after a hypertonic saline solution was injected into volunteers' TLFs. This observation led to the implication that A- and C-nociceptor fibers exist in the TLF, specifically in the overlaying superficial posterior layer of the

TLF compared with the lower response from the underlying muscles (i.e., erector spinae) (Schilder et al. 2014). To confirm this finding, they conducted a further study whereby high-frequency electrical stimulation tests (instead of the previous immunohistochemical test) were used on patients (Schilder et al. 2016). The result was that the fascia stimulus recorded lower thresholds compared with the stimuli induced in muscles.

In fact, another fascia, the tibial anterior fascia located distally on the legs, has been related to pain induced by delayed onset of muscle soreness (DOMS) (Gibson et al. 2009). Mechanical sensitization was confirmed with substantial pain intensity compared with hypertonic sodium solution injections to all other tissues. This alludes to the fact that fascia, rather than muscle, may be the main pain-generating tissue in the case of DOMS. The tensor fascia lata (TFL), another deep fascia invested around the thigh area expanding from the gluteus maximus and inserted between its layers, has been also linked to LBP. Essentially, Lee and Kim (2015) confirmed the tensioning of the anterior fibers of gluteus medius muscle and TFL in patients with

CLBP, whereby strengthening and relaxing these sets tended to relieve pain (Lee and Kim 2015). Plantar fasciitis is the most common cause of heel pain, caused by plantar fascia inflammation and stiffness (Tahririan et al. 2012).

Electrophysiological tests on rat spinal dorsal horn neurons have been previously shown to respond to noxious mechanical and chemical perturbations resulting with stimuli within the noxious range with a low mechanical threshold. Moreover, stimulation of different receptors on different tissue, including the skin and muscle, resulted with clear recordings. Furthermore, studies have shown a variation in the nerve ending distribution within the TLF layers. As such, PLF and MLF layers recorded denser SP-positive free nerve endings (assumed to be nociceptive) (Tesarz et al. 2011). In an attempt to further investigate the sensitivity of fascia to pain, a study on rats showed that new receptive fields appear in deep tissues of the hind-limb when the fascia is pathologically altered. This was concluded as one possible explanation for the spread of pain in patients with nonspecific LBP (Hoheisel and Mense 2015). All these observations have strengthened the argument that TLF is a possible pain source in LBP. Nevertheless, ultrasound elasticity imaging has shown an increased thickness of the perimuscular connective tissues forming the thoracolumbar fascia in the low back in patients with CLBP (Langevin et al. 2009).

LBP has proved to be challenging in diagnosis and medical treatment because of minimal clinical and radiological findings aside from known pathological causes (spinal deformities, trauma, ruptured or degenerative discs, etc.). Wilke et al. presents the hypothesis that the TLF is likely a source of LBP (Wilke et al. 2017). They explain that this consideration would likely open the door for new solutions for treatments and provide potential answers to the cause of LBP. For example, the establishment of treatments such as physical therapy, massage, and heating pads targeted at the TLF could possibly render better treatments. In that sense, CLBP becomes idiopathic with possible causes including the microtearing or inflammation of the fascia. This may be evident in post-surgical recovery times specifically in invasive conventional surgeries via posterior approches whereby patients suffer from persistent LBP after full recovery, hence promoting minimally invasive surgeries as an alternative. Furthermore, patients experience less pain during recovery from anterior approaches that

avoid resecting the TLF. Thus, one may deduce that the TLF, when resected, plays a role in continued pain after surgery (Wilke et al. 2017).

> **KEY POINTS**
>
> Human examinations have shown that respondents to pain tests find that fascial tissue stimuli are more painful than muscle or skin tissue, which may allude to the role of the TLF in LBP.

PERSPECTIVES ON FASCIA IN LOW BACK PAIN

Researchers in different fields have examined LBP treatments with a concentration on thoracolumbar fascia. For instance, in kinesiology, Kineseo-Taping (KT) has been tested on patients suffering from LBP symptoms. Tested on 60 patients with CLBP, results in the Oswestry scale have shown significant improvement within 1 week (Castro-Sánchez et al. 2012). However, several studies have reported that the effect of using KT is minimal, with little to no significant clinical data on the benefits because of the immense methods of application. One study showed that KT limited tissue movements in the subcutaneous zone, particularly in flexion movements. However, the study was not compared with sham taping, which is usually designated as a control test, and no ultrasound imaging was used to test muscle activity, which has previously shown altering effects when applied (Tu et al. 2016). Chiropractic management has been considered to be cost-effective when dealing with common back conditions but may lack concrete translational evidence. Practical techniques tend to breakdown TLF adhesions to promote oxygen and nutriment absorption in areas of muscle and fascial dysfunction due to elevated blood flow. Specifically, the use of deep muscle stimulators (DMS) and radial pulse wave have been previously recommended. A common therapeutic maneuver, pelvic tilt, has also been proven to reduce pain (Minicozzi et al. 2016).

Previously, even though osteopathic manipulative treatment (OMT) showed compelling evidence that OMT aids with back conditions, it is still not enough to make changes to the clinical procedures. However, the American College of Physicians designate spinal manipulation as one of the first methods of treatment in LBP guidelines with the rise in the state of osteopathic clinical research in this area. Myofascial release therapy, a hands-on approach adopted by manual therapists, is when the physician purports to relax and realign the fascia. Literature on this approach has varied greatly from a qualitative standpoint but has positively encouraged its use with its positive outcomes on patients with LBP (Balasubramaniam et al. 2014).

It is evident from biomechanical studies that the TLF plays an important role in transferring loads between the spine and its corresponding muscles (Driscoll 2018). It has been noticed that LBP patients have reduced shear strain passed on because of the connective tissue pathological state (Langevin et al. 2011). Though simplified, a finite-element (FE) study included the TLF with an L4-S1 model and concluded that the spinal stability is effectively provided for by the increase in fascial tension (Choi and

Kim 2017). Moreover, a 2D FE-study of the TLF accompanied with the intraabdominal cavity concluded that the structure (Fig. 5.8.2) tended to reduce the imbalance in postural asymmetry to aid in maintaining spinal integrity (El-Monajjed and Driscoll 2018). Moreover, corresponding results were further supported in a 3-dimensional model inclusive of the thoracolumbar fascia (El-Monajjed and Driscoll 2021). In concert with supporting the role of the thoracolumbar fascia in spine mechanics, this group has validated a numerical model of the spine with very high physiological detail, inclusive of the TLF and volumetric muscles (El-Bojairami et al. 2020). This model was then leveraged to demonstrate the load bearing role the TLF has when a simulated flexion was performed (El-Bojairami and Driscoll 2021). With this model, spine stabilizing tissues were iteratively activated and it was shown that the presence of the TLF can reduce the forces required from paraspinal muscles. Furthermore, the presence of the TLF and activation of the intra-abdominal pressure further reduced these muscle forces. The above studies may suggest that if the synergy between the TLF, paraspinal pressure, intra-abdominal pressures and muscle activation is offset, then one's aspiration towards regular spinal mechanics may be difficult. Furthermore, in addition to its on-off presence or activation, the actual mechanical properties of tissues such as the TLF can have important implications to how loads are distributed or handled, so to speak, within our bodies. Newell and Driscoll showed this in two studies that compared both regular low back pain patients and those with unilateral low back via numerical models to the mechanics of healthy patients. It was shown that if a tissue has an increased elasticity (conventionally referred to as stiffer by clinicians), then it consequently may bear more load (Newell and Driscoll 2021, Newell and Driscoll 2021). This contributes to the notion that Driscoll labels as "Physiological Stress Shielding", which was supported in those and prior studies (Driscoll and Blyum 2010, Driscoll et al. 2009), which could have detrimental short- and long-term influence on spine biomechanics and easily extend into all musculoskeletal biomechanics.

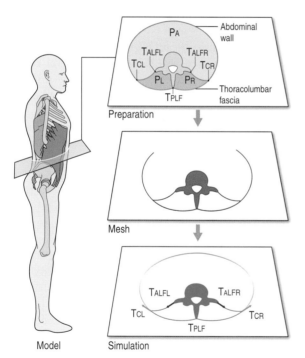

Fig. 5.8.2 Two-dimensional cross-section displaying the fascial envelope of the spine explored via finite-element analysis. PA, abdominal pressure; TALFL: reaction force at the left anterior layer of thoracolumbar fascia; TALFR: reaction force at the right anterior layer of thoracolumbar fascia; TCL: reaction force at the left connection between the thoracolumbar fascia and abdominal wall; PL: left paraspinal muscle compartmental pressure; PR: right paraspinal muscle compartmental pressure; TPLF: reaction force at posterior layer of thoracolumbar fascia; TCR: reaction force at the right connection between the thoracolumbar fascia and abdominal wall.

Summary

LBP is a longstanding problem that is complex, but the TLF and its involvement in LPB is gaining in its attention to pain and biomechanics. This may shine light on explaining old or defining new treatment options.

REFERENCES

Allegri, M., Montella, S., Salici, F., et al., 2016. Mechanisms of low back pain: A guide for diagnosis and therapy. F1000Res. 5, 1530.

Allan, D.B., Waddell, G., 1989. An historical perspective on low back pain and disability. Acta Orthop. Scand., 234, 1–23.

Arnau, J.M., Vallano, A., Lopez, A., et al., 2006. A critical review of guidelines for low back pain treatment. Eur. Spine J. 15, 543–553.

Balasubramaniam, A., Ghandi, V.M., Sambandamoorthy, A.K.C., 2014. Role of myofascial release therapy on pain and lumbar range of motion in mechanical back pain: An exploratory investigation of desk job workers. Ibnosina J. Med. Biomed. Sci. 6, 75–80.

Benzel, E.C., 2005. Spine Surgery: Techniques, Complication Avoidance, and Management, second ed. Churchill Livingstone Elsevier, Philadelphia, PA.

Casazza, B., 2012. Diagnosis and treatment of acute low back pain. Am. Fam. Physician 85, 343–350.

Castro-Sánchez, A.M., Lara-Palomo, I.C., Matarán-Peñarrocha, G.A., et al., 2012. Kinesio Taping reduces disability and pain slightly in chronic non-specific low back pain: A randomised trial. J. Physiother. 58, 89–95.

Choi, H.W., Kim, Y.E., 2017. Effect of lumbar fasciae on the stability of the lower lumbar spine. Comput. Methods Biomech. Biomed. Engin. 20, 1431–1437.

Chou, R., Qaseem, A., Snow, V., et al., 2007. Clinical Guidelines Diagnosis and Treatment of Low Back Pain: A Joint Clinical Practice Guideline from the American College of Physicians and the American. Ann. Intern. Med. 147, 478–491.

Danish Institute for Health Technology Assessment, 1999. Low-Back Pain: Frequency, Management and Prevention from an HTA perspective. Copenhagen, National Board of Health.

Deyo, R.A., Bryan, M., Comstock, B.A., et al., 2015. Trajectories of symptoms and function in older adults with low back disorders. Spine (Phila. Pa. 1976) 40, 1352–1362.

Driscoll, M., 2018. Fascia—The unsung hero of spine biomechanics. J. Bodyw. Mov. Ther. 22, 90–91.

Driscoll, M., Blyum, L., 2010. The presence of physiological stress shielding in the degenerative cycle of musculoskeletal disorders. J. Bodyw. Mov. Ther. 15, 335–342.

Driscoll, M., Aubin, C.-E., Parent, S., et al., 2009. The role of concave-convex biases in the progression of idiopathic scoliosis. Eur. Spine J. 18, 180–187.

El-Bojairami, B., El-Monajjed, K., Driscoll, M., 2020. Development and validation of a novel finite element human spine model for accurate biomechanical simulations. Sci. Rep. Nat. 10, 1–15.

El-Monajjed, K., Driscoll, M., 2021. Objective comparison of mechanical properties of the thoracolumbar fascia in LBP and healthy patients and its biomechanical implication in spine stability. Life 11, 779. 1–9. doi:10.3390/life11080779.

El-Bojairami, I., Driscoll, M., 2021. Coordination between Trunk muscles, thoracolumbar fascia, and intra-abdominal pressure towards static spine stability. Spine (in press), doi: 10.1097/BRS.0000000000004223.

El-Monajjed, K., Driscoll, M., 2018. Mechanical evaluation of the role of intra-abdominal pressure within the thoracolumbar fascia in postural asymmetry: A finite element study. J. Bodyw. Mov. Ther. 22, 854–855.

Erichsen, J.E., 1866. On Railway and Other Injuries of the Nervous System. London, Walton and Moberly.

Farhadi, K., Schwebel, D.C., Saeb, M., et al., 2009. The effectiveness of wet-cupping for nonspecific low back pain in Iran: A randomized controlled trial. Complement. Ther. Med. 17, 9–15.

Gibson, W., Arendt-Nielsen, L., Taguchi, T., Mizumura, K., Graven-Nielsen, T., 2009. Increased pain from muscle fascia following eccentric exercise: animal and human findings. Exp. Brain Res. 194, 299.

Goertz, M., D. Thorson, J. Bonsell, et al., 2012. Adult acute and subacute low back pain. Bloomington, MN, USA, Institute for Clinical Systems Improvement, pp. 1–91.

Hartvigsen, J., Hancock, M.J., Kongsted, A., et al., 2018. What low back pain is and why we need to pay attention. Lancet 391, 2356–2367.

Hoheisel, U., Mense, S., 2015. Inflammation of the thoraco-lumbar fascia excites and sensitizes rat dorsal horn neurons. Eur. J. Pain 19, 419–428.

Hoy, D., Brooks, P., Blyth, F., Buchbinder, R., 2010. The Epidemiology of low back pain. Best Pract. Res. Clin. Rheumatol. 24, 769–781.

Institute of Medicine (US) Committee on Advancing Pain Research, Care, and Education. 2011. Relieving Pain in America: A Blueprint for Transforming Prevention, Care, Education, and Research. National Academies Press, Washington, DC.

Kuslich, S.D., Ulstrom, C.L., Michael, C.J., 1991. The tissue origin of low back pain and sciatica. A report of pain response to tissue stimulation during operations on the lumbar spine using local anesthesia. Orthop. Clin. North. Am. 22, 181–187.

Langevin, H.M., Fox, J.R., Koptiuch, C., et al., 2011. Reduced thoracolumbar fascia shear strain in human chronic low back pain. BMC Musculoskelet. Disord. 12, 203.

Langevin, H.M., Stevens-Tuttle, D., Fox, J.R., et al., 2009. Ultrasound evidence of altered lumbar connective tissue structure in human subjects with chronic low back pain. BMC Musculoskelet. Disord. 10, 151.

Lee, S.W., Kim, S.Y., 2015. Effects of hip exercises for chronic low-back pain patients with lumbar instability. J. Phys. Ther. Sci. 27, 345–348.

Mafi, J.N., McCarthy, E.P., Davis, R.B., Landon, B.E., 2013. Worsening trends in the management and treatment of back pain. JAMA Intern. Med. 173, 1573–1581.

Minicozzi, S.J., Russell, B.S., Ray, K.J., Struebing, A.Y., Owens, Jr., E.F., 2016. Low back pain response to pelvic tilt position: an observational study of chiropractic patients. J. Chiropr. Med. 15, 27–34.

Nasser, M.J., 2005. How to approach the problem of low back pain: An overview. J. Family Community Med. 12, 3–9.

Newell, E., Driscoll, M., 2021. The examination of stress shielding in a finite element lumbar spine inclusive of the thoracolumbar fascia. Med. Biol. Eng. Comput. 59, 1621–1628.

Newell, E., Driscoll, M., 2021. Investigation of physiological stress shielding within the lumbar spinal tissue as a contributor to unilateral low back pain: a finite element study. Comput. Biol. Med. 133, 104351. doi:10.1016/j.compbiomed.2021.104351.

Rizk, M., Nadir, E.A., Karam, C., Ayoub, C., 2012. Low back pain as perceived by the pain specialist. Middle East J. Anesthesiol. 21, 463–482.

Schilder, A., Hoheisel, U., Magerl, W., et al., 2014. Sensory findings after stimulation of the thoracolumbar fascia with hypertonic saline suggest its contribution to low back pain. Pain 155, 222–231.

Schilder, A., Magerl, W., Hoheisel, U., Klein, T., Treede, R.D., 2016. Electrical high-frequency stimulation of the human thoracolumbar fascia evokes long-term potentiation-like pain amplification. Pain 157, 2309–2317.

Schleip, R., Zorn, A., Klingler, W., 2010. Biomechanical properties of fascial tissues and their role as pain generators. J. Musculoskelet. Pain. 18, 393–395.

Tahririan, M.A., Motififard, M., Tahmasebi, M.N., Siavashi, B., 2012. Plantar fasciitis. J. Res. Med. Sci. 17, 799.

Tang, N., Crane, C., 2006. Suicidality in chronic pain: review of the prevalence, risk factors and psychological links. Psychol. Med. 36, 575–586.

Tesarz, J., Hoheisel, U., Wiedenhöfer, B., Mense, S., 2011. Sensory innervation of the thoracolumbar fascia in rats and humans. Neuroscience, 194, 302–308.

Tominaga, M., Numazaki, M., Iida, T., Tominaga, T., 2003. Molecular mechanisms of nociception. Japanese J. Neuropsychopharmacol. 23, 139–147.

Traeger, A.C., Buchbinder, R., Elshaug, A.G., Croft, P.R., Maher, C.G., 2019. Care for low back pain: can health systems deliver? Bull. World Health Organ. 97, 423–33.

Tu, S.J., Woledge, R.C., Morrissey, D., 2016. Does 'Kinesio tape' alter thoracolumbar fascia movement during lumbar flexion? An observational laboratory study. J. Bodyw. Mov. Ther. 20, 898–905.

Vleeming, A., Schuenke, M.D., Danneels, L., Willard, F.H., 2014. The functional coupling of the deep abdominal and paraspinal muscles: the effects of simulated paraspinal muscle contraction on force transfer to the middle and posterior layer of the thoracolumbar fascia. J. Anat. 225, 447–462.

Waddell, G., Feder, G., McIntosh, A., et al., 1998. (1996) Low Back Pain Evidence Review London: Royal College of General Practitioners. J. Man. Manip. Ther. 6(3), 151–153.

Waddell, G., 2004. The Back Pain Revolution, second ed. Churchill Livingstone Elsevier, Edinburgh.

Wilke, J., Schleip, R., Klingler, W., Stecco, C., 2017. The lumbodorsal fascia as a potential source of low back pain: A narrative review. BioMed Res. Int. 2017, 5349620.

Willard, F.H., Vleeming, A., Schuenke, M.D., Danneels, L., Schleip, R., 2012. The thoracolumbar fascia: Anatomy, function and clinical considerations. J. Anat. 221, 507–536.

Wu, A., Dong, W., Liu, S., et al., 2019. The prevalence and years lived with disability caused by low back pain in China, 1990 to 2016: findings from the global burden of disease study 2016. Pain 160, 237–245.

The Role of Fascia in Oncology

Stephanie Otto

CHAPTER CONTENTS

INTRODUCTION

In the past three decades, our approach to understanding the biology of solid tumors has changed tremendously. Cancer is an insidious disease that medical science still considers to be one of the major causes of death. Many cancers are chronic, remitting, relapsing diseases. To understand how it develops and progresses, the biological differences between normal cells and cancer cells need to be investigated. Therefore, the mechanisms underlying fundamental processes such as cell growth, the transformation of normal cells into cancer cells, and their spread in the form of metastases are increasingly becoming the focus of cancer research.

In their pivotal report, Hanahan and Weinberg (2000) defined the characteristic features of tumor cells based on generally accepted cell biological principles from an almost undeniable variety of complex properties. The development of cancer is no longer understood exclusively as a cell-autonomous process but rather as the interaction of the genetically modified malignant cells with their environment, the tumor microenvironment (TME).

Knowledge deepens our understanding of the biology of solid tumors, which are complex organ-like structures and lead to the development of new clinical interventions (Henke et al. 2020). Thus studies on cell signaling pathways in normal cells and cancer cells have essentially contributed to our knowledge of the disease by revealing molecular changes and suggesting possible treatment strategies.

Research has recognized that physical forces can also act on cells (Paluch et al. 2015). Indeed, mechanical stimulation is a potent regulator of anabolic and catabolic cellular metabolism and the physical properties of their synthesized matrix, which are manifested as tissue structures (Ng et al. 2017). Almost every physiotherapeutic intervention introduces mechanical forces, regardless of whether the forces are generated extrinsically by the therapist's intervention or intrinsically within the individual himself through the prescription of movement therapy (Thompson et al. 2016). Even though many patients suffer from the side effects of cancer treatment, they benefit from physical manipulations of connective tissue through body-based treatments, although it is not clear what happens at the cellular and molecular level when these manipulations take place (Fig. 5.9.1).

KEY POINT

At the beginning of this millennium, cancer was recognized as an ultimately genetic disease, but increasingly knowledge appreciates that the environment is of particular importance for the development of tumors.

"Cancer is no more a disease of cells than a traffic jam is a disease of cars. A lifetime study of the internal

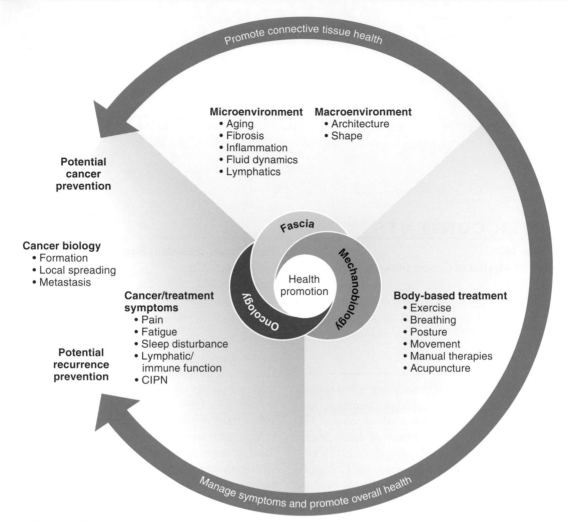

Fig. 5.9.1 Extracellular matrix in the tumor microenvironment and its potential impact on cancer prevention/recurrence to health promotion. The comprehensive role of connective tissue in cancer biology, tumor environment, cancer/treatment symptoms and body-based treatment. CIPN, chemotherapy-induced peripheral neuropathy. *CIPN*, chemotherapy-induced peripheral neuropathy. Modified with permission from Professor Helene Langevin. Diagram from the Joint Conference: Acupuncture, Fascia and Oncology, Osher Center, November 14, 2015. Available at: https://oshercenter.org/oc-event/4569.

combustion engine would not help anyone understand our traffic problems" (Smithers 1962).

Tissue Changes that are Not Cancer

Not all tissue changes in the body are cancer (Fig. 5.9.2). However, if they are not treated, they can deteriorate into cancer. It is called hyperplasia if the cell count increases when a tissue, muscle, or organ is enlarged. Hyperplasia can be caused by chronic irritation or hormonal stimuli and is not malignant. In dysplasia, which

is more serious than hyperplasia, changes in cells, tissues, and organs occur, which are characterized by atypical growth processes and loss of differentiation. If malignant tissue is sealed off from the outside and has not yet spread to the surrounding tissue, the medical term is "carcinoma in situ," an even more serious condition. When this tumor has stopped growing it means that they do not penetrate nearby tissues as cancer cells usually do. Because some carcinomas in situ may become cancer, they are usually treated.

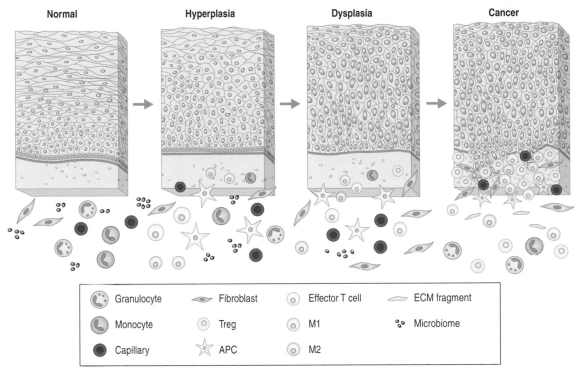

Normal   **Hyperplasia**   **Dysplasia**   **Cancer**

◉ Granulocyte	➤ Fibroblast
◖ Monocyte	◉ Treg
● Capillary	✶ APC

◉ Effector T cell	➤ ECM fragment
◉ M1	❀ Microbiome
◉ M2	

Fig. 5.9.2 From normal cell to cancer cell. Reproduced with permission from Srivastava, S., Ghosh, S., Kagan, J., Mazurchuk, R., Boja, E., Chuaqui, R., Hanlon, S., 2018. The making of a precancer atlas: promises, challenges, and opportunities. Trends in Cancer 4, 523–536.

IDENTIFYING THE MYSTICS OF CANCER BIOLOGY—A BIG CHALLENGE

By the ability to metastasize, mutated cells can travel and implant in distant parts of the body, continuing their abnormal growth. Broadly divided into benign tumors, which are unable to metastasize, or malignant tumors, which are able to invade normal tissues, cancers are further defined and classified by their cell type, tissue, or organ of origin. They are no longer viewed as a collection of genetically altered cells but as aberrant organs with a plastic stroma, matrix, and vasculature. Cancer therapies directed against the tumor environment (TME), which has become the "Achilles' heel" of cancer, are yielding some of the most promising results in years.

The Role of the Tumor Microenvironment (TME)—A Multitasking Player

In 1889, Stephen Paget proposed the "seed and soil" hypothesis to describe the supporting role of the TME (the soil) in promoting the growth and survival of metastatic cancer cells (the seeds). Research has also demonstrated the adverse role of the tumor stroma in carcinogenesis. This means that cancer cells recruit and transform the stromal cells, which in turn remodel the extracellular matrix of the stroma. Thus, cancers are no longer viewed as collections of genetically altered cells but as aberrant organs with a plastic stroma, matrix, and vasculature (Ishiguro et al. 2006; Moinfar et al. 2000; Kurose et al. 2001).

The TME is a complex biochemical network that includes fibroblasts, extracellular matrix (ECM), cytokines, blood vessels, immune cells, hormones, and other components. It differs from the normal tissue environment (NTE) in many aspects, such as tissue architecture, chronic inflammation, level of oxygen and pH, nutritional state of the cells, and tissue firmness. Although TME, despite some anticancer effects, generally promotes the growth of cancer, the NTE can inhibit it. The TME plays a crucial role in the generation and maintenance of cancer stem cells, which are the cause of cancer growth. Because of their capabilities of unlimited self-renewal and apoptosis resistance, cancer stem cells play a central role that is not yet considered in cancer therapy (Zheng and Gao 2019).

Extracellular Matrix (ECM)—A Gatekeeper in Cancer Initiation and Progression?

The ECM in tumors significantly differs in composition and architecture from that in normal tissue. Considering its physical properties, the tumor ECM is more abundant, denser, and stiffer (Henke et al. 2020). Furthermore, it provides a biochemical and biomechanical context within which cancer cells exist. Previously, it was assumed that ECM provides structural information necessary to maintain the physical integrity of tissue (Bonnans et al. 2014). Thus cancer progression depends on the ability of cancer cells to overcome the ECM barrier, gain access to the bloodstream, and form distal metastases. Finally, the importance of the ECM for cancer progression is now well understood, but only little is known about the adaptability of tumor cells to changes in the ECM and their influence on the structure and composition of the ECM (Lim et al. 2010; Jansen et al. 2015).

Cancer Cells on the Move: Along or Across the ECM

The revolutionary idea that a cancer cell is dependent on its environment and does not necessarily develop into a tumor has been pursued by Mina Bissell for decades. The microenvironment and the context that surrounds the cells (ECM) actually are telling the cancer gene and the cancer cell what to do. However, a key factor for the importance of TME is that the environment of the tumor cells influences or restricts the possibilities of cell growth and cell proliferation. Similar insights have been stressed by developmental biologists that have experimentally demonstrated the influence of properties of the ECM on the development of breast cancer (Lochter and Bissell 1995).

It is now established that carcinogenesis involves mutual interactions between cancer cells and components of the surrounding microenvironment (Plava et al. 2019). Finally, there is a close relationship between the signaling pathways that regulate ECM formation and angiogenesis. Because of the common regulation via the hypoxia-response axis, interventions that alter either the tumor ECM or the vascular system are likely to influence each other. In particular, the joint regulation via the hypoxia response axis means that interventions that alter either the tumor ECM or the vascular system will likely also affect the other (Henke et al. 2020).

Everything is Context—Thinking Out of the Box

One of the first to propose and elucidate the important signaling role of the ECM was Mina Bissell. She has been a visionary and pioneer in the ECM and TME area, with special emphasis in breast cancer, and has shown that malignant cells behave much differently in a culture than they do in a body. She recognized the crucial role of the microenvironment surrounding each tissue and organ and of the three-dimensional (3D) tissue structure in differentiation and cancer as factors that determined tissue specificity.

Unraveling the Tumor Microenvironment— the Link to Fibroblasts

Tumor stroma and biomechanical abnormalities that develop during tumor growth are dominant regulators of cancer progression (Jain et al. 2014; Spill et al. 2016; Stylianopoulos et al. 2012). The tumor stroma consists of the ECM, which is composed of immune cells, fibroblasts, capillaries, and fibrillar proteins such as collagen I, elastin and fibronectin, hyaluronan, and other sulfated glycosaminoglycans (Quail and Joyce 2013). Key regulators of the composition and organization of the ECM are fibroblasts that physiologically remain in the quiescent state, with negligible metabolic and transcriptomic activities (Kalluri 2016; Kalluri and Zeisberg 2006). On the other hand, tissue damage promotes the activation of fibroblasts and the overproduction of ECM proteins, mainly collagen I and fibronectin; secrete cytokines and growth factors; and exert contractile forces that alter tissue architecture (Kalluri 2016; Kalluri and Zeisberg 2006).

In response to several growth factors secreted by the highly proliferative cancer cells, they acquire a constantly activated phenotype such as the transforming growth factor-β (TGF-β), epidermal growth factors (EGFs), and bone morphogenetic proteins (BMPs) (Kalluri 2016; Kalluri and Zeisberg 2006). They can differentiate into myofibroblasts when stimulated by transforming growth factor beta 1 (TGF-β1) and other prodifferentiation signals (Bordoni et al. 2018).

The Concert of Cancer Cells, Cancer-Associated Fibroblasts (CAFs), and Macrophages

One of the most abundant and critical components of the tumor mesenchyme in the tumor stroma is activated fibroblasts, commonly known as cancer-associated fibroblasts (CAFs), which cause a chronic wound healing–like response toward cancer cells and lead to desmoplasia, an excessive accumulation of fibrillar ECM proteins (Kalluri 2016). Under this desmoplastic reaction, proinflammatory CAFs continuously produce and remodel tumor ECM and increase tumor stiffness (Jain 2014; Kalluri 2016). Both desmoplasia and ECM stiffening characterize many tumor types, especially breast and pancreatic cancer, and usually promote tumor progression (Jain 2014).

The effect of fibrosis on cancer formation, growth, and progression is controversial, however. The supporting pro- and antitumorigenic roles of fibrosis in cancer initiation, growth, and metastasis is summarized in Fig. 5.9.3 (Chandler et al. 2019).

The Yin and Yang of Inflammation in the Context of Cancer Progression

Inflamed, mechanically altered fascia is at the root of cancer and all sickness and disease. Therefore, research is pointing to inflammation and connective tissue stiffness as contributing to tumor growth, spreading, and metastasis.

Studies during the last two decades have demonstrated that inflammatory immune cells are essential players of cancer-related inflammation (Gonzalez et al. 2018). Generally, inflammation and fibrosis are well-recognized contributors to cancer, and connective tissue stiffness is emerging as a driving factor in tumor growth. Tumor-associated fibrosis is characterized by unchecked profibrotic and proinflammatory signaling (Jiang et al. 2017). Inflammation is the cause of problems in the ECM, which is a highly dynamic structure as well. Thus increasing evidence suggests that ECM proteins establish a physical and biochemical niche for cancer stem cells (CSCs) (Fig. 5.9.4).

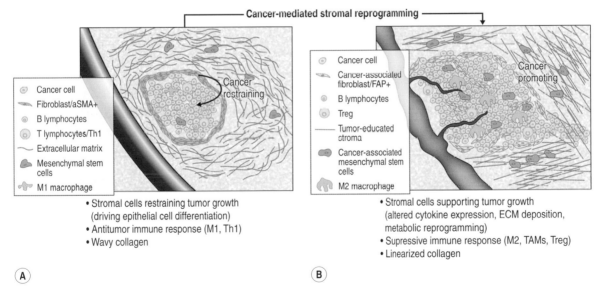

Fig. 5.9.3 **Dual roles of fibrosis in cancer.** (A) Early cancer with tumor-restraining stroma. Fibrosis acts to restrain cancer growth during cancer initiation, however, after a process of cancer-mediated stromal reprogramming. (B) Advanced cancer with reprogrammed protumorigenic stroma. Fibrosis acts to enhance cancer growth with stiffened extracellular matrix (ECM), enhanced angiogenesis, and suppressive immune response. From Chandler, C., Liu, T., Buckanovich, R., & Coffman, L., 2019. The double edge sword of fibrosis in cancer. Translational Research 209, 55–67. Open Access. Distributed under the Creative Commons CC-BY-NC-ND license: http://creativecommons.org/licenses/by-nc-nd/4.0/.

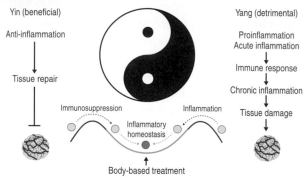

Fig. 5.9.4 The yin and yang of inflammation in connective tissue in the context of cancer progression.

Inflammation is a Double-Edged Sword in Cancer

Chronic inflammation, which is a critical hallmark of cancer, has profound tumor-promoting effects (Hanahan and Weinberg 2011). Indeed, inflammatory cells are the main actors in the immune monitoring of tumors, and it is known that the tumor risk is increased by immunosuppression. Connective tissue disease (CTD)–associated chronic inflammation leads to changes in homeostasis, which favors the development of malignancies, particularly hematological malignancies (Noureldine et al. 2020). But chronic inflammation is a necessary consequence of cancer progression. Different inflammatory conditions can lead to neoplastic transformation. However, most tumors develop into a state of chronic inflammation, enhancing various aspects of tumor progression (Gonzalez et al. 2018).

Are Tumors Nonhealing Wounds?

Tumors are known as wounds that do not heal. Specifically, this means that cells involved in angiogenesis and response to injury play a prominent role in the progression, growth, and spread of cancer (Kalluri and Zeisberg 2006). Indeed, fibroblasts play a key role in orchestrating the healing process, and their structural and functional contributions to this process are beginning to emerge.

> ### ⚑ KEY POINT
> Many interactions of TME, also known as cancer's "Achilles' heel," promote tumor growth and progression—for instance, increased matrix stiffness destabilizes the adhesion of cell junctions and integrins.

MECHANO-ONCOLOGY—CANCER MECHANOBIOLOGY

Cancer research has mainly focused on identifying genetic drivers and understanding the mechanism by which genes and specific signaling pathways in the cell drive tumor formation. From tumor initiation and metastasis to the formation of secondary tumors, cancer primarily involves both genetic changes in a cell and physical changes in tissue structure and cancer cells (Carey et al. 2012). The ability of the cell to modulate its stiffness seems to be a key process in maintaining the balance of forces between a cell and its environment. This determines the elastic nature of the cytoskeleton and so in turn affects a diverse range of cellular processes (Tee et al. 2009).

For this reason, studies have focused on the mechanobiology of tumor progression. Until now, these mechanical aspects of biology have been largely ignored, not least because of the lack of technology that enables complex mechanical measurements. However, better tools are being developed to track mechanical activity in cells and tissues. Creating minimodels of human tissue in the laboratory is only the beginning. Mechanobiology thus integrates the physical sciences into biology and drives the development of new technologies. And because of this visibility, new drugs and treatments are beginning to emerge.

Stiffness Influences Dynamic Interactions between Cancer Cells and Stroma

Abnormal stroma in solid tumors contributes to the development of biomechanical abnormalities (increase in matrix stiffness, accumulation of solid stress) in TME. However, whether matrix stiffness and solid stress are closely related or whether they play different roles in tumor progression remains to be clarified. It is equally important to determine the biological effects of the two anomalies in tumor development and metastasis (Kalli and Stylianopoulos 2018).

The growing awareness that cell–matrix interactions are mechanoregulated has profoundly changed our basic understanding of how the microenvironment determines cell fate (Northcott et al. 2018). The mechanoregulation of structural ECM component interactions among each other and their associated matrix architectures provides another as yet unrecognized paradigm of how forces can affect the mechanobiology of matrix and thereby cell and tissue fate. New therapeutic strategies are emerging to relieve the mechanical stresses that drive the cancer to malignancy. In the metastatic process, tumor cells are exposed to a variety of additional microenvironments and forces. If the tumor cells escape the primary tumor and migrate through the bloodstream, they are exposed to a number of different and fluid forces, many of which trigger shear stresses (Northcott et al. 2018) (Fig. 5.9.5).

It is now well-accepted that mechanical changes in both cells and tissues can contribute to malignancy and metastasis; however, we have yet to fully understand the mechanisms by which mechanics promotes cancer. Engineers have the unique skills to build platforms to measure, probe, and manipulate cell and tissue mechanics to better understand cancer mechanobiology and translate it into the clinic.

 KEY POINT

Physical and mechanical environments can regulate cell behavior and tumor progression at the cellular level. The paradigm of how forces can affect the mechanobiology of matrix and thereby cell and tissue fate is as yet unrecognized.

Are Cells Affected by Physical Forces? Expedition to Discover the Smallest Biological Components

Mechanically, all tumor components interact with each other (e.g., stretching of collagen by cancer cells and CAFs), which leads to the creation of mechanical tension between them and may explain the pathogenesis of the disease (Voutouri et al. 2016). The mechanical forces, in fact, help shape how the cells interact with the ECM and thus shape the overall tissue, and in combination with biochemical factors within the microenvironment, this then influences factors such as tissue differentiation. Therefore, it is possible that mechanobiology also plays a role in the progression of cancer and how it metastasizes (Lim et al. 2010; Jansen et al. 2015).

 KEY POINT

Mechanobiology seems to play a role in the progression and metastasizing of cancer.

BODY-BASED TREATMENT STRATEGIES IN THE CONTEXT OF CANCER

Exercise Oncology—The Paradigm Shift

Physical activity and exercise can have both immediate and long-term health benefits. Therefore, the principle of "use it or lose it" in muscle maintenance is well-established. However, what is the biochemical benefit of physical activity and what physical and mechanical principles are associated with the disease?

The evidence of positive effects of exercise oncology has grown considerably over the past two decades. Currently more than 700 studies have investigated the effects of exercise before, during, and after oncological treatment (Christensen et al. 2018). The data convincingly show that in many disease patterns, highly symptomatic disease- and therapy-related stress can be significantly reduced or even completely prevented by regular physical exercise (Christensen et al. 2018).

The Effect of Exercise on Growth and Progression of Cancer

Growing evidence suggests that physical and mechanical environments can regulate cell behavior and tumor progression at the cellular level, and many patients benefit from physical manipulation of connective tissue, but it is not clear what exactly happens. Nevertheless, there is a great discrepancy between the approaches of cell and connective tissue biology and integrative medicine. Advancing this field will require a coordinated effort combining epidemiology with cancer cellular and ECM biology. To determine whether we can safely influence tumor progression and the underlying biology with active and passive physical manipulation, the considerations of the physical sciences in oncology should be extended to the entire host and possible paths of integrative medicine. Conversely, body-based therapy research should be extended to the underlying matrix, cell, and molecular mechanisms to understand the effects at the tissue level of physical manipulation of the host (Langevin et al. 2016).

The pioneering hypotheses of experimental animal models justifies this relationship by energy metabolism. Studies show that exercise can have protective or cancer-inducing effects, depending on the intensity, duration, and type of exercise. The mechanisms involved in the effects of exercise on tumor growth are still unclear, possibly because of the heterogeneous nature of tumors

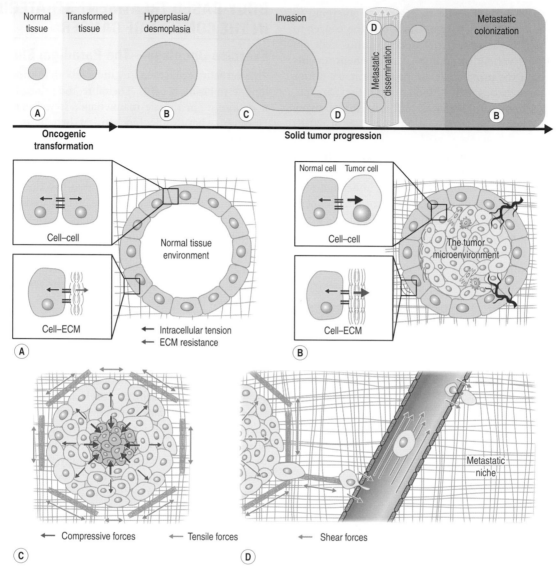

Fig. 5.9.5 Diverse mechanical stimuli act on tumor cells throughout cancer progression. Simplified depiction of oncogenic transformation and solid tumor progression for cancers of epithelial origin (top). Letters indicate the stages of cancer progression focused on in panels (A–D). (A) In homeostatic tissues, the forces between cells and the extracellular matrix (ECM) are balanced. (B) The tumor microenvironment is composed of cancer cells with augmented contractility (increased intracellular tension), surrounded by a progressively stiffening ECM (increased ECM resistance) and a host of stromal cell types, including fibroblasts, immune cells, and vascular cell types. (C) Tumor expansion confined by the surrounding stroma compresses both the tumor and the adjacent stromal tissue, causing increased interstitial pressure. Augmented ECM rigidity increases stromal resistance to compression and exacerbates solid stress. (D) A high interstitial fluid pressure gradient elicits fluid flow from the tumor core to the periphery, promoting metastatic dissemination. After escape from the primary tumor, cancer cells migrate along tension-oriented collagen fibers toward the vasculature. Tumor cells are exposed to high shear stresses as they intravasate/extravasate between endothelial cells and travel through the circulation en route to future secondary tumor sites. From Northcott, J. M., Dean, I. S., Mouw, J. K., Weaver, V. M. (2018). Feeling stress: the mechanics of cancer progression and aggression. Frontiers in Cell and Developmental Biology 6, 17. Open access. Distributed under the terms of the Creative Commons Attribution License (CC BY): https://creativecommons.org/licenses/by/4.0/.

and biological intraindividual variation. This will be the subject of further work (Arab et al. 2017).

Helene Langevin, director of the National Center for Complementary and Integrative Health (NCCIH), authored multiple research papers investigating the link between fascia and cancer. Animal studies, for example, indicate a three-fold increase in breast tumor and tumor metastasis when there is dense breast tissue (Berrueta et al. 2016). Langevin's work has focused on the effects of stretching on inflammation resolution mechanisms within connective tissue (Berrueta et al. 2016).

Effect of Stretching on Tumor Growth

The approach to cancer biology and treatment has changed over time. Helene Langevin suspected that the loss of functional mobility and reduced patient activity might not only contribute to additional tissue stiffening within this network, but that the stiffness of the connective tissue might be associated with the growth, spread, and metastasis of the tumor. Stretching, a gentle, non-pharmacological intervention, could become an important part of cancer treatment and prevention (Langevin et al. 2016). The migration of neutrophils and the increase in tissue RvD1 concentration was reduced by stretching of connective tissue in ex-vivo experiments. In addition, stretching reduces the level of PD-1, a protein that blocks the body's ability to defend itself against cancer cells. These results show that stretching reduces tumor growth in a mouse breast cancer model. This appears to be a direct mechanical influence of stretching on inflammation regulation mechanisms within the connective tissue (Berrueta et al. 2016).

Resistance Training

Resistance training has been shown to reduce mortality and improve quality of life in cancer survivors (Hardee et al. 2014; Cormie et al. 2014). Research studies dealing with the acute response to IGF-1 have proven that circulating IGF-1 and free IGF-1 are increased by intense concentric and eccentric muscle concentrations during resistance training (Kraemer and Ratamess 2005). In contrast, other studies have demonstrated no changes in acute IGF-1 after resistance exercise (Kraemer and Ratamess 2005). Findings by Teixeira and colleagues (2020) showed that resistance training increased plasma levels of IGF-1 in the adult Wistar rat prostate. The research group concluded that physical resistance training can alter lipid metabolism and increase markers of apoptosis in the adult Wistar rat prostate, suggesting physical resistance training as a potential new therapeutic strategy for the treatment of prostate cancer.

Fascia researcher Thomas Findley favors resistance training when the load is mainly in the short length position (Findley 2015a). Oriented toward a 10-repetition maximum (RM), patients performed training sets by applying the first set of 10 at 50% of the 10-RM, the second at 75% of the 10-RM, and the third and final set at 100% of the 10-RM. He showed that the load on the muscles in the longitudinal direction is lower than in middle or long positions when they are loaded near their short position. However, the lateral load—forces transmitted via the epimysium to structures parallel to the working muscle fibers—is much higher (Findley et al. 2015b). He cites preliminary results suggesting that such force distribution leads to a decrease in TGF-1 expression, a substance that is commonly attributed to an aggravating effect on tissue stiffness and cancer progression (Findley 2015).

Effects on Complementary Movement Therapies

Yoga, tai chi, qi gong, and other mind-body-based treatments are frequently used and well-tolerated among cancer patients for managing symptoms and improving mobility and well-being (Cramer et al. 2017; Deng and Cassileth 2014; Greenlee et al. 2017). This is supported by a growing body of research pointing to the importance of mechanical factors in the pathophysiology of many diseases, including cancer (DuFort et al. 2011; Ingber 2003).

Summary

This chapter highlights the biological background of cancer and the importance of mechanical signals on biological tissue. Modern research in cancer biology has created a wide range of knowledge that is essential for progress in the fight against the disease. Thus mechanobiology seems to play a role in the progression of cancer and the metastasis of cancer. By having an understanding of the mechanotransduction and mechanobiological response across length and time scales, physical exercise and gentle mind–body-based treatments can be used to achieve functional restoration of diseased or injured tissues. Therefore collaboration in the field of cancer rehabilitation is urgently needed.

REFERENCES

Arab, C., Crocetta, T.B., Keil, P.M.R., et al., 2017. The pioneering hypotheses of exercise effects on tumour growth: Systematic review. Clin. Oncol. 2, 1–6.

Berrueta, L., Muskaj, I., Olenich, S., et al., 2016. Stretching impacts inflammation resolution in connective tissue. J. Cell. Physiol. 231, 1621–1627.

Bonnans, C., Chou, J., Werb, Z., 2014. Remodelling the extracellular matrix in development and disease. Nat. Rev. Mol. Cell Biol. 15, 786–801.

Bordoni, B., Marelli, F., Morabito, B., Castagna, R., Sacconi, B., Mazzucco, P., 2018. New proposal to define the fascial system. Complement. Med. Res. 25, 257–262.

Carey, S.P., D'Alfonso, T.M., Shin, S.J., Reinhart-King, C.A., 2012. Mechanobiology of tumour invasion: Engineering meets oncology. Crit. Rev. Oncol. Hematol. 83, 170–183.

Chandler, C., Liu, T., Buckanovich, R., Coffman, L., 2019. The double edge sword of fibrosis in cancer. Transl. Res. 209, 55–67.

Christensen JF, Simonsen C, Hojman P (2018) Exercise training in cancer control and treatment. Compr Physiol 9:165–205

Cormie, P., Galvão, D.A., Spry, N., Joseph, D., Taaffe, D.R., Newton, R.U., 2014. Functional benefits are sustained after a program of supervised resistance exercise in cancer patients with bone metastases: Longitudinal results of a pilot study. Support. Care Cancer 22, 1537–1548.

Cramer, H., Lauche, R., Klose, P., Lange, S., Langhorst, J., Dobos, G.J., 2017. Yoga for improving health-related quality of life, mental health and cancer-related symptoms in women diagnosed with breast cancer. Cochrane Database Syst. Rev. 1, CD010802.

Deng, G., Cassileth, B., 2014. Integrative oncology: An overview. Am. Soc. Clin. Oncol. Educ. Book 34, 233–242.

DuFort, C.C., Paszek, M.J., Weaver, V.M., 2011. Balancing forces: architectural control of mechanotransduction. Nat. Rev. Mol. Cell Biol. 12, 308–319.

Findley, T., 2015a. Link between Manual Therapy, Movement, Fascia and Cancer. Video presentation from the 2015 Joint Conference on Acupuncture, Oncology and Fascia. Boston. Available from: https://oshercenter.org/joint-conference-2015-video-presentations/.

Findley, T., Chaudhry, H., Dhar, S., 2015b. Transmission of muscle force to fascia during exercise. J. Bodyw. Mov. Ther. 19, 119–123.

Gonzalez, H., Hagerling, C., Werb, Z., 2018. Roles of the immune system in cancer: from tumour initiation to metastatic progression. Genes Dev. 32, 1267–1284.

Greenlee, H., DuPont-Reyes, M.J., Balneaves, L.G., et al., 2017. Clinical practice guidelines on the evidence-based use of integrative therapies during and after breast cancer treatment. CA Cancer J. Clin. 67, 194–232.

Hanahan, D., Weinberg, R.A., 2000. The hallmarks of cancer. Cell 100, 57–70.

Hanahan, D., Weinberg, R.A., 2011. Hallmarks of cancer: the next generation. Cell, 144, 646–674.

Hardee, J.P., Porter, R.R., Sui, X., et al., (2014). The effect of resistance exercise on all-cause mortality in cancer survivors. Mayo Clin. Proc. 89, 1108–1115.

Henke, E., Nandigama, R., Ergün, S., 2020. Extracellular matrix in the tumour microenvironment and its impact on cancer therapy. Front. Mol. Biosci. 6, 160.

Ingber, D., 2003. Mechanobiology and diseases of mechanotransduction. Ann. Med. 35, 564–577.

Ishiguro, K., Yoshida, T., Yagishita, H., Numata, Y., Okayasu, T., 2006. Epithelial and stromal genetic instability contributes to genesis of colorectal adenomas. Gut, 55, 695–702.

Jain, R.K., Martin, J.D., Stylianopoulos, T., 2014. The role of mechanical forces in tumour growth and therapy. Ann. Rev. Biomed. Eng. 16, 321–346.

Jansen, K.A., Donato, D.M., Balcioglu, H.E., Schmidt, T., Danen, E.H., Koenderink, G.H., 2015. A guide to mechanobiology: Where biology and physics meet. Biochim. Biophys. Acta. 1853, 3043–3052.

Jiang, H., Hegde, S., DeNardo, D.G., 2017. Tumour-associated fibrosis as a regulator of tumour immunity and response to immunotherapy. Cancer Immunol. Immunother. 66, 1037–1048.

Kalli, M., Stylianopoulos, T., 2018. Defining the role of solid stress and matrix stiffness in cancer cell proliferation and metastasis. Front. Oncol. 8, 55.

Kalluri, R., 2016. The biology and function of fibroblasts in cancer. Nat. Rev. Cancer 16, 582.

Kalluri, R., Zeisberg, M., 2006. Fibroblasts in cancer. Nat. Rev. Cancer 6, 392–401.

Kraemer, W.J., Ratamess, N.A., 2005. Hormonal responses and adaptations to resistance exercise and training. Sports Med. 35, 339–361.

Kurose, K., Hoshaw-Woodard, S., Adeyinka, A., Lemeshow, S., Watson, P.H., Eng, C., 2001. Genetic model of multi-step breast carcinogenesis involving the epithelium and stroma: Clues to tumour–microenvironment interactions. Hum. Mol. Genet. 10, 1907–1913.

Langevin, H.M., Keely, P., Mao, J., et al., 2016. Connecting (t) issues: How research in fascia biology can impact integrative oncology. Cancer Res. 76, 6159–6162.

Lim, C.T., Bershadsky, A., Sheetz, M.P., 2010. Mechanobiology. J. R. Soc. Interface 7 (Suppl. 3), S291–S293.

Lochter, A., Bissell, M.J., 1995. Involvement of extracellular matrix constituents in breast cancer. In: Seminars in Cancer Biology, vol. 6, no. LBNL-4097E. Lawrence Berkeley National Lab.(LBNL), Berkeley, CA.

Moinfar, F., Man, Y.G., Arnould, L., Bratthauer, G.L., Ratschek, M., Tavassoli, F.A., 2000. Concurrent and independent genetic alterations in the stromal and epithelial cells of mammary carcinoma: implications for tumourigenesis. Cancer Res. 60, 2562–2566.

Ng, J.L., Kersh, M.E., Kilbreath, S., Knothe Tate, M., 2017. Establishing the basis for mechanobiology-based physical therapy protocols to potentiate cellular healing and tissue regeneration. Front. Physiol. 8, 303.

Northcott, J.M., Dean, I.S., Mouw, J.K., Weaver, V.M., 2018. Feeling stress: the mechanics of cancer progression and aggression. Front. Cell Dev. Biol. 6, 17.

Noureldine, H.A., Nour-Eldine, W., Hodroj, M.H., Noureldine, M.H.A., Taher, A., Uthman, I., 2020. Hematological malignancies in connective tissue diseases. Lupus 29, 225–235.

Paluch, E.K., Nelson, C.M., Biais, N., et al., 2015. Mechanotransduction: Use the force(s). BMC Biol. 13, 47.

Plava, J., Cihova, M., Burikova, M., Matuskova, M., Kucerova, L., Miklikova, S., 2019. Recent advances in understanding tumour stroma-mediated chemoresistance in breast cancer. Mol. Cancer 18, 67.

Quail, D.F., Joyce, J.A., 2013. Microenvironmental regulation of tumour progression and metastasis. Nat. Med. 19, 1423.

Smithers, D.W., 1962. An attack on cytologism. Lancet 10;1(7228), 493–499.

Spill, F., Reynolds, D.S., Kamm, R.D., Zaman, M.H., 2016. Impact of the physical microenvironment on tumour progression and metastasis. Curr. Opin. Biotechnol. 40, 41–48.

Srivastava, S., Ghosh, S., Kagan, J., et al., 2018. The making of a PreCancer atlas: Promises, challenges, and opportunities. Trends Cancer 4, 523–536.

Stylianopoulos, T., Martin, J.D., Chauhan, V.P., et al., 2012. Causes, consequences, and remedies for growth-induced solid stress in murine and human tumours. Proc. Natl. Acad. Sci. 109, 15101–15108.

Tee, S.Y., Bausch, A.R., Janmey, P.A., 2009. The mechanical cell. Curr. Biol. 19, R745–R748.

Teixeira, G.R., Mendes, L.O., Veras, A.S.C., et al., 2020. Physical resistance training-induced changes in lipids metabolism pathways and apoptosis in prostate. Lipids Health Dis. 19, 1–9.

Thompson, W.R., Scott, A., Loghmani, M.T., Ward, S.R., Warden, S.J., 2016. Understanding mechanobiology: Physical therapists as a force in mechanotherapy and musculoskeletal regenerative rehabilitation. Phys. Ther. 96 560–569.

Voutouri, C., Polydorou, C., Papageorgis, P., Gkretsi, V., Stylianopoulos, T., 2016. Hyaluronan-derived swelling of solid tumours, the contribution of collagen and cancer cells, and implications for cancer therapy. Neoplasia 18, 732–741.

Zheng, J., Gao, P., 2019. Toward normalization of the tumour microenvironment for cancer therapy. Integr. Cancer Ther. 18, 1534735419862352.

Diagnostic Procedures for Fascial Elasticity

6.1

Diagnostic Procedures for Fascial Elasticity: An Introduction

Thomas W. Findley

This is the shortest Part of this text, not because it is less important but because the field is the least developed. Given the paucity of evidence on palpation, the first chapter presents a method of assessment that could form the basis for a standardized and then testable palpatory technique for fascial disorders. Spinal palpatory findings differ between examiners, showing low to moderate reliability in the review by Seffinger and colleagues (2004); pain provocation tests were more reliable than soft tissue palpation, which is of course precisely what manual therapists consider to be most important. Inclusion of the clinical context rather than blind assessment of the patient improved reliability in upper extremity examinations (Hickey et al. 2007; Smith et al. 2010). Both Cibere et al. (2008) and Brunse et al. (2010) showed that test standardization improved those examination signs with poor rater agreement. Newer examination tools described in the next chapter provide such an opportunity but await clinical correlations. Kim et al. (2007) found that they were able to identify structural problems, but the results were unfortunately independent of the physical exam or the pain symptoms. Lee et al. (2016) reviewed multiple methods, including Cutometer, to assess skin scars but found quantitative imaging generally too expensive and bulky to be suitable for clinical use. Different subjective and objective measures were directly compared in 55 patients with nonkeloid scars (Lee et al. 2019), in one patient with keloid (Chambert et al. 2019), and at 9 skin sites in 30 patients after modified radical mastectomy and axillary lymph node dissection (De Groef et al. 2018), with little correlation between subjective and objective measures. MyotonPRO was used to measure muscle stiffness in sternomastoid, pectoral, and upper trapezius in 22 patients after breast cancer surgery, but only the pectoralis showed a difference from the uninjured side (An et al. 2018; Yeo et al. 2020). The device approach to measuring soft tissue mechanical properties is critically summarized in Chapter 6.4.

Once a standardized assessment is developed, it can be improved into a psychometrically more sound test (Hunt et al. 2009). As Seffinger et al. (2004) concludes: given that spinal palpatory procedures are a cornerstone of diagnostic and therapeutic interventions across disciplines for patients with low back and neck pain, professional societies and organizations need to enact continuing medical education programs and establish research procedures to address the reliability of spinal palpatory procedures.

Another chapter addresses a vexing problem, hypermobility (HM). Whereas there are multiple techniques for the management of people who have decreased range of motion, there are far fewer options for those with increased range. The *British Medical Journal* has begun a series of articles for physicians on conditions often missed, and one by Ross and Grahame (2011) is highly recommended for your interactions with traditional medical practitioners. It lists a number of clues (besides joint mobility) that suggest the joint hypermobility syndrome, which in adults may include symptoms of pain, arthritis, autonomic dysfunction, and gastrointestinal disorders. A somewhat different set of symptoms are found in children and adolescents, including late walking, ankle sprains, decreased coordination, and widespread pain.

There is not enough research on psychological aspects of fascial disorders to devote a whole chapter to this, but there are some intriguing findings regarding hypermobility. A strong association between hypermobility and anxiety and panic disorder was noted in a case control study by Martín-Santos and colleagues (1998), with 68% of persons diagnosed with anxiety showing hypermobility, compared with 10% of persons with medical or psychiatric diagnoses. That group has continued to find this association in the general population, with increased scores measuring trait anxiety in persons with hypermobility (Bulbena et al. 2004) in a general medical clinic, and increased scores measuring fear in a general population sample with hypermobility, compared with those without (Bulbena et al. 2006). Bulbena and colleagues (2011) reported a 15-year follow-up of a general population recruited at ages 16 to 20; in this population 20% have hypermobility, similar to the population rate in many other places. In the 15 years since entry into their study, an astounding 41% of the persons with hypermobility have developed panic disorder, compared with only 2% of the persons with normal mobility. There was also a significant increase of social phobia (6×), simple phobia (3×), and anxiolytic drug use (4×) in persons with hypermobility.

These findings have been replicated by two other groups: Ercolani et al. (2008) found increased anxiety and somatic symptoms in a case–control study, compared with normal mobility persons and another group of persons with fibromyalgia. García-Campayo et al. (2010) found a similar 20-fold increase in panic disorders in persons with hypermobility (61% compared with only 10% in the general population) and noted a direct correlation ($r = 0.52$) between the Beighton hypermobility score and the panic and agoraphobia scale. For a review of the association between anxiety and hypermobility, see García-Campayo et al. (2011).

The parallel between increased anxiety and panic disorder in HM and in persons with gastrointestinal (GI) disorders was noted by Zarate et al. (2010), who looked more closely at the correspondence between HM and GI disturbances. They found that 50% of new patients in a GI clinic had hypermobility and hypothesize a change in the connective tissue and passive mechanical properties of the gut wall or concurrent changes in the autonomic nervous system as possible etiologies. The same group (Mohammed et al. 2010) looked at persons with rectal evacuation dysfunction and found 32% reported hypermobility symptoms on a simple five-question screening test, compared with 14% of controls. Vounotrypidis et al. (2009) looked at specific types of GI disorders and found joint hypermobility in 70% of clinic patients with Crohn's disease and 35% of patients with ulcerative colitis, compared with 25% of controls.

In all of these studies, patients are given a hypermobility score based on specific numbers of joints involved, without specifying a specific pattern of increased mobility. In my clinical practice, I have noticed patients who have distal hypermobility particularly in the arms, some with excessive but some with reduced straight leg raise. Voermans et al. (2009) nicely categorize the pattern of joint hypermobility found in persons with myopathies, and their findings are instructive as we continue to explore the issue of hypermobility in general. Although they list findings by muscle disease, their joint findings can be categorized by the effect on joints in a fashion of more use to studies of fascia:

I. Conditions with diffuse distal and proximal hypermobility. The elbow joint may start hypermobile but develop contractures—Marfans, Ehlers–Danlos classical type, tenascin-X, and hypermobility type. In central core disease the ankle may develop contractures.

IA. Diffuse distal and less so proximal mobility—multiminicore disease.

II. Distal hypermobility only—Ehlers–Danlos vascular and kyphoscoliotic types.

III. Distal hypermobility and proximal contractures—Ulrich congenital myopathy, Bethlem myopathy, and congenital muscular dystrophy with joint hypermobility (CMDH). The ankle also develops contractures.

IV. Mixed pattern—limb girdle muscular dystrophy shows hypermobility in wrist, proximal interphalangeal joints (PIP), and metacarpophalangeal joints (MCP) joints, but contractures in distal interphalangeal joints (DIP), elbow, and knee.

In many of these conditions the elbow develops contractures. This may reflect a tendency for trauma in this joint. In my residency training 30 years ago, I was taught that physical therapy could aggressively stretch every joint in the body except the elbow, where aggressive stretching usually led to decreasing, not increasing, range of motion. Or perhaps it relates to the muscle–ligament complex at the elbow so elegantly described by Van der Wal (2009): as the joint moves, the ligaments must change length to accommodate the changing distance between the bones, and this change is modulated by muscular connections into the ligament. So attempting to stretch the ligaments without addressing the muscular component is counterproductive.

The diagnosis of hypermobility is primarily done through well-established clinical tests that have demonstrated good reproducibility (kappa scores of 0.75–0.85)

(Remvig et al. 2007; Juul-Kristensen et al. 2007). Clinical tests of skin elasticity have been developed, which show promise for quantifying hypermobility (Delalleau et al. 2008; Remvig et al. 2009; Remvig et al. 2010; Farmer et al. 2010). Physiological changes have been found in motor control, posture, reflexes (Ferrell et al. 2007), force development in muscle (Mebes et al. 2008), proprioception (Fatoye et al. 2009), and these have been reviewed in the context of creating a physical rehabilitation program (Keer and Simmonds 2011). Electromyographic investigation of persons with suspected carpal tunnel syndrome found that hypermobility was more common, the more severe the carpal tunnel findings ($r = 0.6$) (Aktas et al. 2008). Eighty-five percent of those with symptoms who had positive test findings also had hypermobility, whereas only 20% of those with symptoms but negative electrodiagnostic tests had hypermobility. These physiological findings will lead to more targeted research and treatments for persons with hypermobility.

REFERENCES

Aktas, I., Ofluoglu, D., Albay, T., 2008. The relationship between benign joint hypermobility syndrome and carpal tunnel syndrome. Clin. Rheumatol. 27, 1283–1287.

An, S.Y., Yeo, S.M., Cheong, I.Y., Hwang, J.H., 2018. Mechanical properties of muscles around shoulder in breast cancer patients: Intra-and inter-reliability and symmetry using MyotonPRO. Ann. Phys. Rehabil. Med. 61, e455.

Brunse, M.H., Stochkendahl, M.J., Vach, W., et al., 2010. Examination of musculoskeletal chest pain – an inter-observer reliability study. Man. Ther. 15, 167–172.

Bulbena, A., Agulló, A., Pailhez, G., et al., 2004. Is joint hypermobility related to anxiety in a nonclinical population also? Psychosomatics 45, 432–437.

Bulbena, A., Gago, J., Pailhez, G., et al., 2011. Joint hypermobility syndrome is a risk factor trait for anxiety disorders: a 15-year follow-up cohort study. Gen. Hosp. Psychiatry 33 (4), 363–370.

Bulbena, A., Gago, J., Sperry, L., Berge, D., 2006. The relationship between frequency and intensity of fears and a collagen condition. Depress. Anxiety 23, 412–417.

Chambert, J., Lihoreau, T., Joly, S., et al., 2019. Multimodal investigation of a keloid scar by combining mechanical tests in vivo with diverse imaging techniques. J. Mech. Behav. Biomed. Mater. 99, 206–215.

Cibere, J., Thorne, A., Bellamy, N., et al., 2008. Reliability of the hip examination in osteoarthritis: effect of standardization. Arthritis Rheum. 59, 373–381.

De Groef, A., Van Kampen, M., Moortgat, P., et al., 2018. An evaluation tool for myofascial adhesions in patients after breast cancer (MAP-BC evaluation tool): Concurrent, face and content validity. PloS One 13, e0193915.

Delalleau, A., Josse, G., Lagarde, J.M., Zahouani, H., Bergheau, J.M., 2008. A nonlinear elastic behavior to identify the mechanical parameters of human skin in vivo. Skin Res. Tech. 14, 152–164.

Ercolani, M., Galvani, M., Franchini, C., Baracchini, F., Chattat, R., 2008. Benign joint hypermobility syndrome: psychological features and psychopathological symptoms in a sample pain-free at evaluation1. Percept. Mot. Skills 107, 246–256.

Farmer, A.D., Douthwaite, H., Gardiner, S., Aziz, Q., Grahame, R., 2010. A novel in vivo skin extensibility test for joint hypermobility. J. Rheumatol. 37, 1513–1518.

Fatoye, F., Palmer, S., Macmillan, F., Rowe, P., van der Linden, M., 2009. Proprioception and muscle torque deficits in children with hypermobility syndrome. Rheumatology 48, 152–157.

Ferrell, W.R., Tennant, N., Baxendale, R.H., Kusel, M., Sturrock, R.D., 2007. Musculoskeletal reflex function in the joint hypermobility syndrome. Arthritis Rheum. 57, 1329–1333.

García-Campayo, J., Asso, E., Alda, M., 2011. Joint hypermobility and anxiety: the state of the art. Curr. Psychiatry Rep. 13, 18–25.

García-Campayo, J., Asso, E., Alda, M., Andres, E. M., Sobradiel, N., 2010. Association between joint hypermobility syndrome and panic disorder: a case–control study. Psychosomatics 51, 55–61.

Hickey, B.W., Milosavljevic, S., Bell, M.L., Milburn, P.D., 2007. Accuracy and reliability of observational motion analysis in identifying shoulder symptoms. Man. Ther. 12, 263–270.

Hunt, T.N., Ferrara, M.S., Bornstein, R.A., Baumgartner, T.A., 2009. The reliability of the modified Balance Error Scoring System. Clin. J. Sport Med. 19, 471–475.

Juul-Kristensen, B., Rogind, H., Jensen, D.V., Remvig, L., 2007. Inter-examiner reproducibility of tests and criteria for generalized joint hypermobility and benign joint hypermobility syndrome. Rheumatology 46, 1835–1841.

Keer, R., Simmonds, J., 2011. Joint protection and physical rehabilitation of the adult with hypermobility syndrome. Curr. Opin. Rheumatol. 23, 131–136.

Kim, H.A., Kim, S.H., Seo, Y.I., 2007. Ultrasonographic findings of the shoulder in patients with rheumatoid arthritis and comparison with physical examination. J. Korean Med. Sci. 22, 660–666.

Lee, K.C., Bamford, A., Gardiner, F., et al., 2019. Investigating the intra-and inter-rater reliability of a panel of subjective and objective burn scar measurement tools. Burns 45, 1311–1324.

Lee, K.C., Dretzke, J., Grover, L., Logan, A., Moiemen, N., 2016. A systematic review of objective burn scar measurements. Burns Trauma 4, 14.

Martín-Santos, R., Bulbena, A., Porta, M., et al., 1998. Association between joint hypermobility syndrome and panic disorder. Am. J. Psychiatry 155, 1578–1583.

Mebes, C., Amstutz, A., Luder, G., et al., 2008. Isometric rate of force development, maximum voluntary contraction, and balance in women with and without joint hypermobility. Arthritis Rheum. 59, 1665–1669.

Mohammed, S.D., Lunniss, P.J., Zarate, N., et al., 2010. Joint hypermobility and rectal evacuatory dysfunction: an etiological link in abnormal connective tissue? Neurogastroenterol. Motil. 22, 1085–1283.

Remvig, L., Duhn, P., Ullman, S., et al., 2010. Skin signs in Ehlers–Danlos syndrome: clinical tests and para-clinical methods. Scand. J. Rheumatol. 39, 511–517.

Remvig, L., Duhn, P.H., Ullman, S., et al., 2009. Skin extensibility and consistency in patients with Ehlers-Danlos syndrome and benign joint hypermobility syndrome. Scand. J. Rheumatol. 38, 227–230.

Remvig, L., Jensen, D.V., Ward, R.C., 2007. Are diagnostic criteria for general joint hypermobility and benign joint hypermobility syndrome based on reproducible and valid tests? A review of the literature. J. Rheumatol. 34, 798–803.

Ross, J., Grahame, R., 2011. Joint hypermobility syndrome. BMJ 342, c7167.

Seffinger, M.A., Najm, W.I., Mishra, S.I., et al., 2004. Reliability of spinal palpation for diagnosis of back and neck pain: a systematic review of the literature. Spine 29, E413–E425.

Smith, C.K., Bonauto, D.K., Silverstein, B.A., Wilcox, D., 2010. Inter-rater reliability of physical examinations in a prospective study of upper extremity musculoskeletal disorders. J. Occup. Environ. Med. 52, 1014–1018.

Van Der Wal, J., 2009. The architecture of the connective tissue in the musculoskeletal system—an often overlooked contributor to proprioception in the locomotor apparatus. Int. J. Ther. Massage Bodywork 2, 9–23.

Voermans, N.C., Bonnemann, C.G., Hamel, B.C.J., et al., 2009. Joint hypermobility as a distinctive feature in the differential diagnosis of myopathies. J. Neurol. 256, 13–27.

Vounotrypidis, P., Efremidou, E., Zezos, P., et al., 2009. Prevalence of joint hypermobility and patterns of articular manifestations in patients with inflammatory bowel disease. Gastroenterol. Res. Pract. 2009, 924138. Available from: https://www.ncbi.nlm.nih.gov/pmc/articles/PMC2821781/.

Yeo, S.M., Kang, H., An, S., et al., 2020. Mechanical properties of muscles around the shoulder in breast cancer patients: intra-rater and inter-rater reliability of the MyotonPRO. PM R 12, 374–381.

Zarate, N., Farmer, A.D., Grahame, R., et al., 2010. Unexplained gastrointestinal symptoms and joint hypermobility: is connective tissue the missing link? Neurogastroenterol. Motil. 22, 252–278.

Fascial Palpation

Thomas W. Myers

CHAPTER CONTENTS

DEFINING PALPATION

The phenomenon commonly called "touch" actually involves several sense types—somesthetic, proprioceptive, and interoceptive—synthesized via higher-level processing we do not yet fully comprehend (Craig 2015; Bainbridge-Cohen 2018). Neuroanatomists commonly use the terms "somatic sensation" or "somatosensory" to describe this afferent function, which arises from all over the body (Leonhardt et al. 1987).

"Palpation" specifies touching with some form of overt diagnostic intent or therapeutic inquiry. Palpation is usually done with the human hand, an instrument with 6 million years of on-the-job training in detecting subtle differences in other humans' skin. Palpatory information can be gathered actively, finding and checking a particular structure or movement, or it can be gathered passively, allowing a broad spectrum of information to arrive from the subject's tissue to the palpator's somatosensory system. In either active or passive palpation, a thorough and accurate visual picture of the underlying anatomy will always be a major asset to the therapist (Stecco 2015).

"Fascial" palpation is our focus in this chapter, but we must note from the outset that this is a misnomer: it is impossible to palpate fascia without palpating every other form of tissue—epithelial, muscle, and neural—at the same time. So a more accurate statement concerning what follows is palpation of the disposition of fascial tissues and the structures they create, within the broader context of the tissue medium and its rhythms in general.

Manual therapists have recognized the fascial system as a prime target in body pain and movement limitation and have thus focused their attention there (Hoheisel et al. 2012). In fact, several major schools of manual therapy, such as structural integration, fascial stretch therapy, or fascial manipulation, have built their treatment philosophy and rationale around the fascial system (Stecco 2004; Chaitow 2017; Fredrick and Fredrick 2014; Myers 2020).

Though the fascial system has been described as an "endless web," it is far more organized and responsive than the inert "packing material" it was previously imagined to be (Schultz and Feitis 1996). The fascial system can be seen as a continuous organ that surrounds our entire 70 trillion cells—just under the skin as the superficial fascia, and then, as deep fascia, enwrapping and investing all the other tissues and organs (Rolf 1977). It is, as observed by Franscisco Varela, the "organ of form" (Varela and Frenk 1987). But in addition to its anatomical and physical properties, the fascial system is increasingly recognized for its physiological and morphogenic properties (Langevin et al. 2006; Ingber 2003).

ACTIVE VS PASSIVE ASSESSMENT

Palpating a moving structure can produce significant clinical information. Different types of information can be gleaned when the movement is performed actively by the client versus passively, where the practitioner moves the structure for the client. Motion quality, range, and end-feel can all be assessed using this method. In addition, motion against resistance can inform the practitioner as to the relative strength and/or sensitivity of a movement. Some of these approaches are to be found in the exercises later in the chapter.

Any time a therapist makes manual contact, a palpatory experience occurs, and the intention of the palpator affects what is likely to be felt. Palpation is routinely used to assess the condition of the client prior to any therapeutic intervention (whether or not a diagnosis is made). Palpation may be employed during a therapeutic intervention, or used to assess results.

> **KEY POINTS**
>
> Palpation assessments are a tool for the manual or movement professional. Findings from palpation are inherently subjective, and objective evidence is thin for palpatory findings correlated with imaging techniques. Repetition of palpation assessments builds reliability to the findings of any given practitioner. Relaxation and focused attention in the practitioner are important for increased reliability of palpatory findings. Palpatory findings should be confirmed by other means where possible.

PALPATION TOOLS

Although the hand is the primary palpatory tool, manual therapists can occasionally move beyond just the palms of the hands and fingers to use the back of the hand or forearm to assess. The amount of pressure applied by the therapist varies with the depth of the structure being assessed. The direction of the applied pressure depends on whether the practitioner is performing a "direct" or "indirect" technique, that is, pushing toward or away from a motion barrier, respectively, depending on the relative acuteness or chronicity of the involved tissues (Chaitow 2017). Additionally palpation can go across a muscle, tendon, or ligament, depending on the information being gathered. As with treatment, the speed that a palpator's contact moves through the tissues depends on the consistency of the target tissue and the rate of "tissue compliance" that is noted, with slower movements indicated in more tender areas or those areas that are palpably different in texture—for example, denser than surrounding tissue.

Different forms of manual therapy target varying parts of our anatomy. Regardless of the target, the ability to accurately visualize the structures beneath the hands is of utmost importance. If you have no picture of what you are touching, palpation is a frustrating and ultimately useless exercise. Three-dimensional anatomical knowledge coupled with palpation skill allows the practitioner to develop a coherent and sound treatment strategy, that is, where to go next, or in some cases, where not to go next—and when to stop.

Two examples come to mind:

- The organization of the thoracolumbar fascia involves a superficial posterior layer that has a significantly different directionality than the deeper layer. In turn, the middle layer has a significantly different thickness and organization than the other two (Vleeming and Stoeckart 2007). Obviously this speaks to their different functional roles, and knowledge of the anatomy will influence what you can detect, which in turn guides the treatment plan.
- The layered muscles of the posterior neck present an extraordinarily complex pattern with the all-important function of aligning the head and cervical vertebrae such that the eyes are parallel to the horizon. At least a dozen muscles or muscle groups are present on each side of the midline. As the hands and fingers palpate from superficial to deep, different myofascial fiber directions will be encountered as well as different levels of muscle tone. An accurate three-dimensional picture that translates from "the books"—anatomy atlases—to the felt sense is essential to useful clinical palpatory skills.

RELAXED PALPATION

To maximize the information gathered from palpation, it is helpful to minimize the amount of noise in the system. A conscious effort to reduce excess tension in the therapist is fundamental to refined palpation skills to improve the signal-to-noise ratio in his/her own system and get an accurate reading on the client. Ensure as you begin that your body is well-supported from the ground up and that the upper limbs are as relaxed as possible. This is especially true of the muscles of the shoulder girdle and hand, neck, jaw, and face. In addition, most palpation benefits from the breath being slow, deep, and as unrestricted as possible.

LAYERS

Palpation by definition begins with skin-to-skin contact. Here, observations can be made regarding the skin: is it smooth, rough, oily, dry, sweaty; are its characteristics limited to a specific area, etc.? Palpation of the skin can be performed by simply moving the hands lightly along the surface without actually moving the skin.

The layer just deep to the skin is the superficial fascia (Fig. 6.2.1). This layer is of varying depth around the body and can be encountered by applying just enough pressure, such that the skin will move with the hands of the therapist. The skin is backed (as a carpet is backed) by the dermis, a thin and tough "hide"—and always the first layer of fascia encountered—that moves with the skin anywhere on the body.

Deep to the dermis is the hypodermis or subcutaneous layer, a loose, areolar type of connective tissue often invested with adipose. This layer can be thin or thick, denser or very loose, elastic or slow to return, with varying densities of adhesion to the underlying deep fascia. Abnormalities in the subcutaneous layer often point to concerns at a deeper level.

The superficial fascia is specialized in various areas to perform specific functions, such as cushioning the soles of the feet and supporting the lower abdominal wall (Scarpa's fascia). Occasionally, the superficial fascia virtually disappears, leaving the deep fascia very close to the surface. This can happen more widely in the body in a wasting disease—some forms of cancer for example—or commonly in certain areas, for example, the dimples at the posterior superior iliac spines.

Just deep to the areolar fascia is the deep fascia, the first discernible layer of which is a "unitard" covering the entire body from the plantar surface of the foot to the scalp at the top of the head. It is given various names in different segments—the crural fascia, the fascia lata—but this entire layer pulls in like an elastic suit, holding the body in its shape to maintain structural and functional balance. This layer effectively provides another set of muscle attachments and is essential to stability (Stahl and Nichols 2011).

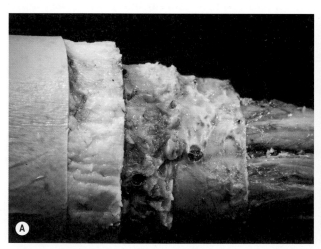
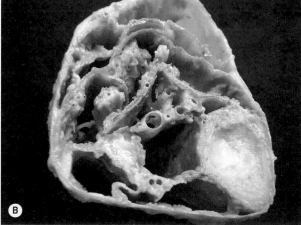

Fig. 6.2.1 (A) Typical fascial layering, dissected and plastinated, from the posterior lower leg. (B) Plastinated slice from the Fascial Net Plastination Project (FNPP). The layers interact in various ways at different levels. Fluids are carried between each layer, large or small. Other areas might contain more or fewer layers between skin and bone. Images reproduced with permission from the Fascial Net Plastination Project (www.FasciaResearchSociety.org/Plastination).

The inner surface of the fascia profundis, the "endless web" described by Schultz and Feitis (1996), surrounds, invests, and supports every other tissue: muscles, nerves, blood vessels, and organs. Muscles can be seen not so much as operating only from origin to insertion but as muscular fish swimming together in a fascial net. The tremulous jelly of the brain is supported by a network of glia within, and the pia and dura mater without. The entire digestive system is wrapped in tunics that are hung to the body wall. The wet surface of the lungs and the constant muscle of the heart are mounted on fascial scaffolding. Only the open lumens of the digestive and respiratory systems are free from some form of the fascial net.

From a developmental point of view, the fascia is derived from the embryonic mesoderm and forms the template in which all other mesenchymal derivatives arise. For example, bones and muscles develop within sheaths of mesodermal tissue, the periosteum and epimysium, respectively. As a result, very rarely do muscles attach directly to bone. Usually there is some form of intervening connective tissue. In fact, each individual muscle cell is encased in the connective tissue endomysium, whereas groups of myofibers, the muscle fascicles, are wrapped in perimysium. Joint capsules, tendons, and ligaments are all specializations of mesodermal connective tissue and are considered "fascial" elements by many practitioners. These specialized tissues are subject to physiological changes based on use (or lack of it), injury, and habit, and such changes are both palpable and actionable.

Accessing the deepest layers of fascia presents a challenge to the therapist. To address these deep layers, it is paradoxically best not only to go slower, but also to lighten the pressure applied. There is sometimes an inverse relationship between pressure and depth, and there is often an inverse relationship between speed and sensitivity.

Palpating deep fascial structures is possible without causing discomfort to the client/patient by allowing the more superficial tissues to "melt" under the hands of the therapist. Moving slowly into the movement endpoint of the tissue and then pausing will usually result in a release and further movement potential.

This releasing phenomenon may relate to a property of the extracellular matrix known as thixotropy, where the ground substance part of the fascia is rehydrated. Or the relaxation may be totally neuromuscular—the evidence is not clear.

KEY POINTS

Palpating specifically for fascial structures requires an accurate three-dimensional picture of the anatomy being assessed. Fiber direction, physiological condition, and adhesion/glide among available layers are all relevant factors specific to fascial treatment. Use palpation to detect abnormal tissue texture, evaluate symmetry, assess variations in range of movement and "end feel," to specify and localize pain symptoms, or to detect and evaluate change—are conditions improving or worsening?

COMMUNICATING WITH THE CLIENT

One problem with palpatory findings is that any interpretation is, by definition, subjective. As reported by the Cochrane group, interoperator reliability for soft-tissue tests is poor. Intraoperator reliability—what might be called "practice-based evidence" or extended clinical experience—is better (Green et al. 2003). If you have felt something similar on a number of clients, you have a better chance of knowing what you are feeling and what to do about it.

How such interpretations are expressed in language is a key element in any therapeutic relationship. The therapist and client are in a partnership that will only function maximally if free lines of communication and trust exist. This entails making sure the client is in control of the situation, where he/she is able to understand the language of the therapist, and that the client is aware of what's going to happen next. The practitioner will benefit from that relationship by palpating kindly and communicating the results in a confident, reassuring, and understandable manner.

It is important to remember that many of the mechanoreceptors in the fascia also double as pain receptors (nociceptors) (Craig 2015). As such, there will be an intensity threshold for every individual where pressure becomes painful. Because each person's experience of the phenomenon is different, it is important to monitor that experience periodically by asking the client about their experience, especially when addressing areas of potential tenderness (e.g., close to bones). Any wince is a bellwether—even the most minor contraction in the corner of the eye should alert the practitioner that they have crossed the line from sensation into pain.

PALPATING FOR INFORMATION

It is axiomatic that practitioners who use their hands to manipulate soft or bony structures should be able, accurately and relatively swiftly, to feel, assess, and judge the state of a wide range of physiological and pathological conditions and parameters relating not only to the tissues with which they are in touch but others associated with these, perhaps lying at greater depth or at some distance.

The information a practitioner needs to gather will vary according to the therapeutic approach, possibly including:

*   range of motion of a given joint or range of movement of a joint complex
*   the feel of joint play and the "end feel" when the joint is taken to end range
*   standing tone, and relative weakness or tightness in muscles
*   the amount of induration, edema, or fibrosis in soft tissues
*   the feel, density, mobility, and ability for adjacent fascial layers to glide
*   identification of regions in which reflex activity is operating
*   noises or palpable "clicks" in tissue
*   the quality of perceived tissue vitality (flaccid, toned, etc.)
*   variations in temperature over regions of the body
*   and many other pieces of acquired information.

Once gathered, the individual practitioner needs to fit the acquired information into his or her own conceptual system to use in accordance with whatever therapeutic methods are seen to be appropriate. The aim is therefore to identify what is under our hands when they are in contact with the patient, and, in the context of this book, what information we can gather regarding fascial structures and behavior in particular.

PALPATION OBJECTIVES

Philip Greenman (1989), in his book *Principles of Manual Medicine*, summarizes the five objectives of palpation. He suggests that the practitioner/therapist should be able to:

1. detect abnormal tissue texture
2. evaluate symmetry in the position of structures, both physically and visually

3. detect and assess variations in range and quality of movement during the range, as well as the quality of the end of the range of any movement
4. sense the position in space of yourself and the person being palpated
5. detect and evaluate change in the palpated findings, whether these are improving or worsening as time passes.

These elements, described by Greenman, with the qualification that fascia is the focus in this chapter, are our major objectives in obtaining palpatory literacy in fascial palpation.

PALPATE BY "FEELING," NOT THINKING

Palpation allows us to "see inside" to interpret tissue function. Different histological make-up influenced by genetics and diet brings differing amounts of inherent pliability and elasticity to each individual. This requires the practitioner to listen closely, because in different patients a muscle's ligaments, bones, and organs can have variable consistencies. Thus there is a "normal" feel when they are healthy, which is different for each tissue. This has to be learned through repeated exploration of "normal" tissue so that the practitioner builds a vocabulary of what "normal" feels like. Once someone is trained to use palpation efficiently, then finer and finer differences between tissues can be noted. Practice, and repetition, is vital in order to be able to differentiate when something has changed from being "normal."

Kappler (1997) has explained this as follows:

The art of palpation requires discipline, time, patience and practice. To be most effective and productive, palpatory findings must be correlated with a knowledge of functional anatomy, physiology and pathophysiology.

It is much easier to identify frank pathological states, a tumor for example, than to describe signs, symptoms, and palpatory findings that lead to or identify pathological mechanisms. Palpation with fingers and hands provides sensory information that the brain interprets as: temperature, texture, surface humidity, elasticity, turgor, tissue tension, thickness, shape, irritability, or motion. To accomplish this task, it is necessary to teach the fingers to feel, think, see, and know. One feels through the palpating fingers on the patient; one sees the structures under the palpating fingers through a visual image based on knowledge of anatomy; one thinks what is normal and abnormal, and one knows with confidence acquired with practice that what is felt is real and accurate. (Kappler 1997)

These words define succinctly the tool we use and the task we perform when we palpate.

Different parts of the human hand are more or less able to discriminate variations in tissue features, such as relative tension, texture, degree of moisture, temperature, and so on. This highlights the fact that overall palpatory sensitivity depends on a combination of different perceptive (and proprioceptive) qualities and abilities.

These include the ability to:

- register temperature variations and the subtle differences that exist in a spectrum of tissue states, ranging from very soft to extremely hard;
- register the existence and size of extremely small entities, such as are found in fibrotic tissue or areas of myofascial trigger point activity;
- sensitively distinguish between many textures and ranges in tone, from flaccid to spastic, and all the variables in between.

KEY POINTS

Building palpation skills involves the ability to detect increasingly subtle differences in tissue and movement, amplify the signal for accurate analysis, and interpret how the palpation findings will be applied in treatment. Palpation exercises (often accompanied by an anatomy atlas) build confidence and certainty in palpatory findings, which in the case of fascial tissue assessment requires feeling for slight but detectable differences.

PHYSIOLOGY OF TOUCH

Palpatory perception also results, in large measure, from variations in the number and type (see summary in Box 6.2.1) of sensory neural receptors found in the skin and tissues of various anatomical regions, because these greatly influence the discriminatory capabilities of those regions.

- Light touch is generally accepted as being achieved via mechanoreceptors (such as Meissner's corpuscle and Merkel's disc, as well as hair-root plexi) lying in the skin, muscles, joints, and organs. They respond to mechanical deformation resulting from pressure,

---

BOX 6.2.1 Receptors and Perception

Mechanoreceptors	
Light touch	Meissner's corpuscle
	Merkel's disc
	Hair-root plexus
Deep pressure	Pacinian corpuscle
Crude touch	Thought to be Krause's end-bulb
	Thought to be Ruffini's ending
Proprioceptors, Body Positioning	
Muscle length	Muscle spindle
Tendon and tissue load	Golgi tendon organ
Joint position	Joint/kinesthetic receptors
Fascial plane shear	Ruffini endings
Pressure and weight	Paciniform corpuscles
Nociceptors	
Pain	Free nerve endings
Thermoreceptors	
Warmth	Thought to be free nerve endings
Cold	Thought to be free nerve endings
Internal temperature	Hypothalamic thermostat

Adapted from Chaitow, L., 2010. Palpation and Assessment Skills, 3rd ed. Churchill Livingstone, Edinburgh.

stretch, or hair movement. It is in the skin that the greatest number of these receptors is found.

- Cruder touch perception and body position sensing is thought to relate to Krause's end-bulb, Ruffini's ending, Golgi tendon organs, and Pacinian corpuscles.
- Sensations of heat and cold are detected by thermoreceptors that are considered to be the free nerve endings in the skin.
- If cold is intense, detection is by nociceptors—specialized pain detectors—that are also free nerve endings.

FILTERING INFORMATION

Fine-touch receptor adaptation may cause the palpator's sensitivity to attenuate, especially if the practitioner maintains a constant position. Even a slight change of hand position can renew the flow of sensory information for the practitioner. At other times too much information is being received, and a degree of discrimination or filtering is required in order to make sense of it. Kappler summarizes this as follows:

A more significant component [of palpation skills] is to be able to focus on the mass of information being perceived, paying close attention to those qualities associated with tissue texture abnormality, and bypassing many of the other palpatory clues not relevant at the time. This is a process of developing mental filters. . . . The brain cannot process everything at once. By concentrating only on the portion you want, it becomes easy and fast to detect areas of significant tissue texture abnormality. (Kappler 1997)

Kappler et al. (1971) tested this concept and found that when they compared student examiners with experienced practitioner examiners, although the students recorded more palpation findings, the practitioners recorded more significant findings.

The experienced practitioners were filtering out the unimportant and focusing on what was meaningful, rather than being "overwhelmed with the mass of palpatory data." The ability to sort palpatory findings into the meaningful and the irrelevant is again a subjective process and points to the importance of the intentions of the assessor in interpreting what is felt.

AN EXPERIENCED PALPATION PERSPECTIVE

Gibbons and Tehan (2001) explain the basis of osteopathic palpation when assessing for somatic dysfunction (their particular focus is on spinal and joint dysfunction):

- *A relates to asymmetry.* DiGiovanna (1991) links the criterion of asymmetry to a positional focus, stating that the "position of the vertebra or other bone is asymmetrical." Greenman (1996) broadens the concept of asymmetry by including functional, in addition to structural, asymmetry. (In some ways, symmetry is a false God often worshipped by manual practitioners. Although symmetry is a good starting place for assessment, some functional asymmetry is always found in those with a dominant hand—or eye, leg, or pattern of mastication.)
- *R relates to range of motion.* Alteration in range of motion can apply to a single joint, several joints, or a region of the musculoskeletal system. The abnormality may be either restricted or increased mobility and includes assessment of quality of movement and "end feel." Be sure your test is isolating the structure or structures you wish to test.

- *T relates to tissue texture changes.* The identification of tissue texture change is important in the diagnosis of somatic dysfunction. Palpable changes may be noted in superficial, intermediate, and deep tissues. It is important for clinicians to distinguish normal from abnormal, and, in the case of fascial assessment, to assess gliding ability between layers.
- *T relates to tissue tenderness.* Undue tissue tenderness may be evident. Pain provocation and reproduction of familiar symptoms are often used to localize somatic dysfunction.

PRACTICAL PALPATION

A series of fascial palpation exercises are described elsewhere (Myers 2010). You are advised, after making contact with the tissues being investigated, to increase the pressure on the palpating fingers just sufficiently to make a contact with the tissues deep in the skin—meeting and matching the tissue tension, not invading it.

As the fingers lightly insinuate themselves through the tissues, various changes may be noted: mobility, tenderness, edema, deep muscle tension, fibrosis, increased density, and interosseous changes. All but fibrosis can be perceived in both acute and chronic lesions.

- *Detection* is a matter of being aware of the possible findings and practicing the techniques required to expose these possibilities.
- *Amplification* requires localized concentration on a specific task and the ability to block out extraneous information.
- *Interpretation* is the ability to relate the information received via detection and amplification.

Questions the palpator could be asking involve the following descriptors, for example:
- superficial/deep
- compressible/rigid
- warm/cold
- moist or damp/dry
- painful/pain free
- local or circumscribed/diffuse or widespread
- relaxed/tense
- able to glide / restricted
- hypertonic/hypotonic
- normal/abnormal

Where fascia is the intent of the palpation, we focus on tissue hydration, texture, the ability to glide, and any adhesion.

CONCLUSION

This chapter is intended to offer only an overview of the rich potential that awaits palpatory exploration of the fascial network.

It is important to caution that palpation assessments are not considered highly reliable means of acquiring information in terms of an "evidence base." The variability of palpation methodology, and the skills employed, alongside the subjective nature of interpretation, combine to raise important questions about such assessment methods. And even if an assessment method is shown to be potentially reliable, the degree of accuracy via interpretation remains questionable.

Until the development of quantitative methods such as ultrasound (see Chapter 8.2) and MRI and elastography (see Chapter 8.3), there were no alternative methods of fascial assessment even for research purposes. Although these tools are barely within the reach of most clinicians, research is increasingly coordinating those results with palpation. Without confirmation, the clinician must constantly consider: What am I feeling? What is its status? What does it mean in diagnostic terms? How accurate are my findings?.

Seffinger (2010) has offered a summary of these considerations as follows:

Precision is the measure of the variability in a [palpation] test, and is often used synonymously with reliability. A palpatory test is precise if it repeatedly measures the same thing with little variation. If a palpation test is precise and accurate, then it is both reliable and has validity.

Seffinger et al. (2004) identify the main element of reliability in palpation when they state that this is determined by comparing the reproducibility and concordance of diagnostic findings from the same examiner, and from different examiners palpating the same subject or group of subjects. And they clearly find that the careful specification inherent in high-quality research is necessary to achieve reliability; those studies that are less well-designed find much less agreement among examiners. In short, interoperator reliability is poor, but intraoperator reliability, especially for the experienced practitioner, is much higher.

It would therefore seem clinically prudent to use palpation methods as *a part* of a general evaluation, rather than relying completely on one means of assessment (i.e., palpation) alone, when formulating a treatment plan. Years of teaching from authors confirm that reliability of palpatory findings is highest when the practitioner has performed the same assessment with a large sample of patients.

Developing palpatory literacy, then, is the task of the clinician who wishes to be able to rely on palpation to complement other findings, signs, and tests. For advanced and reliable palpation skills, continuous practice and frequent self-reflection will be rewarded with sure-footed findings that will inform an effective treatment plan.

Summary

Palpation is a potent tool for the manual therapy professional, when used in conjunction with other assessment tools, and especially in the experienced practitioner. Palpatory findings are subjective and always require interpretation, so repetition of palpatory tests on many subjects is a prerequisite for reliable comparison. Use palpatory tests to detect abnormal tissue texture, evaluate symmetry, assess variations in range of movement and "end feel," to assess tissue layer glide, to specify and localize pain symptoms, and to detect and evaluate therapeutic change. Palpatory findings can help specify treatment plans.

REFERENCES

Bainbridge-Cohen, B., 2018. Basic Neurocellular Patterns. Burchfield Rose Publishers, El Sobrante, CA.

Chaitow, L. (Ed.), 2014. Fascial Dysfunction. Handspring, Edinburgh.

Chaitow, L. (Ed.), 2017. Palpation and Assessment in Manual Therapy, fourth ed. Handspring, Edinburgh.

Craig, A.D., 2015. How do you feel? An Interoceptive Moment with you Neurobiological Self. Princeton University Press, Princeton, NJ.

DiGiovanna, E., 1991. Somatic dysfunction. In: DiGiovanna, E., Schiowitz, S. (Eds.), An Osteopathic Approach to Diagnosis and Treatment. JB Lippincott, Philadelphia, pp. 6–12.

Fredrick, A., Fredrick, C., 2014. Fascial Stretch Therapy. Handspring, Edinburgh.

Gibbons, P., Tehan, P., 2001. Spinal Manipulation: Indications, Risks and Benefits. Churchill Livingstone, Edinburgh.

Green, S, Buchbinder, R., Hetrick, S., 2003. Physiotherapy interventions for shoulder pain. Cochrane Syst. Rev., CD004258.

Greenman, P., 1989. Principles of Manual Medicine. Williams and Wilkins, Baltimore.

Greenman, P., 1996. Principles of Manual Medicine. Williams and Wilkins, Baltimore.

Hoheisel, U., Taguchi, T., Mense, S., 2012. Nociception: the thoracolumbar fascia as a sensory organ. In: Schleip, R., Findley, T., Chaitow, L. et al. (Eds.), Fascia, the Tensional Network of the Body. Churchill Livingstone, Edinburgh.

Ingber, D.E., 2003. Mechanobiology and diseases of mechanotransduction. Ann. Med. 35, 564–577.

Kappler, R., 1997. Palpatory skills. In: Ward, R. (Ed.), Foundations for Osteopathic Medicine. Williams and Wilkins, Baltimore.

Kappler, R., Larson, N., Kelso, A., 1971. A comparison of osteopathic findings on hospitalized patients obtained by trained student examiners and experienced physicians. J. Am. Osteopath. Assoc. 70, 1091–1092.

Langevin, H.M., Konofagou, E.E., Badger, G.J., et al., 2006. Tissue displacements during acupuncture using ultrasound elastography techniques. Ultrasound Med. Biol. 30, 1173–1183.

Leonhardt, H., Töndury, G., Zilles, K. (Eds.), 1987. Rauber/Kopsch Anatomie der Menschen Lehrbuch und Atlas, III: Nervensystem, Sinnesorgane Stuttgart: Thieme Verlag.

Myers, T., 2010. Fascial palpation. In: Chaitow, L. (Ed.), Palpation and Assessment Skills, third ed. Churchill Livingstone, Edinburgh.

Myers, T., 2020. Anatomy Trains, fourth ed. Churchill Livingstone, Edinburgh.

Rolf, I.P., 1977. Rolfing: Reestablishing the Natural Alignment and Structural Integration of the Human Body of Vitality and Well Being. Healing Arts Press, Rochester, VT.

Schultz, R., Feitis, R., 1996. The Endless Web: Fascial Anatomy and Physical Reality. North Atlantic Books. Seattle, WA.

Seffinger, M., 2010. Palpation reliability and validity. In: Chaitow, L. (Ed.), Palpation and Assessment Skills, third ed. Churchill Livingstone, Edinburgh.

Seffinger, M.A., Najm, W.I., Mishra, S.I., et al., 2004. Reliability of spinal palpation for diagnosis of back and neck pain: a systematic review of the literature. Spine 29, E413–E425.

Stahl, V.A., Nichols, T.R., 2011. Short-term effects of muscular denervation and fasciotomy on global limb variables during locomotion in the decerebrate cat. Cells, Tissues, Organs. 193, 325–335.

Stecco, C., 2015. Functional Atlas of the Human Fascial System. Churchill Livingstone, Edinburgh.

Stecco, L., 2004. Fascial Manipulation for Musculo-Skeletal Pain. PICCIN, Padua.

Varela, F., Frenk, S., 1987. The organ of form. J. Soc. Biol. Struct. 10, 73–83.

Vleeming, A., Stoeckart, R., 2007. The role of the pelvic girdle in coupling the spine and the legs: a clinical-anatomical perspective on pelvic stability. In: Vleeming, A., Mooney, V., Stoeckart, R. (Eds.), Movement, Stability, and Lumbopelvic Pain, Integration of Research and Therapy. Elsevier, Edinburgh (Chapter 8).

Hypermobility, Hypermobility Spectrum Disorders, and Hypermobile Ehlers–Danlos Syndrome

Jane Simmonds

CHAPTER CONTENTS

INTRODUCTION

Joint hypermobility (JH) is the universally accepted term used to define the ability of a joint (or a group of joints) to move, passively and/or actively, beyond normally expected limits. Therefore JH is a description rather than a diagnosis (Castori et al. 2017). There are many factors that contribute to JH, including joint shape, muscle tone, physical training, and connective tissue liability. JH may be localized (LGH) or generalized (GJH), and although usually asymptomatic has been shown to predispose to musculoskeletal pain and injury in teenagers (Tobias et al. 2013).

Joint hypermobility is a unifying feature of Ehlers-Danlos syndrome (EDS), Marfan's syndrome (MFS), Loeys-Dietz syndrome (LDS), and osteogenesis imperfecta (OI), a group of heritable disorders of connective tissue (HDCT) that affect the connective tissue matrix proteins (Castori et al. 2017). Joint hypermobility exists on a spectrum, ranging from asymptomatic to symptomatic hypermobility that is previously known as joint hypermobility syndrome (JHS or HMS) or Ehlers-Danlos syndrome hypermobility type or type III (EDS-HT or EDS-III) (Castori et al. 2017). Researchers and clinicians have found it difficult to distinguish between what used to be called JHS and EDS-HT, and therefore in 2017 defined a more detailed diagnostic criteria, now called hypermobile Ehlers-Danlos syndrome (hEDS) (Fig. 6.3.1), and less restrictive diagnosis of hypermobility spectrum disorders (HSD). In creating tighter diagnostic criteria the potential for being able to determine genetic markers will be more likely. The HSD diagnosis is a diagnosis of exclusion. Experts propose that when people present with musculoskeletal signs and symptoms related to joint hypermobility and do not fulfil the criteria for hEDS, or another diagnosis could explain the presentation, they should receive the diagnosis of HSD (Castori et al. 2017).

It is important to remember that joint hypermobility may exist for reasons other than ligamentous laxity, such as myopathies or neurological or skeletal disorders (Castori et al. 2017). The discussions in this chapter refer to both HSD and hEDS (HSD/hEDS), as the management is essentially the same. It should be noted that most research cited used prior diagnostic labels and criteria for JHS or EDS-HT.

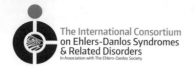

Diagnostic Criteria for Hypermobile Ehlers-Danlos Syndrome (hEDS)

This diagnostic checklist is for doctors across all disciplines to be able to diagnose EDS

The International Consortium on Ehlers-Danlos Syndromes & Related Disorders
In Association with The Ehlers-Danlos Society

Distributed by
The **Ehlers Danlos** Society.

Patient name: _____ DOB: _____ DOV: _____ Evaluator: _____

The clinical diagnosis of hypermobile EDS needs the simultaneous presence of all criteria, 1 **and** 2 **and** 3.

CRITERION 1 – Generalized Joint Hypermobility

One of the following selected:
- ☐ ≥6 pre-pubertal children and adolescents
- ☐ ≥5 pubertal men and woman to age 50
- ☐ ≥4 men and women over the age of 50

Beighton Score: _____ /9

If Beighton Score is one point below age- and sex-specific cut off, two or more of the following must also be selected to meet criterion:
- ☐ Can you now (or could you ever) place your hands flat on the floor without bending your knees?
- ☐ Can you now (or could you ever) bend your thumb to touch your forearm?
- ☐ As a child, did you amuse your friends by contorting your body into strange shapes or could you do the splits?
- ☐ As a child or teenager, did your shoulder or kneecap dislocate on more than one occasion?
- ☐ Do you consider yourself "double jointed"?

CRITERION 2 – Two or more of the following features (A, B, or C) must be present

Feature A (five must be present)
- ☐ Unusually soft or velvety skin
- ☐ Mild skin hyperextensibility
- ☐ Unexplained striae distensae or rubae at the back, groins, thighs, breasts and/or abdomen in adolescents, men or pre-pubertal women without a history of significant gain or loss of body fat or weight
- ☐ Bilateral piezogenic papules of the heel
- ☐ Recurrent or multiple abdominal hernia(s)
- ☐ Atrophic scarring involving at least two sites and without the formation of truly papyraceous and/or hemosideric scars as seen in classical EDS
- ☐ Pelvic floor, rectal, and/or uterine prolapse in children, men or nulliparous women without a history of morbid obesity or other known predisposing medical condition
- ☐ Dental crowding and high or narrow palate
- ☐ Arachnodactyly, as defined in one or more of the following:
  (i) positive wrist sign (Walker sign) on both sides, (ii) positive thumb sign (Steinberg sign) on both sides
- ☐ Arm span-to-height ratio ≥1.05
- ☐ Mitral valve prolapse (MVP) mild or greater based on strict echocardiographic criteria
- ☐ Aortic root dilatation with Z-score >+2

   Feature A total: _____ /12

Feature B
- ☐ Positive family history; one or more first-degree relatives independently meeting the current criteria for hEDS

Feature C (must have at least one)
- ☐ Musculoskeletal pain in two or more limbs, recurring daily for at least 3 months
- ☐ Chronic, widespread pain for ≥3 months
- ☐ Recurrent joint dislocations or frank joint instability, in the absence of trauma

CRITERION 3 - All of the following prerequisites MUST be met

1. Absence of unusual skin fragility, which should prompt consideration of other types of EDS

2. Exclusion of other heritable and acquired connective tissue disorders, including autoimmune rheumatologic conditions. In patients with an acquired CTD (*e.g.* Lupus, Rheumatoid Arthritis, etc.), additional diagnosis of hEDS requires meeting both Features A and B of Criterion 2. Feature C of Criterion 2 (chronic pain and/or instability) cannot be counted toward a diagnosis of hEDS in this situation.

3. Exclusion of alternative diagnoses that may also include joint hypermobility by means of hypotonia and/or connective tissue laxity. Alternative diagnoses and diagnostic categories include, but are not limited to, neuromuscular disorders (*e.g.* Bethlem myopathy), other hereditary disorders of the connective tissue (e.g. other types of EDS, Loeys-Dietz syndrome, Marfan syndrome), and skeletal dysplasias (*e.g.* osteogenesis imperfecta). Exclusion of these considerations may be based upon history, physical examination, and/or molecular genetic testing, as indicated.

Diagnosis: _____

v9

Fig. 6.3.1 2017 Diagnostic criteria for hEDS. Reproduced with permission from the Ehlers-Danlos Society. Available from: https://www.ehlers-danlos.com/heds-diagnostic-checklist/.

Joint hypermobility–related conditions are likely the most common inherited connective tissue disorder. They are more common than rheumatoid arthritis and almost as common as fibromyalgia. In the United Kingdom, where there is more research on the condition, JHS was found in 30% of patients presenting to a primary care clinic (Connelly et al. 2015) and 39% and 37% of pain management and rheumatology clinics, respectively (To et al. 2017). In Oman the incidence of JHS in a female outpatient setting was 60% of all new patients and 55% in returning patients (Clark and Simmonds 2011). Surveys among physical therapists in Europe, the United States, and the United Kingdom have highlighted the lack of knowledge with regard to diagnosis, assessment, and management and the need for education and empirical research (Russek et al. 2016; Rombaut et al. 2015; Lyell et al. 2016; Palmer et al. 2017).

Although genetic abnormalities have been identified for other forms of EDS, no specific genetic abnormality has been associated with HSD/hEDS. This is probably because of the wide heterogeneity. The pathophysiology of HSD/hEDS remains unclear and is likely to be multifactorial. Several defects in the connective tissue proteins have been found, including types I, III, and V collagen and tenascin X (Syx et al. 2017). Although joint hypermobility is often the most visible sign, HSD/hEDS affects connective tissue in many body systems, causing widespread signs and symptoms involving most body systems (Table 6.3.1) (Bulbena et al. 2017; Chopra et al. 2017; Malfait et al. 2017; Tinkle et al. 2017; Simmonds et al. 2019).

CLINICAL PRESENTATION

Patients with HSD/hEDS may present with a wide range of signs and symptoms (Table 6.3.1) (Chopra et al. 2017; Malfait et al. 2017; Tinkle et al. 2017; Simmonds et al. 2019). All individuals with HSD/hEDS have hypermobile joints, either currently or historically. Additional signs and symptoms vary significantly among individuals, with some people affected mostly by pain and musculoskeletal problems, others by fatigue, and yet others by symptoms such as dysautonomia, gastrointestinal, and urogenital problems (Simmonds et al. 2019). Cross-sectional studies, however, suggest that the presentation of HSD/hEDS tends to change over the lifespan. Childhood and adolescence may be characterized by delayed motor development, poor coordination, fatigue, gastrointestinal problems, and intermittent pain often associated with dislocations or sprains. The second and third decades of life tend to be dominated by recurrent muscle, joint, tendon, and peripheral neurogenic pain; sleep disorders; and urogenital problems. Later adulthood tends to be associated with widespread chronic pain, disabling fatigue, central sensitization, and multiple visceral problems. Research suggests that these patients have generalized hyperalgesia and central sensitization (Scheper et al. 2017). It is been hypothesized that the persistent nociceptive input in HSD/hEDS due to joint abnormalities might trigger central sensitization in the dorsal horn neurons, possibly involving the descending modulatory system (Di Stefano et al. 2016).

Severity and complexity can present in a broad spectrum HSD/hEDS, from acute/simple cases with only a few mild complaints to chronic/complex cases in which patients may be completely disabled by hypermobility-related complaints (Keer and Simmonds 2011). Some people with HSD/hEDS experience flare-ups of symptoms, particularly after periods of overactivity or inactivity because of injury, illness, or stressful life events. Any of these triggers can exacerbate muscle weakness due to pain or deconditioning, which further increases joint instability (Keer and Simmonds 2011).

The clinical presentation of HSD/hEDS is further complicated by dysautonomia and sometimes by mast cell activation syndrome (MCAS). The most common form of dysautonomia in HSD/hEDS is postural orthostatic tachycardia syndrome (POTS). The mechanism for POTS in HSD/hEDS is not clear but may be due to both peripheral vascular pooling in hyperelastic vascular structures and abnormal sympathetic activity (De Wandele et al. 2014; Hakim et al. 2017). Regardless of the cause, POTS results in reduced stroke volume and functional capacity. The relationship between MCAS and HSD/hEDS is also not clear; one hypothesis is through an excess of chymase-positive mast cells affecting the connective tissue (Seneviratne et al. 2017).

EXAMINATION OF PATIENTS WITH HYPERMOBILITY SPECTRUM DISORDER

A biopsychosocial approach should be adopted when examining patients (Englebert et al. 2017). It is also essential to ask questions about multisystem involvement typical of HSD/hEDS, because often patients are unaware that nonmusculoskeletal symptoms are associated with HSD/hEDS and might not offer this information unless asked (Keer and Simmonds 2011). The International

TABLE 6.3.1   Common Signs and Symptoms Associated with Hypermobility Spectrum Disorder and Hypermobile Ehlers-Danlos Syndrome

Body System	Signs and Symptoms
Musculoskeletal	• Frequent sprains, subluxations, and dislocations • Chronic joint pain • Scoliosis • Decreased bone density with associated increased fracture rate • Tendinitis, bursitis, synovitis, tenosynovitis, fasciitis, tendon ruptures • Trigger points, muscle tension/spasm, muscle strain
Autonomic	• Dysautonomia with orthostatic hypotension and/or postural orthostatic tachycardia syndrome (POTS)—tachycardia, presyncope/syncope, anxiety, chronic fatigue, sleep disorder, exercise intolerance, dependent edema, mottled purple skin in the periphery, temperature dysregulation, "brain fog" and trouble concentrating, sexual dysfunction
Cardiovascular	• Mitral valve prolapse • Aortic dilatation • Varicose veins
Neurological	• Developmental motor delay • Proprioceptive and motor control deficits • Fibromyalgia/central sensitization, hyperalgesia • Headaches and migraines • Paresthesias and nerve compression disorders • Autistic spectrum disorder
Cognitive	• Anxiety and panic disorder • Attention deficit hyperactivity disorder • Memory or concentration problems • Depression
Gastrointestinal	• Gastroesophageal reflux, chronic gastritis • Irritable bowel syndrome, constipation or diarrhea, bloating, abdominal pain, gastroparesis, food sensitivities • Prolapsed rectum • Hernias
Integumentary	• Hyperextensible skin • Slow healing • Widened scarring and poor wound healing • Easy bruising • Striae
Urogenital	• Overactive bladder • Urinary incontinence • Prolapsed bladder or uterus • Urinary tract infections • Dysmenorrhea, endometriosis, vulvodynia, pelvic pain, painful intercourse
Immune	• Mast cell activation syndrome (MCAS): flushing, rashes, watery eye, environmental sensitivities, medication and food sensitivities, fatigue, trouble concentrating, migratory pain, excessive inflammatory response, anxiety

Chopra, P., Tinkle, B., Hamonet, C., et al., 2017. Pain management in the Ehlers-Danlos syndromes. Am. J. Med. Genet. C Semin. Med. Genet. 175, 212–219; Malfait, F., Francomano, C., Byers, P., et al., 2017. The 2017 international classification of the Ehlers-Danlos syndromes. Am. J. Med. Genet. C Semin. Med. Genet. 175, 8–26; Tinkle, B., Castori, M., Berglund, B., et al., 2017. Hypermobile Ehlers-Danlos syndrome (a.k.a. Ehlers-Danlos syndrome Type III and Ehlers-Danlos syndrome hypermobility type): Clinical description and natural history. Am. J. Med. Genet. C Semin. Med. Genet. 175, 48–69; Simmonds, J.V., Herbland, A., Hakim, A., et al., 2019. Exercise beliefs and behaviours of individuals with Joint Hypermobility syndrome/Ehlers-Danlos syndrome–hypermobility type. Disabil. Rehabil. 41, 445–455.

Classification of Function (ICF) model provides an effective way to integrate body structure and functional impairments with functional restrictions and personal and environmental factors and is advocated in the most current clinical guideline paper (Engelbert et al. 2017). Disability in HSD/hEDS may be due to pain, fatigue, or psychological distress, and therefore each of these domains needs a thorough investigation. Childhood symptoms, such as developmental delay and clumsiness and gastrointestinal problems, are also relevant.

Core components of the new 2017 hEDS diagnostic criteria are assessed through the history. Formal diagnosis of a first-degree relative with hEDS is one of the new diagnostic criteria. History of hernias, organ prolapse, recurrent nontraumatic dislocations, mitral valve prolapse, and aortic dilatation are considered characteristics of a systemic connective tissue disorder (Malfait et al. 2017). The history should also include questions about contributing factors, such as provocative postures and activities, especially when there is no clear traumatic onset. Furthermore the assessment should include questions about periods of inactivity due to illness or life events, as these may also trigger episodes of increased symptoms. Systemic profiling using the Spider,

a multisystem symptom impact scale (De Wandele et al. 2020), can be very helpful for educating patients and guiding treatment (Fig. 6.3.2).

The physical assessment should include key components of diagnostic criteria for hEDS (Fig. 6.3.1). The Beighton score assesses hypermobility at the elbows, knees, thumbs, fifth MCP, and trunk. The required number of hypermobile joints varies with age: at least 6/9 for prepubertal children, at least 5/9 for adolescents to 50 years, and at least 4/9 for individuals over 50 years old. Individuals who are 1 point below the threshold may score 1 additional point by answering yes to at least two questions in the Five-Point Questionnaire, which asks about historical hypermobility (Malfait et al. 2017). Although the Beighton scale is used to make a decision about whether a person has generalized joint hypermobility, it is limited by uniplanar and upper limb biased joint assessment. Therefore clinicians are encouraged to use the Lower Limb Assessment scale, which has been validated for children and adults (Ferarri et al. 2005; Meyer et al. 2017), and the newly described and validated Upper Limb Hypermobility Assessment Tool, which to date has been validated in adults (Nicholson and Chan 2018).

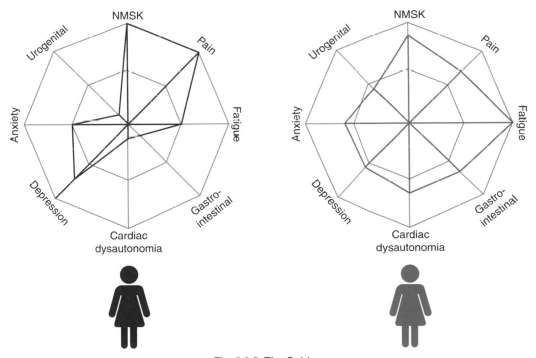

Fig. 6.3.2 The Spider.

The diagnostic criterion for a systemic connective tissue disorder include: soft velvety skin; mild skin hyperextensibility at the volar forearm (1.5 cm); unexplained stretch marks; piezogenic papules in the heel (nodules visible with weight-bearing); and atrophic scarring. Other connective tissue features include umbilical, inguinal, or abdominal hernias and pelvic floor, rectal, or uterine prolapse. Marfanoid signs of arachnodactyly (tested using armspan to height and the Steinberg or Walker signs) and high narrow palate can also be assessed. It should be noted that many of the extrarticular connective tissue features may not present until skeletal maturity and therefore a diagnosis of hEDS may not be able to be made until such time.

Further physical assessments should be based on the patient's reported symptoms to identify functional limitations, symptomatic tissues, and factors contributing to those symptomatic tissues Engelbert et al. 2017; Castori 2016; Chopra et al. 2017). Functional activity limitations can be assessed using standard outcome measures based on the patient's level of function, which can range from high level athlete to profoundly disabled and bed-bound. Particular attention should be given to quality of movement and motor control (Keer and Simmonds 2011). Research has demonstarted that people with HSD/hEDS have proprioceptive deficits in the upper and lower extremities (Hall et al. 2004; Smith et al. 2013; Scheper et al. 2017) whereas other research suggests decreased precision of movement (Clayton et al. 2015). Balance (Schubert-Hjalmarsson et al. 2012) and postural control (Lisi et al. 2017) also appear to be compromised, at least in children.

When examining children with HSD/hEDS the history taking should include a thorough exploration of developmental milestones and onset and triggers for pain, fatigue, and joint instability. As with adults it is important to ask the child/caregiver about complaints in other systems, as multisystem involvement has been shown to predict more disablement (Scheper et al. 2017). The physical examination should include sitting and standing posture, where children may hang on ligaments (e.g., anterior pelvic tilt, genu recurvatum, pes planus) and poor stabilization (e.g., winging scapulae). Upper extremity weight-bearing tests, such as four-point kneeling and the superman test, may demonstrate hyperextension of elbows or wrists and poor trunk control. Functional strength and dynamic control in midrange can be observed during movements such as wall squats, heel raises, single leg stand, Y balance test,

bridging, star jumping, and hopping. Therapists should be aware that although the standardized developmental assessments such as the Movement Assessment Battery for Children (M-ABC), can give quantitive scores on movement capability, they may not reveal poor quality of motion often seen in children with HSD/hEDS. Gait abnormalities are also common and should be explored (Englebert et al. 2017). The examination should also ideally include some aspect of endurance testing, as fatigue can exacerbate instability and poor motor control.

The Bristol Impact of Hypermobility (BIOH) self-report questionnaire is the only disease-specific validated outcome measure for adults (Palmer et al. 2017). The Pediatric Quality of Life Measure (PedsQL) is a valid and reliable generic outcome measure for children as it covers physical function and emotional, social, and school domains, which are relevant to young people aged 5 to 18 years.

KEY POINTS

- The diagnostic criteria for Hypermobile Ehlers-Danlos Syndrome (hEDS) were revised in 2017.
- Hypermobility Spectrum Disorder (HSD) is a diagnosis of exclusion and focuses on musculoskeletal and neurophysiological symptoms.
- Use a biopsychosocial approach when assessing and treating people with hEDS/HSD.
- It is also essential to ask questions about multisystem involvement typical of HSD/hEDS, because often patients are unaware that nonmusculoskeletal symptoms are associated with HSD/hEDS and might not offer this information unless asked.

EVALUATION, DIAGNOSIS, AND MANAGEMENT PLANNING

Current and historical hypermobility should be assessed in patients presenting with complaints typical of HSD/hEDS. Genetic testing is only appropriate if one of the other forms of EDS is suspected. The second most common form of EDS is classical EDS, which has more significant skin involvement. Even though vascular EDS is not common, it is a differential diagnosis that should be considered because of life-threatening risk of aortic or organ rupture. People with vascular EDS typically have translucent skin with prominent veins, easy bruising, and a characteristic facial appearance with prominent eyes (Malfait et al. 2017). The 2017 diagnostic criteria for hEDS (Fig. 6.3.1) have three standards that must all be met: (1) generalized joint hypermobility, (2) systemic manifestations of a connective tissue disorder, and (3) exclusion of other conditions. Criterion 1, generalized hypermobility, has been described previously. Criterion 2 requires that at least two of three subcategories be met (systemic connective tissue involvement, first-degree family history, and musculoskeletal pain or dislocations) (Malfait et al. 2017). Criterion 3 is exclusion of other conditions associated with hypermobility (Fig. 6.3.1) and may require referral for further medical testing. The restrictive diagnostic criteria for hypermobile Ehlers-Danlos Syndrome (hEDS), compared with JHS and EDS-HT, is an attempt to identify a more homogeneous population in an effort to identify a specific genetic etiology (Malfait et al. 2017). Many people who used to meet the diagnostic criteria for JHS or EDS-HT do not meet the criteria for hEDS and are now included in the category of HSD, which is the presence of generalized laxity, and have a few of the characteristics of hEDS but not enough to meet the stricter criteria (Castori et al. 2017).

It is important to identify relevant comorbidities. The diagnostic criteria for POTS are heart rate increase of ≥30 bpm within 10 minutes of a standing or tilt-table test in the absence of orthostatic hypotension (no drop of >20 mmHg systolic blood pressure). Children must demonstrate heart rate increase of ≥40 bpm. Patients should have no other reason for their tachycardia, such as prolonged bedrest or conditions or medications affecting autonomic regulation (Raj 2013; Hakim et al. 2017). The presence of POTS influences therapy interventions, as patients may have poor exercise tolerance, especially with upright activities. Postoperative patients may be particularly vulnerable to syncope episodes.

Fibromyalgia is a common comorbidity of HSD/hEDS and may be misdiagnosed when the actual diagnosis is HSD/hEDS (Chopra et al. 2017). Fibromyalgia should be assessed using the 2016 American College of Rheumatology 2016 diagnostic criteria (Wolfe et al. 2016). One longitudinal study undertaken by Scheper and colleagues in 2017 suggests that multisystem involvement is associated with greater disability and worse prognosis. Consequently other system involvement may justify referral to gastroenterologists, nutritionists/dieticians, immunologists, psychologists, and psychiatrists.

Once identification of HSD/hEDS and possible comorbidities has been completed, evaluation needs to prioritize the patient's problems and determine whether this is an active, stable patient with an acute injury or a deconditioned, unstable patient. Similarly, differentiation between acute/simple cases and chronic/complex cases facilitates a tiered approach to management (Fig. 6.3.3). For example, a "simple" patient might present with a recent

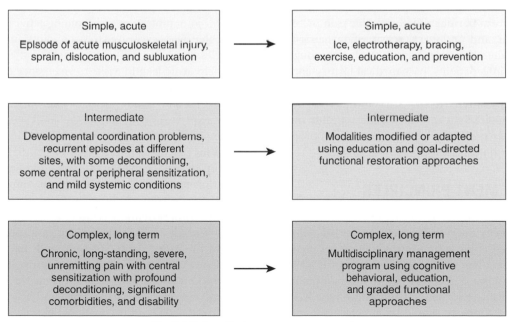

Fig. 6.3.3 Stratified management approach.

history of anterior pain due to pes planus coupled with overpronation at the subtalar joint. A "complex" patient may present with widespread pain of long duration, multiple system involvement, multiple comorbidities, and significant psychiatric and social problems. Although pain, fatigue, multisystem involvement, and psychological distress all contribute to disability, fatigue and distress are more highly correlated with disability than pain (Scheper et al. 2016; Scheper et al. 2017). Consequently, a biopsychosocial multidisciplinary approach is needed to address the multiple issues in these patients.

Children with HSD/hEDS frequently have poorer quality of life than nonhypermobile peers. Factors contributing to quality of life deficits in children include pain, fatigue, stress incontinence, and gastrointestinal disturbance (Pacey et al. 2015). A seminal study in the United Kingdom suggested that 75% of patients develop symptoms prior to age 15. Hypermobile adolescents are twice as likely to develop musculoskeletal problems as nonhypermobile peers. Overweight adolescents with GJH are almost 12 times as likely to experience pain (Tobias et al. 2013).

In addition to identifying symptomatic tissues, therapists need to identify factors contributing to symptoms. Psychosocial factors may also contribute to pain through central sensitization, especially in more complex patients (Castori 2016; Chopra et al. 2017). It is also important to determine the type of pain, as inflammatory and mechanical nociceptive should be managed differently from peripheral neuropathic pain or central sensitization, and peripheral sensitization needs to be addressed when present (Castori 2016). A thorough investigation into patients' past medical history and understanding the severity of their current and potential added complications from other medical conditions and how they interact with their general health and fitness level will help create a plan of care with appropriate time lines and goals (Engelbert et al. 2017).

MANAGEMENT PRINCIPLES

Despite the growing body of literature, there have been few high-quality intervention studies reported, with case studies, expert opinion, and single joint studies predominating. Current best practice management of HSD/hEDS is essentially a problem-solving approach underpinned by the best available evidence and aligned with the ICF. The management approach should be multifactorial and address all of the patient's needs. This may include patient and caregiver education; exercises the patient can consistently tolerate; pain, fatigue, and stress management; self-management techniques; splinting or bracing recommendations; cognitive behavioral strategies; and referral to other providers as appropriate. As noted previously, patients may present as simple/acute, intermediate, or complex/chronic. In general, simple/acute patients may benefit from typical rehabilitation activities such as neuromuscular reeducation, therapeutic exercise, manual therapy, and modalities; patient education about injury prevention, body mechanics, and joint protection are important to minimize future injury. Intermediate patients may also require additional guidance regarding activity modification and pacing. Complex/chronic patients require multidisciplinary care, chronic pain management, and cognitive behavioral approaches with an emphasis on teaching self-management skills.

Condition-specific patient education and goal-oriented shared decision-making forms the basis of empowerment-based self-management models for long-term conditions. Effective communication is essential and patients have expressed in research the importance and value of working in partnership with therapists (Simmonds et al. 2019). Patients who fully understand their condition, triggers and reactions, and self-care strategies can more effectively manage pain and disability and more efficiently recover from a flare-up or injury.

Patients and parents/caregivers need to learn strategies for joint protection and avoiding activities and positions that place excessive stress on joints and stabilizing muscles. Learning self-management and subluxations can help avoid lengthy visits to emergency departments and inappropriate medications. Understanding of body mechanics and ergonomics can minimize stress to the body. Experts suggest that external joint support such as braces and splints can help protect both large and small joints for functional or recreational activities. One of the benefits of bracing may be through providing additional proprioceptive input by enhancing cutaneous sensory input; compression clothing, taping, and orthotics may enhance proprioception (Dupuy et al. 2017). Preliminary research exploring the use of ring splints demonstrates improved grip strength and hand function (Schlepe et al. 2018). Moreover, adaptive utensils and tool modifications may decrease stress on hand joints. Patients need to understand when and how to use such assistive devices, and occupational therapy plays a very important role for this (Engelbert et al. 2017).

Experts recommend gradually progressed exercises guided by motor learning theory to ensure quality movement (Engelbert et al. 2017). There is a tendency for individuals with HSD/hEDS to move quickly and use global, more phasic muscles; exercise therapists are advised to facilitate patients to be mindful and to move slowly to help reduce the risk of injury and to improve motor learning (Boudreau et al. 2010). Closed-chain exercises and augmented or external feedback using biofeedback, tape, and close-fitting clothing may be particularly helpful because of decreased proprioception (Keer and Simmonds 2007) (Fig. 6.3.4). Patients report that a "hands-on" approach to help guide and aid learning is beneficial from the patients' perspective (Simmonds et al. 2017) (Fig. 6.3.5). Proprioceptive training can be beneficial both for improving movement precision and for decreasing kinesiophobia and pain (Sahin et al. 2008) whereas movement education can help prevent fear avoidance strategies that can amplify functional impairments. Both general strengthening and targeted strengthening of injured joints are beneficial in reducing pain. Joint stability can be addressed through postural awareness, learning efficient

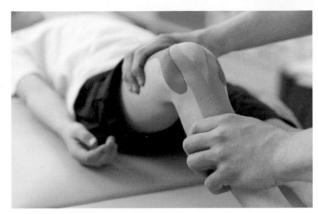

Fig. 6.3.5 Hands-on therapy to correct and facilitate movement. Courtesy iStock.com/Katarzyna Bialasiewicz.

body mechanics, muscle strengthening, and motor control training, and consistent physical activity to improve overall physical fitness (Kemp et al. 2010; Pacey et al. 2013; Palmer et al. 2014; Scheper et al. 2017). Muscle mass in those with hEDS, although comparable in size to the general unaffected population, demonstrates decreased strength, strength endurance, and functional capacity (Rombaut et al. 2012; To and Alexander 2019). Maintaining muscle strength to reinforce joint stability can reduce chronic widespread joint pain or specific deficient joints that are problematic or injured (Palmer et al. 2016). Moreover, spinal stabilization exercises can decrease pain and improve function (Toprak and Ozer Kaya 2017). When implementing strengthening programs, progression should be slow to avoid irritating unstable joints and surrounding easy-to-irritate muscles and tendons, which respond differently to muscle activation than the normal population. This impaired firing pattern may be related to the altered connective tissue found in the extracellular matrix of muscle fiber affecting force transmission of the contraction, along with increased elasticity of the muscle tendon complex to work against during muscle firing (Rombaut et al. 2012).

Patients with HSD/hEDS often report having tight muscles (Simmonds et al. 2019). Although overstretching joints is commonly discouraged in patients with hypermobility, focused stretching can be appropriate if needed to address muscle imbalances with the local joint maintained in a stable position.

Patients report that aquatic therapy can be beneficial (Keer and Simmonds 2011; Simmonds et al. 2019).

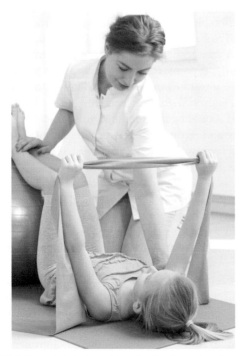

Fig. 6.3.4 Closed-chain exercise using feedback from Theraband. Courtesy iStock.com/Katarzyna Bialasiewicz.

Although joint compression forces are decreased in water, resistance caused by drag forces in water can contribute to strain on the muscles, tendons, and ligaments required to stabilize the joints. Patients with POTS may benefit from improved venous return produced by hydrostatic pressure but may have poor tolerance to prolonged time in warm water.

Fatigue can be addressed through patient education and exercise. Patients should be educated about sleep hygiene, relaxation and stress management, pacing, and prioritizing. A gradually progressed exercise program can address deconditioning but may need to start at very low levels to avoid "boom and bust" cycles (Hakim et al. 2017). Muscle strengthening can also decrease fatigue (Voermans et al. 2011).

When prescribing exercise, clinicians should be aware that physical activity is a demanding task for the circulatory system, which is already functioning at its upper limit in patients with POTS. In this population, a restricted tolerance for exercise is prevalent, with reports of postexertional malaise and symptom aggravation due to exercise (Oldham et al. 2016). First-line management for POTS involves increasing fluids and salt, avoiding triggers such as hot environments, and eating large carbohydrate meals. Patients learn anti-syncope maneuvers such as fist clenching and changing position when standing. Compression garments may help venous return. Experts and emerging research supports slow, progressive programs beginning with recumbent exercises, lower extremity, and core strengthening to facilitate venous return, with a progression of cardiovascular training toward upright exercise. This approach is supported by the growing research evidence base in adults (Fu et al. 2011) and best practice guidelines for adolescents (Kizilbash et al. 2014). Second-line management involves medications to increase blood volume or increase vascular tone. Although medications play an important role in the management of dysautonomia, they should be viewed as part of a wide multisystem approach and reconditioning is essential. Psychological support is recommended for anxiety, pain, and illness behavior (Mathias et al. 2011; Kizilbash et al. 2014).

Recognition of the systemic issues commonly associated with HSD/hEDS by clinicians is instrumental in promoting the best possible treatment outcomes. For example, MCAS signs and symptoms such as skin reactions to adhesives and slow healing of wounds to systemic and local inflammatory reactions and severe fatigue need to recognized, bearing in mind that they can vary daily in intensity (Seneviratne et al. 2017). Patients may also be affected by fragile skin, anxiety, cognitive fatigue, gastrointestinal problems, incontinence, and gynecological issues (Tinkle et al. 2017). It is therefore important to educate patients and families and to refer to other professionals or accommodate these issues within the physical therapy plan of care.

Pain management is often very difficult for these patients and those with flare-ups of uncontrolled pain. Patients with HSD/hEDS frequently report insufficient pain control even when on multiple analgesics (Rombaut et al. 2011). Pain education helps patients understand their pain and how to ultimately self-manage appropriately in a way that works for them. With children, it's important that parents/carers understand how to parent a child in pain. For example, how to use ice, heat, and bracing. Cognitive behavioral approaches targeting both parents and children are helpful in managing pain. Learning to correct body mechanics and slow and steady progression of activities can prevent overuse injuries or an inflammatory response. Cognitive behavioral approaches such as relaxation, coping skills, sleep hygiene, and rest can reduce symptoms (Bathen et al. 2013). There is no current evidence regarding modalities for reducing pain in this population, but manual therapies, heat, ice, electrotherapy, and acupuncture modalities have been reported to be helpful anecdotally (Simmonds and Keer, 2007). A case report demonstrates how manual therapy such as trigger point release and focused joint mobilization might be integrated into a comprehensive program for a patient with HSD/hEDS (Pennetti 2018). Joint mobilizations should be implemented with prudence because of laxity and sensitivity of tissues (Simmonds and Keer 2007). Pharmacological management of pain in HSD/hEDS is beyond the scope of this chapter. For further information about drug management, readers are referred to papers by Castori and colleagues (2016) and a review article by Chopra and colleagues (2017).

Regular physical activity is crucial for long-term management of both musculoskeletal and systemic symptoms. Weight management is important, especially for young people (Tobias et al. 2013). Physical activity needs to include cardiovascular and strengthening activities tailored to the individual's interests and capabilities. High-impact contact sports, such as soccer, rugby, and American football, should be avoided because there is a greater risk of knee injury (Pacey et al. 2010). Importantly acute and chronic training needs careful monitoring to prevent injury. This is of particular importance during the adolescence growth spurt, a time when many hypermobile adolescents present with injury.

Because patients with HSD/hEDS have slow and poor tissue healing, surgical interventions should be avoided if conservative care might be effective (Ericson and Wolman 2017; Tinkle et al. 2017). One study found that only 33.9% of surgical interventions for people with HMS were considered successful, compared with 63.4% success with physical therapy (Rombaut et al. 2011). When surgery is needed, recommendations include minimizing surgical incision size and tissue traction, avoiding skin clips, supplementing sutures with steristrips, and leaving sutures in place for longer than normal (Burcharth and Rosenberg 2012).

In summary, patients with HSD/hEDS are likely to present to medical and health professionals with a variety of complaints involving multiple body systems beyond just musculoskeletal. Treatment provided by health professionals knowledgeable about this condition is key to managing it effectively. Patient and family education is critical so patients can actively engage in self-management and injury prevention. Tissue fragility may decrease patient tolerance to interventions such as exercise or manual therapy, and patients are likely to progress more slowly than nonhypermobile patients. Because research is just beginning to provide evidence regarding optimal interventions for this condition, therapists will need to integrate existing research with clinician expertise and patient preference to maximize the benefit for each individual patient.

Summary

Hypermobility spectrum disorders and hypermobile Ehlers–Danlos syndrome exists on a spectrum. Patients with HSD/hEDS are likely to present to medical and health professionals with a variety of complaints involving multiple body systems beyond just musculoskeletal. Treatment provided by health professionals knowledgeable about this condition is key to managing it effectively. Patient and family education is critical so patients can actively engage in self-management and injury prevention. Tissue fragility may reduce patient tolerance to interventions such as exercise or manual therapy, and patients are likely to progress more slowly than nonhypermobile patients. Because research is just beginning to provide evidence about optimal interventions for this condition, clinicians will need to integrate existing research with clinician expertise and patient preference to maximize the benefit for each individual patient.

REFERENCES

Bathen, T., Hångmann, M., Hoff, L.O., Andersen, L.Ø., Rand-Hendriksen, S., 2013. Multidisciplinary treatment of disability in Ehlers-Danlos syndrome hypermobility type/hypermobility syndrome: A pilot study using a combination of physical and cognitive-behavioral therapy on 12 women. Am. J. Med. Genet. A. 161A, 3005–3011.

Boudreau, S A, Farina, D., Falla, D., 2010. The role of motor learning and neuroplasticity in designing rehabilitation approaches for musculoskeletal pain disorders. Man. Ther. 15, 410–414.

Bulbena, A., Baeza-Velasco, C., Bulbena-Cabré, A., et al., 2017. Psychiatric and psychological aspects in the Ehlers–Danlos syndromes. Am. J. Med. Genet. Part C Semin. Med. Genet. 175, 237–245.

Burcharth, J., Rosenberg, J., 2012. Gastrointestinal surgery and related complications in patients with Ehlers-Danlos syndrome: a systematic review. Dig. Surg. 29, 349–357.

Castori, M., 2016. Pain in Ehlers-Danlos syndromes: manifestations, therapeutic strategies and future perspectives. Expert Opin. Orphan Drugs 4, 1145–1158.

Castori, M., Tinkle, B., Levy, H., Grahame, R., Malfait, F., Hakim, A., 2017. A framework for the classification of joint hypermobility and related conditions. Am. J. Med. Genet. C Semin. Med. Genet. 175, 148–157.

Chopra, P., Tinkle, B., Hamonet, C., et al., 2017. Pain management in the Ehlers-Danlos syndromes. Am. J. Med. Genet. C Semin. Med. Genet. 175, 212–219.

Clark, C., Simmonds, J.V., 2011. An exploration of the prevalence of hypermobility syndrome in Omani women attending an outpatient department. Musculoskeletal Care 9, 1–10.

Clayton, H.A., Jones, S.A., Henriques, D.Y., 2015. Proprioceptive precision is impaired in Ehlers-Danlos syndrome. Springerplus 4, 323.

Connelly, E., Hakım, A., Davenport, S., Simmonds, J.V., 2015. A study exploring the prevalence of Joint Hypermobility Syndrome in patients attending a Musculoskeletal Triage Clinic. Physiother. Pract. Res. 36, 43–53.

De Wandele, I., Rombaut, L., Leybaert, P., et al., 2014. Dysautonomia and its underlying mechanisms in the hypermobility type of Ehlers-Danlos syndrome. Semin. Arthritis Rheum. 44, 93–100.

De Wandele, I., Kazkaz, H., Tang, E., et al., 2020. Development and initial validation of The Spider, a multisystem symptom impact questionnaire for patients with joint hypermobility_part 1. EDS ECHO Summit: A Virtual Scientific Conference on EDS. Oct 2-3. Poster. Abstract.

Di Stefano, G., Celletti, C., Baron, R., et al., 2016. Central sensitization as the mechanism underlying pain in joint hypermobility syndrome/Ehlers -Danlos syndrome, hypermobility type. Eur. J. Pain. 20(8), 1319–1325.

Dupuy, E.G., Leconte, P., Vlamynck, E., et al., 2017. Ehlers-Danlos syndrome, hypermobility type: impact of somatosensory orthoses on postural control (A Pilot Study). Front. Hum. Neurosci. 11, 283.

Engelbert, R.H.H, Juul-Kristensen, B., Pacey, V., et al., 2017. The Evidence-based rationale for physical therapy treatment of children, adolescents and adults diagnosed with joint hypermobility syndrome/hypermobile Ehlers Danlos Syndrome. Am. J. Med. Genet. C Semin. Med. Genet. 175, 158–167.

Ericson, Jr., W.B., Wolman, R., 2017. Orthopaedic management of the Ehlers-Danlos syndromes. Am. J. Med. Genet. C Semin. Med. Genet. 175, 188–194.

Fatoye, F., Palmer, S., Macmillan, F., Rowe, P., van der Linden, M., 2012. Pain intensity and quality of life perception in children with hypermobility syndrome. Rheumatol. Int. 32, 1277–1284.

Fatoye. F.A., Palmer, S., van der Linden, M.L., Rowe, P.J., Macmillan, F., 2011. Gait kinematics and passive knee joint range of motion in children with hypermobility syndrome. Gait Posture 33, 447–451.

Fu, Q., Vangundy, R., Shibata, S., Auchus, R.J., Williams, G.H., Levine, B.D., 2011. Exercise training versus propranolol in the treatment of the postural orthostatic tachycardia syndrome. Hypertension 58, 167–175.

Hakim, A., De Wandele, I., O'Callaghan, C., Pocinki, A., Rowe, P., 2017. Chronic fatigue in Ehlers-Danlos syndrome-hypermobile type. Am. J. Med. Genet. C Semin. Med. Genet. 175, 175–180.

Hakim, A., O'Callaghan, C., De Wandele, I., Stiles, L., Pocinki, A., Rowe, P., 2017. Cardiovascular autonomic dysfunction in Ehlers-Danlos syndrome-hypermobile type. Am. J. Med. Genet. C Semin. Med. Genet. 175, 168–174.

Hall, M.G., Ferrell, W.R., Sturrock, R. D. et al., 1995. The effect of the hypermobility syndrome on knee joint proprioception. Rheumatology 34(2), 121–125.

Keer, R., Simmonds, J.V., 2011. Joint protection and physical rehabilitation of the adult with hypermobility syndrome. Curr. Opin. Rheumatol. 23, 131–136.

Kemp, S., Roberts, I., Gamble, C., et al., 2010. A randomized comparative trial of generalized vs targeted physiotherapy in the management of childhood hypermobility. Rheumatology (Oxford) 49, 315–325.

Kizilbash, S.J., Ahrens, S.P., Bruce, B.K., et al., 2014. Adolescent fatigue, POTS, and recovery: a guide for clinicians. Curr. Probl. Pediatr. Adolesc. Health Care 44, 108–133.

Lisi, C., Monteleone, S., Tinelli, C, et al., 2020. Postural analysis in a pediatric cohort of patients with Ehlers-Danlos Syndrome: a pilot study. Minerva Pediatr. 72(2), 73–78.

Lyell, M., Simmonds, J.V., Deane, J.A., 2016. A study of UK physiotherapists' knowledge and training needs in hypermobility and hypermobility syndrome. Physiother. Pract. Res. 37(2), 101–109. doi:10.323/PPR-160073

Malfait, F., Francomano, C., Byers, P., et al., 2017. The 2017 international classification of the Ehlers-Danlos syndromes. Am. J. Med. Genet. C Semin. Med. Genet. 175, 8–26.

Mathias, C., Lowe, D., Iodice, V., Mathias, C.J., 2011. Postural tachycardia syndrome – Current concepts. Nature 8, 22–34.

Meyer, K.J., Chan, C., Hopper, L., Nicholson, L.L., 2017. Identifying lower limb specific and generalised joint hypermobility in adults: validation of the Lower Limb Assessment Score. BMC Musculoskelet. Disord. 18, 514.

Nicholson, L., Chan, C., 2018. Upper limb assessment tool: A novel validated tool for adults. Musculoskelet. Sci. Prac. 35, 38–45.

Oldham, W.M., Lewis, G.D., Opotowsky, A.R., Waxman, A.B., Systrom, D.M., 2016. Unexplained exertional dyspnea caused by low ventricular filling pressures: results from clinical invasive cardiopulmonary exercise testing. Pulm. Circ. 6, 55–62.

Pacey, V., Nicholson, L., Adams, R.D., Munn, J., Munns, C.F., 2010. Generalized joint hypermobility and risk of lower limb joint injury during sport: a systematic review with meta-analysis. Am. J. Sports. Med. 38, 1487–1497.

Pacey, V., Tofts, L., Adams, R.D., et al., 2013. Exercise in children with joint hypermobility syndrome and knee pain: a randomised controlled trial comparing exercise into hypermobile versus neutral knee extension. Pediatr. Rheumatol. Online J. 11, 30.

Pacey, V., Tofts, L., Adams, R.D., Munns, C.F., Nicholson, L.L., 2015. Quality of life prediction in children with joint hypermobility syndrome. J. Paediatr. Child Health 51, 689–695.

Palmer, S., Bailey, S., Barker, L., Barney, L., Elliott, A., 2014. The effectiveness of therapeutic exercise for joint hypermobility syndrome: a systematic review. Physiotherapy 100, 220–227.

Palmer, S., Terry, R., Rimes, K. A., et al., 2016. Physiotherapy management of joint hypermobility syndrome–a focus group study of patient and health professional perspectives. Physiotherapy 102, 93–102.

Palmer, S., Cramp, F., Lewis, R., Gould, G., Clark, E.M., 2017. Development and initial validation of the Bristol Impact of Hypermobility questionnaire. Physiotherapy 103, 186–192.

Pennetti, A., 2018. A multimodal physical therapy approach utilizing the Maitland concept in the management of a patient with cervical and lumbar radiculitis and Ehlers-Danlos syndrome-hypermobility type: A case report. Physiother. Theory Pract. 34, 1–10.

Raj, S.R., 2013. Postural tachycardia syndrome (POTS). Circulation 127(23), 2336–2342.

Rombaut, L., Malfait, F., De Wandele, I., et al., 2011. Medication, surgery, and physiotherapy among patients with the hypermobility type of Ehlers-Danlos syndrome. Arch. Phys. Med. Rehabil. 92, 1106–1112.

Rombaut, L., Malfait, F., De Wandele, I., et al., 2012. Muscle mass, muscle strength, functional performance, and physical impairment in women with the hypermobility type of Ehlers-Danlos syndrome. Arthritis Care. Res. (Hoboken) 64, 1584–1592.

Rombaut, L., Deane, J., Simmonds, J, et al., 2015. Knowledge, assessment, and management of adults with joint hypermobility syndrome/Ehlers -Danlos syndrome hypermobility type among flemish physiotherapists. Am. J. Med. Genet. Part C. 169C, 76–83.

Russek, L.N., LaShomb, E.A., Ware, A.M., Wesner, S.M., Westcott, V., 2016. United States physical therapists' knowledge about joint hypermobility syndrome compared with fibromyalgia and rheumatoid arthritis. Physiother. Res. Int. 21, 22–35.

Sahin, N., Baskent, A., Cakmak, A., Salli, A., Ugurlu, H., Berker, E., 2008. Evaluation of knee proprioception and effects of proprioception exercise in patients with benign joint hypermobility syndrome. Rheumatol. Int. 28, 995–1000.

Scheper, M., Juul-Kristensen, B., Rombaut, L., et al., 2017. Generalized hyperalgesia in children and adults diagnosed with hypermobility syndrome and Ehlers-Danlos syndrome hypermobility type: a discriminative analysis. Arthritis Care Res. (Hoboken) 69, 421–429.

Scheper, M., Nicholson, L., Adams, R.D., Tofts, L., Pacey, V., 2017. The natural history of children with joint hypermobility syndrome and Ehlers-Danlos hypermobility type: a longitudinal cohort study. Rheumatology (Oxford) 56, 2073–2083.

Scheper, M., Rombaut, L., de Vries, J., et al., 2017. The association between muscle strength and activity limitations in patients with the hypermobility type of Ehlers-Danlos syndrome: the impact of proprioception. Disabil. Rehabil. 39, 1391–1397.

Scheper, M.C., Engelbert, R.R.H., Rameckers, E.A.A., Verbunt, J., Remvig, L., Juul-Kristensen, B., 2013. Children with generalised joint hypermobility and musculoskeletal complaints: state of the art on diagnostics, clinical characteristics, and treatment. Biomed Res. Int. 2013, 121054.

Scheper, M.C., Juul-Kristensen, B., Rombaut, L., Rameckers, E.A., Verbunt, J., Engelbert, R.H., 2016. Disability in adolescents and adults et al. diagnosed with hypermobility-related disorders: a meta-analysis. Arch. Phys. Med. Rehabil. 97, 2174–2187.

Schlepe, N., Rombaut, L., De Wandele, I., 2017. Functional ring silver splints for people with hypermobility of the hand. Poster presentation. Ehlers Danlos Society Medical and Scientific Meeting, Ghent Belgium.

Schubert-Hjalmarsson, E., Öhman, A., Kyllerman, M., Kyllerman, M., Beckung, E., 2012. Pain, balance, activity, and participation in children with hypermobility syndrome. Pediatr. Phys. Ther. 24, 339–344.

Seneviratne, S., Maitland, A., Afrin, L., 2017. Mast cell disorders in Ehlers-Danlos syndrome. Am. J. Med. Genet. C Semin. Med. Genet. 175, 226–236.

Smith, T.O., Jerman, E., Easton, V. et al., 2013. Do people with benign joint hypermobility syndrome (BJHS) have reduced joint proprioception? A systematic review and meta-analysis. Rheumatol. Int. 33, 2709–2716.

Simmonds, J.V., Herbland, A., Hakim, A., Ninis, N., Lever, W., Aziz, Q., et al., 2019. Exercise beliefs and behaviours of individuals with Joint Hypermobility syndrome/Ehlers-Danlos syndrome - hypermobility type. Disabil. Rehabil. 41, 445–455.

Simmonds, J.V., Keer, R.J., 2007. Hypermobility and the hypermobility syndrome. Man. Ther. 12, 298–309.

Syx, D., De Wandele, I., Rombaut, L., Malfait, F., 2017. Hypermobility, the Ehlers-Danlos syndromes and chronic pain. Clin. Exp. Rheumatol. 35 Suppl 107, 116–122.

Tinkle, B., Castori, M., Berglund, B., et al., 2017. Hypermobile Ehlers-Danlos syndrome (a.k.a. Ehlers-Danlos syndrome Type III and Ehlers-Danlos syndrome hypermobility type): Clinical description and natural history. Am. J. Med. Genet. C Semin. Med. Genet. 175, 48–69.

To, M., Alexander, C.A., 2019. Are people with joint hypermobility slow to strengthen? Arch. Phys. Med. Rehabil. 100, 1243–1250.

To, M., Simmonds, J., Alexander, C., 2017. Where do people with joint hypermobility syndrome present in secondary care? the prevalence in a general hospital and the challenges of classification. Musculoskeletal Care 15, 3–9.

Tobias, J.H., Deere, K., Palmer, S., Clark, E.M., Clinch, J., 2013. Joint hypermobility is a risk factor for musculoskeletal pain during adolescence: findings of a prospective cohort study. Arthritis Rheum. 65, 1107–1115.

Toprak, C., Ozer Kaya, D., 2017. Effects of spinal stabilization exercises in women with benign joint hypermobility syndrome: a randomized controlled trial. Rheumatol. Int. 37, 1461–1468.

Voermansa N.C., Knoop, H, Bleijenberg, G., van Engelena, B.G, 2011. Fatigue is associated with muscle weakness in Ehlers-Danlos syndrome: an explorative study. Physiotherapy 97(2), 170–174.

Wolfe, F., Clauw, D.J., Fitzcharles, M.A., 2016. 2016 Revisions to the 2010/2011 fibromyalgia diagnostic criteria. Semin. Arthritis Rheum. 46(3), 319–329.

Mechanical Deformation-Based Assessment Methods

Mark Driscoll and Natasha Jacobson

INTRODUCTION

Palpation, as described in Chapter 6.2, is a qualitative method of in-vivo soft tissue evaluation, with poor inter-relater reliability. The distinction between "unhealthy" and "normal" fascia or, at the other end of the spectrum, "normal" and "performant" fascia, has largely been a matter of perception. Regarding a static and dynamic touch, our fingers can sense very small differences in deformation and surface roughness. Further, it may be perceivable that clinicians inherently have, or gain over time, a more refined sense of touch. However, often one needs to make comparisons before and after treatment, or gauge if a palpated tissue is deemed normal or healthy. Limited information on distinguishing metrics indicates the need for standardized, in-vivo measurement devices. To provide a more objective evaluation of fascia, measurement devices have been developed that allow for quantitative measures to be acquired. Though no "gold standard" has been suggested, the use of such quantitative fascia tooling offers the potential of determining "normal" or "healthy" stiffness values or ranges for select tissues. Thus these tools offer a means for quantitative and objective comparisons to be made.

TERMINOLOGY

Tissue mechanical properties contrast between engineering definitions and their clinical counterparts. As such, distinctions must be made between the two. In engineering, constitutive material properties are divulged from a material's response to applied loading. The stress (σ) to strain (ϵ) curve is a common graphical representation of this response. The slope, or angle of inclination, of a material's σ-ϵ curve is the Young's modulus (also known as elasticity, or modulus of elasticity, E) and describes a material's resistance to strain, or, relative deformation. However, if the σ-ϵ slope changes under different loading rates (i.e., loaded faster or slower) then the material can be termed viscoelastic, presenting both viscous and elastic properties (Ramalingam 2009).

Clinicians may alternatively observe a physiological cavity's pressure-volume (P-V) curve, the illustration of the enveloping tissue's resistance to expansion or contraction. In this case, the slope of the P-V curve represents the tissue's elastance (Stedman 2006).

As fascia is inherently anisotropic (responds to stress differently in each direction), another property of interest is Poisson's ratio (ν): the ratio of material strain in one axis relative to another orthogonal axis. Poisson's ratio can range between 0 and 0.5—perfectly compressible and in-compressible, respectively (Ramalingam, 2009). Ideal incompressible materials ($v = 0.5$) include air or water, such that the density of the material is not changed because of loading. Given the high water content of biological tissues, Poisson's ratio is often considered between 0.3 and 0.5 (Choi and Zheng 2005; Lu et al. 2012; Hayes et al. 1972).

Given contradicting definitions between manual therapists and even within literature at times, Table 6.4.1

is provided to distinguish between engineering terminology and the resulting clinical observation. In some instances, such as for elastance, there does not exist an associated mechanical definition.

DEVICES

Ex vivo measurement methods for tissue characterization cannot accurately replicate a physiological environment, as

TABLE 6.4.1 Common Engineering Terms and their Corresponding Clinical Observations

Term	Symbol	Engineering Definition	Clinical Observation
Bulk Modulus	K	Resistance to strain under hydrostatic conditions (uniform normal stress on entire material surface). For incompressible materials, K tends to infinity (kPa)	N/A
Compliance	C	The inverse of stiffness (m/N)	Measure of tissue expansion (volumetric response) given a change in pressure. The inverse of elastance
Elastance	N/A	N/A	Ability to maintain pressure given a change in volume. Measured by the slope of a tissue's pressure-volume curve
Elasticity	E	(Young's modulus) Resistance to strain under an applied stress. Measured by the slope of a material's stress-strain curve (kPa)	To be elastic/flexible/pliable. Antonym of stiffness
Poisson's Ratio	v	Ratio of material strain in perpendicular directions. Incompressible materials have a v of 0.5	Material compensation; lengthening in one direction shortens in the perpendicular axis
Shear Modulus	G	Resistance to strain under an applied shear stress (stress tangential to applied material surface) (kPa)	Slippage between tissue layers
Stiffness	S	Resistance to deformation under an applied force [N/m]	To be stiff/resist deformation
Strain	ϵ	Material length change per initial unit length (m/m)	Elongation, or shrinkage
Stress	σ	Load per unit area, normal to the applied material surface. Can be in tension (tensile stress) or compression (compressive stress) (kPa)	Pressure (kPa)
Viscoelasticity	N/A	The property of a material to change its elasticity depending on applied strain rate	Combination of viscous and elastic properties in a tissue

Ramalingam, K., 2009. Material properties. In: Ramalingam, K. (Ed.), *Handbook of Mechanical Engineering Terms*, second ed. New Age International, New Delhi, pp. 39–52; François, D., Pineau, A., Zaoui, A., 2012. Elastic behaviour, viscoelasticity. In: Micro- and Macroscopic Constitutive Behaviour, second ed. (Mechanical Behaviour of Materials, vol. 1). Springer, New York, pp. 83–154, 445–505; Stedman, T., 2006. Stedman's Medical Dictionary, twenty-eighth ed. Lippincott Williams & Wilkins, Philadelphia.

tests occur outside living organisms. Thus in-vivo (physiological) alternatives are of greater interest here. Table 6.4.2 lists said alternatives, detailing the advantages and disadvantages of each method.

Given the lack of a "gold standard" measurement technique, it has been suggested to use more than one measurement system for more comprehensive results (Zügel et al. 2018). As such, the following discusses several existing means of mechanically characterizing soft tissues. That said, consensus has been reached among experts that a standardized and portable device is still necessary to establish norms in tissue properties (Zügel et al. 2018).

KEY POINTS

Ex vivo measurement methods for tissue characterization cannot accurately replicate a physiological environment.

STATIC DEFORMATION

Though manual palpation remains the simplest and cheapest form of in-vivo soft tissue evaluation, it is a qualitative and practitioner-dependent method (Chaitow et al. 2012). Alternatively, static, quantitative measurement systems are wide ranging and include indentation (Wilke et al. 2018), myometry (Agyapong-Badu et al. 2018), aspiration (Tarsi et al. 2013), and durometry (Kutz 2015). To measure the mechanical properties of fascia, only indentation, myometry (popularized by the MyotonPro; Peipsi et al. 2012) and aspiration are discussed, as durometers report Shore hardness (resistance to indentation), as opposed to elasticity, a constitutive material property (Ramalingam 2009).

Figure 6.4.1 illustrates each method of static deformation, with corresponding dimensions for mechanical characterization.

Indentation, myometry, and aspiration devices use similar theories to determine stiffness (S): a known normal force (F) is applied to a local tissue, and the resulting linear displacement (δ) is measured (Feng et al. 2018; Zheng and Huang 2016). In its simplified form, this yields the equation $S = F/\delta$. That said, in the case of the MyotonPro a popularized myometric method of measurement (Agyapong-Badu et al. 2018) an impulse, rather than a single, continuous, static force, is applied to the tissue. As a result, stiffness is measured dynamically by

$S = a_{max}m_{probe}/\Delta l$, where a_{max} is the peak acceleration amplitude, m_{probe} is the preload caused by the mass of the probe, and Δl is the peak displacement amplitude (Peipsi et al. 2012). As Newton's law states $F = ma$, stiffness measured by indentation, aspiration, and myometry are mathematically equivalent, despite the static (via indentation/aspiration) versus dynamic (via myometry) means of applied deformation. However, the MyotonPro outputs a second, dimensionless value: elasticity. This term is defined as the logarithmic decrement of probe acceleration (Peipsi et al. 2012), in conflict with the engineering definition for elasticity (see Table 6.4.1). Thus published values of "elasticity" from studies using the MyotonPro should be evaluated critically. Handheld, user-friendly measurement systems are available, such as MyotonPro (Peipsi et al. 2012), Cutometer (Draaijers et al. 2004), Nimble (Müller et al. 2018), or the semi-electronic tissue compliance meter (Wilke et al. 2018). That said, none of the existing static deformation methods can distinguish between tissue layers or provide insight into deeper fascia (Zügel et al. 2018). A novel macrosuction system was proposed that suggests the possibility of measuring elasticity of deeper tissues; however, further research is required to confirm this hypothesis (Jacobson and Driscoll 2021). As such, said techniques are only recommended to evaluate superficial, and not deeper, tissues.

BIOIMPEDANCE

In all materials, there exists a unique impedance, or resistance to electrical current. This also holds true in fascia, thus denoted bioimpedance. Research has explored the possibility of exploiting this characteristic to correlate bioimpedance to mechanical properties, such as elasticity or thickness (David et al. 2018; Bayford and Tizzard 2012). Though simple, noninvasive, and potentially economical, further research must be pursued to provide inter- and intrarater reliability studies against more conventional methods.

ULTRASONOGRAPHY AND ELASTOGRAPHY

Modern technologies, such as ultrasonography (US) and elastography, offer greater detail and information about fascial layers, however, they are not handheld, portable, or widely economical (Zheng and Huang 2016; Zügel et al. 2018). Sonography (McAuliffe et al. 2017)

TABLE 6.4.2 Existing Methods of Soft Tissue Mechanical Measurement. Relative Comparisons Made With the Indenter as a Benchmark

Method	Mechanical Property	Description	Non-invasive	Quanti-tative	Tissue Distinc-tion	Hand-held	Reli-ability	Cost	Anatomy	Reference
Palpation	Relative stiffness	Qualitative evaluation of top layer tissue stiffness.	X			X	−	++	Superficial tissues	Yen 2003
Robotic palpation	Relative stiffness	Qualitative evaluation from machine learning to distinguish between stiff and flexible tissues for use in tumor identification.	X				0	N/A	Superficial tissues	Nichols and Okamura 2015
Myometry	Stiffness, "elasticity," "tone," stress relaxation time. "creep"	An impulse of known force is applied to a soft tissue, and the tissue response in acceleration vs. time and deformation vs. time are mapped.	X	X	X	X	0	−	Superficial tissues	Agyapong-Badu et al. 2018; Feng et al. 2018
Indentometry	Stiffness	Measurement of resulting tissue deformation given an applied, known, point load (indent). Can also be inverse measure tissue response force for given deformation.	X	X	X	X	0	0	Superficial tissues	Wilke et al. 2018; Oflaz and Baran 2014; Williams et al. 2007
Aspiration	Stiffness	The reverse of indentometry. A closed volume of soft tissue is resected using a locally applied negative pressure. Vertical tissue displacement and applied pressure are recorded to determine stiffness.	X	X	X	X	0	0	Superficial tissues	Tarsi et al. 2013; Nava et al. 2004; Müller et al. 2018; Elahi et al. 2019

Continued

TABLE 6.4.2 Existing Methods of Soft Tissue Mechanical Measurement. Relative Comparisons Made With the Indenter as a Benchmark—cont'd

Method	Mechanical Property	Description	Non-invasive	Quantitative	Tissue Distinction	Hand-held	Reliability	Cost	Anatomy	Reference
Torsion/rotary shear	Shear modulus	Linear viscoelastic response of tissues under a vibrating torque. No axial force is applied, and the tissue's response vibrations are captured by electromagnetic transducers.	X	X			N/A	0	Superficial tissues	Valtorta and Mazza, 2005
Durometer	Shore hardness	Measurement of resulting load impression in tissue given applied, known, point load.		X		X	0	0	Skin or ex vivo tissues	Kutz, 2015
Bioimpedance	Geometry	An array of electrodes, placed across the tissue of interest, map tissue impedance given an applied frequency. Results can be mapped to produce a topographical image or correlated to a property of interest.	X				—	—	Superficial tissues	Bayford and Tizzard, 2012
Piezoelectric ceramic material	Young's modulus	The impedance of a soft tissue is measured with a polymer film (PVDF) given a small applied voltage. This can be correlated to mechanical characteristics of the tissue.	X	X		X	N/A	0	Superficial tissues	Narayanan et al. 2006

			Description							
Ultra-sonography (US)	B-mode	Young's modulus, thickness	Standard US can be used to evaluate the thickness of tissues by direct measurement in produced images. If combined with indentometer, can also measure Young's Modulus.	X	X	X	+	–	Superficial to deep tissues	McAuliffe et al. 2017; Sigrist et al. 2017; Lung et al. 2020
	Strain US imaging	Young's modulus	Use of an US to visualize tissue movement given varying normal stresses.	X	X	X	+	–	Superficial to deep tissues	Sigrist et al. 2017
Virtual Imaging	Direct image correlation	Bulk modulus	With 2 cameras, a 3D image can be produced given a tissue with a defined pattern (such as fine, dark paint spray). Inputting images into finite element analysis allows for deformation to be mapped given loading.	X	X	X	N/A	N/A	Superficial tissues	Moerman et al. 2009

Continued

TABLE 6.4.2 Existing Methods of Soft Tissue Mechanical Measurement. Relative Comparisons Made With the Indenter as a Benchmark—cont'd

Method		Mechanical Property	Description	Non-invasive	Quantitative	Tissue Distinction	Hand-held	Reliability	Cost	Anatomy	Reference
	Virtual fields method	Shear modulus	Using an anatomically correct finite element model, the constitutive mechanical properties of soft tissues can be solved for given a known (experimental) applied force and resulting deformation. This is an inverse engineering problem, but only accurate for a given anatomical geometry and study participant.	X	X	X		N/A	N/A	Model-dependent	Zhang et al. 2017
Elastography	US elastography (compression based or shear wave)	Shear modulus/ Young's modulus, thickness	Use of a US to visualize tissue shear strain given shear stress (by applied shear waves). Force or deformation mapping.	X	X	X		+	−	Deep viscera	Feng et al. 2018; Sigrist et al. 2017; Bensamoun et al. 2011
	MRI elastography (compression based or shear wave)	Shear modulus/ Young's modulus, thickness	Use of MRI to visualize tissue shear strain given shear stress (by applied shear waves). Force or deformation mapping.	X	X	X		+	−	Deep viscera	Feng et al. 2018; Sigrist et al. 2017; Bensamoun et al. 2011
	Tomoelastography	Shear modulus/ Young's modulus, thickness	Combination of an elastography method and an analysis system to reduce output noise.	X	X	X		+	−	Deep viscera	Dittmann et al. 2017

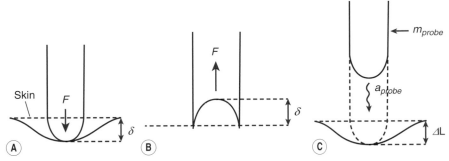

Fig. 6.4.1 Schematics of (A) indentation, (B) aspiration, and (C) myometry methods for mechanical characterization of soft tissues. The applied force (F or ma) and its resulting deformation (δ or Δl) are illustrated. a_{probe} = acceleration of the probe; m_{probe} = preload due to the mass of the probe.

and elastography (Sigrist et al. 2017; Feng et al. 2018) methods have gained popularity owing to their ability to map deep viscera. Geometrical distinctions between fascial layers in sonography provide benchmarks from which to measure thickness. As such, tissue thickness is typically measured with US (McAuliffe et al. 2017).

Elastography is a medical imaging technique that maps stiffness in deep tissue by sending acoustic vibrations, in US, or harmonic vibrations, in magnetic resonance imaging (MRI), through tissue layers. Both systems incur a shear wave such that the faster the shear wave, the stiffer the material (Hirsch et al. 2017). Resulting stiffnesses are then overlaid on MRI or US images to establish an anatomical map of tissue elasticity. All elastography methods determine local tissue properties (i.e., measuring along the length of the respective probe), not global, while assuming linear elastic, homogeneous, isotropic material properties. This is contrary to physiological properties that are viscoelastic, multilayered, and anisotropic (Glaser and Ehman 2014). These limitations must be considered when comparing measurement methods. Further, fatty tissues cause shear waves to change at deeper tissue layers, therefore, this method is less reliable in overweight populations. This is particularly evident in fat deposit areas, including the abdomen or upper legs. Finally, it should be noted that commercial shear wave elastography (SWE) systems output measures of elasticity (E). If shear elasticity (G) is reported, linear elasticity can be calculated using $E = 2G(1 + \nu)$ (Miller et al. 2018). In this case the material's Poisson's ratio (ν) is assumed to be 0.5 (i.e., incompressible), as suggested by modern studies (Miller et al. 2018).

Summary

Clinicians may always find a benefit to manually palpating tissues, but measurement devices offer an opportunity to better understand absolute values of stiffness, elasticity, and viscoelasticity. Furthermore, although these distinct interpretations of material behavior have long been used in the engineering world, clinical training may be required to divulge a medical interpretation of numerical data. What is clear is that for such potential benefits to be derived, two things need to take place: First, the device under consideration must accurately detect a tissue deformation and then apply appropriate equations to derive material properties. Second, the user must be aware of the definition of the material property that is being reported and how to relate that to their clinical practice. Ideally, collaboration between engineers and clinicians may support correlation between engineering measurements and manual palpation.

REFERENCES

Agyapong-Badu, S., Warner, M., Samuel, D., Stokes, M., 2018. Practical considerations for standardized recording of muscle mechanical properties using a myometric device: recording site, muscle length, state of contraction and prior activity. J. Musculoskelet. Res. 21, 1–13.

Bayford, R., Tizzard, A., 2012. Bioimpedance imaging: An overview of potential clinical applications. Analyst 137, 4635–4643.

Bensamoun, S.F., Robert, L., Leclerc, G.E., Debernard, L., Charleux, F., 2011. Stiffness imaging of the kidney and adjacent abdominal tissues measured simultaneously using magnetic resonance elastography. Clin. Imaging 35, 284–287.

Chaitow, L., Coughlin, P., Findley, T.W., Myers, T., 2012. Fascial palpation. In: Schleip, R., Findley, T., Huijing, P. (Eds.), Fascia: The Tensional Network of the Human Body, first ed. Elsevier, London, pp. 269–277.

Choi, A.P.C., Zheng, Y.P., 2005. Estimation of Young's modulus and Poisson's ratio of soft tissue from indentation using two different-sized indenters: Finite element analysis of the finite deformation effect. Med. Biol. Eng. Comput. 43, 258–264.

David, M., Raviv, A., Peretz, A., Berkovich, U., Pracca, F., 2018. Towards a continuous non-invasive assessment of intra-abdominal pressure based on bioimpedance and microwave reflectometry: A pilot run on a porcine model. Biomed. Signal Process. Control 44, 96–100.

Dittmann, F., Tzschätzsch, H., Hirsch, S., et al., 2017. Tomoelastography of the abdomen: Tissue mechanical properties of the liver, spleen, kidney, and pancreas from single MR elastography scans at different hydration states. Magn. Reson. Med. 78, 976–983.

Draaijers, L.J., Botman, Y.A., Tempelman, F.R., et al., 2004. Skin elasticity meter or subjective evaluation in scars: A reliability assessment. Burns 30, 109–114.

Elahi, S., Connesson, N., Chagnon, G., Payan, Y., 2019. In vivo soft tissues mechanical characterization: Volume-based aspiration method validated on silicones. Exp. Mech. 59, 251–261.

Feng, Y.N., Li, Y.P., Liu, C.L., Zhang, Z.J., 2018. Assessing the elastic properties of skeletal muscle and tendon using shearwave ultrasound elastography and MyotonPRO. Sci. Rep. 8, 17064.

François, D., Pineau, A., Zaoui, A., 2012. Elastic behaviour, viscoelasticity. In: Micro- and Macroscopic Constitutive Behaviour, second ed. (Mechanical Behaviour of Materials, vol 1). Springer, New York, pp. 83–154, 445–505.

Glaser, K., Ehman, R., 2014. Perspectives on the development of elastography. In: Venkatesh, S.K., Ehman, R.L. (Eds.), Magnetic Resonance Elastography, Springer. New York, NY, pp. 3–18.

Hayes, W.C., Herrmann, G., Keer, L.M., Mockros, L.F., 1972. Mathematical analysis for indentation tests of articular cartilage. J. Biomech, 5, 541–551.

Hirsch, A., Braun, J., Sack, I., 2017. Introduction. In: Magnetic Resonance Elastography. Wiley-VCH, Weinheim, pp. 1–5.

Jacobson, N., Driscoll, M., 2021. Design synthesis and preliminary evaluation of a novel tool to non-invasively characterize pressurized, physiological vessels. J. Med. Devices,15, 025001.

Kutz, M., 2015. Measurement of material characteristics. In: Kutz, M. (Ed.), Mechanical Engineers Handbook: Materials and Engineering Mechanics, fourth ed. John Wiley, New Jersey, 852–855.

Lu, M.H., Mao, R., Lu, Y., et al., 2012. Quantitative imaging of Young's modulus of soft tissues from ultrasound water jet indentation: A finite element study. Comput. Math. Methods Med. 2012, 979847.

Lung, C.W., Jan, Y.K., Lu, J.H., et al., 2020. The evaluation of mechanical properties of soft tissue on pressure ulcers among bedridden elderly patients. In: Goonetilleke, R.S., Karwowski, W. (Eds.), Volume 967 of the 2019 AHFE: Advances in Physical Ergonomics and Human Factors. Cham: Springer, Washington DC, 360–368.

McAuliffe, S., Mc Creesh, K., Purtill, H., O'Sullivan, K., 2017. A systematic review of the reliability of diagnostic ultrasound imaging in measuring tendon size: Is the error clinically acceptable? Phys. Ther. Sport 26, 52–63.

Miller, R., Kolipaka, A., Nash, M., Young, A. A., 2018. Relative identifiability of anisotropic properties from magnetic resonance elastography. NMR Biomed. 31, e3848.

Moerman, K.M., Holt, C.A., Evans, S.L., Simms, C.K., 2009. Digital image correlation and finite element modelling as a method to determine mechanical properties of human soft tissue in vivo. J. Biomech. 42, 1150–1153.

Müller, B., Elrod, J., Pensalfini, M., et al., 2018. A novel ultra-light suction device for mechanical characterization of skin. PLoS One, 13, e0201440.

Narayanan, N., Bonakdar, A., Dargahi, J., Packirisamy, M., 2006. Design and analysis of a micromachined piezoelectric sensor for measuring the viscoelastic properties of tissues in minimally invasive surgery. Smart Mater. Struct. 15, 1684–1690.

Nava, A., Mazza, E., Kleinermann, F., et al., 2004. Evaluation of the mechanical properties of human liver and kidney through aspiration experiments. Technol. Health Care 12, 269–280.

Nichols, K., Okamura, A., 2015. Methods to segment hard inclusions in soft tissue during autonomous robotic palpation. IEEE Trans. Robot. 31, 344–354.

Oflaz, H., Baran, O., 2014. A new medical device to measure a stiffness of soft materials. Acta Bioeng. Biomech. 16, 125–131.

Peipsi, A., Kerpe, R., Jäger, H., et al., 2012. Myoton Pro: A novel tool for the assessment of mechanical properties of fascial tissues. J. Bodywork Move. Ther. 16 (4), 527.

Ramalingam, K., 2009. Material properties. In: Ramalingam, K. (Ed.), Handbook of Mechanical Engineering Terms, second ed. New Age International, New Delhi, pp. 39–52.

Stedman, T., 2006. Stedman's Medical Dictionary, twenty-eighth ed. Lippincott Williams & Wilkins, Philadelphia.

Sigrist, R.M.S., Liau, J., Kaffas, A.E., Chammas, M.C., Willmann, J.K., 2017. Ultrasound elastography: Review of techniques and clinical applications. Theranostics 7, 1303–1329.

Tarsi, G.M., Gould, R.A., Chung, J.A., et al., 2013. Method for non-optical quantification of in situ local soft tissue biomechanics. J. Biomech. 46, 1938–1942.

Valtorta, D., Mazza, E., 2005. Dynamic measurements of soft tissue viscoelastic properties with a torsional resonator device. Med. Image Anal. 9, 481–490.

Wilke, J., Vogt, L., Pfarr, T., Banzer, W., 2018. Reliability and validity of a semi-electronic tissue compliance meter to assess muscle stiffness. J. Back Musculoskelet. Rehabil. 31, 991–997.

Williams, R., Ji, W., Howell, J., Conatser, R.R., 2007. Device for measurement of human tissue properties in vivo. J. Med. Devices 1, 197–205.

Yen, P., 2003. Palpation sensitivity analysis of exploring hard objects under soft tissue. In: IEEE/ASME International Conference on Advanced Intelligent Mechatronics. IEEE, Kobe, Japan, pp. 1102–1106.

Zhang, L., Thakku, S.G., Beotra, M.R., et al., 2017. Verification of a virtual fields method to extract the mechanical properties of human optic nerve head tissues in vivo. Biomech. Model. Mechanobiol. 16, 871–887.

Zheng, Y., Huang, Y., 2016. Measurement of Soft Tissue Elasticity in Vivo: Techniques and Applications. Taylor and Francis Group, Boca Raton, FL.

Zügel, M., Maganaris, C.N., Wilke, J., et al. 2018. Fascial tissue research in sports medicine: From molecules to tissue adaptation, injury and diagnostics: Consensus statement. Br. J. Sport. Med. 52, 1497.

Fascia-Oriented Therapies

Fascia-Oriented Therapies: Inclusion Criteria and Overview

Carla Stecco

Before starting this Part, I would like to recall the personality of Leon Chaitow, the previous and first editor of this section. I feel responsible for this "heredity" and would like to thank him for everything he did to support the field of fascial concepts, so that they are now known all over the world.

Research into and improved knowledge of connective tissues and fascia have grown in modern times, leading to a deeper understanding of the human body. There has been a demand for evidence-based work, to support the safe use of manual and exercise-based therapeutic modalities. It has become important in establishing which of the many techniques, modalities, systems, and methods currently in use by manual therapists, practitioners, and physicians actually do influence fascial behavior.

In addition, the mechanisms involved when fascial structures are treated, manually or by other means (needling, mechanical force, exercise, etc.), have attracted research interest. What should become clear is that any method that incorporates the application of pressure, shear forces, rhythmic movements, and stretching works with and on fascial structures, whether the therapist is aware of this or not. Intelligent use of manual clinical methods involving fascial structures, as evidenced in many examples in this section, is clearly more desirable than random, virtually accidental influence.

The selection of topics in this chapter therefore reflects a wide spectrum of modalities, and it is sometimes difficult to decide which method to use, according to the patient's state. Although the topics in this section are not definitive of all the therapeutic methods used in manual therapy, they do represent them correctly. We selected techniques to give readers an overview of the various perspectives available in fascial treatments, from movements to passive treatments, from superficial massage to deep manipulation. All these techniques can affect fascia, but in different ways, and some techniques can probably be more accurately focused on the superficial fascia, others on the deep fascia; some are more useful in cases of acute pain, others in chronic patients. The idea for the future is therefore to search for better knowledge of what *affects* fascia, and what *effects* fascial treatment may have. To do this, we must return to anatomy, recalling that there are various types of fasciae, with differing features, depth, etc., and that each manual and physical therapy probably is more effective for a specific fascial structure. In addition, to be able to give the correct indications to our patients, we must understand the biological effect of each of those treatments. We now know that the fascia are much more complex than we thought as little as 10 years ago: it is composed of varying kinds of cells and fibers and, as it is sensitive to pH and various hormones, we must examine all these aspects if we aim at having a true healthy fascia (Fig. 7.1.1). At the same time, as each technique could definitely be better focused on one of these specific aspects, we can consequently decide on one approach or another according to the patient's symptoms (Fig. 7.1.2). For example, we can start with passive treatment to "free" the fascial tissue and, within the range of all possible passive treatments, we must choose the best one for our patient, considering if the symptoms are more closely related to the superficial fascia (e.g., edema, cellulitis, alteration of venous return, skin tropism) or to the deep fasciae (alteration of proprioception, motor coordination, etc.). We can also choose whether it is better to work using our hands, or various kinds of tools. Then, particularly if our patient has chronic problems, we must reinforce and improve the results with active treatment, that is, various types of exercises (Fig. 7.1.3). In this case it is important to

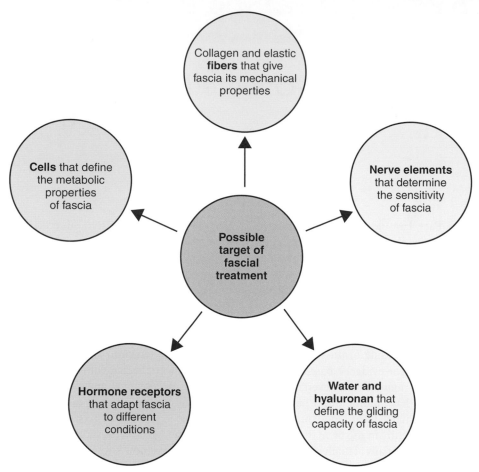

Fig. 7.1.1 The various targets of fascial treatment. The different therapies can affect one or more of these elements.

remember that the fasciae are composed of two key elements: loose connective tissue and dense connective tissue and that, if we aim at a healthy fascia, both must be trained. In reality, the two elements respond to loads and movements in totally different ways: the fibrous component answers better to loading and the loose component to shearing forces, so that exercises will probably differ according to our target. Lastly, some suggestions regarding nutrition, hormonal evaluations, etc., may also be useful in patients with complex difficulties, to understand why myofascial pain always returns, or never goes away.

An integrated approach to the fascia may be necessary in order to manage all these aspects in the best possible way. Thus during this Part, we will attempt to create a scheme in our minds, in which we relate the chronicity of the problem, its location, etc., with the various possible treatments. In this way, for every patient we can create and complete a flowchart to select the best combination of treatments among the various fascial treatments at our disposal, considering the history of our patients and their overall assessment.

To conclude, I would like to note that our work is not devoted to demonstrating which technique is the best, but to care for our patients as well as possible.

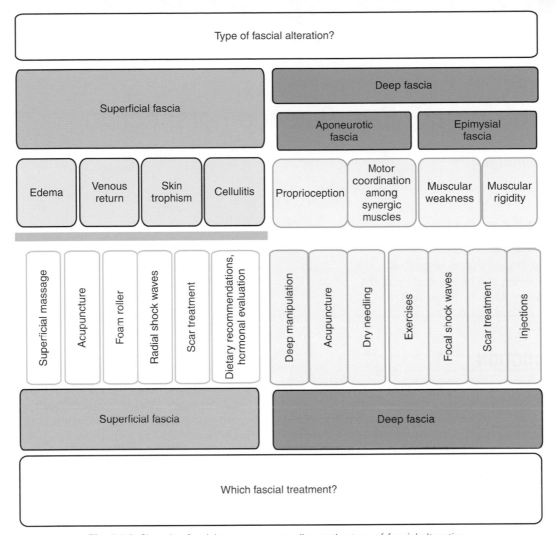

Fig. 7.1.2 Choosing fascial treatment according to the type of fascial alteration.

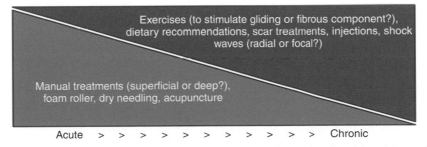

Fig. 7.1.3 Relative suitability of the different treatments according to the chronicity of the problem.

Trigger Point Therapy from a Contemporary Pain Science Perspective

Jan Dommerholt

INTRODUCTION

Myofascial pain continues to be a somewhat controversial topic with, on the one hand, clinicians, researchers, and major medical societies, such as the International Association of Pain, establishing that myofascial pain is a prevalent type of musculoskeletal pain that may contribute to acute and persistent pain syndromes, and, on the other hand, select individuals who have determined that the construct is invented without any scientific evidence, resembling a futile quest for mythical creatures (Weisman et al. 2018). Nevertheless, trigger points (TrPs), the hallmark characteristic of myofascial pain, are located within muscle contractures, commonly referred to as "taut bands." These contractures are thought to be nonelectrogenic, meaning that they occur endogenously within muscle fibers independent of alpha motor neuron electrical activity (Simons and Mense 1998). It is likely that a nonquantal release of acetylcholine from the alpha motor neuron at motor endplates is responsible for the formation of these contractures, but the exact mechanisms are still elusive (Gerwin et al. 2004).

A TrP is defined as "a hyperirritable spot in skeletal muscle that is associated with a hypersensitive palpable nodule in a taut band." Trigger points have been reported in all age groups, except infants (Fernández-De-Las-Peñas and Dommerholt, 2018b, p. 1). Sixty

experts from 12 different countries agreed in a Delphi study that active TrPs refer or reproduce a patient's recognized pain, give local and referred pain, and reproduce any symptoms experienced by the patient. Latent TrPs also produce local and referred pain but are only painful when palpated or needled and do not reproduce the patient-experienced symptoms (Fernández-De-Las-Peñas and Dommerholt 2018b).

The identification of TrPs starts with palpating the local contracture of a taut band perpendicular to the muscle fiber direction. Next, a local hardened or nodular region is identified within the taut band, which is referred to as a TrP. Usually, TrPs develop as a result of local muscle overuse, but they are also frequently associated with other dysfunctions, such as pain diagnoses with peripheral and central sensitization, joint dysfunction, dental or otolaryngic diagnoses, visceral and pelvic diseases and dysfunctions, tension-type headaches and migraines, stress and anxiety, hypothyroidism, systemic lupus erythematosus, infectious diseases, parasitical diseases, systemic side effects of medications, and metabolic or nutritional deficiencies or insufficiencies.

Some professional groups are particularly prone to developing TrPs, especially musicians and computer operators, who perform their duties using low-level muscle contractions for prolonged periods of time (Hoyle et al. 2011). With submaximal contractions, smaller motor units are recruited first and de-recruited last without any rotation and substitution of motor units as expressed through the Cinderella hypothesis, with consideration of Henneman's size principle (Hägg 2003).

Numerous MRI, sonography, elastography, histochemical, electromyography, and microdialysis studies have confirmed the presence of taut bands and TrPs, their relative size, and the chemical composition of the TrP environment. Elastography and spectral Doppler revealed that a TrP region has a 27% lower vibration amplitude compared with normal muscle tissue, which suggests a much greater than normal degree of stiffness (Chen et al. 2016). Electromyography has shown that TrPs feature a specific electrical signature, referred to as endplate noise, which is caused by the excessive release of acetylcholine. There is a direct correlation between the presence of endplate noise and the degree of pain intensity, irritability, and pressure-pain thresholds. Several therapeutic interventions can reduce the degree of endplate noise and improve the patient's status, including calcium blockers, administration of the alpha-adrenergic antagonist phentolamine, dry needling, laser, and injections with botulinum toxin (Dommerholt et al. 2019).

> **KEY POINTS**
>
> Trigger points are an accepted clinical entity linked to dysfunctional motor endplates. Endplate noise is the characteristic feature of trigger points and correlates with the degree of pain experienced by patients.

INTEGRATED TRIGGER POINTS HYPOTHESIS

The current thinking about TrPs is best captured by the evidence-informed integrated trigger point hypothesis (Donnelly 2019). The model is not perfect and has been modified several times to reflect the latest contemporary research. There are other theoretical models, but they lack sufficient experimental support. In summary, according to the updated trigger point hypothesis, TrPs are associated with dysfunctional motor endplates featuring an excess release of acetylcholine attributed to a variety of possible reasons, including an insufficiency of acetylcholinesterase; an increased sensitivity of nicotinic acetylcholine receptors; an acidic pH; hypoxia; a lack of adenosine triphosphate; certain genetic mutations; certain drugs; and particular chemicals, such as calcitonin gene-related peptide, diisopropylfluorophosphate, or organophosphate pesticides (Gerwin et al. 2004; McPartland 2004). Many of these factors behave in an interactive fashion; for example, a low pH inactivates acetylcholinesterase. Calcitonin gene-related peptide also inhibits acetylcholinesterase but also stimulates the release of acetylcholine and sensitizes acetylcholine receptors. The hypothesis maintains that endplate dysfunction is characterized by an abnormal depolarization of the postjunctional membrane that may contribute to autonomic and sensory reflex arcs, which are sustained by complex sensitization mechanisms against the background of a localized hypoxic energy crisis (McPartland and Simons 2006). Numerous human, rabbit, and equine studies offer support for the integrated trigger point hypothesis (Fernández-De-Las-Peñas and Dommerholt 2018a).

Jafri emphasized the importance of reactive oxygen species (ROS) and the critical role of an excessive release of Ca^{2+} (Jafri 2014). Mechanical deformation of the microtubule network leads to the production of ROS, which in turn can oxidize ryanodine receptors, resulting in an increased Ca^{2+} release from the sarcoplasmic reticulum. The pathway that describes the excessive release of Ca^{2+} after mechanical stretch is known as X-ROS signaling. In skeletal muscles, X-ROS triggers increased nociceptive input and inflammatory pain by sensitizing Ca^{2+}-permeable sarcolemmal transient receptor potential (TRP) ion channels, which are expressed by glial cells in the central nervous system. Activating the TRPV1 receptor leads to a quick increase in intracellular Ca^{2+} concentrations (Dommerholt et al. 2019). Jafri speculated that myofascial pain may be due to a combined activation of several ligand-gated ion channels, including acid-sensing ion channels (ASIC3); transient receptor potential cation channels, such as TRPV1; and bradykinin and purinergic receptors, among others (Jafri 2014).

The integrated TrP hypothesis is best viewed within a broader pain neuroscience context. Contemporary views on the experience of pain continue to develop and clinicians should familiarize themselves with Melzack's neuromatrix model, Gifford's mature organism model, and Hodges and Tucker's motor adaptation model in conjunction with the integrated TrP hypothesis (Dommerholt et al. 2019). These models have in common that they view the patient as a whole individual with many interacting systems. Clinicians need to determine which pain mechanisms are dominant in a particular patient's case as a guide to develop the optimal management strategy. From a pain science perspective, TrPs are persistent sources of peripheral nociceptive input, potentially leading to local pain and to peripheral and central sensitization with hyperalgesia, allodynia, and secondary hyperalgesia, which in the myofascial pain literature is often characterized as referred pain (Fernández-de-las-Peñas and Dommerholt 2014). Treatment options to inactivate TrPs are also best offered from a pain science perspective (Fernández-de-Las-Peñas and Nijs 2019), realizing that neither aspect of the treatment is offered as a stand-alone intervention.

KEY POINT

The integrated trigger point hypothesis is continuously being modified and updated with new research insights and different pain models. In the current understanding, trigger points are sources of peripheral nociceptive input, contributing to local pain and peripheral and central sensitization.

FASCIA, MUSCLES, AND MYOFASCIAL PAIN

Although Travell emphasized the importance of including the word "fascia" into the descriptive term "myofascial pain," it would take several decades before researchers and clinicians considered the potential role of fascia in this common clinical problem. The first editions of the Travell and Simons trigger point manuals contained little or no information about fascia and its possible interactions with muscles or as a potential source of persistent nociceptive input (Simons et al. 1999); however, the 2019 edition does include a chapter on the role of fascia in myofascial pain (Dommerholt 2019). Although Travell entertained the notion of the existence of fascial TrPs, this concept was later discarded, and only muscular TrPs are now recognized within the context of myofascial pain (Donnelly 2019). The next update of the integrated TrP hypothesis will also have to include more current fascia research, not only because of the many interconnections between muscles and fascia but also because several

therapeutic strategies overlap with similar underlying mechanisms. What is referred to as TrPs in the myofascial pain literature may occasionally overlap with what in the fascia literature is referred to as densifications, although not all densifications are necessarily TrPs.

After the 2015 fourth Fascia Research Congress in Washington, DC, the "fascial system" was defined as:

The fascial system consists of the three-dimensional continuum of soft, collagen-containing, loose and dense fibrous connective tissues that permeate the body. It incorporates elements such as adipose tissue, adventitia and neurovascular sheaths, aponeuroses, deep and superficial fasciae, epineurium, joint capsules, ligaments, membranes, meninges, myofascial expansions, periostea, retinacula, septa, tendons, visceral fasciae, and all the intramuscular and intermuscular connective tissues including endo-/peri-/epimysium. The fascial system interpenetrates and surrounds all organs, muscles, bones and nerve fibers, endowing the body with a functional structure, and providing an environment that enables all body systems to operate in an integrated manner. (Adstrum et al. 2017)

Based on the multiple interconnections between muscles and fascia, it should be obvious that any discussion of myofascial pain has to take into consideration that fascia and muscles are inseparable. The connections between muscles and fascia are probably quite important in clinical practice and may have certain implications for the biomechanical aspects of TrPs. Not only do many muscles connect directly to other muscles, such as the rhomboid muscles connecting to the serratus anterior muscle (Fig. 7.2.1), or many orofacial muscles, such as the zygomaticus muscles attaching to the orbicularis oris muscle, muscles also connect directly to fascia and, in fact, are enveloped by the epimysium.

Furthermore, each muscle fiber bundle is embedded within the perimysium and each fiber is surrounded by the endomysium. The endomysium, perimysium, and epimysium are aspects of the deep fascia. In muscles that connect to other muscles or to intramuscular connective tissues, epimuscular force transmission involves connective tissues outside the muscle (Huijing and Jaspers 2005). Nearly 40% of muscle force is transmitted through fascia (Huijing 2009). The perimysium, for example, plays a significant role in lateral force transmission in skeletal muscle (Passerieux et al. 2007).

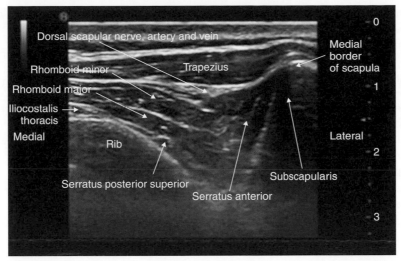

Fig. 7.2.1 Attachments of the rhomboid muscles to the serratus anterior muscle. Courtesy Kris Demanet, MD, Brugge, Belgium.

The connections between muscles and fascia are essential for force transmission, stability, flexibility, and overall mobility. A decrease in the mobility of the layers of the thoracolumbar fascia is associated with restricted mobility and stiffness. Aponeurotic fascia, such as the thoracolumbar fascia, can transmit forces over much greater distances than epimysial fascia (Huijing and Baan 2008). Deep fascia contains many mechanoreceptors and can restrict muscle function and contribute to increased muscle stiffness (Stecco et al. 2013, Passerieux et al. 2007).

It is likely that fibroblasts, located in the extracellular matrix (ECM), are intimately involved in the mechanical force patterns with direct involvement of integrins (Chiquet et al. 2003). Fibroblasts register force-induced deformations of the ECM and stimulate the release of several substances, such as paracrine growth factor (Schleip et al. 2006). When tissues are stretched beyond their capacity and get damaged, fibroblasts differentiate into myofibroblasts and deposit collagen, fibronectin, and glycosaminoglycans (Keane et al. 2018). Fibroblasts have stress fibers and focal adhesions and they are lamellar in shape when being stretched. Under low stress, fibroblasts are more or less rounded structures (Miron-Mendoza et al. 2008). Lamellar fibroblasts can differentiate into intrafascial myofibroblasts complete with a contractile apparatus of actin microfilaments and nonmuscle myosin (Tomasek et al. 2002), which provides a mechanism for altering tissue stiffness. There is no evidence that these cellular contractions contribute much to joint stability in the short term, but in the long term this cellular activity may induce tissue contractures (Schleip and Klingler 2019). Of interest is that the perimysium has a high density of fibroblasts.

Stecco et al. suggested that decreased viscoelasticity is associated with a lack of hyaluronan, a glycosaminoglycan polymer of the ECM found between muscle fibers, nerves, and fascial layers (Stecco et al. 2011). Of interest in this context is that researchers identified increased levels of glycosaminoglycan near TrPs in a rodent model (Margalef et al. 2019). Although they did not determine the particular type of glycosaminoglycan, it is possible that they contribute to the formation of TrPs. There are four main groups of glycosaminoglycans, including heparin/heparan sulfate, chondroitin sulfate/dermatan sulfate, keratan sulfate, and hyaluronan (Zhang et al. 2009). Glycosaminoglycans do contribute to the release of nociceptive substances near active TrPs. They are hygroscopic in nature, and it is conceivable that the nodular nature of TrPs may at least in part be due to the presence of glycosaminoglycans. Manual TrP techniques aimed to inactivate TrPs may reduce their volume and contribute to a decrease in the concentrations of nociceptive substances. Roman et al. developed a mathematical model that showed that tangential oscillation and perpendicular vibration techniques may cause hyaluronan to move near the edges of the fascial area under manipulation and create improved lubrication and perhaps more mobility (Roman et al. 2013).

SOME SENSORY ASPECTS OF FASCIA

Fibroblasts are not only linked to myofascial pain from a mechanical point of view. An immunocytochemical analysis of collagen-I, collagen-III, and fibrillin on fibroblasts isolated from human fascia lata demonstrated that fascial cells can modulate the production of certain components of the extracellular matrix when treated with β-estradiol. Interestingly, adding relaxin-1 to the cell culture stabilized the production of extracellular matrix. The study showed that hormonal dysfunctions can contribute to a dysregulation of the extracellular matrix production in fasciae, which may indirectly contribute to a decrease in the pain threshold (Fede et al. 2019). Perhaps this is part of the reason why women tend to experience more myofascial pain than their male counterparts.

Several studies have shown that fascia contains many nociceptors; for example, the thoracodorsal fascia of rodents had three times as many nociceptors than the back muscles (Taguchi et al. 2008; Barry et al. 2015). When fascia is being stretched, sensitization of fascial nociceptors may contribute to persistent myofascial pain (Deising et al. 2012). In this context, it is noteworthy that especially the perimysium is sensitive to changes in mechanical tension. Injections of nerve growth factor or even hypertonic saline into fascia can cause significant exercise-induced pain, mechanical hyperalgesia, and a prolonged decreased pressure threshold and may result in significantly more pain than similar injections in the subcutis and muscle (Schilder et al. 2014; Weinkauf et al. 2015). Fascia is not only part of the muscular system. The loose connective tissue of the patellar tendon, for example, contains peptidergic sensory nerve endings with antibodies for calcitonin gene-related peptide and substance P (Danielson et al. 2006). Fascia is not a static structure. Under pathological conditions, fascia can produce new nociceptive fibers that are immunoreactive to substance P (Sanchis-Alfonso and Rosello-Sastre 2000). There are nociceptive substance P endings in the outer layer of the thoracolumbar fascia, once again suggesting that fascia may play a significant role in myofascial pain conditions.

KEY POINTS

Travell's early insights that included fascia into the myofascial pain construct are finally being addressed. Fascia cannot be separated from muscles or from the nervous system from a biomechanical point of view and from a pain science point of view. Mechanically, muscles and fascia work together. From a pain perspective, fascia contains many nociceptors and, as such, is a major contributor to acute and chronic pain problems.

TRIGGER POINT THERAPY

Any therapeutic intervention should be evidence-informed and based on scientific evidence, clinicians' judgments, expertise, and clinical decision-making. In a simplified model, clinicians are tasked with decreasing the excitability of muscle nociceptors, reversing hypoxia observed at TrPs, and increasing the local pH. Traditionally, TrP therapy has focused primarily on muscle dysfunction, especially inactivating TrPs, improving the local circulation, and addressing perpetuating factors. Travell and Simons emphasized TrP injections, spray and stretch, manual techniques, and moist heat (Simons et al. 1999).

Dry needling has become a popular treatment option, especially among physiotherapists (Fig. 7.2.2). In addition to dry needling, other current treatment options include invasive and noninvasive approaches, such as manual compression; fascia-focused approaches, including Fascial Manipulation, Myofascial Induction Therapy (MIT), and Rolfing Structural Integration (Fig. 7.2.3);

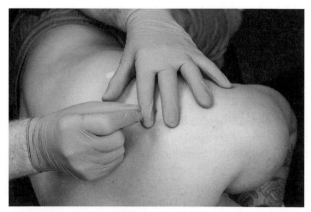

Fig. 7.2.2 Dry needling of the infraspinatus muscle.

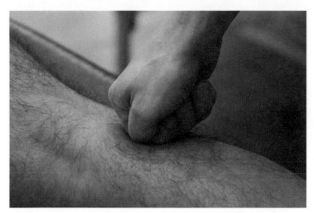

Fig. 7.2.3 Manual compression techniques.

Summary

Myofascial pain is an established clinical entity recognized by major medical societies and supported by a wide range of objective studies. Trigger points are the hallmark characteristic of myofascial pain. In the past, trigger point therapy was administered more or less in isolation of other therapeutic approaches and philosophies. Fascia was never really a consideration even though Travell insisted on calling the syndrome myofascial pain. The fields of fascia research and myofascial research are slowly but steadily merging. Although many questions remain, there is enough known to project that in the foreseeable future, the integrated trigger point hypothesis will need to be updated with a full integration of fascial research. From a therapeutic point of view, it appears that integrating various treatment options with a focus on pain science education appears to be beneficial.

injection therapy, including anesthetics, botulinum toxin, and serotonin antagonists; spray and stretch; laser; ultrasound; electrotherapy; shockwave therapy; and pain science education, among others. Integrating various treatment options within a more biopsychosocial paradigm with a focus on pain science education appears to be beneficial (Fernández-de-Las-Peñas and Nijs, 2019).

It is not necessarily clear whether certain approaches are more effective than others, but it is beyond the scope of this chapter to provide an in-depth review of the various treatment options. Studies comparing dry needling to manual approaches show benefits to both with varying results and many advocate combining different approaches to achieve optimal outcomes (Bağcıer and Yılmaz 2020). A case series of five patients with nonspecific low back pain showed that treating painful fascial spots in other areas of the body was effective, presumably because of the continuity of the thoracolumbar fascia into the deep fascia of the limbs (Casato et al. 2019). Dry needling of the superficial fascia from T2 to T7 along the spine reduced pain and restored range of motion and function (Anandkumar and Manivasagam 2017). Four sessions of myofascial release techniques applied to the lower back significantly improved pain, disability, and the myoelectric activity of the lumbar erector spinae muscles but did not change the lumbar spine kinematics (Arguisuelas et al. 2019). Manual TrP therapy was very effective for the treatment of myofascial pain in the emergency department as an alternative to pharmacological interventions, such as opioids (Grover et al. 2019).

REFERENCES

Adstrum, S., Hedley, G., Schleip, R., Stecco, C., Yucesoy, C.A., 2017. Defining the fascial system. J. Bodyw. Mov. Ther. 21, 173–177.

Anandkumar, S.M., Manivasagam, M., 2017. Effect of fascia dry needling on non-specific thoracic pain–A proposed dry needling grading system. Physiother. Theory Pract. 33, 420–428.

Arguisuelas, M.D., Lison, J.F., Domenech-Fernandez, J., Martinez-Hurtado, I., Salvador Coloma, P., Sanchez-Zuriaga, D., 2019. Effects of myofascial release in erector spinae myoelectric activity and lumbar spine kinematics in non-specific chronic low back pain: Randomized controlled trial. Clin. Biomech. (Bristol, Avon) 63, 27–33.

Bağcıer, F., Yılmaz, N., 2020. The impact of extracorporeal shock wave therapy and dry needling combination on the pain, grip strength and functionality in patients diagnosed with lateral epicondylitis. Turk. J. Osteoporos. 25, 65–71.

Barry, C.M., Kestell, G., Gillan, M., Haberberger, R.V., Gibbins, I.L., 2015. Sensory nerve fibers containing calcitonin gene-related peptide in gastrocnemius, latissimus dorsi and erector spinae muscles and thoracolumbar fascia in mice. Neuroscience 291, 106–117.

Casato, G., Stecco, C., Busin, R., 2019. Role of fasciae in nonspecific low back pain. Eur. J. Transl. Myol. 29, 8330.

Chen, Q., Wang, H.J., Gay, R.E., et al., 2016. Quantification of Myofascial Taut Bands. Arch. Phys. Med. Rehabil. 97, 67–73.

Chiquet, M., Renedo, A.S., Huber, F., Fluck, M., 2003. How do fibroblasts translate mechanical signals into changes in extracellular matrix production? Matrix Biol. 22, 73–80.

Danielson, P., Alfredson, H., Forsgren, S., 2006. Distribution of general (PGP 9.5) and sensory (substance P/CGRP) innervations in the human patellar tendon. Knee Surg. Sports Traumatol. Arthrosc. 14, 125–132.

Deising, S., Weinkauf, B., Blunk, J., Obreja, O., Schmelz, M., Rukwied, R., 2012. NGF-evoked sensitization of muscle fascia nociceptors in humans. Pain 153, 1673–1679.

Dommerholt, J., 2019. The role of muscles and fascia in myofascial pain syndrome. In: Donnelly, J. (Ed.), Travell, Simons & Simons' Myofascial Pain and Dysfunction: The Trigger Point Manual. Wolters Kluwer, Baltimore.

Dommerholt, J., Gerwin, R.D., Courtney, C.A., 2019. Pain sciences and myofascial pain. In: Donnelly, J. (Ed.), Travell, Simons & Simons' Myofascial Pain and Dysfunction: The Trigger Point Manual. Wolters Kluwer, Baltimore.

Donnelly, J., 2019. Travell, Simons & Simons' Myofascial Pain and Dysfunction: The Trigger Point Manual. Wolters Kluwer, Baltimore.

Fede, C., Pirri, C., Fan, C., et al., 2019. Sensitivity of the fasciae to sex hormone levels: Modulation of collagen-I, collagen-III and fibrillin production. PLoS One 14, e0223195.

Fernández-De-Las-Peñas, C., Dommerholt, J., 2018a. Basic concepts of myofascial trigger points (TrPs). In: Dommerholt, J., Fernández-De-Las-Peñas, C. (Eds.), Trigger Point Dry Needling; an Evidenced and Clinical-Based Approach. Churchill Livingstone, Edinburgh.

Fernández-De-Las-Peñas, C., Dommerholt, J., 2018b. International Consensus on Diagnostic Criteria and Clinical Considerations of Myofascial Trigger Points: A Delphi Study. Pain Med. 19, 142–150.

Fernández-De-Las-Peñas, C., Dommerholt, J., 2014. Myofascial trigger points: peripheral or central phenomenon? Curr. Rheumatol. Rep. 16, 395.

Fernandez-De-Las-Penas, C., Nijs, J., 2019. Trigger point dry needling for the treatment of myofascial pain syndrome: current perspectives within a pain neuroscience paradigm. J. Pain Res. 12, 1899–1911.

Gerwin, R.D., Dommerholt, J., Shah, J.P., 2004. An expansion of Simons' integrated hypothesis of trigger point formation. Curr. Pain Headache Rep. 8, 468–475.

Grover, C., Christoffersen, K., Clark, L., Close, R., Layhe, S., 2019. Atraumatic back pain due to quadratus lumborum spasm treated by physical therapy with manual trigger point therapy in the emergency department. Clin. Pract. Cases Emerg. Med. 3, 259–261.

Hägg, G.M., 2003. The Cinderella Hypothesis. In: Johansson, H., Windhorst, U., Djupsjöbacka, M., Passatore, M. (Eds.), Chronic Work-Related Myalgia. Gävle University Press, Gävle.

Hoyle, J.A., Marras, W.S., Sheedy, J.E., Hart, D.E., 2011. Effects of postural and visual stressors on myofascial trigger point development and motor unit rotation during computer work. J. Electromyogr. Kinesiol. 21, 41–48.

Huijing, P.A., 2009. Epimuscular myofascial force transmission between antagonistic and synergistic muscles can explain movement limitation in spastic paresis. In: Huijing, P.A., Hollander, P., Findley, T., Schleip, R. (Eds.), Fascia Research II; Basic Science and Implications for Conventional and Complementary Health Care. Urban & Fischer, Munich.

Huijing, P.A., Baan, G.C., 2008. Myofascial force transmission via extramuscular pathways occurs between antagonistic muscles. Cells Tissues Organs 188, 400–414.

Huijing, P.A., Jaspers, R.T., 2005. Adaptation of muscle size and myofascial force transmission: a review and some new experimental results. Scand. J. Med. Sci. Sports 15, 349–380.

Jafri, M.S., 2014. Mechanisms of Myofascial Pain. Int. Sch. Res. Notices 2014, 523924.

Keane, T.J., Horejs, C.M., Stevens, M.M., 2018. Scarring vs. functional healing: Matrix-based strategies to regulate tissue repair. Adv. Drug. Deliv. Rev. 129, 407–419.

Margalef, R., Sisquella, M., Bosque, M., et al., 2019. Experimental myofascial trigger point creation in rodents. J. Appl. Physiol. (1985) 126, 160–169.

McPartland, J.M., 2004. Travell trigger points-molecular and osteopathic perspectives. J. Am. Osteopath. Assoc. 104, 244–249.

McPartland, J.M., Simons, D.G., 2006. Myofascial trigger points: translating molecular theory into manual therapy. J. Man. Manipulative Ther. 14, 232–239.

Miron-Mendoza, M., Seemann, J., Grinnell, F., 2008. Collagen fibril flow and tissue translocation coupled to fibroblast migration in 3D collagen matrices. Mol. Cell. Biol. 19, 2051–2058.

Passerieux, E., Rossignol, R., Letellier, T., Delage, J.P., 2007. Physical continuity of the perimysium from myofibers to tendons: involvement in lateral force transmission in skeletal muscle. J. Struct. Biol. 159, 19–28.

Roman, M., Chaudhry, H., Bukiet, B., Stecco, A., Findley, T.W., 2013. Mathematical analysis of the flow of hyaluronic acid around fascia during manual therapy motions. J. Am. Osteopath. Assoc. 113, 600–610.

Sanchis-Alfonso, V., Rosello-Sastre, E., 2000. Immunohisto-chemical analysis for neural markers of the lateral retinaculum in patients with isolated symptomatic patellofemoral malalignment. A neuroanatomic basis for anterior knee pain in the active young patient. Am. J. Sports Med. 28, 725–731.

Schilder, A., Hoheisel, U., Magerl, W., Benrath, J., Klein, T., Treede, R.D., 2014. Sensory findings after stimulation of the thoracolumbar fascia with hypertonic saline suggest its contribution to low back pain. Pain 155, 222–231.

Schleip, R., Klingler, W., 2019. Active contractile properties of fascia. Clin. Anat. 32, 891–895.

Schleip, R., Naylor, I.L., Ursu, D., et al., 2006. Passive muscle stiffness may be influenced by active contractility of intramuscular connective tissue. Med. Hypotheses 66, 66–71.

Simons, D.G., Mense, S., 1998. Understanding and measurement of muscle tone as related to clinical muscle pain. Pain 75, 1–17.

Simons, D.G., Travell, J.G., Simons, L.S., 1999 Travell and Simons' Myofascial Pain and Dysfunction; the Trigger Point Manual. Williams & Wilkins, Baltimore.

Stecco, A., Gesi, M., Stecco, C., Stern, R., 2013. Fascial components of the myofascial pain syndrome. Curr. Pain Headache Rep. 17, 352.

Stecco, C., Stern, R., Porzionato, A., et al., 2011. Hyaluronan within fascia in the etiology of myofascial pain. Surg. Radiol. Anat. 33, 891–896.

Taguchi, T., Hoheisel, U., Mense, S., 2008. Dorsal horn neurons having input from low back structures in rats. Pain 138, 119–129.

Tomasek, J.J., Gabbiani, G., Hinz, B., Chaponnier, C., Brown, R.A., 2002. Myofibroblasts and mechano-regulation of connective tissue remodelling. Nat. Rev. Mol. Cell Biol. 3, 349–363.

Weinkauf, B., Deising, S., Obreja, O., et al., 2015. Comparison of nerve growth factor-induced sensitization pattern in lumbar and tibial muscle and fascia. Muscle Nerve 52, 265–272.

Weisman, A., Meakins, A., Rotem-Lehrer, N., 2018. A Delphi Study: Defining a Unicorn. Pain Med. 19, 1295.

Zhang, F., Zhang, Z., Linhardt, R.J., 2009. Glycosaminoglycans. In: Cummings, R.D., Pierce, J.M. (Eds.), The Handbook of Glycomics. Academic Press, Edinburgh.

Structural Integration

Heidi Massa and Monica Caspari

PREMISES OF THE WORK

Structural Integration (SI), developed in the mid-20th century by Ida P. Rolf, PhD, organizes the human being in gravity.[1] It enhances structural and functional integrity, as revealed by proper alignment and coordination. Two foundational premises distinguish SI from other somatic practices: first, that physical balance, fluidity, ease, and grace—and, indeed, personal well-being—all require appropriate adaptation to the field of gravity; and second, that the primary organ of body structure is fascia.

SI practitioners approach misalignments and chronic musculoskeletal complaints from the perspective that symptoms manifest a more generalized dysfunction, and that when overall alignment and movement quality improve, complaints are likely to resolve spontaneously.[2]

Thus SI does not address presenting complaints *per se*, but instead approaches the person as a functional whole.

CHARACTERISTICS OF FASCIA KEY TO STRUCTURAL INTEGRATION

SI works because fascia is:
- physically and functionally continuous
- responsive to gravity
- able to transmit locally registered information throughout the body
- malleable due to its viscoelasticity.

Because fascia forms a continuous web throughout the whole body—surrounding each muscle, bone, nerve, and organ[3]—through the fascia, every body area is affected somewhat by any change in another area. Thus fascial continuity allows the distinctly nuanced and vectored touch of SI to facilitate change in tissues distant from the practitioner's contact point—even tissues that cannot be touched directly.

---

[1]Dr. Rolf's work is now known by her original and preferred term, *structural integration*. "Rolfing structural integration" refers to the work of graduates and members of the Dr. Ida Rolf Institute (DIRI), as Dr. Rolf's original school is now known. The Little Boy logo (Fig. 7.3.1) is a service mark of DIRI, registered in the United States and other countries.

[2]For a sampling of literature on random trials in normal persons, as well as how SI affects conditions such as anxiety, cerebral palsy, and chronic pain and fatigue, see the chapter Bibliography.

[3]As the fascia associated with any body structure typically lacks an anatomical name, here we use the name of the structure itself to refer to its associated fascia.

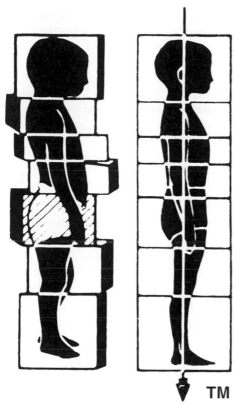

Fig. 7.3.1 The Little Boy logo (a DIRI registered service mark) illustrates progress to orthogonal order in three dimensions. Reprinted with permission from the Dr. Ida Rolf Institute.

KEY POINT

Structural integrators work with an awareness of gravity as the one constant force upon the fascial net—which, in turn, is the primary organ of structure. Structural integration succeeds by exploiting several of fascia's key characteristics.

Fascia responds to gravity—the force to which humans are continuously subjected. As a ship's sail needs the force of wind to function, fascia needs the force of gravity; that is, gravity is a fixed vector against which fascia organizes bodily structure and function.

The fascia, dense with various mechanoreceptors, is a body-wide mechanosensory organ (Schleip 2003), which tells us where we are in space and what our bodies are doing. As they gather local information that is carried through the fascial web (Langevin 2006), the mechanoreceptors enable self-regulation of the neuromotor system.

Finally, to adapt to mechanical and other stresses, the fascial web constantly changes shape, chemical composition, and physical properties. Recognizing fascia's capacity to self-correct over time, SI facilitates limited positional and functional changes to which the body can adapt, and allows adequate time between interventions for the adaptations to occur. After each adaptation, further changes become possible.

FACILITATING INTEGRATED STRUCTURE AND FUNCTION

Much of the work of SI is to balance opposing lengths and tensions within the fascial net. Structurally, practitioners look for a *palintonic* quality of posture (relative segmental arrangement). The Greek *palintonos* refers to the dialog between opposites within an orthogonal order—an order manifest in spatial dimensions, volumes, and planes. An imaginary plumb line through the center of the body expresses occupation and use of space in the sagittal, frontal, and horizontal planes (see Fig. 7.3.1), which both potentiates and limits movement options. Functionally, SI practitioners assess movement for ease and fluidity and for contralateral movement through the limbs, shoulder and pelvic girdles, and spine. Generally, as palintonic right angles are established in the structure, the diagonals and spirals of contralaterality emerge in function.

But preceding movement is orientation to directions in space. Therefore SI reaches beyond fascial patterns to patterns of (1) sensory perception (touch, vision, hearing, and proprioception) and (2) neuromotor coordination (balance between tonic and phasic muscles, and between local and global body stabilizers), as dysfunction in either of these areas limits structural and functional order.

Finally, because SI views both structure and function to be in some sense relational attitudes based on all aspects of experience, the practitioners consider not only the client's perceptions of the social and physical environment, but also awareness of and attribution of meaning to them.

KEY POINT

Structural integration balances span and tonus throughout the fascial net to enhance both structure and function. In addition to optimizing physical patterns, it also addresses perceptual and relational patterns.

What follows is an explication of the traditional 10-session SI series to illustrate how SI exploits key characteristics of fascia. It is descriptive only, and far from comprehensive as to elements or processes.

THE TRADITIONAL STRUCTURAL INTEGRATION 10-SERIES

Though in practice the number and content of sessions are determined by the client's needs and the practitioner's expertise, Dr. Rolf's 10-session protocol is both a teaching tool and a basic strategy to deliver the work. Building on key characteristics of fascia as an organ of structure and communication, the logic of the protocol delivers an orderly and well-supported arrangement of body segments in three-dimensional space along the imaginary plumb line.

Because fascia wraps body parts in layers of varying depths, the protocol starts from the outer layers, first working inward—and then back outward. Since fascia is malleable according to changes in functional demands and over time, the protocol induces changes in an acceptable order—that is, in an order such that the fascia can adapt and integrate them. Also, because the density of mechanoreceptors and other characteristics of healthy fascia make it an information highway (especially for information related to the gravity response), key orienting areas such as the feet and the occiput are addressed early on. Finally, because fascia responds to gravity, the protocol starts from the ground and works up—and then back down—building from an adequate foundation a balanced structure free of cantilever-induced torsions.

KEY POINT

The traditional 10-series protocol is organized around both the anatomy and the functional characteristics of fascia.

The logic of the protocol is functional, too; for example, we begin by freeing the breath, progress through finding the ground, and conclude by integrating the person in his or her surroundings. The sequence facilitates progressive levels of movement integration, manifesting as enhanced contralaterality.

Session 1: Open the Superficial Fascia

SI begins by making space in the superficial fascia, with particular attention to its attachments at bony margins (e.g., the iliac crest and scapular spine) and to regions where it limits the position of major bony segments (e.g., superficial rib fascia and femoral head fascia). This is essentially preparatory, as restriction in this outermost layer limits changes in deeper layers.

Structurally, SI differentiates thorax from shoulder girdle, thorax from pelvis, and pelvis from legs. This differentiation is a precondition for a balanced and palintonic arrangement among these major segments. For example, as femoral rotation approaches neutral, the pelvis has greater independence from the legs and can find better balance over the feet. This, in turn, allows the pelvis to provide greater support for the thorax.

Functionally, Session 1 frees the breath. The ontogenic logic is evident: a newborn's first act is a deep breath. Improving the pelvis as a base of support enables adaptable sagittal plane movement of the upper body's center of gravity (located at approximately T4), called in SI parlance G-prime (G′).

Session 2: Establish a Base of Support

An upright body needs sound and adaptable feet. Loaded with mechanoreceptors, the feet gather much of the information required to maintain overall balance. Because the entire fascial system responds to gravity, better feet allow greater overall ease. Session 2 differentiates and makes adaptable the myofascia and bones of the feet and lower legs and begins to release fascial restrictions of posterior structures, such as hamstrings and spinal erectors.

Structurally, Session 2 balances the feet from front to back, and from the lateral arch to the medial arch (through the transverse arch); restores resilience to the lower leg's interosseus membrane; and organizes the lower leg's various muscle compartments. This brings greater order to G (the lower body's center of gravity, located at approximately L4) by giving the lower body a better place to rest its weight.

Functionally, Session 2 decouples the foot's intrinsic muscles from the extrinsic muscles crossing the ankle, allowing the toes to move independently of the ankles and improving the propulsion phase of the gait. Stimulation of the intrinsic muscles refines contact with the ground and introduces movement in the frontal plane by restoring the interplay between the cuboid and navicular bones. This enhances the ability of the feet (in conjunction with the eyes, inner ear, and temporomandibular joint) (Bricot 2001) to maintain dynamic equilibrium.

Work on the superficial spinal erectors begins the task of optimizing the lumbo-dorsal hinge—the transition point for contralateral spinal movement, located ideally between T8 and T10. Transition at a point more cephalad produces a long or exaggerated lordosis, which dissipates the impulse coming from the legs at the level of the abdomen. This manifests as excessive motion in the pelvic girdle and legs relative to that of the shoulder girdle and arms. Conversely, transition at a point caudad to T8/T10 produces relatively flat lumbars and a long or exaggerated kyphosis. This configuration cannot efficiently transform the impulse from the legs into contralateral movement at the axial level, and the shoulder girdle and arms will compensate with excessive motion relative to that of the pelvic girdle and legs.

Session 3: Balance Fascial Span Along the Lateral Line

Session 3 builds on the volume, adaptability, and support already achieved to address the relative positions of G′ and G along the lateral line of the body. If either G′ or G is displaced forward or backward of the lateral line—that is, if the lateral line between G′ and G deviates from the vertical—the thoracic and abdominal volumes are distorted (see, e.g., Fig. 7.3.2)

Alignment is in one sense an accumulation of relational attitudes, and habitual G′/G positions relative to the lateral line are their physical manifestations. Although there is no universal correlation among relative segmental positions and particular emotional states, each of us can recognize how the body reacts to socioemotional stimulus with small forward or backward displacements of either the thorax or the pelvis.

Session 3 addresses (1) the fascia of the arms and shoulder girdle, which can restrict the position and movements of G′, and (2) the more superficial structures that influence the tilt of the pelvis over the femoral heads and control forward flexion of the torso over the hip joints. Finally, quadratus lumborum and the abdominal flexors—the bridges between the thorax and the pelvis—are balanced to allow differentiated movement between these body segments.

Structurally, Session 3 evokes a palintonic arrangement of major body segments along a lateral line from the joints of Chopart to the glenohumeral joints. It also eases restrictions between the thorax and the pelvis, permitting each of these segments to assume sagittal plane positions approximating horizontal.

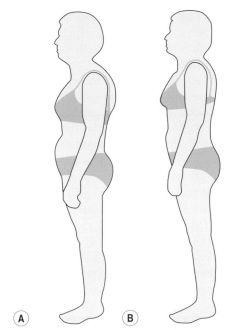

Fig. 7.3.2 These illustrations are based on photos of a client before (A) and after (B) 10 sessions. Observe the normalization of thoracic and abdominal volumes.

Functionally it frees the hip hinge to allow prevertebral length to be maintained in reaching movements. Balance of front-to-back spans from pelvis to ribs—and the horizontals it reveals—sets the stage for diagonal (i.e., contralateral) limb engagement and encourages contralateral movement within the spine itself.

Session 4: Balance the Spans of the Inner and Outer Legs

Session 4 is the first of three sessions on the leg-to-pelvis relationship. It is also the bridge from the lower limbs to the prevertebral space: though the territory of contact is the midline of the legs, fascial continuities among the adductors, pelvic floor tissues, and sacrolumbar prevertebral space allow the adductor work to affect prevertebral structures we cannot touch directly.

Imbalances between the femoral adductors and abductors cause medial or lateral femoral rotation, either of which restricts hip extension and diminishes the fascial organization and function of the pelvic floor, sacroiliac joints, and psoas. Session 4 frees the medial line by differentiating the adductors from the adjacent quadriceps (anterior) and medial hamstrings (posterior). Thanks to fascial continuity, as the adductors become better organized, the pelvic floor benefits, which allows the fascial connection from the inner legs to the front of the spine to become evident.

Structurally, this advances the work of Session 2 to equalize span and create dynamic balance between the inner and outer lines of the legs and feet. It carries the work from the feet to the front of the lumbar spine.

Functionally, Session 4 connects the feet to the spine through the fascia of the medial line, which indirectly affects the location of the lumbo-dorsal hinge, which is key to contralaterality (see Session 2 discussion). Typically, both practitioner and client observe the legs seeming to reach out from the abdomen, yielding a longer stride as the body organizes toward its midline and upward. Clients report a sense of greater torso volume and heightened awareness to the prevertebral abdominal space.

> ### KEY POINT
>
> Thanks to fascial continuity, the effects of local interventions are felt at some distance from the work site. Fascial continuity even allows structural integrators to access and influence tissues that cannot be touched directly.

Session 5: Connect the Legs to the Front of the Spine

When span and tonus are balanced across large joints like the hip, gravity works through those joints. Session 5 addresses structures crossing the hip anteriorly—the quadriceps and iliopsoas. The territory includes the fascia of the abdominal wall, which enhances continuity of the legs with the lumbar spine via the iliopsoas. Parts of this territory that cannot be touched directly are affected through fascial continuity.

Structurally the goal is enough space and length along the anterior thigh and through the prevertebral region for full leg extension, as well as accommodation of the organs that occupy the pelvic/thoracic visceral prevertebral column (Schwind 2006). When the fascia has sufficient length and the deep flexors move freely within the abdominal cavity, the bony pelvis will rebalance over the feet, easing pelvic tilt and shift patterns (Fig. 7.3.3).

Functionally, only when the leg fully extends can the feet (especially the toes) truly propel the body forward and extend the spine. The psoas, which now connects the legs to the spine without interference from the pelvic structures, can stabilize the head of the femur to

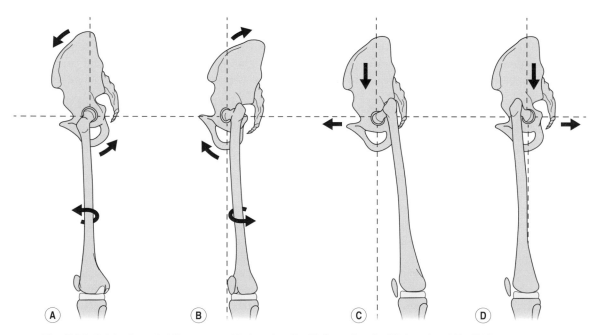

Fig. 7.3.3 Pelvic tilt and shift patterns. (A) Anterior tilt. (B) Posterior tilt. (C) Anterior shift. (D) Posterior shift. Reproduced with permission from Elizabeth Gaggini.

allow contralateral leg motion and the emergence of the functional core. Functional differentiation of the core transversus abdominus from the superficial rectus abdominus is essential. In walking, before the leg swings smoothly forward, gravity appears to release it from the front of the lumbar spine.

Session 6: Establish Posterior Length, Continuity, and Order

Session 6 addresses the posterior body, which is unified by a continuous fascial span from the soles of the feet all the way through the galea aponeurotica. This continuity allows local work to influence the entire posterior surface. Here, SI addresses deeper muscle chains—for example, biceps femoris/transversus abdominus/multifidus—and diagonal spans united by the lumbar fascia, for example, latissimus dorsi/gluteus maximus. This session presents the opportunity to address spinal and sacroiliac torsions and counter-torsions.

Structurally, SI releases pelvic and spinal rotations by rebalancing spans of fascia that influence the relative positions of the bones. Differentiation of myofascial layers encourages discriminated function, and differentiation of the posterior leg structures enhances leg extension.

Functionally, Session 6 enhances the leg-to-spine connection. This connection is key to the functional core, which emerges through the tendency of fascia to sense and communicate: weight or pressure triggers the mechano-sensors embedded in the plantar fascia, activating the deep biceps femoris/transversus abdominus/multifidus chain, which stabilizes the lumbar spine as a fixed point for the iliopsoas. Improved contralateral movement within the spine augments contralateral coordination between the pelvic and shoulder girdles. Finally, despite the tendency toward flexion throughout the entire human life cycle, all vertebrae should be capable of extension.

Session 7: Organize the Upper Pole

Though position potentiates movement, more is needed: preceding any movement is perception of and orientation to the ground through gravity, to three-dimensional space, and finally to objects and others. Several key components of the perceiving and orienting system—the suboccipital muscles, vestibular system, vision, hearing, and temporomandibular joint—are in the head and neck. To paraphrase Dr. Rolf, during neck work, our fingers are as close as they will ever get to the body's control structures.

As neck alignment influences occiput position, SI treats the neck and head together. Hypertonic sterno-cleidomastoids betray absence of core support for the neck; interfere with the deeper scalenes' fine motor activity; and actually reduce peripheral visual and auditory fields. We enhance cervical mobility, especially in extension, because an erect neck requires a balanced relationship among trapezius, SCM, splenius capitis, and longus capitis. Finally, the normal position of the head on the neck requires balanced tonus of the masseter and the supra- and infrahyoid muscles.

Structurally, Session 7 improves conditions for action of the suboccipitals: though they have many times more stretch receptors than any other muscles, their receptors do not activate an internal stretch reflex; instead, they inform the tonic function of the entire body. Thus optimizing suboccipital function touches the whole via the fascial system.

Functionally, because balanced scalene activity is key to free head and neck orientation, SI evokes the function of the prevertebral longus colli, which supports the neck and forms a core-stabilizing gestalt with transversus abdominus, multifidus, and iliopsoas. Working together, the scalenes and longus colli decompress the cervicals and allow deep breathing, whereas working alone, scalenes compress the cervicals into a hyperlordotic position and encourage shallow breathing. Because Session 7 is intimately involved with the senses, the work is more efficient when combined with education in perception and coordination.

Sessions 8 Through 10: Integrate the Girdles Within the Person, and the Person Within the Environment

Dr. Rolf observed, "Anybody can take a body apart . . . but only a few can put one together" (Rolf 1977). This *putting together* happens in Sessions 8 through 10. In differentiating myofascial structures in Sessions 1 through 7, the intent is largely within the body, which responds through better alignment in gravity, and support is essentially static, coming mainly from the ground. By contrast, the final sessions allow the body to integrate not only intrinsically but also within the environment and relative to others. The intent is beyond the body, with dynamic support coming from the hands as they relate through space to the outside.

The more differentiated body segments are, the more easily joints work, but for the segments to act in concert, they need integration as well. In each of Sessions 8 and 9, the practitioner seeks to improve the least integrated body area—often the pelvic girdle and legs in Session 8, followed by the shoulder girdle and arms in Session 9. In any case, one session accesses the *down* direction, mass and gravity, and the other the *up* direction, expansion and space.

The idea is to establish palintonic right angles in both the fascial and spatial planes. As the practitioner positions the fascia, the client moves to facilitate orderly transmission of motion through the joint and associated tissues. This capitalizes on fascia's physiological responses to changes in degree and direction of mechanical load. Because fascia is a body-wide mechanosensitive signaling network (Langevin 2006), it is from those right angles that contralateral movement at progressive levels of limbs, girdles, and spine emerges.

Whereas Sessions 8 and 9 address the pelvic and shoulder girdles to integrate the upper and lower bodies and improve how they relate as parts of a whole, Session 10 facilitates an integrated relationship of the person to objects and others in the environment. Its territory is the whole body. The typical pre-10 client has restrictions at the neck and ankles, which hearken to the initial functional issues of orientation to space and ground. This time, work with the superficial fascia enhances the client's ability to be fully present to the outside, while at the same time accessing support for the inside from the ground through gravity.

For Dr. Rolf, "The job in the 10th hour is a relating job. It's a relating of planes of space, but it is also a relating of planes of fascia. Now you can't get those planes until you get a vertical. You can't get a vertical except as you approximate these planes" (Rolf). Integration is more about conclusion than perfection. *Putting together* relates imperfect segments to constitute the most functional whole possible in the moment. It brings closure to the SI process and sets the client free to integrate changes.

However, SI produces changes not only in fascia but also in the client's perception, coordination, meaning (psychology), and way of being in the world. The effects of restrictions in these realms are often misperceived in terms of biomechanics. Clients who do not integrate these changes, as well, tend over time to reestablish their original tissue fixations.

Summary

Structural integration is grounded in two premises: first, that physical and personal well-being requires appropriate adaptation to the field of gravity, and second, that the primary organ of body structure is fascia. SI works because fascia is: (1) physically and functionally continuous; (2) responsive to gravity; (3) able to transmit locally registered information throughout the body; and (4) malleable due to its viscoelasticity. By exploiting these key characteristics of fascia as an organ of structure and communication, the traditional 10-session SI protocol delivers an orderly and well-supported arrangement of body segments in three-dimensional space along the imaginary plumb line and facilitates progressive levels of movement integration.

REFERENCES

Bricot, B., 2001. A reprogrammation Posturale Globale (Bushatsky, A., trans., second ed.). Posturologia, Ícone, São Paulo.

Langevin, H.M., 2006. Connective tissue: a body-wide signaling network? Med. Hypotheses 66, 1074–1077.

Rolf, I.P., 1977. Rolfing: The Integration of Human Structures. Dennis Landman, Santa Monica, CA.

Schleip, R., 2003. Fascial plasticity – a new neurobiological explanation. J. Bodyw. Mov. Ther. 7, 11–19 (Part 1); 7, 104–116 (Part 2).

Schwind, P., 2006. Fascial and Membrane Technique. Elsevier Ltd, Philadelphia (chap. 6).

BIBLIOGRAPHY

Random Trials in Normal Persons

Cottingham, J., 1988. Shifts in pelvic inclination angle and parasympathetic tone produced by Rolfing soft tissue manipulation. Phys. Ther. 68, 1364–1370.

Cottingham, J., Porges, S.W., Lyon, T., 1988. Effects of soft tissue mobilization (Rolfing pelvic lift) on parasympathetic tone in two age groups. Phys. Ther. 68, 352–356.

Weinberg, R.S., Hunt, V.V., 1979. Effects of structural integration on state-trait anxiety. J. Clin. Psychol. 35, 319–322.

Studies in Specific Patient Populations

Deutsch, J.E., Derr, L.L., Judd, P., Reuven, L.L., 2000. Treatment of chronic pain through the use of Structural Integration (Rolfing). Orthop. Phys. Ther. Clin. North Am. 9, 411–425.

Deutsch, J.E., Judd, P., DeMasi, I., 1997. Structural integration applied to patients with a primary neurologic diagnosis: two case studies. Neurol. Rep. 21, 161–162.

James, H., Castaneda, L., Miller, M.E., Findley, T., 2009. Rolfing structural integration treatment of cervical spine dysfunction. J. Bodyw. Mov. Ther. 13, 229–238.

Perry, J., Jones, M.H., Thomas, L., 1981. Functional evaluation of Rolfing in cerebral palsy. Dev. Med. Child. Neurol. 23, 717–729.

Talty, C.M., DeMasi, I., Deutsch, J.E., 1998. Structural integration applied to patients with chronic fatigue syndrome: a retrospective chart review. J. Orthop. Sports Phys. Ther. 27, 83.

Abstracts of Case Studies Regarding Specific Conditions

Prado P., 2012. The case study method: year two of the ABR/Uniitalo SI Postgraduate Program. Scientific Exploration of Rolfing® SI in the holistic paradigm. Structural Integration. December 2012. Available from: http://www.pedroprado.com.br/imgs/pdf/1242.pdf.

Prado P., 2015. The case study method: the latest from the ABR/Uniitalo SI Postgraduate Program. Scientific Exploration of Rolfing® SI in the holistic paradigm. Structural Integration. March 2015. Available from: http://www.pedroprado.com.br/imgs/pdf/1341.pdf.

The full case studies are available through the Ida P. Rolf Library of Structural Integration. Available from: https://pedroprado.com.br/?lang=en.

Myofascial Induction Approaches

Andrzej Pilat

CHAPTER CONTENTS

INTRODUCTION

Myofascial induction therapy (MIT) is a hands-on, full-body approach focusing on restoration of altered fascial tissue function. During the application, the clinician stretches or compresses the specific body area in order to transmit a low-intensity mechanical input and carries out other procedures aimed at restoring body movement variables (sliding between fascial planes, viscoelasticity, etc.), through transverse and longitudinal sliding applications. These actions modify fascial dynamic restrictions in order to reestablish a mechano-chemical equilibrium in and beyond the fascial network. It is hypothesized that this procedure can restore the ability to move more efficiently and to achieve better functionality with lower energy expenditure.

Fascial restriction is described as any impediment to optimal gliding, at both macroscopic and microscopic fascial organizational levels, between endofascial fibers and interfascial planes. Such restriction can cause anomalous tension and movement disorders.

One possible reason for a restriction of the fascial tissues may be excessive stimulation of collagen production inducing fibrosis, resulting in loss of its smoothness and/ or isotropy and creation of entrapment areas. This suggests that such entrapment areas may alter physiological body movements in relation to amplitude, velocity, resistance, and coordination, altering body homeostasis.

In the presence of long-term restrictions, fascial tissue becomes overloaded and suffers dysfunctional consequences. These changes first affect the loose connective tissues, followed by reorganization of regular or irregular dense connective tissue, such as tendons, ligaments, or capsules, creating excessive density and reorientation of fibers. Fascial restrictions of short durations affect the tissues locally, whereas restrictions of long duration induce a more global dysfunction pattern (Langevin 2006).

Fascial tissue is related to the interchange of body fluids and to mechanoreceptor coordination. In addition, because of the close relationship between the perimysium and the neuromuscular spindles, fascia can operate the excitability of the motoneurons and peripherally coordinate muscle contraction (Stecco et al. 2016). A decrease of fascial mobility can alter the blood circulation and cause ischemia, deteriorating muscle fiber quality. And because many mechanoreceptors are embedded within fascia, altered proprioceptive afferents can change the ability of optimal muscle tonic contraction. As a result, alterations in stabilizing functions and in the coordination of joint movements may occur, with consequent difficulty of joint compression at its optimal point of action, possibly leading to joint overload, inflammation, and/or pain in myofascial structures.

Some theories suggest that the three-dimensional fascial network can be involved in pain transmission, with peripheral pain possibly having an origin in the connective tissue (Liptan 2009). Taguchi et al. (2009) suggest that the thoracolumbar fascia is an important source of nociceptive input in chronic LBP patients.

Various concepts exist related to the manual treatment of fascial system restrictions, with different names used to describe similar treatment approaches. The conceptual bases of most of these are similar. Further clinical research is needed in order to unify and validate these clinical procedures (Remvig 2007). An interesting discussion on this topic published by Leon Chaitow compared both names myofascial release and myofascial induction and concludes: "MFR (MIT) appears to have increasing degrees of evidence, as safe and effective manual therapy approaches, in management of musculoskeletal pain and dysfunction. Returning to the question in the title of this editorial as to whether the method should be called Myofascial Release or Myofascial Induction? The latter would seem to be more appropriate" (Chaitow 2017). MIT aims to be a treatment that focuses on the patient (Pilat 2015).

KEY POINT

"The MFR (MIT) appears to have increasing degrees of evidence, as safe and effective manual therapy approaches, in management of musculoskeletal pain and dysfunction. Returning to the question in the title of this editorial as to whether the method should be called Myofascial Release or Myofascial Induction? The latter would seem to be more appropriate" (Chaitow 2017).

NEUROPHYSIOLOGICAL MECHANISMS FOR RELEASING THE RESTRICTIONS OF THE FASCIAL SYSTEM

The clinical hypothesis of MIT is that it produces a mechanical stimulus in the connective tissue. The effect may occur at micro- or macroscopic levels of fascial organization and may include a group of cells, tissues, organs, or the whole body.

Anatomical analysis in unembalmed specimens confirms continuity of the fascial system through the entire body (Fig. 7.4.1). Benjamin (2009), Stecco et al.

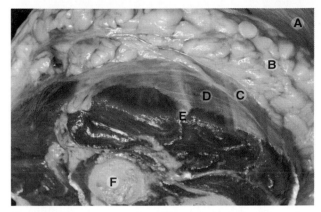

Fig. 7.4.1 Transverse section of forearm. Note fascial continuity from the skin up to the bone. (A) Skin; (B) "honey comb" fascia with the fat nodules, (C) superficial fascia, (D) deep fascia; (E) intermuscular septa; and (F) bone.

(2008), Pilat (2010), van der Wal (2009), and Mass and Sandercock (2010) all demonstrate movement continuity on macroscopic levels, focused not only on the fascia-to-bone connections but also on the direct fascia-to-fascia transmission in both articular and intermuscular links (Fig. 7.4.2). Ingber (Wang et al. 2009) and Langevin (2010), among others, have demonstrated dynamic continuity at the microscopic, intracellular, and intercellular levels.

In 1997, Ingber proposed intercommunication systems based on tensegrity principles (Ingber 1997). This

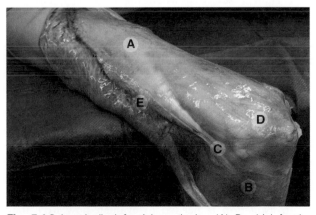

Fig. 7.4.2 Longitudinal fascial continuity. (A) Brachial fascia; (B) antebrachial fascia; (C) fascia-to-fascia connection between brachial and antebrachial deep fascia at the posterior aspect of upper limb; (D) triceps brachii insertion (tendon-to-bone connection); and (E) superficial-to-deep fascia continuity.

suggests a system of shared tensions in the distribution of mechanical forces, at multiple body levels, possibly explaining the global reaction of the fascial system in response to mechanical stimuli. Different studies (for example, Wang et al. 2009) have shown that cell dynamic and active responses of the cytoskeleton, responding to mechanical forces from the extracellular matrix, induce tissue remodeling at both cellular and subcellular levels. Considering that the structure of the body follows the principles of hierarchical assembly, the previously discussed process is not limited to cells but also involves tissues and organs (Huang and Ingber 2000). Ingber (Wang et al. 2009) showed continuity of mechanical stimuli from the cytoskeleton to intranuclear level, and Langevin (2010) demonstrated mechanical impulse continuity from the skin to the nucleus membrane in mouse fibroblasts.

In conclusion, any action performed locally can potentially involve function throughout the body. The correction of myofascial dysfunction can take place in only one, or in different, system segments. Finally, the abundant innervation of the fascial system (of particular importance are the nonmyelinated "C" fibers, polymodal receptors) will also be stimulated by manual impulse. It stimulates the peripheral, medullary, and supramedullary modulation mechanisms and can influence any expression of the nervous system.

It is hypothesized that mechanical stimuli can create at least four types of reactions:

- Piezoelectricity: This is a phenomenon exhibited by certain crystals that, when subject to mechanical tensions, acquire a polarization in their atomic structure, generating a difference of electrical potential and loads at their surface (Pilat 2003). The basic properties of the organism (i.e., elasticity, flexibility, elongation, resistance) depend to a great extent upon the ability to maintain a continuous information flow. Oschman (2003) affirms that information is transmitted electrically through the connective tissue matrix. Because collagen may be interpreted as a semiconductor, it may be capable of forming an integrated electronic network enabling the interconnection of all fascial system components. Further investigation is needed to evaluate how MIT may influence this property of the body network.
- Dynamics of the myofibroblasts response: The dynamic behavior of the fascial tissue depends on the properties of the extracellular matrix and the active (dynamic) remodeling of the fibroblast cytoskeleton (Langevin et al. 2011). The current understanding of the regulation of fascial stiffness seems to be subject to active cellular contraction, which can increase the stiffness of fascial tissues and thus contribute to musculoskeletal dynamics (Schleip et al. 2019). Studies focusing on skin-healing processes and pathologies, such as Dupuytren's contracture, plantar fasciitis, and frozen shoulder, that relate to actin microfilament contraction strongly support this reasoning (Gabbiani 2007). Chaudhry et al. (2008), using a 3-D mathematical model for deformation of human fascia, suggest that mechanical forces applied during manual techniques can create mechanical changes in loose connective tissue (i.e., superficial nasal fascia). Changes in the resting tone of skeletal muscle fibers can transmit their tension force to the fascial tissue.
- Viscoelasticity: This is a property of fascia that describes the characteristics it displays of viscosity and elasticity, when undergoing deformation, during application of, for example, stretching or shear forces. Elasticity describes a process such as stretching in which the structure returns to normal once the stress ceases; viscosity involves the diffusion of atoms or molecules inside an amorphous material, such as the colloidal extracellular matrix (ECM) (Pilat 2018). The viscoelastic properties of fascia have been observed in numerous studies: thoracolumbar fascia (Yahia et al. 1993), subcutaneous fascia of rats (Iatridis et al. 2003), the fascia lata, plantar fascia, and nasal fascia (Chaudhry et al. 2008). Also, it has been established that connective tissue fibroblasts can indirectly influence the stiffness of the matrix (passive remodeling) through the production and degradation of matrix proteins (Prajapati et al. 2000).
- Concepts for practical treatment applications have been defined by Rolf (1994), Cantu and Grodin (2001), and Pilat (2003).
- Interoception remodeling: The remodeling of the environment (the matrix) of the fast conduction and unmyelinic free nerve ending mechanoreceptors present in the fascial tissue could trigger a new homeostatic body attitude, giving rise to a new perceptual body experience (subjective body image). This subjective image of "tension relief" could contribute to a better "sensation of movement," improving the dynamics of body movement (Craig 2003; Tsakiris and Critchley 2016). Researchers report the activation of

the interoceptive homeostatic afferent pathway, the participation of the cannabinoid system (McPartland 2008), the response through the "ideomotor movement" (Dorko 2003), and the involvement of the emotional motor system and pandiculation (Simmonds et al. 2012).

KEY POINT

MIT is a therapeutic concept belonging to manual therapy, aimed at the functional restoration of the altered fascial system. MIT is a process of assessment and treatment in which the clinician transfers a slight force (traction and/or compression) and also other procedures aimed at restoring body movement variables through transverse and longitudinal sliding applications to the target tissue (Pilat 2012), facilitating the recovery of the fascial system quality.

METHOD DESCRIPTION

The term "induction" is related to the facilitation of movement rather than a passive stretching of the fascial system. The result is a reciprocal reaction from the body involving the biochemical, metabolic signaling reaction and, finally, the physiological responses. This process aims to reshape the quality of the extracellular matrix of the connective tissue to facilitate and optimize the transfer of information to and within the fascial system (Chiquet et al. 2003; Pilat 2017). It is a process controlled by the central nervous system in which the practitioner acts as a facilitator (Pilat and Castro, 2018). It is important to note that the approach seeks local corrections but also focuses on the recovery of global dynamic body balance in the relief of pain (Fig. 7.4.3).

The applications of MIT suggested in the next section are based on the clinical experience of the author and his teaching team (Pilat 2003) and are based on the theoretical frameworks discussed previously. MIT may be combined with other manual therapy strategies with therapeutic exercise or an exclusive treatment procedure.

General Observations for Clinical Applications

- The evaluation of fascial dysfunction should be included into clinical reasoning processes. An exhaustive case intake is required, with annotations concerning the duration of symptoms and a visual analog scale (VAS) evaluation.
- We suggest exploration of general posture disorders and local dysfunction testing.
- Biomechanically, the myofascial system responds to compression and traction forces (Chaudhry et al. 2008). These two mechanical strategies can be used when applying MIT.
- The direction of the releasing movement is toward restriction barriers. Arbitrary directions of tissue engagement should be avoided. Restrictions may occur in various directions and planes. They may also occur in different directions in the same plane, or in the same direction in various planes, or in different planes in various directions. See also Chapter 7.5 for discussion of indirect myofascial release methods.
- There is no need for active muscle contraction by the patient, who may be asked to maintain a state of active passivity.

Clinical Procedure Principles

- The therapist applies a slow, three-dimensional compression or traction causing the tissue to become tense. This is referred to as the first restriction barrier (Fig. 7.4.4).
- The applied pressure is constant during the first 60 to 90 seconds. This is the time required for releasing the first restriction barrier according to the viscoelastic response (Chaudhry et al. 2008).
- During the first phase of the technique, the therapist barely causes the tissue to move.
- The impulse of a three dimensional and slowly applied compression or traction force generates tissue remodeling, manifesting itself with movement. The direction of this movement is called "facilitation path."
- Upon overcoming the first restriction barrier, the therapist accompanies the movement in the direction of the facilitation, pausing at each new barrier.
- In each application, the therapist may overcome three to six consecutive barriers. The time required is usually 3 to 5 minutes. Depending on the severity of the lesion, the process may take up to 30 minutes.
- The tension applied to the tissue must be constant, so the pressure (force) applied may need to be modified after overcoming the first barrier. Pressure should be reduced if there is an increase in pain and/or excessive movement or activity.

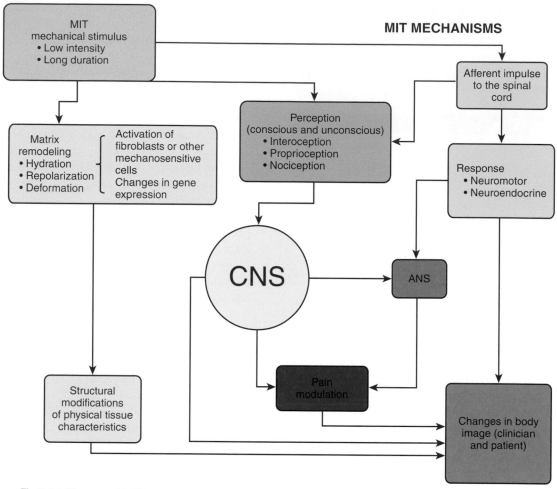

MIT MECHANISMS

Fig.7.4.3 Diagram of MIT´s conceptual reasoning process. Modified from Pilat, A., 2017. Myofascial induction therapy. In: Liem, T., Tozzi, P., Chila, A. (Eds.). Fascia in the Osteopathic Field. Handspring Publishing, Pencaitland, East Lothian. ANS, autonomic nervous system; CNS, central nervous system; MIT, myofascial induction therapy.

SCIENTIFIC EVIDENCE RELATED TO THE RESULTS IN THE MYOFASCIAL APPROACH

Studies have focused on microscopic changes in connective tissue and on clinical reactions, both in pathological and healthy subjects.

- Leonard et al. (2009), studying wound-healing processes in 20 patients with diabetic foot ulcers, concluded that connective tissue manipulation improved peripheral circulation and also enhanced wound healing.

- Significant differences between pre- and postmeasurements of pressure pain thresholds, with decreasing sensitivity of myofascial trigger points, were reported in adductor longus strains (Robba and Pajaczkowski 2009), upper trapezius muscle, and cervical muscles (Hou et al. 2002).

- Arguisuelas et al. (2019) concluded that MFR therapy produced a significant improvement in both pain and disability.

- Marshall et al. (2009) concluded that myofascial release reduced the severity and intensity of muscle pain in people with chronic fatigue syndrome.

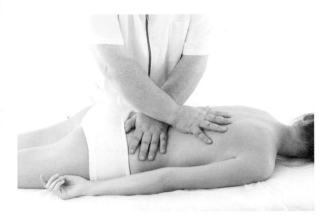

Fig. 7.4.4 Cross hands technique on the thoracolumbar region. The aim is remodeling of connective tissue in order to facilitate gliding movement at intrinsic and extrinsic structure levels. The therapist is standing at the level of the prone patient's back and places crossed hands on the patient's back, pressing with a slight force toward the table and craniocaudally, following the principles of induction movement.

- Hicks et al. (2009) reported that human fibroblasts secrete the soluble mediators of myoblast differentiation, and that myofascial release can regulate muscle development.
- An objective form for evaluating the effect of MIT applications in muscular lesions with dynamic sonoelastography was reported by Martínez (2010) (Fig. 7.4.5).
- Ortiz-Comino et al. (2018) recorded that "One session of myofascial induction treatment increases mandibular opening, cervical mobility, and craniocervical motor control in head and neck cancer survivors compared with a placebo intervention."

- Heart rate variability and blood pressure recovery improved following myofascial release, after physically stressful situations, compared with sham electrotherapy treatment (Arroyo-Morales et al. 2008a).
- Pinheiro et al. (2018) affirmed, "Myofascial Induction of quadratus lumborum II may have an immediate influence in postural orientation of asymptomatic standing subjects by increasing body verticality; nevertheless, the results found deserve further research. This finding highlights the possibility of including fascial system-related approaches in the intervention of individuals with altered postural control."
- Arroyo-Morales et al. (2008b) reported that application of an active recovery protocol using whole-body myofascial treatment reduces EMG amplitude and vigor when applied as a passive recovery technique, after a high-intensity exercise protocol.
- Application of a single session of a manual therapy (including Myofascial Induction) program produces an immediate increase of heart rate variability and a decrease in tension, anger status, and perceived pain in patients with chronic tension-type headache (Toro-Velasco et al. 2009).
- Arroyo-Morales et al. (2009), in a randomized, single blind, placebo-controlled study, reported that myofascial induction may encourage recovery from a transient immunosuppression state induced by exercise, in healthy active women.
- Saíz-Llamosas et al. (2009) concluded that the application of a cervical myofascial induction technique resulted in an increase in cervical flexion, extension, and left lateral-flexion, but not rotation motion in a cohort of healthy subjects. No changes in PPT in either C5 C6

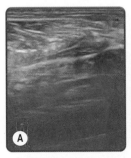 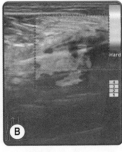 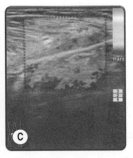

Fig. 7.4.5 Sonoelastography images of a 3-week muscle injury evolution (A, B). Image (C) taken after 30 minutes of MIT application. Note the significant change in local elasticity determined by the color scale. Courtesy Martínez, R., 2010 (unpublished). Presentation II. Scientific Fascia Research Symposium at the EUF (Escuela Universitaria de Fisioterapia), ONCE Universidad Autónoma de Madrid, Madrid.

zygapophyseal joint (local point) or tibialis anterior muscle (distant point) were found.

- In a study involving 41 healthy male volunteers randomly assigned to experimental or control groups, significantly decreased anxiety levels were observed in healthy young adults after the application of myofascial induction treatment. Significantly lower systolic blood pressure values versus baseline levels were also observed (Fernández-Pérez et al. 2008).

In conclusion, MIT has been shown to encourage:

- more efficient circulation of antibodies in the ground substance;
- an increase in the blood supply (release of histamine) in the region of restriction;
- improved orientation in fibroblast mechanics;
- greater blood supply to the nervous system;
- an increase in metabolite flow to and from tissues, facilitating the recovery process.

Castro-Martín et al. (2017) report that a single myofascial induction session decreases pain intensity and improves neck-shoulder range of movement to a greater degree than placebo electrotherapy for breast cancer survivors experiencing pain.

Summary

Myofascial induction therapy (MIT) is a nonstandard treatment approach that, under different names, is currently used by a considerable number of therapists worldwide. MIT meets the criteria that allow its use as a manual treatment modality. The most relevant evidence relates to:
- anatomical fascial continuity;
- intra- and interfascial force transmission;
- scientific validation of treatment parameters;
- definition of possible side effects;
- identification of contraindications, such as aneurysms, systemic diseases, inflammatory soft tissue process in the acute phase, acute circulatory deficiency, advanced diabetes, and anticoagulant therapy.

At present, clinical evidence is limited and unified research criteria should aim to identify:
- more objective evaluation processes;
- classification of strategies (local versus global approach);
- unification of parameters of force, timing, intensity, and frequency of application;
- identification and analysis of responses in different body systems;
- identification and classification of nonresponders;
- analysis of long-term results.

Summary

"MFR (MIT) appears to have increasing degrees of evidence, as safe and effective manual therapy approaches, in management of musculoskeletal pain and dysfunction. Returning to the question in the title of this editorial as to whether the method should be called Myofascial Release or Myofascial Induction? The latter would seem to be more appropriate" (Chaitow 2017). The application of the Myofascial Induction Therapy (MIT) is recommended in therapeutic interventions which focus to the promotion and recovery of well-being and also looking to the benefit of the performance of activities that imply movement as a form of expression.

The term "induction" is related to the facilitation of movement rather than a passive stretching of the fascial system. The MIT aspires to be the patient-focused approach.

REFERENCES

Arguisuelas, M.D., Lisón, J.F., Doménech-Fernández, J., Martínez-Hurtado, I., Salvador Coloma, P., Sánchez-Zuriaga, D., 2019. Effects of myofascial release in erector spinae myoelectric activity and lumbar spine kinematics in nonspecific chronic low back pain: Randomized controlled trial. Clin. Biomech. (Bristol, Avon) 63, 27–33.

Arroyo-Morales, M., Olea, N., Martínez, M., Moreno-Lorenzo, C., Díaz-Rodríguez, L., Hidalgo-Lozano, A., 2008a. Effects of myofascial release after high-intensity exercise: a randomized clinical trial. J. Manipulative Physiol. Ther. 31, 217–223.

Arroyo-Morales, M., Olea, N., Martínez, M.M., Hidalgo-Lozano, A., Ruiz-Rodríguez, C., Díaz-Rodríguez, L., 2008b. Psychophysiological effects of massage-myofascial release after exercise. J. Altern. Complement. Med. 14, 1223–1229.

Arroyo-Morales, M., Olea, N., Ruíz, C., et al., 2009. Massage after exercise-responses of immunologic and endocrine markers. J. Strength Cond. Res. 23, 638–644.

Benjamin, M., 2009. The fascia of the limbs and back – a review. J. Anat. 214, 1–18.

Cantu, T.I., Grodin, A.J., 2001. Myofascial Manipulation: Theory and Clinical Application. Aspen Publishers, Maryland.

Castro-Martín, E., Ortiz-Comino, L., Gallart-Aragón, T., Esteban-Moreno, B., Arroyo-Morales M., Galiano-Castillo, N., 2017. Myofascial induction effects on neck-shoulder pain breast cancer survivors: randomized, single-blind, placebo-controlled crossover design. Arch. Phys. Med. Rehabil. 98, 832–840.

Chaitow, L., 2017. What's in a name: myofascial release or myofascial induction? J. Bodyw. Mov. Ther. 21, 749–751.

Chaudhry, H., Schleip, R., Zhiming, J.I., Bukiet, B., Maney, M., Findley, T., 2008. Three-dimensional mathematical model for deformation of human fasciae in manual therapy. J. Am. Osteopath. Assoc. 108, 379–390.

Chiquet, M., Renedo, A.S., Huber, F., Flück, M., 2003. How do fibroblasts translate mechanical signals into changes in extracellular matrix production? Matrix Biol. 22, 73–80.

Craig, A.D., 2003. Interoception: the sense of the physiological condition of the body. Curr. Opin. Neurobiol. 13, 500–505.

Dorko, B.L., 2003. The analgesia of movement: ideomotor activity and manual care. J. Osteopath. Med. 6, 93–95.

Fernández-Pérez, A.M., Peralta-Ramírez, M.I., Pilat, A., Villaverde, C., 2008. Effects of myofascial induction techniques on physiologic and psychologic parameters. J. Altern. Complement. Med. 14, 807–811.

Gabbiani, G., 2007. Evolution and clinical implications of the myofibroblast concept. In: Huijing, P.A., Hollander, P., Findley, T.W., et al. (Eds.), Fascia Research II. Elsevier GmbH, Munich, pp. 56–60.

Hicks, M., Meltzer, K., Cao, T., Standley, P.R., 2009. Human fibroblast (HF) model of repetitive motion strain (RMS) and myofascial release (FR): potential roles in muscle development. In: Huijing, P.A., Hollander, P., Findley, T.W., et al. (Eds.), Fascia Research II. Elsevier GmbH, Munich, p. 259.

Hou, C.R., Tsai, L.C., Cheng, K.F., Chung, K.C., Hong, C.Z., 2002. Immediate effects of various physical therapeutic modalities on cervical myofascial pain and trigger point sensitivity. Arch. Phys. Med. Rehabil. 82, 1406–1414.

Huang, S., Ingber, D., 2000. Shape-dependent control of cell growth, differentiation, and apoptosis: switching between attractors in cell regulatory networks. Exp. Cell. Res. 261, 91–103.

Iatridis, J.C., Wu, J., Yandow, J.A., Langevin, H.M., 2003. Subcutaneous tissue mechanical behavior is linear and viscoelastic under uniaxial tension. Connect. Tissue Res. 44, 208–217.

Ingber, D., 1997. Tensegrity: the architectural basis of cellular mechanotransduction. Annu. Rev. Physiol. 59, 575–599.

Langevin, H.M., 2006. Connective tissue: a body-wide signaling network? Med. Hypotheses 66, 1074–1077.

Langevin, H.M., 2010. Tissue stretch induces nuclear remodeling in connective tissue fibroblasts. Histochem. Cell. Biol. 133, 405–415.

Langevin, H.M., Bouffard, N.A., Fox, J.R., et al. 2011. Fibroblast cytoskeletal remodeling contributes to connective tissue tension. J. Cell. Physiol. 226, 1166–1175.

Leonard, J.H., Teng, S.C., Gan, J.H., et al., 2009. Physiological effects of connective tissue manipulation on diabetic foot ulcer. In: Huijing, P.A., Hollander, P., Findley, T.W. et al. (Eds.), Fascia Research II. Elsevier GmbH, Munich, p. 95.

Liptan, L., 2009. Fascia: A missing link in our understanding of the pathology of fibromyalgia. J. Bodyw. Mov. Ther. 14, 3–12.

Marshall, R., Paula, L., McFadyen, A.K., Wood, L., 2009. Evaluating the effectiveness of myofascial release to reduce pain in people with chronic fatigue syndrome (CFS): A pilot study. In: Huijing, P.A., Hollander, P., Findley, T.W., et al. (Eds.), Fascia Research II. Elsevier GmbH, Munich, p. 305.

Martínez, R., 2010. [unpublished] Presentation. II Scientific Fascia Research Symposium, at the EUF, ONCE Universidad Autónoma de Madrid, Madrid.

Mass, H., Sandercock, T.G., 2010. Transmission between synergistic skeletal muscles through connective tissue linkages. J. Biomed. Biotechnol. 2010, 575672.

McPartland, J.M., 2008. Expression of the endocannabinoid system in fibroblasts and myofascial tissues. J. Bodyw. Mov. Ther. 12, 169–182.

Ortiz-Comino, L., Martin-Martin L., Castro-Martín, E., et al., 2018. Effects of myofascial induction on mobility and motor control in head and neck cancer survivors: a randomized, crossover, and single blind study. J. Bodyw. Mov. Ther. 22, 861–862.

Oschman, J.L., 2003. Energy Medicine in Therapeutics and Human Performance. Nature's own Research Association Dover, New Hampshire.

Pilat, A., 2003. Inducción Miofascial. MacGraw-Hill, Madrid.

Pilat, A., 2010. Myofascial induction. In: Chaitow, L., Jones, R. (Eds.), Practical Physical Medicine Approaches to Chronic Pelvic Pain (CPP) & Dysfunction. Churchill Livingstone, Elsevier, London.

Pilat A. 2012. Myofascial induction approaches. In: Schleip R., Findley T.W., Chaitow L., Huijing P.A. (Eds.), Fascia: The Tensional Network of the Human Body. Elsevier, Churchill Livingstone, Edinburgh.

Pilat, A., 2015. Myofascial induction approaches. In: Fernández-de-las-Peñas, C., Cleland, J., Dommerholt, J. (Eds.), Manual Therapy for Musculoskeletal Pain Syndromes of the Upper and Lower Quadrants: An Evidence and Clinical Informed Approach. Elsevier, London.

Pilat, A., 2017. Myofascial Induction Therapy. In: Liem, T., Tozzi, P., Chila, A. (Eds.), Fascia in the Osteopathic Field. Handspring Publishing, Pencaitland, East Lothian.

Pilat, A., 2018. Myofascial Induction Approach. In: Chaitow, L. (Ed.), Fascial Dysfunction. Manual Therapy Approaches, second ed. Handspring Pencaitland, East Lothian.

Pilat, A., Castro-Martín, E., 2018. Myofascial Induction approaches in temporomandibular disorders. In: Fernández-de-las-Peñas C, Mesa-Jiménez, J.(eds). Temporomandibular Disorders, p.191. Handspring Publishing. Pencaitland, East Lothian

Pinheiro, A.R., Cunha, C., Fernandes, A.R., et al. 2018. Immediate effects of myofascial induction of quadratus lumborum in postural orientation of standing asymptomatic subjects. J. Bodyw. Mov. Ther. 22, 856.

Prajapati, R.T., Eastwood, M., Brown, R.A., 2000. Duration and orientation of mechanical loads determine fibroblast cyto‚Äêmechanical activation: Monitored by protease release. Wound Repair Regen. 8, 238–246.

Remvig, L., 2007. Fascia research. Myofascial release: An evidence based treatment concept. In: Huijing, P.A., Hollander, P., Findley, T.W., et al. (Eds.), Fascia Research II. Elsevier GmbH, Munich.

Robba, A., Pajaczkowski, J., 2009. Prospective investigation on hip adductor strains using myofascial release. In: Huijing, P.A., Hollander, P., Findley, T.W., et al. (Eds.), Fascia Research II. Elsevier GmbH, Munich, p. 96.

Rolf, I., 1994. La Integración de las Estructuras del Cuerpo Humano. Ediciones Urano, Barcelona.

Saíz-Llamosas, J.R., Fernández-Pérez, A.M., Fajardo-Rodríguez, M.F., Pilat, A., Valenza-Demet, G., Fernández-de-Las-Peñas, C., 2009. Changes in neck mobility and pressure pain threshold levels following a cervical myofascial induction technique in pain-free healthy subjects. J. Manipulative Physiol. Ther. 32, 352–357.

Schleip, R., Gabbiani, G., Wilke, J., et al., 2019. Fascia is able to actively contract and may thereby influence musculoskeletal dynamics: a histochemical and mechanographic investigation. Front. Physiol. 10, 336.

Simmonds, N., Miller, P., Gemmell, H., 2012. A theoretical framework for the role of fascia in manual therapy. J. Bodyw. Mov. Ther. 16, 83–93.

Stecco, A., Stern, R., Fantoni, I., et al. 2016. Fascial disorders: implications for treatment. PM R. 8, 161–168.

Stecco, C., Porzionato, A., Macchi, V., et al., 2008. The expansions of the pectoral girdle muscles onto the brachial fascia. Cells Tissues Organs 188, 320–329.

Taguchi, T., Tesarz, J., Mense, S., 2009. The thoracolumbar fascia as a source of low back pain. In: Huijing, P.A., Hollander, P., Findley, T.W., et al. (Eds.), Fascia Research II. Elsevier GmbH, Munich, p. 251.

Toro-Velasco, C., Arroyo-Morales, M., Fernández-de-Las-Peñas, C., Cleland, J.A., Barrero-Hernández, F.J., 2009. Short-term effects of manual therapy on heart rate variability, mood state, and pressure pain sensitivity in patients with chronic tension-type headache. J. Manipulative Physiol. Ther. 32, 527–535.

Tsakiris, M., Critchley, H., 2016. Interoception beyond homeostasis: affect, cognition and mental health. Phil. Trans. R. Soc. Lond. B Biol. Sci. 371, 20160002.

van der Wal, J., 2009. The architecture of the connective tissue in the musculoskeletal system. Int. J. Ther. Massage Bodywork 2, 9–23.

Wang, N., Tytell, J., Ingber, D., 2009. Mechanotransduction at a distance: mechanically coupling the extracellular matrix with the nucleus. Science 10, 75–81.

Yahia, L.H., Pigeon, P., DesRosiers, E.A., 1993. Viscoelastic properties of the human lumbodorsal fascia. J. Biomed. Eng. 15, 425–429.

Osteopathy and Fascia in Clinical Practice

Hollis H. King

CHAPTER CONTENTS

INTRODUCTION

In virtually every osteopathic evaluation and manipulative procedure, consideration of fascial elements is explicitly acknowledged and in some instances is the primary focus of the evaluation and treatment in osteopathic practice. The founder of osteopathic medicine, Andrew Taylor Still, DO, is noted for writings regarding fascia central and extraordinary properties related to manual treatment and properties of human nature and disease: "I write at length of the universality of the fascia to impress the reader with the idea that this connecting substance must be free at all parts to receive and discharge all fluids, and eject all impurities. . . . A knowledge of the universal extent of the fascia is imperative, and is one of the greatest aids to the person who seeks the causes of disease" (Still 1902, 61).

 KEY POINT

A. T. Still is arguably the first of modern era anatomists and medical clinicians to place fascia in the forefront of medical diagnosis and treatment (Fig. 7.5.1). Still's emphasis on the nature of fascia is seen in virtually all manual medicine and manual therapy traditions extant today.

There is ample evidence that the manipulation techniques predominantly used by Still would currently be considered as articulatory and myofascial release maneuvers (Van Buskirk 2018).

Anticipating an anatomical finding amply explicated in this volume, Brous (1997, 23–24) has stated: "If all other organs and tissues were removed from the body, with the fascia kept intact, one would still have the replica of the human body."

The principle of the continuity of fascia throughout the body is a mainstay of osteopathic manipulative treatment (OMT) and has been adopted by virtually all professions who deliver healthcare service by application of manually guided contact with patients and clients.

To illustrate the central place of fascia in OMT, examples from the major, most frequently used modalities are described. This is followed by brief descriptions of formulations as to the nature of human fascia as it impacts medical and therapeutic considerations of human anatomy and physiology.

FASCIA IN THE PERSPECTIVE OF OSTEOPATHIC MANIPULATIVE TREATMENT

High-Velocity, Low-Amplitude Method or Impulse Techniques

High-velocity, low-amplitude (HVLA) procedure is commonly applied in manual therapy/manual medicine

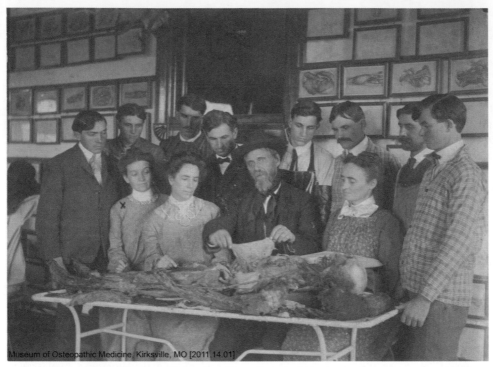

Museum of Osteopathic Medicine, Kirksville, MO [2011.14.01]

Fig. 7.5.1 Andrew Taylor Still in a Dissection Class. Typical of his emphasis on fascia, he appears to be holding abdominal fascia. Circa 1906. Reprinted with permission of the Museum of Osteopathic Medicine.

as well as OMT. From the perspective of OMT, HVLA is defined as "An osteopathic method in which the restrictive barrier is engaged in one or more planes of motion and then a rapid, therapeutic force of brief duration traveling a short distance is applied within the anatomic range of motion" (Educational Council on Osteopathic Principles (ECOP) 2018). Because the "restrictive barrier" almost always involves dysfunctional ligaments and tendons, instruction in how to perform the HVLA method is accompanied by a detailed consideration of the fascia, in and around any joint where the method may be applied.

The restrictive barrier is determined by careful precise palpation of the condition of muscle and fascia derangement, a palpatory skill developed through osteopathic training that requires the ability to distinguish altered conditions of muscle and fascia.

Apropos to the application of HVLA, and any of the following OMT modalities, is the unique approach to musculoskeletal system assessment that originated in osteopathy and the osteopathic medical profession. The osteopathic diagnosis (required in U.S. practice documentation) and evaluation (recorded in patient charts

in countries where osteopaths are registered) is called *somatic dysfunction*, a medical diagnosis described in the *International Classification of Diseases*, tenth ed. (ICD-10) (World Health Organization 2016). The components of somatic dysfunction *that identify changes from the norm by using the mnemonic TART include: (1) Are there palpable tissue texture changes (T)? (2) Is there visually observable asymmetry (A)? (3) Is there restriction of motion (R)? (4) Does the palpatory exam elicit tenderness (T)?* (Giusti and Hruby 2018, 818). In the United States the treatment of somatic dysfunction is by the medical procedure of OMT, designated as such in the American Medical Association's *Current Procedural Terminology* (2020).

Muscle Energy Technique

Muscle energy technique is defined as "a direct treatment method that the patient's muscles are employed upon request, from a precisely controlled position, in a specific direction, and against a distinctly executed physician counterforce. First described in 1948 by Fred Mitchell, Sr, DO." (ECOP 2018).

Because tendons attach to virtually all muscles, fascia is involved in almost all muscle energy manipulative techniques. Ehrenfeuchter (2018) describes the central place of fascia in muscle energy technique: "Golgi tendon organ: a spindle-shaped end organ within a tendon that provides information about muscle tension. It becomes relatively stretched during muscle contraction where the overall length of the muscle does not change. When a critical amount of tension occurs, its increased activity provides a reflex relaxation of the muscle as a whole."

 KEY POINT

In every OMT procedure the anatomical and physiological condition of fascia is an integral part of the process of delivering the manually guided forces in treatment and also is assessed and taken into account in every palpatory evaluation and diagnosis.

Strain/Counterstrain Technique

Also called counterstrain, the OMT procedure developed in 1955 by Jones (1964) is defined as "an osteopathic method of diagnosis and indirect treatment in which the patient's somatic dysfunction, diagnosed by an associated myofascial tender point, is treated by using a position of spontaneous tissue release while simultaneously monitoring the tender point. Developed by Lawrence Jones, DO, FAAO, in 1955 (originally 'spontaneous release by positioning,' it was later termed 'strain-counterstrain)'" (ECOP 2018). Counterstrain technique involves shortening myofascial structures to reduce the nociceptive experience from firm palpation of a tender point.

Glover and Rennie (2018, 866) state, "The location of a specific tender point is constant from one patient to another and can be mapped. These areas of tenderness and/or tissue texture changes can be found in different myofascial structures including tendons, ligaments, fascia and muscle bellies." This suggests a strong anatomical basis for their location. Without description of the involvement of fascia, counterstrain technique could not be adequately explained.

Balanced Ligamentous Tension and Ligamentous Articular Strain Techniques

Developed and first presented by Sutherland in the early 1940s, balanced ligamentous tension (BLT) and ligamentous articular strain (LAS) techniques have

fascial elements at the core of musculoskeletal diagnosis and treatment (Lippincott 1949). The basis of balanced ligamentous tension "Is the precise physiological point in which the proprioceptive information provided by the ligaments allow the body to equalize the stresses exerted on an articulation in all directions. The method involves the minimization of periarticular tissue load and the placement of the affected ligaments in a position of equal tension in all planes so that the body's inherent forces can resolve the somatic dysfunction" (ECOP 2018).

Just as a manual medicine/manual therapy practitioners follow fascial planes in directions of ease of motion, the application of BLT focuses on the ligaments and related fascia holding joints in position, placing these structures into a balanced tension position, so that inherent bodily forces and/or respiratory facilitation complete the articular correction. Carreiro (2003, 917) states, "The physician must skillfully position the joint so that all forces within the articular mechanism converge on one specific point. This point then becomes the fulcrum around which the shift or change will occur. ... The more skilled the operator, the more specific the convergence and the less force needed to correct the dysfunction. Very skilled physicians will merely ask the patient to exhale, or will flex the patient's head to articulate the joint."

The Lippincott (1949) article describes Sutherland's techniques, which would be termed myofascial release, because they were directed toward structures such as diaphragms (respiratory, thoracic inlet, and pelvic) that were not specifically articular. The BLT techniques have been elaborated and expanded based on the work of Rollin Becker, DO, and colleagues, who carried on the teaching of Sutherland's techniques, and the term LAS has come into use because of a teaching manual published with that name (Speece et al. 2009).

Myofascial Release Techniques

As noted previously, attention to fascia has been central to osteopathy and osteopathic medicine since the 1890s. Myofascial release (MFR) is:

a treatment method first described by Andrew Taylor Still, DO, and his early students, which utilizes continual palpatory feedback to alleviate restriction of the somatic dysfunction and its related fascia and musculature. With direct MFR the dysfunctional myofascial tissues are loaded and restrictive barrier is engaged with a constant force. With indirect MFR the dysfunctional myofascial tissues are loaded and then guided toward the position of greatest ease. (ECOP 2018).

As this book amply illustrates, there are a number of different schools of thought and teaching on the subject of myofascial technique. Out of the osteopathic tradition, besides BLT and LAS, there are two other sets of techniques directly focused on the fascia, ligamentous release approach: (1) the indirect approach (Chila 2003) and (2) the integrated neuromusculoskeletal release and myofascial release (Ward 2003). A careful reading of Chila (2003) and Ward (2003) reveals that the underlying principles are very similar, but specific hand placements and areas of body contact are somewhat different. Taken together, the Chila and Ward approaches constitute a comprehensive system of the application of myofascial treatment techniques. In fact, teaching in U.S. osteopathic medical schools draws upon and combines the techniques of BLT and LAS along with integrated neuromusculoskeletal release (INR) and myofascial release (MFR). However, in the context of this book it is helpful to describe techniques associated with different terminologies, because that is how they are identified in texts and teaching as well as in documentation for medical procedure description and coding for reimbursement of healthcare services (particularly in the United States).

O'Connell (2018) reaffirmed the descriptions of the approaches of Chila and Ward to MFR. She goes on to describe her version of MFR based on the bioresponsive electric potentials of the fascia and summarizes the evolution of biomechanical to biodynamic perspective in Still's writings.

Don't believe for one second that this was the limit of his vision. According to many who worked with him and others who spent years studying his works it was his hope that the experience of living, dynamic anatomy would awaken dormant centers of perception in the student. Gradually over a period of years of focused attention, conscious intention of purpose and deep non-judgmental concentration on the experience of life as manifested in the patient, the physician would evolve to higher level of interaction with the dynamic mechanism of the patient. He would evolve into an osteopath. (O'Connell 2018, 844).

Osteopathy in the Cranial Field

Osteopathy in the cranial field (OCF) is the most widely used term to refer to the cranial concept developed by William Garner Sutherland, DO; however, OCF is considered a historic term (ECOP 2018). The descriptive phrase currently used is *osteopathic cranial manipulative medicine* (OCMM), defined as "A system of diagnosis and treatment by an osteopathic practitioner using the primary respiratory mechanism and balanced membrane tension" (ECOP 2018).

Also called cranial osteopathy and cranial manipulation, this set of procedures involves great attention to intracranial dura (Magoun 1966). "It has been stated that Sutherland did for the head that which Still did for the rest of the body, which was to delineate an anatomically based understanding of range and vector of motion and physiologic dynamics of cranial bones and intra-cranial structures" (King 2011). Structures such as the falx cerebri and diaphragma sellae are contiguous with spinal dura mater, presenting a basis for fascial manipulative techniques that can affect brain centers (King 2007).

Although OCF originated in osteopathy, in the context of this book it is important to acknowledge that cranial manipulation has other proponents and perspectives, for example, craniosacral therapy (Upledger and Vredevoogd 1983) and sacro-occipital technique (SOT) (DeJarnette 1967). All cranial manipulation traditions embrace the fascial continuity perspective and its importance in the application of therapy and treatment procedures.

Visceral Manipulation

Visceral manipulation is defined as follows by the ECOP (2018) glossary of osteopathic terminology, "Historically called ventral techniques. A method of diagnosis and treatment directed to the viscera and/or the supportive structures to improve physiologic function." There are two chapters devoted to visceral diagnosis and treatment in the fourth edition of *Foundations of Osteopathic Medicine* (Lossing and Giusti 2018; Lossing 2018). These authors (Lossing and Giusti 2018, 747) describe "visceral dysfunction as impaired or altered mobility or motility of the visceral system and related fascia, neurological, vascular, skeletal and lymphatic elements." Each organ is described as having a unique motility. Abnormal motion tests and changes in distensibility and/or viscoelastic of fascial attachments support the diagnosis of visceral dysfunction. Visceral manipulation has been described and taught since the 1890s in osteopathic training and practice and cannot be successfully applied without the practitioner having a detailed knowledge of anatomy of the viscera and their fascial attachments.

Osteopathic Manipulative Treatment—Summary

The foregoing discussion amply illustrates the central position that fascia holds in the formulation and application of OMT. A similar discussion could describe the attention given to fascia in other OMT techniques such as facilitated positional release, progressive inhibition of neuromuscular structures technique, functional technique, and articulatory technique.

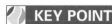

KEY POINT

The concept of the common compensatory pattern is uniquely osteopathic and readily applied clinical practice.

OSTEOPATHIC CONTRIBUTIONS TO THE UNDERSTANDING OF FASCIA

Common Compensatory Pattern

The concept of the common compensatory pattern (CCP) is based entirely on the nature of fascial patterns

of preferred motion (also termed "ease of motion") (Zink and Lawson 1979; Pope 2003). Among the many structural findings in the CCP were a left iliac crest more cephalad than right, superior and slightly lateral left anterior superior iliac spines, the pubic symphysis more cephalad on the left, the left leg appearing longer, and the right leg more externally rotated. Among the descriptions of dynamic palpatory findings, the following is an example with the patient in a standing position: "The palms of the physician's hands are placed on the anterosuperior iliac spines so that the fingers follow the crests. The physician's right hand moves with ease superiorly and laterally over the tissues, while the left hand moves with ease inferiorly and medially, resistance is encountered when the hands are moved in the opposite direction" (Zink and Lawson 1979). "The CCP can be seen as a bias of the fascias of the body along its length, occurring from the ground up. Such that, with respect to the feet, the pelvic girdle is found to be rotated to the right, the lower thoracic outlet to be left, the upper thoracic outlet to the right, and the craniocervical junction to the left" (Pope 2003).

There are four transition zones, the occipito-atlantal (OA), cervical thoracic (CT), thoraco-lumbar (TL), and lumbo-sacral (LS), and the finding in healthy people is that the direction of fascial ease of motion alternates between these areas (Fig. 7.5.2).

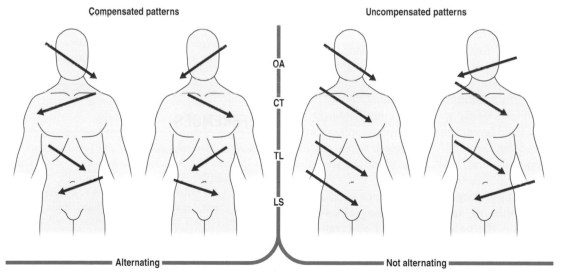

Fig. 7.5.2 Compensated and Uncompensated Patterns. Adapted with permission from Kuchera, W., Kuchera, M., 1994. Osteopathic Principles in Practice. Greyden Press, Columbus, OH.

The reason it is called the CCP is that, according to Zink and Lawson (1979), it occurs in about 80% of individuals; the reverse occurs in 20% and has been named the uncommon compensatory pattern (UCCP). The utility of the CCP concept was that Zink believed that the transition zones between the alternating fascial planes, ease of motion directions, were weak anatomically and should always be treated no matter what else was found to be dysfunctional. If these alternating fascial ease of motion planes were not found to alternate, for example, if all planes seemed to rotate in the same direction, this was called an "uncompensated" pattern and would eventually lead to more serious health problems if not treated.

Treatment of the transitional zones could be done by muscle energy procedure to the OA junction or cranial manipulation procedure to the cranial diaphragm, but more generally followed conventional myofascial manipulation procedures in which the operator's hands contacted the area of concern. The tissues are followed in their preference for side-bending, rotation, and any other vector of motion, such as forward or backward bending, and then held in that position as the patient breathes in and out. The operator follows the tissue preferences until the tissues "release" in a "letting-go" or "softening" palpatory manifestation and approach the midline again.

Although speculative, the theory of the origin of the CCP is worthy of note as it may be related to the birth process, in which the fetal head and body go through a series of positions as the birth canal is traversed, leaving a lifelong fascial motion preference. Evidence for this view is that the majority of fetal presentations are with the left occiput presenting first, and this affects the fascial motion preference as well as the position of the labyrinthine structures in the temporal bones that then maintain postural balance in a compensated manner (Pope 2003). Zink himself felt the CCP was due to injury caused by the many falls a child has during its early development from infant to toddler (Zink 1977). If research can confirm either hypothesis, one implication would be for more awareness to treat infants and toddlers.

As with many concepts, there is often a thread from Greek philosophy or art. An intriguing observation (Quinn 2000) is the possible historical observation of the CCP in art as seen in Greek art, such as the statue *Cidian Aphrodite* (c. 340–330 BCE), and described by the Italian word *contrapposto*, which refers to the natural pose of a figure where "the parts of the body are placed asymmetrically in opposition to each other around a central axis" (Fig. 7.5.3).

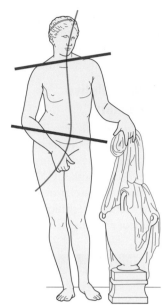

Fig. 7.5.3 In this rendering of the statue *Cnidian Aphrodite* from 340–330 BCE, contrapposto is demonstrated by the S curve of the axial skeleton in relation to the tilt of the hips and shoulders in opposite directions. Adapted with permission from Quinn, A., 2000. The compensatory pattern as seen in art and osteopathy. American Academy of Osteopathy Journal 10, 21–23.

Summary

In osteopathic practice worldwide, fascia has played a central role in the evaluation and treatment of patients. Founder of osteopathy A. T. Still (1902) said "we live in our fascia." Every type of osteopathic intervention specifically refers to the central role of fascia and its response to injury and then the manner in which the intervention is applied to return the body to its optimal structure and function.

REFERENCES

American Medical Association, 2020. Current Procedural Terminology. American Medical Association, Chicago, IL

Brous, N., 1997. Fascia. In: DiGiovanna, E., Schiowitz, S. (Eds.), An Osteopathic Approach to Diagnosis and Treatment. Lippincott-Raven, Philadelphia.

Carreiro, J., 2003. Balanced ligamentous tension techniques. In: Ward, R.C. (Ed.), Foundations for Osteopathic Medicine, second ed. Lippincott, Williams & Wilkins, Philadelphia, pp. 916–930.

Chila, A.C., 2003. Fascial-ligamentous release – indirect approach. In: Ward, R.C. (Ed.), Foundations for Osteopathic Medicine, second ed. Lippincott, Williams & Wilkins, Philadelphia, pp. 908–915.

DeJarnette, M.B., 1967. The Philosophy, Art and Science of Sacral Occipital Ethnic. Privately published, Nebraska City, NE.

Educational Council on Osteopathic Principles (ECOP), 2018. Glossary of Osteopathic Terminology. American Association of Colleges of Osteopathic Medicine, Chevy Chase, MD.

Ehrenfeuchter W.C. 2018. Muscle Energy. In Seffinger, M.A. (ED.) Foundations of osteopathic medicine 4e. Wolters Klumer, Philadelphia, pp. 797-812.

Giusti, R.E., Hruby, R.J., 2018. High-Velocity Low-Amplitude (HVLA) thrust. In: Seffinger, M.A. (Ed.), Foundations of Osteopathic Medicine, fourth ed. Wolters Kluwer, Philadelphia, pp. 813–834.

Glover, J.C., Rennie P.R., 2018. Strain/counterstrain. In: Seffinger, M.A. (Ed.), Foundations of Osteopathic Medicine, fourth ed. Wolters Kluwer, Philadelphia, pp. 864–884.

Jones, L.H., 1964. Spontaneous release by positioning. The DO. 4, 109–116.

King, H.H., 2007. Cranial Fascia: Continuity and motion characteristics. In: Presentation at First International Fascia Research Congress: Basic Science and Implications for Conventional and Complementary Health Care. Harvard, Boston, MA.

King, H.H., 2011. Research on somato-visceral interactions and the impact of manual therapy on systemic disorders. In: King, H.H., Jänig, W., Patterson, M. (Eds.), The Science and Clinical Application of Manual Therapy. Churchill Livingstone Elsevier, London, UK.

Lippincott, H.A., 1949. The osteopathic technique of Wm. G. Sutherland, D.O., Yearbook of the Academy of Applied Osteopathy. American Academy of Osteopathy, Indianapolis, IN, pp. 1-24.

Lossing, K., 2018. Visceral manipulation. In: Seffinger, M.A. (Ed.), Foundations of Osteopathic Medicine, fourth ed. Wolters Kluwer, Philadelphia, pp. 1022–1026.

Lossing, K., Giusti R.E., 2018. Internal organ assessment for visceral motion dysfunction. In: Seffinger, M.A. (Ed.), Foundations of Osteopathic Medicine, fourth ed. Wolters Kluwer, Philadelphia, pp. 747–762.

Magoun, H.I., 1966. Osteopathy in the Cranial Field, second ed. Journal Publishing Company, Kirksville, MO.

O'Connell, J.A. 2018. Myofascial release. In: Seffinger, M.A. (Ed.) Foundations of Osteopathic Medicine, fourth ed. Wolters Kluwer, Philadelphia, pp. 835–863.

Pope, R.E., 2003. The common compensatory pattern: Its origin and relationship to the postural model. Am. Acad. Osteopath. J. 14, 19–40.

Quinn, A., 2000. The compensatory pattern as seen in art and osteopathy. Am. Acad. Osteopath. J. 10, 21–23.

Speece, C.A., Crow, W.T., Simmons, S.L., 2009. Ligamentous Articular Strain, second ed. Eastland Press, Seattle.

Still, A.T., 1902. Philosophy and Mechanical Principles of Osteopathy. Hudson-Kimberly Pub. Co., Kansas City, MO.

Upledger, J.E., Vredevoogd, J.D., 1983. Craniosacral Therapy. Eastland Press, Seattle.

Van Buskirk, R.L., 2018. Still technique. In: Seffinger, M.A. (Ed.), Foundations of Osteopathic Medicine, fourth ed. Wolters Kluwer, Philadelphia, pp. 958–961.

Ward, R.C., 2003. Integrated neuromusculoskeletal release and myofascial release. In Ward, R.C. (Ed.), Foundations for Osteopathic Medicine, second ed. Lippincott, Williams & Wilkins, Philadelphia, pp. 931–968.

World Health Organization, 2016. International Classification of Diseases, tenth ed. World Health Organization, Geneva, Switzerland.

Zink, G.J., 1977. Respiratory and circulatory care: the conceptual model. Osteopath. Ann. 5, 108–112.

Zink, G.L., Lawson, W.B., 1979. An osteopathic structural examination and functional interpretation of the soma. Osteopath. Ann. 7, 433–440.

Connective Tissue Manipulation

Katja Bartsch and Robert Schleip

CHAPTER CONTENTS

HISTORY AND BACKGROUND

Connective tissue manipulation (CTM) is a manual reflex therapy that was developed in the late 1930s by Elisabeth Dicke in Germany. Hede Teirich-Leube and Professor Wolfgang Kohlrausch supported and continued Dicke's work. Originally the German term *Bindegewebsmassage* (BGM) was used and translated to connective tissue massage, as the method was spread throughout Europe (Holey and Dixon 2014). However, this term is misleading. The focus of CTM was never to simply massage the connective tissue, but rather to target the connective tissue in order to take effect through the autonomic nervous system (Teirich-Leube 1968). Thus the term "connective tissue manipulation" was used from the 1980s onward.

The scientific footing for the field is still developing, with current review articles and clinical studies advancing the scientific basis of CTM. We are drawing from overview works of Holey and Dixon (e.g., Holey and Dixon 2014, 2018) in the structure and outline of this chapter.

We describe the applications, contraindications, and technique of CTM treatment and summarize the scientific evidence for physiological effects and clinical benefits.

APPLICATIONS AND CONTRAINDICATIONS

CTM is suited for various clinical applications. Holey and Dixon (2014) categorize these applications into four groups (Table 7.6.1). The authors state that several of the four categories can coexist and that CTM is a suitable intervention where pain has an autonomic component.

Contraindications of CTM include acute inflammation, active infection, malignancy, unstable heart pressure or heart conditions, early- or late-stage pregnancy, menstruation, and the use of anxiolytic drugs (Goats and Keir 1991; Holey and Dixon 2014).

PRINCIPLES OF CONNECTIVE TISSUE MANIPULATION

CTM is based on the assumption and observation that the dysfunction of an organ is reflected in changes of the skin and subcutaneous tissues (Head's zones) and also changes in the tone of superficial muscles (Mackenzie's zones). Such changes and signs are usually found in the dermatomes corresponding to the segmental innervation of the affected organ (Goats and Keir 1991).

TABLE 7.6.1 CTM—Areas of Application	
Type of Clinical Problem	**Examples**
Zonal	e.g., when autonomically induced changes in connective tissue zones are producing symptoms
Hormonal-endocrine	e.g., menstrual or menopausal problems, diabetes
Local mechanical/musculoskeletal	e.g., chronic nerve root pain
Other symptoms	e.g., restlessness, anxiety, resulting from a general autonomic imbalance

Reproduced with permission from Holey, L.A., Dixon, J., 2014. Connective tissue manipulation: A review of theory and clinical evidence. J. Bodyw. Mov. Ther. 18, 112–118.

Assessment

Before starting CTM treatment, questions regarding the extent of autonomic imbalances (such as problems with sleep and relaxation) should be part of the assessment.

Furthermore, the connective tissue is to be inspected for topographical changes such as flattened, indrawn areas surrounded by edemas. Such changes can be found in specific areas known as connective tissue zones in the patient's back and are related to visceral functions and disturbances (Teirich-Leube 1964; Holey and Dixon 2018) (Figure 7.6.1).

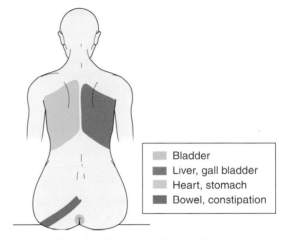

Bladder
Liver, gall bladder
Heart, stomach
Bowel, constipation

Fig. 7.6.1 Connective Tissue Zones.

> ### KEY POINT
>
> ***Connective Tissue Zones***
> - Elisabeth Dicke found the connective tissue zones when pulling and stretching the tissues of her own back skin, aiming to relieve her pain. Such zones are visible when changes in the subcutaneous tissues occur.
> - The English neurologist Sir Henry Head (1861–1940) found changes on the surface of the skin when visceral disturbances were present. Such changes included altered contours and skin temperature.
> - Furthermore, McKenzie (1917) found increased tension and hypersensitivity in muscles of the same segmental innervation with pathologically altered viscera.
> - Head and McKenzie offered an anatomical explanation for the connective tissue zones and the proposed link to visceral effects aimed for with CTM. The inspection of the connective tissue for topographical changes is therefore an integral part of the assessment before treatment.

To screen for changes in the contour of the skin and subcutaneous tissues, the patient is positioned seated so that the therapist can observe and palpate the patient's back. When palpating the respective tissues, small finger pulls or longer pulling strokes over the whole length of the back can help identify and interpret the connective tissue zones (Goats and Keir 1991).

Technique

Treatment is usually applied with the middle and ring fingers through firm lifting strokes, beginning with a series of short strokes over the sacrum, lumbar spine, and posterolateral pelvis (Fig. 7.6.2).

The strokes get progressively longer and can progress to the thoracic and cervical regions, the limbs, and the head. The area around the sacrum is targeted first in order to desensitize the skin, which is reflexively linked to the parasympathetic nervous system as a means of starting to rebalance the autonomic nervous system. Superficial layers should be treated before deep layers to clear excess skin tension or edema so that the later stages of treatment are not painful. As pain would increase sympathetic activity, increasing pain levels throughout the treatment would be

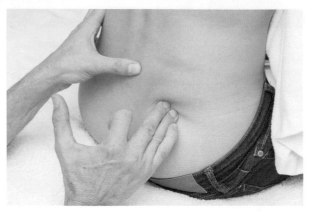

Fig. 7.6.2 The strokes included in the CTM protocol aim to create traction and shear force between the tissue layers. Oftentimes, the pad of the longest finger or thumb will serve as an effective tool. From: https://pixabay.com/de/photos/massage-rand-muskel-hip-bindegewebe-2441817/. Public domain.

detrimental to the overall intention of CTM techniques and are therefore to be avoided. Furthermore, the practitioner should aim to create a shear force between the skin and the deeper tissue layers in order to stimulate mechanoreceptors and mast cell activation. When targeting the deep fascia correctly in this way, a nonpainful "cutting" sensation can be felt by the patient. The effects and progress of the treatment can show with a delay. It is therefore essential to reassess before each consecutive session. If no progress is achieved after three treatments, CTM therapy should not be pursued further. Generally, sessions should be concluded when the practitioner feels that the attained improvements have reached a plateau (Goats and Keir 1991; Holey and Dixon 2014, 2018).

EFFECTS OF CONNECTIVE TISSUE MANIPULATION

CTM aims to obtain suprasegmental (generalized autonomic) and segmental (rather localized mechanical) effects through mechanisms that are distinct from traditional massage techniques.

Suprasegmental Effects

The main mechanisms of CTM are thought to be related to the autonomic nervous system. Although the detailed mechanisms are not yet fully understood, it is believed that through the stimulation of cutaneovisceral reflexes, an autonomic reflex response is induced. The shear force produced through CTM techniques presumably stimulates such reflexes via the nerve endings and horizontal circulatory plexi between dermis and subcutaneous layer and subcutaneous layer and deep fascia, respectively. As most blood vessels do only have sympathetic innervation, this in turn can cause effects on the autonomic nervous system. However, as the knowledge of fascia as a sensory organ has tremendously increased over the last years, it seems likely that targeting the various fascial layers by CTM will stimulate a wide range of receptors and thus give input to the autonomic nervous system through various somatosensory afferents. It is furthermore assumed that problems or imbalances in the connective tissue zones change the discharge frequency of neurons. As synapses can become "irritated" the autonomic nervous system might answer with a heightened state of activity, which in turn can spill over throughout the spinal segment. CTM can rebalance the autonomic nervous system, which oftentimes will mean that the parasympathetic output will be enhanced while the sympathetic output will decrease, presenting for instance with improved energy and sleep patterns as well as feelings of relaxation (Goats and Keir 1991; Holey and Dixon 2014, 2018).

Segmental Effects

CTM techniques presumably create a shear force between the skin and deeper fascial tissue layers. They may also lead to a wider distribution of tissue fluids in the skin and relaxation of the skin fibroblasts (Pohl 2010). Segmental effects constitute an improved functioning of the tissues linked by the same spinal segment of the treated reflex zone. The skin of the treated area will appear better hydrated and show enhanced texture, circulation, muscle tone, and visceral function. In addition, pain and tissue stiffness can improve. Thus the segmental effects of CTM constitute a key element in clinical treatment (Holey and Dixon 2014, 2018).

Evidence Base

The evidence base for the physiological effects of CTM is still developing. The few studies that are available show results related to cardiovascular parameters such as blood pressure and blood flow.

- A study by Akbaş et al. (2019) investigated acute autonomic responses to CTM in healthy young women; 150 participants received CTM, and 60 volunteers did not receive any intervention. Respiratory rate, heart rate, blood pressure, oxygen saturation, and body temperature were measured. Physical activity levels were assessed via questionnaire. Respiratory rate increased, and systolic and diastolic blood pressures were significantly reduced in the CTM group. No significant alterations were observed in the control group. Accordingly, the study showed that CTM has reducing effects on sympathetic activity in healthy young women.

- Holey et al. (2011) used thermography and physiological measurements, such as blood pressure and heart rate, in a group of eight healthy participants before and after a single CTM session. Results showed some small measurable physiological changes, such as an increase in skin temperature. The authors also found that CTM may possibly affect diastolic blood pressure, but not systolic blood pressure or heart rate.
- Kaada and Torsteinbo (1989) studied a group of 12 volunteers who suffered from various types of pain. They found that CTM produces pain relief and an increase of microcirculation in a number of vascular beds. They also reported a 16% increase of β-endorphins lasting for about an hour after treatment, which is assumed to be linked to the reported pain relief and a feeling of warmth and well-being related to CTM treatment.
- Reed and Held (1988) looked at 14 healthy, middle-aged and elderly subjects. Skin temperature, skin resistance, arterial blood pressure, and heart rate did not differ between the CTM group and the control group, which received a sham ultrasound treatment.
- To evaluate sympathetic activity related to CTM treatment, Kisner and Taslitz (1968) looked at heart rate, blood pressure, skin resistance of the palm of the hand, and skin temperatures of the index finger and large toe of nine healthy subjects. The responses in outcome measures reflected a trend of sympathetic activity for CTM: subjects showed an increase in heart rate (after the first 15 minutes of treatment), blood pressure, and peripheral reistance compared with control situations. This trend in cardiovascular parameters can be interpreted as functions of increasd sympathetic activity.
- Horstkotte et al. (1967) determined toe-skin blood flow and toe temperature as outcome measures. Blood flow decreased immediately after CTM treatment and was still below controls 35 minutes later. Two weeks after therapy, however, peripheral blood flow had increased.

Most of these selected studies were carried out with healthy subjects. Clinical groups would presumably benefit more from CTM treatment and would potentially produce greater responses.

However, further research is needed in order to clarify the evidence base for the presence as well as the theoretical model and mechanisms of the physiological effects of CTM.

CLINICAL BENEFITS

The studies evaluating the clinical benefits of CTM are few. Moreover, the explanatory value of the existing studies is limited, as most studies do either apply CTM alongside another treatment or do not include a control group. If CTM is investigated in combination with another mode of treatment, no direct inference about the effects of CTM can be drawn—only the combination of CTM in conjunction with the other treatment can be evaluated. In studies without a control group, one cannot determine whether the impact stems from the CTM treatment or from other factors, such as non treatment-related improvements or regression to the mean. In order to assess systematic differences between groups and conduct ethical studies at the same time, comparing CTM against a control group receiving standard or usual care would be desirable (Holey and Dixon 2014, 2018).

We summarize selected studies examining clinical benefits of CTM in the fields of pain, diabetes, fibromyalgia, constipation, and primary dysmenorrhea later. The mentioned limitations are present in a number of these studies.

Pain

- Celenay et al. (2019) evaluated the effectiveness of CTM for improving pain, mobility, and well-being in chronic low back pain; 60 participants were randomized to three groups: CTM, sham massage, and control groups. They received standardized physiotherapy in addition to their related applications for 15 sessions over the course of 3 weeks. Pain, mobility, and disability improved in all groups, with CTM showing superiority in improving these parameters.
- Celenay et al. (2016) compared the effectiveness of cervical and scapulothoracic stabilization exercises with and without CTM in patients with chronic mechanical neck pain. Outcome measures included pain, anxiety, and quality of life. Sixty volunteers

took part in the study and were randomly assigned to the two groups. The program was carried out for 12 sessions over the course of 4 weeks. Pain intensity and the level of anxiety decreased in both groups. Physical health increased in both groups as well. However, stabilization exercises with CTM seemed to be superior in improving pain intensity at night, pressure pain threshold, state anxiety, and mental health compared with the exercise regimen alone.

- Bakar et al. (2014) evaluated the short-term effects of classical massage and CTM on pain pressure threshold and muscle relaxation response in women with chronic neck pain. Forty-five female volunteers took part in the study. They received one session of either CTM or classical massage. Muscle relaxation response measured by electromyography biofeedback was significantly different for the CTM group, whereas pain pressure threshold measured with an algometer was only differed for the classical massage group.

- The goal of the study by Yagci et al. (2004) was to investigate whether ischemic pain tolerance changed in patients who had undergone treatment for chronic cervical myofascial pain syndrome. Forty subjects were randomly allocated into two groups. One group was treated with vapocoolant spray-stretch technique, the second group with CTM treatments. The only difference that was found between the groups was a lower pain intensity measured by a visual analog scale in the CTM group. Although there was a decrease in pain intensity and number of trigger points, and an increase in range of motion in both groups, there was no significant difference in ischemic pain threshold or tolerance compared with pretreatment measurements.

- In a study by McKechnie et al. (1983): Five patients with pain of varying sorts underwent CTM therapy. Heart rate, frontalis EMG, skin resistance, and forearm extensor EMG were taken before and after treatment. Although no control group was present, some reductions in heart rate were observed.

Diabetes

- Joseph et al. (2016) investigated the therapeutic effects of CTM in diabetic foot ulcer. Twenty participants were randomized into a CTM and a conventional treatment group. The authors looked at percentage wound area reduction (PWAR) and bacterial colonization count (BCC) at baseline and after 6 weeks of treatment. PWAR changed significantly in both groups. BCC showed a significant reduction, with a higher percentage of reduction in the CTM group compared with the conventional treatment group.

- The authors Castro-Sánchez et al. (2011) evaluated the effects of CTM on blood circulation and claudication symptoms in type 2 diabetic patients; 98 participants were randomly assigned to a massage group or a placebo group. Measurements were taken at 30 minutes, 6 months, and 1 year after the 15-week treatment. CTM improved blood circulation in the lower limbs quantified by arterial pressure, skin blood flow, and oxygen saturation. Heart rate and temperature did not change significantly. Some of the outcome measures were still improved after 6 months and 1 year, respectively.

Fibromyalgia

- Celenay et al. (2017) compared the effectiveness of a combined exercise program with and without CTM on pain, fatigue, sleep problems, health status, and quality of life in 40 patients with fibromyalgia syndrome. Participants were randomly allocated to the two groups. The treatments (with and without CTM) were carried out 2 days a week for 6 weeks. The study showed that exercises with CTM might be superior in improving pain, fatigue, sleep problems, and role limitations due to physical health compared with exercise alone.

- A study of Ekici et al. (2009) compared the effects of manual lymph drainage therapy and CTM in women with primary fibromyalgia. Treatments were given five times a week over the course of 3 weeks. Both groups showed a decrease of pain pressure threshold and pain intensity and an increase in quality of life and health status.

- In a study by Citak-Karakaya et al. (2006), short-term and 1-year follow-up results of CTM and combined ultrasound therapy were evaluated. Twenty female patients took part in the prospective cohort study. Intensity of pain, complaint of nonrestorative sleep, and the impact of fibromyalgia on functional activities were assessed by visual analog scales. Measurements were taken before and after 20 treatment sessions. All parameters improved after the treatment program.

- Brattberg (1999) looked at the effect of CTM in the treatment of individuals with fibromyalgia. Although he reported positive effects on quality of life and pain levels, the study is somewhat hard to interpret, as both groups (CTM treatment and reference group) received CTM treatments at some stage during the study. Furthermore, pain had returned to 90% of the baseline values after 6 months.

Constipation

- Orhan et al. (2018) investigated the effects of CTM, Kinesio Taping® on constipation, and quality of life in children with cerebral palsy. Forty children with chronic constipation were randomly assigned to the CTM group, KT group, or control group. Results showed differences regarding changes in defecation frequency and duration and pediatric quality of life for both treatment groups. The study showed that CTM and Kinesio Taping seemed to be equally effective approaches for the treatment of pediatric constipation.
- Gürsen et al. (2015) examined the effects of CTM on the severity of constipation and health-related quality of life in individuals diagnosed with chronic constipation. Fifty patients were randomized to an intervention or control group. Both groups were given lifestyle advice for constipation. The CTM treatment group additionally received 20 CTM treatments in 4 weeks. Measures were taken before and after the 4-week treatment period. Compared with the control group, the CTM group reported greater improvements measured with the constipation severity instruments well as the Constipation Quality of Life questionnaire. Furthermore, frequency and duration of defecation, stool consistency, and the feeling of incomplete evacuation were significantly better than in the control group.
- In a single case study by Holey and Lawler (1995), CTM produced better effects than abdominal massage at reducing constipation and improving the consistency of stool.

Primary Dysmenorrhea

- Özgül et al. (2018) evaluated the short-term effectiveness of CTM for relieving menstrual pain and symptoms in primary dysmenorrhea. Forty-four women were randomized to a treatment or control group. Both groups received advising. The treatment group received additional CTM sessions. Compared with the control group, the treatment group showed significant improvements in pain, medication use, menstrual symptoms, and pain catastrophizing.
- Demirtürk et al. (2016) compared reflexology and DTM in participants with primary dysmenorrhea. CTM was applied to 15 of the participants for 5 days a week, while the other 15 volunteers received foot reflexology treatments for 3 days a week during one cycle. Assessments were performed before treatment, after termination of the treatment, and approximately 1 month after the consecutive menstrual period. Results showed that both treatments provided significant improvements, and no superiority existed between groups.

The direct clinical effects of CTM can only be assessed through a couple of these studies due to the described limitations. Still, the existing scientific base does indicate clinical benefits in the mentioned fields. More research is needed to fully understand the clinical benefits of CTM therapy.

 KEY POINT

Scientific Evidence Base

- There are a number of studies related to the physiological and clinical effects of CTM treatment.
- Regarding the physiological effects, many of the studies are carried out with healthy subjects. Therefore the explanatory power of these studies might be limited, as clinical samples might show bigger physiological effects from CTM treatment.
- In this chapter we summarized selected studies for the fields of pain, diabetes, fibromyalgia, constipation, and primary dysmenorrhea. A number of these studies apply CTM alongside another treatment or do not have a control group. As a result of these limitations, CTM effects cannot be fully evaluated in these studies.

Summary

CTM is a reflex therapy that stimulates the autonomic nervous system, aiming to rebalance the sympathetic and parasympathetic components. Alongside these generalized effects, localized mechanical effects can be a result of the technique.

Very few studies constitute the scientific footing for the mechanisms and clinical benefits of CTM. Although a good number of existing studies has limitations, the evidence base is developing and reviews and clinical studies are shedding further light upon the field.

REFERENCES

Akbaş, E., Ünver, B., Erdem, E.U., 2019. Acute effects of connective tissue manipulation on autonomic function in healthy young women. Complement. Med. Res. 26, 250–257.

Bakar, Y., Sertel, M., Oztürk, A., et al., 2014. Short term effects of classic massage compared to connective tissue massage on pressure pain threshold and muscle relaxation response in women with chronic neck pain: a preliminary study. J. Manipulative Physiol. Ther. 37, 415–421.

Brattberg, G., 1999. Connective tissue massage in the treatment of fibromyalgia. Eur. J. Pain. 3, 235–244.

Castro-Sánchez, A.M., Moreno-Lorenzo, C., Matarán-Peñarrocha, G.A., et al., 2011. Connective tissue reflex massage for type 2 diabetic patients with peripheral arterial disease: randomized controlled trial. Evid. Based Complement. Alternat. Med. 2011, 804321.

Celenay, S.T., Anaforoglu Kulunkoglu, B., Yasa, M.E., et al., 2017. A comparison of the effects of exercises plus connective tissue massage to exercises alone in women with fibromyalgia syndrome: a randomized controlled trial. Rheumatol. Int. 37, 1799–1806.

Celenay, S.T., Kaya, D.O., Akbayrak, T., 2016. Cervical and scapulothoracic stabilization exercises with and without connective tissue massage for chronic mechanical neck pain: A prospective, randomised controlled trial. Man. Ther. 21, 144–150.

Celenay, S.T., Kaya, D.O., Ucurum, S.G., 2019. Adding connective tissue manipulation to physiotherapy for chronic low back pain improves pain, mobility, and well-being: a randomized controlled trial. J. Exerc. Rehabil. 15, 308–315.

Citak-Karakaya, I., Akbayrak, T., Demirtürk, F., Ekici, G., Bakar, Y., 2006. Short and long-term results of connective tissue manipulation and combined ultrasound therapy in patients with fibromyalgia. J. Manipulative Physiol. Ther. 29, 524–528.

Demirtürk, F., Erkek, Z.Y., Alparslan, Ö., et al., 2016 Comparison of reflexology and connective tissue manipulation in participants with primary dysmenorrhea. J. Altern. Complement. Med. 22, 38–44.

Ekici, G., Bakar, Y., Akbayrak, T., Yuksel, I., 2009. Comparison of manual lymph drainage therapy and connective tissue massage in women with fibromyalgia: a randomized controlled trial. J. Manipulative Physiol. Ther. 32, 127–133.

Goats, G.C., Keir, K.A., 1991. Connective tissue massage. Br. J. Sports Med. 25, 131–133.

Gürsen, C., Kerem Günel, M., Kaya, S., Kav, T., Akbayrak, T., 2015. Effect of connective tissue manipulation on symptoms and quality of life in patients with chronic constipation: a randomized controlled trial. J. Manipulative Physiol. Ther. 38, 335–343.

Holey, E., Dixon, J., 2018. Connective tissue manipulation and skin rolling. In: Chaitow, L. (Ed.), Fascial Dysfunction: Manual Therapy Approaches, second ed. Handspring Publishing, Edinburgh.

Holey, L.A., Dixon, J., 2014. Connective tissue manipulation: A review of theory and clinical evidence. J. Bodyw. Mov. Ther. 18, 112–118.

Holey, L.A., Dixon, J., Selfe, J., 2011. An exploratory thermographic investigation of the effects of connective tissue massage on autonomic function. J. Manipulative Physiol. Ther. 34, 457–462.

Holey, L.A., Lawler, H., 1995. The effects of classical massage and connective tissue manipulation on bowel function. Br. J. Ther. Rehabil. 2, 627–631.

Horstkotte, W., Klempien, E.J., Scheppokat, K.D., 1967. Skin temperature and blood flow changes in occlusive arterial disease under physical and pharmacologic therapy. Angiology 18, 1–5.

Joseph, L.H., Paungmali, A., Dixon, J., et al., 2016. Therapeutic effects of connective tissue manipulation on wound healing and bacterial colonization count among patients with diabetic foot ulcer. J. Bodyw. Mov. Ther. 20, 650–656.

Kaada, B., Torsteinbo, O., 1989. Increase of plasma beta-endorphins in connective tissue massage. Gen. Pharmacol. 20, 487–489.

Kisner, C.D., Taslitz, N., 1968. Connective tissue massage: influence of the introductory treatment on autonomic functions. Phys. Ther. 48, 107–119.

McKechnie, A.A., Wilson, F., Watson, N., Scott, D., 1983. Anxiety states: a preliminary report on the value of connective tissue massage. J. Psychosom. Res. 27, 125–129.

McKenzie, J., 1917. Krankheitszeichen und ihre Auslegung. Cited in: Ebner, M. (1980). Conncective Tissue Manipulations, Krieger, Florida.

Orhan, C., Kaya Kara, O., Kaya, S., et al., 2018. The effects of connective tissue manipulation and Kinesio Taping on chronic constipation in children with cerebral palsy: a randomized controlled trial. Disabil. Rehabil. 40, 10–20.

Özgül, S., Üzelpasaci, E., Orhan, C., et al., 2018. Short-term effects of connective tissue manipulation in women with primary dysmenorrhea: A randomized controlled trial. Complement. Ther. Clin. Pract. 33, 1–6.

Pohl, H., 2010. Changes in the structure of collagen distribution in the skin caused by a manual technique. J. Bodyw. Mov. Ther. 14, 27–34.

Reed, B.V., Held, J.M., 1988. Effects of sequential connective tissue massage on autonomic nervous system of middle-aged and elderly adults. Phys. Ther. 68, 1231–1234.

Teirich-Leube, H., 1964. Reflexzonenmassage im bindegwebe - diagnostik und therapie. Hippokrates, 35, 603–605.

Teirich-Leube, H., 1968. Grundsätzliches zu dem begriff bindegewebsmassage. Krankengymnastik 10, 414–417.

Yagci, N., Uygur, F., Bek, N., 2004. Comparison of connective tissue massage and spray-and-stretch technique in the treatment of chronic cervical myofascial pain syndrome. Pain Clin. 16, 469–474.

7.7

Fascial Manipulation

Antonio Stecco and Tiina Lahtinen-Suopanki

CHAPTER CONTENTS

INTRODUCTION

Fascial Manipulation is a manual therapy for the treatment of musculoskeletal pain developed by Luigi Stecco, an Italian physiotherapist. This method, which has evolved since 1980 through anatomical studies and clinical practice, is based on a three-dimensional biomechanical model for the human fascial system (Stecco and Stecco 2017). The key premise of this model is that fascia is not just a uniform membrane, but it presents a specific organization and relationship with the underlying muscles and with respect to internal organs. In particular, the fascia is seen as a:

- coordinating element for motor units (grouped together in myofascial units),
- uniting element between unidirectional myofascial units (myofascial sequences),
- connecting element between body segments via myofascial expansions and retinacula (myofascial spirals),
- unifying element for synergic organs (organ-fascial units), and
- connecting element between organ-fascial units that participate in the same physiological activity (apparatus fascial sequence).

These biomechanical models are supported by in-depth studies of fascial anatomy and physiology.

Numerous dissections of unembalmed human cadavers have evidenced:

- muscular fiber insertions directly onto deep fascia (Stecco et al. 2007b, 2013; Stecco 2015),
- fiber distribution according to precise motor directions (Stecco et al. 2008, 2013, 2019), and
- myotendinous expansions that link adjacent segments (Stecco et al. 2009).

Extensive histological analysis of deep muscular fascia has also provided evidence for hypotheses concerning fascia's role in proprioception and tensional force distribution within the fascial system (Stecco et al. 2006, 2007b).

Treatment modalities specifically addressing these fascial layers have been developed. The Fascial Manipulation method for musculoskeletal dysfunctions is characterized by an analytical procedure that results in personalized treatment for each subject. A combination of codified movement and palpatory tests permits therapists to determine which *fascial points*[1] are involved in any given dysfunction. Each of these *fascial points* has a precise anatomical location within the fascial system, based on a functional interpretation of movement, as provided by the biomechanical model. A fundamental

---

[1]These points/areas are described in depth later in the chapter.

aspect of this method lies in differentiating between the area where the patient actually perceives pain, and the fascial points that require treatment.

 KEY POINTS

Fascial Manipulation was developed by Luigi Stecco more than 40 years. The first book of Luigi Stecco was published in 1987.

THE BIOMECHANICAL MODEL FOR THE MUSCULOSKELETAL SYSTEM

The Fascial Manipulation method considers the myofascial system as a three-dimensional continuum and aims to act upon the deep muscular fascia, including epimysium and retinacula, in the treatment of musculoskeletal pain. This continuum is well-organized and easily analyzable, with an innovative biomechanical model that interprets the fascial system from a functional viewpoint. The base element or functional unit of this biomechanical model is the myofascial unit.

The Myofascial Unit

Each myofascial unit (MFU) is made up of monoarticular and biarticular muscular fibers, the fascial structures, bones, nerve terminations, and the specific portion of a joint involved in moving a body segment in a specific direction. In other words, each MFU is a functional unit composed of three elements that work in unison:
- the force-exerting element—the unidirectional muscle fibers,
- the coordinating element—the deep fascia,
- the perceptive element—the nerve structures, the joint capsule, and the ligaments.

A significant characteristic of each MFU is the presence of both monoarticular and biarticular muscular fibers. The monoarticular fibers in each MFU are generally deeper fibers, specialized in moving a joint on one plane, and these fibers could be involved in the interplay between agonists and antagonists. In almost every MFU, a number of monoarticular fibers insert onto the intermuscular septum that separates two antagonist MFUs on the same plane (Turrina et al. 2013). Whenever the agonist MFU is activated, traction exerted on the intermuscular septum could cause tension in the antagonist MFU, contributing to simultaneous adaptation, according to the inclination of the fibers and the segment involved. Studies of agonist and antagonist interaction by Huijing (2007) support this hypothesis.

The biarticular fibers in each MFU could intervene in synchronizing the activity of two in-series MFUs, modifying the position of the proximal segment in relation to movements of the distal segment, or vice versa, when necessary. At the same time, the monoarticular fibers of the respective MFUs could provide added stability for joints as they move. Different studies evidence the role of monoarticular and biarticular muscle fibers in multiple joint movements (Kurtzer et al. 2006).

Within each MFU, some muscle fibers also insert directly onto the overlying fascia. These insertions could contribute to the maintenance of a basal tension of the fascia and guarantee that fascia is stretched in a specific direction each time these muscle fibers contract (Stecco et al. 2008, 2009, 2019).

Within each MFU, two specific points can be identified (Fig. 7.7.1):
- A *center of perception (CP):* a precise area of the joint where traction exerted by the MFU on the joint capsule, tendons, and ligaments is thought to converge. In a dysfunctional MFU this traction is not aligned along the correct physiological axis, causing joint movement to be incongruent or out of alignment. Over time, this could determine joint conflict, with friction and subsequent inflammation of periarticular soft tissues resulting in sensations of pain or joint instability.
- A *center of coordination (CC):* a small area on the deep muscular fascia where force exerted by the muscular fibers of an MFU converges (the "point," referred to earlier). The resultant myofascial forces could be transmitted to the surface of the deep fascia via its continuity with the endomysium, perimysium, and epimysium. The CC within each MFU is thought to have the role of coordinating the motor units that are contained within that MFU.

Evidence exists regarding reduced coordination of motor units in the presence of joint pain (Mellor and Hodges 2005), although the mechanism is unknown. The Fascial Manipulation model suggests a new neurophysiological basis for the coordinating role of the CC. During any movement, motor units are activated, causing muscle fibers to contract according to the degree and direction of required joint movement. Muscle spindle capsules,

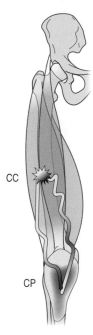

Fig. 7.7.1 Center of coordination (CC) and center of perception (CP) of the antemotion myofascial unit (MFU) of the knee (AN–GE). The CC is over the fascia lata, at the level of the vastus intermedius muscle, the CP over the anterior part of the knee. From Stecco, L., Stecco, C. 2007. Fascial Manipulation for Musculoskeletal Pain. Theoretical Part. Padova, Piccin, with permission.

embedded between muscle fibers, are continuous with surrounding endomysium; therefore when gamma fiber stimulation causes intrafusal spindle fibers to contract, a minimal stretch is propagated throughout the entire fascial continuum, including the fascia at the CC. If the fascia at the CC is elastic, then it will adapt to this stretch, permitting muscle spindles to contract normally, correct activation of alpha motor fibers, and subsequent muscular contraction to proceed smoothly. If fascia at the CC is not elastic, the muscle spindle contraction could interfere with motor unit activation. Incongruent motor unit activation would then result in uncoordinated movement, perceived at the CP either as joint instability or as pain (Stecco et al. 2014b; Kalichman et al. 2016; Pintucci et al 2017).

For each body segment, six MFUs have been identified and each one is specific for one direction. This is also true for those joints that have limited movement on some planes (e.g., frontal plane for the knee or elbow), because these joints always have muscular and fascial components that act as stabilizers on those planes.

Each MFU is located on one of the three spatial planes. The MFUs associated with the movement of antemotion[2] (AN) are located in the anterior region of the limbs and trunk while the MFUs associated with retromotion[3] (RE) are located in the posterior region. The MFUs associated with lateromotion (LA), movement away from the midline, are all located in the lateral region of the limbs and trunk, and those MFUs associated with mediomotion (ME), movement toward the midline, are located in the medial region. The MFUs associated with extrarotation (ER) are located in the retrolateral region of the limbs and trunk, and those associated with intrarotation (IR) in the anterolateral region (Fig. 7.7.2). Each MFU is named according to the segment it moves and the direction in which it moves that segment. There are 14 body segments and 6 directions, making a total of 84 CC and 84 CP (Fig. 7.7.3).

> **KEY POINT**
>
> Myofascial unit is the basic element for the peripheral coordination of the movement.

The Sequences

Myofascial sequences are formed by a succession of unidirectional MFUs positioned in a specific direction. This organization permits single MFUs to synchronize their activity, particularly during forceful movements, and to monitor upright posture in the three spatial planes.

From an anatomical viewpoint, unidirectional MFUs connect to each other via:

- the muscular fascia, which unites them within the same fascial compartment;

---

[2] The authors have chosen the term *antemotion* because it has a precise directional significance. Even the CNS organizes movement according to spatial directions and not according to closure (flexion) or aperture (extension) of joints. The MFUs of *antemotion* (AN) are all implicated in the forward movement of a body segment on the sagittal plane, and these MFUs are always situated in the anterior region of the body. At the knee, for example, the *antemotion* MFU is involved in coordinating the forward movement of the lower limb on the sagittal plane, commonly termed knee extension.

[3] For the same reason as mentioned in note 1, the authors have chosen the term *retromotion* to define all backward movements of a segment on the sagittal plane.

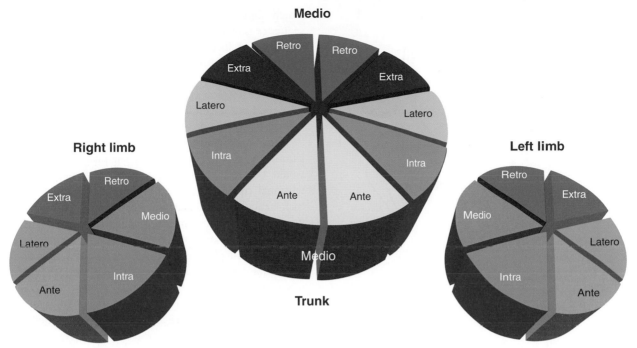

Fig. 7.7.2 Six MFUs are recognized for each section. The different MFUs show a specific spatial disposition; in particular, the MFUs associated with the movement of antemotion (Ante [flexion]) are located in the anterior region of the trunk, the MFUs associated with retromotion (Retro [extension]) are located in the posterior region, the MFUs associated with lateromotion (Latero [lateral side-flexion]) are all located in the lateral region of the trunk, the MFUs associated with mediomotion (Medio [medial side-flexion]) are located in the medial region, the MFUs associated with extrarotation (Extra) are located in the retrolateral region of the trunk, and those associated with intrarotation (Intra) in the anterolateral region.

- the biarticular muscle fibers that extend between two MFUs in series;
- the myotendinous expansions onto the overlying fascia that extend between segments.

The orientation of these myotendinous expansions (Stecco et al. 2007a, 2008, 2013) guarantees that fascia is stretched simultaneously in more than one point, such that even minimal movement in a specific direction is perceived.

One example of a myofascial sequence is the antemotion sequence of the upper limb. It is formed by the following MFUs:

1. AN–SC, forward movement of the scapula, motor units from pectoralis major (biarticular fibers) and pectoralis minor (monoarticular fibers) and their connecting fascia;
2. AN–HU, forward movement of humerus, motor units from the clavicular head of pectoralis major, long head of biceps (biarticular fibers), anterior deltoid, and coracobrachialis (monoarticular fibers) and their connecting fascia;
3. AN–CU, forward movement of elbow, motor units from biceps brachii (biarticular fibers) and brachialis (monoarticular fibers) and their connecting fascia;
4. AN–CA, forward movement of wrist, motor units from flexor carpi radialis (biarticular fibers) and flexor pollicis longus (monoarticular fibers) and their connecting fascia;
5. AN–DI, forward movement of fingers, motor units from flexor pollicis longus (biarticular fibers) flexor and abductor pollicis brevis (monoarticular fibers) and their connecting fascia.

Note that biarticular muscle fibers and deep fascia (brachial and antebrachial), onto which pectoralis major, biceps brachii, and flexor carpi radialis all extend robust myotendinous expansions, unite these MFUs together in one myofascial sequence.

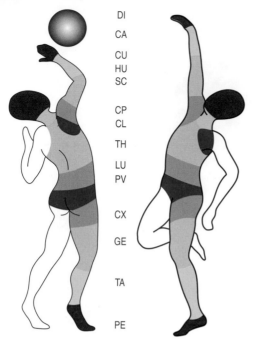

DI
CA
CU
HU
SC

CP
CL

TH

LU
PV

CX

GE

TA

PE

Fig. 7.7.3 Segments of the body. The segments are: DI, digiti/fingers; CA, carpus/wrist; CU, cubitus/elbow; HU, humerus/shoulder; SC, scapula; CP, caput/head; CL, collum/neck; TH, thorax; LU, lumbi; PV, pelvis; CX, coxa/hip; GE, genu/knee; TA, talus/ankle; PE, pes/foot. Redrawn with permission from Stecco, L., 2004. Fascial Manipulation for Musculoskeletal Pain. Piccin, Padova.

All myofascial sequences terminate in the extremities: fingers, toes, and head (Fig. 7.7.4). Tensional compensation beyond these extremities is not possible. Fascial fibrosis along a sequence could culminate in myofascial retraction of the digits and, over time, possibly lead to bony deformation (e.g., hammer toe). According to

which digits are involved, the corresponding myofascial sequence is identifiable.

This overall concept of myofascial sequences can assist in the interpretation of the spread of tensional compensations throughout the fascial system. Some of the more common types of compensations include:

• ascending/descending, and
• homolateral/contralateral.

If the human body were formed by a mere single articulation, then compensation between agonist and antagonist would be sufficient to maintain equilibrium. However, tensional equilibrium involves numerous segments, and each articulation regulates its alignment in relation to proximal and distal segments. In clinical practice, dysfunctions distributed over one spatial plane and, at times, over more than one plane, are much more frequent than pure, segmental dysfunctions. This method stresses the importance of reestablishing equilibrium through the correct interpretation of compensations, working appropriately to distend an entire sequence and restoring balance between agonist and antagonist MFUs (Stecco and Stecco 2017).

KEY POINT

The myofascial sequence are the muscular fascial continuities that we have in our body. It can explain the transmission of force, the coordination between synergic muscle, and some of the Chinese acupuncture meridians.

The Spirals

Each joint commonly moves through intermediate degrees, shifting from one plane to the next. This requires a gradual decrease in the activity of one MFU, simultaneous

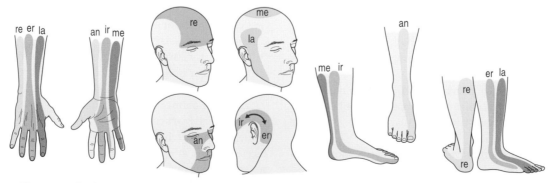

Fig. 7.7.4 Confluence of the sequences in the hands, head, and feet; an, antemotion; re, retromotion; la, lateromotion; me, mediomotion; er, extrarotation; it, intrarotation.

increase of activity in an adjacent MFU, and activation of the appropriate rotatory MFU (in intra- or extrarotation). Furthermore, limb segments often move simultaneously in opposite directions rather than simultaneously in a single direction. Other points on the deep muscular fascia, called centers of fusion (CF), participate with CC in the coordination of these more complex movements. Anatomically, CF are located over the retinacula, which are specialized reinforcements of the muscular fascia in periarticular regions (Stecco et al. 2010; Stecco et al. 2016). Retinacula actually continue from one joint to the next via the oblique collagen fibers within the deep fascia itself, and these oblique fibers create macroscopically visible, extended spiral formations. During complex movements, for example, walking or running, these spiral-form collagen fibers wind and unwind, tensioning the retinacula and thereby activating, deactivating, and synchronizing the CF. At a segmental level, CF are considered to be responsible for monitoring intermediate movements between two directions, whereas when activated in a myofascial spiral, they could monitor movements of adjacent segments in opposite directions.

THE BIOMECHANICAL MODEL FOR THE INTERNAL SYSTEM

In the same way as in the musculoskeletal system, a biomechanical model for the fascial system for internal dysfunctions is introduced.

Visceral fasciae can be divided into two, and they have the same sublayer organization described for the muscular fasciae: investing fascia and insertional fascia (Stecco et al. 2017). The investing fascia that adheres to viscera, glands, and vessels is thin, well-innervated fascia. It is closely related to the individual organ, giving the organ its shape, and supports the organs physiological compliance and movement. Insertional fasciae are thick, less elastic, and less innervated, but they contain large myelinated nerves. They form the compartments and maintain vital spaces around the organs and connect the internal organs to the musculoskeletal system in longitudinal and transverse directions and provide attachments to the trunk wall and muscular fasciae at specific points via mesenteries and internal ligaments. The trunk wall is like a "container" for the internal organs (Stecco et al. 2017; Day 2018).

Fascial Manipulation for Internal Dysfunctions (FMID) can be considered an indirect approach that influences internal organs and systems by acting on key areas on the "container" related to internal fasciae. The functional unit of this biomechanical model is the organ-fascial unit (OFU). Each OFU includes an organ within a trunk segment that performs a specific function and fascia uniting these organs together (Stecco and Stecco 2017).

The organization of the internal fasciae:

- The trunk is formed by four segments: neck, thorax, lumbi, and pelvis.
- Diaphragms subdivide the trunk segments into cavities: cervical, thoracic, lumbar, and pelvic (tensile structures).
- The internal fasciae form three types of fascial compartments in each of the four cavities: one connected to the viscera (visceral OFU), the other to the vessels (vascular OFU), and the third to the glands (glandular OFU).
- Compartments are composed of insertional fasciae that connect OFUs that participate in the same physiological activity (apparatus-fascial sequence).
- Organs that work in synchrony coordinated by their fasciae are found within each of these compartments (OFU).
- Investing fascia coordinate the organs of OFU.

The well-being of any organ or apparatus depends on the balance that exists between its components (Stecco and Stecco 2017). In the normal healthy state the visceral fasciae are relaxed and can stretch and move without restriction. Their pliability can be altered by physical trauma, scarring, infection, or inflammation, and their tightness can produce pain or restriction of motion of the organs (Stecco et al. 2017).

> **KEY POINT**
>
> Fascial Manipulation is able to improve and resolve viscerosomatic and somatovisceral dysfunctions thanks to the connection between the muscular fasciae and the visceral fasciae. Because of these connections, Fascial Manipulation does not have to manipulate the deep part of the abdominal cavity, but its effects appear to restore the mobility and motility of the organs through the normalization of the "containers" and the visceral insertional fasciae.

TREATMENT

Fascial Manipulation method has proven to be effective in reducing subjective pain perception (Guarda-Nardini et al. 2012; Pratelli et al. 2015; Branchini et al. 2015), increasing ROM (Pintucci et al. 2017; Stecco et al. 2014a; Busato et al. 2016) and improving balance (Stecco et al. 2011) and preventing sports injuries (Brandolini et al. 2019).

In the Fascial Manipulation method, it is fundamental to go beyond the idea of treating the site of pain (CP) and to trace the fascial origin in the corresponding CC and/or CF requiring treatment.

Altering the fascia within an MFU could cause:
- inaccurate muscle recruitment,
- nonphysiological joint movement,
- activation of joint nociceptors, and
- joint pain.

Thus it is logical to address the cause of the problem rather than the effect, and a clear understanding of MFU anatomy will assist in this research.

The Fascial Manipulation method has a systematic assessment process for evaluating MFU function. After recording an accurate history, the next step involves specific movement tests to highlight nonfunctional MFUs. Because each MFU performs a single movement, at a single joint and in a specific direction, isotonic or isometric movement tests can reveal which plane of movement is more limited and/or painful. Therefore to test the single MFUs, six specific movement tests have been chosen for each segment.

The next step is comparative palpation of potentially altered CC, as indicated by the movement tests. In this phase, it is important for therapists to know the precise localization of the different CC. The therapist compares sensations perceived by the patient during palpation (e.g., needlelike pain, referred pain) and the quality of the fascial tissue (e.g., fibrotic, lack of elasticity, etc.). Under normal conditions CC and CF are not painful and do not produce referred pain when palpated, because if fascia is elastic it adapts to compression, and embedded receptors are not irritated. Pain on palpation indicates an altered state of the deep muscular fascia, implying that this fascia is unable to accommodate to stretch from underlying muscle fibers, and that embedded receptors, such as free nerve endings, have a lowered pain threshold because of overstimulation.

Accurate compilation of the appropriate evaluation grid will then highlight the degree of involvement of the various MFU, facilitating selection of CC/CF to be treated (Fig. 7.7.5). Single segment problems are relatively rare. Dysfunctions often involve adjacent segments (agonist/antagonist compensation), compensation along fascial compartments (myofascial sequence), or an alternating pattern in different joints (myofascial spiral).

The biomechanical model is useful for interpreting the passage of compensation from one MFU to another, or the evolution from an initial segmental disturbance to a more generalized dysfunction. Evaluation may necessarily extend:
- from one MFU to a distal or proximal CC along the same myofascial sequence,
- to CC in the antagonist sequence, or
- to associated CF.

This investigation process can also include so-called silent CC and CF. These points are not indicated by the specific movement tests and are deduced from the context of the dysfunctional movement or posture. In this way, each individual treatment consists of an individual selection of fascial points.

When the patient presents both musculoskeletal as visceral dysfunctions, Fascial Manipulation level III guides the practitioner to palpate the biomechanical structures that compose the trunk cavities (tensostructure): catenaries, supporting tensors and distal tensors.

If the patient presents also systemic dysfunctions, Fascial Manipulation level IV guideline recommends to add the palpation of superficial fascia to define the treatment plan (Stecco et al. 2016).

The treatment technique consists of a deep friction applied to a precise, limited area (altered CC/CF) (Fig. 7.7.6). The pressure required varies according to the area treated, ranging from 35 to 75 N, with no apparent correlation to body mass index or age (Pedrelli et al. 2009). The aim of treatment is to provoke a localized increase in temperature through mechanical stress over the layers of the deep fascia that are not gliding properly because of densified loose connective tissue.

By limiting the area of treatment, the effects of manual pressure are considered to be deeper and more intense. The direction of the manipulation is also important. It varies from region to region, according to depth of fascia and fiber direction, and indications are given for positioning both patient and therapist to obtain the most effective treatment for each fascial point. Heat, produced by localized friction, could modify the extracellular matrix by decreasing the viscosity (Cowman et al. 2015), restoring the proper sliding between the fascial system. Enhanced fluidity of extracellular matrix would alleviate tension on receptors embedded within the fascial layers restoring their normal threshold of activation. This may account for the sudden "release" sensation perceived by therapists after an average of 3 minutes and until the friction is halved, whereas subjects often report a simultaneous reduction in localized pain and a sensation of

No.	Segments	Location	Side	Duration (acute, 1st time)	T/?	VRS (n–m)	Rec/con	Painful movements:	
SiPa									[logo] Fascial Manipulation – Stecco®
PaConc									
									Name:
Extremities — CP									
Extremities — DI									Surname:
Extremities — PE									
PaPrev								Investigations:	Date of birth:
								Medication:	
Surgery								Internal dysfunction:	Occupation:
Trauma Fracture								Posture:	Sports:

HYPOTHESIS	A	D	SAGITTAL				FRONTAL				HORIZONTAL				Other MoVe:
			ANTE		RETRO		MEDIO		LATERO		INTRA		EXTRA		
SEGMENTS			L	R	L	R	L	R	L	R	L	R	L	R	

		ANTE–MEDIO		RETRO–LATERO		RETRO–MEDIO		ANTE–LATERO	
		L	R	L	R	L	R	L	R
MoVe									
PaVe									

	Outcome	Now
		2nd treatment

Fig. 7.7.5 Fascial Manipulation assessment chart. SiPa, site of pain; PaConc, concomitant pain; PaPrev, previous pain; CP, symptoms related to the head; DI, symptoms related to the hand; PE, symptoms related to the feet; MoVe, movement assessment; PaVe, palpation assessment; A, ascendant; D, descendant; Rec/con, recurrent or constant; T/?, trauma or no trauma; VRS (n–m), verbal rating system (now–maximal).

reduced pressure over the treated point. Reported changes in referred pain experienced during treatment of an altered CC could be due to the normalizing of tension along a myofascial sequence.

This type of treatment produces a localized inflammatory response that is supposed to metabolize the anomalous high viscous extracellular matrix (Cowman et al. 2015). The fasciacyte (Stecco et al. 2018) will then produce the correct hyaluronan for restoring the physiological intrafascial layers' lubrification. However, only a correct tensional balance will guarantee that this occurs according to the physiological direction of movement. Hence, to avoid relapses, treatment should always be aimed at recreating balance within the entire fascial system.

As Fascial Manipulation is applied at a distance from the actual site of joint pain (CP), it has very few contraindications, and this method can be applied safely even during the acute phase of a dysfunction.

Relative contraindications include fever, suspected fracture, or seriously debilitated general health. The most significant drawback is, perhaps, operator inexperience and/or inadequate comprehension of the method. Without a good understanding of all the implications and correlations, restoring a correct equilibrium to the fascial system is rather difficult.

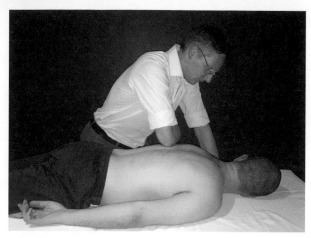

Fig. 7.7.6 Treatment position of the center of coordination of RE-TH (over the fascia of the erector spinae muscles, at the level of the first lumbar vertebra) according to the Fascial Manipulation technique.

Summary

Fascial Manipulation has published more than 30 articles that prove the efficacy and the long-lasting results of the method through many randomized control trials and case series.

These results were possible thanks to a clear understanding of the human fascial system and its disorders, which lead to biomechanical problems such as a decrease in range of motion, pain, and lack of proprioception.

REFERENCES

Branchini, M., Lopopolo, F., Andreoli, E., Loreti, I., Marchand, A., Stecco, A., 2015. Fascial Manipulation® for chronic aspecific low back pain: a single blinded randomized controlled trial. F1000Res. 4, 1208.

Brandolini, S., Lugaresi, G., Santagata, A., et al., 2019. Sport injury prevention in individuals with chronic ankle instability: Fascial Manipulation® versus control group: A randomized controlled trial J. Bodyw. Mov. Ther. 23, 316–323.

Busato, M., Quagliati, C., Magri, L., et al., 2016. Fascial manipulation associated with standard care compared to only standard care postsurgical care for total hip arthroplasty: A randomized controlled trial. PMR 8, 1142–1150.

Cowman, M., Schmidt, T., Raghavan, P., Stecco, A., 2015. Viscoelastic properties of hyaluronan in physiological conditions. F1000Res. 4, 622

Day J., 2018. Fascial Manipulation -Stecco method. The practitioner´s perspective. Handspring, Edinburgh.

Guarda-Nardini, L., Stecco, A., Stecco, C., Masiero, S., Manfredini, D., 2012. Myofascial pain of the jaw muscles: comparison of short-term effectiveness of botulinum toxin injections and fascial manipulation technique. Cranio 30, 95–102.

Huijing, P.A., 2007. Epimuscular myofascial force transmission between antagonistic and synergistic muscles can explain movement limitation in spastic paresis. J. Electromyogr Kinesiol. 17(6), 708–724.

Kalichman, L., Lachman, H., Freilich, N., 2016. Long term impact of ankle sprains on postural control and fascial densification. J. Bodyw. Mov. Ther. 20, 914–919.

Kurtzer, I., Pruszynski, J.A., Herter, T.M., Scott, S.H., 2006. Primate upper limb muscles exhibit activity patterns that differ from their anatomical action during a postural task. J. Neurophysiol. 95, 493–504.

Mellor, R., Hodges, P.W., 2005. Motor unit synchronization is reduced in anterior knee pain. J. Pain 6, 550–558.

Pedrelli, A., Stecco, C., Day, J.A., 2009.Treating patellar tendinopathy with Fascial Manipulation. J. Bodyw. Mov. Ther. 13, 73–80.

Pintucci, M., Simis, M., Imamura, M., et al., 2017. Successful treatment of rotator cuff tear using Fascial Manipulation® in a stroke patient. J. Bodyw. Mov. Ther. 21, 653–657.

Pratelli, E., Pintucci, M., Cultrera, P., et al., 2015. Conservative treatment of carpal tunnel syndrome: comparison between laser therapy and Fascial Manipulation®. J. Bodyw. Mov. Ther. 19, 113–118.

Stecco, A., Gilliar, W., Hill, R., Fullerton, B., Stecco, C., 2013. The anatomical and functional relation between gluteus maximus and fascia lata. J. Bodyw. Mov. Ther. 17, 512–517.

Stecco, A., Macchi, V., Stecco, C., et al., 2009. Anatomical study of myofascial continuity in the anterior region of the upper limb. J. Bodyw. Mov. Ther. 13, 53–62.

Stecco, A., Meneghini, A., Stern, R., Stecco, C., Imamura, M., 2014a. Ultrasonography in myofascial neck pain: randomized clinical trial for diagnosis and follow up. Surg. Radiol. Anat. 36, 243–253.

Stecco, A., Stecco, C., Macchi, V., et al. 2011. RMI study and clinical correlations of ankle retinacula damage and outcomes of ankle sprain. Surg. Radiol. Anat. 33, 881–890.

Stecco, A., Stecco, C., Raghavan, P., 2014b. Peripheral mechanisms contributing to spasticity and implications for treatment. Curr. Phys. Med. Rehabil. Rep. 2, 121–127.

Stecco, A., Stern, R., Fantoni, I., De Caro, R., Stecco, C., 2016. Fascial disorders: implications for treatment. PMR 8, 161–168.

Stecco, C., 2015. Functional Atlas of the Human Fascial System. Elsevier, China.

Stecco, C., Fede, C., Macchi, V., et al., 2018. The Fasciacytes: A New Cell Devoted to Fascial Gliding Regulation. Clin. Anat. 31, 615–757.

Stecco, C., Fede, C., Macchi, V., et al., 2018. The fasciacytes: A new cell devoted to fascial gliding regulation. Clin. Anat. 31, 667–676.

Stecco, C., Gagey, O., Belloni, A., et al., 2007a. Anatomy of the deep fascia of the upper limb. Second part: study of innervation. Morphologie 91, 38–43.

Stecco, C., Gagey, O., Macchi, V., et al., 2007b. Tendinous muscular insertions onto the deep fascia of the upper limb. First part: anatomical study. Morphologie 91, 29–37.

Stecco, C., Macchi, V., Porzionato, A., et al., 2010. The ankle retinacula: morphological evidence of the proprioceptive role of the fascial system. Cells Tissues Organs. 192, 200–210.

Stecco, C., Pirri, C., Fede, C., et al., 2019. Dermatome and fasciotome. Clin. Anat. 32, 896–902.

Stecco, C., Porzionato, A., Macchi, V., et al., 2008. The expansions of the pectoral girdle muscles onto the brachial fascia: morphological aspects and spatial disposition. Cells Tissues Organs 188, 320–329.

Stecco, C., Porzionato, A., Macchi, V., et al., 2006. Histological characteristics of the deep fascia of the upper limb. Ital. J. Anat. Embryol. 111, 105–110.

Stecco, C., Sfriso, M., Porzionato, A., et al., 2017. Microscopic anatomy of the visceral fasciae. J. Anat. 231, 121–128.

Stecco, L., 2004. Fascial Manipulation for Musculoskeletal Pain. Piccin, Padova.

Stecco, L., Stecco, A., 2017. Fascial Manipulation® for Musculoskeletal Pain. Theoretical Part. second ed. Piccin, Padua.

Stecco, L., Stecco, C., 2007. Fascial Manipulation for Musculoskeletal Pain. Theoretical Part. Piccin, Padua.

Turrina, A., Martínez-Gonzáles, M., Stecco, C., 2013. The muscular force transmission system: Role of the intramuscular connective system. J. Bodyw. Mov. Ther. 17, 95–102.

Managing Dysfunctional Scar Tissue

Mariane Altomare

CHAPTER CONTENTS

INTRODUCTION

The wound-healing mechanisms after injury are among the most complex processes occurring in multicellular organisms. In mammals, the typical response to injury is fibrotic scar formation, which reestablishes the tissue integrity and function. The adult human wounds heal with some degree of scar formation that may compromise function and appearance, during the estimated 230 million major surgical procedures performed worldwide each year. After skin injury, the mechanophysiological conditions are drastically changed by wound healing and considerably influence the degree of scarring. The result of the process can be a fine, thin scar, barely perceptible, or an exuberant fibrosis that can be dysfunctional and disfiguring. In this chapter, the author proposes successful treatment based on the effects of mechanical forces and tissue reactions at a microscopic level during wound healing, because these forces play an important therapeutic target in preventing skin fibrosis and ameliorating the quality of scar tissues.

CONNECTIVE TISSUE AND THE EXTRACELLULAR MATRIX

Connective tissue is classified based on the characteristics of its cellular and extracellular components, and it is very important to understand the normal assembly to identify alterations, for example, the presence of fibrosis, adhesions, and scars.

The extracellular matrix (ECM) is a highly dynamic structural network that continuously undergoes remodeling mediated by several matrix-degrading enzymes during normal and pathological conditions (Theocharis et al. 2016).

ECM accumulation and increase in tissue stiffness are common features of fibrosis. This accumulation alters the tissue's mechanical properties, which in turn can deleteriously affect organ function. Cells sense and respond to ECM rigidity, which can regulate cell growth, migration, and differentiation. ECM rigidity also affects other parameters associated with fibrosis, including the deposition and organization of the ECM structure. ECM function is directly associated with its assembly. Alterations of the assembly will affect function. It is now very clear that tissue stiffness may precede fibrosis or at least contribute to ongoing fibrosis. ECM accumulation can also reduce fascial mobilization, clutch nerves, and impair lymphangiogenesis.

WOUND HEALING

Injury to tissue triggers several events to start the healing process. Wound healing is a complex and dynamic process that involves many components of ECM, soluble mediators, and blood and resident cells, orchestrated to restore tissue integrity. Healing happens in three interrelated and interdependent phases: inflammation, granulation tissue formation, and remodeling (Fig. 7.8.1).

KEY POINTS

Wound healing is a dynamic, interactive process involving soluble mediators, blood cells, extracellular matrix, and parenchymal cells. Wound healing occurs in three phases—inflammation, tissue formation, and tissue remodeling—that overlap in time.

The inflammatory phase is the first one, right after injury. Tissue injury causes the disruption of blood vessels and extravasation of blood components that lead to clot formation. The clot provides a provisional extracellular matrix, formed mainly by fibrin and fibronectin that allow the migration of other cells, attracted by the platelets, which also release and activate several vasoactive mediators and chemotactic factors, such as vascular endothelial growth factor, epidermal growth factor, platelet-derived growth factor, and transforming growth factor beta (TGF-β).

During granulation tissue formation (proliferative phase), fibroblasts and endothelial cells proliferate and move into the wound space, leading to extracellular

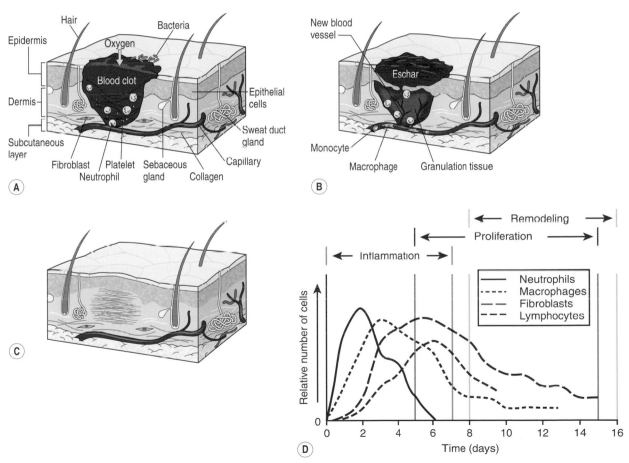

Fig. 7.8.1 Wound-healing process: (A) Inflammation; (B) proliferation (ECM synthesis); (C) remodeling and scar formation; (D) overlapping of the three phases in days. Redrawn from Brown, M. S., Ashley, B., Koh, A., 2018. Wearable technology for chronic wound monitoring: current dressings, advancements, and future prospects. Front. Bioeng. Biotechnol. 6, 47. Open access. https://creativecommons.org/licenses/by/4.0/

matrix deposition and angiogenesis, which are typical features of granulation tissue formation. The provisional ECM is replaced by fibroblasts that participate actively in wound healing, and that is why it is important to know the mechanisms involved in their behavior.

Myofibroblasts

Myofibroblasts are differentiated fibroblasts that are activated in response to tissue injury with the primary task to repair lost or damaged extracellular matrix. Their function includes wound contraction and collagen secretion.

Differentiated myofibroblasts can be distinguished from proto-myofibroblasts by the expression of alpha-smooth muscle actin (alpha-SMA) and the increased expression of ED-A fibronectin, as well as increased assembly of stress fibers and focal adhesions. TGF-β1 has a key role in stimulating all of these characteristics of the differentiated myofibroblast (Tomasek et al. 2002)

Enhanced collagen secretion and subsequent contraction and scarring are part of the normal wound-healing response and crucial to restoring tissue integrity. Because of myofibroblasts' ability to repair but not regenerate, accumulation of scar tissue is always associated with reduced organ performance. After successful repair they vanish, and dysregulation of the process can lead to persistent myofibroblast activation. Pathological/excessive repair leads to the accumulation of stiff collagenous ECM contractures—fibrosis with dramatic consequences for organ function (Hinz 2016).

SCAR TISSUES

Mechanobiology and Neurophysiology

The effect of mechanical forces on tissue fibrosis has been observed as early as the 19th century, but we have only just begun to understand the underlying molecular mechanisms. The effects of mechanical forces on cells and tissues have received greater attention, and experimental models have been developed to systematically analyze these effects. Research in the field of soft tissue mechanobiology has elucidated how mechanical forces regulate cellular organization and behavior.

Mechanotransduction

Mechanotransduction is the study of the mechanisms by which mechanical forces are converted to biochemical changes and has been linked to inflammation and fibrosis formation. It plays a critical role in scarring.

Mechanical forces play important roles in homeostasis and pathogenesis. They can affect cell behavior, including proliferation, differentiation, migration, and gene expression. It is well established how cells respond to mechanical stimuli and has resulted in enhanced interest in the contribution of these forces to pathogenesis, including tissue fibrosis.

Cells can be exposed to diverse types of extrinsic mechanical forces, including mechanical stretch (tension), compression, and shear stress. Alterations in mechanical load in vivo have been known for some time to affect synthesis and deposition of the ECM. Because of accumulation of ECM components and cross-linking of these components, alterations in tissue stiffness are a common feature of fibrosis (Carver and Goldsmith 2013).

Biomechanical properties of the microenvironment can direct the expression of ECM components and ECM-modifying enzymes with stiffer tissue properties contributing to enhanced ECM production. Less rigid matrices appear to promote an antifibrotic environment that includes increased production of matrix-degrading proteases and antifibrotic agents like prostaglandin.

Matrix rigidity affects not only the expression of ECM components but also other parameters associated with fibrosis, including the deposition and organization of these components.

Cutaneous Nerves

The skin is densely innervated with an intricate network of cutaneous nerves, neuromodulators, and specific receptors that influence a variety of physiological and disease processes. There is emerging evidence that cutaneous innervation may play an important role in mediating wound healing. Numerous neuropeptides that are secreted by the sensory and autonomic nerve fibers play an essential part during the distinct phases of wound healing (Ashrafi et al. 2016).

The innervated skin is a vital barrier with direct contact to the central nervous system. These nerves are crucial in influencing physiological and pathophysiological cutaneous functions. Mechanoreceptors, thermoreceptors, and nociceptors are found in the epidermis and dermis. Mechanoreceptors in the epidermis are Merkel discs and free nerve endings. Mechanoreceptors in the dermis are Ruffini, Meissner, and Pacinian corpuscles and free nerve endings (Alvarez and Fyffe 2000).

Cutaneous sensory nerves are classified according to diameter and speed of impulse as Aβ, Aδ, and C nerve fibers. Aβ fibers are fast and large whereas C fibers are slow and small. Aδ fibers constitute 80% of primary sensory nerves emerging from the dorsal root ganglia, whereas C fibers make up 20% of the primary nerves (Caillaud et al. 2019).

It is impossible to mention cutaneous nerves without mentioning Diane Jacobs and her dermoneuromodulation, which is a special manual treatment focused on restoring the nerves' blood flow and drainage, respecting neurophysiology, and so decreasing pain and dysfunction.

KEY POINTS

- Nerves are physical and have biomechanics, called "neurodynamics."
- Neurons are well-protected within nerve walls from compression.
- Skin organ contains thousands of small physical nerve branches.
- Skin organ is easy to move around.
- Moving skin will move these rami PLUS activate low-threshold mechanoreceptors and affect the nervous system and nerve physiology; PLUS it has psychosocial benefits.
- The main goal is to help the entire system relieve pain from pathodynamic effects of nerves that cannot move adequately.

Nerves and Scar Tissues

The nervous system is a very long organ and provides unique features that explain many clinical problems that are not attributable to other systems. During body movements, tension is applied to the nervous system at the site where the force initiated, and this tension is transmitted further along the system. The nerve slide mechanisms depend on the connective tissues around the fibers; thus scar tissues can impair nerve function by blocking the sliding.

Neurodynamics is not only normal movement but is also used as a treatment approach (Shacklock 1995). Compression forces can affect the blood nerve flow and produce neuropathic symptoms; this is called the "Tourniquet effect" (Shacklock 2005).

Scars

A. Cutaneous Scar Classification According to Gold (2014)

Mature

Light-colored, flat scar

Immature

Red, sometimes itchy or painful, and slightly elevated scar in the process of remodeling

Many will mature normally over time, become flat, and assume a pigmentation that is similar to the surrounding skin, although they can be paler or slightly darker.

Linear hypertrophic (e.g., surgical/traumatic)

Red, raised, sometimes itchy scar confined to the border of the original surgical incision. This usually occurs within weeks after surgery.

May increase in size rapidly for 3 to 6 months and then, after a static phase, begin to regress.

Generally mature to have an elevated, slightly rope-like appearance with increased width that is variable. Full maturation process may take up to 2 years.

Widespread hypertrophic (e.g., burn)

Widespread, red, raised, sometimes itchy scar that remains within the borders of the burn injury

Minor keloid

Focally raised, itchy scar extending over normal tissue

May develop up to 1 year after injury and does not regress on its own

Simple surgical excision is often followed by recurrence

May be a genetic abnormality involved in keloid scarring

Typical sites include earlobes

Major keloid

Large, raised (>0.5 cm) scar, possibly painful or pruritic and extending over normal tissue

Often results from minor trauma and can continue to spread over the years.

B. Evaluation: Cutaneous Scar Grading Systems

A variety of measurement tools have been applied to grade scars based on parameters such as pigmentation, vascularity, thickness, pliability, height or depression, patient acceptability, and comfort.

Scar grading systems are used to quantify changes in scar appearance during treatment, typically in a clinical research setting.

C. Dysfunctional Scar Tissues

The presence of scar tissue can induce dysfunction not only in skin but in all surrounding tissues (nerves, fascia, muscles, joints) and can compromise the sliding/gliding fascial system. The loose connective tissue layers that permit micro- and macromovements between interfascial planes dehydrate, generating friction, and can impair normal movement. Furthermore, chronic pain is not rare after surgeries.

Immobilization must be avoided to prevent mobility dysfunctions and chronic pain; this can be achieved with the proper manual therapy treatment followed by active movement to complete function.

D. Fibrosis and Adhesions

First, it is important to clarify the differences between scars, fibrosis, and adhesions, because these differences influence the therapeutic strategy.

Fibrosis is the *excess* of deposition of ECM components, with increased stiffness. The molecular mechanisms that lead to fibrosis formation include (1) differentiation of the fibroblasts in myofibroblasts, (2) permanence of myofibroblasts (delayed apoptosis), (3) activation of TGF- β1, and (4) alteration of a large damaged area (that needs a large amount of scar tissue to be filled).

Normally, if the inflammatory phase is too intense—which happens accordingly to the trauma extension—the proliferative phase will also be intense. Therefore one good option to prevent fibrosis is controlling the wound area in order to decrease the inflammatory response.

Fibrosis can also develop because of a prolonged proliferative phase—bad treatment choices can delay the remodeling phase or cause tissue damage by microtrauma or inappropriate tension, friction, rubbing the tissues, and alterations on the biomechanical environment.

Fibrosis is also a consequence of a fibroproliferative disease but is always associated with excess of the ECM components, mainly collagen. We can say that fibrosis is like a hypertrophic scar, but localized under the skin on subcutaneous tissues and organs.

> **KEY POINT**
>
> Fibrosis is a common pathological process characterized by the excessive accumulation of extracellular matrix proteins, in particular, collagen. The increased deposition of collagen is the result of increased collagen synthesis accompanied by decreased proteinase activity.

It is common to hear that once fibrosis has begun, it cannot be reversed; however, studies have illustrated that fibrosis can be reversed by applying manual therapy (Altomare et al. 2018). ECM biomechanical properties may be important therapeutic targets that are able to

modulate myofibroblast formation and fibrosis (Carver and Goldsmith 2013).

Adhesions are the loss of the loose connective layers' sliding system. This can happen with or without tissue damage. For example, loose connective tissue densification/dehydration can promote adhesions and impair the glide between the layers. Adhesions can also be defined as abnormal bands of fibrous tissue that form between two anatomically different structures, causing adherence and restricted visceral mobility (Awonuga et al. 2011).

Adhesions are an issue in abdominal surgeries, and they are related to chronic pain: "Adhesions from a surgical scar can not only contribute to immediate postoperative pain, but can contribute to the development of local or radiating chronic pain" and "alter the proprioceptive input of the region as a result of compromised tissue tensioning. This faulty afferent input can cause subsequent faulty efferent output, leading to a variety of complications such as protective postural patterns, increased neurovascular activity, and pain syndromes" (Kobesova et al. 2007; 30, 234–238).

THERAPEUTIC APPROACH

Although many treatment modalities are effective as monotherapies for scar revision, in some cases the optimal improvement is achieved by combining multiple treatment strategies, and it is important to work with a multiprofessional team. The first step before any treatment is to evaluate the clinical features of the scar, observing the timing in relation to the initial surgical procedure. During healing, the scar improves in a natural way, affected by the micromechanical environment (Gurtner et al. 2011); the treatment should include the observation (and respect) of clinical features/wound-healing phases and time relative to initial scar formation or subsequent treatment intervention. Routine clinical practice, including evaluation of size, thickness, symptom severity, and patient concerns, is recommended.

For an effective treatment of dysfunctional scar tissues, it is mandatory to respect the wound-healing biological mechanisms and both the mechano- and neurophysiological aspects. Hence we propose a specialized manual treatment based on molecular mechanisms of wound healing, applying concepts to control the biomechanical environment, thus preventing and treating fibrosis, adhesions, and scars. This treatment is called Manual Mechanomodulatory Therapy (see more in Orthopedic Manipulative Physical Therapy, later).

Dermatological/Cosmetic/Surgical Options

This modality of treatment includes: intralesional corticoids; laser therapies; microneedling and fractional needle radiofrequency; use of antifibrotic cytokines; scar revision surgery; cryosurgery; stem cells; and tissue engineering (Berman et al. 2017; Gold et al. 2014).

Massage Therapies/Myofascial Techniques

There are a lot of differing techniques described to release scar tissue (and abdominal scar tissue), including direct and indirect mobilization of the abdominal viscera (Barral and Mercier 2005), pelvic and abdominal diaphragmatic myofascial release (Barnes et al. 1997), and direct scar release (Manheim 2008). The literature suggests scar massage/myofascial techniques for treatment of adhesions and scar pain. Bove and Chapelle demonstrated in rats that interperitoneal lesions can be treated with a technique called MMT—Modeled Manual Therapy (Bove and Chapelle 2012). Shin and colleagues used the Patient and Observer Assessment Scale (POSAS) in a systematic review that revealed scar massage techniques performed on surgical scars show a 90% improvement of the appearance of the scar; however, they noted that the scar massage techniques used lacked standardized, objective measurements, and also the techniques and regimens used were varied (Shin and Bordeaux 2012).

Although the literature shows the use of massage techniques to treat scars and adhesions, it is highly recommended to respect the mechanical forces that control cell metabolism (mechanotransduction) to optimize the results. See the following discussion on the specialized scar tissue approach Manual Mechanomodulatory Therapy.

Orthopedic Manipulative Physical Therapy

Orthopedic manual physical therapy is a specialized area of physiotherapy/physical therapy for the management of neuromusculoskeletal conditions based on clinical reasoning, using highly specific treatment approaches, including special manual techniques and therapeutic exercises. Orthopedic manual physical therapy also encompasses, and is driven by, the available scientific and clinical evidence and the biopsychosocial framework of each individual patient. Because we are evaluating dysfunctional tissues, it is important to note that not only skin suffers the consequences of the presence of scars but also nerves, joints, fasciae, and muscles,

and an appropriate, entire, and specialized therapeutic approach is essential to achieve normal function.

Here in Brazil, we developed a treatment strategy regarding experimental findings with the triad *wound healing x manual therapy x fibrosis, scars, and adhesions* based on the concerns of orthopedic manual physical therapy.

Specialized Manual Therapy for Fibrosis, Scars, and Adhesions: The Manual Mechanomodulatory Therapy

Although there are no randomized controlled trials on this issue, in the author's almost 20 years of physiotherapy clinical practice, always performing criterious evaluations on the mobility of skin, ROM (range of motion) stiffness, and patients' sensations (pain, rigidity, restrictions), the importance of fibrosis prevention and specific treatment by orthopedic manual therapy has been noticed.

Ever since the literature started showing the molecular mechanisms of fibrosis formation, we started using those concepts in our clinical practice. This is done to control the tissue's biomechanical environment while preventing and treating fibrosis (collagen excess) by applying manual mobilization, especially shear stress and compression on skin and subcutaneous tissues, balancing intrinsic and extrinsic forces and also reducing ECM excess to achieve better quality and functional scar tissue formation and prepare the whole body for movement.

In our treatment strategy, Manual Mechanomodulatory Therapy, we apply the concepts of mechanobiological and neurophysiological aspects to prevent and treat fibrosis, and we are currently collecting data for our clinical trial that will soon be published.

Understanding the ECM dynamics involved in fibrosis formation is helpful to develop therapeutic options. Manual myofascial therapies and fascial movement therapies can assist in the process of improving matrix remodeling, but to reach optimal results, the therapeutic option must respect tissue physiology— concepts described in research on mechanobiology and neurophysiology.

When to Use Manual Mechanomodulatory Therapy?

Manual Mechanomodulatory Therapy is recommended to treat fibrosis, adhesions, and scars, thus it is necessary to evaluate tissue mobility (sliding system) and stiffness.

Palpation is one of the options. It is possible to touch the tissues at different depths and feel the hardening if you are a well-skilled therapist.

Several tools have been proposed for the assessment of stiffness, but according to Stecco and colleagues (2019), "ultrasonography appears to be most practical. The reflection of ultrasound waves as it travels through tissue enables assessment of tissue echogenicity, which is influenced by the characteristics of the sound wave as well as the characteristics of the tissue through which it passes, such as the amount of fat and fibrous tissue" (Fig. 7.8.2, p 178).

Once densification and movement dysfunction is detected, Manual Mechanomodulatory Therapy can be used, because the therapeutic indication is to decrease stiffness/densification and fibrosis and recover the sliding system of the tissue interfaces.

Basic Principles of Manual Mechanomodulatory Therapy

- There is no protocol; the approach is ALWAYS according to clinical findings. You cannot determine the approach according to the number of days after the wounding, for example. You need to find the exact location that you need to treat (use palpation and shearing).
- Evaluation is key: where exactly are the glide limitations and stiffness?
- Once you carry out the correct movements, the tissue will melt, and you can feel the restoration of the gliding system.
- Specific treatment for specific indication: if you need to reduce fibrosis, densification and adherences, you will achieve mechanical balance and restore tissue layer sliding.

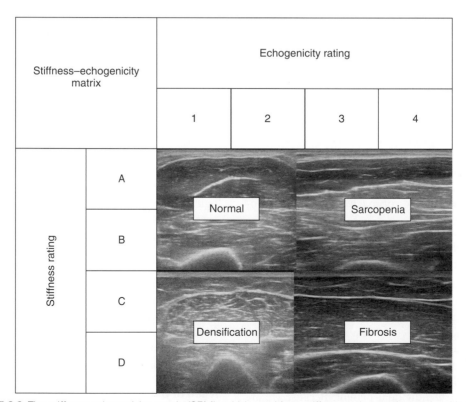

Fig. 7.8.2 The stiffness-echogenicity matrix (SEM), which combines stiffness rating on the y-axis with echogenicity rating on the x-axis: each quadrant of the matrix can represent a wide spectrum of conditions seen in clinical practice. Redrawn with permission from Stecco, A., Pirri, C., De Caro, R., Raghavan, P., 2019. Stiffness and echogenicity: Development of a stiffness-echogenicity matrix for clinical problem solving. Eur. J. Transl. Myol. 29, 178–184.

- Use safe techniques, as it respects physiological and structural parameters.
- MANAGE: never use unnecessary stimuli.

For application, some precautions are essential:

Depth: depends on the tissue you need to reach—subcutaneous/superficial fascia, muscles/deep fascia, viscera, or joints. The pressure of the hands will be heavier to treat deeper layers.

Mobilization: keep the pressure on the layer to be treated while sliding skin over superficial fascia or deep fascia; respect the barriers: (1) structural—bony edges, pressure is lighter when we are over bony edges (thin subcutaneous); and (2) functional—only up to tissue allows, it's only movement without stretching. Just moving the tissues and their interfaces.

KEY POINTS

Manual Mechanomodulatory Therapy "secret" keys:
- NEVER spread the scar edges.
- Don't mobilize between the edges of normal scars: the treatment is performed at surrounding tissues. If you treat between the edges, you take the tensile strength of the scar, and it can widen.
- To a perfect scar: balance the intrinsic and extrinsic forces, off-loading the surrounding tissues by mobilization of the adjacent subcutaneous.
- You can treat recent and belated fibrosis simply by applying movement between tissue layers, but you must respect the functional barriers and put pressure on the fibrosis.
- You can use kinesio tape as a mechanical treatment to shield the edges.
- Patient position: it is mandatory to slack the tissues before accessing them. If you pressure a dense (overloaded) area, you will increase intrinsic tension. For example, to access a C-section scar, you must bend the patient's legs and trunk.
- Repeat the technique in a time interval of about 5 to 10 days. Usually you do not need more than 3 to 5 sessions.
- Do it slowly. To respect nerve fibers and skin receptors, the movement is slow and never produces pain or discomfort.

Another important point in Manual Mechanomodulatory Therapy principles is to always start in superficial layers and proceed deeper as the tissue allows. To treat deep fascia/muscles and viscera make sure there is no stiffness in the subcutaneous layer.

When limiting fibrosis/adhesions/scars are detected, the initial approach must be passive mobilization, and when the tissues are released, the approach involves active movements for a complete functional recovery.

Summary

- During wound healing or chronic pathological conditions—such as fibrosis—tissue stiffness can increase progressively in days to weeks because of the action of mechanical forces and the contractile activity of myofibroblasts.
- The presence of hypertrophic scars close to joints, muscles, and tendons can compromise the functionality and articular movement, requiring appropriate treatment of the adjacent loose connective tissues (responsible for the movement between the tissue interfaces) prior to the articular approach, to avoid overloading scar tissues.
- Though appropriate amounts of intrinsic tension are required for wound closure, an important factor in the degree of healing after injury is extrinsic mechanical strength. The balance of these forces plays a fundamental role in the formation of scars.
- Scars under tension show greater cellularity, vascularization, and number of myofibroblasts, a phenotype that could be avoided by discharging the adjacent/extrinsic tension. Controlling the mechanobiological environment is crucial for the quality of scar formation after injury.
- The intrinsic tension of the tissues influences the skin response to the injury.
- Manually tissue unloading significantly reduces pathological healing.
- Previous studies have suggested that ECM remodeling induced by mobilization is an important natural mechanism that limits excessive healing and fibrosis after injury.
- It is clear in the literature that mechanical forces are crucial in the development, homeostasis, and repair of human skin. Effective approaches to prevent and treat excess scarring are needed.
- The accumulation of extracellular matrix molecules or changes in the proportion of their proteins, as occurs during fibrosis and healing, can directly inhibit the proliferation of lymphatic endothelial cells.
- It is well established that the evolution (remodeling) of granulation tissue in scar tissue implies a massive decrease in cellularity and disappearance of myofibroblasts (apoptosis). High degree of cellularity is a characteristic of hypertrophic scars.
- Do not treat scar tissue with aggressive and/or painful maneuvers.
- Release of neurotransmitters can stimulate matrix synthesis and excessive healing.

REFERENCES

Altomare, M., Monte-Alto-Costa, A., 2018. Manual mobilization of subcutaneous fibrosis in mice. J. Manipulative Physiol. Ther. 41, 359–362.

Alvarez, F.J., Fyffe, R.E., 2000. Nociceptors for the 21st century. Curr. Rev. Pain 4, 451–458.

Ashrafi, M., Baguneid, M., Bayat, A., 2016. The role of neuromediators and innervation in cutaneous wound healing. Acta Derm. Venereol. 96, 587–594.

Awonuga, A.O., Fletcher, N.M., Saed, G.M., Diamond, M.P., 2011. Postoperative adhesion development following cesarean and open intra-abdominal gynecological operations: a review. Reprod. Sci. 18, 1166–1185.

Barnes, M.F., Gronlund, R.T., Little, M.F., Personius, W.J., 1997. Efficacy study of the effect of a myofascial release treatment technique on obtaining pelvic symmetry. J. Bodyw. Mov. Ther. 1, 289–296.

Barral, J.P., Mercier, P., 2005. Visceral Manipulation Eastland Press; Seattle USA Revised ed.

Berman, B., Maderal, A., Raphael, B., 2017. Keloids and hypertrophic scars: pathophysiology, classification, and treatment. Dermatol. Surg. 43, S3–S18.

Bove, G.M., Chapelle, S.L., 2012. Visceral mobilization can lyse and prevent peritoneal adhesions in a rat model. J. Bodyw. Mov. Ther. 16, 76–82.

Caillaud, M., Richard, L., Vallat, J.M., Desmoulière, A., Billet, F., 2019. Peripheral nerve regeneration and intraneural revascularization. Neural Regen. Res. 14, 24–33.

Carver, W., Goldsmith, E.C., 2013. Regulation of tissue fibrosis by the biomechanical environment. Biomed Res. Int. 2013, 101979.

Gold, M.H., McGuire, M., Mustoe, T.A., et al., 2014. Updated international clinical recommendations on scar management: part 2—algorithms for scar prevention and treatment. Dermatol. Surg. 40, 825–831.

Gurtner, G.C., Dauskardt, R.H., Wong, V.W., et al., 2011. Improving cutaneous scar formation by controlling the mechanical environment. Large animal and phase I studies. Ann. Surg. 254, 217–225.

Hinz, B., 2016. Myofibroblasts. Exp. Eye Res. 142, 56–70.

Kobesova, A., Morris, C.E., Lewit, K., Safarova, M., 2007. Twenty-year-old pathogenic "active" postsurgical scar: a case study of a patient with persistent right lower quadrant pain. J. Manipulative Physiol. Ther. 30, 234–238.

Manheim, C.J., 2008. The Myofascial Release Manual, fourth ed. Slack Books, Thorofare, NJ.

Shacklock, M., 1995. Neurodynamics. Physiotherapy 81, 9–15

Shacklock, M., 2005. Clinical Neurodynamics. Butterworth-Heinemann Elsevier, Edinburgh.

Shin, T.M., Bordeaux, J.S., 2012. The role of massage in scar management: a literature review. Dermatol. Surg. 38, 414–423.

Stecco, A., Pirri, C., De Caro, R., Raghavan, P., 2019. Stiffness and echogenicity: Development of a stiffness-echogenicity matrix for clinical problem solving. Eur. J. Transl. Myol. 29, 8476.

Theocharis, A.D., Skandalis, S.S., Gialeli, C., Karamanos, N.K., 2016. Extracellular Matrix Structure, Adv. Drug Deliv. Rev. 97, 4–27

Tomasek, J.J., Gabbiani, G., Hinz, B., Chaponnier, C., Brown, R.A., 2002. Myofibroblasts and mechanoregulation of connective tissue remodeling. Nat. Rev. Mol. Cell Biol. 3, 349–363.

Acupuncture as a Fascia-Oriented Therapy

Dominik Irnich and Johannes Fleckenstein

CHAPTER CONTENTS

HISTORICAL BACKGROUND

Acupuncture has increasingly been used in Western medicine over the last three decades. It originated with Traditional Chinese medicine (TCM) in the early Han period and was described systematically for the first time in the medical compilation *Huangdi Neijing* (*Yellow Emperor's Inner Classic*), whose texts date from the Han period (200 BCE to CE 200) (Zhu 2001). Acupuncture means in its Chinese translation of *zhen jiu* "needling burning." However, before the development of steel needles, acupuncture consisted of skin irritation using sharp objects (e.g., stones), local warming at defined body sites, and minimal surgical interventions like bloodletting (for review, see: O'Connor and Bensky 1981; Cheng 1987).

Nowadays, acupuncture is defined as needling at anatomically defined sites of the body (acupuncture points) or sensitive spots (*ah shi* points) for therapeutic purposes, including so-called moxibustion—that is, heating or warming of the skin at acupuncture points with the help of burning mugwort (*Artemisia vulgaris*) (Fig. 7.9.1).

Acupuncture includes different techniques of needle stimulation, for example, repetitive thrusting, twisting, rotating, or electrical stimulation to achieve different treatment effects according to the theoretical background.

There are different acupuncture-related techniques such as laser acupuncture, injection in acupuncture points, and acupressure. A huge body of further manual or tool-assisted treatment approaches is based on the concept of acupuncture points and meridians.

The theoretical background of acupuncture is based on Chinese, Confucian-legalistic, social, and political philosophy of the first century. Acupuncture can be performed based on the theory of traditional Chinese medicine but also pragmatically and anatomically based (e.g., ear acupuncture, trigger point acupuncture). In general, acupuncture is based on the subjective aspects of disease, in contrast to the diagnostic and therapeutic understanding in Western medicine, which is based on objective measurable pathologies. Acupuncture consists of systematic analogy expressed in the early concepts of yin and yang, qi and the internal organs, and results of detailed observations of nature and life.

KEY POINT

Acupuncture is an ancient technique deriving from philosophical concepts in China. Acupuncture means needling at defined sites of the human body. Nowadays, several stimulation techniques originating from all over the world (besides needling, e.g., warming, cupping, and electrostimulation) are subsumed under the term acupuncture.

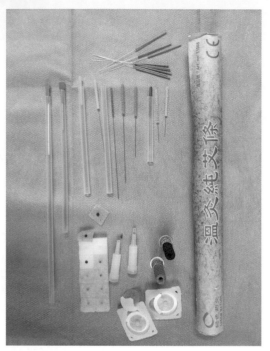

Fig. 7.9.1 Choice of acupuncture instruments: different kinds of needles and mugwort. From J. Fleckenstein's personal collection, with permission.

Yin and Yang

Originally the light and shadow side of a hill, yin and yang are the two opposites of a dual principle as a pattern of organization for the whole cosmos but also for the physiology and anatomy of organisms.

Qi

Qi expresses an energetic concept of vitality circulating in every body, in the beginning more likely as living matter. It might be weak, blocked, accumulated, or misdistributed—all this aiming to describe different subjective symptoms.

Acupuncture Points

Acupuncture points are anatomically defined sites through which the qi of the meridians and zang fu organs (see later discussion) is transported to the body surface. The Chinese characters for an acupuncture point mean, respectively, "transportation" and "hole." From an anatomical and physiological point of view acupuncture points can correlate to myofascial trigger points, overlap zones of segmental innervation,

openings in the fascia for vessel-nerve cords, or sites with easy access to nerves and/or vessels.

Meridians

All 361 classical acupuncture points lie strung together on the body surface according to a yin–yang pattern. They are lined up in three systems (front, back, and lateral aspects of the body). Qi is supposed to circulate within these meridians (Fig. 7.9.2).

Internal Organs (Zang Fu)

The concept of organs is based on the principle of the Five Phases—correlating organ dysfunction to other physiological and psychoemotional conditions. This traditional concept goes far beyond anatomical and physiological considerations. Organs and meridians are internally and externally connected.

> **KEY POINT**
>
> Yin and yang, qi, meridians, acupuncture points, and zang fu are standing concepts in TCM and acupuncture. They are needed in the process of diagnosis and therapy.

TCM holds that there is normally a state of relative equilibrium between the human body and the external environment, on the one hand, and among the internal organs within the body, on the other hand—that is, the equilibrium between protective and pathogenic influences. Pathogenesis may be caused by external (e.g., annual recurrence of hay fever, improper diet) or internal (e.g., emotions, overstrain) factors. The occurrence of any disease is, therefore, according to the philosophical background, due to a relative imbalance of yin and yang. This imbalance may result in different symptoms expressed, for example, as a stagnation of the flow of qi in channels on the body surface or internal organs. Regulation of yin and yang is therefore a fundamental principle in the clinical treatment. To restore health, acupuncturists insert and manipulate needles or heat the skin using moxibustion at prescribed acupuncture points to promote the flow of qi and blood so they can recirculate through the meridians or in the relevant organs.

Patients and the therapist himself may feel a so-called "deqi phenomenon" (needle sensation), which in the framework of TCM is achieved by needling the acupuncture point. This phenomenon can be felt as propagated

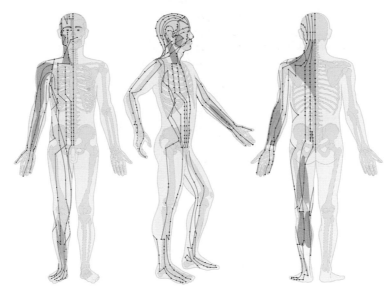

Fig. 7.9.2 Meridian system: front, back, and lateral aspects of the body. From Irnich, D., 2009. Leitfaden Triggerpunkte [Trigger Point Manual]. Elsevier, Urban & Fischer, Munich, with permission.

sensation along the meridians and is described as sore, aching, numb, warm, or radiating. Some acupuncturists consider the eliciting of a deqi response to be a precondition for an effective treatment.

All these concepts described in the *Huangdi Neijing* are still the basis of traditional Chinese acupuncture, but underwent different interpretations and receptions in past centuries, resulting in many different schools of acupuncture today. Even if the traditional Chinese acupuncture system is not comprehensible to many Western people, it is itself logical and thoughtful.

Today, needle acupuncture comprehends a broad range of approaches, including traditional Chinese acupuncture, with different understanding and interpretation in its respective schools; treatment includes microsystem acupuncture (e.g., ear acupuncture [mostly developed in Europe], Yamamoto New Scalp Acupuncture), dry needling of myofascial trigger points, or acupuncture forms further developed in other countries (e.g., Korea, Germany, Japan, Russia, Taiwan, United States).

> ### KEY POINT
> Besides traditional acupuncture at well-defined acupuncture points, there are several other approaches to achieve energetic homeostasis, for example, microsystem acupuncture or dry needling.

ACUPUNCTURE MECHANISM

Acupuncture effects are mediated through different neurophysiological mechanisms: activation of mechano- and nociceptors, descending inhibitory pathways (comprising diffuse noxious inhibitory controls), or spinal and supraspinal modulation form some of the explanations to describe local and distant needling effects. Basic research showed the release of different neurotransmitters (e.g., norepinephrine [noradrenaline], serotonin), hormones (e.g., estrogen, cortisol), and peptides (e.g., endorphin) to be related to acupuncture treatment. Nevertheless, there is no single mechanism that explains the treatment effects of acupuncture in general. On the contrary, it is well accepted that needling activates complex neurophysiological mechanisms as well as contextual and setting factors (e.g. psychological). Acupuncture points have been supposed to be spots characterized by a high density of neural receptors. In addition, acupuncture points have been found to be situated next to vascular, nerve, and ligamentous sheets, despite there being more than 10,000 sheets in the superficial fascia of the human body, most of them not correlating with an acupuncture point. Studies of electrical properties of acupuncture points have shown that the electrical skin resistance at these points can be increased or decreased compared with the surrounding skin area. None of those findings was able to define acupuncture points anatomically.

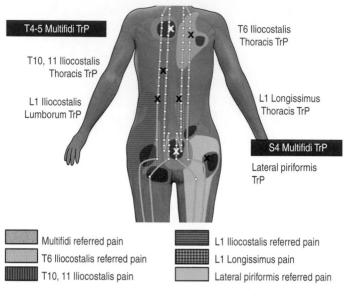

Fig. 7.9.3 Referred pain patterns of myofascial trigger points of the back and their correlation to the bladder meridian and its respective acupuncture points. From Irnich, D., 2009. Leitfaden Triggerpunkte [Trigger Point Manual]. Elsevier, Urban & Fischer, Munich, with permission.

A remarkable observation to explain acupuncture points and meridians comes from myofascial referred pain that was observed to spread along the supposed meridian courses. Dorsher and Fleckenstein (2008a, 2008b) compared the anatomical correspondence of the "common" myofascial trigger point locations described in the *Myofascial Trigger Point Manual* (Travell and Simons 1983, 1992) to the locations of classical acupuncture points (Fig. 7.9.3). Anatomical correspondence of a common myofascial trigger point and a classical acupuncture point means those points are proximate and are demonstrated by acupuncture and anatomy references to enter the same muscle region. There is at least a 93.3% correspondence, if the distance between points on the skin is at most 3 cm; nonetheless, points had to enter the same muscle region. At a maximum skin distance of 1 cm, 37% of points can still be found to correspond. Authors currently presented updated data suggesting the myofascial correlation to be even greater. There are marked clinical correspondences of both the pain indications (up to 97%) and somatovisceral indications (>93%) of anatomically corresponding common myofascial trigger point–classical acupuncture point pairs (classical acupoints that are proximate to *and* enter the muscle region of

their correlated common myofascial trigger points). The spread of deqi along the meridians seems to be the same phenomenon as the physiologically analogous concept of referred pain arising from myofascial trigger points in the myofascial pain tradition. This provides a clinical line of evidence that myofascial trigger points and acupuncture points likely might describe the same physiological phenomena.

These correlations make the explanation of the connecting meridians between acupuncture points more feasible. Speculation in this regard has continued, since acupuncture's earliest days, as to whether acupuncture meridians are conceptual constructs or have an anatomical basis. Connective tissue might mediate acupuncture effects: Langevin and colleagues (Langevin et al. 2002; Langevin and Yandow 2002) showed that rotation after needling activates fibroblast by mechanosensory transduction. These local effects can also be tracked in distant connective tissue. Additionally, some researchers have described a degree of overlap of meridians and the peripheral nervous system in the extremities, whereas others have postulated that the meridians may exist in the myofascial layer of the body, reflecting perceived sensations by stimulating fascial structures. These results have been supported by a study by Maurer and colleagues, showing a large coincidence of the course of acupuncture meridians (i.e., gallbladder and stomach) with the human superficial fascia and extracellular matrix (Maurer et al. 2019). An interesting observation might be that anatomically derived myofascial meridians have distributions similar to those of acupuncture meridians described by TCM (Dorsher 2009; Myers 2001).

However, it remains clear that the target tissue of acupuncture points varies, comprising not only myofascial trigger points but also nerves, bones, ligaments, vessels, and the autonomic nervous system.

> ### KEY POINT
>
> The underlying mechanism of acupuncture effects is of neurophysiological origin. Mechanical and algetic stimuli mediate diverse peripheral, spinal, and supraspinal neurophysiological responses. In addition, stimuli to myofascial and connective tissue have been shown to spread needling stimuli to other parts of the body. Still, there is no single effect that provides a full explanation of the acupuncture mechanism.

TECHNIQUES

Acupuncture has been increasingly used in Western medicine in the last three decades. In Germany, about 30,000 medical doctors apply acupuncture at least occasionally. This chapter will point out an integrative and pragmatic principle of acupuncture treatment, especially for diseases of the locomotor system. It has been systematically used and evaluated in large trials by medical acupuncturists of the Medical School of the Ludwig-Maximilians University of Munich and other members of the German Medical Association for Acupuncture, the oldest and largest medical acupuncture society of the Western world (Irnich et al. 2001, 2002).

The applicable treatment spots range from painful points, meridians, and classical points to extrapoints microsystems and the traditional concept of organ diseases, zangfu. Treatment techniques, among others, might be needling, cupping, and massage techniques. Chinese medicine also comprises herbal medicine and Qi Gong.

We present the basic principle of treatment for diseases of the locomotor system, comprising five steps.

Start with Distant Points and/or Microsystem Points

Classical acupuncture points and microsystem points can have distant effects. Distant points are chosen to achieve immediate pain relief and improve range of motion. Their choice is based on the location of the acupuncture points in the meridian system. If the course of the meridian meets the affected body region its distant points may be used to release the symptoms. Microsystems meet the definition of distant treatment area even if the microsystem is located next to the affected area. Microsystem points are chosen according to their propagated projection zones (Fig. 7.9.4). Distant points and microsystems are known to soften tenderness and might especially be indicated in the first contact with the patient or highly acute conditions of the disease, as they are far away from the tender spots (e.g., SI 3 is known to release pain syndromes of head, neck, and shoulder; Table 7.9.1).

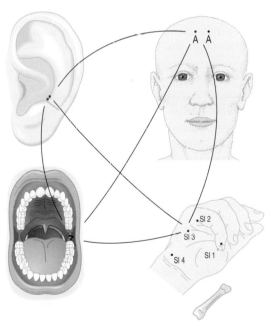

Fig. 7.9.4 Analogies of different microsystems. Analogous points to treat neck pain. Preferable treatment area is the most sensitive microsystem. From Irnich, D., 2009. Leitfaden Triggerpunkte [Trigger Point Manual]. Elsevier, Urban & Fischer, Munich, with permission.

TABLE 7.9.1 Most Effective Distant Points

Indication	Distant Point
Frontal headache	ST 44, ST 36, LI 4
Lateral headache	LIV 3, GB 41, TW 3 or 5
Occipital headache	BL 60 or 62, SI 3
Neck pain	BL 60 or 62, SI 3, Ex-UE 8
Shoulder	ST 38
Elbow	Microsystem ear
Low back pain	BL 40, NP 67, Ex-UE 7, YNSA D-Zone
Knee	Microsystem ear, extraoral incisors (mouth)

This table displays a selection of potentially effective treatment spots in acupuncture.

Look for Tender Regional/Segmental Points

Needling of painful spots (ah shi points) is an ancient concept of TCM. It only requires the localization of painful spots where acupuncture needles are inserted, taking into account anatomical and physiological knowledge of the underlying structures. The choice of segmental points has been described by traditional Chinese acupuncture (i.e., shu points).

Treat Myofascial Trigger Points

Trigger point acupuncture (dry needling) might not only be applied for myofascial trigger points—other structures (myofascial, cutaneous, ligamentous, osseous) are also known to represent trigger points that can be treated similarly, with the difference that local twitch responses may not always occur because of their nature. For further description, please see the remaining discussion.

Supplement with Local Meridian Points or Ah Shi Points

In case treatment of distant and regional points or myofascial trigger points does not produce results, local acupuncture or tender points could be added to the selected treatment points. Treatment techniques range from achieving deqi sensations penetrating acupuncture points to superficial manipulation aiming to evoke reflectory twitching of superficial muscular layers.

Treat Internal Organs in Chronic Diseases

Functional diseases, especially, require comprehensive approaches to understand the patient's situation, comprising biological, mental, social, or spiritual aspects of well-being. According to the traditional concepts (zang fu), illness is understood as an imbalance of physical and mental vitality (qi). The zang fu approach integrates the symptoms, needs, and worries of the patient and surrounding factors, and aims to develop a long-lasting, individualized treatment concept using different kinds of traditional Chinese philosophies and techniques. Acupuncture points, especially, will be chosen according to patterns following rules such as yin and yang in order to balance the patient.

KEY POINT

The basic treatment principle in acupuncture comprises five steps:
1. Start with distant points and/or microsystem points.
2. Look for tender regional/segmental points.
3. Treat myofascial trigger points.
4. Supplement with local meridian points or ah shi points.
5. Treat internal organs in chronic diseases.

DRY NEEDLING: A TECHNIQUE APPROACHING MUSCLE AND FASCIA

In the following section we present a special needling technique applied in the treatment of myofascial disorders (Melzack 1977; Fleckenstein et al. 2010)—myofascial trigger point acupuncture (named dry needling). Dry needling is an invasive procedure in which an acupuncture needle is inserted into the skin and muscle. As the name implies, it is directed at myofascial trigger points. Dry needling does not require fundamental knowledge of TCM and acupuncture, but technical skills are necessary. Precondition for successful treatment is the identification and localization of active myofascial trigger points (Irnich 2013; Fleckenstein 2015; Harden et al. 2000) In addition, clinical experience implies that dry needling integrated in a classical acupuncture treatment is beneficial for the patient's outcome; therefore, both techniques may be combined. This chapter gives practical instruction for fascia treatment. To understand the whole system of TCM comprising acupuncture, meridians, point selection, etc., we suggest the respective textbooks.

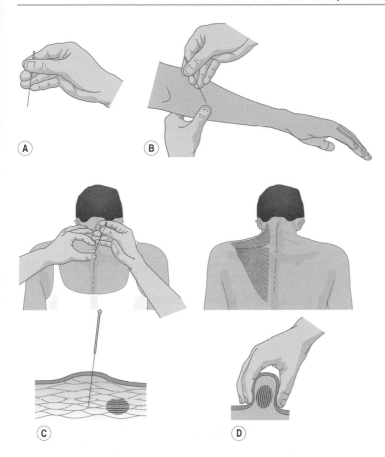

Fig. 7.9.5 Dry needling technique. Holding of needle and injection techniques: (A) holding with three fingers; (B) stretching with soft tissues; (C) needling with thumb pressure; (D) grabbing of muscle. From Irnich; D., 2009. Leitfaden Triggerpunkte [Trigger Point Manual]. Elsevier, Urban & Fischer, Munich, with permission.

Once the skin is prepared and the myofascial trigger point is identified, the overlying skin is grasped or fixed between the thumb and index finger or between the index and middle finger (Fig. 7.9.5). There are three different approaches to perform dry needling.

> ### KEY POINT
>
> Dry needling is a special needling technique aimed at myofascial trigger points. These points are defined as tender spots that are identifiable in muscular taut bands. Pressure on this spot elicits a referred pain pattern that is reproducible and can be recognized by the patient.

Direct Dry Needling

The needle is inserted approximately 1 to 1.5 cm away from the myofascial trigger point to facilitate the advancement of the needle into the myofascial trigger point. The grasping fingers isolate the taut band and

prevent it from rolling out of the trajectory of the needle. The aim is to target the myofascial trigger point and to elicit a local twitch response, a visible or palpable quick twitch of the taut band under the fingertip, while examining the skin above the muscle fibers for this characteristic short and rapid movement (Fig. 7.9.6). The focus for the therapist is the tip of the needle and the texture of the surrounding tissue (fascia, muscle, connective tissue). The trigger point might be felt rubberlike at the tip of the needle. The local twitch response has been shown to predict the effectiveness of the myofascial trigger point needling. A quick removal of the needle outside the muscle is recommended to avoid the needle damaging the muscle fibers or the surrounding tissue, as shearing forces and tension could occur during the contraction of the muscle while twitching. The needle may be withdrawn to the level of the superficial fascia without exiting, and it should be redirected to the myofascial trigger point to repeat the process. The process of entering the myofascial trigger point and

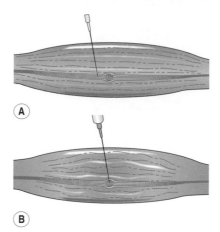

Fig. 7.9.6 Scheme demonstrating the exact targeting of the myofascial trigger point in order to elicit a local twitch response. From Irnich, D., 2009. Leitfaden Triggerpunkte [Trigger Point Manual]. Elsevier, Urban & Fischer, Munich, with permission.

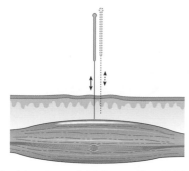

Fig. 7.9.7 Fascial and superficial dry needling. Solid needle is irritating the outer muscular fascia while the spotted needle is only inserted in the connective tissue. From Irnich, D., 2009. Leitfaden Triggerpunkte [Trigger Point Manual]. Elsevier, Urban & Fischer, Munich, with permission.

eliciting local twitch responses should proceed, attempting to extinguish the twitch response of the myofascial trigger points and to contact as many sensitive loci as possible. The grasping finger remains in position till the end of the treatment; besides marking the myofascial trigger point spot, it represents a diagnostic instrument to feel the vegetative response of the patient such as smaller twitch responses (transient contraction) of superficial muscle layers.

> ### KEY POINT
> Direct dry needling aims to irritate the tender spots within the muscular taut band. A successful treatment is indicated by a local twitch response that can be observed while needling.

Dry Needling of the Muscular Fascia

Local twitch responses may be irritating the outer fascia of the corresponding muscle. The needle only touches the fascia, without penetrating and exploring the myofascial trigger point. This technique is especially used when needling larger superficial muscle layers (e.g., M. trapezius, M. levator scapulae). The needle is inserted approximately 1–1.5 cm away from the myofascial trigger point to facilitate the advancement of the needle in the direction of the muscle fascia and is manipulated at high frequency to elicit a local twitch response (Fig. 7.9.7).

Superficial Dry Needling

This special technique only requires insertion of the needle into the connective tissue above the myofascial trigger point. The needle will be removed after approximately 30 seconds; meanwhile, detonization of the myofascial trigger point is proven by palpation. Treatment can be repeated with longer needle-in intervals. The aim of this procedure is not to release a local twitch response but indirect (e.g., neuronal) resolution of the myofascial trigger point (Fig. 7.9.7).

The local twitch response has been shown to predict the effectiveness of myofascial trigger point needling. Patients' responses regarding local twitch responses range from immediate relief to no effect if irrelevant myofascial trigger points are treated or additional trigger points sustain pain and restricted motion. Twitch responses after needling normally appear as short and dull-pulling feelings comparable to a muscular fasciculation. This sensation might continue being apparent after treatment in the form of aching muscles or a posttreatment soreness, both therapeutically reasonable reactions (e.g., due to abnormal posture prior to the treatment).

An integral part of myofascial trigger point therapy is therefore postprocedural stretching. After dry needling, the muscle group that was treated should undergo a stretch.

The choice of an appropriate acupuncture needle, such as for the depth of the muscular region aimed for, depends on the skills of the practitioner. In contrast to injection needles, acupuncture needles possess an atraumatic sharpening: instead of cutting they slide into the tissue, thus reducing the risk of surrounding hematoma. The appropriate choice of needle equates with the principle "as thin as possible and as long as necessary." Guiding tubes have become very helpful in the handling of thin needles. Patients sensitive to pain might more likely tolerate those needles; as the pressure of the tubes on the patient's skin irritates mechanosensitive afferent fibers, their noxious input while needling might be reduced, thus reducing patients' sensations, stress, and defense. The same effect might be released by triggering the skin with palpation of the fingers.

EVIDENCE

There is a huge body of scientific literature showing the physiological and clinical effects of acupuncture and dry needling. Indications—that is, anesthesia, pain relief, mental disorders, and disturbances—in gynecological endocrinology figuring among the most prominent and best investigated conditions. However, there remain many unsolved questions (e.g., specificity of the concepts, indications, optimum dose).

Clinical trials give profound evidence of the analgetic effects of acupuncture, especially for the treatment of chronic musculoskeletal, headache, and osteoarthritis pain (Vickers et al. 2018). Even as myofascial disorders may be subsumed under the term "musculoskeletal," the results of several meta-analyses limiting their evaluations to myofascial disorders only could not yet provide a conclusive statement regarding the effectiveness of acupuncture and dry needling:

1. A network meta-analysis of 33 randomized controlled trials dating from 2017 suggests that most acupuncture therapies are effective in decreasing pain and in improving physical function in myofascial pain syndrome (Li et al. 2017), with acupuncture and dry needling being the techniques mostly applied. Still, included studies present some risk of bias.

2. A systematic review and meta-analysis dating from 2017 states manual acupuncture to be efficacious when stimulating myofascial trigger points in terms of pain relief and reduction of muscle irritability (Wang et al. 2017).

3. Regarding the use of dry needling on its own, there is moderate evidence in patients suffering from low back pain, and acupuncture is thought to be more effective when combined with other therapies (Liu et al. 2018). However, there remains uncertainty regarding its clinical

superiority compared with other standard treatments in improving functional disability and its follow-up effects (Cummings and White 2001). One meta-analysis shows low evidence to treat trigger points in the shoulder region for upper extremity pain or dysfunction (Hall et al. 2018). When explicitly referring to myofascial pain, dry needling compared to sham or placebo has been recommended on a Grade-A level to decrease pain immediately and on a short term in patients with upper-quarter myofascial pain syndrome (Kietrys 2013).

4. A systematic review from 2017 suggests acupuncture and conventional medicine for chronic neck pain to have similar effectiveness on pain and disability (Seo et al. 2017). Adding acupuncture to conventional treatment reduces pain better than on its own. Electroacupuncture was emphasized as being an especially effective acupuncture technique.

5. Authors refer again to the high risk of bias and imprecision of many of the included studies.

KEY POINT

Acupuncture effects have been proven especially for disorders of the locomotor system, whereas the specific needling of myofascial trigger points still lacks convincing evidence, even if clinical experience suggests strong therapeutic effects on muscle and fascia dysfunction.

Summary

The term acupuncture comprises a broad range of different treatment approaches. Their basis can be found in the old textbooks of TCM. Acupuncture, and especially dry needling, are promising treatment options in the therapy of myofascial trigger points and related disorders compared with other tool-assisted approaches but also in comparison with manual therapies. A good relationship between patient and acupuncturist based on empathy and understanding, as well as anatomical and therapeutic skills, are requisites for successful treatment.

REFERENCES

Cheng, X., 1987. Chinese Acupuncture and Moxibustion, Foreign Language Press, Beijing, China.

Cummings, T.M., White, A.R., 2001. Needling therapies in the management of myofascial trigger point pain. Arch. Phys. Med. Rehabil. 82, 986–992.

Dorsher, P.T., 2009. Myofascial referred-pain data provide physiologic evidence of acupuncture meridians. J. Pain 10, 723–731.

Dorsher, P.T., Fleckenstein, J., 2008a. Myofascial trigger points and classical acupuncture points, I: Qualitative and quantitative anatomic correspondences. Dt. Ztschr. F. Akup. 51, 15–24.

Dorsher, P.T., Fleckenstein, J., 2008b. Myofascial trigger points and classical acupuncture points, 2: Clinical correspondences in treating pain and somatovisceral disorders. Dt. Ztschr. F. Akup. 51, 6–11.

Fleckenstein, J., 2015. To the Editor: Diagnostic requirements are necessary prior to dry needling in the treatment of chronic pain. Pain, 156, 1827 (IF 5.56).

Fleckenstein, J., Zaps, D., Rüger, L.J., et al., 2010. Discrepancy between prevalence and perceived effectiveness of treatment methods in myofascial pain syndrome: results of a cross-sectional, nationwide survey. BMC Musculoskelet. Disord. 11:32.

Hall, M.L., Mackie, A.C., Ribeiro, D.C., 2018. Effects of dry needling trigger point therapy in the shoulder region on patients with upper extremity pain and dysfunction: a systematic review with meta-analysis. Physiotherapy 104, 167–177.

Harden, R.N., Bruehl, S.P., Gass, S., Niemiec, C., Barbick, B., 2000. Signs and symptoms of the myofascial pain syndrome: a national survey of pain management providers. Clin. J. Pain 16, 64–72.

Irnich, D., 2009. Leitfaden Triggerpunkte [Trigger Point Manual]. Elsevier, Urban & Fischer, Munich.

Irnich, D., 2013. Myofascial Trigger Points: Comprehensive Diagnosis and Treatment. Churchill Livingstone, Elsevier, London.

Irnich, D., Behrens, N., Gleditsch, J.M., et al., 2002. Immediate effects of dry needling and acupuncture at distant points in chronic neck pain: results of a randomized, double-blind, sham-controlled crossover trial. Pain 99, 83–89.

Irnich, D., Behrens, N., Molzen, H., et al., 2001. Randomised trial of acupuncture compared with conventional massage and "sham" laser acupuncture for treatment of chronic neck pain. BMJ 322, 1574–1578.

Kietrys, D.M., Palombaro, K.M., Azzaretto, E., Hubler, R., Schaller, B., Schlussel, J.M., Tucker, M., 2013. Effectiveness of dry needling for upper-quarter myofascial pain: a systematic review and meta-analysis. J Orthop Sports Phys Ther. 43, 602-634.

Langevin, H.M., Churchill, D.L., Wu, J., et al., 2002. Evidence of connective tissue involvement in acupuncture. FASEB J. 16, 872–874.

Langevin, H.M., Yandow, J.A., 2002. Relationship of acupuncture points and meridians to connective tissue planes. Anat. Rec. 269, 257–265.

Li, X., Wang, R., Xing, X., et al., 2017. Acupuncture for myofascial pain syndrome: a network meta-analysis of 33 randomized controlled trials. Pain Physician 20, E883–E902.

Liu, L., Huang, Q.M., Liu, Q.G., et al., 2018. Evidence for dry needling in the management of myofascial trigger points associated with low back pain: a systematic review and meta-analysis. Arch. Phys. Med. Rehabil. 99, 144–152.

Maurer, N., Nissel, H., Egerbacher, M., Gornik, E., Schuller, P., Traxler, H., 2019. Anatomical evidence of acupuncture meridians in the human extracellular matrix: results from a macroscopic and microscopic interdisciplinary multicentre study on human corpses. Evid. Based Complement. Alternat. Med. 2019, 6976892.

Melzack, R., Stillwell, D.M., Fox, E.J., 1977. Myofascial trigger points and acupuncture points for pain: Correlations and implications. Pain 3, 3–23.

Myers, T.W., 2001. Anatomy Trains: Myofascial Meridians for Manual and Movement Therapists. Churchill Livingstone, Edinburgh.

O'Connor, J., Bensky, D. (Eds.), 1981. Acupuncture: a Comprehensive Text (J. O'Connor, D. Bensky, Trans.). Chicago, Eastland Press, p. 741.

Seo, S.Y., Lee, K.B., Shin, J.S., et al., 2017. Effectiveness of acupuncture and electroacupuncture for chronic neck pain: a systematic review and meta-analysis. Am. J. Chin. Med. 45, 1573–1595.

Travell, J.G., Simons, D.G., 1983. Myofascial Pain and Dysfunction: The Myofascial Trigger Point Manual. Vol. 1. Williams & Wilkins, Baltimore, p. 713.

Travell, J.G., Simons, D.G., 1992. Myofascial Pain and Dysfunction: The Myofascial Trigger Point Manual. Vol 2. The lower extremities. Williams & Wilkins, Baltimore, p. 607.

Vickers, A.J., Vertosick, E.A., Lewith, G., et al., 2018. Acupuncture Trialists' Collaboration. Acupuncture for Chronic Pain: Update of an Individual Patient Data Meta-Analysis. J Pain 19, 455–474.

Wang, R., Li, X., Zhou, S., Zhang, X., Yang, K., Li, X., 2017. Manual acupuncture for myofascial pain syndrome: a systematic review and meta-analysis. Acupunct. Med. 35, 241–250.

Zhu, M., 2001. The Medical Classic of the Yellow Emperor. Foreign Languages Press, Beijing, p. 302.

Gua Sha

Arya Nielsen

CHAPTER OUTLINE

INTRODUCTION

Gua sha is an essential modality of Traditional East Asian Medicine (TEAM), defined as instrument-assisted unidirectional press-stroking of the body surface to intentionally create *transitory therapeutic petechiae* representing extravasation of blood in the subcutis. Gua sha has been used for centuries in Asia, and Asian immigrant communities, as a form of self or familial care and by practitioners of TEAM worldwide in clinical practice (Nielsen 2013; So 1987; Zhang and Hao 2000).[1] TEAM dates from 21st century BCE with earliest known medical texts dated 200 BCE (Lu and Needham 1980). The first acupuncture text was printed in 90 BCE (Epler 1980); the earliest Chinese text linked to Gua sha is the *Shi Yi De Xiao Fang* (1337) (Nielsen 2013). With the advance of TEAM outside of Asia, Gua sha has been used over broad geographical areas, in multiple cultural settings and by millions of people.

This chapter explains Gua sha's relevant terms, indications, and specifics of palpation; contraindications; evidence of effect; biomechanism; physiological relationship to connective tissue; and recommendations for safe practice.

GUA SHA TERMS

Gua sha consists of repeated, closely timed, unidirectional press-stroking with a smooth-edged instrument at a lubricated area of body surface until sha petechiae appear (Fig. 7.10.1). Gua sha can be applied with a simple metal cap with a smooth round-lipped edge. Traditional tools include a (Chinese) soup spoon, coin, honed horn, bone, jade, or stone (Fig. 7.10.2). These blunt tools generate certain discomfort for the patient, which is avoided with the smooth-edged, thinner-gauged metal cap that is also disposable after a single use. Bone or horn tools cannot sustain autoclaving or high-level disinfection required for medical device reuse (Nielsen et al. 2014). Sometimes translated as "scraping," there is no abrasion or bruising with Gua sha, merely short-lived petechiae and ecchymosis in the subcutis.

The term "sha" is polysemous, having several meanings. Sha describes surface "blood stasis" in a symptomatic or presymptomatic state, evident on palpation. Sha also describes the petechiae raised from Gua sha. The literal translation of "sha" from Chinese is "sand, sharkskin, or red, raised, millet-size rash." The fresh petechiae raised

---

[1] Recent adaptations of Gua sha have appeared in the form of Graston Technique and ASTYM (Augmented Soft Tissue Mobilization).

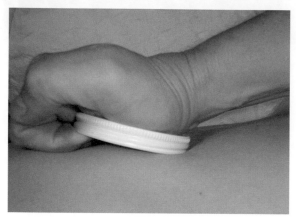

Fig. 7.10.1 A smooth-edged instrument is moved over the surface of the skin as it is pressed into the flesh while maintaining flesh-to-flesh contact of a portion of the practitioner's hand and the patient, press-stroking right to left, producing petechiae and ecchymosis. These simple metal caps have a rounded, smooth-edged lip. Reproduced with permission from Nielsen, A., 2013. Gua sha: A Traditional Technique for Modern Practice, second ed. Churchill Livingstone Elsevier, Edinburgh.

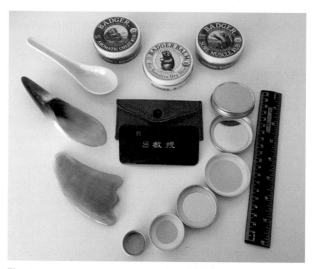

Fig. 7.10.2 Gua sha tools: soup spoon; honed pieces of water buffalo horn; and simple smooth, round-lipped metal caps of various sizes. The warming, cooling, and/or neutral lubricants from Badger Balm (www.badgerbalm.com) are shown at the top. (Image by and with permission, Arya Nielsen, PhD.)

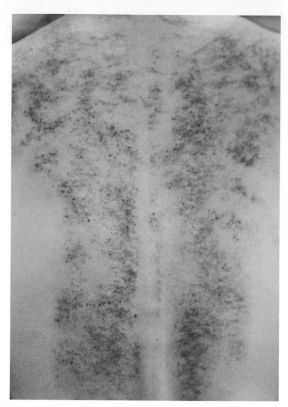

Fig. 7.10.3 Fresh sha petechiae and ecchymosis on the back of a patient treated for chill and aversion to cold with knee pain and swelling. Reproduced with permission from Nielsen, A., 2013. Gua sha: A Traditional Technique for Modern Practice, second ed. Churchill Livingstone Elsevier, Edinburgh.

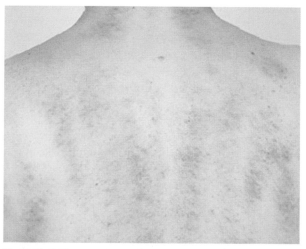

Fig. 7.10.4 Picture taken the day after Gua sha treatment showing the fading of ecchymosis. Reproduced with permission from Nielsen, A., 2013. Gua sha: A Traditional Technique for Modern Practice, second ed. Churchill Livingstone Elsevier, Edinburgh.

from Gua sha immediately begin to fade and blend to ecchymosis. See Figs. 7.10.3 and 7.10.4.

Sha is also translated as cholera, wherein sha blemishes resemble cholera's end-stage rash. Gua sha in the East, like frictioning in early Western medicine (Jackson 1806), was used in the treatment of cholera and cholera-like disorders

(So 1987), mimicking the Hippocratic crisis stage of an illness that produces a cure (Nielsen 1996).

Early translations of Gua sha in the Western medical literature included "coining," "scraping," "spooning," "cao gio," (Vietnamese) and "kerik" (Indonesian) (Nielsen 2009). Steps on how to apply Gua sha are covered elsewhere (Nielsen 2013).

INDICATIONS

Gua sha is indicated for acute or chronic pain, problems with movement or range of motion, and/or disturbed organ or system function, including acute infectious or chronic illness, for reduction of fever and thermal dysregulation, as in potentially life-threatening heat stroke. In TEAM, pain represents a kind of stasis, reflected in the Chinese aphorism: "No free-flow: pain; free flow: no pain" (Nielsen 2013). Sha is a categorical form of *blood stasis* where pain is fixed, persistent, or recurring. This can be also associated with trigger point "loading" or fascial constriction or reflect deeper organ pathology. Palpation can be used to confirm the presence of sha stasis and the need to apply Gua sha (see Fig. 7.10.5A–C and Box 7.10.1).

KEY POINT

Surface ischemia, or sha, is associated with fixed, persistent, and recurring pain. Palpating for surface ischemia is key to palpation literacy. See Fig. 7.10.5A–C.

Palpation

Palpation in myofascial work typically evaluates asymmetry, range of motion, tissue texture changes, and

BOX 7.10.1 Signs of "Blood Stasis" Surface Ischemia and Indications for Gua Sha

- Patient reports pain that is fixed, persistent, or recurring
- Pain on palpation of an area that may or may not propagate to other areas
- Pressing palpation shows blanching that is slow to fade (Fig. 7.10.5A–C)
- Report exposure to wind, cold, or change in temperature
- Report of illness with or without fever, nausea, fatigue, lethargy, pain, digestive, or respiratory symptoms
- Bodywork or hot shower comforts pain that subsequently returns or worsens

tenderness (ARTT) with emphasis on "temperature, texture, surface humidity, elasticity, turgor, tissue tension, thickness, shape, irritability, motion" (Chaitow 2012, p. 131). In TEAM there are additional filters to palpation: indications of surface ischemia called "sha"; focus on patterns of pain trajectory; and "affiliation" and relationship with known points, channels, and organs. Palpating for surface ischemia should be part of palpation literacy because any perfusion restriction can be associated with persistent pain and reduced oxygen and glucose, leading to muscle or relevant tissue "fatigue" (Chaitow and Delany 2011), restriction in tissue stretch, or mobility resulting in myofascial dysfunction (Chaitow 2012). Pressing palpation that creates blanching that is slow to fade (So 1987) confirms sha stasis wherein normal surface perfusion is hindered (see Fig. 7.10.5A–C.)

Causes of dysfunction in myofascial tissues are often reduced to misutilization: overuse, misuse, abuse, or disuse, with exceptions for congenital problems and impact of emotion or psychological stress (Chaitow and Delany 2011). A glaring omission that is based in every

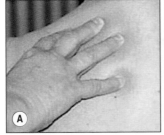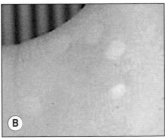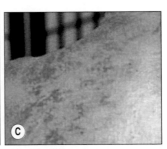

Fig. 7.10.5 Palpation for "sha stasis" surface ischemia. Pressing palpation (A) and top results in blanching (B) that is slow to fade, which indicates sluggish surface perfusion, sha "blood stasis," in traditional East Asian medicine. Image (C) is the same patient after Gua sha. Reproduced with permission from Nielsen, A., 2013. Gua sha: A Traditional Technique for Modern Practice, second ed. Churchill Livingstone Elsevier, Edinburgh.

system of original medicine is the effect of exposure. Exposure to elements of wind, cold, heat, dryness, and dampness beyond the body's ability to compensate, or even because of how the body compensates, can lead to pain and illness. For example, cooling of the feet provokes symptomatic lower urinary tract infection in cystitis-prone women (Baerheim and Laerum 1992).

For decades, researchers held that the rhinovirus was the cause of the common cold and exposure to cold was considered an "old wives' tale." However, exposure to cold can influence the onset of common cold symptoms. A decline in either temperature or humidity and not necessarily low temperature or humidity in the 3 days prior to onset increases the risk of influenza (Jaakkola et al. 2014) and human rhinovirus infections (Ikäheimo et al. 2016) in a cold climate. Increased duration of exposure to cold is associated with greater susceptibility to infection (Mourtzoukou and Falagas 2007). Respiratory epidemics after a period of very cold weather may also be due to conversion of subclinical infections into symptomatic clinical infections (Mourtzoukou and Falagas 2007). Not every exposure results is an illness; every person exposed is not equal in terms of vulnerability to exposure or compounding risks, such as lack of sleep, proper nutrition, immune status, or stress. Still, it is conceded now that exposure is a risk.

Exposure can result in surface ischemia, and this is evident in "sha" palpation. Also interesting to note is that pain stasis related to sha often becomes exacerbated by body work. Patients may feel better with massage, or a hot shower, but will report feeling worse later. These symptoms should also trigger an evaluation and palpation inspection for sha.

A patient may notice pain or tenderness during palpation that may ramify to other areas of the body. Sha may also be accompanied by fatigue. In TEAM, this stasis in the surface tissue is thought to express from, and to, internal organ or system function (Lu and Needham 1980).

The benefits of Gua sha are commonly felt immediately and are sustained, to some degree, over time, though repeating treatment may be indicated to reach maximum benefit. In the language of TEAM Gua sha removes blood stasis, dredges the channels, vents heat, and quickens internal organ function. The recovery of the tissue is expressed not only by immediate improvement in pain status but by changes in pulse, tongue, digestion, urine, stool, sleep, libido, flexibility, and mood as well as other presenting symptoms (Nielsen 2013).

The Chinese language database includes study of Gua sha in internal medicine, surgery, gynecology, pediatrics, musculoskeletal conditions, pain management, and general medicine for acute infectious illness, respiratory conditions, and autoimmune and inflammatory disorders (Nielsen 2013).

Randomized controlled trials (RCTs) published in the Western literature show effective use of Gua sha for neck pain (Braun et al. 2011) and chronic neck and back pain (Lauche et al. 2012) on symptoms and inflammatory biomarkers associated with chronic low back pain (Yuen et al. 2017; Saha et al. 2019), breast engorgement during lactation (Chiu et al. 2010; Mangesi and Zakarija-Grkovic 2016), and diabetic peripheral neuropathy (Xie et al. 2019). A 2017 systematic review and network meta-analysis of 33 RCTs found that compared with placebo-sham, Gua sha combined with warming acupuncture and moxibustion were more effective for decreasing pain intensity in myofascial pain syndrome (Li et al. 2017). A systematic review (six RCTs) with meta-analysis (five RCTs) found that Gua sha combined with Western medicine therapy improved perimenopausal symptoms compared with Western medicine alone (Ren et al. 2018). Significant improvements in serum levels of follicle-stimulating hormone (FSH) and luteinizing hormone (LH) were shown in the combined therapy group. An RCT of Gua sha combined with Chinese herbal therapy effective for perimenopausal symptoms had a significant advantage over the herbal therapy alone for perimenopausal hot flashes, sweating, paresthesia, insomnia, nervousness, melancholia, fatigue, and headache that were not associated with differences in serum estrogen, FSH, or LH (Meng et al. 2017). This is an example of Gua sha venting heat and dredging the channels in East Asian medical terms.

Similarly, Gua sha is used to enhance athletic performance by dredging channels and venting heat associated with extreme or prolonged exertion. Gua sha improved muscle strength of university students performing a bench press (Zhao et al. 1995) and enhanced the performance of weightlifters when a series of Gua sha treatments allowed greater weight to be lifted while the subject's weight sense remained stable (Wang et al. 2014). In Western terms, this benefit may relate to interoception regulation and interstitial matrix hydration, discussed later in this chapter. Gua sha was found to benefit parasympathetic nervous activity and modulate heart rate variability (HRV) in healthy men and weightlifters (Wang et al. 2015). In the latter trial, serum markers showed a sparing of creatinine kinase (CK) and blood urea nitrogen (BUN), which is associated with exertional muscle damage, indicating the potential of Gua sha to facilitate muscle and fascia loading in athletic performance.

CONTRAINDICATIONS

Gua sha is contraindicated where the dermis or flesh is injured or compromised, as in sunburn, abrasion, rash, or contusion (Nielsen 2013). In cases of injury, Gua sha may be applied adjacent, proximal, or distal to but not at the area of trauma. Gua sha, cupping, and acupuncture are contraindicated in areas where a patient has used topical antibiotics or steroid creams, as in eczema, for example (see Safety section). These topicals increase an existing complication of colonization of staphylococcus or even MRSA at the skin (Hon et al. 2013), whereby penetrating treatment can deepen the pathogen into the body causing systemic infection, even death.

Gua sha is:

- *not* contraindicated for patients who are weak or menstruating;
- *not* contraindicated for pregnant women if over limited areas and can be indicated where other medicine is unsafe, as in sinusitis; colds and cough; for headache, neck, shoulder, back, and hip pain; and for sciatica (author's experience); and
- *not* contraindicated in patients with a stable INR (international normalized ratio) who take anticoagulation medication (if properly applied) because the capillary bed is not damaged with Gua sha (Nielsen et al. 2007).[2]

BIOMECHANISM/PHYSIOLOGY

Observation

What a provider observes when applying Gua sha is a gradual expression of small red petechiae (that can sometimes be brown, blue, very deep red, or nearly black). The color of the sha and how it changes can be both diagnostic and prognostic (Nielsen 2013). The patient often feels exhilarated, invigorated, even excited.

---

[2]The author (AN) has used Gua sha on hundreds of patients taking anticoagulation medication. See *Gua Sha Step-by-Step: A Teaching Video* (www.guasha.com).

Acute pain is immediately affected, sometimes completely resolved. Nausea and vomiting cease (So 1987), wheezing and shortness of breath lessen or completely resolve; other acute symptoms are mitigated or resolve completely (Nielsen 2013). The area treated warms, wherein a chilled patient will warm up, but an overheated or fevered patient will cool down.

Research

Research in perfusion, temperature, and serum markers help contextualize the physiology of Gua sha. Gua sha increases surface microperfusion 400% for 7.5 minutes and significantly for 25 minutes after treatment at, but not outside, a treated area while immediately reducing pain locally and distally (Nielsen et al. 2007). Production of nitric oxide (NO) in the process of increased perfusion and vasodilation is one mechanism for immediate pain relief (Nielsen 2013; Mackenzie et al. 2008). Another relates to the innate antiinflammatory ferroheme metabolism.

Sha petechiae change to ecchymosis, blend, and fade over 3 to 5 days. Extravasated blood cells are reabsorbed and metabolized, catalyzing the transformation of ferroheme into biliverdin, carbon monoxide (CO), and free iron with upregulation of genetic expression of heme oxygenase-1 (HO-1) (Xia et al. 2008). One of the most prompt protective and adaptive responses to insult by all tissues is the robust activation of HO-1 that is both antiinflammatory and cytoprotective (Agarwal and Bolisetty 2013). A Harvard study has shown Gua sha upregulates genetic expression of HO-1 at multiple internal organ sites and over a period of days after a single treatment (Kwong et al. 2009).

HO-1 has become a therapeutic target in many inflammatory disease models (Xia et al. 2008) and has been reported to be effective in the control of hepatitis B virus (HBV) infection and decreases hepatitis C virus (HCV) replication (Zhu et al. 2008). A single Gua sha treatment in a patient with active chronic hepatitis reduced levels of liver enzymes, modulated T helper (Th)1/Th2 balance, and enhanced HO-1, which is suggested as responsible for the hepatoprotective effect (Chan et al. 2011). HO-1 can exert a significant antiviral activity against a wide variety of viruses in addition to HBV and HCV, including HIV; "enterovirus 71"; influenza virus; respiratory syncytial virus; dengue and Ebola virus (Espinoza et al. 2017); and acute inflammatory, infectious, and neoplastic gastrointestinal disease (Chang et al. 2015), implying a role for Gua sha related to HO-1 upregulation and immune protection in all but Ebola. A single Gua sha treatment has been shown to increase the immune response to intradermal vaccination (Chen et al. 2016).

> ### 🔑 KEY POINT
>
> HO-1 upregulation provides an antiinflammatory and immune protective effect. Gua sha upregulates HO-1 immediately and for days after a single treatment.

Painful conditions or illnesses may be accompanied by altered or inflamed connective tissue and are observed to respond to manual therapies, including Gua sha, by stimulating fascial mechanoreceptors that trigger tonus changes in connected skeletal muscles, in addition to NO relaxation of skeletal muscles vis-a-vis vasodilation. TEAM was first to propose connective tissue "fascia," called "cou li, li" or "lining," to be an actual organ (Fig. 7.10.6), the San Jiao or Triple Burner (Unschuld et al. 2011; Unschuld 1986)—the only organ that lacked a recognized Western analogous structure until the focus on connective tissue (Langevin 2006). The San Jiao governs the upper, middle, and lower body or "burners," linking the "exterior with the interior" outer flesh to the organs via the channels that reside in the "li" (Epler 1980; Unschuld 1986).

Qi moves vertically through the main channels and horizontally through the "Lo" channels that connect the main channels to each other and to the interior tissue and organs through the "cou li" lining (connective tissue). Langevin and Yandow (2002) have shown that most common acupuncture points exist at cleavage concentrations of connective tissue within and along meridian/fascial layers, suggesting that activation at these sites would, in fact, augment a connective tissue response. Insertion of a needle off site from an acupuncture point might activate a physiological response but less than needling a known acupuncture point. This is borne out by studies comparing acupuncture to control points, where control points demonstrate some therapeutic effect (Haake et al. 2007; Nielsen and Wieland 2019).

Safety

The most significant and consistent complication reported in the Western medical literature for Gua sha is the misattribution of the transitory therapeutic sha petechiae and ecchymosis as a burn, bruise, or dermatitis caused by "abuse," "battery," "torture," or "pseudoabuse" (Nielsen 2009). Physicians may still be taught to discourage use of Gua sha as "harmful" and "unacceptable in our culture." This ignorance and bias represents a risk to patients that can be mitigated by clinicians providing a handout explaining the technique, describing the normal presence and process of therapeutic petechiae and ecchymosis, and providing the clinician's contact information (www.guasha.com).

A report of acute epiglottitis after Gua sha at the trachea represents a negligent use and not a side effect or risk of appropriate Gua sha (Tsai and Wang 2014). Other adverse events inappropriately associated with Gua sha include a report of microhematuria in an infant with an infectious illness and fever; a brain bleed in a female despite symptoms and condition preceding Gua sha; burns caused by fire cupping misattributed to coining; and camphor toxicity from liniments no longer produced, have been disproven (Nielsen 2013).

Universal Precautions and Contamination Risks

Gua sha instruments that are intended for reuse are considered semicritical instruments according to the

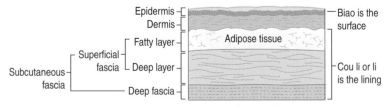

Fig. 7.10.6 Comparative anatomy. In Chinese, the "biao" closely corresponds to the dermal layer and is distinguished from the "cou li" or "li" (lining) (Epler 1980; Unschuld 1986), where the "3 qi steam." The channels communicate through the "li" lining, which corresponds to fascia and connective tissue (Lin and Yu 2009). Redrawn with permission from Nielsen, A., 2013. Gua Sha: A Traditional Technique for Modern Practice, second ed. Churchill Livingstone Elsevier, Edinburgh.

Centers for Disease Control and Prevention (CDC) and must be high-level disinfected or sterilized before reuse (Rutala et al. 2008). Because bone and horn tools cannot sustain high-level disinfection or sterilization required, single-use disposable caps with a smooth edge are recommended (Nielsen et al. 2014). Dedicated instruments intended for specific patients must also be sterilized or high-level disinfected between each use to be compliant with CDC standards.

Preventing risk of exposure to bloodborne pathogens can be accomplished by

- gloving both hands prior to and during Gua sha procedure;
- using single-use disposable press-stroking devices, that is, a smooth-edged metal cap;
- immediately washing and then either autoclaving or high-level disinfecting devices intended for reuse and between each use;
- decanting lubricant onto a paper towel for use with a single patient to prevent cross-contamination, or using lotion from a pump dispenser as lubricant;
- following safe sequencing of palpation, gloving, needling, use of lubricant, application of procedure and clean-up with disposal of gloves and paper towels, and either disposal or processing (washing and then autoclaving or high-level disinfecting) of instruments.

Summary

Gua sha is a healing technique of traditional East Asian medicine, defined as instrument-assisted unidirectional press-stroking of a lubricated area of the body surface to intentionally create transitory therapeutic petechiae called "sha" representing extravasation of blood in the subcutis. Fixed, persistent, and recurring pain and inflammation are indications for Gua sha, with the presence of sha confirmed by pressing palpation that creates blanching that is slow to fade. Modern research shows Gua sha uniquely involves the ferro-heme metabolism and upregulation of HO-1, producing an antiinflammatory and immune protective effect that persists for days after a single Gua sha treatment. HO-1 upregulation contributes to Gua sha's effect on pain, stiffness, fever, chill, cough, wheeze, nausea and vomiting, etc.; enhanced athletic performance; and why Gua sha is effective in acute and chronic internal organ disorders, including liver inflammation in hepatitis. For more information on Gua sha training, see www.guasha.com.

REFERENCES

Agarwal, A., Bolisetty, S., 2013. Adaptive responses to tissue injury: role of heme oxygenase-1. Trans. Am. Clin. Climatol. Assoc. 124, 111–122.

Baerheim, A., Laerum, E., 1992. Symptomatic lower urinary tract infection induced by cooling of the feet. A controlled experimental trial. Scand. J. Prim. Health Care 10, 157–160.

Braun, M., Schwickert, M., Nielsen, A., et al., 2011. Effectiveness of traditional Chinese "Gua sha" therapy in patients with chronic neck pain. A randomized controlled trial. Pain Med. 12, 362–369.

Chaitow, L., 2012. The ARTT of palpation? J. Bodyw. Mov. Ther. 16, 129–131.

Chaitow, L., Delany, J., 2011. Clinical Application of Neuromuscular Techniques, Volume 2: the Lower Body, Churchill Livingstone Elsevier, Edinburgh.

Chan, S.T., Yuen, J.W., Gohel, M.D., Wong, H.C., Kwong, K.K., 2011. Guasha-induced hepatoprotection in chronic active hepatitis B: A case study. Clin. Chim. Acta. 412, 1686–1688.

Chang, M., Xue, J., Sharma, V., Habtezion, A., 2015. Protective role of hemeoxygenase-1 in gastrointestinal diseases. Cell. Mol. Life Sci. 72, 1161–1173.

Chen, T., Liu, N., Liu, J., et al., 2016. Gua Sha, a press-stroke treatment of the skin, boosts the immune response to intradermal vaccination. Peer J. 4, e2451.

Chiu, J.Y., Gau, M.L., Kuo, S.Y., Chang, Y.H., Kuo, S.C., Tu, H.C., 2010. Effects of Gua-Sha therapy on breast engorgement: a randomized controlled trial. J. Nurs. Res. 18, 1–10.

Epler Jr., D.C., 1980. Bloodletting in early Chinese medicine and its relation to the origin of acupuncture. Bull. Hist. Med. 54, 337–367.

Espinoza, J.A., González, P.A., Kalergis, A.M., 2017. Modulation of antiviral immunity by heme oxygenase-1. Am. J. Pathol. 187, 487–493.

Haake, M., Müller, H., Schade-Brittinger, C., et al., 2007. German Acupuncture Trials (GERAC) for chronic low back pain. Arch. Intern. Med. 167, 1892–1898.

Hon, K.L., Luk, D.C., Leong, K.F., Leung, A.K., 2013. Cupping therapy may be harmful for eczema: a PubMed search. Case Rep. Pediatr. 2013, 605829.

Ikäheimo, T.M., Jaakkola, K., Jokelainen, J., et al., 2016. A decrease in temperature and humidity precedes human rhinovirus infections in a cold climate. Viruses 8, 244.

Jaakkola, K., Saukkoriipi, A., Jokelainen, J., et al., 2014. Decline in temperature and humidity increases the occurrence of influenza in cold climate. Environ. Health 13, 22.

Jackson, H., 1806. On the Efficacy of Certain External Applications. Medical College Library Rare Books Room: University of Pennsylvania, New York

Kwong, K.K., Kloetzer, L., Wong, K.K., et al., 2009. Bioluminescence imaging of heme oxygenase-1 upregulation in the Gua Sha procedure. J. Vis. Exp., 1385.

Langevin, H.M., 2006. Connective tissue: a body-wide signaling network? Med. Hypotheses 66, 1074–1077.

Langevin, H.M., Yandow, J.A., 2002. Relationship of acupuncture points and meridians to connective tissue planes. Anat. Rec. 269, 257–265.

Lauche, R., Wübbeling, K., Lüdtke, R., et al., 2012. Randomized controlled pilot study: pain intensity and pressure pain thresholds in patients with neck and low back pain before and after traditional East Asian "gua sha" therapy. Am. J. Chin. Med. 40, 905–917.

Li, X., Wang, R., Xing, X., et al., 2017. Acupuncture for myofascial pain syndrome: a network meta-analysis of 33 randomized controlled trials. Pain Physician 20, E883–E902.

Lu, G.D., Needham, J., 1980. Celestial Lancets. Cambridge University Press, Cambridge.

Mackenzie, I.S., Rutherford, D., MacDonald, T.M., 2008. Nitric oxide and cardiovascular effects: new insights in the role of nitric oxide for the management of osteoarthritis. Arthritis Res. Ther. 10, S3.

Mangesi, L., Zakarija-Grkovic, I., 2016. Treatments for breast engorgement during lactation. Cochrane Database Syst. Rev. (6), CD006946. doi:10.1002/14651858.CD006946.pub3.

Meng, F., Duan, P.B., Zhu, J., et al., 2017. Effect of Gua sha therapy on perimenopausal syndrome: a randomized controlled trial. Menopause 24, 299–307.

Mourtzoukou, E.G., Falagas, M.E., 2007. Exposure to cold and respiratory tract infections. Int. J. Tuberc. Lung Dis. 11, 938–943.

Nielsen, A., 1996. Gua Sha as counteraction: the crisis is the cure. J. Chin. Med. 50, 4–10.

Nielsen, A., 2009. Gua sha research and the language of integrative medicine. J. Bodyw. Mov. Ther. 13, 63–72.

Nielsen, A., 2013. Gua sha, A Traditional Technique for Modern Practice: Churchill Livingstone Elsevier, Edinburgh.

Nielsen, A., Kligler, B., Koll, B.S., 2014. Addendum: Safety standards for Gua sha (press-stroking) and Ba guan (cupping). Complement. Ther. Med. 22, 446–448.

Nielsen, A., Knoblauch, N.T.M., Dobos, G.J., Michalsen, A., Kaptchuk, T.J., 2007. The effect of Gua Sha treatment on the microcirculation of surface tissue: a pilot study in healthy subjects. Explore (NY) 3, 456–466.

Nielsen, A., Wieland, L.S., 2019. Cochrane reviews on acupuncture therapy for pain: a snapshot of the current evidence. Explore (NY) 15, 434–439.

Ren, Q., Yu, X., Liao, F., et al., 2018. Effects of Gua Sha therapy on perimenopausal syndrome: A systematic review and meta-analysis of randomized controlled trials. Complement. Ther. Clin. Pract. 31, 268–277.

Rutala, W.A., Weber, D.J., 2008. Committee HICPA. Guideline for disinfection and sterilization in healthcare facilities, CDC. Centers for Disease Control and Prevention.

Saha, F.J., Brummer, G., Lauche, R., et al., 2019. Gua Sha therapy for chronic low back pain: A randomized controlled trial. Complement. Ther. Clin. Pract. 34, 64–69.

So, J.T.Y., 1987. Treatment of Disease with Acupuncture. Paradigm Publishing, Brookline, MA.

Tsai, K.K., Wang, C.H., 2014. Acute epiglottitis following traditional Chinese gua sha therapy. CMAJ. 186, E298.

Unschuld, P.U. (Unschuld, P., Trans.), 1986. Nan-Ching, the Classic of Difficult Questions. University of California Press, Berkeley, CA.

Unschuld, P.U., Tessenow, H., Zheng, J., 2011. Huang di nei jing su wen : an annotated translation of Huang Di's Inner Classic–Basic Questions. University of California Press, Berkeley, CA.

Wang, X., Chatchawan, U., Nakmareong, S., et al., 2015. Effects of GUASHA on heart rate variability in healthy male volunteers under normal condition and weightlifters after weightlifting training sessions. Evid. Based Complement. Alternat. Med. 2015, 268471.

Wang, X., Eungpinichpong, W., Yang, J., et al., 2014. Effect of scraping therapy on weightlifting ability. J. Tradit. Chin. Med. 34, 52–56.

Xia, Z.W., Zhong, W.W., Meyrowitz, J.S., Zhang, Z.L., 2008. The role of heme oxygenase-1 in T cell-mediated immunity: the all-encompassing enzyme. Curr. Pharm. Des. 14, 454–464.

Xie, X., Lu, L., Zhou X., et al. Effect of Gua Sha therapy on patients with diabetic peripheral neuropathy: A randomized controlled trial. Complement Ther. Clin. Pract. 2019;35:348–352.

Yuen, J.W.M., Tsang, W.W.N., Tse, S.H.M., et al., 2017. The effects of Gua sha on symptoms and inflammatory biomarkers associated with chronic low back pain: A randomized active-controlled crossover pilot study in elderly. Complement. Ther. Med. 32, 25–32.

Zhang, X., Hao, W., 2000. Holographic Meridian Scraping Therapy. Foreign Language Press, Beijing.

Zhao, Z.L., Yin, K.J., Liu, W.B., 1995. The study of Traditional Chinese Medicine to the effect of upper limb function in bench press. Shanxi J. Trad. Chin. Med. 18, 34–35.

Zhu, Z., Wilson, A.T., Mathahs, M.M., et al., 2008. Heme oxygenase-1 suppresses hepatitis C virus replication and increases resistance of hepatocytes to oxidant injury. Hepatology 48, 1430–1439.

Prolotherapy as a Regenerative Injection Treatment

Jeni Saunders

CHAPTER CONTENTS

INTRODUCTION

Prolotherapy is an injection therapy used to treat chronic ligament, joint, capsule, fascial, and tendinous injuries (see Fig. 7.11.1). The goal of this treatment is to stimulate proliferation of collagen at the fibro-osseous junctions to promote nonsurgical soft tissue repair and to relieve pain (see Fig. 7.11.2) (Klein and Eck 1997). Originally defined by Hackett as "the rehabilitation of an incompetent structure (ligament or tendon) by the generation of new cellular tissue," prolotherapy has received a variety of names (Dagenais et al. 2005; Alderman 2007).

Prolotherapy now includes all regenerative methods by injection, including dextrose-based, inflammation-based, platelet-rich plasma, (adult) stem cell-based, and essentially any other injection method in which either growth factors are stimulated or disrepair factors are blocked.

Growth factors are powerful polypeptides that induce wide-ranging effects, including cell migration, proliferation, and protein synthesis. These proteins may be produced by the affected cells or in other cells. These growth factors must avoid the binding proteins that could cause their inactivation, find their way to the area needing growth, and hook onto an appropriate receptor protein (Reeves 2000).

Prolotherapy has been used extensively in the United States since the 1930s (over 450,000 people have undergone prolotherapy treatment) and in other countries around the world. Yet it has not become a mainstream therapy (Mooney 2003). The abundance of case series studies and anecdotal evidence (Yelland et al. 2003; Dagenais et al. 2007) is beginning to be supported by an emerging body of randomized controlled trials (Rabago et al. 2013; Louw et al. 2019).

HISTORY

Hippocrates (460–370 BCE) was the first to describe the intentional provocation of scar tissue formation by searing the shoulder capsules in the unstable shoulders of javelin throwers in Sparta (trans. by Adams 1946). Two millennia later, in 1837, Robert Valpeau of Paris described the use of scar formation for the repair of hernias. One hundred years later, Yeomans (1939) extensively reviewed the genealogy of herniology and a

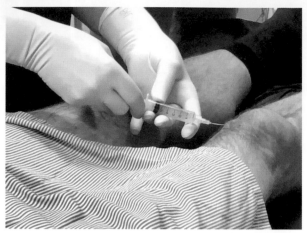

Fig. 7.11.1 Prolotherapy involves injection of carefully chosen liquid substances with the intention of stimulating growth factors and/or inhibiting disrepair factors in the treated tissue.

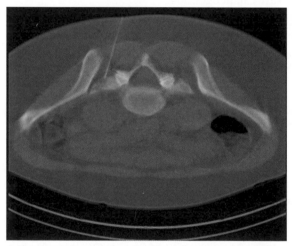

Fig. 7.11.2 CT scan of prolotherapy in the dorsal interosseous ligament of the sacroiliac joint. Radio-opaque contrast can be added to demonstrate correct placement of the hypertonic dextrose solution and local anesthetic. Courtesy H. Van der Wall and L. Wong.

variety of vein sclerosis techniques. Gedney (1937) applied these injection techniques to joints, the first being the sacroiliac joint. He maintained the term sclerotherapy, which remained in use until the 1950s. In that same year, Schultz (1937) described, in the *Journal of the American Medical Association,* a treatment for subluxation of the temporomandibular joint.

In the mid-1950s, George Hackett published a number of articles based on his more than 20 years' experience, culminating in his book *Ligament and Tendon Relaxation*

Treated by Prolotherapy (Hackett 1956), where he claimed an 82% cure rate in a population of 1600 people with back pain (Hackett and Huang 1961). In 1983 Liu confirmed, experimentally, increases in ligament junction strength and diameter of collagen fibrils.

In 1995, prolotherapy was renamed by some as regenerative injection therapy (RIT), or "the injection of growth factor production stimulants to promote regeneration of normal cells and tissue" (Linetsky and Manchikanti 2005; Reeves et al. 2008).

WOUND HEALING, REPAIR, AND REGENERATION

An idea of tissue healing and repair is necessary to better understand the effects of prolotherapy. Wound healing and repair of injured tissues follows four stages (bleeding, inflammation, matrix deposition, and remodeling) in healthy individuals (Hildebrand et al. 2005). Wound healing generally leads to repair, and in many cases allows return to at least partial function of the injured tissue, but not to tissue regeneration. The repair process leads to a loss of function as a result of scar tissue formation. This is an important factor when dealing with connective tissue that functions in a mechanically active environment. The repair of connective tissue by scar formation—ultimately healing by second intention—may restore connective tissue to its preinjury length but will not provide adequate (preinjury) tensile strength in ligaments and tendons (Reeves 2000; Linetsky and Manchikanti 2005).

The Bleeding and Inflammatory Phase

After an acute overt injury there is pain and bleeding. The latter is repaired with the formation of a fibrin clot, which prevents further bleeding and provides a provisional matrix for migrating cells. Blood clotting also releases proinflammatory substances, including components of the clotting cascade, cytokines, and growth factors released from other cells such as platelets. This contributes to the subsequent migration, localization, and proliferation of other cells (mesenchymal cells, fibroblast-like cells, etc.), which sets the stage for the second phase of the repair process.

The Matrix Deposition Phase

Once the fibrin clot is consolidated and the influx of a subset of cells and deposition of these new cells is established, the deposition of matrix molecules can begin.

The purpose of matrix formation is to bridge the damaged area with residual ligamentous tissue. Two points need to be considered:

1. The tissue deposited attempts to bridge the injured area, regardless of the tissue structure it attempts to gap or repair.
2. The changes in the matrix deposited early in the process lead to the organization of deposited matrix that is different from normal tissue. In mechanically active tissues this will result in a severe compromise of the tensile strength of the new tissue formed: scar tissue is not as strong as the original ligamentous tissue.

In addition to matrix deposition in the early stage of healing, there is an increase in cellularity and in vascularity (Bray et al. 1996) due to the release of angiogenic factors in the early postinjury stages. Increased vascularity generates the influx of new microvessels. Those connective tissues with endogenous microvasculature will heal well, whereas those that are poorly vascularized (e.g., menisci) do not heal well. In the early stages of scar tissue formation there are almost no neural elements and therefore minimal regulation of fibroblast-like cells or microvasculature.

The Remodeling Phase

This is a much slower process, which involves not only alterations in the remodeling of the existing matrix but also gene expression, cellularity, vascularity, and innervation (Hildebrand et al. 2005). The material deposited early is reorganized to suit the mechanical demands of the injured tissue. In the case of ligament, the organization of fibrils becomes oriented toward the axis of the ligament, whereas in other tissues such as skin, a more basket-weave arrangement takes place that provides strength in multiple directions. This process may take months or even years, and the composition of the repaired tissue changes with time, as does the gene expression phenotype.

The advent and use of erythrocyte growth factor (erythropoietin) to stimulate red cell proliferation in patients with chronic anemia and even in preparation for acute blood loss in surgery has led to the study of growth factors and their effect in both musculoskeletal medicine and other areas outside medicine, such as endurance sports.

Improved understanding of the role of growth factors in tissue regeneration and healing is compatible with the traditional inflammatory reaction theory and takes it to a new dimension. The definition of prolotherapy now includes the injection of external growth factors—blood, platelet rich plasma (PRP), adult mesenchymal stem cells, or the injection of growth factor stimulators (traditional prolotherapy solutions).

The application of growth factors to stimulate cell proliferation and extracellular matrix synthesis in tendinopathy has been described by Wang and colleagues (2006) and can represent a new look at the mechanism of action of prolotherapy solutions. The transplantation of mesenchymal stem cells into injured tendons has been shown to promote tendon healing in laboratory animal models (Smith and Webbon 2005). The injection of growth factors should produce structural changes in the tissues injected, and these changes result in improved mechanical quality and function. These changes have not been conclusively proven to date, but the possible role of growth factors represents an exciting development pathway. Further systematical study of the topic is required before definite statements can be made.

MECHANISM OF ACTION AND SUBSTANCES INJECTED

Two types of substance are used in prolotherapy. The first is injection of growth factor-containing substances. Examples of this include injection of blood and injection of mass-produced recombinant growth factors, PRP, and mesenchymal stem cells. The second method is stimulation of growth factor production, in which the injected solution initiates production of growth factors (dextrose, inflammatory agents that initiate an inflammatory cascade to produce growth factors), and plasmid DNA (Reeves 2000).

In the classical understanding of the inflammatory reaction theory, there are four types of solutions, grouped according to the suspected mechanism of action (Banks 1991):

1. Osmotic (e.g., hypertonic dextrose) solutions are thought to provoke cell dehydration, with subsequent cell lysis and release of cellular fragments, which in turn attract granulocytes and macrophages. In addition, dextrose could cause glycosylation of cellular proteins.
2. Irritants (e.g., phenol) have a phenolic hydroxyl group that is believed to alkylate surface proteins; these either become antigenic or are damaged and in turn attract granulocytes and macrophages.
3. Chemotactics (e.g., sodium morrhuate) are chemically related to inflammatory mediators such as leukotrienes and prostaglandins, and possibly undergo conversion to these substances to mediate the inflammatory response.

4. Particulate irritants (e.g., pumice flour) are believed to attract macrophages, leading to phagocytosis.

Injections of inflammatory proliferant solutions in connective tissues have demonstrated ligament thickening, hypertrophy of the bone–tendon unit, and the strengthening of tendon and ligament in animal studies (Hackett 1956; Liu et al. 1983; Ongley et al. 1988). The injection of hyper- or hypo-osmolar dextrose induces cells to proliferate and produce a number of growth factors. RIT was coined to reflect currently prevailing anatomical and pathophysiological trends in nomenclature. It stimulates chemomodulation of collagen by repetitive induction of inflammatory and proliferative stages leading to tissue regeneration and repair, thus increasing tensile strength, elasticity, mass, and load-bearing capacity of collagenous connective tissues. This makes RIT a viable treatment for painful chronic enthesopathies, tendinosis, ligament degeneration, and laxity (Linetsky and Manchikanti 2005).

In retrospect, we can say that the original concept of prolotherapy solutions triggering the inflammatory cascade was overly simplistic. The mechanism of action is now considered to be multifaceted and includes any or all of the following components (Klein et al. 1989; Reeves 2000; Yelland et al. 2004; Linetsky and Manchikanti 2005):

1. Cellular and extracellular matrix damage induced by mechanical needle injury stimulates the inflammatory cascade, which in turn governs the release of growth factors.
2. Compression of cells by a relatively large volume of external fluid, as well as cell expansion or constriction caused by osmotic properties of the solution injected that stimulates the release of intracellular growth factors.
3. Chemomodulation of collagen through inflammatory, proliferative, regenerative/reparative responses induced by the chemical properties of the solutions injected and mediated by cytokines and multiple growth factors.
4. Chemoneuromodulation of peripheral nociceptors provides stabilization of antidromic, orthodromic, sympathetic, and axon reflex transmissions.
5. Modulation of local hemodynamics with changes in intraosseous pressure leads to reduction of pain. Empirical observations suggest that a dextrose/lidocaine combination has a much more prolonged action than lidocaine alone.
6. Temporary repetitive stabilization of painful hypermobile joints, induced by inflammatory response to the solutions injected, that provides a better environment for regeneration and repair of the affected ligaments and tendons.
7. Additional possible mechanisms of action include the disruption of adhesions that have been created by the original inflammatory attempts to heal the injury by the large volume of solutions injected. The relatively large volume of chemically nonirritating solution assumes the role of a space-occupying lesion in a relatively tight and slowly equilibrating extracellular compartment of the connective tissue.

INDICATIONS, CONTRAINDICATIONS, COMPLICATIONS, AND RISKS

The general indication for prolotherapy is chronic musculoskeletal pain resistant to other physical therapies: chronic sprains and strains, myofascial syndromes, and arthritis. Whiplash injuries; medial and lateral epicondylitis of the elbow, knee, ankle, shoulder, and other joint pain; tendinosis; and musculoskeletal pain related to osteoarthritis all fall within the three general indications. It is based on the premise that pain results from ligaments or entheses, and that these ligaments or entheses can be strengthened by the injection of irritant proliferant solutions into them. Injection of hypertonic dextrose has also been used to restore ligament function rather than to treat of pain (Cusi et al. 2010).

Contraindications include potential local infection, allergies to the local anesthetic used or to some of the substances injected (allergy to shellfish is a contraindication to sodium morrhuate), injection into prosthetic joints, and patients on anticoagulants who have a high INR (international normalized ratio).

Complications and risks can be patient related, needle related, or substance related.

Patient Related

- Platelet count (range of normal from 150–450 x 10^9/L)
- Platelet function (blood dyscrasias, medications)
- Hypertension
- Mental and physical stress (both exercise and surgery)
- Diet: saturated fats, heavy sugar intake, caffeine, quercetin (found in onions, apples, tea, and wine reduces Pl activation), anthocyanins (cause a decrease in the number of activated platelets and are found in many

fruits—blackberries, blueberries, cranberries, egg-plant, grape juice, plums, prunes) (Kuffler 2018)
- Medications (NSAIDs, aspirin, tamoxifen); alcohol: reduces platelet activation and sensitivity to thrombin; smoking: increases platelet aggregation; SSRIs; tricyclic antidepressants; some antibiotics; antihistamines; quinine (reduces platelet count) (Kuffler 2018).

Needle Related

- Joint sepsis (Gray and Gottlieb 1983; Pal and Morris 1999). Infection rate post-prolotherapy is not greater than postinjection of corticosteroids and is generally accepted at between 1 in 10,000 and 1 in 50,000.
- Spinal headache (for injections near the spinal canal)
- Peripheral nerve injury
- Pneumothorax (injections around the thoracic wall)
- Needle phobia.

Substance Related

- Stiffness or soreness postinjection, which typically can last 1 to 3 days
- Allergies (especially to shellfish in sodium morrhuate injections)
- Chemical arachnoiditis (especially if using phenol in spinal or paraspinal injections).

The adverse effects of prolotherapy injections have been studied by Dagenais et al. (2006). Side effects related to prolotherapy for back and neck pain, such as temporary postinjection pain, stiffness, and bruising were found to be common and benign. Adverse events related to prolotherapy for back and neck pain are similar in nature to other widely used spinal injection procedures, and in general prolotherapy can be considered relatively safe when the more common solutions are used. Further study on this matter is required to replicate Dagenais's findings.

TECHNIQUES

There is a wide variety of injection protocols described in the literature. Usually, tender spots are identified with the palpating finger and the skin marked. The number of sites selected for injection, the composition of the proliferant (dextrose-based or dextrose in combination with other substances, often phenol and glycerin), and the volume of injectate varies but is generally 0.5–1.00 mL per site injected. Injections are repeated regularly at varying intervals until the desired effect is achieved, with a maximum of weekly injections for up to 6 to 12 weeks. Injection may or may not be associated with manipulation. A bleb of local anesthetic is used sometimes, but not always (Reeves 2000).

The use of ultrasound guidance at point of care, to improve accuracy of location of the injection, is also emerging.

OUTCOMES AND CLINICAL EVIDENCE

In a systematic review of prolotherapy for chronic musculoskeletal pain, Rabago et al. (2005) stated in their conclusion that "there are limited high-quality data supporting the use of prolotherapy in the treatment of musculoskeletal pain or sport-related soft tissue injuries." Positive results compared with controls have been reported in randomized and nonrandomized controlled trials. Further investigation with high-quality randomized controlled trials with noninjection control arms in studies specific to sport-related and musculoskeletal conditions is necessary to determine the efficacy of prolotherapy. Literature interpretation is hampered by the variety of solutions and the variety of methods used. Nevertheless, there are several areas of literature in which the unique advantages of prolotherapy are being demonstrated (accessibility and low cost compared with alternative therapies such as surgery), to the point where close observation for follow-up studies is warranted.

A selection of some quality studies published so far follows, regardless of outcome, for specific conditions. There is a much wider body of published research, but its quality is variable and levels of evidence poor.

Lateral epicondylosis. Rabago et al. (2009) have identified strong pilot-evidence supporting the use of dextrose, polidocanol, whole blood, and PRP injections in the treatment of lateral epicondylosis. Prolotherapy in this summary includes under its umbrella all regenerative methods by injection, including dextrose-based, inflammation-based, platelet/WBC-based (platelet-rich plasma), adult stem cell-based, and essentially any other injection method in which either growth factors are stimulated or disrepair factors are blocked (as was mentioned earlier).

Achilles tendinosis. Sweeting and Yelland (2009) have found that prolotherapy alone is more effective than eccentric loading exercises—at present the "gold standard"—for chronic Achilles tendinosis. The combination of both treatments is again superior to either of them individually. A nonrandomized study of 32 consecutive patients treated with intratendinous 25% dextrose injections (four injections on average) identified improvement of pain for activities of daily living (ADL) of 84%, and for sporting activity (71%). Although not a randomized trial, a 94% (30 out of 32) follow-up rate at 12 months (4.5–28) suggests effective treatment (Maxwell et al. 2007).

Groin pain. A study of 24 elite-level athletes (22 rugby, 2 soccer) with chronic groin pain, failure of all standard therapies, and failure to play at high level was reported by Topol et al. (2005). Twenty-two out of 24 returned to full play in sustained fashion. This study was then in essence repeated with 48 additional nonelite athletes, with identical results (Topol and Reeves 2008).

Plantar fasciitis (fasciosis). A small case series of 20 consecutive patients reports good to excellent results in 16 patients, which compares favorably with extracorporeal shock wave therapy (Ryan et al. 2009). However, further larger studies are necessary before confirming its effectiveness.

Low back pain. Most published clinical studies of prolotherapy are for low back pain. They include nonspecific low back pain, sciatica, and sacroiliac disorder. The five randomized control trials published (Mathews et al. 1987; Ongley et al. 1987; Klein et al. 1993; Dechow et al. 1999; Yelland et al. 2004; Dagenais et al. 2007) are of unequal quality and significance, and may be subject to different interpretations. Yelland and colleagues (2004) found that both injections of normal saline and dextrose solution resulted in a significant improvement, but that there was no statistically significant difference between normal saline (placebo) injections and prolotherapy. This highlights the difficulty of finding an appropriate placebo, because dry needling a ligament can cause an inflammatory reaction. It is therefore not a real placebo but a different intervention. Several consecutive case series since then have confirmed the positive clinical effects of prolotherapy (Hooper and Ding 2004; Wilkinson 2005; Cusi et al. 2010). These results need to be confirmed with well-designed randomized clinical trials that compare prolotherapy to a real placebo injection.

Patellar tendinosis. Two pilot studies (Alfredson and Ohberg 2005; Volpi et al. 2007) suggest that either polidocanol or PRP are effective to reduce pain and improve function. Again, this initial work needs to be completed with larger randomized trials.

Knee osteoarthritis. Rabago and colleagues (Rabago et al. 2013) showed that prolotherapy was better than saline or physiotherapy exercise on WOMAC scores at 52 months with a group of 90 adults. Further follow-up at 2.5 years showed that this effect was maintained (Rabago et al. 2015). His group did further studies using cartilage biopsies undertaken at arthroscopy, whereby the surgeon was blinded to whether the patient had received prolotherapy. This showed improvement in cartilage scores (Topol et al. 2016).

Shoulder rotator cuff tears. A controlled study looking at prolotherapy injections for rotator cuff tears present for more than 6 months was also able to show better outcomes in the prolotherapy group than the physiotherapy-only group (Seven et al. 2017). This study compared 60 controls with 60 individuals receiving prolotherapy, showing 92.9% of prolotherapy patients reporting good outcomes at 6 months compared with 56.8% of controls.

FASCIAL NEURAL HYDRODISSECTION FOR ENTRAPMENT NEUROPATHY

This is an emerging treatment using either PRP or Dextrose 5% to hydrodissect fascial planes around peripheral nerves. Deep nerve hydrodissection uses fluid under pressure to separate nerves from possible fascial adhesions. These entrapments are said to occur where the nerve changes direction, enters a fibro-osseous tunnel, or where the nerve passes over a fibrous or muscle band (Kopell and Thompson 1976). Lam and colleagues have published a safety study on the use of dextrose 5% as the fluid for these injections in entrapments of the upper torso (Lam et al. 2017). This paper also looked at efficacy in 26 patients and found good efficacy with diminishment of numeric pain rating scale (NPR) from 8.3 ± 1.3. to 1.9 ± 0.9. at 2 months posttreatment. Each patient received 3.8 ± 2.6 injections to achieve this relief.

FUTURE CHALLENGES

Although there is a considerable body of literature, the standard of the published research is of unequal quality. Techniques vary widely, as do the substance injected, volume, and frequency. Many studies can only be considered initial; however, further RCTs are now becoming available as previously stated.

The clinical expertise already gathered in the practice of prolotherapy is gradually gaining evidence-based research, and experts' consensus to gain acceptance in mainstream medical practice, in keeping with the principles of evidence-based medicine (Sackett and Rosenberg 1995), is for the benefit of all.

Summary

Regenerative techniques for treatment of musculoskeletal pain have been used for over 50 years. Present evidence with inclusion of systematic reviews and randomized and nonrandomized evidence indicates effectiveness of RIT in painful enthesopathies. The role of prolotherapy in "mainstream" medicine is improving with further quality research, including standard protocols, properly conducted randomized trials, patient selection, and defined outcome measures beginning to appear in the literature. The further use of PRP in fascial neural hydrodissection is another emerging use of regenerative techniques.

REFERENCES

Adams F, trans., 1946. The Genuine Works of Hippocrates. Williams & Wilkins, Baltimore.

Alderman, D., 2007. Prolotherapy for musculoskeletal pain. Pract. Pain Manag. 1, 10–15.

Alfredson, H., Ohberg, L., 2005. Neovascularisation in chronic painful patellar tendinosis – promising results after sclerosing neovessels outside the tendon challenge the need for surgery. Knee Surg. Sports Traumatol. Arthrosc. 13, 74–80.

Banks, A., 1991. A rationale for prolotherapy. J. Orthop. Med. 13, 54–59.

Bray, R.C., Rangayyan, R.M., Frak, C.B., 1996. Normal and healing ligament vascularity: a quantitative histological assessment in the adult rabbit medial collateral ligament. J. Anat. 188, 87–95.

Cusi, M., Saunders, J., Hungerford, B., Wisbey-Roth, T., Lucas, P., Wilson, S., 2010. The use of prolotherapy in the sacro-iliac joint. Br. J. Sports Med. 44, 100–104.

Dagenais, S., Haldeman, S., Wooley, J.R., 2005. Intraligamentous injection of sclerosing solutions (prolotherapy) for spinal pain: a critical review of the literature. Spine J. 5, 310–328.

Dagenais, S., Ogunseitan, O., Haldeman, S., Wooley, J.R., Newcomb, R.L., 2006. Side effects and adverse events related to intraligamentous injection of sclerosing solutions (prolotherapy) for back and neck pain: A survey of practitioners. Arch. Phys. Med. Rehabil. 87, 909–913.

Dagenais, S., Yelland, M.J., Del Mar, C., Schoene, M.L., 2007. Prolotherapy injections for chronic low-back pain. Cochrane Database Syst. Rev. 2007 (2), CD004059.

Dechow, E., Davies, R.K., Carr, A.J., Thompson, P.W., 1999. A randomized, double-blind, placebo-controlled trial of sclerosing injections in patients with chronic low back pain. Rheumatology 38, 1255–1260.

Gedney, E.H., 1937. Hypermobile joint. Osteopath. Prof. 4, 30–31.

Gray, R.G., Gottlieb, N.L., 1983. Intra-articular corticosteroids. An updated assessment. Clin. Orthop. Relat. Res., 235–263.

Hackett, G.A. (Ed.), 1956. Ligament and Tendon Relaxation Treated by Prolotherapy, third ed. vol. 1. C.C. Thomas, Springfield, IL, 99.

Hackett, G.S., Huang, T.C., 1961. Prolotherapy for sciatica from weak pelvic ligaments and bone distrophy. Clin. Med. (Northfield) 8, 2301–2316.

Hildebrand, K.A., Gallant-Behm, C.L., Kidd, A.S., Hart, D.A., 2005. The basics of soft tissue healing and general factors that influence such healing. Sports Med. Arthrosc. 13, 136–144.

Hooper, R.A., Ding, M., 2004. Retrospective case series on patients with chronic spinal pain treated with dextrose prolotherapy. J. Altern. Complement. Med. 10, 670–674.

Klein, R.G., Dorman, T.A., Johnson, C.E., 1989. Proliferant injections for low back pain: histologic changes of injected ligaments and objective measurements of lumbar spine mobility before and after treatment. J. Neurol. Orthop. Med. Surg. 10, 123–126.

Klein, R.G., Eck, B., 1997. Prolotherapy: an alternative approach to managing low back pain. J. Musculoskelet. Med. 14, 45–49.

Klein, R.G., Eek, B.C., DeLong, W.B., Mooney, V., 1993. A randomized double-blind trial of dextrose glycerine-phenol injections for chronic low back pain. J. Spinal Disord. 6, 23–33.

Kopell, H., Thompson, W., 1976. Peripheral Entrapment Neuropathies. Baltimore, Williams and Wilkins.

Kuffler, D.P., 2018. Variables affecting the potential efficacy of PRP in providing chronic pain relief. J. Pain Res. 12, 109–116.

Lam, K.H., Reeves, K.D., Cheng, A.N., 2017. Transition from deep regional blocks toward deep nerve hydrodissection in the upper body and torso: method description and results from a retrospective chart review of the analgesic effect of 5% dextrose water as the primary hydrodissection injectate to enhance safety. BioMed Res. Int. 2017, 7920438.

Linetsky, F.S., Manchikanti, L., 2005. Regenerative injection therapy for axial pain. Tech. Reg. Anesth. Pain Manag. 9, 40–49.

Liu, Y.K., Tipton, C.M., Matthes, R.D., Bedford, T.G., Maynard, J.A., Walmer, H.C., 1983. An in situ study of the influence of a sclerosing solution in rabbit medial collateral ligaments and its junction strength. Connect. Tissue Res. 11, 95–102.

Louw, W.F., Reeves, K.D., Lam, S.K.H., Cheng, A.L., Rabago, D., 2019. Treatment of temporomandibular dysfunction with hypertonic dextrose injection (prolotherapy): a randomized controlled trial with long-term partial crossover. Mayo Clin. Proc. 94, 820–832.

Mathews, J.A., Mills, S.B., Jenkins, V.M., et al., 1987. Back pain and sciatica: controlled trials of manipulation, traction, sclerosant and epidural injections. Br. J. Rheumatol. 26, 416–423.

Maxwell, N.J., Ryan, M.B., Taunton, J.E., Gillies, J.H., Wong, A.D., 2007. Sonographically guided intratendinous injection of hyperosmolar dextrose to treat chronic tendinosis of the Achilles tendon: a pilot study. Am. J. Roentgenol. 189, W215–W220.

Mooney, V., 2003. Prolotherapy at the fringe of medical care, or is it the frontier? Spine J. 3, 253–254.

Ongley, M.J., Dorman, T.A., Klein, R.G., Eek, B.C., Hubert, L.J., 1987. A new approach to the treatment of chronic low back pain. Lancet 2, 143–146.

Ongley, M.J., Dorman, T., Eck, B., 1988. Ligament instability of knees: a new approach to treatment. Man. Med. 3, 152–154.

Pal, B., Morris, J., 1999. Perceived risks of joint infection following intra-articular corticosteroid injections: a survey of rheumatologists. Clin. Rheumatol. 18, 264–265.

Rabago, D., Best, T.M., Beamsley, M., Patterson, J., 2005. A systematic review of prolotherapy for chronic musculoskeletal pain. Clin. J. Sport Med. 15, 376–380.

Rabago, D., Best, T.M., Zgierska, A.E., Zeisig, E., Ryan, M., Crane, D., 2009. A systematic review of four injection therapies for lateral epicondylosis: prolotherapy, polidocanol, whole blood and platelet-rich plasma. Br. J. Sports Med. 43, 471–481.

Rabago, D., Mundt, M., Zgierska, A., Grettie, J., 2015. Hypertonic dextrose injection (prolotherapy) for knee osteoarthritis: Long term outcomes. Complement. Ther. Med. 23, 388–395.

Rabago, D., Patterson, J.J., Mundt, M., et al., 2013. Dextrose prolotherapy for knee osteoarthritis: a randomized controlled trial. Ann. Fam. Med. 11, 229–237.

Reeves, K.D., 2000. Prolotherapy: basic science, clinical studies, and technique. In: Lennard, T.A. (Ed.), Pain Procedures in Clinical Practice. Hanley & Belfus, Philadelphia, pp. 172–190.

Reeves, K.D., Topol, G.A., Fullerton, B.D., 2008. Evidence-based regenerative injection therapy (prolotherapy) in sports medicine. In: Seidenberg, P.H., Beutler, P.I. (Eds.), The sports Medicine Resource Manual. Saunders Elsevier, Philadelphia, PA, pp. 611–619.

Ryan, M.B., Wong, A.D., Gillies, G.H., Wong, J., Taunton, J.E., 2009. Sonographically guided intratendinous injections of hyperosmolar dextrose/lidocaine: a pilot study for the treatment of chronic plantar fasciitis. Br. J. Sports Med. 43, 303–306.

Sackett, D.L., Rosenberg, W.M.C., 1995. On the need for evidence-based medicine. J. Public Health 17, 330–334.

Schultz, L., 1937. A treatment for subluxation of the temporomandibular joint. JAMA 109, 1032–1035.

Seven, M., Ersen, O., Akpancar, S., et al., 2017. Effectiveness of prolotherapy in the treatment of chronic rotator cuff lesions. Orthop. Traumatol. Surg. Res. 103, 427–433.

Smith, R.K.W., Webbon, P.K., 2005. Harnessing the stem cell for the treatment of tendon injuries: heralding a new dawn? Br. J. Sports Med. 39, 582–584.

Sweeting, K., Yelland, M., 2009. Achilles tendinosis: How does prolotherapy compare to eccentric loading exercises? J. Sci. Med. Sport 12, S19.

Topol, G.A., Podesta, L.A., Reeves, K.D., et al., 2016. Chondrogenic Effect of Intra-articular Hypertonic-Dextrose (Prolotherapy) in Severe Knee Osteoarthritis. PM R. 8, 1072–1082.

Topol, G.A., Reeves, K.D., 2008. Regenerative injection of elite athletes with career–altering chronic groin pain who fail conservative treatment: a consecutive case series. Am. J. Phys. Med. Rehabil. 87, 890–902.

Topol, G.A., Reeves, K.D., Hassanein, K.M., 2005. Efficacy of dextrose prolotherapy in elite male kicking- sport athletes with chronic groin pain. Arch. Phys. Med. Rehabil. 86, 697–702.

Volpi, P., Marinoni, L., Bait, C., De Girolamo, L., Schoenhuber, H., 2007. Treatment of chronic patellar tendinosis with buffered platelet rich plasma: a preliminary study. Med. Sport (Roma) 60, 595–603.

Wang, J.H., Losifidis, M.I., Fu, F.H., 2006. Biomechanical basis for tendinopathy. Clin. Orthop. Relat. Res. 443, 320–322.

Wilkinson, H.A., 2005. Injection therapy for enthesopathies causing axial spine pain and the "failed back syndrome": a single blinded, randomized and cross-over study. Pain Physician 8, 167–173.

Yelland, M.J., Del Mar, C., Pirozzo, S., Schoene, M.L., Vercoe, P., 2004. Prolotherapy injections for chronic low-back pain. Cochrane Database Syst. Rev. 2004 (2), CD004059.

Yelland, M.J., Glasziou, P.P., Bogduk, N., McKernon, M., 2003. Prolotherapy injections, saline injections, and exercises for chronic low-back pain: a randomized trial. Spine 29, 9–16.

Yeomans, F.C., 1939. Sclerosing Therapy: The Injection and Treatment of Hernia, Hydrocele, Varicose Veins and Hemorrhoids. Williams & Wilkins, Baltimore.

Neural Therapy

Rainer Wander and Christl Kiener

CHAPTER CONTENTS

THERAPY WITH LOCAL ANESTHETICS

Neural therapy is considered to be a regulatory and system-resetting therapy in which local anesthetics (LA) are injected in defined regions of the body. Homeostasis is thought to be reestablished by extinguishing peripheral irritation and stimulating regulatory processes (Perschke 1989; Gross 1986, 1988; Heine 2006).

LAs are commonly applied in surgery for local, regional, and nerve block anesthesia. However, they are also applied in segment therapy, trigger point therapy, interference-field therapy, and ganglion anesthesia.

LAs block the sodium-potassium channel in the cell membrane and interrupt nerve impulses (Fleckenstein 1950). This is the well-known anesthetic effect in neurogenic sympathicolysis. Since the discovery of cellular G-proteins and the receptors coupled with them, it has been found that the expression of the inflammatory mediators from the defense cells by LAs is reduced or eliminated (Hollmann and Durieux 2000). The interleukins IL1, IL2, IL6; TNFα; prostaglandins; and NO are excreted by the defense cells, but these cells have no sodium-potassium channels, so the antiinflammatory effect seems not to be bound to the anesthetic effect. The excreted cytokines induce the production of corticotropin releasing hormone (CRH) in the hypothalamus.

This hormone activates the two stress axes: the sympatho-adreno-medullar axis (SAM) and the hypothalamic-pituitary axis (HPA) (Rensing et al. 2005). This central sympatheticotonic effect induces peripherally a chronic inflammation with structural alteration of proteins.

The fast SAM axis excites the initial nuclei of the sympathetic system in the lateral horn of the spinal cord from C8 to L2. From there, the stimuli go to the sympathetic trunk and divergently accompany the trigeminal branches, all the spinal nerves, and the blood vessels (Wancura-Kampik 2009).

The cytokines (peripheral) in combination with CRH (central) also activate the HPA axis. The pituitary gland excretes ACTH, FSF, and TSH—just to name a few of the hormones. It is an attempt to correct the duration of stress activity on the adrenal cortex with cortisone release and to optimize the energy metabolism. However, the LA must be injected directly into the inflamed area to stop its cytokine production there.

Procaine is the preferred LA because of its short duration of action and its positive effect on tissue perfusion; the latter also probably due to its metabolites (para-aminobenzoic acid and di-ethyl-amino-ethanol). It is also assumed to influence cytokine metabolism (IL1, IL6, TNF-alpha, CRP) and activate the endocannabinoid system (Travell and Simons 1983; Heine 2006).

The antiinflammatory effect of LA has been discovered by Hollmann and Durieux (2000). The antiinflammatory effect is independent from the sodium channel action of LA, and it lasts much longer than the anesthesia induced by LA.

This is perhaps one of the most important explanations of the therapeutic properties of LAs. This mechanism also explains their relaxing effect on muscular trigger points (Heine 2006). In addition, LAs reduce neurogenically induced inflammation by influencing neurotransmitters (Tracey 2009; Oke and Tracey 2009). LAs also seem to have remarkable effects on the immune system (Cassuto et al. 2006; Rosas-Ballina and Tracey 2009).

The application of neural therapy is recommended only after the relevant knowledge of anatomy, physiology, and pharmacology has been acquired, and after a thorough training in the application of the therapy (for standards, see Weinschenk 2020 [HUNTER group University of Heidelberg] and Fischer 2007; training standard of the German society for acupuncture and neural therapy [DGfAN]).

NEUROANATOMY, NEUROPHYSIOLOGY

All LAs inhibit conduction of all nerves and therefore have a sympathetic inhibitory effect. These properties are connected with their influence on protein structures in the extracellular matrix (intercellular substance) (Pischinger and Heine 2007; Papathanasiou 2010).

The extracellular matrix is produced by the fibrocytes and also dissolved again. Increased sympathetic activity leads to increased collagen formation. The matrix becomes less diffusible and the fascia becomes hardened and painfully glued. The regional tissue is acidified and the nociceptive activity increased.

Neural therapy is further based on segmental reflex mechanisms: all impulses coming from the periphery (peripheral nervous system) converge in the dorsal horn of the spinal cord (the central nervous system). Impulses originating from the cutis and subcutis; from joint structures, tense muscles, and affected organs; and from scars or injuries may become pathological. In the dorsal horn, they are normally eliminated by descending inhibitory systems and the patient remains symptom free. If these impulses become too strong, or if the inhibitory systems are impaired, there is a relay in three directions:
- via the anterolateral tract for the cortical perception of pain,

- via the motor anterior horn for the muscles, and
- via the sympathetic neurons in the lateral horn and the sympathetic trunk, which has connections to the peripheral nervous system and to the blood vessels and thus to all tissue structures.

The anatomical interconnection of these pathways causes a positive feedback of the impulses through several segments (Jänig 1987).

These horizontal segmental projections may also be projected vertically beyond the segments by the muscular, fascial, vasal, sympathetic, and parasympathetic systems as well as the so-called functional chains, which can be biomechanical, myofascial, fascial, and neuromuscular.

From the sympathetic trunk, the sympathetic fibers accompany the trigeminal branches and all spinal nerves and blood vessels. The blood vessels are sympathetically supplied twice, once by the spinal nerve and once by the sympathetic ganglia (Wancura-Kampik 2017). The dorsal branch of the spinal nerve is accompanied by a blood vessel in each segment. This sympathetic-vascular supply remains dorsally as a subcutaneous projection, for example, in the vertebral body plane.

The ventral and lateral branches of the spinal nerve increasingly shift caudally, projecting sympathetic, nociceptive, and proprioceptive stimuli of the internal organs into the Head zones (Head 1898), which are hypersensitive to irritation. Palpating the skin on the back we find segmental proliferation zones (Kibler fold) and laterally and ventrally sensitive organ zones (Figs. 7.12.1 and 7.12.2).

Examples of functional chains transmitting functional disorders are:

Biomechanical chain: stimuli from the paranasal sinuses, teeth, and tonsils ipsilateral increase the tone of the deep neck muscles. The atlas gets into a sideways displacement, which is followed by the axis with a rotation to the opposite side. The result is scoliosis. The S-shaped scoliosis affects the organs innervated by these segments because of their deformation. The consequence of this functional scoliosis is a functional leg length difference with pain in the sacroiliac joint, that is, the sacral segments S1–S3 with sciatic symptoms (Fig. 7.12.3).

Myofascial chain: disorders in the area of the paranasal sinuses, teeth, and tonsils irritate the segments C1 to C4 (C7). The trapezius muscle is supplied C2 through C4 (Fig. 7.12.4). Its caudal fibers reach the spinous processes of thoracic vertebras 12, 11, 10, so the stimulus reaches the segments Th12, Th11, and

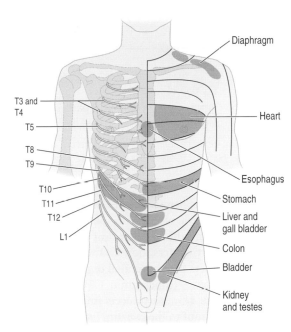

Fig. 7.12.1 Head zones: projection of the internal organs on the skin of the trunk and the abdomen.

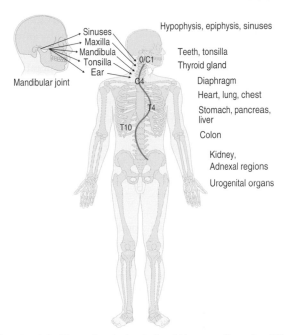

Fig. 7.12.3 Biomechanical chain (Wancura-Kampik 2017; Wander 1992).

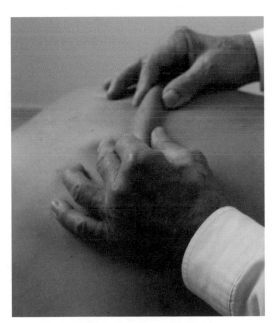

Fig. 7.12.2 Segmental proliferation or swelling zone: Kibler fold.

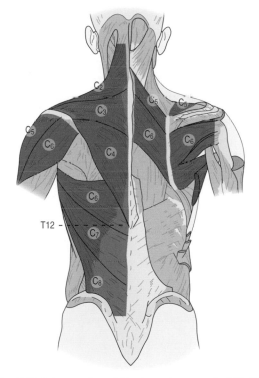

Fig. 7.12.4 Innervation of the trapezius muscle (C2–C4).

Th10. The dermatome Th12 is located above the spinous process of lumbar vertebra 5, so the stimulus also affects the subcutaneous tissue of L5 and leads to lumbalgia and eventually to the degeneration of the disc nucleus.

Fascial chain: disorders in the range of the paranasal sinuses and teeth segments C1 to C4 and tonsils (C4 to C8) irritate the cervical segments, the latter via the autochthonous dorsal muscles. The caudal fiber parts of the M. latissimus dorsi are supplied by C8. They radiate into the thoracolumbar fascia and irritate the opposite iliac crest and the sacroiliac joint (Fig. 7.12.5).

Neuromuscular chain: It is important to consider a chronic, silent inflammation of the tonsils. The tonsils belong to the segment C4 (C3 to C7). The phrenic nerve, originating in the neck (C2 to C5) and passing down between the lung and heart, innervates the diaphragm.

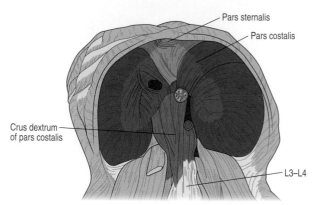

Fig. 7.12.6 The three portions of the diaphragm are innervated by three cervical nerves C3–C5 and are connected to the thoracic nerves Th6–L3/4.

The sternal part (innervation C3) of it communicates with the segments Th6 to Th8 and affects the thoracic organs and the costal part of the stomach.

The costal part (innervation C4) with the segments Th8 to Th12 affects the abdominal organs.

The lumbar part (innervation C5) extends to the lumbar vertebrae 4/5 and projects impulses along the anterior ligamentum to the sacrum. From there, stimuli project into the subcutaneous tissue (subcutome) and promote disc degeneration with lumbago and sciatica (Wancura-Kampik 2021). The innervation of the diaphragm is shown in Fig. 7.12.6.

These paths of the stimulus vary individually; they may omit some segments or be shifted up or down over several segments.

> ### KEY POINT
>
> Myofascial or vertebral irritations can be improved by manual procedures. But the root cause of the phenomenon—the chronic inflammation of the tonsils—can only be resolved by neural therapy.

THERAPEUTIC PRINCIPLES

Local Therapy

In order to treat local inflammation, LAs can be administered at the site of tenderness or inflammation. Typical indications are: skin inflammation, wasp bites, prolonged wound healing, muscle injury, tissue damage due to chemicals, and keloidal scars.

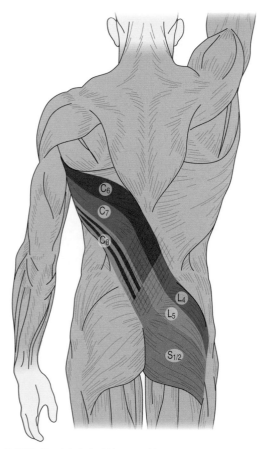

Fig. 7.12.5 Fascial chain (Wancura-Kampik 2021; Wander 1992).

Segment Therapy

The focus here is the neurologically defined segment of the spinal and cranial nerves (Hansen and Schlack 1962). A segment consists of all structures innervated by one spinal nerve: cutis, subcutis, joints (also spinal joints), joint capsules, muscles, fascia, bones, and viscera. Every part of the segment reacts simultaneously on external stimuli of any other part, probably due to the convergence of all segmental impulses on the spinal level (Sessle et al. 1986). A therapeutic stimulus applied in one segment can affect another part of the segment. The easiest way to apply a stimulus is by intracutaneous injection in the corresponding dermatome, thereby producing a small papule or wheal. The weal simultaneously reaches the sympathetic-sensory dermatome and the sympathetic-vasal subcutaneous tissue, which are projected into different segments of the spinal nerves. This is because the sensory-sympathetic dermatome arose embryonically from the ectoderm; the underlying capillary sympathetic subcutome has a mesodermal origin.

In addition, the therapist may infiltrate scars, trigger points, fascia, the periosteum, or joint capsules (in particular, vertebral joint capsules), and related blood vessels in the respective segment.

Example 1 Patient with shoulder pain (dermatome C4 and C5): two intracutaneous routes of papules (weals); the first route goes from the C7 spinous process to the acromion and to the base of the deltoid muscle (segments C4 → C5/6) and the second goes from the anterior axillary fold on the acromion to the posterior axillary fold (segments Th2 → C5 → C4). In this way, adjacent segments with ancillary function to the shoulder joint (acromioclavicular joint, sternoclavicular joint, clavicle, first and second rib) may also be included (Fig. 7.12.7).

Example 2 Patient with gastrointestinal symptoms in the upper abdomen: injections of intracutaneous papules/wheals and subcutaneous injections in the area of the costal arch (so-called Vogler points, Fig. 7.12.8) and the fascia of the abdominal muscles. The xyphoid process (a rudiment of the seventh rib) is of special significance in this region and belongs to the T7 segment.

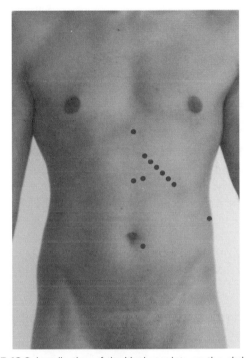

Fig. 7.12.8 Localization of the Vogler points on the abdomen.

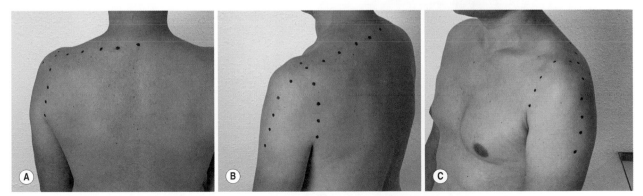

Fig. 7.12.7 Injection routes in a patient with shoulder pain. Internal organs can be influenced using the knowledge of the cuti-visceral and viscero-motoric reflex arcs.

The duodenum and the pancreas belong to the same segment. Because of the segmental organization of skin, muscle, fascia, and periosteum there is a connection between these structures and the stomach, the pancreas, and the small intestine through which these organs can in turn be influenced.

Intracutaneous and deeper prefascial injection can also be applied in the anterior midline at acupuncture point CV12/Th8 (see Fig. 7.12.9). This point is connected with the celiac ganglion, which controls the sympathetic abdominal organs (Heine 2006; Wancura-Kampik 2021).

Acupuncture points are considered by some authors to be passage points in the fascia (Heine 2006) through which nerves, blood, and lymphatic vessels come to the surface. It is suggested that these structures can be influenced by injecting procaine at one of these points as well. Neural therapists also choose acupuncture points for treatment (Heine 2006).

Extended Segment Therapy, Ganglia Therapy

If the segmental injections are not sufficient to improve the patient's symptoms, the clinician may block the afferent stimulus at the level of the spinal nerves, the plexus, the vessels, and the sympathetic or parasympathetic ganglia (so-called extended segment therapy). By eliminating the afferent and efferent impulses and simultaneously activating the descending endogenous inhibitory systems, the auto-organization of the peripheral nervous system can recover (see also Oke and Tracey 2009).

In the patient with shoulder pain (*Example 1*), this could be achieved by an injection into the stellate ganglion or the axillary plexus. In the patient with gastric problems (*Example 2*), extended segment therapy would consist of injection into the sympathetic celiac ganglion. In addition, an injection into the associated vertebral facet joints in the vicinity of the sympathetic trunk can be applied (indirect injection to the sympathetic trunk) (Kupke 2010), which affects 80% of the sympathetic afferent and efferent nerve fibers of the corresponding segment. This procedure practically corresponds to an indirect injection into the sympathetic trunk, which can affect up to 80% of all sympathetic afferent and efferent fibers in the segment. The internal organs and the musculoskeletal system can be influenced via the segments C8 to L2. Above and below these segments, facet infiltration affects mainly the musculoskeletal system.

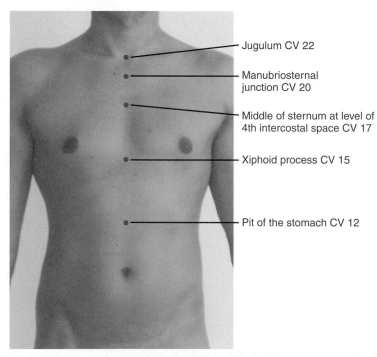

Fig. 7.12.9 Points on the frontal middle line (CV meridian) with acupuncture point CV 12.

The *cranial parasympathetic* ganglia (ciliary, pterygo-palatine, and otic) can be easily and safely accessed by injection. Their fibers accompany the trigeminal branches and their associated ganglia. Trigeminal irritation due to pathological processes in the sinuses, the teeth, local inflammation (e.g., granulomas), jaw disorders (e.g., TMJ syndrome), the tonsils, and the ears can be treated in this way.

The *sacral parasympathetic* nuclei are located in the lateral horn of the sacral cord (S2 to S4) and accompany the pudendal nerve. Thus gynecological disorders or sacral irritations can be positively influenced by injecting the sacral parasympathetic ganglia, for example, the inferior hypogastric plexus (Frankenhäuser plexus; Wander 2003).

Frequently, sacral parasympathetic stimuli from, for example, episiotomy scars, hysterectomy scars, and chronic prostatitis are directed cranially, where they are switched parasympathetically cranially and projected trigeminally. With trigeminal neuralgia, this path should always be considered and also treated via the sacral parasympathetic ganglia.

Therapy via the Interference Field (Störfeld)

An interference field is defined as an oligo- or asymptomatic region of the body that causes irritation in another remote location.

If a morphological substrate of the interference field can be found, it is also called "focus" (Mastalier and Weinschenk 2010). Interference fields, for example, can be scars or inflammatory or infectious tooth disorders. Many mechanisms have been postulated to explain these remote effects. A neuroanatomic explanation is segmental irritation, which is processed into the posterior horn. By projection to neighboring segments, it can cause secondary disorders. A cross-connection from trigeminal nuclei to their adjacent vagal nerve nuclei might also play an important part in projection disorders (Sessle et al. 1986; Hülse et al. 2005).

> #### KEY POINT
> The site of interference fields itself is asymptomatic, but its altered stimulus triggers autonomic dysregulation (e.g., increased tonicity of muscles or the sympathetic system), of which the patient may be aware. Their major effect, however, is the pathological irritation of a remote area.

More than 70% of the interference fields are located in the cranial region (sinuses, teeth, tonsils, ear) (Mastalier and Weinschenk 2010). Their stimuli cause characteristic changes in the neck area with its complex musculature. These changes are palpable—the so-called neck reflex points (NRP) or Adler–Langer pressure points.

NRP are easily detectable by their tenderness and sometimes swelling and are strictly associated with interference fields in the corresponding segment of the frontal head (Weinschenk and Langer 2020). Projections of stimuli of the cervical spinal segments are not transferred to the corresponding segmental dermatomes but almost exclusively to the myotomes of the same segment (Neuhuber 2007). They are no longer palpable after successful neural therapy of the corresponding interference field. Epidemiology and the importance of the NRP in the detection of interference fields are subject to current research.

Example 3 NRP 4 (= tonsils) is palpable as a painful swelling (Fig. 7.12.10). After the injection into the tonsils, the NRP 4 together and the accompanying muscular tension (Mm. recti capitis, Mm. obliqui capitis, Mm. interspinales) is no longer palpable.

Therapy via Functional Chains

The existence of NRP demonstrates the close relationship between structures of the facial region, the "inner organs"

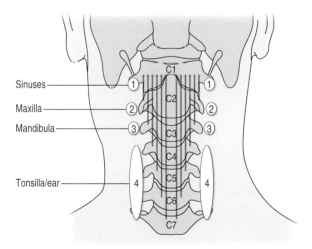

Fig. 7.12.10 Neck reflex points (Adler-Langer points) are painful points in the cervical muscles in patients with interference fields in the ENT and dental area.

of the face/head (paranasal sinuses, teeth, tonsils, and ears), and the segments of the cervical spine. The resulting changes of muscles and ligaments of the neck can be further transferred to lower parts of the spine. Asymmetrical tension of the neck region may be conducted to the thoracic and lumbar regions of the spine, resulting in their countermotion and possibly a functional scoliosis.

This close relation between cervical, thoracic, and lumbar spine and the sacroiliac joints is well-known in many medical specialties, for example, osteopathy (craniosacral therapy) (see Fig. 7.12.3). Blockades of certain vertebral joints are part of this functional scoliosis and can easily be diagnosed by a trained manual therapist. Major diagnostic signs of the functional scoliosis will be found at cervical vertebrae 1 and 4, thoracic vertebrae 4 and 10, and lumbar vertebra 5/sacrum (sacroiliac joint). A link between a functional scoliosis and functional variation of the leg length can be observed.

Vertebral blockades can cause sympathetic stimulation of the respective vertebral segments and might lead to disorders of the associated internal organs (Wander 2010).

Almost always, the functional chains run cranial (segments C1–C3/C4) to caudal (segments L5, S1, sacroiliac joint). The palpation of the neck reflex points; the subsequent injection of local anesthetics onto the paranasal sinuses, teeth, or tonsils; and the controlled extinction of the neck reflex points are prerequisites for further therapeutic steps. In the pain regions of the cervical, thoracic, and lumbar spine, which are indicated by the patient, weals should be raised or injections made at facet joints, trigger/tender points, or painful spinous processes. The spinous processes of the cervical vertebrae 2 and 7, the thoracic vertebrae 6 and 12, the lumbar vertebra 5, and the sacroiliac joint are often painful. Injections in ganglia or blood vessels are only indicated if there is no therapeutic effect.

Systemic Therapy

The vascular supply to the tissues is not only segmentally organized. Blood vessels have their own "vascular zones," which can maintain skin and muscle pain beyond the corresponding spinal segmental organization (Gross 1986, 1988). All vessels (arterial, venous, and lymphatic) are accompanied by sympathetic fibers. In response to lesions, the vessels contract and cause disorders in both directions of flow, with corresponding pain symptoms. Injection of LA into the affected or other vessels will bring pathological contraction back to a normal state. For example, a painful sensation in the dorsal thigh underneath the buttock fold can be caused by fascial radiation from the thoracic fascia into the lumbar fascia. But it can also be caused by a vasal projection of the internal iliac artery and thus as a sign of disorder/inflammatory process of the pelvic organs. This would implicate a different therapeutic approach (LA injection onto pelvic organs).

Common routes of intravasal application of neural therapy are intravenous, intraarterial, and infusion therapy. A well-known example is LA infusion in the treatment of tinnitus (Shea and Emmett 1981).

INDICATIONS, CONTRAINDICATIONS, COMPLICATIONS

Indications: More than 100 years of clinical experience (Spiess 1902) indicates that neural therapy can be successfully applied in all functional and regulatory disorders, with and without pain, including headache, vertigo, tinnitus, spinal disorders, musculoskeletal pain, neuralgia, chronic inflammation, thoracic and abdominal diseases, circulatory disorders, and other diseases (for an overview, see Weinschenk 2020; Hollmann and Herroeder 2010).

Contraindications for neural therapy are: advanced structural damage of organ systems (e.g., cirrhosis), genetic diseases, deficiency disorders, coagulation disorders, and mental disorders. Structural changes and defects prevent neural therapy's beneficial effects (as in acupuncture and osteopathy).

Complications very rarely occur in neural therapy. The rule is: care reduces risk! The following complications can occur:
- allergic reactions (rare; Weinschenk et al. 2017),
- injuries (e.g., bleeding, hematoma),
- infection,
- patient's overreaction after injection, e.g., collapse due to fear, stress, vago-vasal orthostasis,
- reaction due to additional medication or a secondary disorder (beta-blockers, tranquillizers, anticholinergic syndrome),
- central toxic or cardiac symptoms due to overdose (30–50 mg/day = 30–50 mL 1% solution).

PRACTICAL PROCEDURE

The steps in neural therapy are:
- Segment therapy: Segments are assigned to the area supplied by a spinal nerve. The therapeutic measures include:
  - Weals in the dermatome, if dorsally, preferably paravertebral at the inner branch of the bladder meridian
  - Injections into the myotome: trigger points, acupuncture points, origin, and attachment of the muscles
  - Preperiosteal infiltration of the sclerotome: spinous processes, ligaments, or large and small joints.

The enterotome can be reached directly or indirectly by means of:
- Ganglio-therapy: if this segmental therapy is not successful, the sympathetic and parasympathetic ganglia, and possibly the blood vessels, should be flooded.
- Interference-field therapy: if these segmental and oversegmental injections are unsuccessful, consideration must be given to remote effects caused by interference fields. The diagnosis of the neck reflex points shows us the way to the injection of the paranasal sinuses, teeth, or tonsils, or also abdominal organs and scars, old fractures, or surgical scars.

Summary

Local anesthetics have various pharmacological properties that make them potential drugs for neural therapy in the treatment of a variety of functional and pain disorders. Therapy follows the principle of "as little harm as possible." Beginning with simple injections, many beneficial results can be achieved.

Neural therapy extinguishes irritating peripheral stimuli. Thus the neurogenic stress in various tissues can be decreased and therefore serve as a preparation for the successful application of further treatment methods (e.g., osteopathy). This combination potentiates the effect of the various procedures.

RESEARCH

Although LAs have been used therapeutically since they were discovered in the late 1880s, almost all the scientific literature that has been published is on their anesthesiological application in surgery.

After the important results on the antiinflammatory effects of LAs were revealed, more and more reports on their therapeutic effects have been published (for review, see Cassuto et al. 2006; Hollmann and Herroeder 2010). Studies on the clinical effects of LAs often cannot be found under the term "neural therapy." They have been published widely in different areas of medicine.

However, neural therapy has been integrated as a discipline in various universities worldwide, especially in Central America, Switzerland (University of Bern), and Germany (University of Heidelberg). This provides a platform for future research in this field. There are various research projects in progress at the University of Bern (Egli et al. 2010, cited in Fischer 2014): for example, on the effect of neural therapy in patients resistant to conventional therapies, on the neuronal regulation of blood vessels, on the importance of the sympathetic system in the development of chronic pain and inflammation, and a prospective study on pain and neural therapy.

At the University of Heidelberg, major projects are addressing the molecular mechanisms of the antiinflammatory effect of LAs, NRP, and their clinical importance in diagnosis and therapy; the correlation of neural therapeutic effects to vegetative parameters; and the quantification of side effects and complications of neural therapy. All these studies provide a promising platform for future research in this field.

ACKNOWLEDGMENTS

The authors are very grateful to Christl Kiener, M.D., and her husband Paul Crichton, M.D., for their support in preparing the manuscript. They would like to thank Dr. Wancura-Kampik for the illustrations.

REFERENCES

Cassuto, J., Sinclair, R., Bonderovic, M., 2006. Anti-inflammatory properties of local anesthetics and their present and potential clinical implications. Acta. Anaesthesiol. Scand. 50, 265–282.

Fischer, L., 2007. Neuraltherapie nach Huneke. 3. Aufl. Hippokrates, Stuttgart.

Fischer, L., 2014. Neuraltherapie: Neurophysiologie, Injektionstechnik und Therapievorschläge. (Studie von Egli et al. 2010, Seite 179). 4. Auflage, Haug, Stuttgart. Egli S, Pfister M, Ludin SM, Busato A, Fischer L. 2010. Können Lokalanästhetika (Neuraltherapie) bei überwiesenen, therapieresistenten, chronischen Schmerzpatienten einen Circulus vitiosus durchbrechen? Dissertation an der Universität Bern.

Fleckenstein, A., 1950. Mechanismen der Lokalanästhesie. Klinische Wochenschrift 1950;28(25-26) 452–453.

Gross, D., 1986. Therapeutische Lokalanästhesie. 3. Aufl. Hippokrates, Stuttgart.

Gross, D., 1988. Therapeutische Lokalanästhesie Band II. Anwendung in Klinik und Praxis, Hippokrates, Stuttgart.

Hansen, K., Schliack, H., 1962. Segmentale Innervation. Stuttgart: Thieme.

Head, H., 1898. Die Sensibilitätsstörungen der Haut bei Visceralerkrankungen. (Übersetzt von W. Seiffer). Hirschwald, Berlin.

Heine, H., 2006. Lehrbuch der Biologischen Medizin. 3. Aufl. Hippokrates, Stuttgart.

Hollmann, M.W., Durieux, M.E., 2000. Local anesthetics and the inflammatory response: a new therapeutic indication? Anesthesiology 93, 858–875.

Hollmann, M.W., Herroeder, S., 2020. Alternative Wirkmechanismen von Lokalanästhetika. In: Weinschenk, S. (Hrsg.) (Ed.), Handbuch Neuraltherapie. 2. Auflage. Thieme, Stuttgart, pp 104–109.

Hülse, M., Neuhuber, W., Wolff, H.D., 2005. Die obere Halswirbelsäule. Springer, Heidelberg.

Jänig, W., 1987. Neuronal mechanisms of pain with special emphasis on visceral and deep somatic pain. Acta. Neurochir. Suppl. (Wien) 38, 16–32.

Kupke, T., 2010. Fecettengelenke der Wirbelsäule. In: Weinschenk, S. (Ed.), Handbuch Neuraltherapie. Elsevier, München, pp. 628–633.

Mastalier, O., Weinschenk, S., 2010. Fokus und Herdgeschehen. In: Weinschenk, S. (Ed.), Handbuch Neuraltherapie. Elsevier, München, pp. 137–168.

Neuhuber, W., 2007. Anatomie, funktionelle Neuroanatomie der oberen Halswirbelsäule. Manuelle Medizin 4, 227–231.

Oke, S.L., Tracey, K.J., 2009. The inflammatory reflex and the role of complementary and alternative medical therapies. Ann. N. Y. Acad. Sci. 1172, 172–180.

Papathanasiou, G., 2010. Bindegewebe, Matrix und Neuraltherapie. In: Weinschenk, S. (Ed.), Handbuch Neuraltherapie. Elsevier, München, pp. 131–137.

Perschke, O., 1989. Kombination von Akupunktur, Neuraltherapie, Manualtherapie bei Gelenkerkrankungen. Dt. Z. Akup. 32, 34–40.

Pischinger, A., Heine, H., 2007. The Extracellular Matrix and Ground Regulation: Basis for a Holistic Biological Medicine. North Atlantic Books, Berkeley, CA.

Rensing, L., Koch, M., Rippe, B, Rippe, V., 2005: Mensch im Stress, Springer Spektrum, München.

Rosas-Ballina, M., Tracey, K.J., 2009. The neurology of the immune system: neural reflexes regulate immunity. Neuron 64, 28–32.

Sessle, B.J., Hu, J.W., Amano, N., Zhong, G., 1986. Convergence of cutaneous, tooth pulp, visceral, neck and muscle afferents onto nociceptive and non-nociceptive neurones in trigeminal subnucleus caudalis (medullary dorsal horn) and its implications for referred pain. Pain 27, 219–235.

Shea, J.J., Emmett, J.R., 1981. The medical treatment of tinnitus. J. Laryngol. Otol. Suppl. 4, 130–138.

Spiess, G., 1902. Die Heilwirkung der Anästhetics, Med. Welt Zbl. Inn. Med. 23: p. 222-223.

Tracey, K.J., 2009. Reflex control of immunity. Nat. Rev. Immunol. 9, 418–428.

Travell, J.G., Simons, D.G., 1983. Myofascial pain and dysfunction: the trigger point manual. Williams & Wilkins, Baltimore.

Wancura-Kampik, 2009. Segmentan-Anatomie, Urban & Fischer, München, p. 93–122.

Wancura-Kampik, I., 2017. Segment-Anatomie. 3. Aufl. Elsevier, Urban & Fischer, München. (English edition: 2012, Segmental Anatomy, Elsevier, Urban & Fischer, München).

Wancura-Kampik, I., 2021. Segment-Akupunktur. 2. Aufl. KIENER, München

Wander, R., 1992. Neuraltherapie der Wirbelsäule und Gelenke. Ärzte Z. Naturheilverfahren 33, 927–975.

Wander, R., 2003. Anatomie und Physiologie des vegetativen Nervensystems. Dt. Ztschr. f. Akup 45, S. 34–40.

Wander, R., 2010. Diagnostik über Muskelfunktionsketten. In: Weinschenk, S. (Hrsg.) (Ed.), Handbuch Neuraltherapie. Elsevier, München, pp. 302–310.

Weinschenk, S. (Ed.), 2020. Handbuch Neuraltherapie. 2. Auflage. Thieme, Stuttgart.

Weinschenk, S., Langer, H., 2020. Examination of neck reflex points (Adler-Langer Points). In: Weinschenk, S. (Hrsg.) (Ed.), Handbuch Neuraltherapie. Thieme, Stuttgart.

Weinschenk, S., Mergenthaler, C., Armstrong, C., Göllner, R., Hollmann, M.W., Strowitzki. T., 2017. Local Anesthetics, Procaine, Lidocaine, and Mepivacaine Show Vasodilatation but No Type 1 Allergy: A Double-Blind, Placebo-Controlled Study. Biomed Res. Int. 2017, 9804693.

Instrument-Assisted Soft Tissue Mobilization: Emphasizing the Fascia

Warren I. Hammer

CHAPTER CONTENTS

INTRODUCTION

This chapter is intended for manual therapists and clinicians who use their hands directly on the body to achieve therapeutic results. Many manual therapists believe that nothing can enhance or improve human touch, although there is considerable evidence that the use of instrument-assisted soft tissue mobilization (IASTM) is making a major difference for clinicians and their patients. A major obstacle in the life of clinicians who use their hands is the development of repetitive trauma injury to their hands and upper extremities over time (Snodgrass et al. 2003). There have been many peer reviewed papers on IASTM (Hammer and Pfefer 2005; Loghmani and Warden 2009; Melham et al. 1998) just to mention a few. IASTM researched in the early 1990s, and Graston Technique was introduced formally in 1994 (Graston Technique Manual). The original patented technology Graston Technique (GT-IASTM) incorporates the use of stainless steel instruments. At present, numerous varieties of stainless steel instruments have become available.

Subjects discussed in this chapter are new information about the structure and function of fascia, the how, when, and where IASTM—elbows, knuckles, etc.—should be applied. How deep should we penetrate tissue, what exactly should we be palpating for, how do we recognize when to stop applying load, how do symptoms relate to the layers of soft tissue depth, and where should the load be applied? It is necessary to determine whether our applied mechanical load is treating a local pathological area or a local proprioceptive area or both (Hammer 2018). Also included are IASTM contraindications, and the importance of creating a tissue glide. Densification versus fibrosis. The concept that the proprioceptive system is treated over particular fascial areas containing mechanoreceptors. A global approach may also be necessary over what are called quadrants or even over any restricted fascial locations throughout the body.

NORMAL MUSCLE FUNCTION REQUIRES NORMAL FASCIAL GLIDING

Most receptors that report to the central nervous system (CNS) on the status of muscles are in the fascia. Most all mechanoreceptors, in order to provide the central nervous system with maximum information about muscle function, are required to stretch with movement. It is so important that mechanoreceptors stretch that the chief function of the Gamma neuron from the CNS representing 31% of efferent motor supply to our muscles is to stretch the intrafusal fibers in the spindle cell. This stimulates 1a and 2 sensory nerves that allow the CNS to determine how each muscle functions. If, because of trauma, surgery, or overuse, fascia becomes restricted during motion, the feedback to the CNS is altered, resulting in decreased coordination (Mense and Schneider 2010), causing eventual muscle weakness and pain in the associated joint. An important way of detecting diminished mechanoreceptor stretching is through the palpation of the quality of a gliding sensation at specific fascial points (see Chapter 7.7: Fascial Manipulation).

RELATION OF HYALURONAN TO THE GLIDING OF FASCIA AND MUSCLE FIBERS

One of the key elements that define fascial gliding is hyaluronan (HA). HA is a high-molecular-weight glycosaminoglycan polymer of the extracellular matrix. HA in the muscle system is located between the sublayers of aponeurotic fascia and between the deep fascia and underlying muscles (Stecco 2015) (Fig. 7.13.1; also see Chapter 7.7). Besides functioning to protect muscles from injury and stimulating satellite cell proliferation, HA is the principal GAG that allows gliding of muscles, fascia, and joints. It is present in the loose connective tissue and because of injury, overuse, or surgery can become concentrated, fragmented, and entangled, preventing or diminishing receptor glide during movement. It is hypothesized that an increase in viscosity of HA is an underlying reason receptors, especially spindle cells, Pacinian, and Ruffini receptors, are prevented from normal stretching, resulting in abnormal muscle function (Stecco et al. 2016). With increasing concentration, HA chains begin to entangle, conferring distinctive hydrodynamic properties (Stecco et al. 2011). Fascial treatment may be mostly effective because of the breaking of HA entanglements in the loose connective tissue between muscles and fascia.

Stecco and colleagues (2013) did an ultrasonography on the diagnosis of myofascial chronic neck pain (CNP more than 3 months), without radiculopathy, comparing the thickness of the collagen (type 1 fibers) to the thickness of the loose connective tissue (LCT) that contains GAGs and HA. The patients with increased thickening of the LCT experienced increased pain and stiffness versus the patients with normal loose connective tissue. The data support the hypothesis that loose connective tissue inside the fasciae plays a significant role in the pathogenesis of chronic neck pain (CNP). In particular, the value of 0.15 cm of the sternocleidomastoid fascia was considered as a cut-off value, which allows the clinician to make a diagnosis of myofascial disease in a subject with CNP. The variation of thickness of the fascia correlated with the increase in quantity of the loose connective tissue but not with an increase in dense connective tissue (Fig. 7.13.2). The role of HA in providing a substance for the smooth gliding between surfaces and between the different motor units within muscle has also been described by McCombe and colleagues (2001).

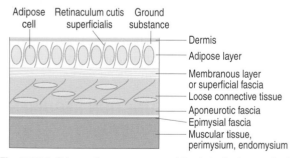

Adipose cell Retinaculum cutis superficialis Ground substance
— Dermis
— Adipose layer
— Membranous layer or superficial fascia
— Loose connective tissue
— Aponeurotic fascia
— Epimysial fascia
— Muscular tissue, perimysium, endomysium

Fig. 7.13.1 Schematic arrangement of fascia in the human body. Redrawn with permission from Stecco, L., Stecco, A., 2018. Fascial Manipulation – Practical Part: First Level, second. ed. Piccin Nuova Libraris S.p.A., Padova, Italy.

KEY POINTS

- Muscle receptors located in the fascia require the ability to stretch.
- Palpation of specific fascial points that do not glide may inhibit normal proprioception.
- An increase in viscosity of hyaluronan in the loose connective tissue will prevent normal gliding and therefore normal fascial stretching.

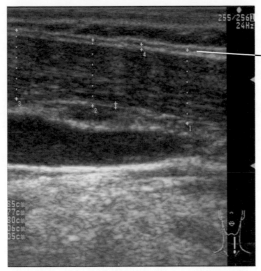

Increased thickening (HA) in loose connective tissue

Fig. 7.13.2 Increase in loose connective tissue space in patient with neck pain. HA, hyaluronan. Reproduced with permission from Stecco, A., Meneghini, A., Stern, R., Stecco, C., Imamura, M., 2013. Ultrasonography in myofascial neck pain: randomized clinical trial for diagnosis and follow-up. Surg. Radiol. Anat. 36, 243–253.

SUPERFICIAL FASCIA

In brief, superficial fascia (SF) is present throughout the body and formed by interwoven collagen fibers, which are loosely packed and intermixed with abundant elastic fibers. SF is the fibrous layer between the superficial adipose tissue (SAT) that connects to the skin and the deep adipose layer (DAT) that connects to the deep fascia (Fig. 7.13.1). SF is thicker in the trunk than in the limbs and gradually becomes thinner in the limbs. SF contains superficial veins and lymphatic vessels. Inside the superficial fascia, the subcutaneous plexus is present, which functions in thermoregulation. The structure of the layer dictates the symptoms of the patient and the amount of manual load necessary. For example, symptoms related to dysfunction of the lymphatic system, superficial circulatory system, and thermoregulation are closely related to dysfunction involving superficial fascia. SF helps ensure the patency of the veins (Stecco 2015). Consequently, effective treatment can be achieved with light massage (Fig. 7.13.3) over local areas or over larger quadrant areas on the superficial subcutis layers. The disposition of the collagen and elastic fibers inside the superficial fascia could guide lymphatic flux in the correct direction. If the superficial fascia is altered, the lymphatic drainage becomes compromised (Stecco et al. 2016). Edema responds to SF treatment both manually and with IASTM.

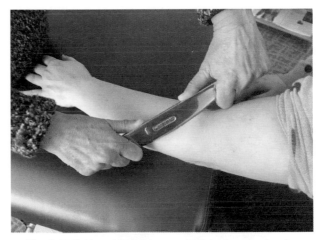

Fig. 7.13.3 Use of IASTM on superficial forearm fascia.

Palpation and Treatment of SF with IASTM

Instruments made of stainless steel have a significant ability to palpate the consistency of soft tissue. Superficially a fibrous granular type of sensation is easily palpated (Fig. 7.13.3). Most authorities recommend treatment in the direction of the tissue barrier. With the use of instruments the area to be treated should first be palpated with fingers, knuckles, and even with elbows depending on the involved site and then similarly reevaluated posttreatment. Palpation by hand also reveals temperature, swelling, and patient sensitivity. Friction of superficial fascia causes modifications in small arterioles, veins, and capillaries in the superficial plexus, resulting in subsequent superficial redness that resolves over a time-span of 15 minutes (Stecco and Stecco 2018).

In the treatment of Achilles tendon problems, the use of IASTM should pay more attention to the paratenon, a superficial structure, rather than the tendon itself. The paratenon is highly vascularized and innervated, whereas the tendon is not innervated, leading to the conclusion that a well-vascularized paratenon is very important for the nutrition of the tendon. Recurring microtrauma of the paratendinous tissue may cause ischemia and degenerative processes of the tendon itself, supporting the hypothesis that it is the origin of pain in tendinopathy (Stecco et al. 2014; Tan and Chan, 2008) (Fig. 7.13.4; see also Retinacula later in this chapter.

DEEP FASCIA

Deep fascia (DF) (Fig. 7.13.1) consists of "all the well-organized dense, fibrous layers that interact with muscles. The deep fascia connects different elements of the musculoskeletal system and transmits muscular force over a distance" (Stecco 2015, p. 51). Deep fascia refers to the three layered aponeurotic fascia (covers all extremities and parts of the trunk) and glides on the epimysial fascia

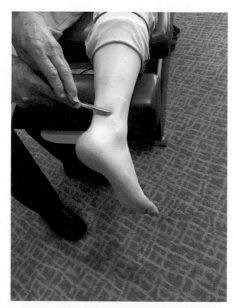

Fig. 7.13.4 Use of IASTM superficially along the paratenon.

that covers muscles. The epimysial fibers connect to the gliding perimysium that covers muscle bundles, and the perimysium connect to the gliding endomysium that cover the muscle fibers (Fig. 7.13.1). Obviously, to reach the deep fascia and muscles a deeper pressure is necessary. It is the deep fascia that contains mechanoreceptors responsible for proprioception, coordination, balance, and myofascial pain (Stecco et al. 2016).

FASCIAL DENSIFICATION/FIBROSIS

A fascial "densification" represents an abnormal functional tissue change compared with a pathological fibrotic-like tissue change (Hammer 2018). Palpation for densification is evaluating for the sensation of fascial gliding rather than pathological ligamentous, tendinous, or muscular-type restrictions. Fascial points require a very local deep contact that does not break the skin surface. Attention to fascial densification includes evaluation and treatment of fascial kinetic chains usually proximal or distal to the site of pain (see Chapter 7.7: Fascial Manipulation). Pathological areas refer to a "fibrosis-like problem similar to the process of scarring, with the deposition of excessive amounts of fibrotic connective tissue, reflective of a reparative or reactive process such as a tendinosis" (Pavan et al. 2014, p. 441). A pathological area can be a fascial fibrosis or a chronic densification affecting the gliding between collagen fibrous bundles and within the fibrous layers rather than in loose connective tissue. It is doubtful that treating an actual scar would benefit from the reparative response obtained treating a chronic tendonitis/tendinosis. Fibrosis or scarring usually relates to a past trauma or surgery, that is, an actual response to tearing of tissue. It obliterates the architecture and function of the involved tissue. It is at times also possible for a pathological area to include a functional mechanoreceptor area.

On palpation, treatment of a lack of normal gliding (densification) at a local receptor point is characteristic of a functional approach. Chronic nonspecific back pain would be more related to fascial densification and its abnormal proprioceptive effect (Casato et al. 2019). Practitioners often misuse the words "scar tissue" for densification.

Palpation of Deep Fascia

For functional points it is necessary to restore a sensation of gliding. You have to select the most restricted direction with enough pressure to reach the deep fascia.

A patient's description of deep fascial pain can be important. According to Schilder and colleagues (2014, p. 222), fascial pain is usually described as "a stabbing, irritating, stinging, sharp or a beating sensation." Muscle pain on the other hand is described as a more dull and deep aching type of pain.

A study by Roman and colleagues (2013) on the best direction of friction massage to stimulate the ideal HA flow was by using a perpendicular compression vibration and tangential oscillation (an angular back and forth movement) rather than an ischemic compression or perpendicular vibration alone. This movement created a higher pressure and greater lubrication of HA. It is usually recommended to use IASTM—elbows, knuckles, etc.—against the direction that a barrier is palpated. The palpation of the examiner always takes precedence over the patient's expression of pain. If a painful area is not necessarily densified or fibrotic, then there is no apparent reason to use any form of mechanical load.

Unfortunately most colleges today do not teach about the fascial system in their core curriculum, and the majority of practitioners using IASTM are devoting their treatment mainly to the site of pain and outlying areas, for example, IASTM of acromial clavicular ligament (Fig. 7.13.5). There is a distinct difference between using mechanical load on functional versus pathological areas (Hammer 2018). Most practitioners do look around the painful site for other restrictions. A minority (fascial trained in identifying mechanoreceptors) look specifically elsewhere considering the fascial kinetic chain (Chapter 7.7). A primary question for practitioners who treat soft tissue is whether the patient's complaint area is the source of the pain or an area compensating for a previous distal or proximal aggravation of the fascial system. One of the basic tenets gleaned from knowledge of the fascial system is to determine particular fascial pathways that may be responsible for local pain (see Chapter 7.7: Fascial Manipulation). Palpation often reveals local, painful, minimal, nodular-like restricted areas along specific fascial pathways that may refer to the site of pain.

> ### KEY POINTS
>
> - It is necessary upon palpation to distinguish between superficial and deep fascia.
> - Each of these layers have their own structure and function: the superficial fascia is more related with exteroception (the perception of stimuli originating outside or at a distance from the body) and the deep fascia associated with proprioception.
> - Each layer exhibits its own particular symptoms and requires a different type of loading.
> - It is necessary to distinguish between a functional densification area versus a pathological (degenerative, tendinosis) area.

Treatment of Deep Fascia: IASTM versus Noninstrument

No matter what type of manual load on soft tissue is used, it is assumed that prior to treatment, some functional tests (passive, resistive, active) are used to determine the most painful movements. It is possible, therefore, if one or several points or areas are to be treated, that after each treated location some improvement in functional testing should occur. Otherwise, one may have to rethink their hypothesis as to where to treat. Although the use of instruments can certainly reach the deep fascia, the treatment of some local areas of deep fascia may be more conducive to the use of elbows or knuckles than instruments, especially when looking for a densification. For both modalities the deep fascia should be treated with the local area in a relaxed position without any undue tension. Although instruments can reach deep fascia, a large amount of operator pressure may be necessary, and attempting to create a local compression with a back-and-forth motion can more easily result in bruising. Some locations of fascia are particularly deep, for example, laterally between the pelvis

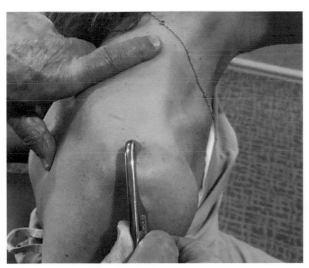

Fig. 7.13.5 Use of IASTM on acromial-clavicular ligament. Patient's arm behind back.

and 12th rib near the quadratus lumborum, where there is a large amount of deep adipose tissue. The use of the elbow offers a stable pressure that penetrates more easily and deeply (Fig. 7.13.6). Patients usually experience more pressure and penetration with an elbow than with a sharp-edged instrument. It is easier at this location (with experience) to use an elbow to determine a lack of fascial gliding than with a metal instrument. The flatness of the distal elbow or the flatness of the second phalanx of the second finger helps to provide a more stable type sensory surface. Other areas where it appears easier to create compression with motion to determine fascial gliding without instruments are the glutei and abdomen.

Alleviation of a densification takes from 3 to, rarely at times, 10 minutes. Most often these areas are normalized—that is, gliding—in one or two visits. An important concept is when to stop treating an area. Of course the immediate answer is a return to painless function. Although there does not seem to be studies on this concept, it also makes sense to restore tissue to its most normal state based on palpation using IASTM or hands.

The treatment time using IASTM is discussed later under Instruments. Treatment of pathological areas (tennis elbow, collateral ligaments, etc.) require repeated

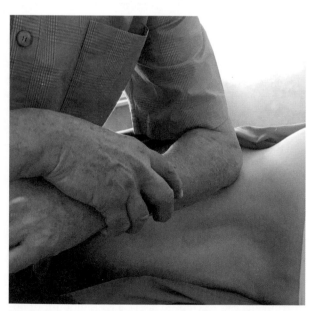

Fig. 7.13.6 Patient sidelying with their upper limb raised above their head. Deep pressure against fascia of quadratus lumborum, between ribs and the iliac crest, transversally in direction of iliac crest, toward the erector spinae.

visits 2 to 3 days apart for several weeks depending on the condition. Often just treating the proprioceptive component in just a few visits is enough to create full painless function. There are situations when, depending on the pathological irregularity, both approaches are required.

RETINACULA

An excellent target of treatment by IASTM are the retinacula (see also Chapter 1.5: Deep Fascia of the Limbs). Retinacula are the whitish tissue surrounding areas such as wrists, elbows, knees, and ankles. They are "local thickenings of the deep fascia with broad insertions into bones, muscles and tendons" (Fig. 7.13.7A) (Stecco 2015, p. 76). Considering that they are especially rich in free nerve endings (Ruffini, Pacini, and Golgi tendon organs), they continually report on joint mechanical deformation and angle change and have a very important proprioceptive role (Stecco et al. 2010). If their three sliding layers (Stecco et al. 2011) are inhibited from gliding as with other receptors, inaccurate proprioceptive afferentation will result. They are activated with motion and sense tension from the tissues to which they are attached (Stecco et al. 2011). Retinacula is a superficial structure, and deep pressure is not necessary. The treatment using IASTM could be local or over a broad bandlike area (Fig. 7.13.7B).

Normally, twisting an ankle into inversion causes the lateral ligaments, muscles, and fibular retinacula to be stretched by inversion of the ankle joint, activating reflex contraction of the fibular muscles. The stretching causes the retinacula receptors (Pacini, Ruffini, Golgi, spindle cells) to fire off action potentials that travel up the spinal cord via afferents where they synapse directly onto gamma motor neurons and alpha motor neurons in the cord associated with the fibularis muscles. With increased tautness there will be more facilitation of the spindle cells leading to alpha motor neuron firing, causing the fibularis muscle to contract and counteract the inversion at the ankle. But a past injury to the ankle might have created fascial restrictions, preventing full receptor stimulation (diminished stretch) resulting in incoordination of the extremity. This explains why an old ankle sprain with lack of suitable communication with the CNS can be an original cause of distal knee, hip, or lumbar involvement (McVey et al. 2005; Bullock-Saxton et al. 1994).

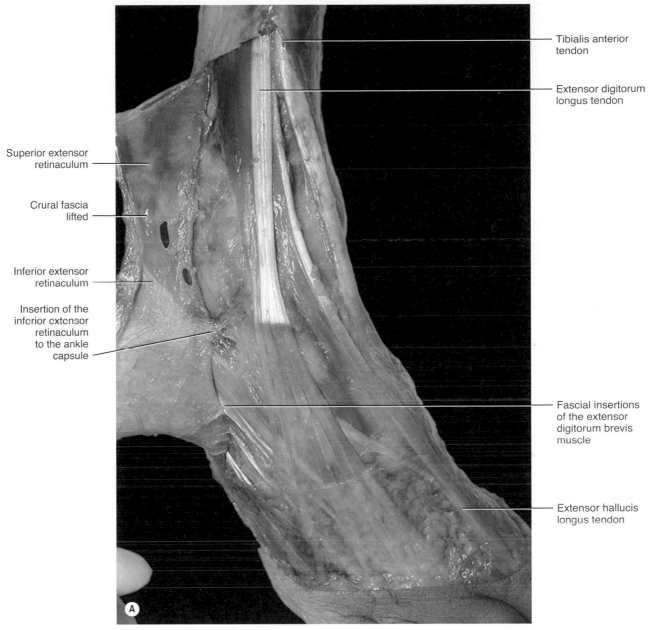

Fig. 7.13.7 (A) View of retinaculum of foot that are local thickenings of the deep fascia with broad insertions into bones, muscles, and tendons. Reproduced with permission from Stecco, C., 2015. Functional Atlas of the Human Fascial System. Elsevier, p. 77, Fig. 3.28.

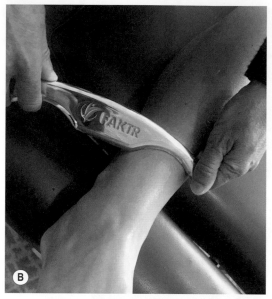

Fig. 7.13.7, cont'd (B) Use of IASTM on the superior extensor retinaculum within the crural fascia.

THICKER AREAS OF FASCIA MAY BE NORMAL TISSUE

It is necessary when using mechanical load to realize that particular areas when palpated may palpate thicker but not necessarily be densified or fibrotic. There are areas of the body where the deep adipose tissue between the superficial and deep fascia is either absent or very thin, resulting in a thickened palpable area where the superficial fascia adheres to the deep fascia. These types of areas may palpate slightly hard or nodular but will normally maintain a gliding sensation (Stecco 2015).

Some of these common areas are the palms of the hands and plantar fascia of the feet, along the spinous processes, along the middle line of the anterior and posterior region of the thigh, along the tibial crest, along the middle line of the posterior region of the leg, along the intermuscular septa of the upper limbs, lateral to the rectus sheath, along the lateral raphe (near middle of quadratus lumborum), at the angle of the mandible, along the occipital tuberosities, at the level of the sixth rib, over the inguinal ligament, along the inferior border of the trapezius muscle, along the iliac crest, and around all the joints of the upper and lower limbs. These areas are definitely thicker and at times almost nodular, especially on the multifidus along the spine.

KEY POINTS

- Decisions about using instruments versus noninstruments must be based on the depth, thickness, and location of the tissue.
- The retinacula contain the most populated receptors in the body, and where they are distally located (wrists, elbows, knees, and ankles) exists a strong possibility of them being responsible for proximal compensatory problems.

SO WHERE DO WE TREAT?

If treating one or two densifications or pathological areas relieves a painful motion, then the practitioner is probably on the correct pathological area or sequence of points. This book emphasizes that the fascial system is the tensional network of the human body. Fascia represents, especially within the musculoskeletal system, the kinetic chain. A lumbar problem can originate from a connective tissue point of view locally by the cervical, scapular, thoracic, pelvis, hip, and distally by the upper and lower extremities. Most notably, the case history is the most important vehicle for determining where to begin treatment. A major question to answer is whether the patient's complaint is a local traumatic event with no other history or is it compensating for a past injury, surgery, or past incident that lasted for a substantial period of time. Treating only the site of pain is often not the answer for obtaining a long-term result.

INSTRUMENTS

Stainless steel empirically seems to be superior to other materials, such as aluminum, wood, or ceramic, for sensory palpation. These instruments serve as levers, increasing the mechanical advantage of the practitioner. They come in a variety of shapes that can easily be applied to different regions of the body. There is no doubt that instruments are very useful for palpation and treatment. They can feel an irregularity or gristle-like tissue compared with normal tissue. With experience one learns that particular tissues such as tendons versus a muscle belly, for example, have their own individuality. An emollient-covering tissue is always necessary for IASTM.

IMPORTANT INFORMATION REGARDING INSTRUMENT-ASSISTED SOFT TISSUE MOBILIZATION

It is thought that IASTM may be more effective if used in combination with movement, thereby helping to translate mechanical forces into chemical signals (mechanotransduction) essential for homeostasis within the extracellular matrix and the cellular level (Sarasa-Renedo and Chiquet 2005). There is some solid evidence (Hyde 2nd Fascial Conference poster, November 2009) and anecdotal evidence that using the instruments on a painful site with movement and additional proprioceptive stimulation will be more effective than static treatment. For example, if a patient flexes forward and feels pain over the posterior lumbar myofascial area, the patient is then asked to point to the painful area. The painful area is treated as he/she repeatedly flexes forward into the pain. The area of pain will frequently disappear and may even refer to an adjoining location where the procedure is repeated (Fig. 7.13.8).

Contraindications
Red Flags
- Patient intolerance
- Hematoma/osteomyelitis/hemophilia
- Unhealed wounds
- Uncontrolled hypertension
- Thrombophlebitis

- Injections: corticosteroids, platelet rich plasma (PRP)
- Prolotherapy, trigger point (for all, wait several weeks)

Yellow Flags
- Anticoagulants
- Varicose veins
- Kidney dysfunction
- Acute inflammation
- Inflammations secondary to infections
- Rheumatoid arthritis
- Cancer

Additional Information
Pretreatment: not mandatory: cardiovascular warm-up, 1 to 3 30-second stretches.

Posttreatment: ice only if necessary. Do not want to interfere with induced healing inflammation, which can last from 2 days to 1 week.

Treatment angle: 30 to 60 degrees to body surface.

Instrument use on body parts: convex instrument on concave body surface, concave instrument on convex body surface. Many instruments have angular areas allowing the practitioner to reach difficult locations (Fig. 7.13.9)—for example, beneath patellar to improve patellar glide. Practitioner presses on the opposite side of patellar to open treatment side.

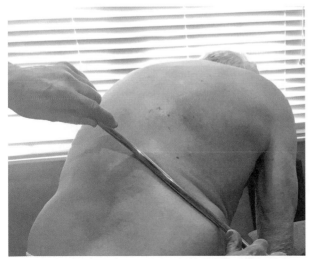

Fig. 7.13.8 IASTM using a broad fascial contact against thoracolumbar fascia either statically or with forward flexion movement.

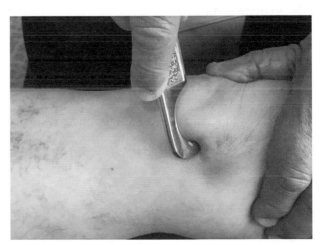

Fig. 7.13.9 Practitioner presses on lateral border of patellar to open restricted medial border to use IASTM to free up retinaculum and associated restrictions. Can pretest patellar by sliding it medial to lateral and lateral to medial, plus all other directions.

Frequency of Treatment (Graston Technique Manual, 2005)

Frequency should be 2 times per week with 2 to 3 days in between.

Duration of Treatment

Per session: 8 to 10 minutes
Per lesion: 30 to 60 seconds
Per region/muscle group: 3 to 5 minutes
Per episode: between 4 and 12 days
Larger regions such as the ITB may take longer.

The author is familiar with two recognized companies teaching and selling instruments: www.graston-technique.com and https://faktr-store.com/. There are, of course, other quality companies.

Summary

1. IASTM is a valuable tool that becomes more valuable with experience.
2. The areas we treat should first be confirmed by functional testing and palpation.
3. It is reasonable that treating pathological areas usually at the site of pain should relieve the patient. But it is also beneficial to evaluate and treat the fascial system. (see Chapters 1.5 and 7.7).

REFERENCES

Bullock-Saxton, J.E., Janda, V., Bullock, M.I., 1994. The influence of ankle sprain injury on muscle activation during hip extension. Int. J. Sports Med. 15, 330–334.

Casato, G., Stecco, C., Busin, R., 2019. Role of fasciae in nonspecific low back pain. Eur. J. Transl. Myol. 29, 8330.

Hammer, W., 2018. Differentiating a pathological from a functional point: potential treatment modifications. In: Day, J.A. (Ed.), Fascial Manipulation®, Stecco® Method, The Practitioner's perspective. Handspring Publishing, Pencaitland, East Lothian, Scotland, pp. 117–127.

Hammer, W.I., Pfefer, M.T., 2005. Treatment of a case of subacute lumbar compartment syndrome using the Graston technique. J. Manipulative Physiol. Ther. 28, 199–204.

Ierna, G.F., 2005. Graston Technique Instruction Manual. TherapyCare Resources, 9–12.

Loghmani, M.T., Warden, S.J., 2009. Instrument-assisted cross-fiber massage accelerates knee ligament healing. J. Orthop. Sports Phys. Ther. 39, 506–514.

McCombe, D., Brown, T., Slavin, J., Morrison, W.A., 2001. The histochemical structure of the deep fascia and its structural response to surgery. J. Hand Surg. Br. 26, 89–97.

McVey, E.D., Palmieri, R.M., Docherty, C.L., Zinder, S.M., Ingersoll, C.D., 2005. Arthrogenic muscle inhibition in the leg muscles of subjects exhibiting functional ankle instability. Foot Ankle Int. 26, 1055–1061.

Melham, T.J., Sevier, T.L., Malnofski, M.J., Wilson, J.K., Helfst Jr., R.H., 1998. Chronic ankle pain and fibrosis successfully treated with a new noninvasive Augmented Soft Tissue Mobilization Technique (ASTM): a case report. Med. Sci. Sports Exerc. 30, 801–804.

Mense, S., Schneider, M., 2010. Personal communication. Addressing the Myofascial Component of Musculoskeletal Pain. University of Pittsburg, Department of Physical Therapy.

Pavan, P.G., Stecco, A., Stern, R., Stecco, C., 2014. Painful connections: densification versus fibrosis of fascia. Curr. Pain Headache Rep. 18, 441.

Roman, M., Chaudhry, H., Bukiet, B., Stecco, A., Findley, T.W., 2013. Mathematical analysis of the flow of hyaluronic acid around fascia during manual therapy motions. J. Am. Osteopath. Assoc. 113, 600–610.

Sarasa-Renedo, A., Chiquet, M., 2005. Mechanical signals regulating extracellular matrix gene expression in fibroblasts. Scand. J. Med. Sci. Sports 15, 223–230.

Schilder, A., Hoheisel, H., Magerl, W., Benrath, J., Klein, T., Treede R.D., 2014. Sensory findings after stimulation of the thoracolumbar fascia with hypertonic saline suggest its contribution to low back pain. Pain 155, 222–231.

Snodgrass, S.J., Rivett, D.A., Chiarelli, P., Bates, A.M., Rowe, L.J., 2003. Factors related to thumb pain in physiotherapists. Aust. J. Physiother. 49, 243–250.

Stecco, A., Meneghini, A., Stern, R., Stecco, C., Imamura, M., 2013. Ultrasonography in myofascial neck pain: randomized clinical trial for diagnosis and follow-up. Surg. Radiol. Anat. 36, 243–253.

Stecco, A., Stecco, C., Macchi, V., et al., 2011. RMI study and clinical correlations of ankle retinacula damage and outcomes of ankle sprain. Surg. Radiol. Anat. 33, 881–890.

Stecco, A., Stern, R., Fantoni, I., De Caro, R., Stecco, C., 2016. Fascial Disorders: Implications for Treatment. PM R. 8, 161–168.

Stecco, C., 2015. Functional Atlas of the Human Fascial System. Churchill Livingstone, Edinburgh.

Stecco, C., Cappellari, A., Macchi, V., et al., 2014. The paratendineous tissues: an anatomical study of their role in the pathogenesis of tendinopathy. Surg. Radiol. Anat. 36, 561–572.

Stecco, C., Macchi, V., Porzionato, A., et al., 2010. The ankle retinacula: Morphological evidence of the proprioceptive role of the fascial system. Cells Tissues Organs 192, 200–210.

Stecco, C., Stern, R., Porzionato, A., et al., 2011. Hyaluronan within fascia in the etiology of myofascial pain. Surg. Radiol. Anat. 33, 891–896.

Stecco, L., Stecco, A., 2018. Fascial Manipulation Practical Part, First Level, second ed. Piccin Nuova Libraris S.p.A., Padova, Italy.

Tan, S.C., Chan, O., 2008. Achilles and patellar tendinopathy: current understanding of pathophysiology and management. Disabil. Rehabil. 30, 1608–1615.

The Fascial Distortion Model

Georg Harrer

THE PATIENT AS EXPERT—THE TYPALDOS APPROACH

Mainstream medicine takes little advantage of the most complex information network provided by the body-wide fascial net. Physicians increasingly ignore it and instead use technological investigation devices. The more imaging technologies are available, the less interesting the perception of the patient. The patient perceives the impression that his perception and description of pain or discomfort disturbs, rather than supports, the diagnostic process. Accordingly, in the industrialized countries magnetic resonance imaging (MRI) scans are currently used to locate the disorder even though key studies suggest that MRI scans are, in spite of their spectacular resolution, questionable tools to locate the source of pain (Jensen et al. 1994; Chou et al. 2009; Matsumoto et al. 2013; Nakashima et al. 2015; Ramadorai et al. 2014).

In most contemporary medical treatment approaches, it is the expert practitioner who makes a diagnosis because of his extensive training and skills. The patients in general are unable to become involved in these deliberations because of the lack of a common language and the impression that their knowledge is inferior. This mismatch was the origin of Stephen Typaldos's fascial distortion model (FDM) (Typaldos 2002).

For Stephen Typaldos, an osteopath and emergency physician, it was a frustrating experience to learn how little medical and osteopathic treatments enable practitioners to help patients suffering from so-called soft tissue injury. Conditions such as sprained ankles, lower back pain, and neck pain seemed to be almost unresponsive to the treatments he could offer within the settings of an emergency department. According to his observation, improving his manipulation skills or increasing the diagnostic effort (MRI, ultrasound, nerve conduction time, etc.) did not improve the outcome.

Typaldos instead started to ask his patients what kind of treatment they themselves considered to bring relief, and, to the patients' surprise, he applied the treatments they proposed. For instance, he pressed on a particular spot in a patient's back, which she was unable to reach by herself, or he pulled on the arm or on the skin of a patient as they suggested. In many cases these procedures had better results than any other therapy these patients had undergone previously. This again was a big surprise to Dr. Typaldos and puzzled him. This method of diagnosis and treatment planning was unknown in both the mainstream medicine and osteopathy that he trained in at Osteopathic University. Also the symptoms reported and the observed improvement could not be explained by conventional diagnoses.

Typaldos's impression was that the proprioceptive and nociceptive network of their fascia gave the patients a subconscious understanding of the nature of their condition and of possible solutions. The patients were only unable to communicate these perceptions and had learned that their attempts were of minor benefit for the cooperation with the medical system. Studying the patients' stories and gestures, he found recognizable entities for which he saw fascia as the common denominator. Typaldos postulated specific three-dimensional deformations of the fascial arrangement that could apparently be repaired by the maneuvers and techniques he had successfully performed under the guidance of his patients. In 1992 and 1993, Typaldos discovered six "fascial distortions," as he called these new diagnoses (Table 7.14.1). Although maintaining his observational approach, he did not find further distortion types but always assumed that there might have been more.

KEY POINT

The fascial distortion model is a fresh perspective on human complaints. In the model, these complaints are caused by specific fascial distortions.

THE FASCIAL DISTORTIONS

KEY POINT

All six distortions are different and highly specific pathologies. Even though there may be more than one fascial distortion present in a certain condition, each single distortion can be identified. The distortions may interact with each other but remain distinct entities.

The six distortions are listed in the order they were discovered by Typaldos in 1992 and 1993. He published his new theory in detail in the *AAOJ (Journal of the American Association of Osteopathy)* (Typaldos 1993, 1994, 1995).

Trigger Band

One type of connective tissue is banded fascia. Banded fascia is an arrangement in which almost all fibers are aligned in the same direction in order to resist forces along this direction. Because of their architecture, these fascial bands are prone to injury caused by shearing forces. Once a shearing force is applied to the banded fascia, the long fibers lose their coherence and a longitudinal crack occurs in the band. The band then becomes shorter and the edges along the crack become twisted. The best analogy to envision the trigger band (TB) concept is probably the Ziploc bag.

Herniated Trigger Point

All compartments of the human body are separated by fascia. The main purpose of this fascial arrangement is to seal the cavities and prevent enclosed tissue from protruding out of the cavity. In general, the pressure gradient makes tissue prone to protrude out of the cavity as soon as a gap in the sealing fascia opens (herniation). Some of these herniations (e.g., inguinal hernia) are well explored, and there are successful, mainly surgical treatments available. Others are less well-known, and the complaints are not understood as herniation of tissue in the current medical models. Only the concerted occurrence of an opening of the canal, a pressure peak, and the protrusion of tissue out of the compartment can be identified as a pathology. Each component occurring on its own is physiological.

Once a herniated trigger point (HTP) is formed, it is maintained by the pressure gradient and by the impinging

TABLE 7.14.1 Fascial Distortion types as Described by Typaldos	
Fascial Distortion Type	**Description**
Trigger band (TB)	Longitudinal crack within a band
Herniated trigger point (HTP)	Gap opening within a sealing fascia, with resultant protrusion
Continuum distortion (CD)	Shift of minerals within transition zone between bone and ligament
Folding distortion (FD)	Overstretching of folds in accordion-like structure
Cylinder distortion (CyD)	Entanglement of cylindrical coils in skin
Tectonic fixation (TF)	Loss of gliding ability in a joint

forces in the orifice of protrusion. Spontaneous healing is not expected but reduction leads to immediate repair. A surgical closure of the physiological aperture is not strictly necessary but might help in some cases to avoid a relapse.

In the FDM, herniations within the musculoskeletal system play a major role in explaining patients' complaints, and entirely new treatment options use the concept of reduction, which would be deemed impossible in other models. In current medical models the very same complaints are interpreted very differently; therefore, reduction is not an option in these approaches (Cooperman and Ackerman 1947; Dittrich 1953, 1957).

Continuum Distortion

In order to understand continuum distortion (CD) (see Fig. 7.14.1), it is necessary to look into the nature of bone and ligament in a fundamental way. In the traditional anatomical model, the point where bone and ligament come together is defined as "insertion." A junction of two obviously different structures is postulated. This is contradictory to the enormous stability of this junction. In the continuum theory, which is part of the FDM, bone and ligament are envisioned as one structure. Ligament is accordingly considered to be nonmineralized bone and bone a calcified ligament. Bones as single entities are not considered to be components of "in-vivo anatomy" and only come into existence as artifacts after collagen biodegradation, or in medical dissection studies. The same principle applies to ligaments.

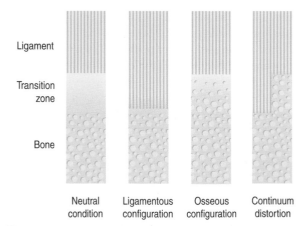

Fig.7.14.1 Continuum distortion. Reproduced with permission from Liem, T., Dobler, T.K., 2009. Leitfaden Osteopathie. Elsevier Urban & Fischer, Munich.

As a ramification of this theory the majority of fibrous pathways are embedded in bone. This suggests an important role for collagen fibers in bone stability. Fascial fibers can be considered as the highly tensile component of this compound, analogous to the steel in ferroconcrete. A purely mineral-based material cannot be resistant to bending forces. Minerals are exclusively resistant to compression forces. The FDM postulates that the tissue in the transition zone has the ability to shift between two states called osseous and ligamentous configuration. Depending on the demands, the transition zone can become ligamentous or osseous by shifting calcium matrix out of or into the zone. Because the calcium concentration is high in the bone and low in the ligament, the soluble mineral is prone to spread into the ligamentous zone driven by the force of entropy. Physical activity forces the calcium back into the bone by triggering osteoblast activity in the bone and mechanical stress on calcium that has shifted into the ligament. The opposite (calcium shifts from bone to ligament) is a common finding in immobilized patients with a lack of physical activity in intensive care units. Osteoporosis in the bones and exostosis in the ligament are the manifestations of this, as seen on X-ray.

According to the FDM, this phenomenon occurs several times per day on a small scale as soon as physical activity leads to a small shift of the transition zone toward its ligamentous configuration, and inactivity leads to a small shift toward osseous configuration. This shift is only possible if synchronized in the entire "insertion." As soon as one part of the transition zone shifts in the osseous configuration while the rest shifts into the ligamentous configuration, continuum distortion occurs, leading to immediate loss of functional ability. The pathology of CD is envisioned as a pathological step in the transition zone between bone and ligament. Osseous and ligamental configuration are present at one time in one location. To envision bones and ligaments as one structure (the continuum) with calcified and noncalcified zones, allow an entirely new perspective on injury and complaints located in or adjacent to "insertions."

Folding Distortion (FD)

In the body there are numerous flexible junctions (see Fig. 7.14.2). These flexible junctions, commonly called joints, are surprisingly durable, even with repetitive movement. A knee joint, for instance, can be bent and straightened without damage or resistance against the

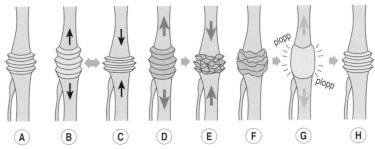

Fig. 7.14.2 Folding distortion. (A–C) Physiological folding, joint stabilization against traction and compression, smoothing of folds at excessive traction. (D–F) Subsequent compression after excessive traction creates knitted folds that remain. (G, H) A "plopping" traction treatment recreates the natural folds. Reproduced with permission from Liem, T., Dobler, T.K., 2009. Leitfaden Osteopathie. Elsevier Urban & Fischer, Munich.

movement. The motion appears to be well-guided by multiple structures. In FDM the sum of all these protective structures are envisioned to work as a bellows. In technical engineering the demand for minimal wear and tear without disturbing flexibility is often met by the utilization of bellows. Examples for the use of bellows vary from the accordion to respiratory tubes in intensive medicine. The bellows or accordion model allows entirely new perspectives on joint complaints.

In neutral position the folds always unfold and refold in the correct pattern. The bellows analogy inevitably leads to the following specific pathologies. As soon as the accordion is overstretched the folds disappear. When now returning toward the neutral position there is no guiding pattern for the folds to refold properly and so they wrinkle. This phenomenon is defined as unfolding distortion (uFD) because the extreme unfolding initially caused the pathology. In this crumpled state the bellows can no longer function properly and the joint is poorly guided. This accordion analogy suggests the opportunity to restore the bellows and its folds by controlled traction. Once the wrinkles of the bellows are restored, the folds can unfold and refold properly again.

If the forces are in the opposite direction, we are facing a refolding distortion. Extreme traction with consecutive compression leads to unfolding distortion uFD and can be restored by controlled traction. Extreme compression leads to refolding distortion (rFD) and can be restored by controlled compression.

Cylinder Distortion

The most superficial connective tissue of the body is the skin. It is tensile in all directions. Different than other manifestations of connective tissue, the specific arrangement of the skin's collagen fibers allows far more elasticity. In the FDM this fascial arrangement is envisioned as a system of spiral cylindrical coils of fascial fibers surrounding the entire body with neither beginning nor end. The cylindrical coils are arranged in virtually all directions. Hence in histological studies of the skin a predominant direction of fascial fibers is not observed.

This arrangement leads to equal resistance in all directions. Although the coils are interwoven, the fibers have to move separately to allow equal distribution of tension to all coils in any movement. If these coils become entangled in one another the ability to move separately decreases, leading to disturbed proprioception in the entire region. In the FDM this condition is defined as cylinder distortion (CyD) (see Fig. 7.14.3). The entanglement might possibly be caused by adhesions attached to the fibers of the coils, or by lateral stress to the skin. The geometry of entanglement is very complex and therefore prognosis and duration of the condition vary significantly. Unlike the other fascial distortions, it is difficult to predict the progression and prognosis of CyD.

Tectonic Fixation

All slide bearings in the body consist of fascia. Some of these slide bearings possess special features such as cartilage or synovial fluid and are therefore termed joints. Other slide bearings lack these features but have similar functional ability. All slide bearings of the body show a similar construction. They consist of two corresponding sliding faces and a layer of lubricant in between. In so-called joints, these sliding faces are cartilage and the lubricant is synovial fluid. In other slide bearings, such

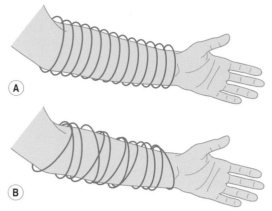

Fig. 7.14.3 Cylinder distortion. Reproduced with permission from Liem, T., Dobler, T.K., 2009. Leitfaden Osteopathie. Elsevier Urban & Fischer, Munich.

as the scapula–thoracic articulation, the lubricant is interstitial fluid. These work the same way and perform a tectonic movement, a horizontal gliding.

In the FDM, tectonic fixation (TF) is defined as the loss of this ability to glide. The production of synovial fluid is triggered by movement. It needs only a short immobilization to omit the production of synovial fluid. This causes stiffness of the joint. As soon as the joint is moved again the production of synovial fluid commences again. This restores the ability to glide. The phenomenon can be observed in every single application of cast, as nonsurgical treatment for fractures in the joints immobilized.

Apart from joints there are numerous slide bearings surrounding tendons or between scapula and the thorax. In these slide bearings the interstitial fluid is the lubricant and the same rules apply. A lack of fluid leads to stiffness. Movement leads to more fluid. TF is always secondary either to other fascial distortions or immobilization due to external reasons. Once the reason for the immobilization is eliminated, children need only a few days to get back to their normal mobility, but in elderly people it may take much longer. The correction of the TF will only lead to sustainable results once the causative fascial distortion (one or more out of the other five) is eliminated.

THE DIAGNOSIS OF FASCIAL DISTORTIONS

General Considerations

As stated previously, the essential hypothesis for any diagnostics in FDM is the supremacy of the patient's refined proprioception and nociception compared with any diagnostic tool from the exterior, whether based on palpation or technology. Because each of the six distortions causes specific mechanical information for the nociceptive-proprioceptive system, they are felt differently by the patient. Usually the patients lack only the vocabulary to communicate these perceptions to the practitioner, and the skills or self-confidence to correct the distortion on their own. Verbal language is a poor tool to communicate pain and discomfort. Depending on the language, there are only a few words for pain and discomfort, far too few to explain these complex impressions. Another obstacle to communication is the fact that patients and physicians think that medical knowledge and terminology improve these communication skills, but in fact the opposite seems to apply. The more the patients are knowledgeable of medical terminology and envision medical models for their condition, the more they are estranged from their own perception.

Diagnostics according to the FDM is based on the following sources of information:

- Nonverbal description of the complaints. Patients use specific gestures to communicate their pain/discomfort (Stechmann 2011; Anker 2011).
- Verbal description of the complaints. Patients use specific expressions to communicate their pain/discomfort.
- Mechanism of injury as far as this is obtainable.
- Objective findings, such as local edema or pain on pressure, mobility and stability tests.
- Palpation (only to facilitate the location of the diagnosed distortion).

Trigger Band

The patient runs the tips of his fingers along a distinct line. In general only the most painful section of the TB is shown with the fingers, not the entire pathway.

Described as "burning," "pulling" pain. Worse in the morning. Restricted motion in one or more than one plane.

The entire pathway is painful on pressure.

Herniated Trigger Point

The patient presses more than one finger or the thumb firmly onto one spot, generally located on soft tissue.

Described as a "dull," "constant" ache in a specific area. Restricted motion in all adjacent joints.

Severe pain on pressure can be well-distinguished from the surrounding tissue. Palpable "ball" in the tissue.

Continuum Distortion

The patient points decisively to a singular spot on a bone, in general close to a joint, using the very tip of the index or middle finger.

Patients complain of pinpoint pain on a bone. Painfully restricted motion in a singular plane, often only in one direction.

Very small spot highly painful on pressure.

Folding Distortion

The patient holds a joint with the hand.

Described as "pain in the joint" or "in the center of the joint," impression of instability, remains unchanged for a long period of time. No significant restrictions in motion.

Palpation is insignificant.

Cylinder Distortion

The body language is a wiping motion with the palm of the hand along a limb or the torso. Also repetitive squeezing of a nonjointed area is presented.

The patients complain about severe, deep pain, which cannot be explained by the objective findings. The pain is difficult to reproduce. The maximum pain is experienced at night-time. Different to TB, the CyD responds poorly to antiinflammatory drugs, morphine, and other medications. The patient also complains of bizarre symptoms such as the impression of swelling, tourniquet, tingling, numbness, and other symptoms, which are in general assigned to the realm of neurology but do not correspond to nerve or spinal root distribution or to other neurological explanations. Reports of very painfully restricted motion but hard to reproduce. Range of motion might appear as normal at the very time of testing.

Palpation insignificant, no tenderness on pressure.

Tectonic Fixation

The patient tries to move the stiff joint forcefully.

TF does not hurt! If there is pain involved it is caused by one or more of the other five fascial distortions. Significant reproducibly restricted motion in all planes. No passive motion possible.

Palpation insignificant.

This proposed patient-guided diagnostic system inevitably leads to a redefinition of the patient–practitioner relationship. It is no longer the qualified, experienced, and highly educated practitioner who makes a diagnosis in a process that cannot be reproduced by the patient. Rather, we see a role reversal, with the patient in the supreme position due to the natural advantage of innervation, which enables the patient to present the diagnosis. The practitioner is only the interpreter and does not only accept the patient's signals but also takes actions that the patient subconsciously suggests but for whatever reason is unable to perform sufficiently on their own. Verbal language, maybe the most striking feature that differentiates us from other animals, is strongly influenced by the intellect, and so all verbal statements might be reflections of the multiple information sources to which the patient was exposed, such as other physician's opinions, X-ray reports, internet research, and so on. Hence, the degree of medical knowledge of the patient is inversely proportional to the value of information that is achieved in history taking. Therefore in FDM the observation is focused on the specific pain gestures, because this language is independent from the intellect. Furthermore, it is international and all ethnicities worldwide can be assessed the same way.

TREATMENT OF FASCIAL DISTORTIONS

FDM leads to a very specific understanding of the particular pathology on the level of fascia. Accordingly, the therapy has to be as specific. Basically, there are many approaches possible. Because Stephen Typaldos had a professional background in osteopathy, the current treatment concentrates on manual approaches to correct fascial distortions. The techniques are highly specific and so only suitable for the correction of specific fascial distortions (Fig. 7.14.4). In manual maneuvers a directed vector of force must always have a specific effect on the particular fascia, so there is no "general fascia technique" in the FDM. Accordingly, the force has to be highly specific for every single fascial distortion. In principle, all fascial distortions are considered to be reversible. As soon as the type of distortion is diagnosed, specific manual techniques are used in order to correct the distortion. After every single step, the complaints and restrictions are reevaluated to guide the treatment.

The FDM as a concept allows many treatment approaches, whether they be surgical or pharmacological. At the present the main treatment is applied manually, until other, possibly even more successful approaches, will be developed.

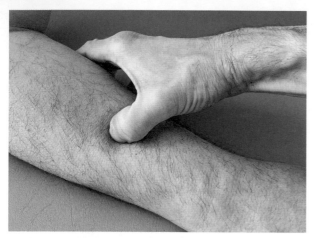

Fig. 7.14.4 Trigger band technique.

Summary

Applying the fascial distortion model, perhaps the most striking difference to other approaches is the reversibility of all pathologies (fascial distortions) by restoring the shape, or arrangement of the fascia. A lack of success in a specific patient is seen as failure of the specific technique applied, not as a failure of envisioning the pathology as a fascial distortion.

In order to apply FDM successfully, various skills such as the power of observation and finesse in the manual techniques are required. Only the patients can judge whether the treatment was successful, because it is their perception of pain, restriction, instability, or weakness that leads to the decision to seek professional help. According to FDM, it can only be considered a success when all these complaints are sustainably eliminated. Clinical experience, as well as a first clinical trial, shows that this result can be achieved in a surprisingly high percentage (Fink et al. 2012).

REFERENCES

Anker, S., 2011. Is a patient's body language, interpreted according to the Fascial Distortion Model, a reliable parameter in the choice of treatment? Master's thesis, Danube University, Krems, Vienna/Austria.

Chou, R., Fu, R., Carrino, J.A., Deyo, R.A., 2009. Imaging strategies for low-back pain: systematic review and meta-analysis. Lancet 373, 463–472.

Coperman, W.S.C., Ackerman, W.L., 1947. Edema or herniations of fat lobules as a cause of lumbar and gluteal "fibrositis." Arch. Int. Med. 79, 22–35.

Dittrich, R.J., 1953. Low back pain-referred pain from deep somatic structures of the back. Lancet 73, 63–68.

Dittrich, R.J., 1957. The role of soft tissue lesions in low back pain. Br. J. Phys. Med. 20, 233–238.

Fink, M., Schiller, J., Buhck, H., 2012. Efficacy of a manual treatment method according to the fascial distortion model in the management of contracted ("frozen") shoulder. Z. Orthop. Unfall. 150, 420–427.

Jensen, M.C., Brant-Zawadzki, M.N., Obuchowski, N., Modic, M.T., Malkasian, D., Ross, J.S., 1994. Magnetic resonance imaging of the lumbar spine in people without back pain. NEJM 331, 69–73.

Liem, T., Dobler, T.K., 2009. Leitfaden Osteopathie. Elsevier Urban & Fischer, Munich.

Matsumoto, M., Okada, E., Toyama, Y., Fujiwara, H., Momoshima, S., Takahata, T., 2013. Tandem age-related lumbar and cervical intervertebral disc changes in asymptomatic subjects. Eur. Spine J. 22, 708–713.

Nakashima, H., Yukada, Y., Suda, K., Yamagata, M., Ueta, T., Kato, F., 2015. Cervical disc protrusion correlates with severity of cervical disc degeneration: a cross sectional study on 1211 relatively healthy volunteers. Spine (Phila PA 1976) 40, E774–E779.

Ramadorai, U., Hire, J., DeVine, J.G., Brodt, E.D., Dettori, J.R., 2014. Incidental findings on magnetic resonance imaging if the spine in asymptomatic pediatric population. A systematic review. Evid. Based Spine Care J. 5, 95–100.

Stechmann, K., 2011. Inter-tester reliability analysis of the classifications of distortion based on body language according to the fascial distortion model. Bachelor's thesis, HAWK University for Applied Sciences and Art, Hildesheim.

Typaldos, S., 1994. Introducing the Fascial Distortion Model. AAOJ 4, 14–18, 33–36.

Typaldos, S., 1994. The Triggerband technique. AAOJ 4, 15–18, 28.

Typaldos, S., 1995. Continuum technique. AAOJ 5, 15–19.

BIBLIOGRAPHY

Anker, S., 2015. Die Schmerzgestik ALS Diagnosekriterium: Interrater-Reliabilität bei der Beurteilung der Körpersprache nach dem Fasziendistorsionsmodell FDM, Akademiker Verlag, Einbeck, Germany.

Typaldos, S.P., 2002. FDM, the Clinical and Theoretical Application of the Fascial Distortion Model, within the Practice of Medicine and Surgery. Orthopathic Global Health Publications, Brewer, ME.

Fascial Treatment of Axillary Web Syndrome After Breast Cancer Surgery

Kyra De Coninck

CHAPTER CONTENTS

INTRODUCTION

Breast cancer is the most common cancer in women in the Western world, with a lifetime risk estimated at one in seven in the United Kingdom (Cancer Research UK 2016). Fifty years ago, 4 in 10 women diagnosed with breast cancer survived beyond 10 years; now it is 8 in 10 women (Cancer Research UK 2016). Because of advances in diagnosis and treatment, the mortality rate for breast cancer in women has fallen by 44% since 1989 (Smittenaar et al. 2016). Surgery remains the most common treatment; 81% of patients diagnosed with breast cancer have surgery to remove the tumor as part of their primary cancer treatment (Cancer Research UK 2016). Despite improvements in surgical techniques, pain and dysfunction remain common morbidities, with more than 60% of women experiencing side effects at 6 years postdiagnosis (Schmitz et al. 2012). Upper limb edema, decreased shoulder movement, and both sensory and motor dysfunction are all well described in the literature (Cheville and Tchou 2007; Schmitz et al. 2012; Rietman et al. 2002; Jung et al. 2003). Axillary web syndrome (AWS), also known as "cording," is a common complication causing arm pain and shoulder dysfunction after breast cancer surgery. The term "axillary web syndrome" was first coined by Alexander Moskowitz in 2001. AWS is characterized by fibrotic bands—"cords" or "vascular

strings"—which develop in the axilla of patients between 1 and 5 weeks after axillary lymphatic node dissection (Moskowitz et al. 2001) (Fig. 7.15.1A). The fibrotic bands are tender and become more prominent, taut, and painful, particularly during shoulder abduction.

> ### KEY POINT
>
> Patients with AWS typically present with pain in the axilla and reduced shoulder mobility. The typical fibrotic "cords" look like guitar strings under the skin and become more prominent, taut, and painful during shoulder abduction. These "cords" start from the axilla, often near the site of surgical scarring, and extend along the medial side of the arm, in some cases continuing to the wrist.

ETIOLOGY

An exact etiology is not known; however, the literature suggests a lymphatic origin. A pioneering biopsy of AWS cords showed dilated lymphatics, fibrin clots, venous thrombosis, inflammation, and fibrosis of veins and lymphatic vessels (Moskowtiz et al. 2001). In one study, Leduc et al. (2009) analyzed the cords of 15 women with AWS and found that the pattern of cords followed the distribution of the brachial lymphatic system (Fig. 7.15.2). Damage to veins as a result of thrombophlebitis and damage to

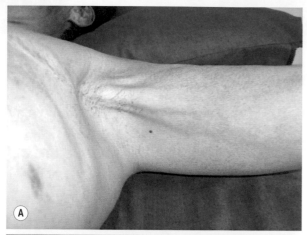

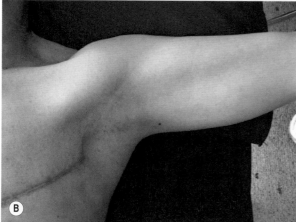

Fig. 7.15.1 (A) Visible cording and tightness in the axilla and upper arm on day 24 postmastectomy and axillary lymph node removal. (B) The axilla with complete resolution of all cords after 11 soft tissue treatments over a period of 26 days. Reproduced with permission from Fourie, W.J., Robb, K.A., 2009. Physiotherapy management of axillary web syndrome following breast cancer treatment: Discussing the use of soft tissue techniques. Physiotherapy 95, 314–320.

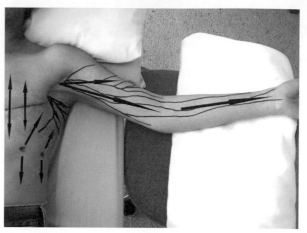

Fig. 7.15.2 Arrows showing direction of skin and superficial fascia tightness on chest wall and arm from surgical scarring, drain sites, and tight cords in the axilla. Visible and palpable cords drawn in red on patient's skin. Reproduced with permission from Fourie W.J., Robb, K.A., 2009. Physiotherapy management of axillary web syndrome following breast cancer treatment: Discussing the use of soft tissue techniques. Physiotherapy 95, 314–320.

lymphatic ducts have also been mentioned as possible causative factors (Fourie and Robb 2009).

The axilla consists of layers of deep and superficial fascia, merging from the arm and the brachial fascia, the pectoralis major and coracoclavicular fascia, and latissimus dorsi and subscapularis fasciae (Stecco et al. 2008). Fat and fibrous tissue binds the numerous axillary structures while simultaneously allowing movement. These fatty tissues protect the neurovascular bundles in the axilla while allowing a substantial degree of movement. If this protective connective tissue is damaged, resulting adhesions or scarring are thought to

contribute to restrictions in shoulder mobility (Fourie and Robb 2009). Surgical removal of lymph nodes requires careful dissection of a number of lymph nodes that reside in the fatty connective tissue of the axilla. When lymph nodes are removed, imaging studies demonstrate that the normal flow of lymph fluid is discontinued and the segment of the lymphatic drainage pathway running from the upper to the subclavicular vein is disrupted (Suami et al. 2018). Despite evidence of regeneration of lymphatics after axillary dissection in animal studies (Suami et al. 2018), human studies demonstrate that lymphatic pathways do not regenerate across scar tissue, which may further contribute to the pathogenesis of AWS (Smith and Ryan 2016). Reported risk factors are invasive and extensive axillary surgery, including an increased number of nodes removed at surgery and administration of radiotherapy or chemotherapy (Leidenius et al. 2003; Suami et al. 2018). Young age and lean body mass have also been noted as risk factors (Dinas et al. 2019; Mullen and Harvey 2019).

KEY POINT

Adhesions, tissue fibrosis, and loss of tissue glide between structures can be identified as the source of pain and restriction of movement and function in up to 72% of patients after surgery for breast cancer (Lee et al. 2009).

AWS has been reported to resolve spontaneously between 3 months and 1 year postsurgery, although some evidence suggests that the condition is not self-limiting, with "cords" still present 12 months and 3 years postsurgery (Johansson et al. 2020; Wyrick et al. 2006). AWS is a distressing and often debilitating condition. Although specific treatment guidelines have not yet been established, soft tissue treatments and physical therapy have been shown to be beneficial (Yeung et al. 2015) (Fig. 7.15.1).

Treatment

Active assisted forward flexion, horizontal abduction, and passive internal and external rotation have been recommended in mild cases of AWS (Cheville and Tchou 2007). However, Moskovitz et al. (2001) did not find any benefit from end-of range-exercises. Soft tissue stretching and myofascial soft tissue techniques have been shown to be beneficial in the management of AWS (Fourie and Robb 2009). Other studies have found manual lymph drainage in combinations with compression bandaging and active assisted shoulder exercisers to be an effective treatment (Koehler et al. 2014).

However, management is frequently required to reduce pain and improve shoulder mobility. Nonsteriodal antiinflammatory drugs or further surgical interventions are not helpful (Dinas et al. 2019). Stretching and soft tissue treatments have shown to shorten the duration on AWS (Fourie and Robb 2009).

Vigorous therapy used too early can stimulate inflammation and edema, prolong the inflammatory phase, or disrupt the wound. Forceful mobilization aimed at breaking established scar tissue may create a new inflammatory response, ultimately causing further scar formation. A secondarily inflamed wound results in additional collagen deposition, compounding existing morbidity.

KEY POINT

When treating AWS, the therapist should have a clear understanding of how deep and firmly to work. A depth-of-touch grading scale of 1 to 10 can be used, with only grades 1–4 being used in myofascial release techniques in AWS (Fourie and Robb 2009).

Grading of techniques and depth of touch:
- Grade 1 to 3: mild and superficial touch with no discomfort
- Grade 4 to 6: Moderate to firm with mild discomfort

- Grade 7 to 8: Deep firm pressure with discomfort, but tolerable (not to be used for myofascial release of AWS
- Grade 9 and 10: Deep, painful, and potentially damaging pressure (not to be used for myofascial release of AWS).

With less fibrosis and better tissue glide, less effort will be needed to produce normal movement and overcome tissue resistance. By being gentle early on, rehabilitation can progress faster at later stages.

The Barrier Phenomenon

Similar to joints, soft tissue has a specified range of available movement that can be divided into a physiological and an anatomical range of movement:
- Physiological range is necessary for smooth, unrestricted movement of underlying structures during normal movement (active range of movement).
- Anatomical range refers to where tissue can be stretched beyond the physiological range and before coming to a stop without discomfort or pain (passive range of movement).
- The distance between physiological and anatomical limits constitutes a "safety zone" protecting the body from damage should external forces be applied.

As in joints, there is a range within which minimal resistance to stretch or shift is encountered. When resistance is met, the anatomical barrier is reached. Under normal conditions, the barrier has a soft, elastic end-feel and can be moved easily, accompanied by a sensation that no unnecessary tension is present in the target tissue.

In a *pathological* barrier, the anatomical (passive) tissue range is reached prematurely. This barrier characteristically has a tense, restrictive feel, with an abrupt, hard, or leathery end-feel. Normal physiological movement may still be present with no apparent movement restriction, but there will be reduced protection when the tissue is strained. Observation of visible axillary cords, which may extend along the medial surface of the upper arm toward the wrist, could become evident only when the arm is moved away from the body (Fig. 7.15.1A)

Assessment of Tissue Movement and Glide

An advantage of manual techniques is that the hand is a sensitive instrument that establishes a feedback relationship with the manipulated tissue.
- Quality refers to the perceived end-feel—a normal soft elastic or an abnormal solid abrupt end-feel.

- The extent of the barrier refers to *where* in the available range resistance is encountered, and how large an area is involved.
- The depth of the tissue barrier may be subjective, but an attempt should be made to distinguish between *which tissue layers* restrictions are felt: superficial between dermis and deep fascia, deep restrictions between muscles, organs or between a tendon and its sheath.
- Three layers of fascial glide need assessment:
  - Skin and superficial fascia manually glide the skin ON the deep fascia. Move hand and skin as a unit to the end of available tissue glide using a pressure grading of 2 to 3.
  - Deep fascia and myofascial interfaces move one deep structure ON another. Change hand or finger position accordingly and glide tissue at a firm pressure grading of 3 to 4.

This is an assessment of tissue *movement*, not of painful areas within the soft tissue. Palpation is for tissue mobility, flexibility, and freedom of tissue glide. The position and direction of tight, hypomobile, or inflexible tissue should be documented.

Principles

- Treatment is directed at the mechanical restriction identified by evaluation.
- The goal is to move the tissue barrier toward a normal end-feel and amplitude.
- Approach treatment in a layered fashion, clearing one layer or compartment of restrictions before moving to a deeper or adjacent layer.
- Techniques are performed at or just before the palpable tissue barrier, at varying angles to the restriction.
- Approaches to engage and move the tissue barrier include (Lewit and Olsanska 2004; Manheim, 2001; Stecco L. and C., 2009):
  - Engage the barrier directly and wait with a sustained pressure until the tissue releases and the barrier shifts after a short delay.
  - Use a sustained stretch of the scarred tissue. Stretch could be uni- or multidirectional.
  - Apply slow, rhythmic mobilizations toward and into the tissue barrier. Movement direction could be perpendicular to, at an angle to, or away from the tissue barrier.

MYOFASCIAL TECHNIQUES

Gross Stretch

This is the most superficial and least painful technique, a longitudinal tissue stretch to strain the cords with the patient's arm in pain-free abduction (Fig. 7.15.3A–B). By using finger or full-hand contact, take up all the tissue slack and apply a gentle stretch along the length of the cord. Hold, wait for release, and stretch again. Change hand position and repeat the stretch perpendicular to the original stretch. Repeat the stretch sequence diagonal

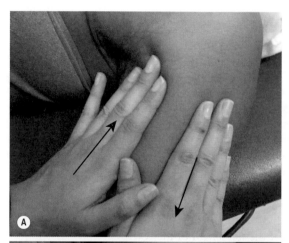

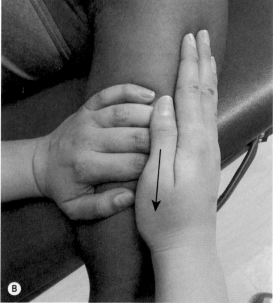

Fig. 7.15.3 (A, B) Gross stretch with full hand contact.

to the previous position. Continue to stretch across the cord in a radiating pattern until no further stretch is possible. Cords may "give way" or "pop," resulting in an increase of available abduction. It has been suggested that this painless "popping" is associated with a release of fascial adhesions under strain (Fourie and Robb, 2009) or a rupture of weak connective tissue in newly forming lymphatics (Koehler et al. 2019). Care should be taken regarding cord "snapping" in the early phases of healing, as this may be related to disruption to newly formed, weak lymphatic connections. A systematic review of 37 studies reported one case study that described a sense of burning followed by a rebound tightening and soreness that occurred within 48 hours after the session of cord release (Yeung et al. 2015).

Gentle Circles

With this technique, the fingers move the skin ON the deep fascia. Tissue movement is of an engaged shearing nature. Rest the fingers on the part to be treated. The heel of the hand may also rest on the body. Starting at 6 o'clock, push the skin around in a circle with the middle three fingers as if following the arms of a clock. Slowly move the skin toward the cord to engage and shear the tissue barrier while keeping the circle round and the pressure and pace even. Change hand position, repeat the circle, and release. Treat the full length of the cord and repeat several times in a session, if needed. Alternatively, start the circle at 12 o'clock and pull down and stretch the skin.

Subsequent treatments:

- Further mobilization and stretching of restricted tissue, touch grades 2 and 4.
- Address any tightness on the chest wall.
- Gentle stretching of restrictive cords.

Vertical Lifts

Vertical lifts (Fig. 7.15.4) are used to treat any cord that can be gently gripped between thumb and fingers. Grip an area of the cord and gently apply a vertical stretch. Hold, wait for release, and increase the stretch. When no further stretch is available, change the angle of stretch while maintaining the vertical lift. Repeat the lift sequence from different angles until no further stretch is available.

Skin Rolling

For adhesions between skin, superficial subcutaneous fascia, and older established cords, lift the skin between

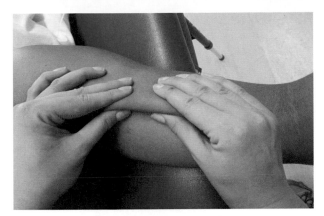

Fig. 7.15.4 Vertical stretch.

thumb and fingers and gently roll the skin over the area or scar. It may be necessary to repeat the rolling technique a few times over the same area in order to release any long-term adhesions.

The selection of technique, direction, and depth is based on the level of dysfunction revealed during the assessment. This approach gives the therapist the flexibility to adapt treatment to the person rather than treating the "diagnosis." Further, based on the treatment response, treatment can be modified in line with the patient's improvement or lack of progress (Fourie and Robb 2009).

When understanding the basic layered arrangement of tissue and how to grade touch, any manual therapy or massage technique can be modified to achieve the aims of restoring tissue mobility, glide, and flexibility.

Treatment is discontinued when the release has been completed in all directions and layers and mobility has been restored. This may not happen in a single treatment and might even take several months, especially in long-standing AWS. Care should be taken not to create an inflammatory response to tissue mobilization.

Summary

The etiology and development of AWS remain poorly understood; however, evidence suggests it is of a lymphatic and venous origin. It is still not clear why some patients develop AWS and others do not. Myofascial release principles can be adapted to treat AWS. There is a definite need for more clinical guidance; more research is now needed to investigate the pathophysiology of AWS and to investigate treatment options.

REFERENCES

Cancer Research UK, 2016. UK Breast Cancer Incidence Statistics [online] Available from: https://www.cancerresearchuk.org/health-professional/cancer-statistics/statistics-by-cancer-type/breast-cancer#heading-Four.

Cheville, A.L., Tchou, J., 2007. Barriers to rehabilitation following surgery for primary breast cancer. J. Surg. Oncol. 95, 409–418.

Dinas, K., Kalder, M., Zepiridis, L., Mavromatidis, G., Pratilas, G. 2019. Axillary web syndrome: Incidence, pathogenesis, and management. Curr Probl Cancer. 43: 100470.

Fourie, W.J., Robb, K.A., 2009. Physiotherapy management of axillary web syndrome following breast cancer treatment: Discussing the use of soft tissue techniques. Physiotherapy 95, 314–320.

Johansson, K., Ingvar, C., Albertsson, M., Ekdahl, C. 2009. Arm Lymphoedema, Shoulder Mobility and Muscle Strength after Breast Cancer Treatment? A Prospective 2-year Study. Advances in Physiotherapy 3, 55–66.

Jung, B.F., Ahrendt, G.M., Oaklander, A.L., Dworkin, R.H., 2003. Neuropathic pain following breast cancer surgery: proposed classification and research update. Pain 104, 1–13.

Koehler, L.A., Haddad, T.C., Hunter, D.W., Tuttle, T.M., 2019. Axillary web syndrome following breast cancer surgery: Symptoms, complications, and management strategies. Breast Cancer: Targets Ther. 11, 13–19.

Koehler, L.A., Hunter, D.W., Haddad, T.C., Blaes, A.H., Hirsh A.T., Ludewig P.M., 2014. Characterizing axillary web syndrome: ultrasonographic efficacy. Lymphology 47, 156–163.

Leduc, O., Sichere, M., Moreau, M., et al., 2009. Axillary web syndrome: nature and localization. Lymphology 42, 176–181.

Lee, T.S., Kilbreath, S.L., Refshange, K.M., Herbert, R.D., Beith, J.M., 2009. Prognosis of the upper limb following surgery and radiation for breast cancer. Breast Cancer Res. Treat. 110, 19–37.

Leidenius, M., Leppänen, E., Krogerus, L., Von Smitten, K., 2003. Motion restriction and axillary web syndrome after sentinel node biopsy and axillary clearance in breast cancer. Am. J. Surg. 185, 127–130.

Lewit K, Olsanska S. 2004. Clinical importance of active scars: abnormal scars as a cause of myofascial pain. J Manipulative Physiol Ther. 27: 399-402.

Manheim, C.J., 2001. The Myofascial Release Manual, third ed. Slack, New York.

Moskovitz, A.H., Anderson, B.O., Yeung, R.S., Byrd, D.R., Lawton, T.J., Moe, R.E. 2001. Axillary web syndrome after axillary dissection. The American Journal of Surgery 181, 434–439

Mullen, L.A., Harvey, S.C. 2019. Review of axillary web syndrome: What the radiologist should know. Eur. J. Radiol 113, 66–73.

Rietman, J.S., Dijkstra, P.U., Hoekstra, H.J., et al. 2002. Late morbidity after treatment of breast cancer in relation to daily activities and quality of life: a systematic review. Eur. J. Surg. Oncol. 29, 229–238.

Schmitz, K.H., Speck, R.M., Rye, S.A., DiSipio, T., Hayes, S.C., 2012. Prevalence of breast cancer treatment sequelae over 6 years of follow-up: the Pulling Through Study. Cancer 118, 2217–2225.

Smith, N.K., Ryan, C., 2016. Burns, mastectomies and other traumatic scars in: traumatic scar tissue management. Handspring, East Lothian, pp. 122–123.

Smittenaar, C., Petersen, K., Stewart, K., Moitt, N., 2016. Cancer incidence and mortality projections in the UK until 2035. Br. J. Cancer 115, 1147–1155.

Stecco, C., Porzionato, A., Macchi, V., et al., 2008. The expansion of the pectoral girdle muscles onto the brachial fascia: morphological aspects and spatial disposition. Cells Tissues Organs 188, 320–329.

Stecco, L., Stecco, C., 2009. Fascial Manipulation. Practical Part. Piccin Nuova Libraria S.p.A, Padova.

Suami, H., Koelmeyer, L., Mackie, H., Boyages, J., 2018. Patterns of lymphatic drainage after axillary node dissection impact arm lymphedema severity: A review of animal and clinical imaging studies. Surg. Oncol. 27, 743–750.

Wyrick, S.L., Waltke, L.J., Ng, A.V. 2006. Physical therapy may promote resolution of lymphatic coding in breast cancer survivors. Rehabilitation Oncology 24, 29–34.

Yeung, W.M., McPhail, S.M., Kuys, S.S., 2015. A systematic review of axillary web syndrome (AWS). J. Cancer Surviv. 9, 576–598.

Temperature Effects on Fascia

Werner Klingler and Katharina Helbig

CHAPTER CONTENTS

INTRODUCTION

In this chapter, the influence of temperature on the myofascial system under physiological and pathological conditions is addressed. Perspectives of therapeutic use and the effect on resting muscle tone are given.

TEMPERATURE-DEPENDENT TISSUE COMPONENTS

Under physiological conditions the skeletal muscle and the fascial components interact closely. The key elements of this interplay are nerval input, muscle metabolism, and connective and, notably, fascial tissue properties. The sophisticated motor system enables humans to lift heavy weights and be able to perform fast and graceful movements, such as playing the piano. A motion sequence is initiated in the brain and translated into electric impulses of the upper and lower motoneuron. The lower motoneuron, that is, alpha-motoneuron, activates the motoric endplates of skeletal muscle fibers. The myofibers are organized as a functional syncytium formed by several confluent and differentiated muscle cells. In contrast to the cell-rich muscle compartment, fascial tissue has less cells. The main components of fascial tissue are extracellular matrix (ECM) and collagen fibers. Properties are influenced by changing of water content, electrolyte composition, pH of the ECM and likewise altered chemical bonding, alignment, and twisting or undulation of collagen fibers. All previously mentioned components (innervation, muscle fibers, fascia) are temperature sensitive, and differences of several degrees strongly effect function, as elucidated in the following paragraphs. Original traces of force measurements in muscle and fascia are displayed in Fig. 7.16.1, and the effect on myofascial tonus regulation is schematically illustrated in Fig. 7.16.2.

KEY POINTS

- Skeletal muscle fibers require input from the alpha-motoneuron for activation.
- Fascial tissue works as a scaffold, aligning and retaining optimum overlap of the contractile elements.

TEMPERATURE CHANGES ARE RELEVANT

At first sight, skeletal muscle and adjacent fasciae seem to have conflicting features regarding temperature dependence. However, from a physiological point of view, the combination makes sense. At lower temperatures—that is, at rest—the viscoelastic properties are adapted

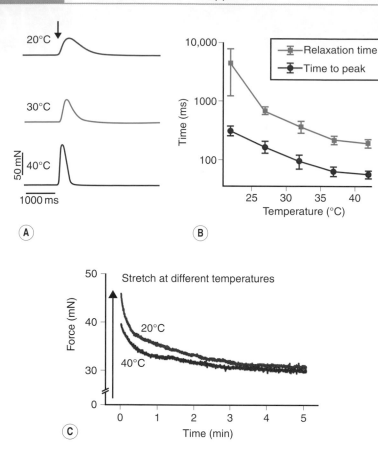

Fig. 7.16.1 Contraction and relaxation parameters of skeletal muscle. (A) Freshly dissected muscle strips from human *m. gastrocnemius* were placed in a physiological organ bath. Force registrations were performed under electrical stimulation of the tissue (0.1 Hz; 1 ms; 25 V). Twitching is clearly temperature dependent. (B) The contraction and relaxation parameters of skeletal muscle (human *m. gastrocnemius,* mean ± SEM, n = 10) obey the logarithmic kinetics of biological reactions. (C) Stretch response of fascia shows at different temperatures. This original force registration shows a response of 4% stretch in *fascia thoracolumbalis*. In a cold environment (20°C), the fascia has a higher peak force and slowed relaxation compared with 40°C. In other words, fascia shows a heat relaxation behavior.

to serve stabilization and load-bearing function (Fig. 7.16.1). Notably, temperature distribution in the body is nonuniform and shows significant differences throughout the body. The outer shell of the body may be 5°C to 8°C cooler in comparison to the body core temperature. Likewise, resting muscle in the outer shell or extremity muscle are significantly colder compared with the core temperature, which is defined as 37°C to 38.5°C. During muscle activity, temperature increases by several degrees. Locally in muscle tissue, temperature physiologically may exceed 38.5°C and even lead to an exercise-induced elevation of core temperature.

KEY POINTS

- Temperature distribution in the body is nonuniform.
- The outer shell and extremity muscles may have temperatures as low as 30°C to 33°C.
- Temperature may vary significantly, comparing resting conditions and muscle activity.

MYOFASCIAL TONUS REGULATION IS TEMPERATURE DEPENDENT

Alpha-motoneurons are big nerve fibers, which predominantly work with a so-called saltatoric conduction system. The nerve conduction speed is temperature dependent and is faster in warm conditions compared with cold environments. Muscle contraction as well is faster in warm conditions. Muscle contraction is initiated by calcium (Ca^{2+}) release from internal stores (sarcoplasmic reticulum), which activates the contractile proteins. Myosin is an enzyme, which acts as an adenosine triphosphate phosphatase (ATPase) and generates force by cross-bridge cycling against the actin filaments. Muscle relaxation is mediated by Ca^{2+} reabsorption into the sarcoplasmic reticulum by an ATP-consuming pump (sarcoplasmic reticulum Ca^{2+} reuptake ATPase, or SERCA). The energy is replenished by glycolysis and the respiratory chain. All these enzymatic processes are temperature

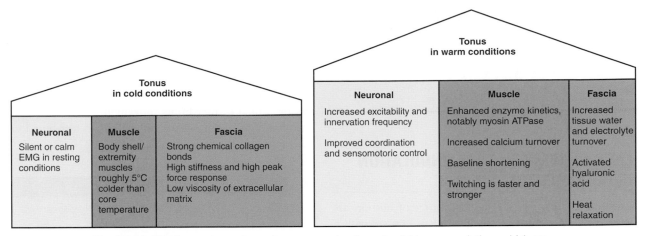

Fig. 7.16.2 The figure shows the main components of myofascial tonus regulation, which are neuronal input and muscle and fascial tissue tension. These elements show different temperature dependence, which is illustrated by unscaled broadening or narrowing of the columns. At rest, muscle tissue in the body shell—that is, extremities—can have temperatures as low as 32°C to 34°C. Electromyography (EMG) shows that there is no or rare electrical activity in muscle in cold conditions (left drawing). Activation may lead to a significant increase in temperature, thereby lowering neuronal excitability and enhancing skeletal muscle kinetics by at least a factor of 2 (see Fig. 7.16.1 for logarithmic dependence of muscle kinetics). In other words, in cold conditions fascia can effectively maintain tension and unburden muscle. In static postures, this mechanism helps saving energy. In contrast, during muscle activity the increased myoplasmic calcium turnover with activation of contractile proteins leads to elevated baseline muscle tension. The temperature is a byproduct of the increased myoplasmic calcium metabolism and results in a temperature-induced relaxation of fascial tissue. Thereby tonus regulation in warm conditions is shifted toward the muscle component (illustrated as broad red column in the drawing on the right). In summary, tonus regulation is a sophisticated interplay of innervation and fascial and muscle properties. The processes are strongly temperature dependent and effect energy efficiency, movement coordination, and regulation of range of motion.

dependent and obey the logarithmic Arrhenius law (Fig. 7.16.1B).

Isolated fascia has a lower metabolic activity and contains fewer cells and mitochondria than muscle bundles. The viscoelasticity is determined by the specific composition and properties of the filaments, the chemical bonds, and other factors such as hydration and hyaluronic acid (Cowman et al. 2015). Several studies show that the viscoelastic properties of fascia are temperature dependent, although assessment is not easy because of technical pitfalls (Lam et al. 1990). Temperature increase in fascia of up 40°C leads to reduced stiffness and more rapid elongation of the tissue, which in part can be attributed to a higher extensibility of collagen and increased slippage of collagen fibers as mediated by, for example, hyaluronic acid (Lehmann et al. 1970; Warren et al. 1971; Ciccone et al. 2006; Bass et al.

2007; Huang et al. 2009; personal data). In other words, there is a heat-induced fascial relaxation. Vice versa, passive cooling leads to an increase in stiffness (Muraoka et al. 2005). Spinal ligaments extend with temperature, as well. In sheep, this thermal expansion has been quantified to roughly 0.5 mm per lumbar segment (Hasberry and Pearcy 1986).

In a nutshell, working muscle produces heat, which facilitates metabolism in terms of a positive feedback loop. Most notably, Ca^{2+} turnover is actuated, which enhances muscle excitability and contraction. An increase of several degrees Celsius, for example, in limbs from roughly 33°C to 39°C, leads to significantly higher viscoelasticity of fascia. In this case muscle is less limited by fascial resistance, and range of motion is increased. Hence, in most situations, this resembles a gain of function during exercise.

KEY POINTS

- Nerve conduction is higher with elevated temperature.
- Parameters of skeletal muscle contraction are faster with elevated temperature.
- Fascial tissue exhibits a reduction of peak force and stiffness with elevated temperature.

LACK OF TEMPERATURE UNDULATION IS DETRIMENTAL

Painful contractures and reduced range of motion are frequently associated with rigid collagenous tissue within and surrounding skeletal muscle, as well as other connective tissue involved in force transmission. The fascial function, such as in joint capsules, tendons, or epi- and endomysium, may be disrupted by trauma and/or inflammation. Although mediated differently, fascial dysfunction can also be caused by central nervous lesions, for example, stroke. Undamped firing of the lower motoneuron leads to a perpetual overstimulation of dependent motor units and secondarily to fascial injuries.

In both cases the myofascial imbalance results in tissue remodeling. Histologically, these areas show an involution of myofibers, an increase of connective tissue, an altered composition of elastin/collagen, and invasion of myofibroblasts. These cells are typically found in scar tissue and exhibit contractile properties. The forces are strong enough to adapt wounds. There are several syndromes that describe fascial contractures, for example, frozen shoulder, Dupuytren´s disease, Peyronie's disease, and many others (Schleip et al. 2005).

In contrast to myofibers (skeletal muscle), the contractile properties of myofibroblasts are slow and smooth muscle-like. The activation of myosin light-chain kinase (MLCK), via a Ca^{2+}–calmodulin complex, is rudimentary and subordinate in myofibroblasts. The main biochemical pathway involves Rho-kinase, which is Ca^{2+} independent and inhibits myosin phosphatase. This, in turn, leads to a sustained and energy-saving contraction. The temperature dependence of myofibroblasts has not yet been evaluated systematically.

Under pathological conditions the portion of connective tissue increases. The viscoelastic properties determine range of motion, myofascial (im)balance, and painful contractions. Under these circumstances it is unlikely that an individual could exercise the affected limb in a manner in which muscular activity could lead to significant heat generation. The lack of the physiological benefits of temperature-induced relaxation might support the beginning of a vicious circle. Unused skeletal muscle disappears and is replaced by connective tissue, which further limits movements. Increased susceptibility of fascial injuries, in the cold, is attributed to more rigid tissue response (Bass et al. 2007).

KEY POINTS

- Heat-induced fascial tissue relaxation is necessary for full range of movement.
- Restricted movement leads to failure of physiological heat production.
- Abnormal remodeling further reduces movement and physiological warm-up.

THERAPEUTIC USE OF HEAT

The use of heat is a common tool in the treatment of muscular disorders such as stiffness or myalgia. Early reports of heat-induced relaxation in connective tissue date back more than half a century (Rigby et al. 1959). Clinical data and in-vitro experiments demonstrate that heat in the therapeutic range leads to a temperature-dependent myofascial relaxation (Lehmann et al. 1970; Warren et al. 1971; Muraoka et al. 2005). Temperature elevation has been shown to alter viscoelastic properties of fascial tissue by changing hyaluronic acid function (Cowman et al. 2015).

Applying heat in the therapeutic range, which means up to 40°C, may be one means by which to prevent the negative feedback loop. It has been shown that external application of heat increases the range of motion after development of a knee joint contracture (Usuba et al. 2006). In addition, the internal thermal effects generated by ultrasound may lead to an increased range of motion (Draper and Ricard 1995). Technically, there are many other ways of warming up myofascial tissue, for example, hot bathtub, short wave diathermy, or the transdermal application of pharmaceuticals, which increase regional blood flow.

The contraindications to heat application include acute inflammatory diseases, skin lesions, and peripheral neuropathy because of the risk of burns. Heat effects are not confined to the biomechanical properties. There is also an influence on the central nervous system and peripheral nociceptors. However, the interaction between thermal and nociceptive pathways, and the relationship to pain perception, is a complex topic that remains controversial (Green 2004). Because of the heat-induced relaxation of fascial tissue, mechanical tension on fascial nociceptors is reduced, thereby altering the activation threshold of these multiquality receptors. In other words, in warmed-up conditions pain receptors may be less sensitive because of a lack of mechanical preload.

Taken together, heat in the therapeutic range leads to relaxation of many fascial contractures associated with myofascial dysfunction. In patients with low back pain, ruptures of the *fascia thoracolumbalis* with prolapse of fatty tissue and muscle have been observed (Dittrich 1963; Faille 1978). Thickened fascia in patients with low back pain may be the correlate of fascial scarring (Langevin et al. 2009). Again, external heat application has been shown to be beneficial in low back pain in a Cochrane review (French et al. 2006). Warming up the "frozen lumbars" may help the individual to stay active and reduce disability.

 KEY POINT

Application of heat in the therapeutic range may have beneficial effects, which in part can be attributed to the heat-induced relaxation of fascia and desensitization of fascial nociceptors.

THERAPEUTIC USE OF COLD

Application of cold is commonly referred as cryotherapy. In contrast to case reports, the previously mentioned Cochrane analysis (French et al. 2006) did not find substantial evidence for beneficial effects of cryotherapy in low back pain. However, summary and comparison of studies is limited because protocols differ substantially and include topical use of cold or, less frequently, whole-body cooling. Short-term icing may help desensitize painful tissue reactions, for example, after sports or after trauma. The underlying mechanism is a reduction of excitability of nociceptors and reduction of nerve conduction velocity and frequency. Beyond this obvious effect, icing may affect tissue regeneration. On

a morphological level, posttraumatic or postexercise tissue remodeling includes the activation of an enzymatic cascade, phagocytes, and other cells of the leukocytic lineage. The time course of the inflammatory response is faster for the metabolically active skeletal muscle compared with the rather bradytrophic fascial tissue. Hence, catabolic enzymes and phagocytosis predominantly affect apoptotic myotubes whereas the fascial collagen fibers stay intact. Teleologically this makes sense, because in defective skeletal muscle, strong collagen fibers maintain biomechanical stability. The inflammatory response goes along with chemotaxis of growth hormones, such as insulin-like growth factor (IGF-1) or transforming-growth factor (TGF beta), which in turn activate proliferation and differentiation of muscle satellite cells (Zullo et al. 2017). Icing can substantially influence this regeneration by slowing muscle regeneration. In an animal model it has been shown that icing for 20 minutes results in a significant and persistent increase of collagen content in skeletal muscle (Takagi et al. 2011).

 KEY POINT

Application of cold may influence nociception and tissue regeneration.

Summary

The lesson we learn from the differential temperature effects on fasciae and myofibers also helps explain passive muscle tone (Simons and Mense 1998). Warmth leads to enhanced skeletal muscle excitability, faster contraction, and relaxation parameters, as well as increased force generation. On the other hand, higher temperature leads to heat relaxation and reduced myofascial stiffness in vitro. Given that there is no voluntary innervation, this effect can also be observed in vivo. Hence, the regulation of fascial stiffness plays a major role in resting muscle tone.

REFERENCES

Bass, C.R., Planchak, C.J., Salzar, R.S., et al., 2007. The temperature-dependent viscoelasticity of porcine lumbar spine ligaments. Spine 32, E436–E442.

Ciccone, W.J., Bratton, D.R., Weinstein, D.M., Elias, J.J., 2006. Viscoelasticity and temperature variations decrease tension and stiffness of hamstring tendon grafts following anterior cruciate ligament reconstruction. J. Bone Joint Surg. Am. 88, 1071–1078.

Cowman, M.K., Schmidt, T.A., Raghavan, P., Stecco, A., 2015. Viscoelastic properties of hyaluronan in physiological conditions. F1000Res. 4, 1–11.

Dittrich, R.J., 1963. Lumbodorsal fascia and related structures as factors in disability. Lancet 83, 393–398.

Draper, D.O., Ricard, M.D., 1995. Rate of temperature decay in human muscle following 3 MHz ultrasound: the stretching window revealed. J. Athl. Train 30, 304–307.

Faille, R.J., 1978. Low back pain and lumbar fat herniation. Am. Surg. 44, 359–361.

French, S.D., Cameron, M., Walker, B.F., Reggars, J.W., Esterman, A.J., 2006. A Cochrane review of superficial heat or cold for low back pain. Spine 31, 998–1006.

Green, B.G., 2004. Temperature perception and nociception. J. Neurobiol. 61, 13–29.

Hasberry, S., Pearcy, M.J., 1986. Temperature dependence of the tensile properties of interspinous ligaments of sheep. J. Biomed Eng. 8, 62–66.

Huang, C.Y., Wang, V.M., Flatow, E.L., Mow, V.C., 2009. Temperature-dependent viscoelastic properties of the human supraspinatus tendon. J. Biomech. 42, 546–549.

Lam, T.C., Thomas, C.G., Shrive, N.G., Frank, C.B., Sabiston, C.P., 1990. The effects of temperature on the viscoelastic properties of the rabbit medial collateral ligament. J. Biomech. Eng. 112, 147–152.

Langevin, H.M., Stevens-Tuttle, D., Fox, J.R., et al., 2009. Ultrasound evidence of altered lumbar connective tissue structure in human subjects with chronic low back pain. BMC Musculoskelet. Disord. 10, 151.

Lehmann, J.F., Masock, A.J., Warren, C.G., Koblanski, J.N., 1970. Effect of therapeutic temperatures on tendon extensibility. Arch. Phys. Med. Rehabil. 50, 481–487.

Muraoka, T., Omuro, K., Wakahara, T., Fukunaga, T., Kanosue, K., 2005. Influence of muscle cooling on the passive mechanical properties of the human gastrocnemius muscle. Conf. Proc. IEEE Eng. Med. Biol. Soc. 2006, 19–21.

Rigby, B.J., Hirai, N., Spikes, J.D., Eyring, H., 1959. The mechanical properties of rat tail tendon. J. Gen. Physiol. 43, 265–283.

Schleip, R., Klingler, W., Lehmann-Horn, F., 2005. Active fascial contractility: Fascia may be able to contract in a smooth muscle-like manner and thereby influence musculoskeletal dynamics. Med. Hypotheses 65, 273–277.

Simons, D.G., Mense, S., 1998. Understanding and measurement of muscle tone as related to clinical muscle pain. Pain 75, 1–17.

Takagi, R., Fujita, N., Arakawa, T., Kawada, S., Ishii, N., Miki, A., 2011. Influence of icing on muscle regeneration after crush injury to skeletal muscles in rats. J. Appl. Physiol. 110, 382–388.

Usuba, M., Miyanaga, Y., Miyakawa, S., Maeshima, T., Shirasaki, Y., 2006. Effect of heat in increasing the range of knee motion after the development of a joint contracture: an experiment with an animal model. Arch. Phys. Med. Rehabil. 87, 247–253.

Warren, C.G.T., Lehmann, J.F., Koblanski, J.N., 1971. Elongation of rat tail tendon. Effect of load and temperature. Arch. Phys. Med. Rehabil. 50, 465–474.

Zullo, A., Mancini, F., Schleip, R., Wearing, S., Yahia, L., Klingler, W., 2017. The interplay between fascia, skeletal muscle, nerves, adipose tissue, inflammation and mechanical stress in musculo-fascial regeneration. J. Geront. Geriatr. 65, 271–283.

Neurodynamics: Movement for Neuropathic Pain States

Michel W. Coppieters, Ricardo J. Andrade, Robert J. Nee, and Benjamin S. Boyd

CHAPTER CONTENTS

INTRODUCTION

The nervous system is a remarkable organ system. In many ways, it is well-protected and strong. On average, 50% of a peripheral nerve consists of connective tissue (ranging from 22% to as high as 80%) (Sunderland and Bradley 1949). In addition, there are many other design features that enable the nervous system to handle the significant mechanical demands that are placed upon it during activities. It has the ability to: (1) slide longitudinally and transversely relative to surrounding structures; (2) absorb strain; and (3) distribute loads over long sections of the nervous system thanks to its continuous structure. Complete nerve lesions, such as nerve root avulsions, are rare and typically require a high impact or high velocity trauma.

This macroscopic robustness is however somewhat deceptive. Relatively small pressures may trigger a cascade of immune-inflammatory responses, resulting in peripheral neuropathic pain (Schmid et al. 2013). Certain parts of the nervous system are less protected and more vulnerable to injury. The nerve root, for example, lacks some of the connective tissue layers of the peripheral nerve (epineurium and perineurium, as discussed later), which reduces its protection against compression and inflammation associated with disc or joint pathology. Certain locations predispose the nervous system to

injury as well. Neuropathies, such as carpal tunnel syndrome, cubital tunnel syndrome, and tarsal tunnel syndrome, indicate that the nervous system is more vulnerable in confined spaces, where an increase in pressure will result in nerve compression. However, studies have also suggested that nerves have the capacity to undergo large deformations during physiological joint movements while maintaining their functional integrity (Fleming et al. 2003; Mahan et al. 2015; Phillips et al. 2004; Robinson and Probyn 2019).

Thanks to the advances in neurosciences and immunology, we have a much better understanding of the pathophysiology of entrapment neuropathies, including neuroimmune responses and how neurodynamic and other exercises may influence these responses. These insights are of cardinal importance to understand common symptoms of entrapment neuropathies, such as widespread pain, and their management. However, considering the topic of this textbook, we will first focus on the mechanical aspects of the nervous system and its connective tissues.

KEY POINT

The peripheral nervous system is designed to slide, twist, bend, absorb strain, and distribute mechanical loads over long sections of the nervous system in order to be able to perform its primary function—namely, impulse conduction.

STRUCTURES OF THE PERIPHERAL NERVOUS SYSTEM AND THEIR FUNCTIONS

Neurons are the core components of the nervous system and typically consist of a cell body, dendrites, and an axon. Approximately every 1 to 2 mm, myelinated fibers possess unmyelinated gaps (nodes of Ranvier) where many ion channels are embedded in the membrane. These channels enable electrically charged atoms to transfer across the axolemma and give neurons the property of excitability. The action potential can jump from node to node, resulting in a faster, saltatory conduction. In the peripheral nervous system, myelin is produced and wrapped around the axons by Schwann cells. These cells also contribute to the immune response by the release of immune compounds, such as proinflammatory cytokines, which may contribute to pain and inflammation. In unmyelinated fibers, Schwann cells wrap around a single axon or group of axons, forming Remak bundles.

A peripheral nerve consists of multiple neurons, blood vessels, and various connective tissue sheaths. The endoneurial tubule is the connective tissue sheath that surrounds an individual myelinated fiber or group of unmyelinated fibers. Several tubules are surrounded by perineurium to form fascicles. Fascicles are embedded in and surrounded by epineurium. The mesoneurium is the thin outermost layer of loose connective tissue that surrounds the peripheral nerve and contains adipose tissue. It surrounds the peripheral nerve and helps the nerve to slide relative to neighboring tissues. The collagen fibers in the connective tissue sheaths interlace in all directions to form a strong and irregular network.

The distinct structure and ultrastructure of the collagen network within each layer suggests these connective tissues have different and specific mechanical properties (Georgeu et al. 2005; Tillett et al. 2004). Although the endoneurium provides a trivial amount of tensile strength (Sunderland 1990; Thomas 1963), the perineurium dissipates tensile compressive forces (Haftek 1970; Rydevik et al. 1990) and is considered the primary (multidirectional) load-bearing structure of the nerve (Rydevik et al. 1990; Sunderland 1990). The mesoneurium forms the interface of the peripheral nerve with its surroundings. Studies demonstrated the role of the mesoneurium in modulating regional epineurial strain along the nerves and facilitating low-friction nerve gliding during joint motions, including guiding its trajectory (Foran et al. 2018; Millesi et al. 1995; Sung et al. 2019). Overall, the hierarchical structural organization of the connective tissue layers and the intrinsic mechanical properties of each layer, and their interactions, contribute considerably to the tensile response of nerves under tension.

A new model of nerve layer connections has been proposed to explain the nerve response to stretch (Sung et al. 2019). This model suggests that the mesoneurium, epineurium, and perineurium are tightly coupled by viscoelastic physical connections and interact with a loosely coupled perineurium and endoneurium, which allows axons to glide and unravel throughout the length of the nerve. Such a decoupled mechanism between axons and connective tissue layers suggests that axons may be well-protected from external forces.

The connective tissue sheaths are innervated by the nervi nervorum (Sauer et al. 1999). The nerve trunk is also sympathetically innervated via the perivascular plexuses of the blood vessels that enter the nerve (Bove and Light 1997). The nervi nervorum are predominantly unmyelinated, and some function as nociceptors. As a result, the connective tissues may contribute to a pain experience, theoretically irrespective of pathological changes in conductive nerve fibers. Increased mechanosensitivity of the connective tissue layers may well be an important contributor to a positive neurodynamic test response.

A very well-developed system of extraneural and intraneural blood vessels supplies the nerve. The blood vessels pierce the different connective tissue sheaths to provide oxygen and essential nutrients to the cells. The endothelium cells that line the interior surface of the endoneurial capillary bed together with the perineurium to form the blood–nerve barrier (Mizisin and Weerasuriya 2011). Similar to the blood–brain barrier, it is designed to keep unwanted substances out of the perineurial space. Compression and intraneural ischemia (Yayama et al. 2010) and intraneural activated immune cells (Spies et al. 1995) may cause focal breakdown of the blood–nerve barrier, resulting in intraneural edema and ischemia. Because no lymphatic vessels cross the blood–nerve barrier, reabsorption of this edema within the perineurium and endoneurium may be hampered (Rempel et al. 1999). Lymphocytes, fibroblasts, and macrophages will become activated and intrude as a reaction to previously shielded antigens contained within the perineurial space, resulting in an inflammatory response.

 KEY POINT

A positive neurodynamic test may reflect increased mechanosensitivity of the nervous system more closely than a true neuropathic pain state.

MOVEMENT FOR NEUROPATHIC PAIN STATES

For centuries, movement has been proposed to restore or maintain a healthy (peripheral) nervous system. In this section, the focus will be on neurodynamic exercises, also called "neural mobilization". Neural mobilization facilitates movement between neural structures and their anatomical surroundings, and potentially between fascicles, through manual techniques or exercises. Neuro dynamic exercises are an intervention aimed at restoring the altered homeostasis in and around the nervous system by mobilization of the nervous system itself or the structures that surround the nervous system.

 KEY POINT

The beneficial effects of neurodynamics are not limited to mechanical effects and are probably more closely related to restoration of the altered homeostasis in and around the nervous system.

Neurodynamic Exercises: Sliding and Tensioning Techniques

Historically, the first mobilization techniques for the nervous system resembled neurodynamic tests, or neural "tension tests," as they were initially called. Several biomechanical studies revealed that the nervous system slides considerably relative to its surrounding structures and that strain in the nervous system increases substantially during neurodynamic tests or individual components of the test (Andrade et al. 2016; Coppieters et al. 2001; Gilbert et al. 2007; Lohman et al. 2015). Because of the increase in strain, these initial mobilization techniques are now often referred to as "tensioning techniques" (Butler 2000). Examples of tensioning techniques for the median nerve are elbow extension combined with wrist extension (Fig. 7.17.1B), elbow extension with cervical contralateral side bending (Fig. 7.17.2B), or the combination of wrist and finger extension (Fig. 7.17.3). Obviously, exercises can include various combinations of movements and can be much more functional than the techniques mentioned here, which have been evaluated biomechanically (see below). For example, a classic Frisbee backhand throw (involving elbow and wrist extension) is a nice example of a functioning (and fun and distracting) tensioning technique for the median nerve. Although nerve biomechanics have not been evaluated for these more functional movements, similar "biomechanical principles" apply throughout the human body (e.g., upper limb [Coppieters and Alshami 2007; Coppieters et al. 2009] and lower limb [Coppieters et al. 2015]), and load on the nervous system can therefore be estimated through sound clinical reasoning. The "biomechanical principle" can help clinicians design progressive exercise programs for people with increased peripheral nerve mechanosensitivity.

Even when movement-based management strategies are indicated, the increase in nerve strain associated with tensioning techniques may not be deemed suitable (Coppieters and Butler 2008). For this reason, techniques consisting of a combination of movements in which elongation of the nerve bed at one joint is simultaneously counterbalanced by a reduction in the length of the nerve bed at an adjacent joint have been promoted (Butler 2000; Coppieters et al. 2004, 2009, 2015; Coppieters and Alshami 2007; Coppieters et al. 2015; Coppieters et al. 2009). These techniques were labeled "sliding techniques" because the clinical assumption is that, compared with tensioning techniques, sliding techniques result not only in a larger longitudinal excursion of the nerve relative to surrounding structures but are also associated with significant less strain.

A series of studies support these clinical assumptions (Coppieters and Alshami 2007; Coppieters et al. 2015; Coppieters and Butler 2008; Coppieters et al. 2009). Figs. 7.17.1 and 7.17.2 clearly demonstrate that different types of nerve-gliding exercises have very different mechanical effects on the nervous system. Longitudinal excursion and nerve strain associated with a particular joint movement were strongly influenced by the position or simultaneous movement of an adjacent joint. This biomechanical insight is valuable when designing progressive exercise programs for patients with neuropathic

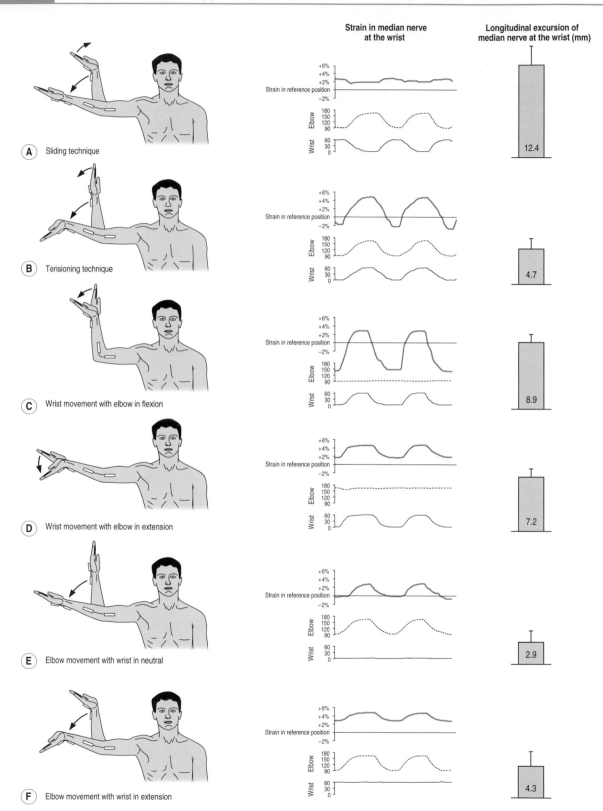

Strain in median nerve at the wrist

Longitudinal excursion of median nerve at the wrist (mm)

A Sliding technique

12.4

B Tensioning technique

4.7

C Wrist movement with elbow in flexion

8.9

D Wrist movement with elbow in extension

7.2

E Elbow movement with wrist in neutral

2.9

F Elbow movement with wrist in extension

4.3

Fig. 7.17.1 Strain and longitudinal excursion of the median nerve at the wrist during combined elbow and wrist movements (A, B) and single joint movements of the elbow or wrist (C–F). For each of the six conditions, the corresponding diagrams in the middle column consist of three waveforms: the top waveform represents the change in nerve strain; the middle and bottom waveforms show the angle at the elbow and wrist as recorded from two electrogoniometers. For the elbow, 180 degrees corresponds with full extension; for the wrist, 60 degrees represents extension. The sliding technique was associated with the largest nerve excursion (mean: 12.4 mm; $p < 0.001$). Also note that the high peaks in nerve strain in the tensioning technique (when both the elbow and wrist are in extension) do not occur in the sliding technique. In the sliding technique, the increase in strain associated with elbow extension is counterbalanced by the simultaneous reduction in nerve strain at the wrist by moving the wrist from extension to neutral. The amplitude through which joints were moved was identical for the different conditions. (Modified with permission from Coppieters, M.W., Butler, D.S., 2008. Do 'sliders' slide and 'tensioners' tension? An analysis of neurodynamic techniques and considerations regarding their application. Man. Ther. 13, 213–221.)

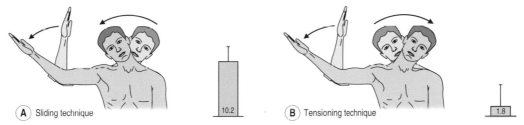

Fig. 7.17.2 Example of a sliding (A) and tensioning technique (B) for the median nerve involving the elbow and neck. Longitudinal excursion (in mm) of the median nerve in the upper arm (as indicated by the bar charts) was largest for the sliding technique ($p < 0.0001$), compared with the tensioning technique or single joint movements of elbow or neck (not shown). In the sliding technique, the distal movement of the median nerve associated with elbow extension is facilitated by the relaxation of the brachial plexus as a result of cervical ipsilateral side bending. In the tensioning technique, the distal movement of the median nerve is impeded by an increased tension in the nervous system, resulting from cervical contralateral side bending. The gray shaded areas show the starting position; the arrows indicate the movement to reach the end position (unshaded). Modified with permission from Coppieters, M.W., Hough, A.D., Dilley, A., 2009. Different nerve-gliding exercises induce different magnitudes of median nerve longitudinal excursion: an in vivo study using dynamic ultrasound imaging. J. Orthop. Sports Phys. Ther. 39, 164–171.

pain. Sliding techniques are considered less aggressive and may be more appropriate for more acute injuries, in postoperative management, and even for conditions characterized by inflammation around the nerve, where large excursions may help disperse some of the intraneural edema (Schmid et al. 2012) and may reduce the concentration of inflammatory mediators (Lutke Schipholt et al. 2021). Again, if we think about more functional movements, the Frisbee backhand throw is a tensioning technique for the median nerve but a sliding technique for the ulnar and radial nerve.

Although tensioning and sliding techniques are biomechanically different, this doesn't imply that sliding techniques are clinically superior to tensioning techniques.

Many activities of daily life and sports activities are associated with substantial increases in nerve strain, and once rehabilitation becomes more functional and more sport-specific, the nervous system may benefit from moderate tension in the system. Although excessive strain impairs neuronal function, animal studies revealed that moderate strain promotes neuronal growth (Love et al. 2017). Animal models also revealed that structural and functional measures of regeneration were equal or even enhanced after end-to-end surgical repairs of nerve lesions under tension compared with tension-free repairs (Howarth et al. 2019; Mathieu et al. 2019; McDonald and Bell 2010). Also, most animal studies that evaluated and reported positive effects of nerve mobilizing exercises

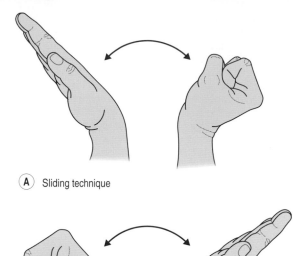

(A) Sliding technique

(B) Tensioning technique

Fig. 7.17.3 Example of a sliding and tensioning technique for the median nerve for the hand and wrist. In the sliding technique (A), the increase in nerve strain associated with finger extension (top left image) or wrist extension (top right image) is compensated by wrist flexion (top left image) or finger flexion (top right image), respectively. In the tensioning technique (B), the hand and wrist are moved from a position of minimal nerve strain (wrist and finger flexion, bottom left image) to a position of maximal nerve strain (wrist and finger extension; bottom right image). The sliding technique is suggested as a nonaggressive mobilization technique in the nonsurgical or postoperative management of patients with CTS. Modified with permission from Coppieters, M.W., Hough, A.D., Dilley, A., 2009. Different nerve-gliding exercises induce different magnitudes of median nerve longitudinal excursion: an in vivo study using dynamic ultrasound imaging. J. Orthop. Sports Phys. Ther. 39, 164–171.

(see Underlying Mechanisms and Clinical Efficacy) have used tensioning techniques rather than sliding techniques. However, we like to reiterate words of wisdom from Robert Elvey, who pioneered the neurodynamic assessment (Elvey 1997) and management (Elvey 1986) of the upper limb: dosage of neurodynamic techniques should be much (much!) lower than techniques directed to other structures, such as muscles or joints (personal communication). As for other domains of therapeutic exercise

prescription, little is known about optimal dosage for neural mobilization exercises. Readers are encouraged to consult published clinical trials (e.g., Ferreira et al. 2016; Nee et al. 2012), prospective cohort studies (Schäfer et al. 2011), and case reports (e.g., Coppieters et al. 2004; Farrell and Lampe 2017) to gain insight on dosage and apply sound clinical reasoning principles to decide on neurodynamic exercises and dosage.

Immobilization and Unloading

The fact that strain and nerve movement are transmitted along long sections of the nervous system and well beyond the proximity of the moving joint also demonstrates that it is virtually impossible to immobilize the nervous system by restricting movement at one or more joints. Wearing a wrist splint at night and/or during aggravating activities is commonly advocated for certain entrapment neuropathies, such as carpal tunnel syndrome. Partial immobilization of the nervous system may indeed result in temporary relief in certain situations. Depending on the clinician's treatment philosophy though, this partial immobilization can also be considered as controlled mobilization and as a first step in a progressive exercise program if symptoms are severe. A more current development is to also consider offloading or unloading neural structures, especially in acute or more irritable stages, to avoid further irritation. With a good understanding of nerve biomechanics and functional anatomy, clinicians and patients can together identify positions that optimally unload the affected peripheral nerve to achieve functional pain relief.

Neighboring Structures

The health of structures that surround the nervous system, such as fascia, muscles, joints, tendons, and bone, is of crucial importance in patients with peripheral neuropathies. Abnormalities in these surrounding structures may negatively affect the health of the nervous system and may obstruct or delay recovery. Assessment and possibly treatment of surrounding structures has long been an integral part of movement-based treatment strategies for patients with peripheral neuropathies (Hall and Elvey 1999). Mobilization of the cervical spine at the level of a relevant segmental motion restriction has shown to be beneficial in patients with neuropathic cervicobrachial pain (Coppieters et al. 2003). Compared with a control intervention, cervical contralateral lateral glides resulted in a reduction in pain intensity and symptom distribution, and improved range of movement. Management of surrounding structures is now an integral part of the conservative management of painful entrapment neuropathies (Ferreira et al. 2016; Nee et al. 2012; Schafer et al. 2011).

Underlying Mechanisms and Clinical Efficacy

Animal studies revealed that neural mobilization positively influence multiple underlying mechanisms (Lutke Schipholt et al. 2021). It lowered mechanical hypersensitivity and concentrations of proinflammatory cytokines in the affected nerve. Furthermore, neural mobilization prevented or reversed interaxonal fibrosis and maintained or restored myelin sheaths at the nerve entrapment site (da Silva et al. 2015). Proximal to the entrapment site, mobilization of surrounding structures reduced the glia cell concentration in the dorsal root ganglia (Song et al. 2006). Nerve mobilization techniques also reduced glia cell activity at the dorsal root ganglion, and additionally in the spinal cord and brain (Santos et al. 2012; Giardini et al. 2017). Neural mobilization also facilitated pain relief via endogenous analgesic modulation by influencing opioid receptors in the midbrain (Santos et al. 2014).

 KEY POINT

Even for a peripheral entrapment neuropathy, normalization of the altered homeostasis may occur not only locally at the entrapment site, but also in the dorsal root ganglia, spinal cord, and brain.

Because invasive assessment, such as a biopsy of neural tissues, is not feasible in humans, far fewer mechanistic studies are performed in people with neuropathies. Studies have shown however that neural mobilization exercises are safe, even in people with diabetes (Boyd et al. 2017) who have traditionally been excluded from clinical trials that evaluate neurodynamic exercises. Furthermore, these exercises reduce intraneural edema (Schmid et al. 2012) and positively influence endogenous pain modulation (Fernández-Carnero et al. 2019).

Although understanding underlying treatment mechanisms are important, the evaluation of the long-term clinical effectiveness of neurodynamic exercises in patients with neuropathic pain is more important.

Several systematic reviews have been published (e.g., Basson et al. 2017; Neto et al. 2017). The largest systematic review summarized the findings from 40 human studies (Basson et al. 2017). The authors concluded that considering the pathophysiology after nerve entrapment, neural mobilization is a biologically plausible intervention and seems effective for various neuromusculoskeletal conditions. The review revealed that neurodynamic techniques are associated with an improvement in pain and disability in patients with nerve-related low back pain. They also improve pain in nerve-related neck-arm pain and plantar heel pain/tarsal tunnel syndrome. The effect of neural mobilization in cubital tunnel syndrome, lateral epicondylalgia (with or without radial nerve involvement), and post-lumbar surgery remains uncertain because of the small number of studies. The review could not make recommendations regarding carpal tunnel syndrome. However, since the publication of the review, several large randomized clinical trials have shown positive effects of neurodynamic exercises for people with carpal tunnel syndrome (Fernández-de-Las-Peñas et al. 2017; Lewis et al. 2020; Wolny et al. 2017).

Whether the effectiveness of neural mobilization depends on the condition, selection criteria, or on the way neural mobilization is delivered (e.g., dosage, technique/exercise selection, etc.) remains uncertain. More high-quality trials are needed to improve the strength of the conclusions and gain better insight into how neurodynamics should optimally be delivered. Judicious clinical reasoning should continue to guide clinical practice and future research so that neural mobilization can be appropriately targeted to maximize efficacy.

THE BIGGER PICTURE

This chapter focused on several aspects of the peripheral nervous system that are relevant to understanding compression neuropathies and a possible management strategy, using movement to restore the altered homeostasis in and around the nervous system. Although important, these are only a few pieces of the complex puzzle of neuropathic pain after nerve compression. We argue that nerve-gliding exercises can be useful, but that these exercises—just as other management strategies—have to be meaningful to the patient and integrated in a much wider approach, possibly including pharmacological treatment options, although great care is needed with stronger neuropathic pain medications. By "meaningful" we mean that the patient must understand the factors that contribute to increased sensitivity of the nervous system. This is likely to require a basic knowledge of neuroscience and pain mechanisms, an understanding of the effect of beliefs, expectations, threats, fear, and stress, and an awareness of maladaptive behaviors. Painless compressed nerves remind us about the complexity of painful entrapment neuropathies.

Summary

In this chapter, we highlight how the structure of the nervous system is designed to accommodate the substantial mechanical demands that are placed on the peripheral nervous system during movement. We describe various treatment possibilities to encourage movement for neuropathic pain states. We propose that a modern view of neurodynamics is an intervention aimed at restoring the altered homeostasis in and around the nervous system, by mobilization of the nervous system itself or the structures that surround the nervous system. This chapter summarizes the efficacy of neurodynamic exercises for various musculoskeletal conditions characterized by peripheral nerve involvement. We highlight the underlying treatment mechanisms with a focus on neuro-immunological effects.

REFERENCES

Andrade, R.J., Nordez, A., Hug, F., et al., 2016. Non-invasive assessment of sciatic nerve stiffness during human ankle motion using ultrasound shear wave elastography. J. Biomech. 49, 326–331.

Basson, A., Olivier, B., Ellis, R., Coppieters, M., Stewart, A., Mudzi, W., 2017. The effectiveness of neural mobilization for neuromusculoskeletal conditions: a systematic review and meta-analysis. J. Orthop. Sports Phys. Ther. 47, 593–615.

Bove, G.M., Light, A.R., 1997. The nervi nervorum. Pain Forum 6, 181–190.

Boyd, B.S., Nee, R.J., Smoot, B., 2017. Safety of lower extremity neurodynamic exercises in adults with diabetes mellitus: a feasibility study. J. Man. Manip. Ther. 25, 30–38.

Butler, D.S., 2000. The Sensitive Nervous System, first ed. Noigroup Publications, Unley, Australia.

Coppieters, M.W., Alshami, A.M., 2007. Longitudinal excursion and strain in the median nerve during novel nerve gliding exercises for carpal tunnel syndrome. J. Orthop. Res. 25, 972–980.

Coppieters, M.W., Andersen, L.S., Johansen, R., et al., 2015. Excursion of the sciatic nerve during nerve mobilization exercises: an in vivo cross-sectional study using dynamic ultrasound imaging. J. Orthop. Sports Phys. Ther. 45, 731–737.

Coppieters, M.W., Bartholomeeusen, K.E., Stappaerts, K.H., 2004. Incorporating nerve-gliding techniques in the conservative treatment of cubital tunnel syndrome. J. Manipulative Physiol. Ther. 27, 560–568.

Coppieters, M.W., Butler, D.S., 2008. Do 'sliders' slide and 'tensioners' tension? An analysis of neurodynamic techniques and considerations regarding their application. Man. Ther. 13, 213–221.

Coppieters, M.W., Hough, A.D., Dilley, A., 2009. Different nerve-gliding exercises induce different magnitudes of median nerve longitudinal excursion: an in vivo study using dynamic ultrasound imaging. J. Orthop. Sports Phys. Ther. 39, 164–171.

Coppieters, M.W., Stappaerts, K.H., Everaert, D.G., Staes, F.F., 2001. Addition of test components during neurodynamic testing: effect on range of motion and sensory responses. J. Orthop. Sports Phys. Ther. 31, 226–235; discussion 236–227.

Coppieters, M.W., Stappaerts, K.H., Wouters, L.L., Janssens, K., 2003. The immediate effects of a cervical lateral glide treatment technique in patients with neurogenic cervicobrachial pain. J. Orthop. Sports Phys. Ther. 33, 369–378.

da Silva, J.T., Santos, F.M., Giardini, A.C., et al., 2015. Neural mobilization promotes nerve regeneration by nerve growth factor and myelin protein zero increased after sciatic nerve injury. Growth Factors 33, 8–13.

Elvey, R.L., 1986. Treatment of arm pain associated with abnormal brachial plexus tension. Aust. J. Phys. 32, 225–230.

Elvey, R.L., 1997. Physical evaluation of the peripheral nervous system in disorders of pain and dysfunction. J. Hand Ther. 10, 122–129.

Farrell, K., Lampe, K., 2017. Addressing neurodynamic irritability in a patient with adhesive capsulitis: a case report. J. Man. Manip. Ther. 25, 47–56.

Fernández-Carnero, J., Sierra-Silvestre, E., Beltran-Alacreu, H., Gil-Martinez, A., La Touche, R., 2019. Neural tension technique improves immediate conditioned pain modulation in patients with chronic neck pain: a randomized clinical trial. Pain Med. 20, 1227–1235.

Fernández-de-Las-Peñas, C., Cleland, J., Palacios-Cena, M., et al., 2017. Effectiveness of manual therapy versus surgery in pain processing due to carpal tunnel syndrome: A randomized clinical trial. Eur. J. Pain 21, 1266–1276.

Ferreira, G., Stieven, F., Araujo, F., et al., 2016. Neurodynamic treatment did not improve pain and disability at two weeks in patients with chronic nerve-related leg pain: a randomised trial. J. Physiother. 62, 197–202.

Fleming, P., Lenehan, B., O'Rourke, S., McHugh, P., Kaar, K., McCabe, J.P., 2003. Strain on the human sciatic nerve in vivo during movement of the hip and knee. J. Bone Joint Surg. Br. 85, 363–365.

Foran, I.M., Hussey, V., Patel, R.A., Sung, J., Shah, S.B., 2018. Native paraneurial tissue and paraneurial adhesions alter nerve strain distribution in rat sciatic nerves. J. Hand Surg. Eur. 43, 316–323.

Georgeu, G.A., Walbeehm, E.T., Tillett, R., Afoke, A., Brown, R.A., Phillips, J.B., 2005. Investigating the mechanical shear-plane between core and sheath elements of peripheral nerves. Cell Tissue Res. 320, 229–234.

Giardini, A.C., Dos Santos, F.M., da Silva, J.T., de Oliveira, M.E., Martins, D.O., Chacur, M., 2017. Neural mobilization treatment decreases glial cells and brain-derived neurotrophic factor expression in the central nervous system in rats with neuropathic pain induced by CCI in rats. Pain Res. Manag. 2017, 7429761.

Gilbert, K.K., Brismee, J.M., Collins, D.L., et al., 2007. 2006 Young Investigator Award Winner: lumbosacral nerve root displacement and strain: part 2. A comparison of 2 straight leg raise conditions in unembalmed cadavers. Spine, 32, 1521–1525.

Haftek, J., 1970. Stretch injury of peripheral nerve. Acute effects of stretching on rabbit nerve. J. Bone Joint Surg. Br. 52, 354–365.

Hall, T.M., Elvey, R.L., 1999. Nerve trunk pain: physical diagnosis and treatment. Man. Ther. 4, 63–73.

Howarth, H.M., Alaziz, T., Nicolds, B., O'Connor, S., Shah, S.B., 2019. Redistribution of nerve strain enables end-to-end repair under tension without inhibiting nerve regeneration. Neural Regen. Res. 14, 1280–1288.

Lewis, K.J., Coppieters, M.W., Ross, L., Hughes, I., Vicenzino, B., Schmid, A.B., 2020. Group education, night splinting and home exercises reduce conversion to surgery for carpal tunnel syndrome: a multicentre randomised trial. J. Physiother. 66, 97–104.

Lohman, C.M., Gilbert, K.K., Sobczak, S., et al., 2015. 2015 Young Investigator Award Winner: cervical nerve root displacement and strain during upper limb neural tension testing: part 1: a minimally invasive assessment in unembalmed cadavers. Spine (Phila, PA 1976), 40, 793–800.

Love, J.M., Bober, B.G., Orozco, E., et al., 2017. mTOR regulates peripheral nerve response to tensile strain. J. Neurophysiol. 117, 2075–2084.

Lutke Schipholt, I.J., Coppieters, M.W., Meijer, O.G., Tompra, N., de Vries, R.B.M., Scholten-Peeters, G.G.M., 2021. Effects of joint and nerve mobilisation on neuroimmune responses in animals and humans with neuromusculoskeletal conditions: A systematic review and meta-analysis. Pain Rep. 6, e927.

Mahan, M.A., Vaz, K.M., Weingarten, D., Brown, J.M., Shah, S.B., 2015. Altered ulnar nerve kinematic behavior in a cadaver model of entrapment. Neurosurgery 76, 747–755.

Mathieu, L., Pfister, G., Murison, J.C., Oberlin, C., Belkheyar, Z., 2019. Missile injury of the sciatic nerve: observational study supporting early exploration and direct suture with flexed knee. Mil. Med. 184, e937–e944.

McDonald, D.S., Bell, M.S., 2010. Peripheral nerve gap repair facilitated by a dynamic tension device. Can. J. Plast. Surg. 18, e17–e19.

Millesi, H., Zöch, G., Reihsner, R., 1995. Mechanical properties of peripheral nerves. Clin. Orthop. Relat. Res. (314), 76–83.

Mizisin, A.P., Weerasuriya, A., 2011. Homeostatic regulation of the endoneurial microenvironment during development, aging and in response to trauma, disease and toxic insult. Acta Neuropathol. 121, 291–312.

Nee, R.J., Vicenzino, B., Jull, G.A., Cleland, J.A., Coppieters, M.W., 2012. Neural tissue management provides immediate clinically relevant benefits without harmful effects for patients with nerve-related neck and arm pain: a randomised trial. J. Physiother. 58, 23–31.

Neto, T., Freitas, S.R., Marques, M., Gomes, L., Andrade, R., Oliveira, R., 2017. Effects of lower body quadrant neural mobilization in healthy and low back pain populations: A systematic review and meta-analysis. Musculoskelet. Sci. Pract. 27, 14–22.

Phillips, J.B., Smit, X., De Zoysa, N., Afoke, A., Brown, R.A., 2004. Peripheral nerves in the rat exhibit localized heterogeneity of tensile properties during limb movement. J. Physiol. 557 (Pt 3), 879–887.

Rempel, D., Dahlin, L., Lundborg, G., 1999. Pathophysiology of nerve compression syndromes: response of peripheral nerves to loading. J. Bone Joint Surg. Am. 81, 1600–1610.

Robinson, L.R., Probyn, L., 2019. How much sciatic nerve does hip flexion require? Can. J. Neurol. Sci. 46, 248–250.

Rydevik, B.L., Kwan, M.K., Myers, R.R., et al., 1990. An in vitro mechanical and histological study of acute stretching on rabbit tibial nerve. J. Orthop. Res. 8, 694–701.

Santos, F.M., Grecco, L.H., Pereira, M.G., et al., 2014. The neural mobilization technique modulates the expression of endogenous opioids in the periaqueductal gray and improves muscle strength and mobility in rats with neuropathic pain. Behav. Brain Funct. 10, 19.

Santos, F.M., Silva, J.T., Giardini, A.C., et al., 2012. Neural mobilization reverses behavioral and cellular changes that characterize neuropathic pain in rats. Mol. Pain 8, 57.

Sauer, S.K., Bove, G.M., Averbeck, B., Reeh, P.W., 1999. Rat peripheral nerve components release calcitonin gene-related peptide and prostaglandin E2 in response to noxious stimuli: evidence that nervi nervorum are nociceptors. Neuroscience 92, 319–325.

Schäfer, A., Hall, T., Müller, G., Briffa, K., 2011. Outcomes differ between subgroups of patients with low back and leg pain following neural manual therapy: a prospective cohort study. Eur. Spine J. 20, 482–490.

Schmid, A.B., Coppieters, M.W., Ruitenberg, M.J., McLachlan, E.M., 2013. Local and remote immune-mediated inflammation after mild peripheral nerve compression in rats. J. Neuropathol. Exp. Neurol. 72, 662–680.

Schmid, A.B., Elliott, J.M., Strudwick, M.W., Little, M., Coppieters, M.W., 2012. Effect of splinting and exercise on intraneural edema of the median nerve in carpal tunnel syndrome-an MRI study to reveal therapeutic mechanisms. J. Orthop. Res. 30, 1343–1350.

Song, X.J., Gan, Q., Cao, J.L., Wang, Z.B., Rupert, R.L., 2006. Spinal manipulation reduces pain and hyperalgesia after lumbar intervertebral foramen inflammation in the rat. J. Manipulative Physiol. Ther. 29, 5–13.

Spies, J.M., Westland, K.W., Bonner, J.G., Pollard, J.D., 1995. Intraneural activated T cells cause focal breakdown of the blood-nerve barrier. Brain 118, 857–868.

Sunderland, S., 1990. The anatomy and physiology of nerve injury. Muscle Nerve 13, 771–784.

Sunderland, S., Bradley, K.C., 1949. The cross-sectional area of peripheral nerve trunks devoted to nerve fibers. Brain 72, 428–449.

Sung, J., Sikora-Klak, J., Adachi, S.Y., Orozco, E., Shah, S.B., 2019. Decoupled epineurial and axonal deformation in mouse median and ulnar nerves. Muscle Nerve 59, 619–628.

Thomas, P.K., 1963. The connective tissue of peripheral nerve: an electron microscope study. J. Anat. 97, 35–44.

Tillett, R.L., Afoke, A., Hall, S.M., Brown, R.A., Phillips, J.B., 2004. Investigating mechanical behaviour at a core-sheath interface in peripheral nerve. J. Peripher. Nerv. Syst. 9, 255–262.

Wolny, T., Saulicz, E., Linek, P., Shacklock, M., Myśliwiec, A., 2017. Efficacy of manual therapy including neurodynamic techniques for the treatment of carpal tunnel syndrome: a randomized controlled trial. J. Manipulative Physiol. Ther. 40, 263–272.

Yayama, T., Kobayashi, S., Nakanishi, Y., et al., 2010. Effects of graded mechanical compression of rabbit sciatic nerve on nerve blood flow and electrophysiological properties. J. Clin. Neurosci. 17, 501–505.

Stretching and Fascia

Thomas W. Myers and Chris Frederick

CHAPTER CONTENTS

INTRODUCTION

Active or passive soft-tissue stretch is routinely applied in:

- manual therapies (massage, myofascial release, active release, muscle energy)
- rehabilitative physiotherapy protocols (pre- / postsurgical, posttraumatic)
- performance enhancement (athletic, dance, Pilates, active isolated stretching)
- self-help methods (yoga, exercise warm-up/cool down routines, tool-assisted self-myofascial release [SMR]), and
- integrative pattern resolution (osteopathy, structural integration).

Much remains unresolved, however, as to the actual mechanics of stretching and what might be the lasting effects of protocols involving such variables as:

- intensity
- amplitude
- duration
- speed
- direction
- repetition (i.e., pulsed, ballistic or cyclic stretching).

Additional variables can pertain, particularly the age, conditioning, tissue health, and genetic predispositions of the patient.

In other words: how much, how fast, and how long for each stretch, as well as how often, in which order, and with what intent?

Variations among these factors produce many types of stretching, generally categorized (with overlaps) as: ballistic, dynamic, static, active, passive, resistive, and broad categories of neuromuscular facilitation (e.g., PNF, muscle energy, strain–counterstrain).

Most studies have concentrated on the effects of stretch on muscular tissue and neuromotor response. Here, we review general concepts, focusing on evidence for the effects of stretching on connective tissue.

DEFINITION

Therapeutic stretching takes an area of tissue to the end of its accustomed range of movement (ROM) and then applies either self- or therapist-assisted additional lengthening. This ROM varies according to the type of joint and soft tissues crossing that joint. ROM may be significantly reduced because of disease, injury, or surgery. Stretching is often applied to restore normal ROM and function in these common clinical scenarios.

Unlike commonplace materials, human tissue when tensioned responds by thickening and widening at

90 degrees to its center instead of thinning (Gatt et al. 2015). Additionally, a linear stretch will be converted in the complexities of fibrous connections to bending, shear, torsion, and other forces due to transmissions in surrounding or "downline" tissues (Franklyn-Miller et al. 2009; Huijing 2002). Increasing evidence indicates that human cells, tissues, organs, and systems assume their structural form and perform all of their functions within a prestretched tensional network (see other chapters on tensegrity or visit www.Biotensegrity.com) (Scarr 2008). Tensegrity is essential to understanding how the body regulates form and function (Ingber 2006, 1998). Tensile prestress is essential for mechanical stability in our structure and in the physiological systems it supports.

Any additional lengthening that either extends into a restricted tissue barrier or beyond the accustomed range meets the traditional definition of "stretching" in manual and movement therapies. Movements within the subject's usual range of motion (ROM) merit the term "movement therapy" or conditioning but not "stretching."

What constitutes a "tissue barrier" varies with patients and the type of stretching applied. Some methods, particularly those focused on proprioceptive change, will be "listening" for the slightest of tissue resistance. Other methods, more focused on tissue lengthening, will hover nearer a strong or even painful challenge to tissue resistance. Both methods can be valid in differing situations.

To be therapeutic, however, stretching should stay within the physiological range of the individual (which varies greatly from very "stiff" to "lax ligaments"); overstretching can produce injury (Swain and McGwin 2016). Indeed, many soft-tissue injuries are seen as the sequelae of local tissues being stretched excessively and too rapidly.

Stretching can be usefully applied to any soft tissue, from the skin, through superficial fasciae, fascia profundis, myofasciae, septa, aponeuroses, tendons, or ligaments, but not cartilage or bone. Thus fascial stretching, intended or inadvertent, occurs in many of the approaches described in this book, and some fascial stretch will occur in the application of most manual or movement therapies.

KEY POINT

Fascial stretching, intended or inadvertent, occurs in many of the approaches described in this book, and some fascial stretch will occur in the application of most manual or movement therapies.

MIXED EVIDENCE

Despite ubiquitous therapeutic and performance-based stretching, research is still divergent regarding its efficacy (Bovend'Eerdt et al. 2008). Although there are many more studies, few of these are of high quality, because they limit themselves to one or two types of stretching techniques, using limited parameters of intensity and duration (Law et al. 2009). Even then, practical application with favorable outcomes are limited.

An analysis of the current literature on the short-term effects of dynamic stretching (DS) showed that, "there is a substantial amount of evidence pointing out the positive effects on range of motion (ROM) and subsequent performance" as determined by the measured production of force and power in the sprint and jump (Opplert and Babault 2018; p. 1).

After years of spirited debate concerning whether stretching is even appropriate for athletes, growing numbers of studies are pointing to benefits. DS is now considered an essential element of athletic preparation (Haff and Triplett 2016), despite a systematic review finding minimal evidence presented as to the mechanism by which DS actually affects the neuromuscular system (Behm et al. 2016).

Countering substantial amounts of evidence favorable to stretching are numerous studies reporting no alteration or even performance impairment (Behm et al. 2016). Additional factors such as stretch intensity, frequency, and tempo may also be relevant, as it, of course, relates to the target population studied.

Contradictory advice therefore informs the daily practice of the how, when, and why of practical myofascial stretching. Few consistent guidelines exist for practitioners or movement educators as to optimal measures of intensity, duration, or frequency. Obtaining evidence-based parameters remains the basis for further research; nevertheless, some studies cited later in this chapter point toward guidelines for positive connective tissue stretch responses.

Another factor in the lack of consistency in stretching research is that the organized study of the biomechanical properties of the various topologies and histologies of connective tissues is still nascent. Little is definitively known about lengthening and remodeling responses in vivo in anatomically intact tissues, as opposed to single structures isolated for testing in vitro (Standley 2009; Solomonow 2009).

Additionally, the broad emphasis on single-unit muscle stretching needs to be reconsidered in terms of newly updated definitions of fascia and novel anatomical models linking muscles, fascia, and ligaments in dynamic series, rather than distinct parallel units that can be treated in isolation (Vleeming 2007; van der Wal 2009; Myers 2020). The evidence is quite clear: the use of the word "isolated" in conjunction with the word "stretching" is difficult to justify when a straight leg lift test—long used as a measure of hamstring compliance—produces nearly two-and-one-half times more strain in the iliotibial tract than it does in the hamstrings (Fig. 7.18.1) (Franklyn-Miller et al. 2009).

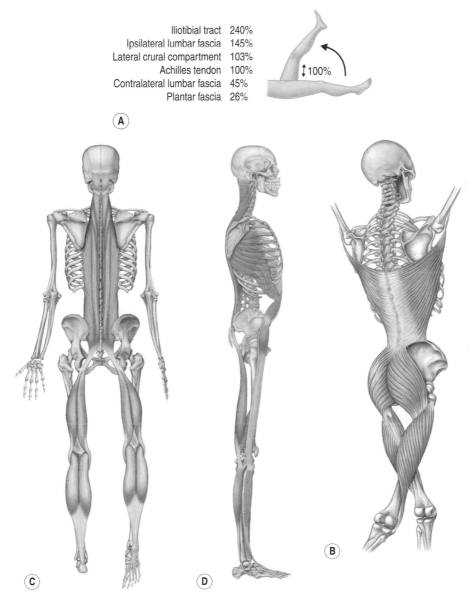

Iliotibial tract	240%
Ipsilateral lumbar fascia	145%
Lateral crural compartment	103%
Achilles tendon	100%
Contralateral lumbar fascia	45%
Plantar fascia	26%

↕100%

(A)

(B)

(C)

(D)

Fig. 7.18.1 Presumptions about stretching, for instance, that the force from a stretch is transmitted from insertion to origin, are challenged by research findings: strain transmission from a straight-leg-lift test (A) shows up in many other tissues beyond the hamstrings. Parts (B), (C) and (D) show possible routes of strain transmission along selected myofascial lines. Parts B, C, and D reproduced with permission from Myers, T., 2020. Anatomy Trains, fourth ed. Churchill Livingstone, Edinburgh.

STRETCHING: THE EVIDENCE FOR TISSUE CHANGE

Fascial stretching is here briefly considered in terms of four potential and interrelated benefits.
- Mechanical lengthening (and resulting segmental realignment)
- Tissue hydration
- Proprioceptive stimulation
- Direct stimulation of connective tissue cells, notably fibroblasts.

MECHANICAL LENGTHENING

All mammals display inflammatory responses to a wide range of trauma or infection, and part of that involuntary response can be neuromyofascial tissue contraction (Grinnel 2009). Humans also respond to stress and distress via skeletal and smooth muscle contraction. Long-term problems arise not so much from reflexive or attitudinal hypertonic responses, but rather because of a lack of postresponse return to normal states of tone and tissue relaxation, even after the threat, trauma, or stress has passed. The subsequent cascade of soft-tissue and skeletal compensations automatically ensues to adapt to what can become a chronic state of myofascial contraction, increased myofibroblast activity, and fascial tissue contracture (Langevin et al. 2011; Pavan et al. 2014).

Many clinicians and researchers propose that chronic "below the voluntary" muscle contraction eventually results in fascial "thickening" (Langevin et al. 2011) or "densification" (Stecco and Stecco 2009) or binding among layers that should slide on each other (Fourie 2009) in various parts of the ECM. These patterns result in chronic eccentric or concentric tissue loading, which taken together form body-wide "soft tissue holding patterns" (Myers 2020). We can also see evidence of the stretch-dependent tensegrity model at work—sometimes working not so well—in the aforementioned clinical scenarios.

In many cases, practitioners approach a body burdened with neuromyofascial imbalance via a stretching protocol that seeks to differentiate, decompress, release, and lengthen areas of hypomobility, to give more space and movement. This approach is felt to have the immediate effect of decreasing the stress of tissues under excessive pulling forces or tension and dampening the effects of hypermobility in joints that compensate for hypomobility elsewhere.

The question remains, however, how far various connective tissues can be stretched, how long various topological and histological areas of connective tissue will retain such length when induced, and which cytokines or other chemical factors could be responsible for retention of such benefits. These complex questions are still being framed, let alone answered.

In general, less deformation occurs in connective tissue that is loaded more quickly than the same tissue loaded at a slower rate, suggesting that a slower stretch will be more effective in tissue lengthening than one that is rapidly applied (Solomonow 2009).

The areolar tissue between the skin and the "unitard" of the fascia profundis shows significant viscoelastic properties, allowing for immediate changes in architecture to accommodate changing forces (Guimberteau 2012). This tissue demonstrates many interesting effects in direct cellular signaling and is easily accessible for, and accommodative of, lengthening in response to an applied uniaxial stretch (Iatrides et al. 2003; Wang et al. 2009).

Within and around the muscle, the fasciae can be histologically divided into the endomysium around myofibrils, the perimysium around fiber bundles, and the epimysium around the muscle itself. Distribution of each of these varies widely between muscles (Purslow 2002). The dual needs for force transmission through the "myofascial unit" while accommodating the vascular supply to the muscle cells dictate that both shear and longitudinal strains through the muscle will not be uniform through different phases of contraction and loading. This suggests that most of the "release" felt in myofasciae during manual therapy is due to muscular relaxation rather than actual lengthening of the fascial elements. To the degree that some mechanical lengthening is available in the myofasciae, research suggests the perimysium may be the most easily adaptable of these three layers (Purslow 2002).

Tendons must stretch in order to serve their primary function—recycle, store, and release energy. Likened to a catapult, tendons are biological springs activating an intrinsic feedforward series elastic mechanism that bridges into the connecting muscle. This mechanism goes beyond the simple actions of a mechanical spring by serving diverse functions including "metabolic energy conservation, amplification of muscle power output, attenuation of muscle power input, and rapid mechanical feedback that may aid in stability" (Roberts, T.J., Azizi, E., 2011, p. 1). In locomotion, "it has been demonstrated that elastic mechanisms are essential for the effective function of the muscle motors that power movement" (Roberts, T.J., Azizi, E., 2011, p. 1; Roberts and Azizi 2011). Consequently, lengthening contraction training (for eccentric strengthening), where it is crucial for tissue to be able to stretch under load, is considered essential when rehabilitating many tendon surgeries, injuries, and conditions (Murtaugh and Ihm 2013).

Ligaments vary in their composition, depending on how elastic they need to be, but ligaments with less elastin have been shown to respond elastically to short-term displacement (as in barefoot running), and with creep to long-term loading (as in chronically hyperextended knees), but there is no evidence to show that ligaments will accept a permanent length change with the forces applied in short-term manual therapy (Solomonow 2009).

In dense connective tissue structures such as the iliotibial tract and plantar fascia, it is now evident that the clinician's feeling of "fascial lengthening" is not coming from actual elongation in the fascial sheet itself, as the forces necessary to lengthen these dense fasciae are far beyond what can be generated therapeutically (Chaudhry et al. 2011). A more likely mechanism is that via neurological feedback, muscles in series with the fascia treated are relaxing from mechanoreceptor stimulation to produce the feeling of release.

Whatever is being "released," it occurs within a stretch-dependent system of tensegrity, as indicated by the following:

- Golgi (load) receptors found throughout dense connective tissues "respond to slow stretch by influencing the alpha motor neurons via the spinal cord to lower their firing rate, i.e. to soften related muscle fibers." However, "such a stimulation happens only when the muscle fibers are actively contracting" (Schleip, R., 2003, p. 14).
- Ruffini type II (shear) receptors are found in "tissues associated with regular stretching" and associated with decreasing muscle tone via "inhibition of sympathetic activity" (Schleip, R., 2003, p. 15).
- The majority of sensory nerves to muscles are types III and IV (free terminals) and occur abundantly in the Interstitium and myofasciae. "The majority of these interstitial receptors function as mechanoreceptors, which means they respond to mechanical tension [or stretch] and/or pressure" (Schleip, R., 2003, p. 16).

A "map" of the architecture of the ECM requires knowing where each structure "should" be tied down to surrounding structures, and where it should slide relative to others (Fourie 2009). In addition to mechanical lengthening of tissues, dysfunction (and apparent "shortness") is surmised to come from adjacent fasciae losing serous lubrication between layers and the establishment of cross-linkages that disallows movement between those layers. Thus stretching can be applied not only to "length" problems but also to "stuck layer" problems. By fixing one layer and requiring stretching movement of the adjacent layer, shear stress is created that allows the influx of hyaluronan and restoration of increased relative movement between the adjacent planes of fascia (Fede et al. 2018).

Muscles attach to and function within connective tissue structures such as ligaments primarily in series rather than the traditionally assumed parallel arrangement (van der Wal 2009) (Fig. 7.18.2). Because each muscle slip attaches to fascial expansions that then attach to periosteum-ligament-joint capsules, which ultimately attach to bone, a stretch designed to target a supposedly "isolated" muscle can be directed laterally, obliquely, or longitudinally to other nearby structures (Franklyn-Miller et al. 2009). This evidence lends support for multidirectional, multiplanar therapeutic stretching after specific local and global tissue evaluation by the practitioner.

Evidence for sustainable viscoelastic change using therapeutic forces in our densest fascia is unlikely. There may be some sustainable change in areolar or other "loose" soft tissues, but further evidence is required to sustain the idea of "fascial lengthening" using manual or stretch therapy.

TISSUE HYDRATION

Stretching is thought to increase circulatory flow to dehydrated tissues and reduce edema by squeezing excess fluid from the intercellular space into lymphatic vessels. The value of tissue hydration is best appreciated when considering how dependent protein interactions are on water. As well as being the essential medium of cell metabolism, surface hydration is essential to proteins' structural stability and flexibility (Chen et al. 2008a).

Water around proteins can be divided into three categories, each with different functions: (1) bulk water surrounding the protein molecule, (2) bound water inside the protein, and (3) hydration directly interacting with the protein at the surface. Bulk water moves freely, assisting in protein diffusion. Hydration water forms

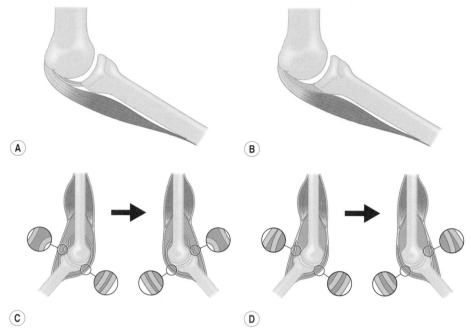

Fig. 7.18.2 Ligaments, thought to run parallel with overlying muscles (A, B), can more accurately be viewed as acting in series with nearby muscles (C, D). From van der Wal, J., 2009. The architecture of the connective tissue in the musculoskeletal system. In: Huijing, P.A., Hollander, P., Findley, T.W., Schleip, R. (Eds.). Fascia Research II: Basic Science and Implications for Conventional and Complementary Health Care. Elsevier GmbH, Munich.

aqueous networks around the protein surface to keep protein in solution. Individually bound water has multiple contacts that stabilize the protein structure from within (Chen et al. 2008b).

Nuclear magnetic resonance (NMR) imaging has demonstrated that water is extruded from tendons when loaded during stretching (Helmer et al. 2006). Some fraction of tendon hydration water then becomes NMR-visible, upon loading with stretch. This might occur as a result of water unbinding from macromolecules in response to load. This mobilizing and extruding/ resorbing process might serve a role in lubricating the tendon during loading, or to increase the stiffness of the tendon in response to loading, as well as aiding in any necessary repair or restoration process.

Ligament creep behavior seems related to the initial state of hydration, decreasing with lower hydration and increasing with higher hydration (Thornton et al. 2001). This knowledge has influenced donor preparation and rehabilitation protocols of ACL and other graft reconstructions (Reinhardt et al. 2010).

In viscoelasticity, the "elasticity" component generally refers to the collagen and elastin chains in fibrils, whereas the "visco" component generally refers to the dynamic interaction of water with the hydrophilic proteins. The viscoelastic response in intramuscular connective tissue originates from gliding between collagen fibrils during stretch (Purslow 2002).

Research of fascia under tension and stretch has described simple modeling of the system as coupled time-dependent molecular gliding within fibrils and between fibrils within a fiber that produces an overall viscoelastic response (Puxkandl et al. 2002).

Klingler and colleagues (2004) examined the water-binding capabilities of ground substance after stretching porcine fascial tissue. The water content was initially reduced, but after 30 minutes rest the water content surpassed the original and continued to increase up to 3 hours after the stretch, producing an increase in elastic stiffness of the tissue. The authors concluded that fascia seems to adapt hydrodynamically in response to mechanical stimuli, possibly because of a sponge-like mechanical squeezing and refilling effects in the bioarchitecture of hydrophilic glycosaminoglycans and proteoglycans.

To summarize, the colloidal nature of connective tissue means that hydrodynamics is a crucial element in the results of tissue stretching, both in reducing edema and in increasing the water supply to underserved proteins, hence increasing the extensibility of the tissue.

> ## KEY POINT
>
> The colloidal nature of connective tissue means that hydrodynamics is a crucial element in the results of tissue stretching, both in reducing edema and in increasing the water supply to underserved proteins, hence increasing the extensibility of the tissue.

PROPRIOCEPTIVE STIMULATION

Deep fascia holds a variety of both free and encapsulated nerve endings, especially Ruffini and Pacini corpuscles, suggesting a proprioceptive capacity of the deep fascia (Stecco et al. 2006). All the ECM displays a range of proprioceptors that respond to various stretch, pressure, vibration, and shear forces, with a hundred million or more receptive endings within the ECM (Grunwald 2017).

There are 10 times as many receptor endings in the ECM as within the muscle itself, with endings located in muscle tissue, possibly better described as "listening" to the fascia within the muscle (van der Wal 2009). Of course, these muscle spindles tend to reflexively re-shorten muscle that has been lengthened, especially if that lengthening occurs quickly—as in the doctor striking your subpatellar tendon. The role of these receptors in stretching is a complex dance that is still being teased out (Craig 2015). These receptors mediate muscle response via spinal cord and higher center mechanisms.

Treatment methods involving stretching and compression are thought to involve responses from these receptors; for example, in proprioceptive neuromuscular facilitation (PNF) (Moore and Hutton 1980) and muscle energy technique (Chaitow 2006). Such reflex mechanisms suggest that the intensity often employed during stretching may be excessive.

Functional reeducation of links in appropriately stretched myofascial chains has been shown to counteract habitual dysfunctional patterns (Richardson et al.

2004). On a global scale, synchronizing breathing with stretching movements has been shown to produce better outcomes for pain reduction, probably through increasing parasympathetic responses (Vagedes et al. 2009).

It has been shown that, along with these proprioceptors, the myofascial tissues are also studded with interoceptors that report to a part of the brain more associated with motivation and purposive movement (Craig 2015). Thus we must now distinguish between proprioceptive sensing (where am I in space?) versus interceptive sensing (how do I feel about that and shall I do something about it?).

This phenomenon is easily observed by holding an arm abducted out straight at 90°. Close your eyes—your proprioceptors are telling you where your arm is in space, and these signals are without judgment or emotional content. They will continue to do that job, but if you continue to hold your arm out for several minutes, the proprioceptors' message will become more insistent: Please take your arm down. Whatever your motivation—to be the last one to quit, or to save damage to your joint (there is none, in fact)—you will eventually be motivated to bring it back down.

The dance between proprioception and interoception is a constant hum under our conscious perception of movement, causing us to shift in our seat at the theater, adjust the chair to a seated task, and set the limits of endurance for any given position.

DIRECT CELLULAR EFFECTS

The effect of stretching on connective tissue cells themselves produces functional changes that in turn affect remodeling changes on the matrix itself. These changes appear to be direct mechanobiological effects (Langevin et al. 2011).

It has been generally supposed that increased tension on the ECM stimulates fibroblasts to create more collagen, increasing the thickness of the matrix. And indeed, cells and their fibrous products do reorient and show changes in function and gene expression in response to tensional loads. This is, however, a self-limiting process. Once the matrix is sufficiently dense, the cells no longer "feel" an applied stretch and thus reduce the production of new collagen to maintenance level (Bouffard et al. 2008) (Fig. 7.18.3). Cyclical mechanical stretching of fascia demonstrates morphological changes in gene expression and protein synthesis that affect both the

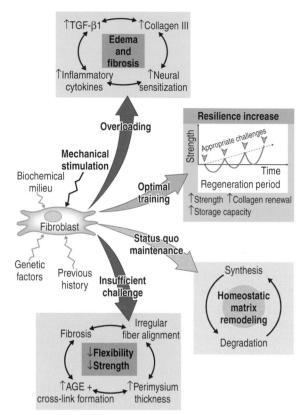

Fig. 7.18.3 Fibroblasts respond to stimulus (chemical, or mechanical from stretch or load) in predictable ways. This diagram shows the vicious cycles involved in either chronic over- or understimulation of the fibroblasts at the top and bottom, with the endless cycle of homeostasis and the virtuous cycle of building strength and resilience in the middle. Courtesy fascialnet.com. Reproduced with kind permission from Robert Schleip.

intracellular and extracellular matrices (Chen et al. 2008b). It is not clear that therapeutic stretching lasts long enough to initiate these effects, but sufficient repetition of a stretch may produce such an effect (Standley 2009).

When cells are put under linear stretch, over lengthy durations (days and weeks) in response to wounds, postural set, and repeated activities in sport or work, they tend to reproduce to try to fill the tensional gap. Cells that are compressed from every direction tend to commit suicide to avoid tumor formation (Ingber 2003). The duration of therapeutic stretches is too short to produce such effects.

In myofibroblasts, found primarily in large sheets of fascia and aponeuroses, the response to a mechanical stretch is to increase the amount and alignment of the contractile actin molecules within the cell and hook

them through the cell membrane integrins to the matrix, exerting a palpable force to prestiffen the sheet of matrix in which the cell resides (Gabbiani 2003).

In the most clinically applicable study, Standley found that 90 seconds of simulated "manual therapy" (pressure and shear on the cell) strongly reduced the effect of 8 hours of "repetitive strain" through the matrix in which the cell lived (Standley 2009).

More research will refine knowledge of how fascia responds to mechanical forces. This newly discovered "communicating system," which rivals the neural system and vascular system in complexity and importance, is "listening" to the cues provided by inadvertent and deliberate stretching to remodel itself accordingly.

KEY POINT

Connective tissues respond differently, depending on their density and composition, to the various forms of stretch via a combination of mechanical lengthening, tissue dehydration and rehydration, proprioceptive feedback, and cellular responses modulated by both mechanical signaling and cytokine feedback.

Summary

Fascial therapies cannot avoid stretch, and stretching cannot avoid affecting various types of tissues. There is insufficient evidence to clarify whether tissues of all ages or genetic dispositions respond similarly to various types of stretch; it is likely that they do not.

Research design is an unfortunate limitation on the usefulness of the voluminous studies on stretching. The high-quality research is too thin to offer precise enough guidelines for practitioners to plan complete valid and reliable assisted stretch therapy or self-stretch programs for their patients and clients. This statement is not designed to discourage stretching protocols, as stretching in particular and movement in general have such anecdotally positive effects.

Although precise guidelines lie in our future, studies on micro- and nanostretching of cells and tissues (much of it about fascial tissues) are gathering specific data that will eventually evolve future design of high-quality macrostretch studies. In the meantime, the conclusions are: (1) "stretch" is a term that is used ubiquitously with many meanings that depend on method and context; (2) in general, stretching can be seen to have salutary effects on local physiology; and (3) precise guidelines for differing forms of stretch in the variety of patients before us lies at the end of further research.

REFERENCES

Behm, D., Blazevich, A.J., Kay, A.D., McHugh, M., 2016. Acute effects of muscle stretching on physical performance, range of motion, and injury incidence in healthy active individuals: a systematic review. Appl. Physiol. Nutr. Metab. 41, 1–11.

Bouffard, N.A., Cutroneo, K.R., Badger, G.J., et al., 2008. Tissue stretch decreases soluble TGF-beta1 and type-1 procollagen in mouse subcutaneous connective tissue. J. Cell. Physiol. 214, 389–395.

Bovend'Eerdt, T.J., Newman, M., Barker, K., Dawes, H., Minelli, C., Wade, D.T., 2008. The effects of stretching in spasticity. Arch. Phys. Med. Rehabil. 89, 1395–1406.

Chaitow, L., 2006. Muscle Energy Techniques. Churchill Livingstone, Edinburgh.

Chaudhry, H., Schleip, R., Ji, Z., et al., 2011. Three dimensional mathematical models for deformation of human fascia. J. Am. Osteopath. Assoc. 108, 379–390.

Chen, X., Weber, I., Harrison, R.W., 2008a. Hydration water and bulk water in proteins. J. Phys. Chem. B. 112, 12073–12080.

Chen, Y.J., Huang, C.H., Lee, I.C., Lee, Y.T., Chen, M.H., Young, T.H., 2008b. Effects of cyclic mechanical stretching on the mRNA expression of tendon/ligament-related and osteoblast-specific genes in human mesenchymal stem cells. Connect. Tissue Res. 49, 7–14.

Craig, A.D., 2015. How Do You Feel?: An Interoceptive Moment with You Neurobiological Self. Princeton University Press, Princeton, NJ.

Fede, C., Angelini, A., Stern, R., et al., 2018. Quantification of hyaluronan in human fasciae: variations with function and anatomical site. J. Anat. 233, 552–556.

Fourie, W., 2009. The fascia lata of the thigh more than a "stocking." In: Huijing P.A., Hollander P., Findley, T.W., Schleip, R. (Eds.) Fascia Research II: Basic Science and Implications for Conventional and Complementary Health Care. Elsevier GmbH, Munich.

Franklyn-Miller, A., Falvey, E.C., Clark, R., Bryant, A.L., Brukner, P., 2009. The strain patterns of the deep fascia of the lower limb. In: Huijing P.A., Hollander P., Findley, T.W., Schleip, R. (Eds.) Fascia Research II: Basic Science and Implications for Conventional and Complementary Health Care. Elsevier GmbH, Munich.

Gabbiani, G., 2003. The myofibroblast in wound healing and fibrocontractive diseases. J. Pathol. 200, 500–503.

Gatt, R., Wood, M.V., Gatt, A., et al., 2015. Negative Poisson's ratios in tendons: An unexpected mechanical response. Acta Biomater. 24, 201–208.

Grinnel, F., 2009. Fibroblast mechanics in three-dimensional collagen matrices [abstract]. In: Huijing P.A., Hollander P., Findley, T.W., Schleip, R. (Eds.) Fascia Research II: Basic Science and Implications for Conventional and Complementary Health Care. Elsevier GmbH, Munich.

Grunwald, M., 2017. Homo Hapticus: Warum wir ohne Tastsinn nicht leben können. Droemer, Munich.

Guimberteau, J., 2012. The subcutaneous and epitendinous tissue behavior of the multimicrovacuolar sliding system. In: Schleip, R., Findley, T.W., Chaitow, L., Huijing P.A., (Eds.). Fascia: The Tensional Network of the Human Body. Churchill Livingstone, Edinburgh, 143–146.

Haff, G.G., Triplett, N.T., 2016. Essentials of Strength Training and Conditioning, NSCA, fourth ed. Human Kinetics, Champaign.

Helmer, K.G., Nair, G., Cannella, M., 2006. Water movement in tendon in response to a repeated static tensile load using one-dimensional magnetic resonance imaging. Biomech. Eng. 128, 733–741.

Huijing, P.A., 2002. Intra-, extra-, and intermuscular myofascial force transmission of synergists and antagonists: effects of muscle length as well as relative position. Int. J. Mech. Med. Biol. 2, 1–15.

Iatrides, J., Wu, J., Yandow, J., Langevin, H.M., 2003. Subcutaneous tissue mechanical behavior is linear and viscoelastic under uniaxial tension. Connect. Tissue Res. 44, 208–217.

Ingber, D., 2006. Mechanical control of tissue morphogenesis during embryological development. Int. J. Dev. Biol. 50, 255–266.

Ingber, D., 2003. Mechanobiology and the diseases of mechanotransduction. Ann. Med. 33, 564–577.

Ingber, D., 1998. The architecture of life. Sci. Am. 278, 48–57.

Klingler, W., Schleip, R., Zorn, A., 2004. European Fascia Research Project Report. 5th World Congress Low Back and Pelvic Pain, Melbourne.

Langevin, H.M., Bouffard, N.A., Fox, J.R., Palmer, B.M., Wu, J., Iatridis, J.C., Barnes, W.D., Badger, G.J., Howe, A.K. 2011. Fibroblast cytoskeletal remodeling contributes to connective tissue tension. J. Cell Physiol. 226 (5), 1166–1175.

Law, R.Y., Harvey, L.A., Nicholas, M.K., Tonkin, L., De Sousa, M., Finniss, D.G., 2009. Stretch exercises increase tolerance to stretch in patients with chronic musculoskeletal pain: a randomized controlled trial. Phys. Ther. 89, 1016–1026.

Moore, M.A., Hutton, R.S., 1980. EMG investigation of muscle stretching techniques. Med. Sci. Sports Exerc. 12, 322–329.

Murtaugh, B., Ihm, J.M., 2013. Eccentric training for the treatment of tendinopathies. Curr. Sports Med. Rep. 12, 175–182.

Myers, T., 2020. Anatomy Trains, fourth ed. Churchill Livingstone, Edinburgh.

Opplert, J., Babault, N., 2018. Acute effects of dynamic stretching on muscle flexibility and performance: an analysis of the current literature. Sports Med. 48, 299–325.

Pavan, P.G., Stecco, A., Stern, R., Stecco, C., 2014. Painful connections: densification versus fibrosis of fascia. Curr. Pain Headache Rep. 18, 441.

Purslow, P., 2002. The structure and functional significance of variations in connective tissue within muscle. Comp. Biochem. Physiol. A Mol. Integr. Physiol. 133, 947–966.

Puxkandl, R., Zizak, I., Paris, O., et al., 2002. Viscoelastic properties of collagen—synchrotron radiation investigations and structural model. Philos. Trans. Roy. Soc. Lond. B Biol. Sci. 357, 191–197.

Reinhardt, K.R., Hetsroni, I., Marx, R.G., 2010. Graft selection for anterior cruciate ligament reconstruction: a level I systematic review comparing failure rates and functional outcomes. Orthop. Clin. North. Am. 41, 249–262.

Richardson, C., Hodges, P., Hides, J., 2004. Therapeutic Exercise for Lumbopelvic Stabilization, second ed. Churchill Livingstone, Edinburgh.

Roberts, T.J., Azizi, E., 2011. Flexible mechanisms: the diverse roles of biological springs in vertebrate movement. J. Exp. Biol. 214, 353–361.

Scarr, G., 2008. A model of the cranial vault as a tensegrity structure, and its significance to normal and abnormal cranial development. Int. J. Osteopath. Med. 11, 80–89.

Schleip, R., 2003. Fascial plasticity – a new neurobiological explanation: Part 1. J. Bodyw. Mov. Ther. 7(1), 14–16.

Schleip, R., Baker, A., 2015. (Eds.), Fascia in Sport and Movement. Handspring Publishing, Pencaitland, East Lothian.

Solomonow, M., 2009. Ligaments: a source of musculoskeletal disorders. J. Bodyw. Mov. Ther. 13, 136–154.

Standley, P.R., 2009. In vitro modeling of repetitive motion strain and manual medicine treatments. In: Huijing P.A., Hollander P., Findley, T.W., Schleip, R. (Eds.) Fascia Research II: Basic Science and Implications for Conventional and Complementary Health Care. Elsevier GmbH, Munich.

Stecco, C., Porzionato, A., Macchi, V., et al., 2006. A histological study of the deep fascia of the upper limb. It. J. Anat. Embryol. 111, 2.

Stecco, L., Stecco, C., 2009. Fascial Manipulation. Practical Part, Piccin, Padua.

Swain, T.A., McGwin, G., 2016. Yoga-related injuries in the United States from 2001 to 2014. Orthop. J. Sports Med. 4, 2325967116671703. doi:10.1177/2325967116671703.

Thornton, G.M., Shrive, N.G., Frank, C.B., 2001. Altering ligament water content affects ligament pre- stress and creep behaviour. J. Orthop. Res. 19, 845–851.

Vagedes, J., Gordon, C., Beutinger, D., et al., 2009. Myofascial release [abstract]. In: Huijing P.A., Hollander P., Findley, T.W., Schleip, R. (Eds.) Fascia Research II: Basic Science and Implications for Conventional and Complementary Health Care. Elsevier GmbH, Munich, pp. 248–249.

van der Wal, J., 2009. The architecture of the connective tissue in the musculoskeletal system. In: Huijing P.A., Hollander P., Findley, T.W., Schleip, R. (Eds.) Fascia Research II: Basic Science and Implications for Conventional and Complementary Health Care. Elsevier GmbH, Munich.

Vleeming, A., Mooney, V., Stoeckart, R., 2007. Movement, Stability, and Lumbopelvic Pain. Elsevier, Edinburgh.

Wang, P., Yang, L., You, X., et al., 2009. Mechanical stretch regulates the expression of matrix metalloproteinase. Connect. Tissue Res. 50, 98–109.

Yoga and Fascia

Bernie Clark

CHAPTER CONTENTS

WHAT IS YOGA?

The term *yoga*, from the Sanskrit "*yug*," is cognate with the English word "yoke." Thus for many people, yoga is translated as "union"; however, what is being united depends on which yoga philosophy one follows. In reality, the term yoga has many meanings. It can be both a noun and a verb: the yoke and the act of yoking (White 2012). In the early Upanishads, circa 500 to ~200 BCE, yoga was a psychospiritual practice leading to liberation (*mukti*) of one's consciousness or soul (*purusha*) from the cycles of birth, death, rebirth, and redeath (*samsara*). Depending on the particular philosophy espoused, this liberation could only occur at the moment of death (*videha mukti*), such as described in the early Upanishads and classical yoga practices, or while still alive and embodied (*jivan mukti*), as described in the Tantric philosophies and Vedanta (Feuerstein 2001).

Yoga has never been one practice, or a practice performed by only one spiritual or religious tradition or in only one culture or country (Eliade 2009). It comprises a variety of tools and views used by many South Asian philosophies, ranging from Buddhism to Jainism to Vedanta (White 2012). In the classic text the *Bhagavad Gita* (circa 200 BCE) three particular yogic practices are described: *karma yoga*, the yoga of selfless work; *bhakti yoga*, the yoga of devotion to god; and *jnana yoga*, the yoga of wisdom or knowledge (Clark 2014). But most of the yoga practiced in these ancient times was done by forest-dwelling ascetics, who shunned normal social mores and lifestyles, or by mercenaries (White 2009). Several yoga techniques were summarized in a celebrated text called the *Yoga Sutra*, attributed to a sage named Patanjali (circa CE 300), which includes a brief and early mention of the word *asana*, which means a "seat" upon which one could meditate (White 2014).

Around CE 800 to ~900, a new form of yoga was codified in India called *hatha yoga*, which can be translated as the forceful, physical, or fierce yoga. In this style, which flourished in the 13th century, cultivation of the body became an important part of the practice: only with a strong, healthy body can a yogi master the higher practices of meditation (*dhyana*) and enstatic absorption (*samadhi*) (Singleton 2010). It is in the state of samadhi that one can achieve ultimate liberation. The earliest texts of hatha yoga described a variety of physical practices: breathwork (*pranayama*), energetic locks (*bandhas*), gestures or physical attitudes (*mudras*), and physical postures (*asanas*) (Saraswati 1999). The asanas portion of the practice was usually secondary to the other practices, and there were few postures described: from 2 to 84, depending on the text (Rosen 2012). However, by the late 1800s the emphasis on asana had greatly expanded, as had the number of postures prescribed (Singleton 2010).

KEY POINT

For millennia there have been a wide variety of yoga styles and traditions practiced in South Asia. Over the last 150 years, a new form of yoga was developed out of the hatha yoga tradition focused predominately on physical fitness and well-being. This new form has been called modern postural yoga.

By the early 1900s, several pioneering yoga teachers began abstracting from the traditional hatha teachings and applied the resulting practice as a health-cure. Riding a worldwide wave of interest in health and wellness ("physical culture"; Singleton 2010), these teachers combined Western calisthenics, gymnastics, and health sciences with the traditional asana and pranayama practices of hatha yoga. (A current appellation for this new form of yoga is modern postural yoga because of its focus primarily on asanas.) Downplayed in this new form of yoga practice were the fiercely ascetic lifestyles and moral commandments of the traditional schools. Yoga was being commodified and made available in group settings. Yoga classes became possible and popular (Goldberg 2016).

Throughout the 20th century both Indian teachers and Western adherents brought the physical practices of yoga to the West (Singleton 2010). With the growth in popularity came variations in the way asanas were practiced, with health and wellness remaining the primary intention for the practice. Classes today can run the gamut from slow, restorative practices where postures are held for long periods of time, with a minimal amount of load on the tissues, to high-intensity, flowing classes in heated rooms to load the muscular and cardiovascular systems. In between are many styles whose intentions range from cultivating mindfulness and calm (reducing psychological stress) to enhancing range of motion, sometimes to extreme degrees (Fig. 7.19.1).

Characteristics of Modern Postural Yoga Practices

The physical practices of hatha yoga create stresses or loads on the tissues in a variety of ways depending on the style chosen (see Table 7.19.1). These stresses can be directed at the muscles, the joints, the organs, or the

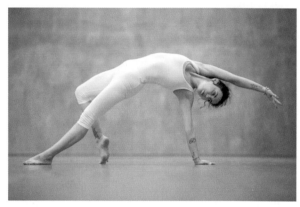

Fig. 7.19.1 In the power yoga and Iyengar styles of physical practice, postures are statically held for 20 seconds to 2 minutes. This particular pose is known as the "wild thing" (camatkarasana). Courtesy Fizkes/Shutterstock.com.

TABLE 7.19.1　Different Yoga Styles Will Create Stress in Different Ways

	Stress Type	Yoga Style
A	Minimal or no stress	Common in restorative yoga practices where there are minimal physical loads and mental relaxation is pronounced.
B	Repetitive, transient, dynamic stresses: stresses in motion, coming into and leaving postures frequently	Common in the power yoga practices, which go by many names: flow, vinyasa, ashtanga, and vinyasa krama. May also arise in kundalini yoga developed by Yogi Bhajan.
C	Bouncy, repetitive (plyometric) stresses	Commonly employed in the rhythmic movements in kundalini yoga developed by Yogi Bhajan, but sometimes included briefly in other yoga classes.
D	Short, static stresses: positions held for 20 to ~120 seconds	Common in basic hatha classes including the Iyengar, Sivananda, Desikachar, and Bikram traditions and their derivatives.
E	Long, static stresses: positions held for 2 to ~10 minutes	Common in yin yoga, although these can also be employed as part of the other styles.

fascia, but in reality all these tissues are affected to some degree regardless of the intention.

The environment for the practice is also highly variable and can affect the body. Yoga studios can be heated (Bikram yoga and hot yoga), sometimes to 40.5°C (Hunter et al. 2018), or left at normal room temperatures. In power yoga and similar (see stress type B in Table 7.19.1) styles, the rooms are often heated, although not to the level of a hot yoga class. The students rely upon movement to generate internal heat (Swenson 2007). Music is often used as well to set a mood (*bhava*) for the class, but the style of music can range from quiet and contemplative (for A, D, and E) to bouncy, loud, and stimulating (for B and C).

KEY POINT

While there are many different styles of modern postural yoga practices, they can be categorized into five groups according to the types and duration of physical stresses employed.

All of the previously mentioned styles of modern postural yoga practices may include and emphasize breathwork (*pranayama*) and mindfulness or meditation (*dhyana*). These techniques can lead toward psychosocial and physical benefits for the student. An evaluation of the energetic effects of the practice is beyond the scope of this chapter; however, breathwork can affect CO_2 levels, thus acidity levels in the blood and tissues, and the vagus nerve, improving vagal tone and heart rate variability (Bernardi et al. 2017; Bernardi et al. 2001). Whether these effects are achieved during a yoga class is uncertain (Tyagi and Cohen 2016). Mindfulness can affect nociception (Zeidan et al. 2011) and psychological stress levels (Jain et al. 2007) and delay cognitive decline (Ramírez-Barrantes et al. 2019).

YOGA'S EFFECTS ON FASCIA

Fascia can be described as a three-dimensional body stocking that winds its way throughout the body, investing and enveloping all other tissues. Thanks to the interconnectedness of the fascia, stresses spread throughout the body. This is shown in Fig. 7.19.2A, where a student is performing a basic seated forward fold (*paschimotta-nasana*). Although the targeted area may be the spine or the hamstrings, stress arises all along the backside of the body and is quite noticeable. By flexing the head and

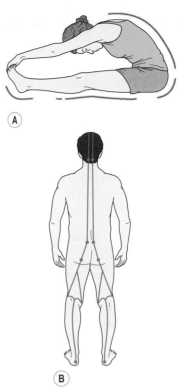

Fig. 7.19.2 (A) During a forward fold (paschimottanasana) the sensation of stress can be felt along the full posterior fascial train. (B) The sensation follows the superficial back line (SBL) as defined by Tom Myers.

neck, stronger sensations may arise in the hamstrings. By dorsiflexing the feet, stronger sensations may occur along the spine. Although the neck does not have muscles that extend to the back of the thighs, nor do the feet have muscles that extend up to the spine, there is a fascial connection between these areas. This particular train of fascial continuity has been described as the superficial back line (SBL), as shown in Fig. 7.19.2B (Myers 2014). Twelve fascial meridians have been postulated (Myers 2014). Three of these have been independently verified: the SBL, the front functional line (FFL), and the back functional line (BFL)[1] (Wilke et al. 2016).

---

[1]The front functional lines (FFL) and back functional lines (BFL) run somewhat helically. They are involved in many yoga postures that use twisting, which can create tensile stresses along the lines. Twisting will stress the ipsilateral FFL and contralateral BFL. Flexion poses of the spine and hips also create tensile stress along the BFL, while extension poses will create tensile stress along the FFL (Myers 2014).

Yoga students can easily attest to the existence of these lines. They feel the continuity (Clark 2018).

Tension in fascia, in its many manifestations, is a major factor in reducing range of motion. Tension can arise in the meridians proposed by Myers; the fascia enveloping and permeating the muscles (epimysium, perimysium, and endomysium); the tendons; the ligaments; and the joint capsules. On a global level, the physical practice of yoga creates stress throughout all these tissues, and this stress is not limited to one particular targeted area. On a local level, however, these physical stresses have different effects on the fascia depending on the nature of the stress.

Variations in Stress Types and their Effect on Fascia

The types of yoga described earlier vary in their physiological effects on fascia, as indicated in Table 7.19.2. (The styles are abbreviated to the first name mentioned in the last column of Table 7.19.1.) Linear forces are created during the static postures that may reinforce the fibrous connections between various segments of the body. This could be important for the coordination of peripheral motor control. Dynamic movements during the practice may affect the viscosity of the fascia, allowing for better gliding between adjacent facial layers or between fascia and the underlying muscles. This could

be important in generating elastic recoil facilitating plyometric movements.

Restorative Yoga

In a restorative yoga class the student spends the majority of the time in a state of comfort and relaxation, both physically and mentally (Lasater 1995). Physical stress is minimized through the use of supporting props. Although there is little to zero stress on the fascial systems, there is still an effect on the fascia. As described by Schleip in Chapter 4.2, the autonomic nervous system can affect fascial tone through cytokine messengers (TGF-B1) and increasing pH levels in the ground substance, thus reducing tension within the fascia. Also, as described earlier, calming breathwork (*pranayama*) can also affect the nervous system, pH levels, and thus the fascial system. Although these effects can arise in the other styles of yoga, the restorative state is usually reserved until the very end of the practice, during a refractory period called *shavasana*.

Power Yoga and More

In these active, dynamic practices movement is used to heat up the body. Interspersed between the movements are short periods of static stresses. The postures may be held from 20 seconds up to 2 minutes. Each movement is linked to the next via the breath, which is slow, deliberate,

TABLE 7.19.2	**Different Styles of Yoga Will Affect Fascia Differently**	
	Yoga Style	**Effects On Fascia**
A	Restorative yoga	Effect is mainly through breathwork and relaxation, which can activate the parasympathetic nervous system and reduce the cytokine TGF-B1, thus decreasing tension within the fascia.
B	Power yoga and similar styles (Fig. 7.19.1)	This style includes dynamic, transient stresses. Because of its viscoelasticity, fascia is less compliant when stressed quickly. These stresses are likely to stimulate stress-generated electrical potentials and piezoelectricity, which may trigger a healing response. These dynamic movements may also improve gliding between fascial layers. This style also includes short static stresses, which may affect the neurological status of muscle tone and produce mechanotransduction signals within cells.
C	Kundalini yoga	Plyometric stresses will help improve the stiffness and elasticity of the fascia, thus building power and speed of movements.
D	Iyengar yoga et al. (Fig. 7.19.1)	Short static stresses may affect the neurological status of muscle tone and produce mechanotransduction signals within cells.
E	Yin yoga (Fig. 7.19.3)	Long-held static stresses will induce collagen creep and stress relaxation, increasing range of motion; change water state from gel to sol, promoting reduction in inflammation; and produce mechanotransduction signals within cells.

and through the nostrils. Certain movements are performed during an inhalation, whereas other movements are done on exhalation (Ramaswami 2005). The quick entry into postures and out of them at the end, along with the flowing movements, may generate electrical currents through both piezoelectricity and stress-generated electrical potentials. As suggested by Oschman in Chapter 2.5, these electrical potentials may spread through the fascia and the cells it envelopes, providing information on the levels of stress, loads, or other events happening elsewhere in the body. Additionally, mechanical forces within the fascial network have been shown to affect the cell's inner skeleton and nucleus (Chen and Ingber 2007). Indeed, all the forms of yoga described in this chapter may stimulate these effects.

The final aspect to note is the value of heat in this style of practice, whether internally generated through movements or externally generated in a heated room. As discussed by Klingler in Chapter 7.16, higher temperatures can reduce fascial stiffness and increase collagen elongation, generate faster muscular contraction, and increase force generation. Hyaluronic acid (HA) becomes liquid at 40°C, which may help disaggregate HA blocks that can inhibit movement or cause pain[2] (Stecco et al. 2013). Thus practitioners of this style of yoga may obtain these heat-related benefits.

Kundalini Yoga

Like most forms of hatha yoga, this style may incorporate mudras, bandhas, meditation, chanting, and asanas. The asanas are grouped into sessions (*kriyas*) in which movement is rhythmic, quick, and enduring; the session may last up to several minutes (Khalsa 2001). The dynamic bouncing movements may facilitate fascial remodeling as described by Schleip in Chapter 7.22. This is the only style of yoga where quick, thrusting, bouncing (plyometric) movements are standard; however, some teachers may briefly include plyometric movements in other styles of yoga classes.

Iyengar Yoga I

In this style of asana practice (Fig. 7.19.1), the postures are usually held for about 1 minute but occasionally can be much longer (Iyengar 1966). These short, static stresses can cause mechanical relaxation, tissue hydration, proprioceptive stimulation, and direct cellular effects as described by Myers in Chapter 7.18. As noted by Myers, a longer lasting stretch is more effective in tissue lengthening than the quicker stresses of the more dynamic, power yoga styles, possibly because of muscle tone relaxation rather than fascial elements lengthening.

Most yoga asanas involve static periods of stress with either an eccentric or isometric activation of the muscles. (There are very few postures in yoga where the muscles are concentrically contracted and then statically held.) Eccentric exercises have been noted to create greater stimulation of fibroblasts, increasing their production of collagen, which may quicken healing and improve the alignment of the fibers in tendons (Stecco 2015).

Yin Yoga

This style incorporates long-held, passive, static stresses (Fig. 7.19.3). Occasionally in the Iyengar yoga styles, postures are maintained passively for up to 15 minutes (Iyengar 1966), but in the yin yoga style, the whole class is designed around these longer stresses. Holding a pose for 4 minutes or longer allows time for the fascia to experience significant creep and maximum relaxation (Stecco 2015). This will have an effect on range of motion and mobility. Yin yoga uses a similar approach to stressing a joint as is used in a form of therapy called static progressive stretch, which uses an orthosis to gradually increase range of motion in a damaged joint (Sodhi et al. 2019). Thus it is speculated that yin yoga may similarly enhance range of motion of joints that are not at their optimal capacity.

> **KEY POINT**
>
> The duration and strength of the stresses applied in the various styles of physical yoga practice will have different therapeutic effects on the fascia.

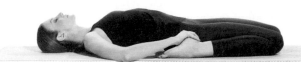

Fig. 7.19.3 In the yin yoga and restorative styles of physical practice, postures are passively and statically held for 2 to 10 minutes. This particular pose is known as the "saddle pose" (suptavirasana). Courtesy Edvard Nalbantjan/Shutterstock.com.

---

[2]While normally HA facilitates gliding between fascial layers, if there is too much, it aggregates and prevents movement (Stecco 2013).

It has been noted that unloaded ligaments undergo contracture and atrophy, partly because of the absence of stress-generated electrical potentials (Dahners and Lester n.d.). Thus the stresses applied in most yoga classes may help avoid contracture of the joints and fascia.

The slow stressing and releasing of the fascia, as found in a yin yoga practice, can affect the state of water, leading to greater tissue hydration after a period of rest (Schleip and Klingler 2007). Free radicals can accumulate over time in the fascial fluids, which can interfere with healing processes, leading to a state of chronic inflammation. When water changes from the normal solid state (gel) to the solution state (sol) through long-held stresses, inflammation-generating free radicals can flow into the lymph system and be eliminated (Schleip 2013).

Fibroblasts subjected to long-held stresses, similar to those applied in yin yoga, undergo shape changes (Langevin 2013). Indeed there is an antiinflammatory effect in the fascia after long-held, static stresses (Corey et al. 2012), which may lead to significant reductions in cancer tumor proliferation (Berrueta et al. 2018). These long-held yogic stresses may act in a similar fashion to acupuncture needles (Langevin 2013).

Additionally, long-held but not maximal stresses can improve wound healing through reducing the size of the wound. Low magnitude loads applied for longer durations are more effective in reducing wound size than larger loads or less time. A 5-minute stress creating a 3% strain in bioengineered tendons reduced wound size by 40% within 24 hours (Cao et al. 2015). This is the main prescription for yin yoga, where it is said that "time is more important than intensity" (Clark 2019).

FASCIA RESEARCH'S EFFECT ON YOGA

The growing knowledge of what fascia is and does can inform the way a student practices yoga. Variety is key: students are advised to vary the duration and direction of the stresses, including angle, tempo, and load (Huijing 2007). All of this may not be practical to include in one particular yoga class but over the space of a week, through multiple practices, it is possible. Ideas to include are:

- Vary the directions of stresses so that movements are not always in straight lines. Incorporate circular motions (circumduction of the joints).

- Vary the time that the stresses are applied. This can range from short, bouncy, dynamic stresses to medium-held static stresses and long-held static stresses.
- For fast, bouncy movements, incorporate countermovements to build the elastic recoil abilities of the fascia. (But, avoid jerky movements or abrupt changes of directions.)
- Include whole body movements.
- Vary the intensity of the stresses from mild or passive to active, larger loads.
- Increase the heat of the body through warming up the muscles or increasing the ambient temperature or both.
- Take a long-term view. Collagen does not turnover quickly. It can take years to be replaced, depending on where it is.
- Feel the fascia! Try to sense tissues other than the muscles (Myers 2011).

More than focusing on *what* we do, it is important to focus on *how* we do what we do. Thus almost any physical practice or exercise can be adapted to and included in modern postural yoga, including the previously mentioned fascial training suggestions as long as they are performed with attention and intention.

Summary

Modern physical yoga practices have evolved from the earlier hatha yoga traditions but are distinct from their predecessors, with much more focus on physical well-being and far less on spiritual transformation. The nature of the physical stresses vary from short, dynamic, and intense to long, static, and mild depending up the style of yoga being practiced. In all cases, however, there are potentially beneficial effects on the body, including to the fascial tissues. These effects range from stimulating the cells within fascia to changing the nature of the extracellular matrix. Discoveries about the importance and malleability of fascia have begun to change the way yoga is taught and practiced.

REFERENCES

Bernardi, L., Sleight, P., Bandinelli, G., et al., 2001. Effect of rosary prayer and yoga mantras on autonomic cardiovascular rhythms: comparative study. BMJ 323, 1446–1449.

Bernardi, N., Bordino, M., Bianchi, L., Bernardi, L., 2017. Acute fall and long-term rise in oxygen saturation in response to meditation. Psychophysiology 54, 1951–1966.

Berrueta, L., Bergholz, J., Munoz, D., et al., 2018. Stretching reduces tumor growth in a mouse breast cancer model. Sci Rep. 8, 7864.

Cao, T.V., Hicks, M.R., Zein-Hammoud, M., Standley, P.R., 2015. Duration and magnitude of myofascial release in a 3-dimensional bioengineered tendons: effects on wound healing. J. Am. Osteopath. Assoc. 115, 72–82.

Chen, C.S., Ingber, D.E., 1999. Tensegrity and mechanoregulation: from skeleton to cytoskeleton. Osteoarthritis Cartilage. 7 (1), 81–94. doi:10.1053/joca.1998.0164.

Clark, B., 2014. From the Gita to The Grail: Exploring Yoga Stories and Western Myths. Blue River Press, Indianapolis, IN.

Clark, B., 2018. Your Spine, Your Yoga: Developing Stability and Mobility for Your Spine. Wild Strawberry Productions, Vancouver, Canada.

Clark, B., 2019. The Complete Guide to Yin Yoga, second ed. Wild Strawberry Productions, Vancouver, Canada.

Corey, S.M, Vizzard, M.A., Bouffard, N.A., Badger, G.J., Langevin, H.M., 2012. Stretching of the back improves gait, mechanical sensitivity and connective tissue inflammation in a rodent model. PLoS One 7, e29831.

Dahners, L., Lester, G., On Changes in Length of Dense Collagenous Tissues: Growth and Contracture. Unpublished. Available from: https://laury.dahners.com/assets/documents/orthopedic/KD%20paper%20for%20web%202020.pdf.

Eliade, M., 2009. Yoga: Immortality and Freedom. Princeton University Press, Princeton, New Jersey.

Feuerstein, G., 2001. The Yoga Tradition: Its History, Literature, Philosophy and Practice. Holm Press, Prescott, Arizona.

Goldberg, E., 2016. The Path of Modern Yoga: The History of an Embodied Spiritual Practice. Inner Traditions, Rochester, VT.

Huijing, P., 2007. Epimuscular myofascial force transmission between antagonistic and synergistic muscles can explain movement limitation in spastic paresis. J. Biomech. 17, 708–724.

Hunter, S.D., Laosiripisan, J., Elmenshawy, A., Tanaka, H., 2018. Effects of yoga interventions practised in heated and thermoneutral conditions on endothelium-dependent vasodilatation: The Bikram yoga heart study. Exp. Physiol. 103, 391–396.

Iyengar, B., 1966. Light on Yoga. Allen & Unwin, New York.

Jain, S., Shapiro, S.L., Swanick, S., et al., 2007. A randomized controlled trial of mindfulness meditation versus relaxation training: effects on distress, positive states of mind, rumination, and distraction. Ann. Behav. Med. 33, 11–21.

Khalsa, S., 2001. Kundalini Yoga. Dorling Kindersley, London, UK.

Langevin, H., May 1, 2013. The science of stretch. The Scientist Magazine.

Lasater, J., 1995. Relax and Renew. Rodmell Press, Berkeley, CA.

Myers, T., 2011. Fascial fitness: training the neuromyofascial web. IDEA Fit. J. 8, 4.

Myers, T., 2014. Anatomy Trains: Myofascial Meridians for Manual & Movement Therapists, third ed. Churchill Livingstone Elsevier, Edinburgh.

Ramaswami, S., 2005. The complete book of Vinyasa Yoga. Marlowe and Company, New York.

Ramírez-Barrantes, R., Arancibia, M., Stojanova, J., Aspé-Sánchez, M., Córdova, C., Henríquez-Ch, R.A., 2019. Default mode network, meditation, and age-associated brain changes: what can we learn from the impact of mental training on well-being as a psychotherapeutic approach? Neural Plast. 2019, 7067592.

Rosen, R., 2012. Original Yoga: Rediscovering Traditional Practices of Hatha Yoga. Shambhala Publications, Boston.

Saraswati, S.S., 1999. Asana Pranayaman Mudra Bandha. Bihar School of Yoga, Munger, Bihar, India.

Schleip, R., 2013. Lumbar Fasciae: A Frequent Generator of Back Pain. Latest Research Findings and Clinical Implication, paper presented at the Europäisches Symposium der traditionellen Osteopathie, Chiemsee, Germany.

Schleip, R., Klingler, W., 2007. Fascial strain hardening correlates with matrix hydration changes. In: Findley, T.W., Schleip, R. (Eds.) Fascia Research: Basic Science and Implications for Conventional and Complementary Health Care. Elsevier GmbH, Munich.

Singleton, M., 2010. Yoga Body: The Origins of Modern Posture Practice. Oxford University Press, Oxford.

Sodhi, N., Yao, B., Anis, H.K., et al., 2019. Patient satisfaction and outcomes of static progressive stretch bracing: a 10-year prospective analysis. Ann. Transl. Med. 7, 67.

Stecco, A., Gesi, M., Stecco, C., Stern, R., 2013. Fascial components of the myofascial pain syndrome. Curr. Pain Headache Rep. 17, 352.

Stecco, C. 2015. Functional Atlas of the Human Fascial System. Churchill Livingstone, UK.

Swenson, D., 2007. Ashtanga Yoga: The Practice Manual. Ashtanga Yoga Productions, Sugar Land, TX.

Tyagi, A., Cohen, M., 2016. Yoga and heart rate variability: a comprehensive review of the literature. Int. J. Yoga 9, 97–113.

White, D.G., 2009, Sinister Yogis. University of Chicago Press, Chicago, IL.

White, D.G., 2012, Yoga in Practice. Princeton University Press, Princeton, New Jersey.

White, D.G., 2014, The Yoga Sutra of Patanjali: A Biography. Princeton University Press, Princeton, New Jersey.

Wilke, J., Krause, F., Vogt, L., Banzer W., 2016. What is evidence-based about myofascial chains? A systematic review. Arch. Phys. Med. Rehabil. 97, 454–461.

Zeidan, F., Martucci, K.T., Kraft, R.A., Gordon, N.S., McHaffie, J.G., Coghill, R.C., 2011. Brain mechanisms supporting the modulation of pain by mindfulness meditation. J. Neurosci. 31, 5540–5548.

Pilates and Fascia: The Art of "Working In"

Marie-José Blom

CHAPTER CONTENTS

INTRODUCTION

Pilates is regarded by its proponents as a comprehensive method of exercise and total body conditioning, created and pioneered by Joseph H. Pilates (1880–1967). The integrity of the method strongly rests on six basic principles: concentration, control, centering, precision, flowing movement, and breathing (Pilates 1945, 1998).

Pilates's methodology and approach to fitness and health took shape from 1914 to 1918 while he was detained on the Isle of Man as a prisoner of war. While living in the camp, he taught other residents the series of exercises that he had developed for personal use over the preceding decades, both in Germany and England (Redfield 2009). He created makeshift equipment from bed springs and frames to support and supplement his movement repertoire. Pilates immigrated to the United States in 1926 (Pilates 1927).

THE BLEND OF EASTERN AND WESTERN PHILOSOPHIES

The design of the Pilates exercise sequences was strongly based on yoga and the principles of Zen (Pilates 1945, 1998). Zen, as an established sect of Buddhism, means meditation, "waking up" to the moment. This mindfulness and awareness is integrated in the Pilates movement with the objective of uniting the body and mind. Pilates's goal is a well-balanced body, with equal importance placed on both internal and external development. He established this balance by creating movement sequences that focus on rhythmic breath, stimulating both circulation and lung capacity. The movements that followed directly involved the spine.

This proves a great advantage to the coupling of fascia and muscle function of the deep abdominal and paraspinal muscles, a biomechanical concept of a fascial "container" that contributes to a thoracic and lumbar girdling system (Vleeming, et al. 2014).

The dynamic, protective function of this fascia-derived girdling system is stimulated by the integration of breathing and movement. The breath itself supports the innermost movement of the respiratory diaphragm. The inner space is divided into two cavities, the thoracic and the abdominal cavity, by which the diaphragmatic movement facilitates stability through its descent by pressurization of the abdominal cavity. During the same phase, the fascia of the lungs (parietal pleura) and the fascia of the heart (pericardium) are gently pulled. The thorax itself is connected via the pleurae of the lungs and via the pericardium to the diaphragmatic fascia (central tendon). The abdominal cavity is connected to the respiratory diaphragm by the peritoneum and thereby connects the two cavities.

The function of integrated breathing aims to cause elastic movements of both the thoracic and abdominal cavities, and therefore via the fascial connections, to affect the motility and circulation of the internal organs within the thorax and in the abdomen and pelvic floor (Calais-Germaine 2005). Pilates movements, choreographed with the breath, are designed to stimulate movement originating from within (the art of "working in"), with the effect of breathing as described in yoga principles (Pranayama) to control the mind (Iyengar 1966).

KEY POINT

The design of the Pilates exercises is strongly based on yoga and the principles of Zen (Pilates 1945, 1998). Mindfulness and awareness underbuilds the objective of uniting the body and mind, currently to benefit interoception, an important neurofascial property (Schleip, Jäger).

FUSION AND INTEGRATION OF VARIOUS DISCIPLINES

Pilates early connections and collaborations involved the New York dance community and its leading figures, including Ted Shawn, Ruth St. Denis, and George Balanchine. Pilates "contrology" (explained later in this chapter) teachings became heavily influenced by dance movement and the vocabulary of both classical and modern dance. This, coupled with his athletic background as a boxer and gymnast, is reflected in all Pilates exercises (Eismen and Friedman 2004).

For many years this integrated approach existed as a well-preserved "secret formula" of conditioning, rehabilitation, and cross-training. By word of mouth, groups of dancers, actors, and athletes would frequent Pilates studio in pursuit of a better-performing body. Originally created as one method or system, different models and approaches have been adapted over time within its teachings. These adaptations serve skill-specific training, as well as therapy and rehabilitation. Examples of these different models can be referred to as contemporary Pilates and may include Pilates for the aging, pre- and postnatal

Pilates, and various sport skill-specific adaptations. Contemporary Pilates is known for its infusion with modifications, therapeutic adaptations, and integration of other disciplines, such as Feldenkrais, yoga, or dance.

One commendable example of therapeutic adaptation is a program that is essential to mention in this chapter: "Heroes in Motion", a specialized program to improve the rehabilitation of wounded soldiers. This program was pioneered by Elizabeth Larkam in 2010. Elizabeth was awarded the Medal of the Danish Society of Military Medicine.

Movement compliant with fascia, especially in forms of therapeutic Pilates, uses the interoceptive properties of the fascia to restore embodiment. As Andrew Taylor Still noted, "Not being embodied is a form of trauma itself" (Andrew Taylor Still MD, 1828-1917).

KEY POINT

A refined model of Pilates technique evolved, benefitting dancers, athletes, and actors in pursuit of an optimal-performing and healthy body. This formed the foundation of the various classifications of Pilates technique—that is, Pilates for the aging, pre- and postnatal Pilates, and important therapeutic adaptations such as "Heroes in Motion" (Larkam 2010).

FASCIA, BOUND BY LIFESTYLE

The Pilates method focuses on postural symmetry (alignment), breath control, center/core strength, spine-pelvis and shoulder stability, well-balanced muscle tone, and joint mobility through its complete range of motion (Pilates 1945, 1998). Extensive research in fascia reveals dense and irregular connective tissue continuity through the entire body that envelops and connects every muscle, myofibril, and internal organ (Schleip 2003; Huijing and Langevin 2009). It functions as a flexible "soft tissue skeleton," offering support, form, and tensile tone through the entire body. The second nature of this mechanical fascial matrix involves neuro-communication. The ability to adapt, change, and influence other systems in the body relates to the presence in fascia of a variety of mechanoreceptors and the presence of smooth muscle cells (myofibroblasts). The integrated system communicates tension and compression through movement stimulation, thereby affecting cellular function (Ingber 1998). Because Pilates movement emphasizes control by creating oppositional length tension of the movement managed during every

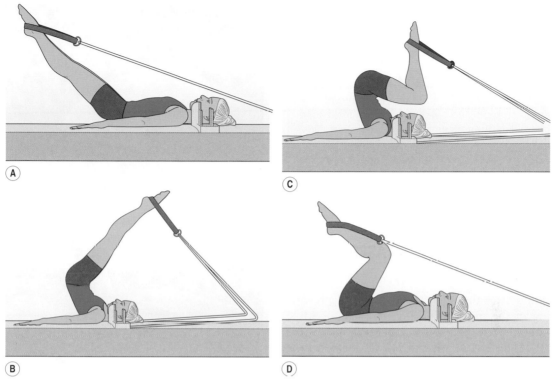

Fig. 7.20.1 (A) Short spine massage, preparation and posturing—this addresses and loads the deep fascial front line (DFL). (B) Short spine massage, phase 2—this is an extension of the full superficial backline (SBL). (C) Short spine massage, phase 3—this phase eccentrically loads the lateral line (LL) and both functional lines (BFL and FFL). (D) Short spine massage, phase 4—this is the resting and control phase. ©1998 Marie-Jose Blom, www.pilatesinspiration.com.

phase of that movement, it challenges and stimulates the tensegrity geometry (Fuller 1961) of the entire body, promoting biomechanical health and strength (Myers 2009).

Fascia, through the presence of myofibroblasts, forms an indirect link to the autonomic nervous system, further affecting the quality and tone of the muscular system, which may be influenced by breathing disorders (pH changes), emotional stress, or diet (Myers 2009; Oschman 2003). In contemporary life, movement and range of motion that support a healthy body may be compromised by stressful environments. For example, a desk-bound lifestyle and lack of activity may lead to a fascial-bound, stagnating structure (Beach 2010). Rather than isolating muscle groups, the focus in Pilates rests on whole-body integration as a possible means to restoring myofascial length, healthy texture, and optimal tissue hydration and resilience.

Myers (2009) (see also Chapter 7.19) has described how yoga movements can be seen to specifically affect and apply to fascial tracts (meridians). Similar parallels can be made with Pilates, for example, in exercises such as the "short spine massage" or a traditional Pilates exercise performed through optimal length tension and omnidirectional and full-range articulated control, affecting the different myofascial "lines" (Fig. 7.20.1). Pilates achieves this effect by positioning and placement of the body. Unlike yoga, Pilates dynamically takes the body into specific repetitive movement patterns, ideally performed through full range, uniting breath control and precision. The movements are performed in a manner that reinforces full oppositional length tension, emphasizing eccentric control, which affects tensile stimulation through the entire network. Within the Pilates paradigm, this effect is thought to transfer into other areas of life, with measurable results of coordination, strength, mobility, posture, grace, and self-confidence (Pilates 1945, 1998; Eismen and Friedman 2004).

> ## KEY POINT
>
> Pilates technique focus: postural symmetry, breath control, center strength, and well-balanced muscle tone. This underbuilds the refinement and energy that aligns with and challenges the fascial infrastructure. Pilates exercises are performed emphasizing oppositional length tension and omnidirectional and full-range articulation control, which affect the different myofascial lines (Myers 2009).

PILATES PRINCIPLES AND FASCIA

Concentration

Pilates emphasizes the importance of "being present" and being in the moment during the exercises while paying attention to every detail of each movement (Pilates 1945, 1998). Attention to detail is considered to promote an openness to explore and experience—that is, to stimulate the learning process (Doidge 2007). Through focused practice, this cognitive learning practice is viewed as contributing to change and "remodeling" of the neuro myofascial structures and influenced mainly by interoceptive neural communication. This interoceptive refinement goes hand-in-hand with a calibration of the parasympathetic nervous system, therefore offering a true mind-body approach. Schleip (2003) indicated that the fascial field not only reacts to verbal instruction but also responds effectively to tactile corrective or directive instruction (Fig. 7.20.2). Reinforcement by imagery, or "ideokinesis," has also been observed to produce similar physical changes in the motor system (Franklin 1996; Doidge 2007). As Andrew Taylor Still noted, "When you deal with the fasciae you are doing business with the branch offices of the brain." (Andrew Taylor Still MD, 1828-1917).

This contemporary motor-learning model is intended to provide the environmental conditions for training of the feed-forward, or core, system and to enhance timing and motor skill coordination, which in turn stimulates neuro-plasticity (Doidge 2007). Over time, this process is thought to lead to new motor patterns that override established compensatory movements that may cause biomechanical strain. Concentration and

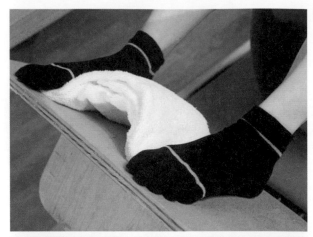

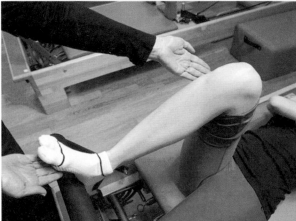

Fig. 7.20.2 Optimizing proprioception through positional correction with touch or props. ©2007 Robert Reiff, www.magiclight.com.

embodiment of the movement in Pilates is considered to enhance coordination of the neuromuscular system with the myofascial system (Oschman 2003; Myers 2009). The emphasis on concentration on the entire body, through each movement, as opposed to compartmentalization, parallels the contemporary science-based anatomy models of a "myofascial" or "neural-myofascial skeletal" continuum, organized and stimulated by directed movement patterns (van der Wal 2009; Myers 2009).

Movement patterns that are sequenced to follow the organization of the densely innervated fascial system are considered both to render deep structural support and to provide position-sense of the body and its movement in space. Pilates proponents posit that this result forms an integrated memory bank and communication system for retraining healthy movement. That is, optimal movement leads to a healthy structure—"form follows function" (Wolff 1986). For example, in the Pilates footwork on the universal reformer, the correct placement of the feet will transfer the movement along the entire kinetic chain via fascial pathways.

When optimal foot positioning is not achieved in these movements, proprioceptive communication and retraining may be compromised (Myers 2009). Positional correction with touch or props (towel) has been observed to optimize proprioception and improve concentration through embodiment (interoception).

> **KEY POINT**
>
> Directed focus or "being present" during the exercises, with attention to every movement detail (Pilates 1945,1998) is regarded a requirement of cognitive learning .This is viewed as contributing to change and remodeling of the neuromyofascial structure and influenced mainly by the interceptive neural communication (Oschman 2003; Myers 2009).

Control or Contrology

Contrology is a term coined by Joseph Pilates to indicate a form of mastery and precision in the smaller, deeper aspect of every movement. Contrology introduces the working of "inner movement" or micromovement. Attention to such detail is believed to stimulate activity on a deeper level where true sensing and connectivity are often lost (Richardson et al. 2004). In this approach, "working in" first rather than working out (superficially) forms the foundation of "core-ability," leading to deep postural support, true strength, and graceful movement.

Precision

Within the Pilates model, striving for the best possible performance renders every movement significant. As each movement is performed with precision, close attention is paid to the physical form, the connectedness and feel of the whole body, which is organized by a mental blueprint of the movement. First-hand observations by the author, and others, indicate that precision might be reinforced by movement imagery. It has been proposed that the union of mental and physical effort stimulates and recovers new neural pathways, a result of neuroplasticity (Doidge 2007).

Centering

In the concept of centering, the following three questions prove significant throughout any movement.
- Where is the movement initiated?
- Where is the movement stabilized ?
- Where is the directional oppositional length-tension (inner tensegrity/preparatory countermovement)?

Centering in Pilates work has become known as core control or movement control (Pilates 1945, 1998; Eien and Friedman 2004; Richardson et al. 2004). Centering involves focus on the development of deep postural endurance leading to core control or "core ability" rather than core strength. Fascial tissue structurally and mechanically differs from muscular tissue in that it is stiffer with less give and therefore reacts through the pull of the attached muscles, contributing to stability of the lumbar spine (Richardson et al. 2004). The Pilates concept of centering may contribute to the prestress theory of tensegrity, where the pull of tension is distributed through all structures surrounding the spine and beyond (Ingber 1998; Myers 2009). This effect is believed to create a more resilient stability model, forming a girdling system (Vleeming 2007) of dynamic support through all movement, omnidirectional.

> **KEY POINTS**
>
> Besides concentration, the following principles are a staple of the Pilates technique.
> - Contrology (coined by J.H. Pilates), an "inner-movement" approach that forms the foundation of "core-ability."
> - Precision, with close attention to the physical form. It has been proposed that the union of mental and physical effort stimulates new neural pathways (Doidge 2007).
> - Centering, currently known as core control or movement control (Pilates 1945, 1998; Eismen and Friedman 2004; Richardson et al. 2004). A new functional model of centering as dynamic support is explained as a "fascial girdling system" (Vleeming 2007).

A Well-Designed Corset of Support

The lumbar fascia does fit this design profile. Current research (Vleeming et al. 2014) revealed a new model of the common tendon of the transversus abdominis (CTrA) that divides the tendon in two, an anterior and a posterior "split" to merge respectively with the medial layer of the lumbar fascia and the posterior layer of the lumbar fascia. This formed (fascial) triangle is referred to as: lumbar inter fascial triangle (LIFT). This model reveals a significant codependent mechanism involving balanced tension between the deep abdominals and lumbar paraspinal muscles.

The LIFT serves as a junction of equal tension between the paraspinal muscles, the TrA, and the internal oblique muscles acting through the CTrA.

KEY POINT

The "girdling system" is a well-designed corset of support. This multilayered fascial system reveals a significant codependent mechanism (LIFT) involving balanced tension between the deep abdominals and the lumbar paraspinal muscles (Vleeming et al. 2014).

CORE ABILITY, A FASCIA-RELATED GIRDLING CONCEPT

This multilayered deep corset functions as a stability amplifier, with feed-forward action that can be learned or relearned with centered "focus." Relearning to connect the corset layers is part of the neural communication skill of the deeper muscles, which is considered to lead to contrology, movement control, and core control—three definitions supporting the same meaning. Within the Pilates paradigm, success in optimizing the full function of the core corset lies in the connection and functional relation of the respiratory system (the diaphragm), the multifidus, and TrA in close synergy with the pelvic floor. In keeping with this new understanding of "girdling," a more functional strategy of core up-training may be in order. A protocol of core up-training is an optimal-aligned, seated position, using tactile and verbal cuing to address multifidus and TrA into coactivation prior to a protocol in the supine position, which may then render embodiment of core ability in supine position more likely. Pilates integrates a specific breathing pattern into the movement repertoire and practices to reinforce this synergy. Breathing and the concept of centering form the underpinnings of core control.

KEY POINT

This multilayered deep corset functions through the LIFT as a stability amplifier. Relearning to connect or to restore the corset layers may offer a new approach of tactile to verbal to neural communication skills achieving "core ability."

THE BREATH IN PILATES

Movement combined with specific integration of the breath is viewed as promoting circulation, oxygenation, and diaphragmatic movement. This concept has been reinforced by accounts of respiratory physiology (Chaitow 2002). It has been proposed that specific and directed integration of breathing with movement can encourage enhanced circulation and elimination of metabolic by-products while promoting connective tissue hydration.

A breath-specific Pilates exercise, The Hundred, is taught in Pilates floor work as first in the sequence of movements. The goal of this supine-positioned exercise is a five-count inhalation followed by a five-count exhalation, performed in a staccato rhythm. This is a sequence of ten, hence the name of this exercise. The upper torso flexes slightly forward to ensure ease in diaphragmatic movement within. Extended legs just clear the floor while the extended arms rhythmically beat within small range. I practice a different version of this classic Pilates exercise and named it "The Inner Hundred." Upper torso passively supported into slight flexion with a pillow. The legs are in hook-lying position, arms are still.

The breathing rhythm here is performed long and smooth. Inhalation over five counts, exhalation over five counts, again the same ten breathing cycles. This enhances and amplifies the movement of the inner respiratory structures and its interconnecting fascia. This variation promotes focus and emphasizes the parasympathetic nervous system.

Instruction on better breathing is a key ingredient to fascial health and health in general. Such instruction is considered to be an important therapeutic tool in Pilates. In support of this position, extensive dissections, specifically directed to the fascial systems, have revealed the significance of the respiratory system via the fascia of the deep front fascial line (Myers 2009). Optimal movement of the breath is visible in the spine and sacrum as a breathing wave, which might also reveal movement stagnation, abnormal movement patterns, or abnormal breathing patterns (Chaitow 2002).

KEY POINT

It has been proposed that specific and directed integration of the breath with movement can encourage enhanced circulation and elimination of metabolic by-products while promoting connective tissue hydration. See the previous description and explanation of the "Inner Hundred," a fascial adaptation of the Pilates breath-specific exercise The Hundred.

WELL-CONNECTED

Starting with the diaphragm, the fascial connections functionally relate the lungs via the parietal pleura and the heart via the pericardium, with the central tendon of the diaphragm.

The crux of the diaphragm below merges with the fascia of the iliopsoas, thereby connecting the diaphragm to the lower quarter and influencing the movement of the hips (walking). The descending psoas then connects its inferomedial fascia with the pelvic floor fascia, linking with the conjoint tendon and internal obliques (Gibbons et al. 2002). This fascial connection links the diaphragm mechanically and functionally to the TrA and the pelvic floor.

The attention to detail and supported alignment, facilitated by Pilates exercises, is viewed as creating the space and length tension of these fascial structures that elongate and decompress through movement of the breath.

From the "Soul" of the Foot to the Core of the Body

The posterior pelvic floor fascial connections form a link via the continuing intramuscular septum of adductor magnus and posterior tibialis into the foot. Here, the fascia aids in load distribution, transmission of forces, and elastic rebound, influencing the postural behavior of the entire body. These fascial connections are materialized and emphasized through specific attention to detail in foot placement during the Pilates footwork and in all foot-supported positions during the work.

biomechanical connection of the foot and the core system of the body.

ALIGNMENT SUPPORT FROM WITHIN

Unlearning poor habits is often more challenging than learning new habits. This problem is particularly true for posture and movement, which require an internal physical sensing or feel for the movement, as well as a feel for positioning. The Pilates perspective proposes that with more refinement a person may also learn to sense the mechanics of the movement. This ability of sensory awareness, or proprioception, is facilitated throughout the body by the highly proprioceptive fascia, among others (Schleip 2003). What is considered important is that feeling is introduced first (i.e., embodiment). Direct observations indicate that such feeling is greatly facilitated by assisting the body in a passive, supported, neutral alignment, which appears by one's own observation to be an essential condition for proprioceptive learning. For example, using a posture support pillow brings the upper body slightly forward, so that the upper and mid back are "opened" to facilitate optimal diaphragmatic excursion and even the smallest space in the lumbar area and the space between the lumbar spine and the floor (when in supine position) are filled, aiming for the passive supported neutral position (Fig. 7.20.3). The author's long-term observations confirm that this passive neutral support can release an otherwise habitual holding pattern and support cognitive learning.

> ### KEY POINT
>
> Intricate and detailed fascial relationships reveal an inner- and interrelationship in function affected by movement (fascial pull) and pressurization through breathing.

These fascial continuities ultimately form a link in function via the intramuscular fascia into the foot (Myers 2009). Specific placement attention through the known Pilates foot and leg sequence awakens these continuities from the bottom upward in the body.

From the "soul" of the foot to the core of the body, is a metaphor created by this author to address the

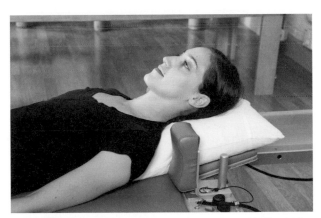

Fig. 7.20.3 A passive supported neutral thoracic positioning, using the SmartSpine Pilates Posture Pillow (www.smartspine.com).

"As Within, So Without": Movement Perceived from the Inside Reflects what Happens on the Outside

Within the Pilates perspective, movement and posture on the outside often reflect a person's internal state. This correspondence relates to the tensional balance of length tension, made continuous via the neuromyofascial system, an omnidirectional fascial system from deep to superficial. Motivating oppositional length tension made visible via the fascial system can provide continuous and dynamic stability in all directions, with optimal mobility and flexibility, very much like a tensegrity system (Fuller 1961). The application of the theory of tensegrity to human anatomy was introduced by Levine (2002), who coined the word biotensegrity, relating the tensegrity concepts to structural integrity in nature, as well as in human movement. Many Pilates movements, with or without equipment support, are performed with the concept of creating space "within" or imagined as creating, moving and shaping space within the body (Fig. 7.20.4).

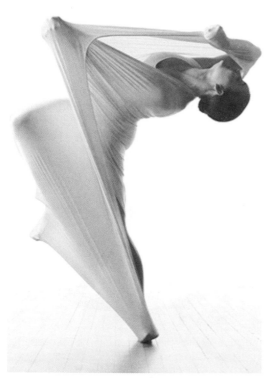

Fig. 7.20.4 This image suggests the internal blueprint of movement, space, and support. ©1992 Lois Greenfield, www. loisgreenfield.com.

Observations indicate that this inner space can be rearranged within the same movement by reversing the breathing pattern and cuing oppositional length tension during the movement. To reinforce the diagonal and tensional connectivity, a light two-point diagonal touch during the movement appears to self-correct and improve innermost movement control.

This Pilates approach to movement is envisioned as a whole body event with an integrated wellness component.

SPECIALIZED EQUIPMENT: REFORMER OR TRANSFORMER

A focal point in the Pilates technique is the designed and technically evolved Pilates equipment, especially the Universal Reformer. The Universal Reformer is a long frame that accommodates a platform that runs in a track. The padded platform is connected by springs to the frame and offers variable resistance. The choice of spring resistance is considered to be particularly appropriate, as the myofascial system behaves similarly to springs. Muscles control and resist deformation resulting from internal and external joint loading, returning to their resting position after lengthening (Richardson et al. 2004). A coiled spring takes time to lengthen and return to its initial position after loading, not unlike the spring-like quality of the muscle. The spring-equipped reformer thus functions as an external coach, guiding internal graduated control. A pulley system is designed to allow for variation, fine-tuning, and integration of proprioceptive challenges using the upper or lower extremities. The equipment is designed to allow the body to be supported in the most productive postural position while introducing movement.

Depending on the movement and the individual, the equipment is intended to function as a tool that can provide more challenge or support for optimal movement learning. The use of variable spring resistance allows for uniform controlled loading, in optimal alignment, through full range of motion of the joint. Direct observations indicate that this resistance offers a similar effect to myofascial tissue release by taking advantage of low load and long duration stress to the fascial tissue via deceleration. In keeping with the Fascia Fitness model, the essential and natural elastic rebound quality of the fascial tissue is a cross-training component in the Pilates technique. A specialized jump board/foot plate attachment facilitates a cross-training such as lower as well as upper body plyometrics that are performed in a variety of arm positions with variable resistance and/or rhythm to address both muscle and fascia during training or conditioning (Larkam 2017).

REFORMER VERSUS MACHINE

The Pilates reformer allows the body to move up through the intended functional sequence, addressing the 3-D neuromyofascial web. As such, Pilates can be used as an exercise modality in the therapeutic environment to mobilize, restore, and stabilize and can be used to remodel fascia to its optimal tension length. On a practical level, the potentiality of the reformer rests in the skills of the teacher, who conveys the process of an exercise, "the how," rather than the event of an exercise, "the what." In the author's experience, teaching the "how" renders the machine a "Reformer" (transforming the body), whereas teaching only the "what" relegates it to remaining a machine creating a robot. Through continued scientific developments, fresh understandings of functional anatomy, removed from compartmentalization in favor of a whole body approach to movement and wellness, have finally emerged in Pilates therapeutic environments (van der Wal 2009).

Summary

Certain cautions and contraindications exist for traditional Pilates. Special care and caution should be taken in cases of:

- Osteoporosis—avoid movements of flexion and flexion/rotation combinations.
- Spinal stenosis—avoid hyperextension and external rotation combination.
- Spondylosis—avoid hyperextension and external rotation combination.
- Idiopathic scoliosis—this requires a specialized approach of curve management, with attention to decompression, balance, and optimal length tension. The modifications needed differ with each individual case and require a well-trained clinical eye.

Any of these potential contraindications may be minimized by positional and postural support, with or without the use of the specialized Pilates equipment, and the changes brought forth by the movement-restoring myofascial continuity. In terms of research and documentation of Pilates technique, its fascial compliancy, and its benefits, commendable progress has been made.

Elizabeth Larkam (2017) researched and authored an extensive body of work in her book *Fascia in Motion: Fascia-focused movement for Pilates.* In her book, Larkam presents and researches all components of the Pilates technique and the individual exercises and protocol with a fascia-focused mind and accordance.

REFERENCES

Beach, P., 2010. Muscles and Meridians: The Manipulation of Shape. Churchill Livingstone, Edinburgh.

Calais-Germaine, B., 2005. Anatomy of Breathing. Editions DesIris, Seattle.

Chaitow, L., 2002. Multidisciplinary Approaches to Breathing Pattern Disorders. Churchill Livingstone.

Doidge, N., 2007. The Brain that Changes Itself. Penguin Group, New York.

Eismen, P., Friedman, G., 2004. The Pilates Method. Warner Books, New York.

Franklin, E., 1996. Dynamic Alignment through Imagery. Human Kinetics, Champaign, IL.

Fuller, R.B., 1961. Tensegrity. Books LLC, Memphis Tennessee, USA.

Gibbons, S., Comerford, M., Emerson, P., 2002. Rehabilitation of the stability function of the psoas major. Orthop. Div. Rev. 7–16.

Huijing, P., Langevin, H., 2009. Communicating about fascia: history, pitfalls and recommendations. Int. J. Ther. Massage Bodywork. 2, 3–8.

Ingber, D., 1998. The Architecture of Life. Scientific American Magazine. January, 278, 48–57.

Iyengar, B., 1966. Light on Yoga. Schocken Books, New York.

Larkam, E., 2010. Heroes In Motion http://www.pilatesmethodalliance.org/heroes" www.pilatesmethodalliance.org/heroes in motion/.

Larkam, E., 2017. Fascia in Motion Fascia-Focused Movement for Pilates. Handspring Publishing, Edinburgh, Scotland.

Levine, S., 2002. The tensegrity-truss as a model for spine mechanics: Biotensegrity. J. Mech. Med. Biol. 2, 375–388.

Myers, T., 2009. Anatomy Trains. Churchill Livingstone, Edinburgh.

Oschman, J., 2003. Energy Medicine in Therapeutics and Human Performance. Butterworth-Heinemann, New York.

Pilates, J.H., March 15, 1927. US Patent 1621477.

Pilates, J.H., 1945, 1998 Return to life through contrology, Reprinted, Pilates Method Alliance, New York.

Redfield, S., 2009. Chasing Joe Pilates. http://www.pilates-pro.com/pilates-pro/2009/10/6/chasing-joe-pilates.html.

Richardson, C., Hodges, P., Hide, J., 2004. Therapeutic Exercises for Lumbopelvic Stabilization. Elsevier, Philadelphia, PA.

Schleip, R., 2003. Fascial plasticity – a new neurobiological explanation. J. Bodyw. Mov. Ther. 7, 11–19.

van der Wal, J., 2009. The architecture of the connective tissue in the musculoskeletal system. Int. J. Ther. Massage Bodywork 2, 9–23.

Vleeming, A., 2007. Movement, Stability and Lumbopelvic Pain. Churchill Livingstone, Edinburgh.

Vleeming, A., Schuenke, M.D., Danneels, L., Willard, F.H., 2014. The functional coupling of the deep abdominal and paraspinal muscles: the effects of simulated paraspinal muscle contraction on force transfer to the middle and posterior layer of the thoracolumbar fascia. J. Anat. 225, 447–462.

Wolff, J., 1986. The Law of Bone Remodeling. Springer, Berlin, Heidelberg, New York.

Nutrition and Fascia: An Antiinflammatory Model

Mary Therese Hankinson and Elizabeth A. Hankinson

CHAPTER CONTENTS

MUSCULOSKELETAL CONDITIONS AND INFLAMMATION

 KEY POINT

Musculoskeletal diseases (MSK) are the leading contributors to global disability across the life course, accounting for 17% of all years lived with disability (YLDs) in 2019. Nutrition offers a nontoxic, long-term approach for management of musculoskeletal conditions by reducing pain and inflammation and supporting optimal musculoskeletal function.

Musculoskeletal diseases (MSK) are the leading contributors to global disability across the life course, accounting for 17% of all years lived with disability (YLDs) in 2019 (Briggs et al 2021). The 2016 global burden of disease (GBD) data identified the profound burden of disease associated with musculoskeletal health. Disability adjusted life years (DALYs) for musculoskeletal conditions increased by 61.6% between 1990 and 2016, with an increase of 19.6% between 2006 and 2016 (Hay et al. 2017). Back pain is the condition causing most disability across the globe. MSK conditions include joint diseases such as osteoarthritis and rheumatoid arthritis; back and neck pain; osteoporosis and fragility fractures; soft tissue rheumatism; injuries due to sports and in the workplace; and trauma commonly related to road traffic accidents. The Global Alliance for Musculoskeletal Health (G-MUSC), formerly known as the Bone and Joint Decade, is an independent global nonprofit organization working to improve the health-related quality of life for people with MSK conditions throughout the world. Many MSK conditions can be effectively prevented and controlled therefore reducing the pain and disability experienced by individuals (Global Alliance for Musculoskeletal Health).

The main feature of osteoarthritis (OA) involves damage to cartilage, a highly specialized connective tissue. Chondrocytes produce inflammatory mediators able to drive cartilage damage and adjacent joint tissue alterations, thus establishing a vicious cycle leading to the progression of OA (Houard et al. 2013). Whatever the primary determinant of OA—aging, genetic predisposition, metabolic syndrome, or trauma—an activation of the inflammatory pathways occurs in cartilage (Berenbaum 2013). Conventional treatment for inflammation includes long-term use of narcotic analgesics, nonsteroidal antiinflammatory drugs (NSAIDS), corticosteroids, and opioid drugs, which have well-established adverse effects and safety risks. Although providing relief from pain, none of these drugs has been shown to inhibit cartilage breakdown or to inhibit the progression of disease; they also potentiate varying degrees of gastrointestinal toxicity, ulcers, and cardiovascular adverse effects (Wang et al. 2015). Novel, safe, and nontoxic anti-OA therapies are needed to retard disease progression at an earlier stage and delay or prevent the need for joint replacement (Rasheed 2016). Nutrition offers a nontoxic long-term approach to chronic disease management, reduces pain and inflammation, and supports optimal musculoskeletal function. Weight loss for treatment of OA results in clinically significant improvements in pain and delays the progression of joint structural damage. Data were obtained from 142 sedentary, overweight, and obese older adults with self-reported disability and radiographic evidence of knee OA who underwent three-dimensional gait analysis. Results indicated that each pound of weight lost results in a four-fold reduction in the load exerted on the knee per step during daily activities (Messier et al. 2005). Weight loss improves inflammation in terms of both the inflammatory (C-reactive protein, TNF-alpha, IL-6 and leptin) and antiinflammatory (adiponectin) obesity-related inflammatory markers (Forsythe et al. 2008).

INFLAMMATORY RESPONSE

KEY POINT

Inflammation contributes to painful and persistent joint damage. The modulation of Nrf2 in response to NF-κB activation can act as a protective mechanism against inflammation. Food and dietary supplements exert a role in Nrf2 activation.

The inflammatory response includes activation of white blood cells and release of immune system chemicals, inflammatory mediators, and prostaglandins. Acute inflammation is the initial response of the body to harmful stimuli mediated by interleukins. Interleukin 1 (IL-1) and interleukin 6 (IL-6) activate neutrophils that recruit macrophages to injured tissue. Neutrophils also release cytotoxic and cytolytic molecules that cause destruction through lysis of muscle cells, fascia, and surrounding tissue. IL-6 contributes to painful and persistent joint

damage and chronic inflammation in rheumatoid arthritis. The most important group controlling OA involves inflammatory cytokines, including IL-1β, TNFα, IL-6, IL-15, IL-17, and IL-18 (Wojdasiewicz et al. 2014). Nuclear factor (erythroid-derived 2)-like 2 (Nrf2) and nuclear factor NF-κB signaling pathways regulate the fine balance of cellular redox status and responses to stress and inflammation. Nuclear factor-κB (NF-κB) serves as a central inflammatory mediator that responds to a large variety of immune receptors and plays a pathogenic role in various inflammatory diseases. Proinflammatory cytokines such as tumor necrosis factor (TNF)α, interleukin (IL)-1β, and bacterial lipopolysaccharide (LPS) are among the most potent NF-κB activators. The modulation of Nrf2 in response to NF-κB activation can act as a protective mechanism against the consequences of inflammation. Intensive research into the antiinflammatory properties of Nrf2 have identified it as a promising strategy for treatment of several inflammatory diseases by blocking NF-κB activity (Wardyn et al. 2015). During the early phase of inflammation-mediated tissue damage, activation of Nrf2 might inhibit the production or expression of proinflammatory mediators including cytokines, chemokines, cell adhesion molecules, matrix metalloproteinases, cyclooxygenase-2 (COX-2), and inducible nitric oxide synthase (iNOS) (Kim et al. 2010). Nrf2 protein remains dormant in a cell until activated by drugs, foods, dietary supplements, or exercise. Sulforaphane found in cruciferous vegetables (broccoli, cabbage, cauliflower, and kale) and curcumin from turmeric root influence Nrf2 activation. Phytochemical components of garlic, tomatoes, grapes, green tea, coffee, and berries have been shown to have Nrf2-activating properties, supporting the possibility that dietary means of Nrf2 activation might be a simple but effective strategy for prevention or treatment of illnesses (Cardozo et al. 2013).

FATTY ACIDS: ANTIINFLAMMATORY PROPERTIES

KEY POINT

Fatty acids influence inflammation through a variety of mechanisms associated with changes to the fatty acid composition of cell membranes. Omega-6 and omega-3 polyunsaturated fatty acids cannot be made by humans and must be derived from diets. Dietary intervention and agricultural practices can be implemented to change the fatty acid composition of inflammatory cells.

Omega-6 and omega-3 polyunsaturated fatty acids (PUFAs) are the two classes of essential fatty acids that must be derived from the diet as they cannot be made by humans, and other mammals, because of the absence of endogenous enzymes for omega-3 desaturation. Omega-6 fatty acids are represented by linoleic acid (LA) and omega-3 fatty acids by alpha-linolenic acid (ALA). Cells involved in the inflammatory response are high in the omega-6 fatty acid arachidonic acid (AA), a precursor for eicosanoid production, present in phospholipids and membranes of the body's cells. Eicosanoid products derived from AA (prostaglandins, prostacyclins, thromboxanes, and leukotrienes) are more potent mediators of inflammation compared with similar products derived from omega-3 (prostaglandin E3 and leukotriene B5) synthesized from eicosapentaenoic acid (EPA). AA is obtained predominantly in the phospholipids from grain-fed animals, dairy, and eggs, or synthesized from LA. LA is found in vegetable oils such as corn, soy, safflower, sunflower, cottonseed, sesame and grape seed, and some nuts and seeds of most plants except for coconut, cocoa, and palm. Polyunsaturated omega-3 fatty acids (PUFAs) include short chain ALA and long-chain molecules, EPA, docosapentaenoic acid (DPA), and docosahexaenoic acid (DHA). ALA is found in the chloroplasts of green leafy vegetables and seeds of flax, rape, chia, perilla, and walnuts. Food sources for long-chain omega-3 fatty acids EPA and DPA include oily fish from cold northern waters, such as salmon, mackerel, sardines, herring, black cod (sable fish or butterfish), fish oil, algae, and DHA-rich eggs (Simopoulos 2016).

Long-chain fatty acids influence inflammation through a variety of mechanisms; many of which are mediated by, or at least associated with, changes in fatty acid composition of cell membranes. AA and omega-3 fatty acids EPA and DHA in cells can be altered through oral administration of EPA and DHA. EPA and DHA increase newly discovered resolvins, which are antiinflammatory and inflammation resolving. Changing the fatty acid composition of inflammatory cells affects production of peptide mediators of inflammation such as cytokines (Calder 2010). Long-chain omega-3 fatty acids oppose inflammation by competing with AA for conversion to proinflammatory cytokines IL-1 and TNFα and compete with COX and lipoxygenase (LOX) enzymes that are upregulated in the inflammatory process. PUFAs, especially total omega-3 fatty acids, are

independently associated with lower levels of proinflammatory markers (IL-6, IL-1ra, TNFα, CRP) and higher levels of antiinflammatory markers (soluble IL-6r, IL-10, transforming growth factor beta TGF-β) independent of confounders, supporting the opinion that omega-3 fatty acids are beneficial in treating diseases characterized by active inflammation (Ringbom et al. 2001).

Western diets are deficient in omega-3 fatty acids and have excessive amounts of omega-6 fatty acids compared with the diet on which human beings evolved and genetic patterns established. Agribusiness and modern agriculture have resulted in Western diets that contain excessive levels of omega-6 PUFAs but very low levels of omega-3 PUFAs, leading to an unhealthy omega-6/omega-3 ratio of 20:1, instead of 1:1 present during human evolution. Modern agriculture practices include changing animal feeds that decrease the omega-3 fatty acid content of animal meats and eggs; aquaculture that produces fish with less omega-3 than fish grown naturally in ocean, rivers, and lakes. Foods from edible wild plants contain a good balance of omega-6 and omega-3 fatty acids. Purslane, an edible wild plant, provides higher amounts of alpha-linolenic acid, antioxidant vitamins C and E, and phenolic compounds compared with cultivated plants (spinach, red leaf lettuce, buttercrunch lettuce and mustard greens) (Simopoulos 2004). Strategies to decrease omega-6 fatty acids include changing dietary vegetable oils high in omega-6 fatty acids to oils high in omega 3s; increasing ingestion of monounsaturated oils such as olive oil, macadamia nut oil, hazelnut oil, or the new high monounsaturated sunflower oil; and increasing fish intake to 2 to 3 times per week while decreasing meat intake (Simoupoulos 2016).

Excess consumption of saturated fatty acids such as palmitic and stearic increases inflammatory signaling through activation of macrophages, neutrophils, and bone marrow-derived dendritic cells, leading to inflammation, impaired insulin signaling, and insulin resistance in white adipose tissue and muscle (Kennedy et al. 2009). Trans-fatty acids are unnatural fat species formed after hydrogenation from naturally occurring cis–fatty acids in margarines and shortenings.

In cross-sectional studies, intake of industrially produced trans-fatty acids (IP-TFA) is positively associated with systemic concentrations of various inflammatory markers such as C-reactive protein (CRP), tumor necrosis factor (TNF) α, and interleukin (IL) 6

(Mozaffarian et al. 2004; Lopez-Garcia et al. 2005). Similar associations with inflammatory markers were associated with intake of partially hydrogenated vegetable oil, which is the primary source of IP-TFA (Esmaillzadeh and Azadbakht 2004).

FATTY ACID DIETARY SUPPLEMENTS

 KEY POINT

Marine n-3 fatty acids (fish oils), avocado/soybean unsaponifiables (ASU), and gamma-linolenic acid (GLA) are associated with treatment of musculoskeletal conditions. The antiinflammatory mechanisms associated with these fatty acid dietary supplements include the decreased production of proinflammatory cytokines and other proinflammatory proteins induced via the NF-κB system and protection against cartilage degeneration. Suggestions are provided for consumers to investigate product information and consult with providers to prevent adverse side effects.

The antiinflammatory effects of marine n-3 fatty acids (fish oils) decreases production of proinflammatory cytokines and other proinflammatory proteins induced via the NF-κB system (Calder 2010). Patients (n = 250) diagnosed with nonsurgical neck or back pain were asked to take 1200 mg per day of ω-3 EFAs (eicosapentaenoic acid and docosahexaenoic acid) found in fish oil supplements. Results demonstrated the use of ω-3 EFA fish oil supplements appear to be a safer alternative to NSAIDs for treatment of nonsurgical neck or back pain in this selective group as sixty percent reported an improvement in overall pain and joint pain with no significant side effects (Maroon and Bost 2006).

Concentrated omega-3 fatty acids found in fish oil supplements offer benefits associated with fish consumption without exposure to harmful environmental toxins such as mercury, polychlorinated biphenyls (PCB), and organochlorine (OC) that can accumulate in fish. Consumers should investigate product information from companies who manufacture fish oil supplements regarding those who employ sustainable fishing practices, molecular distillation to minimize mercury and other toxins, content labeling to identify omega-3, potential for contamination, and product storage.

Schizochytrium microalgae is a DHA-rich fish oil alternative containing small amounts of EPA and negligible AA. Neptune krill oil (NKO) is a phospholipid carrier of omega-3 fatty acids EPA and DHA and includes antioxidants, astaxanthin, and a flavonoid, offering an alternative regimen for management of chronic inflammatory conditions. NKO is extracted from Antarctic krill (*Ephausia superba*), a zooplankton at the bottom of the food chain. Ingestion of NKO at a daily dose of 300 mg significantly inhibits inflammation and reduces arthritic symptoms within 7 to 14 days (Deutsch 2007). Patients should consult with healthcare providers because fish oil supplements taken at certain dosages can cause inhibition of platelet aggregation and require monitoring for patients on anticoagulant drugs and aspirin or impending surgery.

Avocado/soybean unsaponifiables (ASU) contain sterols that are antiinflammatory and provide protection against cartilage degeneration. The biologically active compounds found in avocado and soybean oils are classified as unsaponifiable lipids and include phytosterols beta-sitosterol, campesterol, and stigmasterol (Lippiello et al. 2008). ASU modulates osteoarthritis (OA) pathogenesis by inhibiting several molecules and pathways implicated in OA, including inflammatory cytokines such as interleukin (IL)-1, IL-6, IL-8, tumor necrosis factor, and prostaglandin E2. Other benefits from ASU include reduction of pain and stiffness while improving joint function, resulting in decreased dependence on analgesics (Christiansen et al. 2015). Several clinical trials have confirmed that gamma-linolenic acid (GLA), an omega-6 fatty acid found in borage seed oil, evening primrose oil, and blackcurrant oil, reduces inflammation, tender joint scores, morning stiffness, and requirement for NSAIDs (Kapoor and Huang 2006).

CULINARY SPICES AND HERBS

 KEY POINT

Culinary spices and herbs modulate inflammation through a multitude of pathways versus inhibition of a single enzyme along the inflammatory cascade. Table 7.21.1 provides the antiinflammatory components and associated pathways for numerous culinary spices and herbs.

The health benefits associated with herbs and spices require identification of specific bioactive substances that oppose inflammation. Unlike their pharmaceutical

TABLE 7.21.1 Culinary Herbs and Spices: Antiinflammatory Properties

Culinary Herbs/Spices and Botanical Name	Antiinflammatory Components	Antiinflammatory Properties
Red pepper: chilli, cayenne pepper, pimiento, cherry pepper (*Capsicum frutescens*)	Capsaicin	Potent inhibitor of substance P, neuropeptide associated with inflammatory processes and pain transmission
Ginger (*Zingiber officinale*)	Gingerol Paradol Zingerone	Inhibits COX-1, COX-2, 5-LOX, TNFα, interleukin-1β; suppresses prostaglandin and leukotriene biosynthesis; upregulates NrF2 pathway
Turmeric (*Curcuma longa*)	Curcumin	Inhibits COX-2; upregulates NrF2 pathway; downregulates NF-kB and TNFα
Rosemary (*Rosmarinus officinalis*)	Carnosol Rosmarinic acid Ursolic acid	Decreases inflammatory cytokines, chemokines, and TNFα; suppresses nuclear factor-kappa B (NF-kB)
Clove (*Syzygium aromaticum*)	Carvacrol Thymol Eugenol Cinnamaldehyde	Inhibits COX 1, COX-2, 5-LOX, TNFα, and interleukin-1β
Nutmeg (*Myristica fragrans*)	Myristicin Eugenol	Inhibits TNFα and prostaglandin production
Cinnamon (*Cinnamomum zeylanicum*)	Eugenol Humulene Cinnamaldehyde	Inhibits COX-1, COX-2, 5-LOX, TNFα, and interleukin-1β
Thyme	Ursolic acid	Suppresses nuclear factor-kappa B (NF-kB); inhibits TNFα
Marjoram	Ursolic acid	Suppresses nuclear factor-kappa B (NF-kB)
Oregano	Ursolic acid	Suppresses nuclear factor-kappa B (NF-kB); inhibits TNFα

counterparts, many plants modulate inflammation via a multitude of pathways versus inhibition of a single enzyme along the inflammatory cascade. Ursolic acid (UA) is a natural triterpene compound isolated from the leaves of various plants (rosemary, marjoram, lavender, thyme, and oregano), vegetables, and fruits (berries and apple fruit). UA exerts antiinflammatory effects through suppression of nuclear factor-kappa B (NF-κB) signaling in various tissues and organs (Seo et al. 2018). Antiinflammatory actions are reported for spices and herbs including ginger, turmeric, saffron, curcumin, bromelain, German chamomile, licorice, and capsaicin ginger have been used to treat arthritis since ancient times (Tapsell et al. 2006; Aggarwal et al. 2009; Seo et al. 2018). Patients should consult with healthcare providers regarding herb ingestion, as large doses can be toxic, promote adverse medical consequences, or interfere with medications (see Table 7.21.1).

FRUITS AND VEGETABLES

KEY POINT

Plant-based foods contain phytochemicals such as carotenoids and flavonoids that exert antioxidant and antiinflammatory properties, decreasing the risk of chronic diseases. Table 7.21.2 provides the antiinflammatory components and associated pathways for numerous fruits and vegetables.

Plant-based foods contain phytochemicals such as carotenoids and flavonoids that exert antioxidant and antiinflammatory properties, decreasing the risk of chronic diseases. Flavonoids are responsible for the deep color of fruits and vegetables, which is concentrated in skins and peels. Several mechanisms have been proposed to explain the in-vivo antiinflammatory action of

TABLE 7.21.2 Fruits and Vegetables: Antiinflammatory Properties

Food/Botanical Name	Phytochemicals	Antiinflammatory Properties
Garlic (Allium sativum)	Ajoene and allicin	Inhibits TNFα and inflammatory interleukins
Allium family: onions, garlic, green onions, leeks, shallots, and chives Apples, broccoli, berries, parsley, grapes	Flavones: quercetin	Inhibits COX and 5-LOX pathways; reduces release of arachidonic acid; downregulates NF-kB and TNFα; upregulates NrF2 pathway
Cruciferous vegetables such as broccoli, cabbage, cauliflower, and kale	Sulforaphane	Upregulates NrF2 pathway; downregulates NF-kB and TNFα
Citrus fruit and peel	Flavanones	Inhibits eicosanoid biosynthesis
Guavas, red (cooked) tomatoes, watermelon, pink grapefruit, papaya, sweet red peppers, persimmon, asparagus, red cabbage, and mangos and other red fruit and vegetables	Carotenoids: lycopene	Limits inflammatory damages; upregulates NrF2 pathway
Broccoli, Brussels sprouts, cabbage, and cauliflower	Indoles and isothiocyanates	Enhances downregulation of inducible nitric oxide synthase, COX-2, and TNFα expression
Berries, cherries, red grapes, pomegranate, eggplant	Anthocyanins	Inhibits eicosanoid biosynthesis
Berries (raspberries, strawberries, blackberries, cranberries), grapes, pomegranate, guava	Ellagic acid Ursolic acid	Upregulates NrF2 pathway; suppresses nuclear factor-kappa B (NF-kB)
Apple fruit peel	Ursolic acid	Suppresses nuclear factor-kappa B (NF-kB)

flavonoids. One mechanism involves inhibition of eicosanoid-generating enzymes such as phospholipase A_2, COX, and LOX, which reduce concentrations of prostaglandins and leukotrienes. Some flavonoids, especially flavone derivatives, express their antiinflammatory activity at least in part by modulation of proinflammatory gene expression for COX-2, iNOS, and several pivotal cytokines (Havsteen 2002; Kim et al. 2004). Researchers have shown that a standardized pomegranate fruit extract (PFE) is highly effective for OA management, as PFE exerts human cartilage-sparing effects and is nontoxic to human cartilage cells (Akhtar and Haqqi 2012; Zafar et al. 2009). Crude extract of blueberries (*Vaccinium corymalosum*) is rich in phenolic acids, flavonoids, and anthocyanins, displaying antinociceptive and antiinflammatory activity, which may be helpful in the treatment of inflammatory disorders (Torri et al. 2007). Dietary antioxidants, such as the carotenoids betacryptoxanthin and zeaxanthin, in addition to vitamin C, protect against the development of inflammatory polyarthritis. A modest increase in β-cryptoxanthin (carotenoid) intake equivalent to one glass of freshly squeezed orange juice per day is associated with a reduced risk of

developing inflammatory disorders such as rheumatoid arthritis (Pattison et al. 2005). Bromelain, an aqueous extract obtained from both the stem and fruit of the pineapple plant, contains several proteolytic enzymes associated with antiinflammatory and analgesic properties demonstrated in clinical osteoarthritis trials (Brien et al. 2004) (see Table 7.21.2).

BEVERAGES: GREEN TEA AND EPIGALLOCATECHIN-3-GALLATE

 KEY POINT

Epigallocatechin-3-gallate (EGCG) is the most abundant of the polyphenolic compounds found in green tea. Studies demonstrate EGCG is nontoxic to human OA chondrocytes and exerts cartilage-preserving and chondroprotective activities by blocking proinflammatory events.

Tea contains catechin, a polyphenolic antioxidant plant metabolite that quenches free radicals, protects against oxidative cell damage, and demonstrates other health benefits in vitro and in vivo. Green tea (*Camellia sinensis*) polyphenols such as epicatechin, epigallocatechin, epicatechin-3-gallate, and epigallocatechin-3-gallate are potent antioxidants. Epigallocatechin-3-gallate (EGCG) is the most abundant of the polyphenolic compounds, accounts for 30% to 40% of the dry weight of green tea, and possesses the greatest antioxidant activity (Sutherland et al. 2006). Studies demonstrate EGCG is nontoxic to human OA chondrocytes and exerts cartilage-preserving and chondroprotective activities by blocking proinflammatory events. EGCG inhibits the IL-1β-induced expression of iNOS and production of nitric oxide (NO) by inhibiting the activation of NF-κB inflammatory signaling events in human OA chondrocytes. Additionally, EGCG also inhibits excessive production of prostaglandin E_2 (PGE_2) by blocking of COX-2 activity in human chondrocytes. Furthermore, a wide range of biological effects of EGCG has also been reported that provide evidence of EGCG-induced protective effects on OA cartilage via blocking of various proinflammatory events (Rasheed 2016).

The amount of green tea consumption required to achieve an antiinflammatory response is difficult to quantify because of inconsistent catechin values in various brands and differences in reported product purity (Sutherland et al. 2006).

GLUTEN AND INFLAMMATION

 KEY POINT

Zonulin is a protein that modulates intestinal permeability. Key ingredients in the pathogenesis of inflammation, autoimmunity, and cancer involve disregulation of the zonulin pathway in genetically susceptible individuals, loss of intestinal barrier function through zonulin pathway activation by food-derived environmental triggers and changes in gut microbiota. After removal of gluten from the diet, serum zonulin levels decrease, the autoimmune process shuts off, and small intestine resumes baseline barrier function.

An important function of the gastrointestinal tract is to regulate the transfer of macromolecules between the environmental host through a barrier mechanism. Zonulin, a protein synthesized in intestinal and liver cells, is the physiological modulator of intercellular

tight junctions that regulates intestinal permeability. Key ingredients in the pathogenesis of inflammation, autoimmunity, and cancer involve disregulation of the zonulin pathway in genetically susceptible individuals, loss of intestinal barrier function through zonulin pathway activation by food-derived environmental triggers and changes in gut microbiota. The gliadin fraction of wheat gluten and alcohol-soluble proteins of barley and rye in genetically susceptible individuals leads to small bowel inflammation as the immune system perceives gluten as a foreign substance. After removal of gluten from the diet, serum zonulin levels decrease, the small intestine resumes its baseline barrier function, autoantibody titers are normalized, autoimmune process shuts off, and intestinal damage heals completely (Fasano 2011).

Fibromyalgia (FM) is a commonly recognized syndrome characterized by musculoskeletal pain, sleep disturbance, and fatigue combined with a general increase in medical symptoms (memory problems, thought processes, and psychological distress). Gluten sensitivity that does not fulfill the diagnostic criteria for celiac disease (CD) is increasingly recognized as a frequent and treatable condition with a wide spectrum of manifestations that overlap with the manifestations of FM, including chronic musculoskeletal pain. In one study, patients with severe longstanding FM and duodenal intraepithelial lymphocytosis, in whom CD was ruled out, followed a gluten-free diet. Results demonstrated a reduction in the level of pain and improvements in asthenia and gastrointestinal and neurological symptoms, suggesting a common underlying cause related to gluten (Isasi et al. 2014).

NUTRITION: AN ANTIINFLAMMATORY MODEL

 KEY POINT

The "perfect diet" for decreasing inflammation requires additional evidence-based research. Studies demonstrate that adherence to a Mediterranean-type diet and gluten-free diet can reduce inflammation. The antiinflammatory nutrition model (Fig. 7.21.1) offers a comprehensive approach, using knowledge of nutrigenomics, biochemistry, and culinary arts as an integrative health approach to reduce inflammation in clinical practice.

An antiinflammatory nutrition approach provides a natural and nonpharmacological approach for decreasing pain and inflammation associated with chronic musculoskeletal diseases. Nutrition might also be an aid in improving bone and cartilage structure and function, and in immune modulation (Iolascon et al. 2017). The holistic and natural approach afforded by whole food becomes less natural and less safe when specific nutrients are isolated, packaged, and sold as a single antiinflammatory product. The "perfect diet" for chronic low-grade inflammation is still unclear and additional evidence-based research is warranted. Antiinflammatory diets emphasize plant-based foods including adequate fruit and vegetables; omega-3 fatty acids such as fish, fish oil supplements, and walnuts; whole grains; lean protein; reduction in saturated fatty acids; elimination of trans-fatty acids and refined and processed foods; consumer alcohol in moderation; and a variety of spices, especially ginger and curry (Marcason 2010).

Adherence to a Mediterranean-type diet, determined by a simple questionnaire of 14 questions, was inversely related to CRP levels. Lower levels of CRP were associated with a greater consumption of some typical components of Mediterranean diet (vegetables, fruits, and fish) and dairy products. In a systematic review of 52 clinical trials investigating inflammatory markers in relation to the consumption of dairy products, researchers suggested that dairy products, in particular fermented products, have antiinflammatory properties in humans not suffering from allergy to milk, in particular in subjects with metabolic disorders (Bordoni et al. 2017; Lahoz et al. 2018). Reduced concentrations of inflammatory markers were reported for individuals who adhere to the traditional Mediterranean diet that is abundant in olive oil (Chrysohoou et al. 2004). Oleocanthal, a compound found in olive oil, prevents the production of proinflammatory COX-1 and COX-2 enzymes similarly to the mechanism of action for NSAIDs, decreasing inflammation and pain sensitivity. The highest oleocanthal levels are found in stronger-flavored oils from Tuscany and regions using the same olive varietal. The consumption of 50 mL (3.5 tbsp) of olive oil is equivalent to 200 mg ibuprofen. Weight management is required if olive oil is used as a nutritional intervention to enhance antiinflammatory properties, as 50 mL olive oil ($\approx$400 kcal) yields a high caloric density (Beauchamp et al. 2005).

Adherence to a gluten-free diet offers the potential to decrease inflammation in individuals with gluten sensitivity and associated musculoskeletal pain. Gluten is a glue-like protein found in grains such as wheat, barley, pasta, beer, pastries, and cereals. When water and flour are mixed, the hydration proteins, glutenin and gliadin, form a very elastic substance that is a commodity food ingredient used in baked goods and processed meat products. Wheat gluten can also be processed into texturized vegetable protein for meat application.

Nutritional education and counseling enhance consumer competency related to food purchasing, storage, preparation and enrichment, modifications for various food cultures, dietary restrictions, and allergic reactions. Dietary fats and oils must be properly stored to prevent lipid peroxidation (rancidity) or chemical decomposition, which can promote inflammation, premature aging, and degenerative changes in cells and tissues. Heat and light accelerate oxidation of fats and oils; however, the rate of rancidification can be decreased by refrigeration, or storage in a cool, dark place with little exposure to oxygen or free radicals. Although the omega-3 fatty acid content of farm-raised and wild salmon is nearly equivalent, the higher overall fat content of farm-raised salmon increases exposure to a higher level of PCB contamination. PCB exposure can be reduced by trimming the fat on fish and using dry cooking methods, which enable the PCB content in fat to dissipate.

Although ALA intakes of vegetarians and vegans are similar to those of nonvegetarians, dietary intakes of long-chain n-3 fatty acids EPA and DHA are lower in vegetarians and typically absent in vegans. The clinical relevance of reduced EPA and DHA status among vegetarians and vegans is unknown. ALA is endogenously converted to EPA and DHA, but the process is somewhat inefficient and affected by sex, dietary composition, health status, and age. High intakes of LA may suppress ALA conversion. A ratio of LA/ALA not exceeding 4:1 has been suggested for optimal conversion. The Dietary Reference Intake for ALA is 1.6 g/day and 1.1 g/day for men and women, respectively. For vegetarians and vegans, it may be prudent to ensure higher intakes of ALA. Low-dose microalgae-based DHA supplements are available for all vegetarians with increased needs (e.g. pregnant or lactating women) or with reduced conversion ability (e.g., those with hypertension or diabetes) (Saunders et al. 2013; Sarter et al. 2015; The Academy of Nutrition and Dietetics 2016).

The antiinflammatory nutrition model (Fig. 7.21.1) offers a comprehensive approach, using knowledge of

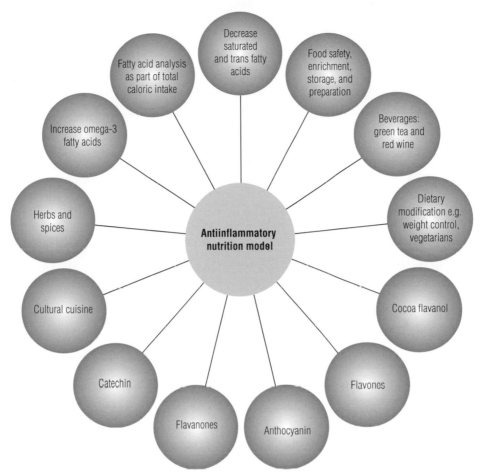

Fig. 7.21.1 Antiinflammatory nutrition model. The antiinflammatory nutrition model offers a comprehensive approach to using knowledge of nutrigenomics, biochemistry, and culinary arts as an integrative health approach to reduce inflammation in clinical practice.

nutrigenomics, biochemistry, and culinary arts as an integrative health approach to reduce inflammation in clinical practice. Nutrigenomics investigates how nutrients and bioactive compounds in food interacts with our genes to affect health. A key component of the antiinflammatory model includes culinary arts or skills required for the preparation, cooking, and presentation of food. The term "culinary genomics" is the revolutionary union of genomics and nutrition science (nutritional genomics) with the culinary arts. Culinary genomics is the art of choosing, preparing, and cooking ingredients in a language recognized by your DNA with the goal of reducing the primary causes of chronic disease and

accelerated aging (Archibald 2019). Antiinflammatory mechanisms associated with culinary genomics target CRP, TNFα, and IL6/6R cascade. A genomic intervention to reduce inflammation includes the balance of omega-3; omega-6; upregulation of NrF2 through quercetin and sulforaphane; and downregulation of NF-kB and TNF-α through curcumin and quercetin.

General recommendations for increasing specific food groups such as fruits and vegetables may not assure a clinical response because of molecular and pharmacological variances of antiinflammatory components. Fruit and plant extracts are a complex mixture of various constituents; however, it is not clear whether a single compound or mixture of compounds is responsible for the antiinflammatory response. Ellagic acid and quercetin, which are both found in pomegranate, exert a more pronounced effect against cancer than either compound alone (Seeram et al. 2005).

REFERENCES

Aggarwal, B., Van Kuiken, M., Iyer, L., Harikumar, K.B., Sung, B., 2009. Molecular targets of nutraceuticals derived from dietary spices: potential role in suppression of inflammation and tumorigenesis. Exp. Biol. Med. 234, 825–849.

Akhtar, N., Haqqi, T.M., 2012. Current nutraceuticals in the management of osteoarthritis: a review. Ther. Adv. Musculoskelet. Dis. 4, 181–207.

Archibald, A., 2021. The Genomic Kitchen, Your Guide to Understanding and Using the Food-Gene Connection for a Lifetime of Health. Available from: https://www.genomickitchen.com/culinary-genomics.

Beauchamp, G.K., Keast, R., Morel, D., et al., 2005. Ibuprofen-like activity in extra-virgin olive oil. Nature 437, 45–46.

Berenbaum, F., 2013. Osteoarthritis as an inflammatory disease (osteoarthritis is not osteoarthrosis!) Osteoarthritis Cartilage 21, 16–21.

Bordoni A., Danesi F., Dardevet D., et al., 2017. Dairy products and inflammation: a review of the clinical evidence. Crit. Rev. Food Sci. Nutr. 57, 2497–2525.

Brien, S., Lewith, G., Walker, A., Hicks, S.M., Middleton, D., 2004. Bromelain as a treatment for osteoarthritis: a review of clinical studies. Evid. Based Complement. Alternat. Med. 1, 251–257.

Briggs, A.M., Slater, H., Jordan, J.E., et al., 2021. Towards a global strategy to improve musculoskeletal health. Global Alliance for Musculoskeletal Health, Sydney, Australia. Global Alliance for Musculoskeletal Health. https://gmusc.com/wp-content/uploads/2021/07/Final-report-with-metadata.pdf.

Calder, P., 2010. Omega-3 fatty acid and inflammatory processes. Nutrients. Mar. 2, 355–374.

Cardozo L.F., Pedruzzi L.M., Stenvinkel, P., et al., 2013. Nutritional strategies to modulate inflammation and oxidative stress pathways via activation of the master antioxidant switch Nrf2. Biochimie 95, 1525–1533.

Christiansen, B., Bhatti, S., Goudarzi, R., Emami, S., (2015). Management of osteoarthritis with avocado/soybean unsaponifiables. Cartilage 6, 30–44.

Chrysohoou, C., Panagiotakos, B., Pitsavos, C., Das, U.N., Stefanadis, C., 2004. Adherence to the Mediterranean Diet attenuates inflammation and coagulation process in healthy adults: The ATTICA Study. J. Am. Coll. Cardiol. 44, 152–158.

Deutsch, L., 2007. Evaluation of the effect of Neptune Krill Oil on chronic inflammation and arthritic symptoms. J. Am. Coll. Nutr. 26, 39–48.

Esmaillzadeh, A., Azadbakht, L., 2004. Home use of vegetables oils, markers of systemic inflammation and endothelial dysfunction among women. Am. J. Clin. Nutr. 88, 913–921.

Fasano, A., 2011. Zonulin and its regulation of intestinal barrier function: the biological door to inflammatory, autoimmunity and cancer. Physiol. Rev. 91, 151–175.

Forsythe, L.K., Wallace, J.M., Livingstone, B.E., 2008. Obesity and inflammation: the effects of weight loss. Nutr. Res. Rev. 21, 117–133.

Global Alliance for Musculoskeletal Health. Available from: https://gmusc.com/.

Havsteen, B.H., 2002. The biochemistry and medical significance of the flavonoids. Pharmacol. Ther. 96, 67–202.

Hay, S.I., Abajobir, A.A., Abate, K.H., GBD 2016 DALYs and HALE Collaborators. 2017. Global, regional, and national disability-adjusted life-years (DALYs) for 333 diseases and injuries and healthy life expectancy (HALE) for 195 countries and territories, 1990-2016: a systematic analysis for the Global Burden of Disease Study 2016. Lancet 390, 1260–1344.

Houard, X., Goldring, M., Berenbaum, F., 2013. Homeostatic mechanisms in articular cartilage and role of inflammation in osteoarthritis. Curr. Rheumatol. Rep. 15, 375–376.

Iolascon, G., Gimigliano, R., Bianco, M. et al., 2017. Are dietary supplements and nutraceuticals effective for musculoskeletal health and cognitive function? A scoping review. J. Nutr. Health Aging 21, 527–538.

Isasi, C., Colmenero, T., Casco, F., et al., 2014. Fibromyalgia and non-celiac gluten sensitivity: a description with remission of fibromyalgia. Rheumatol. Int. 34, 1607–1612.

Kapoor, R., Huang, Y.S., 2006. Gamma linolenic acid: an antiinflammatory omega-6 fatty acid. Curr. Pharm. Biotechnol. 7, 531–534.

Kennedy, A., Martinez, K., Chuang, C., LaPoint, K., McIntosh, M., 2009. Saturated fatty acid-mediated inflammation and insulin resistance in adipose tissue: mechanisms of action and implications. J. Nutr. 139, 1–4.

Kim, H., Son, K.H., Chang, H.W., Kang, S.S., 2004. Antiinflammatory plant flavonoids and cellular action mechanisms. J. Pharmacol. Sci. 96, 229–245.

Kim, J., Young-Nam, C., Young-Joon, S., 2010. A Protective role of nuclear factor-erythroid 2-related factor-2 (Nrf2) in inflammatory disorders. Mutat. Res. 690, 12–23.

Lahoz, C., Castillo, E., Mostaza, J., et al. 2018. Relationship of the adherence to a Mediterranean Diet and its main components with CRP levels in the Spanish population. Nutrients 10, 379.

Lippiello, L., Nardo, J., Harlan, R., Chiou, T., 2008. Metabolic effects of avocado/soy unsaponifiables on articular chondrocytes. Evid. Based Complement. Alternat. Med. 5, 191–197.

Lopez-Garcia E., Schulze M. B., Meigs J. B., et al., 2005. Consumption of trans fatty acids is related to plasma biomarkers of inflammation and endothelial dysfunction. J. Nutr. 135, 562–566

Marcason, W., 2010. What is the antiinflammatory diet? J. Acad. Nutr. Diet. 110, 11, 1780.

Maroon, J.C., Bost, J.W., 2006. Omega-3 fatty acids (fish oil) as an antiinflammatory: an alternative to nonsteroidal antiinflammatory drugs for discogenic pain. Surg. Neurol. 65, 326–331

Messier, S., Gutekunst, D., Davis, C., DeVita, P., 2005. Weight loss reduces knee-joint loads in overweight and obese older adults with knee osteoarthritis. Arthritis Rheum. 52, 2026–2032.

Mozaffarian, D., Pischon, T.T., Hankinson, S.E., et al., 2004. Dietary intake of trans fatty acids and systemic inflammation in women. Am. J. Clin. Nutr. 79, 606 612.

Pattison, D., Symmons, D., Lunt, M., et al., 2005. Dietary beta cryptoxanthin and inflammatory polyarthritis: results from a population-based prospective study. Am. J. Clin. Nutr. 82, 451–455.

Rasheed, Z., 2016. Green tea bioactive polyphenol epigallocatechin-3-O-gallate in osteoarthritis: Current status and future perspectives. Int. J. Health Sci. (Qassim) 10, V–VIII.

Ringbom, T., Huss, U., Stenhold, A., et al., 2001. Cox-2 inhibitory effects of naturally occurring and modified fatty acids. J. Nat. Prod. 64, 745–749.

Saunders, A.V., Davis, B.C., Garg, M.I., 2013. Omega-3 polyunsaturated fatty acids and vegetarian diets. Med. J. Aust. 199, S22 S26.

Sarter, B., Kelsey, K.S., Schwartz, T.A., Harris, W.S., 2015. Blood docosahexaenoic acid and eicosapentaenoic acid in vegans: associations with age and gender and effects of an algal-derived omega-3 fatty acid supplement. Clin. Nutr. 34, 212–218.

Seeram, N.P., Adams, L.S., Henning, S.M., et al., 2005. In vitro antiproliferative apoptotic and antioxidant activities of pugicalaginellagic acid and a total pomegranate tannin extract are enhanced in combination with other polyphenols as food in pomegranate juice. J. Nutr. Biochem. 16, 360–367.

Seo, D., Lee, S., Heo, J., et al., 2018. Ursula acid in health and disease. Ursolic J. Physiol. Pharmacol. 22, 235–248.

Simopoulos, A., 2004.Omega-3 fatty acids and antioxidants in edible wild plants. Biol. Res. 37, 263–277.

Simopoulos, A., 2016. An increase in the Omega-6/Omega-3 fatty acid ratio increases the risk for obesity. Nutrients 8, 128–134.

Sutherland, B., Rahman, R., Appleton, I., 2006. Mechanisms of action of green tea catechins with a focus on ischemia-induced neurodegeneration. J. Nutr. Biochem. 17, 291–306.

Tapsell, L.C., Hemphill, I., Cobiac, L., et al., 2006. Health benefits of herbs and spices: the past, the present, the future. Med. J. Aust. 185, S1–S24.

The Academy of Nutrition and Dietetics, 2016. Position of the American Academy of Nutrition and Dietetics: vegetarian diets. J. Acad. Nutr. Diet. 116, 1970–1980.

Torri, E., Lemos, M., Caliari, V., Kassuya, C.A., Bastos, J.K., Andrade, S.F., 2007. Antiinflammatory and antinociceptive properties of blueberry extract (Vaccinium corymbosum). J. Pharm. Pharmacol. 59, 591–596.

Wang, K., Xu, J., Hunter, D.J., Ding, C., 2015. Investigational drugs for the treatment of osteoarthritis. Expert. Opin. Investig. Drugs 24, 1539–1556.

Wardyn, J., Ponsford, A., Sanderson, C., 2015. Dissecting molecular cross-talk between Nrf2 and NF-kB response pathways. Biochem. Soc. Trans. 43, 621–626.

Wojdasiewicz, P., Poniatowski, L., Szukiewicz, D., 2014. The role of inflammatory and antiinflammatory cytokines in the pathogenesis of osteoarthritis. Mediators Inflamm. 2014, 1–19.

Zafar, R., Akhtar, N., Anbahagan, A., et al., 2009. Polyphenol-rich pomegranate fruit extract (OMx) suppresses PMACI-induced expression of proinflammatory cytokines by inhibiting the activation of MAP Kinases and NF-kB in human KU812 cells. J. Inflamm. 2009, (Online) Available from: http://www.journal-inflammation.com/content/6/1/1.

BIBLIOGRAPHY

Magesh, S., Chen, Y., Hu, L., 2012. Small molecule modulators of Keap1-Nrf2-ARE pathway as potential preventive and therapeutic agents. Med. Res. Rev. 32, 687–726.

Fascial Fitness: Suggestions for a Fascia-Oriented Training Approach in Sports and Movement Therapies

Robert Schleip, Divo G. Müller, and Katja Bartsch

CHAPTER CONTENTS

INTRODUCTION

Whenever a football player is not able to take the field because of a recurrent calf spasm, a tennis star gives up early on a match because of knee problems, or a sprinter limps across the finish line with a torn Achilles tendon, the problem is most often neither in the musculature nor the skeleton. Instead, it is the structure of the connective tissue—ligaments, tendons, joint capsules, etc.—that has been loaded beyond its capacity (Wilke et al. 2019). A focused training of the fascial network could be of great importance for athletes, dancers, and other movement advocates. If one's fascial body is well-trained, that is to say optimally elastic and resilient, then it can be relied on to perform effectively and at the same time to offer a high degree of injury prevention (Kjaer et al. 2009). Until now, most of the emphasis in sports has been focused on the classic triad of muscular strength, cardiovascular conditioning, and neuromuscular coordination (Jenkins 2005). Some alternative physical training activities—such as Pilates, yoga, Continuum Movement, and martial arts—are already taking the connective tissue network into account. Here the importance of the fasciae is often specifically discussed, though modern insights in the field of fascia research have often not been specifically included. We suggest that in order to build up an injury-resistant and elastic fascial body network it is essential to translate current insights in the field of fascia research into a practical training program (Schleip et al. 2020). Our intention is to encourage physical therapists, sports trainers, and movement enthusiasts to incorporate the principles presented in this chapter and to apply them to their specific context.

FASCIAL REMODELING

A recognized characteristic of connective tissue is its impressive adaptability: when regularly put under increasing yet physiological strain, it changes its architectural properties to meet the demand. For example, through our everyday biped locomotion the fascia on the lateral side of the thigh develops a palpable firmness. If we were instead to spend that same amount of time with our legs straddling a horse, then the opposite would happen, that is, after a few months the fascia on the inner side of the legs would become more developed and strong (EI-Labban et al. 1993).

The varied capacities of fibrous collagenous connective tissues make it possible for these materials to continuously adapt to the regularly occurring strain, particularly in relation to changes in length, strength, and ability to shear. Not only the density of bone changes, for example, as happens with astronauts who spend time in zero gravity wherein the bones become more porous (Ingber 2008); fascial tissues also react to their dominant loading patterns. With the help of the fibroblasts, they react to everyday strain and to specific training, steadily remodeling the arrangement of their collagenous fiber network (Kjaer et al. 2009). For example, with each passing year half the collagen fibrils are replaced in a healthy body (Neuberger and Slack 1953). The intention of fascial fitness is to influence this replacement via specific training activities that will, after 6 to 24 months, result in a "silk-like bodysuit," which is not only strong but also allows for a smoothly gliding joint mobility over wide angular ranges.

Interestingly, the fascial tissues of young people show stronger undulations within their collagen fibers, reminiscent of elastic springs, whereas in older people the collagen fibers appear as rather flattened (Staubesand et al. 1997). Research has confirmed the previously optimistic assumption that proper exercise loading—if applied regularly—can induce a more youthful collagen architecture, which shows a more wavy fiber arrangement (Wood et al. 1988; Järniven et al. 2002) and which also expresses a significant increased elastic storage capacity (Fig. 7.22.1) (Reeves et al. 2006).

However, it seems to matter which kind of exercise movements are applied: a controlled exercise study using slow-velocity and low-load contractions only demonstrated an increase in muscular strength and volume; however, it failed to yield any change in the elastic storage capacity of the collagenous structures (Kubo et al. 2003). Furthermore, long-term exposure to a specific activity, such as a specific sport, seems to result in corresponding functional adaptations of mechanical tendon properties. When comparing the biomechanical tendon properties between athletic ski jumpers, runners, swimmers, and nonathletic controls, a lower hysteresis (i.e., time-dependent loss of kinetic energy) was found in the patellar tendon and Achilles of ski jumpers and runners compared with nonathletic controls. Correspondingly, the recovered strain energy of the patellar tendon and Achilles tendon—when normalized to body mass—was ~40% to ~50% higher in ski jumpers than in swimmers and controls (Wiesinger et al. 2017). The authors concluded that a specific type of sport and the respective training and loading patterns can change the mechanical properties of tendons so that the use of their elastic energy can be optimized (Wiesinger et al. 2017).

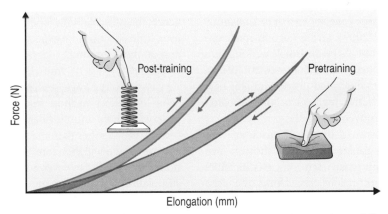

Fig. 7.22.1 Increased elastic storage capacity. Regular oscillatory exercise, such as daily rapid running, induces a higher storage capacity in the tendinous tissues of rats, compared with their nonrunning peers. This is expressed in a more spring-like recoil movement, as shown on the left. The area between the respective loading versus unloading curves represents the amount of "hysteresis": the smaller hysteresis of the trained animals (gray) reveals their more "elastic" tissue storage capacity, whereas the larger hysteresis of their peers signifies their more "viscoelastic" tissue properties, also called inertia. Illustration modified from Reeves, N.D., Narici, M.V., Maganaris, C.N., 2006. Myotendinous plasticity to ageing and resistance exercise in humans. Exp. Physiol. 91, 483–498.

THE CATAPULT MECHANISM: ELASTIC RECOIL OF FASCIAL TISSUES

Kangaroos can jump much farther than can be explained by the force of the contraction of their leg muscles. Under closer scrutiny, scientists discovered that a spring-like action is behind the unique ability—the so-called catapult mechanism (Kram and Dawson 1998). Here, the tendons and the fascia of the legs are tensioned like elastic bands. The release of this stored energy is what makes the amazing jumps possible. The discovery soon thereafter, that the same mechanism is also used by gazelles was hardly surprising. These animals are also capable of impressive leaping as well as running, though their musculature is not especially powerful. On the contrary, gazelles are generally considered to be rather delicate, making the springy ease of their incredible jumps all the more interesting.

The possibility of high-resolution ultrasound examination made it possible to discover similar orchestration of loading between muscle and fascia in human movement. Surprisingly, it has been found that the fasciae of humans have a similar kinetic storage capacity to that of kangaroos and gazelles (Sawicki et al. 2009). This is not only made use of when we jump or run but also with simple walking, as a significant part of the energy of the movement comes from the same springiness described previously. This new discovery has led to an active revision of long-accepted principles in the field of movement science.

In the past, it was assumed that in a muscular joint movement, the skeletal muscles involved shorten and this energy passes through passive tendons, which results in the movement of the joint. This classic form of energy transfer is still true—according to recent ultround examinatiions—for steady movements such as bicycling. Here, the muscle fibers actively change in length, and the tendons and aponeuroses scarcely grow longer. The fascial elements remain quite passive. This is in contrast to oscillatory movements with an elastic spring quality, in which the length of the muscle fibers changes little. Here, the muscle fibers contract in an almost isometric fashion (they stiffen temporarily without any significant change of their length) while the fascial elements function in an elastic way with a movement similar to that of a yo-yo (Fig. 7.22.2). It is this lengthening and shortening of the fascial elements that "produces" the actual movement (Fukunaga et al. 2002; Kawakami et al. 2002).

It is of interest that the elastic movement quality in young people is associated with a typical two-directional lattice arrangement of their fasciae, similar to a woman's stocking (Staubesand et al. 1997). In contrast, as we age and usually lose the springiness in our gait, the fascial architecture takes on a more haphazard and multidirectional arrangement. Animal experiments have also shown that lack of movement quickly fosters the development of additional cross-links in fascial tissues. The fibers lose their elasticity and do not glide against one another as they once did; instead, they become stuck together and form tissue adhesions, and in the worst cases they actually become matted together (Fig. 7.22.3) (Järvinen et al. 2002).

The goal of the fascial fitness training is to stimulate fascial fibroblasts to lay down a more youthful and gazelle-like fiber architecture. This is done through movements that load the fascial tissues over multiple extension ranges while using their elastic springiness.

Fig. 7.22.4 illustrates different fascial elements affected by various loading regimens. Classic weight-training loads the muscle in its normal range of motion, thereby strengthening the fascial tissues, which are arranged in series with the active muscle fibers. In addition, the transverse fibers across the muscular envelope are stimulated as well. However, little effect can be expected on extramuscular fasciae and on those intramuscular fascial fibers that are arranged in parallel to the active muscle fibers (Huijing 1999).

Classic Hatha yoga stretches, on the other hand, will show little effect on those fascial tissues that are arranged in series with the muscle fibers, because the relaxed myofibers are much softer than their serially arranged tendinous extensions and will therefore "swallow" most of the elongation (Jami 1992). However, such stretching provides good stimulation for fascial tissues that are hardly reached by classic muscle training, such as the extramuscular fasciae and the intramuscular fasciae oriented in parallel to the myofibers. Finally, a dynamic muscular loading pattern in which the muscle is both activated and extended promises a more comprehensive stimulation of fascial tissues. This can be achieved by muscular activation (e.g., against resistance) in a lengthened position while requiring small or medium amounts of muscle force only.

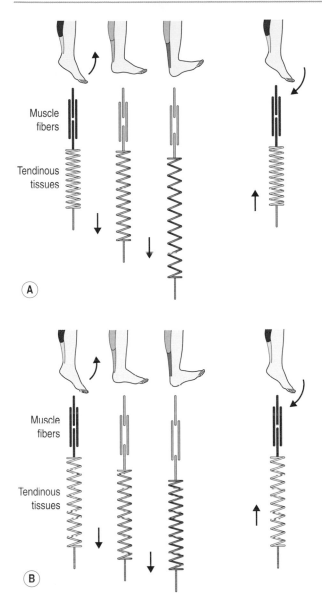

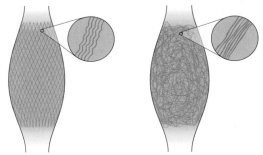

Fig. 7.22.3 Collagen architecture responds to loading. Fasciae of young people—shown on the left—express more often a clear two-directional (lattice) orientation of their collagen fiber network. In addition, the individual collagen fibers show a stronger crimp formation. In contrast, fasciae from older persons show a more irregular alignment with less crimp formation. As evidenced by animal studies, application of proper exercise can induce an altered architecture with increased crimp formation. Lack of exercise, on the other hand, has been shown to induce formation of a multidirectional fiber network and a decreased crimp formation.

Soft elastic bounces in the end ranges of available motion can also be used for that purpose. Repetitive hopping training has been shown to improve the mechanical properties as well. A group of physically active elderly men (mean age 72 years) practiced a carefully orchestrated hopping training for three times a week over a 11-week period. After a warm-up, the training sets included only 15 to 20 hops with short contact time and a 1-minute resting period between sets. In the first week, four such sets were performed per session only, which was slowly increased toward a maximum of seven sets in the last week. Although no strain injury was reported by any of the jumping elder men, their jumping height and tendon use was clearly improved after this carefully controlled hopping training (Hoffren-Mikkola et al. 2015).

The following guidelines are developed to make such training more efficient.

Fig. 7.22.2 Length changes of fascial elements and muscle fibers in an oscillatory movement with elastic recoil properties (A) and in conventional muscle training (B). The elastic tendinous (or fascial) elements are shown as springs, the myofibers as straight lines above. Note that during a conventional movement (B) the fascial elements do not change their length significantly whereas the muscle fibers clearly change their length. During movements like hopping or jumping, however, the muscle fibers contract almost isometrically whereas the fascial elements lengthen and shorten like an elastic yo-yo spring. Redrawn with permission from Kawakami, Y., Muraoka, T., Ito, S., Kanehisa, H., Fukunaga, T., 2002. In vivo muscle fiber behavior during countermovement exercise in humans reveals a significant role for tendon elasticity. J. Physiol. 540, 635–646.

> ### KEY POINT
>
> The capacity of elastic storage in human fasciae is surprisingly high. Especially in oscillatory movements, the fascial elements contribute to the movement much more than previously assumed. Dynamic muscular loading patterns such as soft elastic bounces at the end range of motion can support fascial stimulation to train the elastic recoil of fascial tissue.

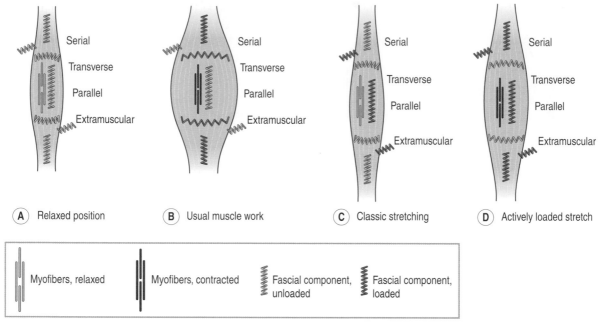

Fig. 7.22.4 Loading of different fascial components. (A) Relaxed position: the myofibers are relaxed and the muscle is at normal length. None of the fascial elements are being stretched. (B) Usual muscle work: myofibers contracted and muscle at normal length range. Fascial tissues, which are either arranged in series with the myofibers or transverse to them, are loaded. (C) Classic stretching: myofibers relaxed and muscle elongated. Fascial tissues oriented parallel to the myofibers are loaded as well, as are extramuscular connections. However, fascial tissues oriented in series with the myofibers are not sufficiently loaded, because most of the elongation in that serially arranged force chain is taken up by the relaxed myofibers. (D) Actively loaded stretch: muscle active and loaded at long end range. Most of the fascial components are being stretched and stimulated in that loading pattern. Note that various mixtures and combinations between the four different fascial components exist. This simplified abstraction therefore serves as a basic orientation only.

TRAINING PRINCIPLES

Preparatory Countermovement

Here, we make use of the catapult effect described previously. Before we perform the actual movement, we start with a slight pretensioning in the opposite direction. This is comparable with using a bow to shoot an arrow; just as the bow has to have sufficient tension in order for the arrow to reach its goal, the fascia becomes actively pretensioned in the opposite direction. In a sample exercise called "the flying sword," the pretensioning is achieved as the body's axis is slightly tilted backward for a brief moment, while at the same time there is an upward lengthening (Fig. 7.22.5). This increases the elastic tension in the fascial bodysuit and as a result allows the upper body and the arms to spring forward and down like a catapult as the weight is shifted in this direction.

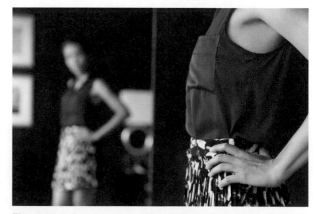

Fig. 7.22.5 Fascia-oriented movement training can induce a positive shift in the internal body image; that is, in the way a person feels about their body from the inside. Photo courtesy shutterstock.com/maridav.

The opposite is true for straightening up—we activate the catapult capacity of the fascia through an active pretensioning of the fascia of the back. When standing up from a forward-bending position, the muscles on the front of the body are first briefly activated. This momentarily pulls the body even further forward and down, and at the same time the posterior fascia is loaded with greater tension. The energy that is stored in the fascia is dynamically released via a passive recoil effect as the upper body "swings" back to the original position. To be sure that the individual is not relying on muscle work, but rather on dynamic recoil action of the fascia, requires a focus on timing—much the same as when playing with a yo-yo. It is necessary to determine the ideal swing, which is apparent when the action is fluid and pleasurable.

The Ninja Principle

This principle is inspired by the legendary Japanese warriors who reputedly moved as silently as cats and left no trace. When performing bouncy movements such as hopping, running, and dancing, special attention needs to be paid to executing the movement as smoothly and softly as possible. A change in direction is preceded by a gradual deceleration of the movement before the turn and a gradual acceleration afterward, each movement flowing from the last; any extraneous or jerky movements should therefore be avoided (Fig. 7.22.6).

Normal stairs become training equipment when they are used appropriately, employing gentle stepping. The production of "as little noise as possible" provides the most useful feedback—the more the fascial spring effect is used, the quieter and gentler the process will be. It may be useful to reflect on the way a cat moves as it prepares to jump. The feline first sends a condensed impulse down through its paws in order to accelerate softly and quietly, landing with precision.

Dynamic Stretching

Rather than a motionless waiting in a static stretch position, a more flowing stretch is suggested. In fascial fitness there is a differentiation between two kinds of

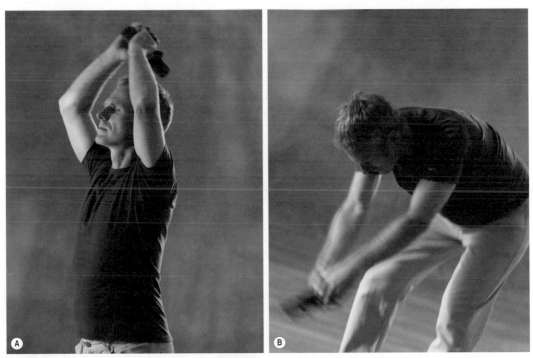

Fig. 7.22.6 Training example: the flying sword. (A) Pre-streching the bow: the preparatory countermovement initiates the elastic-dynamic spring in an anterior and inferior direction. Free weights can also be used. (B) To return to an upright position, the "catapulting back fascia" is loaded as the upper body is briefly bounced dynamically downward followed by an elastic swing back up. The attention of the person doing the exercise should be on the optimal timing and calibration of the movement in order to create the smoothest movement possible.

dynamic stretching: fast and slow. The fast variation may be familiar to many people as it was part of physical training in the past. For several decades, this bouncing stretch was considered to be generally harmful to the tissue, but the method's merits have been confirmed in research. Although stretching immediately before competition can be counterproductive, it seems that long-term and regular use of such dynamic stretching can positively influence the architecture of the connective tissue in that it becomes more elastic when correctly performed (Decoster et al. 2005). Muscles and tissue should first be warmed up, and jerking or abrupt movements should be avoided. The motion should have a sinusoidal deceleration and acceleration shape in each direction turn; this goes along with the perception of a smooth and "elegant" quality of movement. Dynamic, fast stretching has even more effect on the fascia when combined with a preparatory countermovement, as was previously described (Fukashiro et al. 2006). For example, when stretching the hip flexors, a brief backward movement should be introduced before dynamically lengthening and stretching forward.

The long myofascial chains are the preferred focus when doing slow dynamic stretches. Instead of stretching isolated muscle groups, the aim is finding body movements that engage the longest possible myofascial chains (Myers 1997). This is not done by passively waiting, as in a lengthening classic Hatha yoga pose, or in a conventional isolated muscle stretch. Multidirectional movements with slight changes in angle are utilized; this might include sideways or diagonal movement variations and spiraling rotations. With this method, large areas of the fascial network are simultaneously involved (Fig. 7.22.7).

Proprioceptive Refinement

The importance of proprioception for movement control is made clear by the case of Ian Waterman, a man

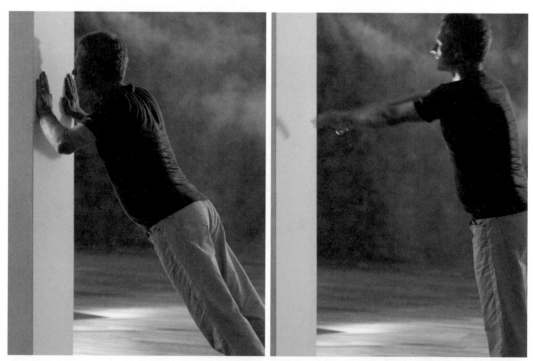

Fig. 7.22.7 Training example: elastic wall bounces. Imitating the elastic bounces of a gazelle, soft-bouncing movements off a wall are explored in standing. Proper pretension in the whole body will avoid any collapsing into a "banana posture." Making the least sound and avoiding any abrupt movement qualities are imperative. Only with the mastery of these qualities can a progression into further load increase—for example, bouncing off a table or window sill instead of a wall—eventually can be explored by stronger individuals. For example, this person should not yet be permitted to progress to higher loads, as his neck and shoulder region already show slight compression on the left picture.

repeatedly mentioned in scientific literature. This impressive man contracted a viral infection at the age of 19 that resulted in a so-called sensory neuropathy. In this rare pathology, the sensory peripheral nerves that provide the somatomotor cortex with information about the movements of the body are destroyed, and the motor nerves remain completely intact. This meant than Mr. Waterman could move, but he could not "feel" his movements. After some time, this giant of a man became virtually lifeless. Only with an iron will and years of practice did he finally succeed in making up for these normal physical sensations, a capacity that is commonly taken for granted. He did so with conscious control that primarily relies on visual feedback. He is currently the only person known with this affliction who is able to stand unaided and able to walk (Cole 2016).

The way Waterman moves is similar to the way patients with chronic back pain move. When in a public place, if the lights unexpectedly go out, he clumsily falls to the ground. Springy, swinging movements are possible for him only with obvious and jerky changes in direction. If doing a "classic" stretching program with static or active stretches, he would appear normal. As for the dynamic stretching that is part of our fascial training, he is clearly not capable, as he lacks the proprioception needed for fine coordination.

Two sisters were found in North America with a proprioceptive impairment similar to that of Ian Waterman. In their case a dysfunction in the newly discovered PIEZO2 receptor found together with a rare genetic disorder led to the altered expression of this highly mechanosensitive receptor channel in the cell membrane of fascial fibroblasts (Chesler et al. 2016). Interestingly, both of them express an idiopathic (juvenile) scoliosis in their posture and both of them report delayed walking development in their childhood (achieving independent walking between 6 and 7 years of age), and early impairments of fine motor skills.

Proprioceptive training has been shown to be effective in reducing the frequency of injuries in athletes (Rivera et al. 2017). It is interesting to note that the classic "joint receptors"—located in joint capsules and associated ligaments—seem to be of lesser importance for normal proprioception, because they are usually stimulated at extreme joint ranges only and not during physiological motions (Lu et al. 2005; Ianuzzi et al. 2011). On the contrary, proprioceptive nerve endings located in the more superficial layers are more optimally situated, as here even small angular joint movements lead to relatively distinct shearing motions. Findings indicate that the superficial fascial layers of the body are, in fact, more densely populated with mechanoreceptive nerve endings than tissue situated more internally (Stecco et al. 2008; Tesarz et al. 2011).

For this reason, we encourage a perceptual refinement of shear, gliding, and tensioning motions in superficial fascial membranes. In doing this, it is important to limit the filtering function of the reticular formation, as it can markedly restrict the transfer of sensations from movements that are repetitive and predictable. To prevent such a sensory dampening, the idea of varied and creative experiencing becomes important. In addition to the slow and fast dynamic stretches noted previously, as well as using elastic recoil properties, we recommend (based on experience) inclusion of "fascial refinement" training in which various qualities of movement are experimented with, for example, extreme slow-motion and very quick micromovements that may not even be visible to an observer, and large macromovements involving the whole body. To this end, it is common to place the body into unfamiliar positions while working with the awareness of gravity, or possibly through exploring the weight of a training partner.

The micromovements are inspired by Continuum Movement (Conrad 2007). Such movement is active and specific and can have effects that are not possible with larger movements. In doing these coordinated fascial movements, it appears possible to specifically address adhesions, for example, between muscle septa deep in the body. In addition, such tiny and specific movements can be used to illuminate and bring awareness to perceptually neglected areas of the body (Fig. 7.22.8). Thomas Hanna uses the label "sensory-motor amnesia" when referring to such places in the body (Hanna 1998).

Hydration and Renewal

The video recordings of fascia by Dr. Guimbertau (see Chapter 3.6) have helped our understanding of the plasticity and changing elasticity of the water-filled fascia. This awareness has proven to be especially effective when incorporated into the slow dynamic stretching and fascial refinement work. An essential basic principle of these exercises is the understanding that the fascial tissue is predominantly made up of free-moving and bound water molecules. During the strain of stretching, the water is pushed out of the more stressed zones,

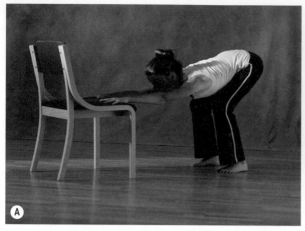
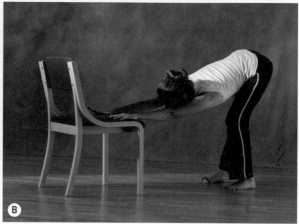

Fig. 7.22.8 Training example: the big cat stretch. (A) This is a slow stretching movement of the long posterior chain, from the fingertips to the sitbones, from the coccyx to the top of the head and to the heels. The movement goes in opposing directions at the same time—think of a cat stretching its long body. By changing the angle slightly, different aspects of the fascial web are addressed with slow and steady movements. (B) In the next step one rotates and lengthens the pelvis or chest toward one side (here shown with the pelvis starting to rotate to the right). The intensity of the feeling of stretch on that entire side of the body is then gently reversed. Note the feeling of increased length afterward.

similar to squeezing a sponge (Schleip and Klingler 2007). With the release that follows, this area is again filled with new fluid that comes from surrounding tissue and the lymphatic and vascular network. The sponge-like connective tissue can lack adequate hydration at neglected places. The goal of exercise is to refresh such places in the body with improved hydration through specific stretching to encourage fluid movement (Schleip et al. 2020).

Proper timing of the duration of individual loading and release phases is very important. As part of modern running training, it is often recommended to frequently interrupt the running with short walking intervals (Galloway 2002). There is good reason for this: under strain, the fluid is pressed out of the fascial tissues and these begin to function less optimally as their elastic and springy resilience slowly decreases. The short walking pauses then serve to rehydrate the tissue, as it is given a chance to take up nourishing fluid. For an average beginning runner, for example, the authors recommend walking pauses of 1 to 3 minutes every 10 minutes. More advanced runners with more developed body awareness can adjust the optimal timing and duration of those breaks based on the presence (or lack) of that youthful and dynamic rebound: if the running movement begins to feel and look more dampened and less

springy, it is likely time for a short pause. Similarly, if after a brief walking break there is a noticeable return of that gazelle-like rebound, then the rest period was adequate.

This cyclic training, with periods of more intense effort interspersed with purposeful breaks, is recommended in all facets of fascia training. The person training then learns to pay attention to the dynamic properties of their fascial "bodysuit" while exercising, and to adjust the exercises based on this new body awareness. This also carries over to an increased "fascial embodiment" in everyday life. Preliminary anecdotal reports also indicate a preventative effect of a fascia-oriented training in relation to connective tissue overuse injuries.

Special foam rollers can be a useful tool for inducing a localized sponge-like temporary tissue dehydration with resultant renewed hydration. However, the firmness of the roller and application of the body weight needs to be individually monitored. If properly applied, and incorporating finely tuned directional changes, the tissue forces and potential benefits could be similar to those of manual myofascial release treatments (Chaudhry et al. 2008). A frequently asked question concerns the velocity of foam rolling. A temporary alteration of water content in the compressed tissue as described previously can have an effect on tissue stiffness. A study by Wilke et al. (2019) suggests that rolling velocity has no clear effect on tissue stiffness, at least when it comes to the acute effects of rolling in healthy adults. This novel finding regarding rolling velocity also holds true for joint mobility measures (range of motion). However, future studies will have to look into the relationship between rolling velocity and parameters such as collagen-synthesis, rehydration or sensory measures, as they have not yet been investigated experimentally.

In addition, the localized tissue stimulation might serve to stimulate and fine-tune possibly inhibited or desensitized fascial proprioceptors in more hidden tissue locations (Fig. 7.22.9).

FASCIAL FITNESS AND BODY IMAGE

Fascial fitness might also promote a more positive attitude toward one's own body as it can have an effect on psychological factors such as body image. A study by Baur et al. (2017) investigated the influence of fascial fitness on body image (Fig. 7.22.5). Eighteen participants performed three sessions of fascial fitness over the course of 3 weeks. This training was shown to induce a significant improvement in the body image—how participants evaluated their physical appearance and how comfortable they felt inside their bodies.

Sustainability: The Power of a Thousand Tiny Steps

An additional and important aspect is the concept of the slow and long-term renewal of the fascial network. In contrast to muscular strength training in which big gains occur early on and then a plateau is quickly reached wherein only very small gains are possible, fascia changes more slowly and the results are more lasting. It is possible to work without a great deal of strain—so that consistent and regular training pays off. When training the fascia, improvements in the first few weeks may be small and less obvious on the outside. However, improvements have a lasting cumulative effect that, after years, can be expected to result in marked improvements in the strength and elasticity of the global fascial net (Fig. 7.22.10) (Kjaer et al. 2009). As the fascial proprioception becomes refined, improved coordination is probable.

It is suggested that training should be consistent, and that only a few minutes of appropriate exercises, performed once or twice per week, is sufficient for collagen remodeling (Fig. 7.22.11). The related renewal process will take between 6 months and 2 years and will yield a lithe, flexible, and resilient collagenous matrix. For those who do yoga or martial arts, such a focus on a long-term goal is nothing new. For the person who is new to physical training, such knowledge of fascial properties can go a long way in convincing them to

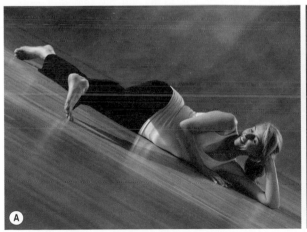
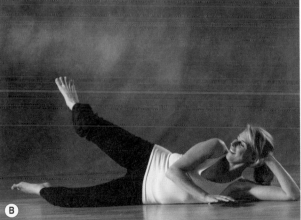

Fig. 7.22.9 Training example: octopus tentacle. With the image of an octopus tentacle in mind, a multitude of extensional movements through the whole leg are explored (A & B) in slow motion. Through creative changes in muscular activation patterns, the tensional fascial proprioception is activated. This goes along with a deep myofascial stimulation that aims to reach not only the fascial envelopes but also into the septa between muscles. While avoiding any jerky movement, the action of these tentacle-like micromovements leads to a feeling of flowing strength in the leg.

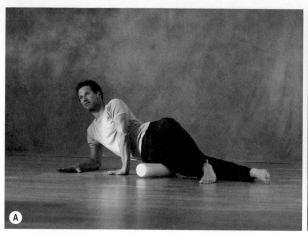
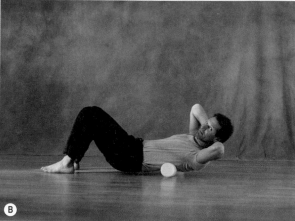

Fig. 7.22.10 Training example: fascial release. The use of particular foam rollers may allow the application of localized tissue stimulations with similar forces and possibly similar benefits as in a manual myofascial release session. However, the stiffness of the roller and application of the body weight needs to be adjusted and monitored for each person (A & B). To foster a sponge-like tissue dehydration with subsequent renewed local hydration, subtle changes in the applied forces and vectors are recommended.

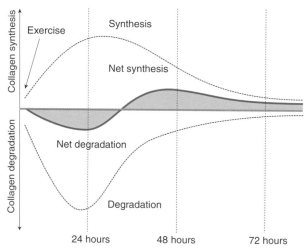

Fig.7.22.11 Collagen turnover after exercise. The upper curve shows collagen synthesis in tendons is increasing after exercise. However, the stimulated fibroblasts also increase their rate of collagen degradation. Interestingly, during the first 1 to 2 days after exercise, collagen degradation outweighs the collagen synthesis, whereas afterward this situation is reversed. To increase tendon strength, the proposed fascial fitness training therefore suggests an appropriate tissue stimulation 1 to 2 times per week only. Although the increased tendon strength is not achieved by an increase in tendon diameter, examinations by Kjaer and colleagues (2009) indicated that it is probably the result of altered cross-link formations between collagen fibers. Courtesy Magnusson, S.P., Langberg, H., Kjaer, M., 2010. The pathogenesis of tendinopathy: balancing the response to loading. Nat. Rev. Rheumatol. 6, 262–268.

train their connective tissues. Of course, fascial fitness training should not replace muscular strength work, cardiovascular training, and coordination exercises; instead, it should be thought of as an important addition to a comprehensive training program (Fig. 7.22.11).

Summary

Fascial fitness aims to support the remodeling of the fascial network by improving the collagen architecture through specific training activities. The training principles of fascial fitness include preparatory countermovements, the Ninja principle, dynamic stretching, and proprioceptive refinement. Implementing these principles into one's existing training routine should be a long-term endeavor. A successful renewal process of the "fascial bodysuit" will take months to years of consistent training efforts.

REFERENCES

Baur, H., Gatterer, H., Hotter, B., Kopp, M., 2017. Influence of structural integration and fascial fitness on body image and the perception of back pain. J. Phys. Ther. Sci. 29, 1010–1013.

Chaudhry, H., Schleip, R., Ji, Z., Bukiet, B., Maney, M., Findley, T., 2008. Three-dimensional mathematical model for deformation of human fasciae in manual therapy. J. Am. Osteopath. Assoc. 108, 379–390.

Chesler, A.T., Szczot, M., Bharucha-Goebel, D., et al., 2016. The Role of PIEZO2 in Human Mechanosensation. N. Engl. J. Med. 375, 1355–1164.

Cole, J., 2016. Losing touch: a man without his body. Oxford University Press, Oxford, U.K.

Conrad, E., 2007. Life on Land. North Atlantic Books, Berkeley, CA.

Decoster, L.C., Cleland, J., Altieri, C., Russell, P., 2005. The effects of hamstring stretching on range of motion: a systematic literature review. J. Orthop. Sports Phys. Ther. 35, 377–387.

El-Labban, N.G., Hopper, C., Barber, P., 1993. Ultrastructural finding of vascular degeneration in myositis ossificans circumscripta (fibrodysplasia ossificans). J. Oral Pathol. Med. 22, 428–431.

Fukashiro, S., Hay, D.C, Nagano, A., 2006. Biomechanical behavior of muscle-tendon complex during dynamic human movements. J. Appl. Biomech. 22, 131–147.

Fukunaga, T., Kawakami, Y., Kubo, K., Kanehisa, H., 2002. Muscle and tendon interaction during human movements. Exerc. Sport. Sci. Rev. 30, 106–110.

Galloway, J., 2002. Galloway's Book on Running. Shelter Publications, Bolinas, CA.

Hanna, T., 1998. Somatics: Reawakening the Mind's Control of Movement, Flexibility, and Health. Da Capo Press, Cambridge, MA.

Hoffrén-Mikkola, M., Ishikawa, M., Rantalainen, T., Avela, J., Komi, P.V., 2015 Neuromuscular mechanics and hopping training in elderly. Eur. J. Appl. Physiol. 115, 863–877.

Huijing, P.A., 1999. Muscle as a collagen fiber reinforced composite: a review of force transmission in muscle and whole limb. J. Biomech. 32, 329–345.

Ianuzzi, A., Pickar, J.G., Khalsa, P.S., 2011. Relationships between joint motion and facet joint capsule strain during cat and human lumbar spinal motions. J. Manipulative Physiol. Ther. 34, 420–431.

Ingber, D.E., 2008. Tensegrity and mechanotransduction. J. Bodyw. Mov. Ther. 12, 198–200.

Jami, A., 1992. Golgi tendon organs in mammalian skeletal muscles: functional properties and central actions. Physiol. Rev. 72, 623–666.

Järvinen, T.A., Józsa, L., Kannus, P., Järvinen, T.L., Järvinen, M., 2002. Organization and distribution of intramuscular connective tissue in normal and immobilized skeletal muscles. An immunohistochemical, polarization and scanning electron microscopic study. J. Muscle Res. Cell Motil. 23, 245–254.

Jenkins, S., 2005. Sports Science Handbook: Volume 1: The Essential Guide to Kinesiology, Sport & Exercise Science. Multi-Science Publishing Co. Ltd., Essex, UK.

Kawakami, Y., Muraoka, T., Ito, S., Kanehisa, H., Fukunaga, T., 2002. In vivo muscle fibre behaviour during countermovement exercise in humans reveals a significant role for tendon elasticity. J. Physiol. 540, 635–646.

Kjaer, M., Langberg, H., Heinemeier, K., Bayer, M.L., Hansen, M., Holm, L., et al., 2009. From mechanical loading to collagen synthesis, structural changes and function in human tendon. Scand. J. Med. Sci. Sports 19, 500–510.

Kram, R., Dawson, T.J., 1998. Energetics and biomechanics of locomotion by red kangaroos (Macropus rufus). Comp. Biochem. Physiol. B. Biochem. Mol. Biol. 120, 41–49.

Kubo, K., Kanehisa, H., Miyatani, M., Tachi, M., Fukunaga, T., 2003. Effect of low-load resistance training on the tendon properties in middle-aged and elderly women. Acta Physiol. Scand. 178, 25–32.

Lu, Y., Chen, C., Kallakuri, S., Patwardhan, A., Cavanaugh, J.M., 2005. Neural response of cervical facet joint capsule to stretch: a study of whiplash pain mechanism. Stapp Car Crash J. 49, 49–65.

Magnusson, S.P., Langberg, H., Kjaer, M., 2010. The pathogenesis of tendinopathy: balancing the response to loading. Nat. Rev. Rheumatol. 6, 262–268.

Myers, T.W., 1997. The "anatomy trains." J. Bodyw. Mov. Ther. 1, 91–101.

Neuberger, A., Slack, H., 1953. The metabolism of collagen from liver, bones, skin and tendon in normal rats. Biochem. J. 53, 47–52.

Reeves, N.D., Narici, M.V., Maganaris, C.N., 2006. Myotendinous plasticity to ageing and resistance exercise in humans. Exp. Physiol. 91, 483–498.

Rivera, M.J., Winkelmann, Z.K., Powden, C.J., Games, K.E, 2017. Proprioceptive training for the prevention of ankle sprains: an evidence-based review. J. Athl. Train. 52: 1065–1067.

Sawicki, G.S., Lewis, C.L., Ferris, D.P., 2009. It pays to have a spring in your step. Exerc. Sport Sci. Rev. 37, 130–138.

Schleip, R., Klingler, W., 2007. Fascial strain hardening correlates with matrix hydration changes. In: Findley, T.W., Schleip, R. (Eds.), Fascia Research: Basic Science and Implications to Conventional and Complementary Health Care. Elsevier GmbH, Munich, p. 51.

Schleip, R., Wilke, J., Baker, A. 2020. Fascia in Sport and Movement, second ed. Handspring Publishing, Edinburgh, UK.

Staubesand, J., Baumbach, K.U.K., Li, Y., 1997. La structure fine de l'aponévrose jambiæÆre. Phlebol 50, 105–113.

Stecco, C., Porzionato, A., Lancerotto, L., et al., 2008. Histological study of the deep fasciae of the limbs. J. Bodyw. Mov. Ther. 12, 225–230.

Tesarz, J., Hoheisel, U., Wiedenhöfer, B., Mense, S., 2011. Sensory innervation of the thoracolumbar fascia in rats and humans. Neuroscience 194, 302–308.

Wiesinger, H.P., Rieder, F., Kösters, A., Müller, E., Seynnes, O., 2017. Sport-specific capacity to use elastic energy in the patellar and Achilles tendons of elite athletes. Front. Physiol. 8, 132.

Wilke, J., Hespanhol, L., Behrens, M., 2019. Is it all about the fascia? A systematic review and meta-analysis of the prevalence of extramuscular connective tissue lesions in muscle strain injury. Orthop. J. Sports Med. 7, 2325967119888500.

Wilke, J., Niemeyer, P., Niederer, D., Schleip, R., Banzer, W., 2019. Influence of foam rolling velocity on knee range of motion and tissue stiffness: a randomized, controlled crossover trial. J Sport Rehabil. 28, 711–715.

Wood, T.O., Cooke, P.H., Goodship, A.E., 1988. The effect of exercise and anabolic steroids on the mechanical properties and crimp morphology of the rat tendon. Am. J. Sports Med. 16, 153–158.

Hydrorelease of Fascia

Tadashi Kobayashi, Hiroaki Kimura, Yoshihiro Zenita, and Hidetaka Imagita

CHAPTER CONTENTS

INTRODUCTION

Hydrorelease (HR) is an injection therapy using physiological saline or other solutions that targets various types of fascia. Although local injections using physiological saline have conventionally been regarded as a placebo, more precise injections under high-performance ultrasound guidance have aided in the understanding of their utility.

HISTORY OF INJECTIONS WITH PHYSIOLOGICAL SALINE

In 1955, a scientific report was presented by Sola and Kuitert on physiological saline injections for the treatment of myofascial pain in 100 cases of neck and shoulder pain (Sola and Kuitert 1955). Since the late 1950s, the development of long-acting local anesthetics has progressed rapidly, and local injection therapy for myofascial pain syndrome (MPS) has focused on local anesthetics. In 1980 a randomized controlled trial by Frost and colleagues demonstrated that the saline solution was superior to local anesthetics in the treatment of MPS (Frost et al. 1980). In contrast, a review concluded that the therapeutic effects of local injections on MPS were equivalent to local anesthetics, steroids, botulinum toxin A, and physiological saline (placebo). The review reinforced the negative considerations of society and the scientific field on local injections as treatment for MPS; although, one interpretation is that physiological saline is truly as effective (i.e., not a placebo) as other drug solutions (Staal et al. 2008). The suggestion in Western medicine that saline is a placebo has been prevalent. Conversely, most research underpinning this review considers local injections to be blind injections, and their accuracy has been a substantial concern. Over time, the resolution of ultrasonographic images has rapidly improved and physiological saline injections, such as hydrorelease (HR), can be precisely performed with ultrasound guidance.

HISTORY AND DEFINITION OF HYDRORELEASE

In 2008, Kimura proposed interfascial block with local anesthetic as a novel treatment procedure for MPS

(Kimura 2008). In April 2010, Matsuoka and colleagues reported this technique to a Japanese journal on pain medicine (Matsuoka et al. 2010). In May 2011, Domingo and colleagues reported on the gross anatomy and clinical effectiveness of ultrasound-guided interfascial injection with local anesthetics (Domingo et al. 2011). Additionally, in 2012, Kimura proposed that the injection of physiological saline instead of a local anesthetic could relieve the symptoms caused by abnormal fascia (Kimura 2012).

In June 2014, Kimura devised a novel procedure termed "ultrasound-guided myofascial release injection," which was defined as a technique for the release (separation in structural view and relaxation in functional view) of stacking fasciae as hyperechoic strip-shaped lesions on ultrasound images, akin to peeling off thin stacking papers and separating fasciae themselves (Kimura 2014)

(Fig. 7.23.1). The word "stacking" originates from poly-acrylamide gel electrophoresis (Chrambach et al. 1971). This injection aims to improve the extensibility of fasciae or to slide between fasciae in addition to having analgesic effects. In 2015 the target of treatment expanded from myofascia to fascia, which included the deep fascia, myofascia, paraneural sheath, tendon, ligament, retinaculum, and fat pads (Kimura 2015).

KEY POINT

Ultrasound-guided fascia release injection was devised by Dr. Kimura of Japan in 2014, and then the term "fascia hydrorelease" was adopted in 2017, which was defined as a technique for the release (separation and relaxation) of abnormal fasciae to improve the extensibility and sliding in addition to having analgesic effects.

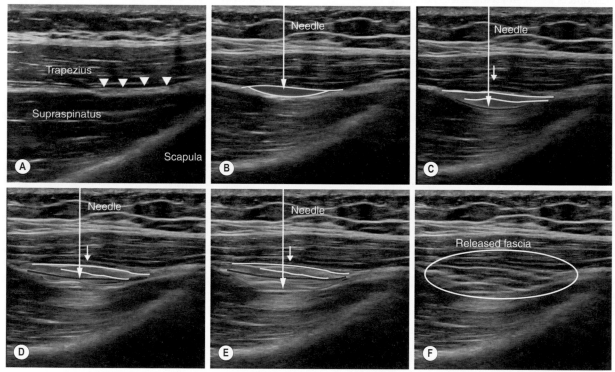

Fig. 7.23.1 Hydrorelease (HR) of Deep Fascia Between the Trapezius and Supraspinatus Muscle and the Injection Technique. (A) Ultrasound image before the injection. White arrowhead shows stacking fascia. Blue area shows injected solution. (B–E) Ultrasound image while injecting. Slightly moving the needle releases fascial layers in sequence from (B) through (C) and (D) to (E). First the yellow line (B) was released followed by the red line (C); green line (D); and light blue line (E). The blue area shows the injected solution. (F) Ultrasound image after the injection of HR. The stacking fascia is released, forming the so-called mille-feuille sign or layer cake sign. The volume of the injected solution is approximately 3 to 5 mL (1–2 mL at each layered fascia of B–E).

In 2016, Kobayashi and colleagues reported two double-blind, randomized controlled studies comparing three types of solutions (physiological saline, local anesthetic, and bicarbonate Ringer's solution) on ultrasound-guided interfascial (fascial release injection for deep fascia) injection for MPS (Kobayashi et al. 2016).

Fascia release includes various therapeutic techniques, such as physical therapy, dry needling, injections, and surgery. In March 2017, researchers adopted the term "fascia HR" for fascial release injections (JNOS 2019). Ultrasound-guided HR was introduced in the academic journal of the Japanese Society of Ultrasound after the publication of an article and textbooks on

fascial release techniques (Matsuzaki 2017; Kimura et al. 2017, 2019). Today, clinical cases of HR are being increasingly reported in various Japanese academic societies, such as orthopedics (Kimura et al. 2018; Nagano 2018), pain medicine, and rehabilitation medicine, and has spread in Asia.

DIFFERENCES BETWEEN HYDRORELEASE AND HYDRODISSECTION

Hydrodissection (HD) is similar to HR; however, it should not be confused with HR. The fundamental differences between HR and HD are shown in Table 7.23.1.

TABLE 7.23.1	Differences Between Hydrorelease and Hydrodissection	
	Hydrorelease (HR)	**Hydrodissection (HD)**
Solution	Any chemical solution Saline Dextrose Low concentration local anesthetic (e.g., 0.1%) Bicarbonate Ringer's solution Hyaluronic acid solution, etc.	Saline Dextrose (5%, 10%; sometimes implemented as prolotherapy) Platelet-rich plasma (PRP)
Needle	30 gauge (19 mm length): more precise HR 27 gauge (38 mm length): standard 25 gauge (60 mm length): deep site	21–23 gauge (25- or 38-mm length): standard 20–22 gauge (60- or 70-mm length): deep site 18 gauge (15 mm length): high volume HD
Dosage	One injection: 1–5 mL Up to 10 mL (hip, etc.)	One injection: 10–20 mL (median nerve, etc.) High-volume HD: 40–50 mL (Achilles tendon, Patella tendon, etc.)
Target structure	Fascia such as superficial fascia, deep fascia, myofascia, retinaculum, ligament, tendon and tendon sheath, joint capsule, fat pad, nerve (paraneural sheath and fascia around the nerve), fascia near vessel, dura complex, etc.	Nerves and ligaments (currently as high-volume HD)
Method of technique	Inject solution to release stacking fasciae akin to peeling off thin stacking papers by moving the needlepoint little-by-little on the ultrasound image to create the so-called mille-feuille sign or layer cake sign	Inject solution around the object to create the so-called doughnut sign or halo sign for the nerve
Presumptive mechanism	Rehydration (electrolyte such as Na+, Cl-) of matrix Washing effect of pain substances Mechanical and chemical effects of fascia and extracellular matrix Stimulation of free nerve endings Improvement of extensibility of fascia and sliding between fasciae	Decompression of peripheral nerves Decrease of abnormal neovascularization and newly formed nerve structure

Reproduced with permission from JNOS homepage. 5–3 The difference between hydrorelease (HR) and hydrodissection (HD). https://www.jnos-global.org/for-medical#5-3_The_difference_between_hydrorelease_HR_and_hydrodissection_HD.

HR aims to treat fascia, whereas HD targets compressed or entrapped peripheral nerves and tendinopathy.

The term "release" of HR indicates separation in both structural or morphological views and relaxation in functional views regarding the fasciae and the fascial system. In contrast, the term "dissection" of HD indicates morphological expression of tissue separation on ultrasound images.

The technical concepts of these methods also differ. Nerve HR is performed with the goal of producing the "mille-feuille sign" or "layer cake sign" as an injection technique akin to peeling off thin stacking papers and separating fasciae themselves on or around peripheral nerves, as well as connective tissue among fascicles, epineurium, and perineurium (JNOS 2019). Nerve HR is performed directly on stacking fasciae (e.g., 3 o'clock side of the nerve) if the stacking fascia is not observed in the entire nerve. Conversely, nerve HD aims to create a "doughnut sign" or "halo sign" on ultrasound images and places peripheral nerve blocks using local anesthetics.

The amount of solution used in HR (1–5 mL is often injected) tends to be much smaller than that in HD (10–20 mL is often injected), especially for the technique known as high-volume HD (high-volume image-guided injection [HVIGI], where 40 to 50 mL is often injected) (Alfredson 2011; Maffulli et al. 2016; Wheeler et al. 2016). Some studies employing blind injections have reported that when greater volumes of physiological saline are injected, the effectiveness of the injections becomes more similar to that of local anesthesia in fibromyalgia patients (Staud et al. 2009; Staud et al. 2014). However, we have reported in macroscopic anatomical studies that if only 1 mL solution is injected accurately using ultrasound guidance, the solution spreads widely into the deep fasciae of multiple layers (Kimura et al. 2019). As the volume of medical solution increases, injection-related complications may occur (e.g., injection-related pain or side effects from contents of the solution). The optimal dose remains controversial.

Various types of medical solutions are used. For example, for HR of fascia, bicarbonate Ringer's solution may be the optimal choice. In 2016 two double-blind, randomized controlled studies by Kobayashi and colleagues compared drug solutions using ultrasound-guided interfascial injections (fascia release injections for deep fascia) for MPS (Kobayashi et al. 2016). The first study (physiological saline versus local anesthetic) revealed that physiological saline was more effective than local anesthetics for pain relief, whereas physiological saline was associated with more injection-related pain than that from local anesthetics. The second study (physiological saline versus bicarbonate Ringer's solution) revealed that bicarbonate Ringer's solution had similar analgesic effects as those of physiological saline but less injection-related pain than physiological saline. Besides, HD using 5% dextrose has been implemented as part of prolotherapy (Lam et al. 2017). HD with platelet-rich plasma (Wu et al. 2019) has been reported, but further studies are needed to compare solutions used for fascia release injections.

MECHANISMS OF ACTION OF HR AND HD

The mechanisms of action of HR have not been fully elucidated and are still being developed; however, some perspectives are introduced in Table 7.23.1. The mechanism of HR is based on the viewpoint that the fascia itself is the cause of pain or various symptoms (e.g., numbness, tingling, pricking , stiffness, fatigue, dizziness, cold sensation), which is different from HD (aims to remove fasciae and decrease abnormal neovascularization and newly formed nerve structures) or prolotherapy (aims to promote soft-tissue repair through inflammatory reactions by injection; discussed in detail in Chapter 7.11: Prolotherapy).

HR of fascia may contribute to various effects, such as the washing effect of pain substances (e.g., substance P, bradykinin, nerve growth factor); fluid replacement (rehydration) effects with injections of water, electrolytes (e.g., sodium or chloride ions), or other substances; mechanical and chemical effects of fascia and extracellular matrix; and electrophysiological effects on free nerve endings, nervi nervorum (Bove et al. 1997), and glio-neural complex (Abdo et al. 2019) on fascia, which can improve the extensibility of fasciae or sliding between fasciae in addition to analgesic effects (Kobayashi et al. 2016; Kimura et al. 2017; Evers et al. 2018). Furthermore, abnormal fascia has been reported to be thicker on ultrasound images (Stecco et al. 2014; Langevin et al. 2011). Therefore we expect that HR will contribute to treatment of abnormal fascia by helping to release stacking fascia.

KEY POINT

The mechanism of hydrorelease is based on the viewpoint that the fascia itself is the cause of pain or various symptoms, which is different from that of hydrodissection (aims to decompress entrapped peripheral nerves, etc.) or prolotherapy (aims to promote soft-tissue repair through inflammatory reactions by injection).

INDICATIONS OF HR

HR targets abnormal fascia. We performed HR on the viewpoints of: fascial pain syndrome (FPS) (Box 7.23.1), which was proposed as a classification criterion concerning the diagnostic criteria of MPS and classification criteria for rheumatoid arthritis, and the guide for selecting the appropriate treatment (e.g., injection, physical therapy such as manipulation, dry needling, or surgery) (Fig. 7.23.2) (JNOS 2019).

The most prominent, clinically relevant indication for HR as local therapy is the precise identification of the source of pain and exacerbating factors associated with patients' symptoms. Additionally, the sharing of these assessments among medical staff facilitates inter-professional collaboration for better patient treatment. It is desirable to perform a medical interview, physical examination (i.e., palpation, motion-analysis at pain motion, range of motion, and special tests for orthopedic examination), and diagnostic imaging such as ultrasonography based on various clinical methods, including dermatomes, osteotome, fasciatomes (Stecco et al. 2019), angiosomes (Taylor et al. 1987), venosomes (Taylor et al. 1990), pattern of referred pain (Donnelly, 2018), and clinical anatomy such as peripheral nerves, vessels, muscles, tendons, ligaments, and fascia.

KEY POINT

After the precise identification of the source of pain and exacerbating factors through a medical interview, physical examination, diagnostic imaging, dermatomes, fasciatomes, angiosomes, venosomes and clinical anatomy, we perform hydrorelease on the viewpoints of fascial pain syndrome (FPS) and the guide for selecting the appropriate treatment.

BOX 7.23.1   The Classification Criteria for Fascial Pain Syndrome (FPS)

FPS is defined as the sensory, motor, and autonomic symptoms caused by abnormal fascia, and the specific fascia and fascial group that causes the symptoms should be identified.

These classification criteria are made available when one or more obvious abnormal fascia is identified that cannot be explained by another diagnosis. FPS is classified when all essential criteria are fulfilled and at least one more confirmatory observation is made. After FPS is classified, the precise intervention for abnormal fascia (e.g., ultrasound-guided intervention) is performed to relieve symptoms of FPS significantly (relief of restrictive range of motion and 75% or more of the pain intensity as per the criterion standard). (JNOS homepage, 3–1 Fascial Pain Syndrome (English). https://www.jnos.or.jp/for_medical#Fascial_Pain_Syndrome_English.

Essential Criteria

- Exquisite spot tenderness if the abnormal fascia is accessible
- Identification of high echoic strip-shaped lesions (stacking fascia) as high-density, adhesive, or cohesive fascia on ultrasound findings on/in the same tenderness spot
- Restricted passive range of motion or a painful limit to a full passive stretch caused by abnormal fascia

Confirmatory Observations

- Low extensibility of fascia and/or sliding between fasciae caused by abnormal fascia
- Visual, tactile, or ultrasonographic identification of local twitch response induced by needle penetration of abnormal fascia
- Observation of increase of arterial pulse pressure near the abnormal fascia released by a procedure
- Patient's recognition of current complaint induced by needle stimulation to abnormal fascia.

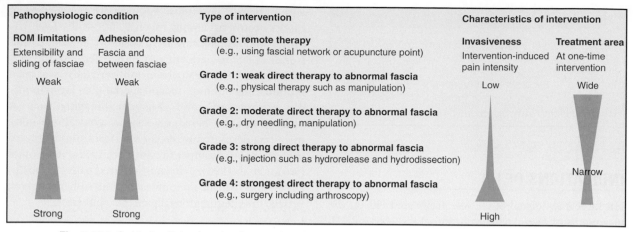

Fig. 7.23.2 Guide for Selecting the Appropriate Treatment: Injection, Physical Therapy, Dry Needling, or Surgery. ROM, range of motion. Modified with permission from Kimura, H., Kobayashi, T., Namiki, H., Takagi, K., 2017. Fundamentals and Clinical Practice of Fascia Release Based on Anatomy, Motion, and Ultrasound: Myofascia Release Developing to Fascia Release. Bunkodo, Tokyo, pp. 22–28.

CONTRAINDICATIONS, COMPLICATIONS, AND RISKS OF HR

Although local anesthetics are not used, local infections or a small amount of local bleeding may occur. Complications and risks are similar to those of prolotherapy (see Chapter 7.11: Prolotherapy).

TECHNIQUES OF HR

Ultrasound-guided HR aims to release stacking fascia as hyperechoic strip-shaped lesions that could be adhesive and cohesive. Slightly moving the needle releases fascial layers in sequence. Physicians release stacking fasciae as if peeling off thin stacking papers to create a "mille-feuille sign" or "layer cake sign" (Kimura et al. 2017; JNOS 2019) (Fig. 7.23.1). Further, it is essential to adjust the direction of the needle bevel for insertion into the space between the fascial layers to be injected. Thinner needles enable proper separation of fascial layers, and by bending the needle, many sites can be treated through a single injection. In contrast, ultrasound-guided HD aims to separate the surrounding tissue of the nerve and generates a "doughnut sign" or "halo sign." Physicians often perform the technique using a needle tip to cut the tissue, excluding peripheral nerves (e.g., scraping, fenestration). Next we discuss the representative HR of fascia for typical targets as of 2018; there are over 300 types of HR techniques, occasionally compared with HD.

KEY POINT

On ultrasound image, hydrorelease aims to create the "mille-feuille sign" or "layer cake sign"; in contrast, hydrodissection does the "doughnut sign" or "halo sign."

MYOFASCIA

The myofascia includes epimysium, perimysium, and endomysium. A typical HR of myofascia targets epimysium and deep fasciae between tissues. Modern ultrasound equipment with high-resolution images enables fine visualization of the level of perimysium. Here, we present an example of ultrasound-guided HR for the myofascia and deep fascia between the trapezius and supraspinatus muscles (Fig. 7.23.1).

NERVE (PARANEURAL SHEATH AND FASCIA AROUND PERIPHERAL NERVES)

The outer fibrils of peripheral nerves is continuous with fasciae (Stecco et al. 2020). For HR, abnormal fascia is treated, which is considered to be an abnormal condition on/around the nerve, such as paraneural sheath and connective tissue among fascicles, epineurium, and perineurium that forms the peripheral nerve. Ultrasound-guided HR aims to spread the injected solution to release stacking fascia in, on, or around the peripheral nerve (Kimura et al. 2017). HR with thinner needles enables proper and safer separation of connective tissue among fascicles. This technique applies to the treatment of fascia, which constitutes the brachial plexus, cervical nerve root, and lumbar nerve root. In contrast, for HD, dissection of fascia, including retinaculum and ligaments, using thicker needles is important to decompress peripheral nerves (Wu et al. 2019).

RETINACULUM

The retinaculum is close to joints of the extremities and thin fascia that reinforces the deep fascia. It has a fibrous connection with surrounding tissues such as bones, muscles, and tendons. It maintains a stable position and transmits mechanical force in various directions. Proprioceptors are abundant and are essential in deep sensation. Clinically, it is crucial as a treatment target of HR for carpal tunnel syndrome. We present here an example of HR of retinaculum for de Quervain disease (Fig. 7.23.3).

TENDON AND TENDON SHEATH

The tendon sheath has a two-layered structure consisting of an inner bursa and outer fibrous tissue. For local injections for tendonitis or tendinopathy, a solution of local anesthetics and steroids is often injected into the tendon sheath. A technique known as high-volume HD

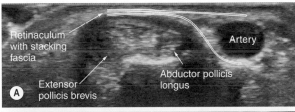
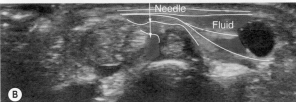

Fig. 7.23.3 Hydrorelease (HR) of Retinaculum. (A) Ultrasound images before HR. (B) Ultrasound images after HR to release the stacking fascia on retinaculum with the injected fluid spread around the artery and in the fascia between extensor pollicis brevis and abductor pollicis longus.

is usually performed for tendinopathies, such as Achilles tendinopathy (Alfredson 2011) and patellar tendinopathy (Maffulli et al. 2016). Its purpose is similar to that of tendon detachment surgery. From the viewpoint of HR, it is essential to carefully release the tendon sheath itself and fascia surrounding the tendon (e.g., in the case of a trigger finger, not only the tendon sheath but also the pully and volar plate) (Kimura et al. 2017). In patellar tendinopathy, the careful release of the tendon itself and surrounding tissues, such as subcutaneous tissue and infrapatellar fat pad, is essential.

JOINT CAPSULE AND SURROUNDING TISSUES

The joint capsule has a two-layered structure consisting of an outer fibrous structure and inner synovium. The outer fibrous structure is continuous with muscles and tendons. HR is performed with cognizance of the continuous structure of muscles, tendons, and joint capsules. When considering moderate to severe injection-related pain, local anesthetics are often used because of the strong injection resistance. Physicians should perform the HR of the joint capsule and its attached tissue.

FASCIA IN FAT PADS

Fat pads are classified from anatomically strong (dense) to soft (loose) and are mixed in one fat pad body. The functions of fat pads include protection of nerves and blood vessels, sliding with surrounding tissues and acting as a pain sensor. When adhesion or cohesion occurs in the fat pad, the range of motion of the joint is limited and pain occurs. We present here an example of ultrasound-guided HR of fascia, nerves, and vessels in, on, or around the fat pad body under the infraspinatus muscle, which is particularly performed if limited range of motion of horizontal adduction of the shoulder is confirmed (Fig. 7.23.4).

LIGAMENTUM FLAVUM/DURA COMPLEX

Abnormalities in the ligamentum flavum/dura complex (LFD) can cause pain (Benditz et al. 2019). Clinically, physicians should consider stubborn pain in the midline, particularly along the spinous processes. Traditional epidural blocks with local anesthetics could also form an aspect of HR of the LFD. Physicians should

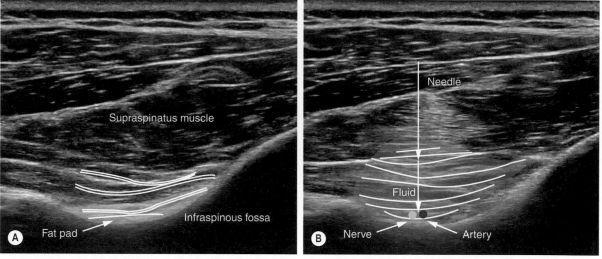

Fig. 7.23.4 Hydrorelease (HR) of Fascia in Fat Pads. (A) Ultrasound images before HR. Stacking fasciae is shown in the muscle and fat pad. (B) Ultrasound images after HR to release the stacking fasciae with the injected fluid spread into fat pad. The artery and nerve in the fat pad appear to be decompressed.

release the ligamentum flavum at the superficial site of LFD to avoid dural puncture. This technique could be performed instead of percutaneous epidural neuroplasty (Holstein et al. 2016) for the removal of adhesive tissues surrounding the spinal cord and LFD (Kimura et al. 2017).

Summary

The history of HR is brief. HR is necessary for basic and clinical research on fascia. HR to target fasciae is different from HD to target peripheral nerves. In clinical practice, it is crucial to assess the precise identification of the source of pain and exacerbating factors associated with symptoms and to share these assessments for interprofessional collaboration.

ACKNOWLEDGMENTS

We would like to thank Takashi Horaguchi, MD, PhD (Division of Sports Medicine, B&J Clinic Ochanomizu / Department of Orthopaedic Surgery and Sports Medicine, Nihon University Hospital) for their thoughtful comments; Ryoya Asaka (Kimura Pain Clinic) for editing figures and tables; and the academic board members of the Japanese Nonsurgical Orthopedics Society (JNOS) for academic advice. We would like to thank Editage (www.editage.com) for English language editing.

REFERENCES

Abdo, H.L., Calvo-Enrique, J.M., Lopez, J.S., et al., 2019. Specialized cutaneous Schwann cells initiate pain sensation. Science 365, 695–699.

Alfredson, H., 2011. Ultrasound and Doppler-guided mini-surgery to treat midportion Achilles tendinosis: results of a large material and a randomised study comparing two scraping techniques. Br. J. Sports Med. 45, 407–410.

Benditz, A., Sprenger, S., Rauch, L., Weber, M., Grifka, J., Straub, R.H., 2019. Increased pain and sensory hyperinnervation of the ligamentum flavum in patients with lumbar spinal stenosis. J. Orthopaed. Res. 37, 737–743.

Bove, G.M., Light, A.R., 1997. The nervi nervorum: missing link for neuropathic pain? Pain Forum 6, 181–190.

Chrambach, A., Rodbard, D., 1971. Polyacrylamide gel electrophoresis. Science 172, 440–451.

Domingo, T., Blasi, J., Casals, M., Mayoral, V., Ortiz-Sagristá, J.C., Miguel-Pérez, M., 2011. Is interfascial block with ultrasound-guided puncture useful in treatment of myofascial pain of the trapezius muscle? Clin. J. Pain 27, 297–303.

Donnelly, J., 2018. Travell, Simons & Simons' Myofascial Pain and Dysfunction: The Trigger Point Manual. Lippincott Williams & Wilkins, Philadelphia, PA.

Evers, S., Thoreson, A.R., Smith, J., Zhao, C., Geske, J.R., Amadio, P.C., 2018. Ultrasound-guided hydrodissection decreases gliding resistance of the median nerve within the carpal tunnel. Muscle Nerve 57, 25–32.

Frost, F.A., Jessen, B., Siggaard-Andersen, J., 1980. A control, double-blind comparison of mepivacaine injection versus saline injection for myofascial pain. Lancet 1, 499–500.

Holstein, S., Center, F.P., Park, C., 2016. Percutaneous and endoscopic adhesiolysis in managing low back and lower extremity pain: a systematic review and meta-analysis. Pain Physician 19, E245–281.

JNOS., 2019. Online academic information for medical staff (Japanese Non-surgical Orthopedics Society, JNOS). Available from: https://www.jnos.or.jp/for_medical.

Kimura, H., 2008. Interfascial injection with a local anesthesia (in Japanese). In: 2nd Conference of Japanese Society for the Study of Myofascial Pain Syndrome (JMPS), Tokyo.

Kimura, H., 2012. SUKIMA block (interfascial block) with physiological saline: new procedure for myofascial pain syndrome. In: 10th Conference of Japanese Society for the Study of Myofascial Pain Syndrome (JMPS).

Kimura, H., 2014. A new injection technique of ultrasound-guided myofascial release (in Japanese). In: 13th Conference of Japanese Society for the Study of Myofascial Pain Syndrome (JMPS).

Kimura, H., 2015. Myofascial release developing to fascial release (in Japanese). In: 15th Conference of Japanese Society for the Study of Myofascial Pain Syndrome (JMPS).

Kimura, H., Kobayashi, T., Namiki, H., 2018. Fascia Release for Shoulder Pain and Stiffness: Focusing on Scapulo-humeral Periarthritis and Adhesive Capsulitis of Shoulder (in Japanese). Bunkodo, Tokyo.

Kimura, H., Kobayashi, T., Namiki, H., Takagi, K., 2017. Fundamentals and Clinical Practice of Fascia Release Based on Anatomy, Motion, and Ultrasound: Myofascia Release Developing to Fascia Release (in Japanese). Bunkodo, Tokyo.

Kimura, H., Kobayashi, T., Zenita, Y., Kurosawa, A., Aizawa, S., 2019. Expansion of 1 mL solution by ultrasound-guided injection between the trapezius and rhomboid muscle: a cadaver study. Pain Med. 21, 1018–1024.

Kobayashi, T., Kimura, H., Ozaki, N., 2016. Effects of interfascial injection of bicarbonated Ringer's solution, physiological saline and local anesthetic under ultrasonography for myofascial pain syndrome. Two prospective, randomized, double-blinded trials. J. Juzen. Med. Soc. 125, 40–49.

Lam, S.K.H., Reeves, K.D., Cheng, A.L., 2017. Transition from deep regional blocks toward deep nerve hydrodissection in the upper body and torso: method description and results from a retrospective chart review of the analgesic effect of 5% dextrose water as the primary hydrodissection injectate to enhance safety. BioMed Res. Int. 2017:7920438. doi:10.1155/2017/7920438.

Langevin, H.M., Fox, J.R., Koptiuch, C., et al. 2011. Reduced thoracolumbar fascia shear strain in human chronic low back pain. BMC Musculoskel. Disord. 12, 203.

Maffulli, N., Del Buono, A., Oliva, F., Testa, V., Capasso, G., Maffulli G., 2016. High-volume image-guided injection for recalcitrant patellar tendinopathy in athletes. Clin. J. Sport Med. 26, 12–16.

Matsuoka, H., Obata, H., Saito, S., et al. 2010. The new nerve block to myofascial pain syndrome (MPS): Interfascial block (SUKIMA block) (in Japanese). Pain Clinic 31, 497–500.

Matsuzaki, M., 2017. The latest technology of musculoskeletal ultrasonography: iterative revolution. J. Med. Ultrason. 44, 223–236.

Nagano, T., 2018. Ultrasound-guided C8 nerve root hydrorelease for C8 nerve radiculopathy: a case report. J. Japan Soc. Orthoped. Ultrason. 30, 230–235.

Sola, A.E., Kuitert, J.H., 1955. Myofascial trigger point pain in the neck and shoulder girdle; report of 100 cases treated by injection of normal saline. Northwest Med. 54, 980–984.

Staal, J.B., de Bie, R., de Vet, H.C., Hildebrandt, J., Nelemans, P., 2008. Injection therapy for subacute and chronic low-back pain. Cochrane Database Syst. Rev., CD001824.

Staud, R., Nagel, S., Robinson, M.E., Price, D.D., 2009. Enhanced central pain processing of fibromyalgia patients is maintained by muscle afferent input: a randomized, double-blind, placebo-controlled study. Pain 145, 96–104.

Staud, R., Weyl, E.E., Bartley, E., Price, D.D., Robinson, M.E., 2014. Analgesic and anti-hyperalgesic effects of muscle injections with lidocaine or saline in patients with fibromyalgia syndrome. Eur. J. Pain 18, 803–812.

Stecco, A., Meneghini, A., Stern, R., Stecco, C., Imamura, M., 2014. Ultrasonography in myofascial neck pain: randomized clinical trial for diagnosis and follow-up. Surg. Radiol. Anat. 36, 243–253.

Stecco, C., Giordani, F., Fan, C., et al. 2020. Role of fasciae around the median nerve in pathogenesis of carpal tunnel syndrome: microscopic and ultrasound study. J. Anat. 236, 660–667.

Stecco, C., Pirri, C., Fede, C., et al., 2019. Dermatome and fasciatome. Clin. Anat. 37, 896–902.

Taylor, G.I., Caddy, C.M., Watterson, P.A., Crock, J.G., 1990. The venous territories (venosomes) of the human body: experimental study and clinical implications. Plast. Reconstr. Surg. 86 (2), 185–213.

Taylor, G.I., Palmer, J.H., 1987. The vascular territories (angiosomes) of the body: experimental study and clinical applications. Br. J. Plast. Surg. 40, 113–141.

Wheeler, P.C., Mahadevan, D., Bhatt, R., Bhatia, M., 2016. A comparison of two different high-volume image-guided injection procedures for patients with chronic noninsertional Achilles tendinopathy: a pragmatic retrospective cohort study. J. Foot Ankle Surg. 55, 976–979.

Wu, Y.T., Chen, S.R., Li, T.Y., et al., 2019. Nerve hydrodissection for carpal tunnel syndrome: a prospective, randomized, double-blind, controlled trial. Muscle Nerve 59:174–180.

Fascia and Traditional Chinese Medicine

Ling Guan

CHAPTER CONTENTS

INTRODUCTION

There are two kinds of treatment in traditional Chinese medicine (TCM). One is the use of herbal medicine. Doctors feel the patient's pulse and prescribe herbs by assessing the patient's constitution. The other is to adjust the human body structure and mobilize the human body to heal itself by acupuncture, moxibustion, massage, scraping, cupping, and other acupoint stimulation. The latter is called nonpharmaceutical therapy. In China, acupuncture and moxibustion are general terms of TCM nonpharmaceutical therapy. It is represented by acupuncture and moxibustion, including but not limited to acupuncture, moxibustion, scraping, cupping, auricular acupressure, acupotomology, acupoint heating, acupoint percutaneous electrical stimulation, acupoint percutaneous magnetic stimulation, acupoint laser, and other acupoint stimulation. Through deep study and careful arrangement of TCM classics, we find that the function of acupuncture and moxibustion is based on skin, veins, flesh, muscles, and bones (Huangdi Neijing 2015),which are called Five Ti (five body structures). In fact, nonpharmaceutical therapy of TCM is to give different stimulation on different body structures to adjust the balance of human body structure and promote functional rehabilitation through direct or indirect effects. The basic theory and technique

of these treatments are closely related to fascia. There are also many studies based on the physiological characteristics of fascia to explore the mechanism of acupuncture and moxibustion. Based on the anatomical structure of the human body, contemporary Chinese acupuncture doctors developed a deeper understanding of traditional acupuncture knowledge and greater technical progress. The new techniques have been called "structure-based medical acupuncture" (Guan et al. 2017). Some important points of this chapter are excerpted from the fascia discussion of structure-based medical acupuncture.

 KEY POINT

Acupuncture is the representative of nonpharmaceutical therapy in traditional Chinese medicine, including many other body surface stimulation techniques in addition to acupuncture.

THE BASIC ELEMENTS OF ACUPUNCTURE AND FASCIA

Meridian

Meridian is one of the most important concepts of acupuncture and moxibustion. Meridian and collaterals systems consist of the meridians—12 main meridians, 8 extrameridians, and 12 divergent meridians—and the collaterals, which include 15 big collaterals, many minute collaterals, and superficial collaterals. In addition, it includes 12 out connection meridians named 12 meridian sinew (the fascia, muscle, and joints connected by the 12 meridians), 12 cutaneous regions (the function of the 12 meridians is reflected in the body surface), and 12 zang-fu organs connected inwardly by meridians (Fig. 7.24.1).

Contemporary scholars believe that the 12 meridians are a high-level generalization of the longitudinal relationship of the human body (Huang 2016). This relationship includes the mechanical relationship of the musculoskeletal system, the electrical relationship of nerves, the chemical relationship of the fluid system, etc. The structural essence of the mechanical relationship is muscle, bone, and fascia.

Meridian Sinew

In classical Chinese meridian theory, muscle and fascia are called "meridian sinew", which means the muscle, tendon, and fascia along the meridian. Meridian sinew is equivalent to the modern myofascial chain to some degree. Some studies have shown that the myofascial meridians in Anatomy Trains (Myers 2014) are highly correlated with acupuncture meridians and some lines overlap (Dorsher 2004). But there are many differences in the details. Modern research believes that the generation of acupuncture meridians is related to the human movement lines observed by ancient doctors (Yan 2016). Researchers (Xie et al. 2019) have found that the meridian sinew theory is consistent with the theory of the myofascial chain in many aspects. But clinically, meridian sinew therapy does not only treat diseases of the muscle and nervous system but also has a good therapeutic effect on diseases related to viscera, whereas

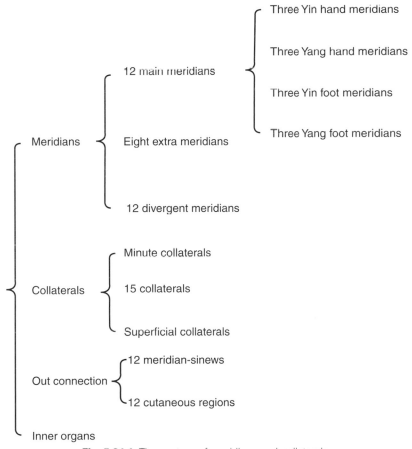

Fig. 7.24.1 The system of meridians and collaterals.

the myofascial chain shows more advantages in posture evaluation and exercise guidance.

Many doctors in China use the theory of meridian sinew to treat diseases; typical examples are Ligong Xue and Jingwei Huang. According to Chinese classics and meridian sinew theory, Ligong Xue (Xue 2009) found that some points along the tendons are more likely to be injured biomechanically. Xue treated the disease by piercing the fascia with a slanted acupotomy needle (type Chang Yuan Zhen) (Fig. 7.24.2). Professor Xue thought that most of these points, which are located near the ligaments of the joints, were bursa. Therefore the treatment has a very good effect on diseases of the motor system.

Jingwei Huang (Huang 1996) thought that the meridians will have corresponding responses when the human body faces internal and external stimulation. When this response exceeds a threshold, it will cause the meridian sinews to produce some pathological "nodule." Huang finds these nodules by palpation, pinches them by needle or softens them by manipulation. The treatment has a wide range of applications, including musculoskeletal pain and many viscera diseases.

Fascia is also concentrated in the scalp. There are many schools of head needle and different acupuncture point positions. Some points are in accordance with the TCM meridian acupoints, some with brain function (Shunfa 2019), and some with holographic theory (Mingjun et al. 2014). In general, the top of the head is the highest and commanding point of the whole body fascia network and a point of mechanical convergence. Acupuncture adjustment in the head can adjust the fascia network of the whole body.

Acupoints

According to Chinese acupuncture theory, there are more than 360 acupoints on the main meridians and nearly 100 acupoints, called extraordinary points, that are not on the main meridians. In addition, there is another kind of acupoint called A-shi acupoint, which changes along with the disease and has no fixed location or quantity. Some classical acupoints, such as GB34 (Yang Ling Quan), are featured by fascia. TCM considers it to be the place where fascia meets and helps to treat systemic fascia diseases. Other acupoints are located near the wrist and ankle, where the fascia is concentrated and can be connected to treat distant diseases. The treatment zone of wrist and ankle needle (Zhang 1978; Ling et al. 2017) divide the subcutaneous tissue around the wrist and ankle into six zones, which converge along the extremities toward trunk and head and connect them, thus treating distant diseases. The theory of the umbilical needle (Qi 2015) is based on the book *I Ching* and the eight diagrams, and the calculation is complicated. Because the navel is a place where fascia is concentrated, the needle placement here also has a regulating effect on the abdominal fascia. Some doctors choose the insertion site based entirely on palpation of the fascia.

ACUPUNCTURE AND MOXIBUSTION TECHNIQUES WITH FASCIA

Acupuncture and Myofascia

In ancient China, many classic acupuncture techniques are related to muscle fascia. One of the most important is the Fen Rou Ci Fa (inserting the needle in the tissues between the muscles), which is one of the nine techniques in the operation specification. The description of acupuncture in the *Huang Di Nei Jing* (Inner Canon of Huangdi) includes not only the principle of treatment but also descriptions of acupuncture tools, acupuncture sites, and acupuncture methods. For example, in the principle of treatment, it says "if the evil qi is in full, you should discharge it; if the positive qi is deficient, you should replenish it; if the patient's feeling is tight and painful, you should needle the Intermuscle." On the

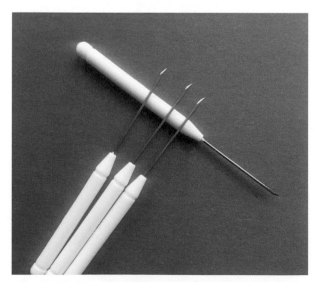

Fig. 7.24.2 Chang Yuan Zhen (slanted acupotomy needles).

acupuncture tools and points, Huang Di Nei Jing says: "the Round Needle, with round body and blunt tip, is 1.5 inches long. It is used to treat Qi of Fen Rou (tissues between the muscles) . . . if the disease is in Fou Rou, use the Round Needles to discharge it." The operation is: "use the Round Needle rub the tissues of Fen Rou, do not injure the muscles so that the Qi of disease will leak out." The place of treatment is *inter-flesh,* which is fascia.

In modern acupuncture treatment, increasing numbers of doctors have found that acupuncture in subcutaneous tissue can effectively relieve musculoskeletal pain, for example, the wrist and ankle needling, the intradermal needling (Dan 2018), the floating needles (Fu 2000, 2016) and the Jin needling (Liu and Liu 2016). Despite the different names, they all have one thing in common: the needles are placed under the skin and above the muscles. This area is called the Fen Rou of traditional Chinese medicine, and it corresponds to the space of human fascia—connective tissue.

Additionally, in the 1970s, Dinghou Lu (Dinghou 1993), a physiology professor in Beijing Sports University, found that chronic strain may cause skeletal muscle cramps. Doctors may find a hard muscle bundle of cords through palpation, which they thought was the "A-shi acupoint" in TCM. To find the "A-shi acupoint," the way is to press it, and the patient will feel pain and say "Ah! Yes! It is here!" When pressing the "A-shi acupoint," the patient feels hard but not necessarily painful. Therefore Professor Lu used a long needle to insert diagonally through the induration to deal with these hard muscle cramps. The method can quickly relieve musculoskeletal pain, and his method was known as the "long needle oblique piercing A-shi acupoint method."

> ### KEY POINT
>
> Acupuncture and moxibustion treatment is characterized by the focus not only on local lesions, but also on the overall changes. The fascia connects the various parts of the human body into a whole. Therefore fascia theory can be used to explain some of the effects of acupuncture. By analyzing the effect, experience, and mechanism of acupuncture and moxibustion, we will find that it is inextricably linked to the fascia.

Moxibustion and Myofascia

Moxibustion entails using burning moxa sticks or other materials to heat the acupoint on the human body in order to treat diseases. In ancient times, people mainly heated with moxa sticks. Nowadays there are many new materials, such as coconut shell, smokeless charcoal, and electric and magnetic heating. Heating can soften stiff fascia, improve circulation of the blood, and increase the mobility between tissues to relieve pain. Moxibustion is effective for many diseases, including musculoskeletal pain, visceral and endocrine diseases, and even cancer.

Scraping and Myofascia

Scraping involves using a smooth plate (Fig. 7.24.3) to push and pull the skin and superficial fascia. Scraping can adjust the tension of the superficial fascia layer; it can also cause subcutaneous congestion, which promotes tissue regeneration during the process of blood absorption. Scraping is used to treat pain in the skeletal muscle system, soft tissue damage, and certain symptoms such as chest tightness, abdominal distension, and dizziness.

Cupping and Myofascia

Cupping therapy involves absorbing the cup on the skin through negative pressure, congesting loose connective tissue under the skin, and repairing tissue in

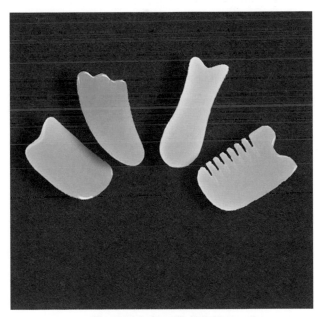

Fig. 7.24.3 Scraping plates.

the process of absorption and reconstruction. Research (Shu and Guan 2019) has proved that cupping therapy can boost the release of β-EP and reduce the release of inflammatory factors such as Il-6, Il-8, and TNF-α in serum, so as to improve the body environment, increase metabolism, and promote the recovery of cells. Cupping can significantly improve the local pain tolerance threshold and improve the pain-induced dysfunction. It can also improve the phagocytosis ability of white blood cells and reticular cells in order to strengthen the body's resistance (Li et al. 2014), increase the local pain tolerance threshold, and alleviate the pain-induced dysfunction (Farhadi et al. 2009).

Warm Needle Moxibustion and Myofascia

In the 1960s, Zhenren Xuan, a famous orthopedic surgeon in Shanghai, found that a large part of low back pain was caused by aseptic inflammatory lesions of soft tissue outside the lumbar spinal canal that stimulated the peripheral nerves, rather than mechanical compression of the herniated disc. Therefore he adopted a procedure called *soft tissue surgery,* which only deals with the muscle to treat severe back pain. The procedure worked very well. Then Xuan changed it to a technique called the *silver needle heating* for tissue release, which is now popular in China. In the early days, the needle was heated by burning moxa balls (Fig. 7.24.4), which originated from the traditional Chinese technique named warm needle moxibustion. Later, an electric heating cap was used for a heating needle (Fig. 7.24.5). Xuan's main academic thoughts were published in *Soft Tissue Theory and Practice* (Xuan 1994) and *Soft Tissue Surgery* (Xuan 2020).

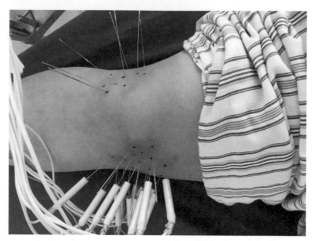

Fig. 7.24.5 Electrically heated silver-needle and silver-needle release technique.

Acupotomy and Fascia

Professor Hanzhang Zhu invented acupotomy (Fig. 7.24.6). The acupuncture needle has a small knife edge on the tip; therefore, it has the function of cutting as well as puncturing and is able to treat some diseases caused by fascia adhesion and scar tissue. This tool can be applied to fascia, muscles, and muscle attachment points and was mainly used for the treatment of muscle, bone, and joint pain, as well as some visceral diseases. The acupotomy

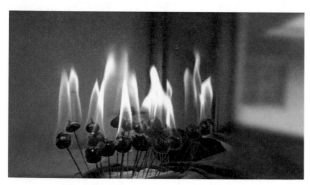

Fig. 7.24.4 Heated-needle moxibustion.

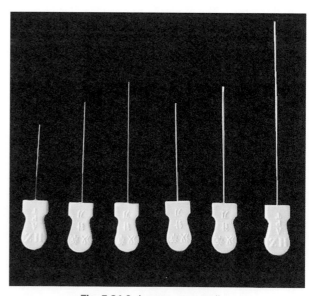

Fig. 7.24.6 Acupotomy needles.

technique is popular in China. Not only acupuncture doctors but also some surgeons like it and regard it as a micro closed surgery or TCM minimally invasive technique. For the mechanism, many studies show that acupotomy can control the inflammatory reaction, improve the microcirculation, inhibit the production of the pain factors, and reduce the muscular cellular apoptosis (Zhang et al. 2019; Kim et al. 2019; Ma et al. 2017). Hanzhang Zhu's main academic thoughts were written in the books *Acupotomy Therapy* (Zhu 1992) and *Acupotomology* (Zhu 2004).

Bo-Needling and Fascia

A new type of needle has appeared in China. It can loosen and stimulate the shallow and middle layers of superficial and deep fascia (Zhao et al. 2019; Gong et al. 2019). This kind of needle has a round blunt tip (Fig. 7.24.7), which can separate the fascia blunt according to patients with different conditions. It can be used not only for the treatment of some stubborn painful disease but also for some chronic diseases such as diabetes, asthma, and gastroenteritis, through activating mesenchymal stem cells of the middle of the superficial fascia, stimulating the body's own immune and repair ability (Wang and Wang 2017).

Manipulation and Fascia

In traditional Chinese practices, many doctors treated osteoarthropathy and even internal diseases using fascia manipulation. There is a saying, "put the bone in the right place, let the myofascial soft, energy and blood will flow naturally perfusion." Youming Luo, famous in China, is a typical doctor of this practice. She started to treat patients in the 1920s and continued to do so until

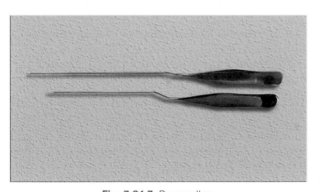

Fig. 7.24.7 Bo-needles.

the 2000s, at the age of 100 years old. Although she had excellent medical skills, she was illiterate and did not write any books. However, she trained a large number of students for medical institutions in China, among which Tianyou Feng (Feng 2002) and Xihuan Yan are two typical representatives. The former is good at osteopathy, whereas the latter is better at toning fascia. Xihuan Yan is known for manipulation of "dredging the myofascia and open the collaterals," which mainly smooths the fascia folds and restores the force line, and then blood (Qi) will operate automatically.

Professor Zheren Xuan, mentioned previously, later also changed the technique of heating the silver needle into a manipulation in his later years. In his proposed strong stimulation massage the main operating site was still on the periosteum, specifically at the attachment areas of skeletal muscles. Years later, his student, Jianmin Li, changed the technique to a weak stimulation periosteum compression. Xuan and his students have had great influence in China, but no matter how the technique develops, the main operating site is on the periosteum, which is part of the fascia.

ACUPUNCTURE RESEARCH AND FASCIA

There has been a lot of research on acupuncture and fascia. A team, led by professor Lin Yuan, has been working on acupuncture and fascia. Lin believes that the anatomical basis of meridians is human fascia framework, and the histological structure of meridians is nonspecific connective tissue (including loose connective tissue and adipose tissue). He also believes that acupoints are the parts of fascia that can produce strong biological information when stimulated. His representative book is *Fasciology* (Lin et al. 2011). Professor Lin Yuan's team has done a lot of research about fascia. For example, Chunlei Wang (Wang 2008) conducted a digital anatomy study on the correlation between acupuncture meridian points and fascia convergence areas. Jun Wang's research (Wang 2008a, 2008b) shows that some important acupoints of human limbs are closely related to the connective tissue. Therefore acupoints may be where the biological receptors in connective tissue produce strong information, and the connective tissue framework of the human body is the anatomical material basis of meridians.

Xiaolei Guan adopted a variety of linear stimulations on fascia tissue to induce meridian phenomena and related transmission phenomena (Guan 2015). Xueme Jiang proved that acupuncture may regulate the body by affecting the connective tissue framework of fascia, causing deformation of tissue cells, affecting the expression of proteins in cell signaling pathways, and leading to biochemical reactions in the body (Jiang 2009).

Helene M. Langevin, of the Harvard Medical School, observed some tissue sections after acupuncture (Langevin et al. 2001). Langevin found that: (1) there was a mechanical connection between the needle and connective tissue, which was caused by the winding of the surrounding tissue during the twisting process; and (2) the acupuncture operation transmits mechanical signals to the connective tissue cells through mechanical force transduction. This mechanism could explain the local and distal effects of acupuncture and the long-term effects of acupuncture. Another article by Langevin pointed out that when manipulated, the body of the needle may send a powerful mechanical signal to the tissue through its entanglement with the connective tissue. The mechanical signaling of these cells and molecules is extensive and powerful, involving processes ranging from cell contraction to signaling pathway activation to gene expression (Langevin et al. 2002).

CONCLUSION: THE CONTRIBUTION OF FASCIA TO ACUPUNCTURE AND MOXIBUSTION

Acupuncture and moxibustion has a history of over 2000 years. The more comprehensive our understanding of fascia, the more profound our understanding of acupuncture and moxibustion will be. In the concept of traditional Chinese medicine, a person is considered as a whole, and doctors should treat patients from the whole body. When they treat patients, Chinese doctors usually do not treat the local acupuncture points, but more distant parts related to them. It seems incredible, which is why people think acupuncture is amazing. Continuous research on fascia allows us to have a better understanding of acupuncture.

Acupuncture and moxibustion is a simple and efficient treatment method discovered by ancient doctors. It makes full use of the human body's structural characteristics to promote self-adjustment. This treatment idea is undoubtedly advanced even in modern society.

Although ancient Chinese doctors did not describe fascia as accurately as we do today, or because of ancient language, we are not able to fully understand what they meant. It is clear that they were aware of the existence of this structure in the human body and found ways to adjust it functionally. A large number of medical classics recorded the experience of Chinese doctors in treating fascia. In contemporary China, there are also many acupuncturists constantly innovating tools, developing treatment methods, and expanding acupuncture indications. These experiences are extremely valuable for the study and use of fascia, and acupuncture makes a great contribution to the research of fascia.

Fascia not only connects the human body, but also Chinese medicine and Western medicine.

Summary

There is a close relationship between acupuncture and fascia. Ancient Chinese doctors realized the structure of fascia and found a series of methods to treat disease by using fascia. It is just not named the fascia. This chapter describes the relationship between acupuncture therapy and fascia and discusses some studies on the correlation between acupuncture and fascia. It is shown that the experience of acupuncture can greatly promote the research of fascia, and the research of fascia is also helpful to deepen our understanding of acupuncture.

REFERENCES

Dan, Z., 2018. Graphic Intradermal Needling Therapy. Chinese Medicine Technology Publishing House, Beijing.

Dinghou, L., 1993. Etiology and Treatment of Skeletal Muscle Injury. Beijing Sport University Press, Beijing.

Dorsher, P.T., 2004. Poster 196 myofascial pain: rediscovery of a 2000-year-old tradition? Arch Phys Med Rehabil, 85, e42.

Farhadi, K., Schwebel, D.C., Saeb, M., Choubsaz, M., Mohammadi, R., Ahmadi, A., 2009. The effectiveness of wet-cupping for nonspecific low back pain in Iran: a randomized controlled trial. Complement. Ther. Med. 17, 9–15.

Feng, T., 2002. Clinical Study on the Treatment of Soft Tissue Injury with the Combination of Traditional Chinese Medicine and Western Medicine. Science and Technology Publishing House, Beijing.

Fu, Z., 2000. Fu's Subcutaneous Needling. People's Military Medical Publishing House, Beijing.

Fu, Z., 2016. The Foundation of Fu's Subcutaneous Needling. People's Medical Publishing House, Beijing.

Gong, G., Sun, S., Wang, X., Dong, H., 2019. Clinical Observation on 42 Cases of Gluteal Muscle Injury Treated by Needles. World Latest Med. Inf. 19, 127–131.

Guan, L., Yu, Y., Du, J.L., 2017. Structure-based Acupuncture. People's Medical Publishing House, Beijing.

Guan, X., 2015. Study on the Meridian Attachment Organization from the Upper Limb's Meridian Sensation and Stretching Meridian. Henan Chinese Traditional Medicine College, Zhengzhou, Henan.

Huang Di Nei Jing (2013). People's Medical Publishing House, Beijing.

Huang, J., 1996. Treatment of Meridian Sinew. Chinese Medicine Publishing House, Beijing.

Huang, L., 2016. Outline of Reduction and Reconstruction of Meridian Theory. People's Medical Publishing House, Beijing.

Jiang, X., 2009. Study on the Role of Fascia in Signal Conduction of Acupuncture and its Relationship with MAPK Pathway. Southern Medical University, Guangzhou, Guangdong.

Kim, S.Y., Kim, E., Kwon, O., Han, C.H., Kim, Y.I., 2019. Corrigendum to "Effectiveness and Safety of Acupotomy for Lumbar Disc Herniation: A Randomized, Assessor-Blinded, Controlled Pilot Study." Evid. Based Complement. Alternat. Med. 2019:4538692.

Langevin, H.M., Churchill, D.L., Cipolla, M.J. 2001. Mechanical signaling through connective tissue: A mechanism for the therapeutic effect of acupuncture. FASEB Journal: official publication of the Federation of American Societies for Experimental Biology, 15, 2275–2282.

Langevin, H.M., Churchill, D.L., Wu, J., et al., 2002. Evidence of connective tissue involvement in acupuncture. FASEB J., 16, 872–874.

Li, D., Meng, X, Lin, H., Zhu, C., 2014. Shengai Piao Research overview on Mechanism of Cupping Therapy. Liaoning J. Tradit. Chin. Med. 41, 2506–2508.

Lin, Y., Bai, Y., Huang, Y., 2011. Anatomical discovery of meridians and collaterals and the theory of Fasciaology. Shanghai J. Acupunct. Moxibustion. 30, 1–5.

Ling, C., Zhou, Q., Gu, W., 2017. Wrist Ankle Acupuncture. Shanghai science and Technology Publishing House, Shanghai.

Liu, N., Liu, Z., 2016. Sinew Needling. People's Medical Publishing House, Beijing.

Ma, S.N., Xie, Z.G., Guo, Y., et al., 2017. Effect of Acupotomy on FAK-PI3K Signaling Pathways in KOA Rabbit Articular Cartilages. Evid. Based Complement. Alternat. Med. 2017:4535326.

Mingjun, A., Huang, L., Fang, Y., 2014. Clinical Experience, Shaanxi Science and Technology Publishing House, Xi'an, Shaanxi.

Myers T.W. 2014. Anatomy Trains: Myofascial Meridians for Manual and Movement Therapists, third ed., Churchill Livingstone Elsevier, Edinburgh.

Qi, Y., 2015. Umbilical Needle Therapy Introduction. People's Medical Publishing House, Beijing.

Shu, M., Guan, L., 2019. Curative effects of moving cupping therapy on chronic back pain and related changes in IL-2 and IL-8. Academic Journal of Chinese PLA Medical School 40, 958–961.

Shunfa, J., 2019. Shunfa Jiao's Scalp Acupuncture. Chinese Medicine Publishing House, Beijing.

Wang, C., 2008a. Digital Anatomic Study on the Relationship between Meridians and Acupuncture Points and Fascia Converging Areas. Southern Medical University, Guangzhou, Guangdong.

Wang, J., 2008b. Medical Imageological Study on the Fasciological Basis for Channels and Points in Human Extremities. Southern Medical University, Guangzhou, Guangdong.

Wang, J., Wang, Z., 2017. Fasciology and Traditional Chinese Medicine. Science and Technology Publishing House, Beijing.

Wilhelm, R. and Baynes, C.F. (translators), 1967. The I Ching, or Book of Changes. Princeton University Press.

Xie, J., Wu, A., Cheng, Y., 2019. On the relevance between meridian and fascial chain theory of traditional Chinese medicine, Hunan J. Tradit. Chin. Med. 35, 113–114.

Xuan, Z., 1994. Theory and Practice of Soft Tissue Surgery. People's Military Medical Publishing House, Beijing.

Xuan, Z., 2020. Soft Tissue Surgery. Wenhui Publishing House, Shanghai.

Xue, L.G., 2009. Chinese Meridian Sinews. Traditional Chinese Medicine Ancient Books Publishing House, Beijing.

Yan, F., 2016. Research and Clinical Applications of Jein-Chin System (twelve human athletic lines). Shandong Chinese Traditional Medicine University, Jinan, Shandong.

Zhang, R., Li, L., Chen, B., et al. 2019. Acupotomy versus nonsteroidal anti-inflammatory drugs for knee osteoarthritis: protocol for a systematic review and meta-analysis. Medicine 98, e17051.

Zhang, X., 1978. Wrist Ankle Acupuncture. Shanghai science and Technology Publishing House, Shanghai.

Zhao, X., Kang, S., Zhang, Z., et al. 2019. Seventy-five cases of lumbosacral fascial fat hernia treated by Z-needling. Chinese J. Tradit. Med. Traumatol. Orthop. 27, 52–54.

Zhu, H., 1992. Acupotomy Therapy. Chinese Medicine Publishing House, Beijing.

Zhu, H., 2004. Acupotomology. Chinese Medicine Publishing House, Beijing.

Extracorporeal Shockwave Therapy Applied to Myofascial Tissue

Hannes Müller-Ehrenberg and Federico Giordani

CHAPTER CONTENTS

INTRODUCTION

Extracorporeal shockwave therapy (ESWT) is a treatment method that was introduced for the therapeutic destruction of kidney stones (lithotripsy) more than 40 years ago (Chaussy et al. 1980). In the past three decades, ESWT has further been implemented for the treatment of musculoskeletal disorders (Moya et al. 2018). Basic studies and clinical trials have shown that ESWT is a safe and effective method for treating diverse musculoskeletal diseases (d'Agostino et al. 2015; Ioppolo et al. 2014).

Initially, mainly bone and calcified structures were the target of ESWT in orthopedics, but other types of tissue, such as skin, nerves, and myofascial tissue were discovered as target tissues for medical interventions (Ramon et al. 2015).

SHOCKWAVE BASICS

A shockwave (SW) is an acoustic energy that is generated from outside of the body and therefore is called extracorporeal shockwave (ESW) (Chaussy et al. 1980; Moya et al. 2018). Its mechanism of action is based on acoustic mechanical waves that act at molecular, cellular, and tissue levels to generate a biological response (Cheng and Wang 2015). For medical use two types of energy are used as shockwaves: the focused ESWT (fESWT) and the so-called radial shockwave, which is a radial pressure wave (RPW). Both technologies differ in their generation devices, physical characteristics, and mechanisms of action.

The mechanical energy of RPW is a pressure wave that applies most of the energy on the surface and then expands radially into the tissue (see Fig. 7.25.1). RPW lacks the physical features of a shockwave because the rise times of the pressure pulses are too long and the pressure outputs are too low (Cleveland et al. 2007). The limitation of RPW is mainly the shorter penetration depth, with maximum intensity at the point of entry, and the lower efficacy of stimulation at the cellular level (Novak 2019).

The mechanisms of action and the biological effects of RPW on living tissue may differ from those of

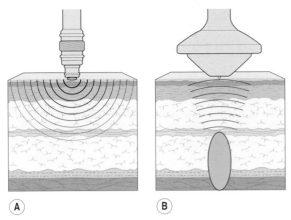

Fig. 7.25.1 Schematic visualization of the distribution of radial pressure waves (A) and focused shockwaves in human tissue (B).

focused shockwaves because biological effects are related to the pressure waveform. The use of RPW is indicated for superficial pain treatment of larger areas. Focused shockwaves can also reach deeper tissue layers with a concentrated energy (d'Agostino et al. 2015; Novak, 2019). Focused SW (fSW) are sonic pulses characterized by a high peak pressure up to more than 100 MPa (500 bar), rapid rise in pressure (<10 ns), short duration (<10 ns), and a broad range of frequency. FSW are produced by an electrohydraulic, piezoelectric, or electromagnetic type generator (Ogden et al. 2001).

MECHANISMS OF ACTION OF EXTRACORPOREAL SHOCKWAVE THERAPY ON TISSUE

There is consensus that the applied shockwave energy (0.01–0.5 mJ/mm^2) does not cause a mechanically destructive effect on the musculoskeletal system but rather affects the function and metabolism of tissue and cells. These are either positively regulated or stimulated. This biological effect is referred to as mechanotransduction (d'Agostino et al. 2015; Wang 2012].

EFFECTS OF ESWT ON TENDONS AND MYOFASCIAL TISSUE

The advancing research on the histology and pathophysiological behaviors of connective tissues indicate that the definition of the fascial system includes tendons and the intra- and intermuscular connective tissues (Adstrum et al. 2017).

Tendinous tissue, which belongs to the family of fascial tissue, has been treated successfully with extracorporeal shockwaves (ESWT) for more than 25 years (Loew et al. 1995). In this time, numerous fundamental studies and clinical trials in this field have been conducted (Moya et al. 2018). This research allows us to extrapolate the effects of ESWT on the entire family of fascial tissue, not only on tendons.

ANTIINFLAMMATORY EFFECTS AND PAIN REDUCTION OF ESWT

> ### KEY POINT
> Clinically significant pain reduction can be achieved with ESWT by decreasing vasonociceptive-active substances.

An acute inflammatory response is a crucial part of the regeneration process. Importantly, the phase of inflammation should be short-lived and reversible for healing to occur (Zügel et al. 2018). In the following text, many factors of the inflammatory and regenerative process that can be modulated by ESWT to support the healing process are introduced.

Macrophages play a key role in the inflammatory phase, but prolonged macrophage activity can lead to an impairment of the healing process. It has been shown that ESWT application can modulate macrophage activity by stimulating a shift in macrophage phenotype from M1 to M2 and increasing T-cell proliferation (Khan and Scott 2009). Thus ESWT application aiming at macrophages reduces prolonged inflammation and aids the healing process (Sukubo et al. 2015). In addition, it was shown that ESWT further regulates inflammation via toll-like receptor 3 (TLR3) pathways by early induction of a proinflammatory reaction (mediated by IL6 and cyclophilin A), followed by an antiinflammatory effect in later phases (mediated by IL10) (Holfeld et al. 2014; Sukubo et al. 2015).

In fundamental research studies it was shown that vasonociceptive-active substances that are part of the inflammatory response, such as substance P, COX-2, prostaglandin-E2, CGRP, and others have been reduced by the application of low- to middle-energy ESWT (Maier et al. 2003; Hausdorf et al. 2008). Importantly, the significant reduction of substance P by ESWT application further leads to a decrease of pain (Hausdorf et al. 2008).

These findings from basic research in animal models can explain the positive effects found in clinical studies, with application of ESWT leading to reduction of myofascial pain (Gleitz and Hornig 2012; Hausdorf et al. 2008; Muller-Ehrenberg and Licht 2005). In support of this, in-vivo studies in humans found elevated levels of substance P, CGFP, bradykinin, and other pain-related vasonociceptive-active substances in myofascial tissue, more specifically in myofascial trigger points (MTrP) (Shah et al. 2005).

ANTIFIBROTIC EFFECTS OF ESWT ON MYOFASCIAL TISSUE

 KEY POINT

ESWT enhances tissue regeneration by acceleration of the inflammatory phase and has an antifibrotic effect on tissue by positive modulation of fibroblast activity.

Fibroblasts are considered to be the major mechanoresponsive cells in the connective tissue (Klingler et al. 2012). With their function of organizing and synthesizing connective tissue, fibroblasts are indispensable for remodeling the extracellular matrix (ECM).

Studies in vitro and in vivo confirmed that ESW treatment enhances fibroblast proliferation and differentiation by activation of gene expression for transforming growth factor β1 (TGF-β1) and collagen types I and III (Frairia and Berta 2011). Research by Fede and colleagues (in preparation) further indicates that collagen cell generation after fESW is enhanced 24 and 48 hours after stimulation (see Fig. 7.25.1). In addition, an increase of nitric oxide (NO) release is reported in an early stage of treatment and the subsequent activation of endothelial nitric oxide synthase (eNOS) and of vascular endothelial growth factor (VEGF) are related to TGF-β1 rise (Frairia and Berta 2011). Furthermore, the increase of angiogenesis observed in ESW-treated tendons is an additional factor in accelerating the repairing process (Frairia and Berta 2011).

Direct effects of ESWT on the ECM have been described (Gollmann-Tepeköylü et al. 2018); therefore, it is assumed that ESWT can modulate these actions with a positive effect on myofascial tissue regeneration and healing processes. Multiple in-vivo and in-vitro studies have confirmed an enhancement of fibroblast proliferation after ESWT (Frairia and Berta 2011; Moortgat et al. 2018).

Further, in the treatment of many diseases in which fibrous tissue is involved (e.g., Dupuytren´s), it was shown that focused ESWT reduced the fibrotic load by modulating the pro- and antifibrotic proteins TGF-β and MMP-2, which lead to an antifibrotic effect (Knobloch et al. 2011; Zhang et al. 2008). This antifibrotic effect can also be explained on a histopathological level, with ESWT down regulating alpha-SMA expression, collagen type I, and myofibroblast phenotype (Rinella et al. 2016; Saggini et al. 2016).

PROMOTION OF HEALING PROCESSES AND EFFECTS OF ESWT ON MYOFASCIAL TISSUE

Among the first reported effects of ESWT on the healing process was the induction of angiogenesis in the treated tissue (Wang et al. 2007), for example, through upregulation of NO and VEGF (Yan et al. 2008), vasodilation, increase in vascular and capillary density, and increased local blood flow (d'Agostino et al. 2015; Frairia et al. 2016; Mittermayr et al. 2011; Romeo et al. 2014; Yan et al. 2008). In-vitro studies deepen our understanding of the observed healing effects in showing that ESWT mechanotransduction activates stem cell mobilization, migration, homing, and differentiation (Suhr et al. 2013; Wang et al. 2002).

A few studies were done on muscle tissue so far with the aim of reducing the muscle tone in spasticity with good results (Lohse-Busch et al. 1997; Manganotti and Amelio 2005).

Myofascial tissue, especially myofascial trigger points, has come more and more into the focus of ESWT (Ramon et al. 2015; Gleitz and Hornig 2012; Hong et al. 2017; Muller-Ehrenberg and Licht 2005; Jeon et al. 2012). Even in acute myofascial pain like muscle soreness, fESWT has shown to have immediate effects on pain relief (Fleckenstein et al. 2017).

THERAPEUTIC APPROACH

 KEY POINT

fESWT can be used as a diagnostic tool for the diagnosis of myofascial pain. For this purpose, fESWT is more accurate than other methods.

A thorough clinical examination should precede any medical treatment with ESW. This includes basic diagnostics such as neurological-orthopedic examination and an overview of the mobility and range of motion (mobility scores, sensomotoric testing, specific stretching test, etc.). An examination including myofascial chains, in addition to testing agonists and antagonists of the motoric system, is favorable.

Although palpation is still the gold standard for the clinical examination of muscles and fascia, adding fESW has several diagnostic advantages. fESW is more precise, does not necessarily activate nociceptors of the skin, can target deeper tissue levels, and does not cause hematomas to develop. Possibly the greatest advantage of fESW lies in the superior diagnostic and therapeutic accuracy. The main diagnostic criteria of pain, the so-called referred pain and the pain recognition, can be evoked by fESW more often than by palpation (Hong et al. 2017; Muller-Ehrenberg and Licht 2005).

Imaging diagnostics, for example, x-ray and ultrasound, are indicated to exclude severe diseases. Further, ultrasound examination with high-definition imaging is gaining attention for a better understanding of myofascial tissue. High-resolution MRI scans are used in scientific studies but so far have no relevance for clinical use.

The indication for ESWT has to be given by an expert physician. The exact application of ESWT, even in deeper tissue layers, allows patients to give direct feedback on the precision of the application. The intensity should be chosen based on patient feedback, preferably near the pain threshold. A combination with other myofascial techniques such as muscle and fascial release techniques, fascial manipulation therapies, relaxation techniques, and physiotherapy is reasonable. ESWT can be further combined with needling techniques such as injection or dry needling in the same session.

The patient should be informed about possible therapy pain (20–30%, usually similar to "sore muscle pain"), and possible vegetative reactions (e.g., sweating, circulatory reaction). NSAID medication can be given if necessary.

ESWT should be applied by a physician who is qualified by means of specialist knowledge. ESW application should be documented accurately, considering locus of application (e.g., treated muscle); diagnostic criteria (e.g., "recognition" and "referred pain" [feedback]); and number of SW pulses and intensity (Energy Flux Density).

No local anesthetics are used and the intensity of ESWT is adapted to the pain, as indicated by the patient. Post-treatment noxious activity should be suspended, and pain-adapted movement is advised.

Contraindication: malign tumor in focus zone

Complications: temporary pain, hematoma (RPW).

Although the application of ESWT for the treatment of myofascial pain, especially for the treatment of MTrPs, has increased over the past years, no standardized protocols have been developed so far. Efforts to standardize treatment protocols have been made by the DIGEST and ISMST, which have stated the following guidelines (see Table 7.25.1).

Treatment Principles

fEWST is not only applied directly to the locus of pain but is also extended to the source of the functional impairment (e.g., fascial densification, MTrP, etc.). "Pain recognition" and "referred pain" are the main diagnostic criteria that indicate a relevant zone for treatment (see Fig. 7.25.2).

TABLE 7.25.1	**Overview of Treatment Parameters for Focused ESWT and Radial Pressure Wave**	
	Focused ESWT	**Radial Pressure Wave (RPW)**
Intensity	EFD: 0.05–0.35 mJ/mm^2	Energy: up to 2.5 bar
Interval	1–2x per week	1–2x per week
Frequency	FSW 4–5 Hz	Up to 10 Hz
Impulses per session	2000–5000	2000–5000
Impulses per MTrP	300–400	300–400
Total number of treatments	3–8	3–8

ESWT, extracorporeal shockwave therapy; EFD, energy flux density; FSW, focused shockwaves; MTrP, myofascial trigger point.

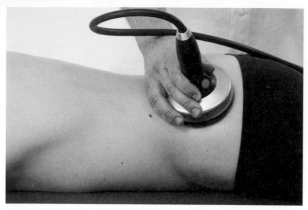

Fig. 7.25.2 Application of focused extracorporeal shockwave therapy (fESWT) to the myofascial tissue of the gluteal region.

In addition to treating solely the locus of pain, research has shown the benefits of extending the application of ESWT to myofascial points and tissue densifications causing the impairment. This aims at restoring the correct biomechanical function of the musculoskeletal system and preventing recurrences by solving the primary cause of pain (Giordani et al. 2019; Moghtaderi et al. 2014).

CLINICAL EXAMPLE OF ESW APPLICATION FOR MYOFASCIAL PAIN IN A MUSCULOSKELETAL DISEASE

 KEY POINT

fESWT can reach myofascial trigger points, densifications, and functional impairment in deep tissue layers.

Research by Giordani and colleagues (2019) investigated the correlation between a global myofascial impairment and plantar fasciitis. The rationale of the treatment was based on the concept of myofascial continuity: the plantar fascia as part of a more complex unit named "Achilles–calcaneus–plantar system." There is a functional connection between the Achilles tendon and the plantar fascia through the posterior trabecular system of calcaneus that works as a hypomochlion (pivotal point), transmitting the force from the tendon to the fascia. It was observed that during ESWT, referred heel pain was often evoked while treating the myofascial altered points in the lower limb. This confirms the relation between proximal impairment and distal pain. Therefore plantar fasciitis

should be considered an epiphenomenon of the tensional disequilibrium in the myofascial system of the lower limb.

In this study, fESWT was applied in the impaired myofascial points that were selected after the Fascial Manipulation method. In each session, three to four points of stiffness and tenderness in the altered lower limb, within the same myofascial sequence or the antagonist one, were chosen; 1500 shocks (PiezoWave 2; 5 Hz, 0.167 mJ/mm²) for each point were given. This protocol has been chosen because it has been observed that this amount of energy is needed to loosen the densification in the fascial point. The treatment aimed at restoring the correct gliding and the physiological tensional relations between myofascial structures.

In addition, it is suggested that ESWT may have a two-stage effect on the tissue; the immediate response is mediated by modification in HA viscoelastic properties, whereas the delayed effect derives from intracellular signal transduction. Indeed, fibroblast stimulation by fESWT results in renewed production of collagen fibers (climax in 48 h) that are arranged in accordance with the tensional line of forces already present in the myofascial system (see Fig. 7.25.3). Thus restoring the correct functional activity of the lower limb is important to obtain stable, long-term pain relief.

In conclusion, a global approach to the musculoskeletal diseases will allow physicians to solve the primary cause of the tensional impairment preventing recurrences. It also helps to avoid direct application of fESWT on the inflamed zone by applying it proximally.

PERSPECTIVES

Although a growing body of fundamental research and first clinical trials have aimed at investigating ESWT effects on healing processes and regeneration of myofascial tissue, randomized controlled trials are needed to explore and understand clinical effects in musculoskeletal diseases.

Previous work has shown the beneficial effect of fEWST application prior to expected tissue damage. The mechanisms suggested are a preconditioning of the tissue on the one hand (Mittermayr et al. 2011; Tobalem et al. 2013) and an attenuation of the apoptosis on the other hand (Zhao et al. 2012; Zhang et al. 2018). Based on these findings, ESWT preconditioning is already used in sports medicine, for example, to the myofascial tissue before a stressful event (e.g., tennis match) to minimize tissue damage and improve regeneration.

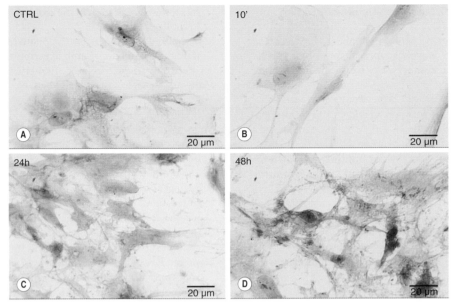

Fig. 7.25.3 Sirius Red staining for collagen fibers in fibroblast cells isolated from human fascia. Collagen fibers generated after focused extracorporeal shockwave therapy (fESTW) stimulation: images of control cells (not treated) (A), and taken 10 minutes, 24 hours, and 48 hours (B, C, D) after stimulation. Courtesy Caterina Fede.

Another promising direction for future investigation is the effect ESWT may have on restoring the correct gliding between myofascial layers. The mechanism of action is suggested to be the mechanical stimulus that rebuilds the physiological viscoelasticity of hyaluronic acid (HA) needed for gliding (Matteini et al. 2009; Stecco et al. 2013). In this context, ESWT effects on fasciacytes—fibroblast-like cells in fasciae specialized for the biosynthesis of the HA-rich matrix—should be a target of future research (Stecco et al. 2018).

Summary

For more than 30 years ESWT has been applied in several musculoskeletal disorders. Mechanotransduction has been described as the main mechanism of action of ESWT, and it is associated with a large number of modifications of cellular processes necessary for the promotion of healing. Many of the described effects play an important role in the regeneration of myofascial tissue. Therefore ESWT is used for the treatment and also diagnosis of myofascial pain. fEWST is applied directly to the locus of pain and also extended to the source of the functional impairment. Guidelines for treatment have already been proposed (ISMST), but standardized protocols need yet to be established.

REFERENCES

Adstrum, S., Hedley, G., Schleip, R., Stecco, C., Yucesoy, C.A., 2017. Defining the fascial system. J. Bodyw. Mov. Ther. 21, 173–177.

Chaussy, C., Brendel, W., Schmiedt, E., 1980. Extracorporeally induced destruction of kidney stones by shock waves. Lancet 316, 1265–1268.

Cheng, J.H., Wang, C.J., 2015. Biological mechanism of shockwave in bone. Int. J. Surg. 24, 143–146.

Cleveland, R.O., Chitnis, P.V., McClure, S.R. 2007. Acoustic field of a ballistic shock wave therapy device. Ultrasound Med. Biol. 33, 1327–1335.

d'Agostino, M., Craig, K., Tibalt, E., Respizzi, S., 2015. Shock wave as biological therapeutic tool: from mechanical stimulation to recovery and healing, through mechano-transducton. Int. J. Surg. 24, 147–153.

Fleckenstein, J., Friton, M., Himmelreich, H., Banzer, W., 2017. Effect of a single administration of focused extracorporeal shock wave in the relief of delayed-onset muscle soreness: results of a partially blinded randomized controlled trial. Arch. Phys. Med. Rehabil. 98, 923–930.

Frairia, R., Berta, L., 2011. Biological effects of extracorporeal shock waves on fibroblasts. A review. Muscles Ligaments Tendons J. 1, 138.

Frairia, R., D'Agostino, M.C., Romeo, P., et al., 2016. Extracorporeal shockwaves as regenerative therapy in orthopedic traumatology: a narrative review from basic research to clinical practice. J. Biol. Regul. Homeost. Agents 30, 323–332.

Giordani, F., Bernini, A., Müller-Ehrenberg, H., Stecco, C., Masiero, S., 2019. A global approach for plantar fasciitis with extracorporeal shockwaves treatment. Eur. J. Transl. Myol. 29, 8372.

Gleitz, M., Hornig, K. 2012. Trigger Points–Diagnosis and treatment concepts with special reference to extracorporeal shockwaves. Orthopade 41, 113.

Gollmann-Tepeköylü, C., Lobenwein, D., Theurl, M., E., et al., 2018. Shock wave therapy improves cardiac function in a model of chronic ischemic heart failure: evidence for a mechanism involving VEGF signaling and the extracellular matrix. J. Am. Heart Assoc. 7, e010025.

Hausdorf, J., Lemmens, M.A., Kaplan, S., et al., 2008. Extracorporeal shockwave application to the distal femur of rabbits diminishes the number of neurons immunoreactive for substance P in dorsal root ganglia L5. Brain Res. 1207, 96–101.

Holfeld, J., Tepeköylü, C., Kozaryn, R., et al., 2014. Shockwave therapy differentially stimulates endothelial cells: implications on the control of inflammation via toll-like receptor 3. Inflammation 37, 65–70.

Hong, J.O., Park, J.S., Jeon, D.G., Yoon, W.H., Park, J.H., 2017. Extracorporeal shock wave therapy versus trigger point injection in the treatment of myofascial pain syndrome in the quadratus lumborum. Ann. Rehabil. Med. 41, 582.

Ioppolo, F., Rompe, J.D., Furia, J.P., Cacchio, A., 2014. Clinical application of shock wave therapy (SWT) in musculoskeletal disorders. Eur. J. Phys. Rehabil. Med. 50, 217–230.

Jeon, J.H., Jung, Y.J., Lee, J.Y., et al., 2012. The effect of extracorporeal shock wave therapy on myofascial pain syndrome. Ann. Rehabil. Med. 36, 665.

Khan, K.M., Scott, A. 2009. Mechanotherapy: how physical therapists' prescription of exercise promotes tissue repair. Br. J. Sports Med. 43, 247–252.

Klingler, W., Jurkat-Rott, K., Lehmann-Horn, F., Schleip, R., 2012. The role of fibrosis in Duchenne muscular dystrophy. Acta Myol. 31, 184.

Knobloch, K., Kuehn, M., Vogt, P.M., 2011. Focused extracorporeal shockwave therapy in Dupuytren's disease–a hypothesis. Med. Hypotheses 76, 635–637.

Loew, M., Jurgowski, W., Mau, H.C., Thomsen, M., 1995. Treatment of calcifying tendinitis of rotator cuff by extracorporeal shock waves: a preliminary report. J. Shoulder Elbow Surg. 4, 101–106.

Lohse-Busch, H., Kraemer, M., Reime, U. 1997. A pilot investigation into the effects of extracorporeal shock waves on muscular dysfunction in children with spastic movement disorders. Schmerz 11, 108–112.

Maier, M., Averbeck, B., Milz, S., Refior, H.J., Schmitz, C., 2003. Substance P and prostaglandin E2 release after shock wave application to the rabbit femur. Clin. Orthop. Relat. Res. 406, 237–245.

Manganotti, P., Amelio, E., 2005. Long-term effect of shock wave therapy on upper limb hypertonia in patients affected by stroke. Stroke 36, 1967–1971.

Matteini, P., Dei, L., Carretti, E., Volpi, N., Goti, A., Pini, R., 2009. Structural behavior of highly concentrated hyaluronan. Biomacromolecules 10, 1516–1522.

Mittermayr, R., Hartinger, J., Antonic, V., et al., 2011. Extracorporeal shock wave therapy (ESWT) minimizes ischemic tissue necrosis irrespective of application time and promotes tissue revascularization by stimulating angiogenesis. Ann. Surg. 253, 1024–1032.

Moghtaderi, A., Khosrawi, S., Dehghan, F., 2014. Extracorporeal shock wave therapy of gastroc-soleus trigger points in patients with plantar fasciitis: A randomized, placebo-controlled trial. Adv. Biomed. Res. 3, 99.

Moortgat, P., Van Daele, U., Anthonissen, M., et al., 2018. Shockwave therapy for wound healing and scar treatment. In: Knobloch, K. (Ed.), ESWT in Aesthetic Medicine, Burns & Dermatology. Level10, Heilbronn, pp. 289–302.

Moya, D., Ramón, S., Schaden, W., Wang, C.J., Guiloff, L., Cheng, J.H., 2018. The role of extracorporeal shockwave treatment in musculoskeletal disorders. J. Bone Joint Surg. Am. 100, 251–263.

Muller-Ehrenberg, H., Licht, G., 2005. Diagnostik und Therapie von myofaszialen Schmerzsyndromen mittels der fokussierten Stosswelle (ESWT). Medizinisch Orthopadische Technik, 125, 75.

Novak, P., 2019. The history of ESWT in medicine. In: Knobloch, K. (Eds.), ESWT in Hand Surgery. Level10, Heilbronn, pp. 16–19.

Ogden, J.A., Tóth-Kischkat, A., Schultheiss, R., 2001. Principles of shock wave therapy. Clin. Orthop. Relat. Res. 387, 8–17.

Ramon, S., Gleitz, M., Hernandez, L., Romero, L.D., 2015. Update on the efficacy of extracorporeal shockwave treatment for myofascial pain syndrome and fibromyalgia. Int. J. Surg. 24, 201–206.

Rinella, L., Marano, F., Berta, L., et al., 2016. Extracorporeal shock waves modulate myofibroblast differentiation of adipose-derived stem cells. Wound Repair Regen. 24, 275–286.

Romeo, P., Lavanga, V., Pagani, D., Sansone, V., 2014. Extracorporeal shock wave therapy in musculoskeletal disorders: a review. Med. Princ. Pract. 23, 7–13.

Saggini, R., Saggini, A., Spagnoli, A.M., et al., 2016. Extracorporeal shock wave therapy: an emerging treatment modality for retracting scars of the hands. Ultrasound Med. Biol. 42, 185–195.

Shah, J.P., Phillips, T.M., Danoff, J.V., Gerber, L.H., 2005. An in vivo microanalytical technique for measuring the local biochemical milieu of human skeletal muscle. J. Appl. Physiol. 99, 1977–1984.

Stecco, A., Gesi, M., Stecco, C., Stern, R., 2013. Fascial components of the myofascial pain syndrome. Curr. Pain Headache Rep. 17, 352.

Stecco, C., Fede, C., Macchi, V., Porzionato, A., Petrelli, L., Biz, C., 2018. The fasciacytes: a new cell devoted to fascial gliding regulation. Clin. Anat. 31, 667–676.

Suhr, F., Delhasse, Y., Bungartz, G., Schmidt, A., Pfannkuche, K., Bloch, W., 2013. Cell biological effects of mechanical stimulations generated by focused extracorporeal shock wave applications on cultured human bone marrow stromal cells. Stem Cell Res. 11, 951–964.

Sukubo, N.G., Tibalt, E., Respizzi, S., Locati, M., d'Agostino, M.C., 2015. Effect of shock waves on macrophages: a possible role in tissue regeneration and remodeling. Int. J. Surg. 24, 124–130.

Tobalem, M., Wettstein, R., Pittet-Cuénod, B., et al., 2013. Local shockwave-induced capillary recruitment improves survival of musculocutaneous flaps. J. Surg. Res. 184, 1196–1204.

Wang, C.J., 2012. Extracorporeal shockwave therapy in musculoskeletal disorders. J. Orthop. Surg. Res. 7, 11.

Wang, F., Yang, K.D., Chen, R.F., Wang, C.J., Sheen-Chen, S.M., 2002. Extracorporeal shock wave promotes growth and differentiation of bone-marrow stromal cells towards osteoprogenitors associated with induction of TGF-β1. J. Bone Joint Surg. Br. 84, 457–461.

Wang, J.H.C., Thampatty, B.P., Lin, J.S., Im, H.J., 2007. Mechanoregulation of gene expression in fibroblasts. Gene 391, 1–15.

Yan, X., Zeng, B., Chai, Y., Luo, C., Li, X., 2008. Improvement of blood flow, expression of nitric oxide, and vascular endothelial growth factor by low-energy shockwave therapy in random-pattern skin flap model. Ann. Plast. Surg. 61, 646–653.

Zhang, A.Y., Fong K.D., Pham, H., Nacamuli, R.P., Longaker, M.T., Chang, J., 2008. Gene Expression Analysis of Dupuytren's Disease: The Role of TGF-β 2. J. Hand Surg. Am. 33, 783–790.

Zhang, Y., Shen, T., Liu, B., et al., 2018. Cardiac shock wave therapy attenuates cardiomyocyte apoptosis after acute myocardial infarction in rats. Cell. Physiol. Biochem, 49, 1734–1746.

Zhao, Z., Ji, H., Jing, R., et al., 2012. Extracorporeal shock-wave therapy reduces progression of knee osteoarthritis in rabbits by reducing nitric oxide level and chondrocyte apoptosis. Arch. Orthop. Trauma Surg. 132, 1547–1553.

Zügel, M., Maganaris, C.N., Wilke, J., et al., Fascial tissue research in sports medicine: from molecules to tissue adaptation, injury and diagnostics: consensus statement. Br. J. Sports Med. 52, 1497.

Bowen Therapy

Kelly Clancy

CHAPTER CONTENTS

WHAT IS BOWEN THERAPY?

Bowen therapy is a unique soft tissue mobilization technique that employs light touch to treat a wide range of complaints. Originally developed in Australia in the 1950s, Bowen is now taught and practiced throughout the world. Bowen therapy is most often provided for specific musculoskeletal complaints but may also be utilized for more systemic issues. The core practice involves movements of the practitioner's fingers and thumbs performed over precise locations, generally in particular sequences, throughout the patient's body (Fig. 7.26.1). These light touch maneuvers are called "moves," which, unique to Bowen, are followed by prescribed periods of waiting called "pauses."

Pauses and somatic reflection on the part of patients are integral to Bowen treatments. After the completion of the move or series of moves at specific locations, the practitioner will remove their hands, stepping away from the table or leaving the room, to wait. During this time, an emphasis is placed upon the client's somatic attending and interoceptive awareness in response to the definitive therapeutic input provided by the practitioner. Throughout the session, clients are encouraged to notice the location of sensations, which may be local or distant to the touch provided. After the designated wait period, the therapist will then determine whether further intervention is warranted at the same location or at a different anatomical site. The sequence of moves are continued at various regions of the body until the desired global tissue tension state or autonomic response is achieved. In addition to emphasizing the somatosensory experience during the wait period and throughout the session, clients are encouraged to continue this interoceptive awareness practice after the treatment has been completed.

> ### KEY POINT
>
> Bowen therapy is minimal in nature, with one of the dominant precepts in Bowen philosophy being "less is best." Bowen asserts that the body will respond more strongly when less input is given to the system. Because of this philosophy, it has sometimes been termed "the homeopathy of bodywork."

Each clinical Bowen session typically lasts from 30 minutes to 1 hour, depending on distinct variables that may include the client's presenting symptoms, how they are receiving and integrating the input, and the particular diagnosis being addressed. Sessions can be

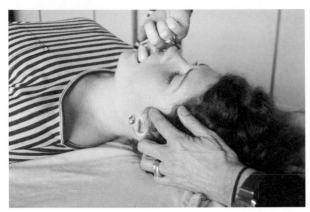

Fig. 7.26.1 Temporomandibular Joint (TMJ) Procedure.

performed directly on skin or over clothing. The treatments are typically performed with the client lying down (Fig. 7.26.2), but can also be modified to accommodate any body limitation or therapeutic situation, such as wheelchair positioning, sporting postures, or active functional movement.

The client is typically instructed to wait 5 to 10 days before they receive any further follow-up treatments, including other forms of bodywork. This period allows the global nervous and fascial systems to respond fully to the input provided and allows for the integration of potential changes within the global structure. During this 5- to 10-day interval, the client is instructed to monitor both subtle and not so subtle responses as a means to increase their bodily awareness and to determine the effects of the session on the body. Typical areas

of change may include connective-tissue tension changes, improved postural alignment, improved sleep, normalized respiration, improvement of appetite and elimination, improved mood, and subsequently an overall increased ease in functioning.

Traditionally, clients seeking out Bowen therapy have done so to address musculoskeletal dysfunctions, including structural imbalances, orthopedic, and neurological conditions. Others have sought this type of therapy to address autoimmune- and endocrine-related dysfunctions. It is not uncommon for a client to come in for a structural issue only to find relief from the targeted condition while subsequently also reporting changes in sleep, mood states, digestion, and an overall sense of well-being. Clients being seen with chronic autoimmune issues also often report Bowen therapy to be beneficial in managing symptoms related to their condition while increasing their function.

> ### KEY POINT
>
> A global shift in the autonomic state is often the fundamental effect experienced by the client and observed by the practitioner during and after a Bowen session.

This may present as a relaxation response with a shift in breathing patterns, reduction in tissue tension, improved peristalsis, mood state changes, sleep improvements, and postural alignment alterations. The effects of these shifts appear to create a more balanced state of homeostasis and regulation within the global structure. As a result of these systemic effects, practitioners may offer Bowen therapy as a preventative intervention or for general relaxation. Bowen applied in this manner can facilitate an experience of stress reduction, decreased connective tissue tension, and the potential for maintenance of general equilibrium and optimal functioning of global bodily systems (Fig. 7.26.3).

The duration of a Bowen treatment varies based on the individual's complaints and goals, as well as their overall health and vitality. For some seeking a site-specific orthopedic or peripheral nerve-related condition, the duration of treatment would typically be between 2 and 8 visits. For those being seen for systemic issues or chronic conditions, regular weekly, bimonthly, or monthly sessions may offer a means to manage symptoms and maximize functioning.

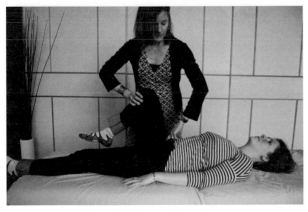

Fig. 7.26.2 Pelvic Procedure.

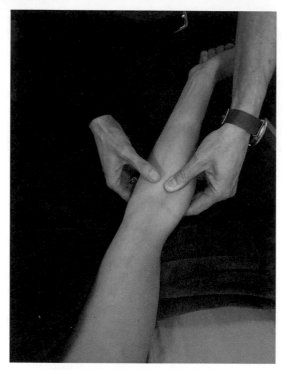

Fig. 7.26.3 Forearm Procedure.

HOW PREVALENT IS BOWEN THERAPY?

Professional organizations and associations devoted to the Bowen technique exist in multiple countries, including Australia, New Zealand, Switzerland, Germany, Austria, Japan, Greece, India, Italy, Ireland, Denmark, Norway, Romania, Bulgaria, Slovenia, Sweden, South Africa, Turkey, the United Kingdom, Canada, and the United States.

A large number of schools and centers educate therapists on some form of Tom Bowen's legacy work. These include Bowtech, The Border College of Natural Therapies (BCNT), The College of Bowen Studies/ The Bowen Technique, Bowen Akademie Europa, The Bowen College, Bowen Seminars, The International School of Bowen Therapy (ISBT), Neuromuscular Integration Technique (NST), Fascia Bowen, and Fascial Kinetics. In addition, there are schools that rely heavily on the Bowen methodology combined with other progressive formats and techniques to create their own unique training programs. Such programs include The Emmett Technique, Smart Bowen,

Tensegrity Medicine, College of Applied Myoskeletal Therapy, Neural Touch, The McLoughlin Scar Tissue Release Technique, and Functional Bowen. These, along with the more traditional Bowen trainings, continue to gain in popularity because of the successful therapeutic effects within a wide variety of diagnoses and medical conditions, as well as the growing and emerging validation among the scientific community around light touch therapies. In addition to the expanding interest in Bowen therapy's benefit for humans, several schools have also introduced this technique into their equine and small animal training programs. Given the proliferation of interest and clinical use of this unique modality, a desire for rigorous scientific explanations has emerged, leading to attempts to understand how this light touch might create local and systemic change.

FOUNDATIONS

Bowen practitioners have reached consensus that this holistic approach follows closely many of the principles of osteopathy. Some of the primary foundational osteopathic precepts consistent with Bowen philosophy include:

- The person is a unit of body, mind, and spirit.
- The body is capable of self-regulation, self-healing, and health maintenance.
- Structure and function are reciprocally interrelated.
- Rational treatment is based upon an understanding of the basic principles of body unity, self-regulation, and the interrelationship of structure and function (American Osteopathic Association 2019).

> **KEY POINT**
>
> A typical client may seek the assistance of a Bowen therapist for the alleviation of somatic dysfunction impairing or altering function, including orthopedic, autoimmune, vascular, lymphatic, or organ dysfunction conditions.

Areas of restriction may be characterized by hyper- or hypomobility, postural restrictions, pain, connective tissue tension, reflex changes, and vasomotor or visceromotor impairments. Assessing the client with any of these conditions represents the first step in formulating a successful Bowen treatment plan.

Unfortunately, there is no global consensus or uniform assessment strategies for the application of Bowen intervention. Some Bowen practitioners, strongly influenced by the chiropractic and osteopathic traditions, believe that the critical aspect of a Bowen assessment and treatment should be a focus on creating structural symmetry. Other practitioners depend on the use of palpation skills, temperature, and observation of the client's responses in guiding their care, whereas still others, trained in Eastern philosophy, may perform assessments and treatment based on the meridian pathways. Therapists have incorporated myokinetic chains and concepts related to biotensegrity as their roadmap.

Assessment is an area of continued discussion, debate, and growth within the Bowen community, now augmented by the plethora of new fascial research and the growth of the popularity of biotensegrity.

BOWEN PRACTICE: THE CLASSIC MOVE

The traditional classic Bowen move has four distinct components that are universally accepted among the schools. The variation that exists in Bowen practice relates to the application, pressure, direction, and location of the moves (Fig. 7.26.4).

The *classic move* is comprised of four distinct steps:

1. **Glue**—Light touch tissue contact is made on the skin on a designated location.
2. **Slack**—The superficial tissue, including the epidermis and superficial fascial layer, is "pulled" to its end range position using light touch pressure without sliding (shear).
3. **Challenge**—The depth of pressure is increased into the tissue while maintaining the shearing of the superficial tissue and is held for a minimum of one breath cycle.
4. **Move**—This pressure is maintained while the tissue is moved back in the opposite direction toward the original location (countershear).

Other types of moves beyond the classic move exist within Bowen therapy and involve firm tapping, rocking of joints, or the distraction or compression of the joint structures. For example, in the *ankle procedure*, the mortis joint is distracted while the practitioner applies cross fiber moves over the ankle retinaculum, the deltoid, and

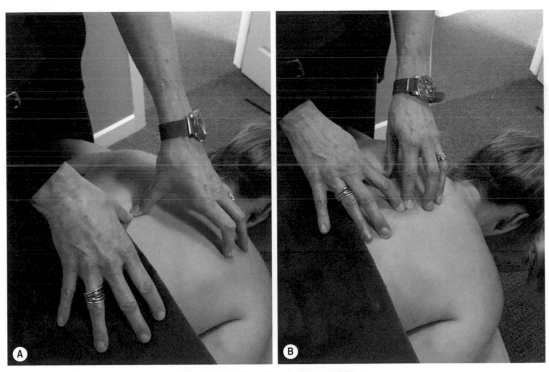

Fig. 7.26.4 The Classic Bowen Move.

calcaneofibular ligaments. A compressive mobilization is then performed at the joint.

In other locations, such as with the *hamstring procedure,* a firm compressive tap is performed over the ball of the foot after strongly mobilizing the tendinous origin and insertion of the hamstring and its muscle bellies (Fig. 7.26.5).

While addressing the shoulder, a Bowen therapist may apply classic moves to the deltoid muscle, which are followed by a passive stretch of the joint into horizontal adduction followed by a firm tap performed over the lateral glenohumeral joint structure.

In all of these cases, it is hypothesized that these adjunctive techniques provide tactile input to the low threshold mechanoreceptors, affecting the muscle spindles and Golgi tendon organs. Such examples of the variation of tissue input demonstrate the complex and comprehensive nature of this simple light touch modality.

Bowen moves are often performed over acupressure points, trigger points, Chapman's neurolymphatic points, joints, and tendinous insertions. The distinct steps outlined previously result in tissue stretching, at different depths with sustained pressure, followed by a

continuous sustained pressure in the opposite direction, using a shearing type action without sliding. Many moves remain at the superficial fascial layer, or the interface between superficial and deep fascial regions, whereas others will penetrate to the deep fascia and sometimes to the periosteal layer.

An experienced Bowen practitioner may apply moves through clothing or directly on the skin. The client can be positioned in varying postures based on comfort level and environmental factors. For these reasons, Bowen therapy offers versatility in its application in multiple settings. Given its light touch nature, Bowen is usually well-tolerated by persons of all ages and with a wide variety of conditions, including those with chronic pain conditions and autoimmune dysfunction.

BOWEN PRACTICE: THE PAUSE

A move or series of moves will typically be followed by a pause of a minimum of 2 minutes, allowing the system to respond.

> ### KEY POINT
>
> The pause within the treatment is one of the signature characteristics of the Bowen technique. The pause can vary in length based on the bodily response of the client and the interoceptive awareness expressed during the session.

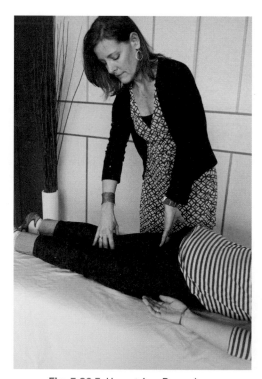

Fig. 7.26.5 Hamstring Procedure.

This time of "hands off" is theorized to allow the mechanosensitive signaling network of the fascial system and the peripheral nervous system to respond to the external input received from the practitioner. During this critical time in the session, the client is instructed to pay close attention to bodily sensations. Utilizing interoceptive awareness, the moment-to-moment representation process of sensations coming from the body may play a key factor in improving the client's physical state. Because interoception can also be considered as a multidimensional construct, including how people evaluate and react to sensations, the scope of interoceptive research has broadly expanded. Chronic pain, posttraumatic stress disorders, affective disorders, addiction, eating disorders, somatoform disorders, and dissociative disorders all appear to be linked to the lack of sensation awareness (D'Alessandro et al. 2016). Growing clinical evidence demonstrates the importance of incorporating sensory experiences and body awareness strategies into mental health and chronic pain management (Schulz and Vogele 2015).

Fostering this awareness during the pause is an integral part of the Bowen session. The verbalization of sensations by the client to the skilled practitioner can facilitate a dialogue that can then guide the therapist in determining where subsequent moves will be applied and when the treatment intervention has reached its completion.

Furthermore, sensations arising from the application of therapeutic pressure or stroking may have an impact on the brain, which in turn can modify an individual's perception. The concept of a cortical body matrix, or virtual body map in the brain, suggests that there is a dynamic neural representation within the brain that integrates sensory data with homeostatic and motor function (Moseley et al. 2011). The pause, then, allows the engagement of the patient's mind in the process of healing.

HYPOTHESIZED MECHANISM OF ACTION

Because of the light touch nature and the pressure changes in the shearing forces, it would be reasonable to assume that a Bowen move could be affecting the fascial adhesions that may be present in densified regions.

According to Findley at the 2015 International Fascial Symposium, changes in the density of fascial tissue may be sufficient to entrap nociceptive nerve endings and cause pain. It is widely held that adhesions between the fascia and adjacent tissues may become painful, possibly because nociceptive nerve endings are trapped in the fibrotic adhesion and excited by shear forces between the tissues involved (Findley 2015).

The shearing force produced by the technique may create a transduction of biochemical responses in the tissue matrix, resulting in physiological change globally in the body. Mechanotransduction is the process of cells sensing physical forces from the external environment and transducing the information into biochemical and biological responses. The fascial network, under continuous tension, is capable of transmitting mechanical forces throughout the system. Forces applied to the cytoskeleton produce biochemical changes on the cellular level by means of mechanochemical transduction (Langevin et al. 2011).

Tension is transmitted from the extracellular matrix through the cytoskeleton to the nucleus, and deformation of the nucleus mediates changes in gene expression that regulate cell cycle progression (Huang and Ingber 1999).

Because the fibroblast would be responding to the mechanical tensioning during the move, the cell environment will theoretically be influenced by the external forces created by the practitioner during Bowen moves. This local tissue tensioning will likely influence the global tissue tension in the system following the biotensegrity paradigm. Research presented at the International Fascial Congress 2015 noted that:

tension modulation by fibroblasts is suggested to regulate interstitial fluid pressure and flow by altering the permeability (pore size) of the extracellular matrix, and thus the movement of water toward the normally underhydrated glycosaminoglycans. Movement of water in or out of the tissue also serves as the mechanism by which fibroblasts sense a change in osmotic pressure and accordingly adjust their shape to control fluid movement. These cytoskeletal responses appear to be unique to loose connective tissues, such as those forming interfaces between subcutaneous and perimuscular layers, and do not occur in other more densely packed connective tissues. (Findley 2015)

CLINICAL RESEARCH

Only a limited number of controlled clinical trials have evaluated Bowen therapy. In 2011, Hansen and Taylor-Pillae performed a systematic review of Bowen therapy, finding that of the 309 citations mentioning Bowen, only 15 articles met the reviewer's inclusion criteria of providing quantifiable or qualitative information reporting on a meaningful clinical outcome. Over half of these reports (53%) concluded that Bowen was effective for pain reduction and 33% reported improved mobility. An additional five studies reported the effectiveness of Bowen therapy on the relief of symptoms experienced by persons living with a chronic illness (Hansen and Taylor-Pillae 2011).

Over the last several years, additional Bowen studies have been published:

A 2011 pilot study enrolled people ($n = 14$) with chronic symptoms related to stroke. Each received 13 sessions of Bowen therapy over a 3-month period. The gross motor assessments and neuromuscular function improved, but there was no control group in this report (Duncan et al. 2011).

A 2011 uncontrolled study on the effects of Bowen on hamstring flexibility ($n = 120$) found increased flexibility levels observed over a 1-week period, with participants receiving a single Bowen session (Marr et al. 2011).

Winter and MacAllister (2011) reported a large, uncontrolled study ($n = 778$) of Bowen therapy in occupational medicine. Presenting conditions were classified into the following five "illness categories": musculoskeletal and rheumatic conditions, mental health and behavioral disorders, injury, and nervous system conditions. Significant clinical improvement was reported in the client's occupational abilities after Bowen treatment. Improvement in general health and well-being with high client satisfaction in regards to the treatment was also reported.

Hipmair et al. (2012) evaluated the effectiveness of Bowen therapy in pain management after total knee replacement ($n = 91$) in a randomized controlled trial. The results revealed a decreased pain score in the early postoperative period in the Bowen-treated group. They concluded that Bowen therapy may be an effective additional treatment tool for pain reduction.

A 2013 randomized controlled study examined the occupational performance improvements of 28 patients receiving Bowen therapy for shoulder pathologies, with inclusion criteria being stiffness, pain, tendon tears, fractures, and neurological involvement. All patients who received Bowen therapy had improvement in their occupational performance, pain, and range of motion (Wan et al. 2016).

A 2016 Portuguese study reported on the immediate effects of pressure pain thresholds and postural sway, following a cross-over, randomized, double-blind study on 34 healthy participants. Each participant attended two sessions and received Bowen therapy and a sham procedure. The results showed a significant increase in the anteroposterior displacement ($p < 0.04$), a significantly lower decrease in the mean velocity ($p < 0.01$) of the center of pressure, and a significant increase in the pressure pain thresholds of 2 out of the 10 body sites in the group receiving Bowen therapy compared with the group receiving the sham. The findings suggest that Bowen therapy has inconsistent immediate effects on postural control and pain threshold in healthy subjects (Félix et al. 2016).

A 2016 uncontrolled study examined the effects of Bowen therapy on the quality of life, functional status, perceived pain, mobility, and edema of 21 women who had undergone breast cancer resection surgery. Each received four Bowen sessions with home exercises. The women reported improved mental health, breast cancer–related functional scores, increased ROM, and reduced edema (Argenbright et al. 2016).

A 2019 pilot study in the *Journal of Bodywork and Movement Therapies* examined the role of Bowen therapy on motor functioning in ten 8- to 11-year-old dyspraxic boys. Significant improvements in both performance and subjective questionnaire measures were noted, with 6 of the children no longer meeting the classification of movement difficulties on the MABC-2 after treatment (Morgan et al. 2019).

In short, although Bowen therapy has been reported to be beneficial in a variety of disorders, the quantity and quality of clinical research has been limited to date.

Summary

Bowen therapy is a form of manual therapy characterized by sequential moves and pauses that can be adapted and implemented into a wide variety of treatment settings. Bowen is currently practiced throughout the world in settings such as sports clinics, hospitals, orthopedic centers, pain clinics, spas, and home health. The Bowen technique may effect change by affecting the mechanotransduction of the extracellular matrix while also influencing the mechanoreceptors through pressure and shearing forces. Though limited in scope, clinical research thus far supports the claims of benefit of Bowen therapy for a variety of maladies.

REFERENCES

American Osteopathic Association. The Tenets of Osteopathic Medicine. Available from: https://osteopathic.org/about/leadership/aoa-governance-documents/tenets-of-osteopathic-medicine/.

Argenbright, C., 2016. Bowenwork for symptom management of women breast cancer survivors with lymphedema: a pilot study. Complement Ther. Clin. Pract. 25,142–149.

D'Alessandro, G., Cerritelli, F., Cortelli, P., 2016. Sensitization and interoception as key neurological concepts in osteopathy and other manual medicines. Front. Neurosci. 10, 100.

Duncan, B., McHugh, P., Houghton, F., Wilson, C., 2011. Improved motor function with Bowen therapy for rehabilitation in chronic stroke. J. Prim. Health Care 3, 53–58.

Félix, G.J.S., Black, L., Rodrigues, M., Silva, A.G., 2016. The acute effect of Bowen therapy on pressure pain thresholds and postural sway in healthy subjects. J. Bodyw. Mov. Ther. 21, 804–809.

Findley, T., 2015. Fascia Research 2015 – State of the Art [online]. Available from: http://fasciacongress.org/pdfs/FasciaConferenceBook_Introduction2015.pdf.

Hansen, C., Taylor-Pillae, R.E., 2011. What is Bowenwork? A systematic review. J. Altern. Complement Med. 17, 1001–1006.

Hipmair, G., Ganser, D., Bohler, N., Schimetta, W., Polz, W., 2012. Efficacy of Bowen therapy in postoperative pain management – a single blinded (randomized) controlled trial. (Translated from German.) In: Wilks, J., Knight, I., Using The Bowen Technique To Address Complex and Common Conditions-Singing Dragon Press, 2014, London, England.

Huang, B., Ingber, D., 1999. The structural and mechanical complexity of cell-growth control. Nat. Cell Biol. 1, E131–E138.

Langevin, H.M., Bouard, N.A., Fox, J.R., et al. 2011. Fibroblast cytoskeletal remodeling contributes to connective tissue tension. J. Cell. Physiol. 226, 1166–1175.

Marr, M., Baker, J., Lambon, N., Perry, J., 2011. The effects of the Bowen technique on hamstring flexibility over time: a randomised controlled trial. J. Bodyw. Mov. Ther. 15, 281–290.

Morgan-Jones, M., Knott, F., Wilcox, H., Ashwin, C., 2019. A Pilot study of fascia Bowen therapy for 8-11 year-old boys with developmental coordination disorder. J. Bodyw. Mov. Ther. 23, 568–574.

Moseley, G.L., Gallace, A., Spence, C., 2011. Bodily illusions in health and disease: physiological and clinical perspectives and the concept of a cortical body matrix. Neurosci. Biobehav. Rev. 36, 34–46.

Schulz, A., Vogele, C., 2015. Interoception and stress. Front. Psychol. 6, 993, ecollection 2015.

Winter, A., MacAllister, R., 2011. An Evaluation of health improvements for Bowen therapy clients. Available from: https://bowenworks.org/downloads/health-improvements-from-bowen.pdf.

Wan, S.L.Y., Chan, E.W.C., Cheng, S.W.C., et al., 2016. Effectiveness of Bowen Therapy performed by Occupational Therapists in Improving Occupational Performance of People with Shoulder Injury – Interim Result of Randomized Control Trial. https://www.scribd.com/doc/306360691/Interim-Results-Shoulder-Study-ISBT-HK.

7.27

Fascia and Mental Imagery: Can the Two Walk Together?

Amit Abraham and Eric Franklin

CHAPTER CONTENTS

INTRODUCTION

Over the past few years, scientific discoveries about the diverse constructions and functions of fascia have shed light on its complex nature and diverse roles in movement, posture, and pathologies. Such new insights are leading to additional innovative questions regarding fascia's interactions with other body tissues (e.g., bones, muscles, and nerves) and with the mind's brain functions and cognition that effect performance outcomes (e.g., speed, accuracy, range of motion, etc.). This chapter considers the bidirectional interactions between fascia and mental imagery (MI), a cognitive process of the mind, to consider how mental imagery of fascia might influence human performance, including in the experiences of daily living.

What might be possible if fascia and MI agreed to "walk together"? Could a person's mental awareness of the nature of fascia facilitate fascia's structures and functions? Might a person's imagery of fascia as "watery" or "happy" affect motor and cognitive capabilities? These

ideas are worth considering, particularly in light of MI's low-cost and ready availability. Sound too good to be true? Well, not so sure . . .

The extent to which fascia and MI interlink may be greater than previously imagined (double meaning). Given gaps in current knowledge and understanding of these phenomena, we take a step-by-step approach to our exploration in this chapter. We identify similarities and connections between fascia and mental imagery. We then present fascial dynamic neurocognitive imagery (fDNI) as an exemplary mental imagery approach that specifically addresses fascia. We conclude with examples of exercises illustrating how fascial dynamic neurocognitive imagery (fDNI) brings to life the ideas presented in this chapter.

 KEY POINT

Both fascia and mental imagery (MI) are emerging fields of research and practice that have been considered to date as distinct areas.

MENTAL IMAGERY: DEFINITIONS AND ROLES

"Mental imagery" is a term used to describe a large array of cognitive processes involved in imagining content, as varied as motor tasks (e.g., lifting the arm or turning the head), sensory experiences (e.g., the smell of a flower or the taste of a food dish), or novel fantasy (Guillot and Collet 2010). Mental imagery typically incorporates at least one of the human senses, such as imagining feeling (kinesthetic), seeing (visual), hearing (auditory), smelling (olfactory), and tasting (gustatory), or any combination of them. Mental images often depict an actual experience stored in memory, available to be retrieved and used as part of the mental imagery process (Guillot and Collet 2010). However, mental images can also move beyond known (or previously experienced) contents to include more "imaginary" ideas or contents (Franklin 2012, 2014a). Mental imagery can employ metaphors to represent a desired borrowed quality that is not necessarily real in order to suggest the ways certain content should be considered (Franklin 2012, 2014a). For example, one can mentally image their spine being a chain of soap bubbles to facilitate a soft, mobile spinal movement (see Fig. 7.27.1). The qualities and ideas reflected by the metaphor (e.g., lightness, subtlety, and agility of the soap bubbles) are being

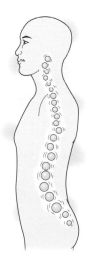

Fig. 7.27.1. Metaphorical mental imagery of the spine as a chain of bubbles. Redrawn from an original drawing by Mr. Eric Franklin.

borrowed and used for the spinal vertebrae for the purpose of promoting ease and variability in the spine.

Mental imagery is considered an innate human capacity and has been referred to as long as 2500 years ago. In modern times, mental imagery has been mainly used in sports, performing arts, and rehabilitation as a tool for obtaining various goals. For example, Mariel Zagunis, the four-time Olympic medalist and the most decorated athlete in the history of US fencing, said she used mental imagery as a way of practicing possible scenarios on the strip: "In sabre fencing, points happen literally in split seconds, and tides can change and turn very, very quickly. So part of visualization is preparing yourself for every situation, so when it shows itself, you're ready for it" (Maese 2016). For some athletes, visual imagery is only part of it. Emily Cook, ski jumper, said she practiced smelling, hearing, and feeling herself at the brink of her aerial maneuvers: "I'm standing on the top of the hill. I can feel the wind on the back of my neck. I can hear the crowd." For Cook, imagery was also available to her even when she was injured and imagined seeing and feeling her bones heal. In addition, she imagined her fear to be "a big red balloon that she popped with a pin" (Clarcy 2014).

Scientific theories and studies to date about how mental imagery enhances performance have mostly been limited to considerations of its effects on muscle tissue (Clark et al. 2014; Guillot et al. 2007). Given fascia's affinity with muscle tissue, links between mental imagery and fascia may also exist. Let us, therefore, begin to invite them to walk together by considering ways in which fascia and mental imagery may be similar and even interlinked.

SIMILARITIES BETWEEN FASCIA AND MENTAL IMAGERY

Although fascia and mental imagery may seem to be two completely distinct phenomena, they share several similarities. Both are complex, multifaceted, and serve a connecting function. Fascia connects different body tissues and organs, and mental imagery connects different cognitive and neural processes. Both have a history of neglect in science and clinical practice over the years, and both are emerging as important components of human functioning. The former conceptualization of fascia as a mere wrapping for bones and muscles is dramatically evolving into an understanding of its essential role in living processes. Similarly, the traditional reference of mental imagery as primarily useful to "see" desired outcomes or anticipated movements (Abraham et al. 2016, 2017) is now being expanded to include multiple senses, in combination with movement (Guillot et al. 2013; Heiland et al. 2012; Heiland and Rovetti 2013), and more kinds, such as anatomical, biomechanical, emotional, and metaphorical imagery (Abraham et al. 2018, 2019a, 2019b; Franklin, 2006, 2012, 2014a).

> ### 🕹 KEY POINT
>
> Identified similarities between fascia and MI include their roles in connecting, articulating, changing, and encompassing motor and cognitive components of movement. Based on these similarities and on MI's effects on motor and cognitive aspects of performance, fascia and MI may be interacting with each other through various mechanisms, such as proprioception, body schema, and movement.

Both fascia and mental imagery affect motor and cognitive functions in daily life, from movement and posture to problem-solving and self-confidence. As such, both are "everywhere" (fascia in the physical sense and mental imagery in the cognitive sense). Both are potentially malleable, and both can get stuck. Experience affects both fascia (Schultz 1996) and mental imagery (Kraeutner et al. 2018; Overby 1990), with traumatic or chronic negative experiences potentially impeding functioning and contributing to pain. For example, in fascia, scar tissue (made of connective tissue) could reflect a prior experience (i.e., a cut, injury, or emotional stress or trauma) that resulted in fascial shortening or inflexibility. At the same time, trauma may often be associated with repetitive intrusive or stuck mental images associated with the traumatic experience (Clark and Mackay 2015).

From a definitional perspective, fascia's interconnected nature and less anatomically bounded structure, and mental imagery's nonphysical and varied character, have contributed to challenges associated with scientifically studying their actions and interactions. Such research challenges could explain in part the historical lack of scientific research into these phenomena individually, and perhaps doubly so regarding research into their interrelationship. Moving forward, new models tying together these two phenomena are beginning to promote innovative research paths for discovering the mysteries within each individually and within their interactions.

SUGGESTED ASSOCIATIONS BETWEEN FASCIA AND MENTAL IMAGERY

After pointing at "why" fascia and mental imagery could "walk together," let us move on to the "how" part of this walk. Although scientific research on both fascia and mental imagery is relatively in early stages, we find clues to their possible interactions in scientific literature from related fields (e.g., neurophysiology, cognitive neuroscience, etc.). Given the connecting functions of both fascia and mental imagery, we find it appropriate to suggest some of the potential paths and associations, both direct or indirect (i.e., through mediating factors or phenomena). The mechanisms of effect through which fascia and mental imagery affect movement are not fully understood to date. However, it may be that at least some of these suggested mechanisms are common to both phenomena, in which case they might serve as channels through which mental imagery and fascia could communicate with each other. These associations could be represented by the metaphorical image of the brain "massaging" the fascia and vice versa, thus nourishing both and facilitating their elasticity and plasticity (see Fig. 7.27.2).

- *Proprioception and Kinesthesis.* Both unconscious (aka proprioception) and conscious (aka kinesthesia) felt sensations of one's own body position and movement rely on sensory information that originates from body

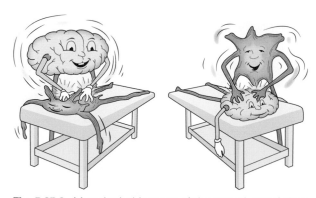

Fig. 7.27.2. Metaphorical imagery of the mutual associations between mental imagery and fascia. Redrawn from an original drawing by Mr. Eric Franklin.

tissues and organs (Bosco and Poppele 2001). Given the sensory information derived from fascia throughout the body, mental imagery's reliance on sensory information in general might be able to use the sensory information coming from fascia to improving the body's proprioception and kinesthesis (see Exercise 1, later).

- *Body Schema.* Body schema is the mental representation of one's body and its parts in space and in relation to each other (de Vignemont 2010). As such, body schema involves both mental imagery (Shenton 2004) and sensory information derived from the body tissues, including fascial. An example of how mental imagery plays a role in body schema is in imagining whether one's body will pass safely through a doorway before actually trying to do so (aka passability judgment). Mental imagery focused on fascia therefore could promote awareness and direct attentional focus to yield an increased amount and/or quality of information from fascia with which to create a more detailed and accurate body schema formation.

- *Nociception (Pain).* Mental imagery has been shown to be useful in diminishing pain sensations (Bowering et al. 2013; Moseley 2004). When fascia is the source of nociception (i.e., painful sensation), mental imagery focused on fascia could possibly be used for treating pain of fascial origin. For example, insofar as pain is one of the symptoms of hypomobile or traumatized fascia, mental imagery targeted at kinematic and rehabilitative aspects of fascia could be useful for regaining mobility and helping to restore pain-free movement.

- *Psychology.* Fascia and mental imagery bilaterally intertwine with psychological emotions and self-confidence (Callow et al. 2006). Psychological components can affect fascia and mental imagery either directly or indirectly, through posture for example. A lack of confidence might show up in a person's rounded shoulders and kyphotic posture. Chronic holding of such a posture can over time result in a shortening and tightening of the interpectoral fascia accompanied by increased inability to imagine alternatives. Practicing mental imagery, such as with positive self-talk and uplifting visuals, could uplift mood and levels of self-confidence. As fascia-targeted mental imagery cues a softening and expanding of the interpectoral fascia, a physical uplift and experience of improved well-being could result. Fascia-targeted manual manipulation on a shortened or contracted area could also promote all three interrelated areas: a better psychological state,

easier engagement in mental imagery, and freer postural habits.

- *Posture and Movement.* Static postures and lack of movement might both negatively affect fascia through mechanical and physiological avenues (Avila Gonzalez et al. 2018; Schleip and Muller 2013; Zügel et al. 2018). For example, a joint held in one position (as in the case of a pathological contracture) may eventually result in shortening, thickening, and reduced mobility of the fascial tissues within and around it. Positive effects of movement on fascia (Schleip and Muller 2013; Zügel et al. 2018) are likely to also apply to mental imagery, given that movement typically characterizes the real-life experiences that serve as a foundation for mental imagery processes, including imagination and creativity. Dancers, for example, often have enhanced mental imagery skills (Pavlik and Nordin-Bates 2016). Movement, essential for both fascia and mental imagery, could be therefore useful to improving both (see Exercise 2, later).

- *Touch.* Fascia has been shown to benefit from touch, including brushing, squishing, vibrating, and stretching, via receptors within the fascia. Mental imagery can affect touch, such as by promoting a more "thoughtful touch," so fascia-targeted touch could facilitate a more discrete image of the fascia in one's mind (see Exercise 3, later).

- *Physiology.* Mental imagery has been hypothesized to positively affect physiological properties of tissues, including those of fascia (Franklin 2016). Given mental imagery's role in switching mindset, and the role of dynamicity in fascial health, mental imagery might encourage fascial mobility, particularly when supported by other factors, such as touch, posture, and movement, as discussed earlier.

Considering these interconnecting pathways and mediators between fascia and mental imagery supports the growing interest in interactive, holistic approaches to human function and movement. As fascia and mental imagery begin to walk together, further exploration of additional mind-body connections is likely to provide insights into integrative, multisystem therapies. These mind-body therapies available through mental imagery could include its feed-forward mechanisms, imagining how one wants to feel, to help override existing sensory information and provide improved sensations and capabilities. We briefly outline some ways that fascia and mental imagery have "walked together" for mutual benefit.

FASCIAL DYNAMIC NEUROCOGNITIVE IMAGERY: A BRIEF HISTORY

The idea of merging fascia with mental imagery emerged approximately 20 years ago, as part of the "Franklin Method" (Franklin, 2004, 2005, 2006, 2012, 2014a, 2019). As a dancer, Eric Franklin noticed that cues and instructions often did not align with human anatomy and correct biomechanics. Being aware of the power of mental imagery from his interaction and training with experts in the field of mental imagery and somatics, including Mabel Todd, Lulu Sweigard, and André Bernard, and influenced by others, including Moshe Feldenkrais, Franklin grew to appreciate the important role of mental imagery in correct, functional movement. He applied his insights into a codified set of practices combining mental imagery, touch, movement, and anatomical knowledge for promoting embodiment and biomechanical understanding. Franklin applied these aspects to fascia, building on fascial discoveries by Carl Toldt, Raymond Dart, Ida Rolf, and others. The resulting dynamic neurocognitive imagery (DNI) is a codified and ongoing mental imagery approach for movement and postural retraining. Fascial DNI (fDNI) specifically includes the integration of cognitive elements with fascial ones to provide an experience of mindful movement (Franklin 2014b). Combining knowledge about the human fascia's structures and functions with mental imagery, touch, movement, and cognitive knowledge facilitates self-awareness, attentional focus, and optimal movement and function.

 KEY POINT

Fascial dynamic neurocognitive imagery (fDNI) is a codified MI training approach for fascia. As such, it holds potential for affecting fascial structure and function.

FASCIAL DYNAMIC NEUROCOGNITIVE IMAGERY EXERCISES FOR MENTAL IMAGERY AND FASCIA

Constantly evolving, fDNI integrates up-to-date scientific discoveries about human movement and function along with fascia's structure and functional role in three-dimensional, whole body movements. A wide variety of ways are offered for students to internally experience mental and physical sensations of fascia's diverse locations, dimensions, compositions, and functions. Anatomical and metaphorical drawings support the ability to visualize the different fascial structures. To address the various receptors in fascia, fDNI cues students to notice how they feel before, during, and after each exercise that typically combines mental imagery with different types of self-touch, such as squishing or sponging, vibrating, applying pressure, and/or brushing, with moving or stretching the body part under consideration. To address fascia's connective function, students are cued to image its structure, such as fascial slings' anatomical and kinetic connections between the triceps and the latissimus dorsi. The imaging of sliding and slippery fascial interfaces during the movement and self-touch reinforces the "packaging" and "differentiating" functions of fascia, not only between muscles but also between organs and their wrappings (see Exercise 4, later).

By addressing what fascia does and how it behaves and works during basic movements of daily living as walking, turning, bending, and reaching, fDNI reinforces fascia's functionality. By comparing movement before and after the exercise, students can assess how much the fascial imagery beneficially affected their range of motion and stability. After every combination of mental imagery, self-touch, and movement, students are cued to pause and take a moment to feel inward for any changes in mind (e.g., mood, sensations, mindfulness) and body (balance, posture). In this way, fascial mental imagery serves a training effect. Anecdotal reports of students and clients describe fDNI's physical effects as better range of motion, balance, flexibility, and coordination, as well as increased presence of mind and belief in their ability to improve fascial functioning.

Following are examples of fDNI exercises demonstrating how fascia and mental imagery's interactions can be experienced to enhance physical and mental clarity, ease, and adaptability. Along with touch and movement experiences, fDNI offers functional mental imagery cues of anatomical, biomechanical, and metaphorical aspects of fascia. Readers are encouraged to try them out for yourself and see whether they work for you!

EXERCISE 1: FASCIAL CONCENTRATION AND AWARENESS

1. Stand in a relaxed, neutral posture. Notice your posture and any sensations from your body. Notice any thoughts about your body you may have.

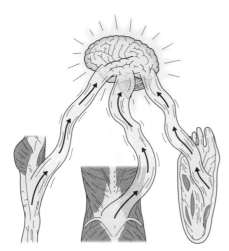

Fig. 7.27.3. A fascial river flowing information to the brain. Redrawn from an original drawing by Mr. Eric Franklin.

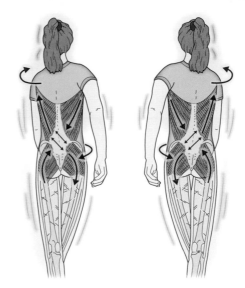

Fig. 7.27.4. Walking while imaging opposing stretchy myofascial slings. Redrawn from an original drawing by Mr. Eric Franklin.

2. Focus on the different fascia in your body (e.g., plantar fascia, thoraco-lumbar fascia, fascia lata, etc.). Mentally see and feel sensations and perceptions arising from your fascia.
3. Image information continuously flowing from the fascia through the nervous system to your brain. Enrich the information with imaged sensations of water flowing in rivers from all over your body. Focus on the image as you continue to breath and relax (Fig. 7.27.3).
4. Let go of your thoughts and notice your awareness of physical sensations. Do you detect any differences from the beginning of the exercise? If so, try to mentally verbalize these differences (e.g., more vivid, awake, alive, dynamic, etc.).

EXERCISE 2: FASCIAL CONCENTRATION AND AWARENESS

1. Walk back and forth, then stop and notice how your body feels.
2. Focus on your thoraco-lumbar fascia (TLF) as you step forward with your right leg, allowing your left arm to swing forward, and image the increasing stretch/lengthening across the posterior crossed myofascial sling from the left shoulder's latissimus dorsi fascia to the right pelvic half's gluteus fascia (Fig. 7.27.4).
3. Taking a step with your left leg, with the right arm swinging forward, image the opposite posterior crossed myofascial sling stretching/lengthening.

4. Integrate this mental image into walking while gradually increasing your gait speed until walking in a normal pace.
5. Stop and notice your body: How did it feel? How was the quality of movement?
6. Go for an integrated walk and notice any changes in your gait pattern and associated feelings/thoughts.

EXERCISE 3: FASCIAL SLIDING INTEGRATED TOUCH AND MENTAL IMAGERY

1. Stand relaxed and reach forward and backward with your right hand.
2. Put your left palm on your right pectoralis major muscle, with your fingertips pointing toward your right shoulder, and continue reaching forward and backward with your right hand. Note changes in the length and orientation of the muscle underneath your left palm.
3. While moving, image pectoral fascia surrounding the muscle as a large net that slackens and expands/stretches while you are reaching forward and backward, respectively (Fig. 7.27.5). Do 5 to 6 repetitions.
4. Let go of the hands and notice any differences between the right and left chest and shoulder areas.
5. Switch sides and repeat the process.

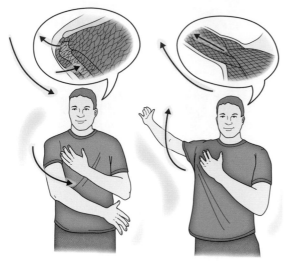

Fig. 7.27.5. The pectoral fascial net. Redrawn from an original drawing by Mr. Eric Franklin.

EXERCISE 4: LUNGS' FASCIAL SLIDING

1. In standing or sitting, side-bend to the right a few times.
2. Notice your movement (range of motion, ease, smoothness, breathing, etc.).
3. Side-bend to the right, and image the right lung and its visceral pleura sliding down on the parietal pleura, as the left lung and its visceral pleura are

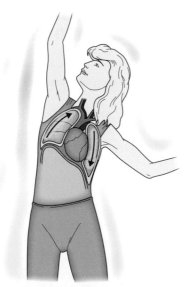

Fig. 7.27.6. Sliding lung fascia. Redrawn from an original drawing by Mr. Eric Franklin.

sliding up (Fig. 7.27.6). As you move back into standing upright, image the lung and pleura sliding back to their original, balanced locations. Repeat a few times.
4. Compare the right and left sides, noting any differences in sensations, posture, and ease of breathing.
5. Repeat the process while side-bending to the left.
6. Take a moment to notice your breathing and posture on both sides as well as your mindset.

Summary

After many years, fascia and mental imagery are beginning to receive the scientific and clinical attention they deserve. Fascia-specific mental imagery, such as that provided by fDNI, offers a way toward understanding how the body and the mind interrelate in movement and personal well-being. Our take-home message is that processes that allow fascia and mental imagery to interact, such as those used by fDNI, show promise in supporting a variety of benefits for motor, cognitive, and psychological functions. We hope that our descriptions of fascia and mental imagery's interrelationships will support further clinical and research studies into more ways that the two can walk together toward improved human functioning.

ACKNOWLEDGMENTS

The authors would like to thank Dr. Rita Durant for her assistance with this chapter.

REFERENCES

Abraham, A., Dunsky, A., Dickstein, R., 2016. Motor imagery practice for enhancing elevé performance among professional dancers: a pilot study. Med. Probl. Perform. Art. 31, 132–139.

Abraham, A., Dunsky, A., Dickstein, R., 2017. The effect of motor imagery practice on elevé performance in adolescent female dance students: a randomized controlled trial. J. Imagery Res. Sport Phys. Activ. 12, 20160006.

Abraham, A., Gose, R., Schindler, R., Nelson, B.H., Hackney, M.E., 2019a. Dynamic neurocognitive imagery (DNI) improves developpé performance, kinematics, and mental imagery ability in university-level dance students. Front. Psychol. 10, 382.

Abraham, A., Hart, A., Andrade, I., Hackney, M.E., 2018. Dynamic neurocognitive imagery (DNI)™ improves mental imagery ability, disease severity, and motor and cognitive functions in people with Parkinson's disease. Neural Plast. 2018, 6168507.

Abraham, A., Hart, A., Dickstein, R., Hackney, M.E., 2019b. "Will you draw me a pelvis?" Dynamic neurocognitive imagery improves pelvic schema and graphic-metric representation in people with Parkinson's disease: a randomized controlled trial. Complement. Ther. Med. 43, 28–35.

Avila Gonzalez, C.A., Driscoll, M., Schleip, R., et al., 2018. Frontiers in fascia research. J. Bodyw. Mov. Ther. 22, 873–880.

Bosco, G., Poppele, R.E., 2001. Proprioception from a spinocerebellar perspective. Physiol. Rev. 81, 539–568.

Bowering, K.J., O'Connell, N.E., Tabor, A., et al. 2013. The effects of graded motor imagery and its components on chronic pain: a systematic review and meta-analysis. J. Pain 14, 3–13.

Callow, N., Roberts, R., Fawkes, J.Z., 2006. Effects of dynamic and static imagery on vividness of imagery, skiing performance, and confidence. J. Imagery Res. Sport. Phys. Activ. 1. doi:10.2202/1932-0191.1001.

Clarey, C., Feb. 22, 2014. Olympians use imagery as mental training. *New York Times.*

Clark, B.C., Mahato, N.K., Nakazawa, M., Law, T.D., Thomas, J.S., 2014. The power of the mind: the cortex as a critical determinant of muscle strength/weakness. J. Neurophysiol. 112, 3219–3226.

Clark, I.A., Mackay, C.E., 2015. Mental imagery and post-traumatic stress disorder: a neuroimaging and experimental psychopathology approach to intrusive memories of trauma. Front. Psychiatry 6, 104.

de Vignemont, F., 2010. Body schema and body image—pros and cons. Neuropsychologia 48, 669–680.

Franklin, E., 2004. Pelvic Power. Princeton Book, Hightstown, NJ.

Franklin, E., 2005. Beautiful Body Beautiful Mind: The Power of Positive Imagery. Princeton Book Company, Hightstown, NJ.

Franklin, E., 2006. Inner Focus Outer Strength. Princeton Book Company, Hightstown, NJ.

Franklin, E., 2012. Dynamic Alignment through Imagery. Human Kinetics, Champaign, IL.

Franklin, E., 2014a. Dance imagery for Technique and Performance. Human Kinetics, Champaign, IL.

Franklin, E., 2014b. Fascia Release and Balance: Franklin Method Ball and Imagery Exercises. OPTP, Minneapolis, MN, USA.

Franklin, E., 2016. Grow Young Daily: The Power of Imagery for Healthy Cells and Timeless Beauty. Dog Ear, Indianapolis, IN.

Franklin, E., 2019. Conditioning for Dance. Human Kinetics, Champaign, IL.

Guillot, A., Collet, C., 2010. The Neurophysiological Foundations of Mental and Motor Imagery. Oxford University Press, New York.

Guillot, A., Lebon, F., Rouffet, D., Champely, S., Doyon, J., Collet, C., 2007. Muscular responses during motor imagery as a function of muscle contraction types. Int. J. Psychophysiol. 66, 18–27.

Guillot, A., Moschberger, K., Collet, C., 2013. Coupling movement with imagery as a new perspective for motor imagery practice. Behav. Brain Funct. 9, 8.

Heiland, T.L., Rovetti, R., Dunn, J., 2012. Effects of visual, auditory, and kinesthetic imagery interventions on dancers' plié arabesques. J. Imagery. Res. Sport Phys. Activ. 7, 5.

Heiland, T., Rovetti, R., 2013. Examining effects of Franklin Method metaphorical and anatomical mental images on college dancers' jumping height. Res. Dance Educ. 14, 141–161.

Kraeutner, S.N., McWhinney, S.R., Solomon, J.P., Dithurbide, L., Boe, S.G., 2018. Experience modulates motor imagery-based brain activity. Eur. J. Neurosci. 47, 1221–1229.

Maese, R., July 28, 2016. For Olympians, seeing (in their minds) is believing (it can happen). *The Washington Post.*

Moseley, G.L., 2004. Graded motor imagery is effective for long-standing complex regional pain syndrome: a randomized controlled trial. Pain 108, 192–198.

Overby, L.Y., 1990. A comparison of novice and experienced dancers' imagery ability. J. Mental Imagery 14, 173–184.

Pavlik, K., Nordin-Bates, S., 2016. Imagery in dance - a literature review. J. Dance Med. Sci. 20, 51–63.

Schleip, R., Muller, D.G., 2013. Training principles for fascial connective tissues: scientific foundation and suggested practical applications. J. Bodyw. Mov. Ther. 17, 103–115.

Schultz, L., Feitis, R., 1996. The Endless Web Fascial Anatomy and Physical Reality. North Atlantic Books, Berkeley, CA.

Shenton, J.T., Schwoebel, J., Coslett, H.B., 2004. Mental motor imagery and the body schema: evidence for proprioceptive dominance. Neurosci. Lett. 370, 19–24.

Zügel, M., Maganaris, C.N., Wilke, J., et al. 2018. Fascial tissue research in sports medicine: from molecules to tissue adaptation, injury and diagnostics: consensus statement. Br. J. Sports Med. 52, 1497.

Foam Rolling

Michele Bond

CHAPTER CONTENTS

INTRODUCTION

History

The use of the foam roller as an educational and therapeutic tool was first introduced by Dr. Moshe Feldenkrais. Before then, he was using wooden rollers to reduce movement friction as part of his somatic education method. When he came to America in the 1970s, he came across cylindrical rollers made of high-density foam used for packing and started using them in his work (Feldenkrais 2009). Practitioners of his method continued the use of the foam roller and by the mid-1990s, foam rolling as a self-massage tool was introduced to the performing artist community as a comprehensive warm-up and conditioning program (Gamboa and Gallagher 1996). It was around this time that the term "self-myofascial release" (SMFR) was introduced by physical therapist Mike Clark, and foam rolling became popular among the weight lifting community as a way to reduce muscle soreness and improve gym performance (Clark 2001). In 2004 a variation of the typical cylindrical roller was registered in the United States. From that time, foam rollers made their way to commercial gym floors, athletics, and the therapeutic community. Since that time, various practitioners have used this modality to develop programs

(e.g., MELT method) to alleviate chronic pain, release tension, and restore mobility. Though a foam roller cannot replace the hands of a skilled practitioner, the foam roller is considered an ideal alterative or adjunct method because of its portability, low cost, and general ease of use (Latella et al. 2018). The research on foam rolling has expanded in many directions to investigate how to improve various performance parameters, increase flexibility and range of motion (ROM), enhance postexercise muscle recovery, and reduce pain sensitivity.

Myofascial Release

In order to examine the concept of SMFR as it pertains to the foam roller, it is important to briefly review the premise behind myofascial release (MFR) itself. MFR, rooted in osteopathic medicine in the early 1900s, is a system of diagnosis and treatment that achieves myofascial release through continuous palpatory feedback. Direct MFR involves loading the tissue with constant force until a release is detected, and indirect MFR involves guiding tissues along the path of least resistance until free movement is achieved (Educational Council on Osteopathic Principles 2009). Myofascial restrictions may occur from injury, inactivity, inflammation, overload, and disease (Behm and Wilke 2019). Myofascial release stimulates the muscles, tendons, and mechanoreceptors of the fascia and biomechanically loads the soft tissues (Remvig et al. 2008). Because MFR involves direct pressure and/or movement over the skin and underlying structures, it is assumed that SMFR will produce similar results due to a stationary direct pressure or a rolling motion that can be created. A continually increasing amount of literature regarding foam rolling (FR) has revealed that SMFR and FR seem to be interchangeable terms (Behm and Wilke 2019). However, it is important to distinguish between the momentum of something that becomes popular and the actual science behind that momentum. It is of great importance in this realm of colliding therapy, exercise/sport, and research worlds to clarify the underlying mechanisms that result in changes in human performance or perception of sensory in the body. The concept of FR as a way to affect many conditions of the body is no different. Taking into account the previous explanation of MFR, it is important to ascertain if SMFR with a foam roller achieves this goal of releasing restricted fascial layers.

Self-Myofascial Release

The popularity of foam roller use among athletes, fitness enthusiasts, and therapists may be caused by its ability to improve flexibility and range of motion, alleviate pain from various sources, and restore performance-related abilities. However, if the intention is to replicate the manual effect of a therapeutic session, a specific protocol must be used (Kopec et al. 2016). A literature review examining the validity of SMFR using the foam roller (Behm and Wilke 2019) discussed ample research that attributed possible other mechanisms to explain the beneficial outcomes of FR. Their research concluded that although many articles attribute FR as a way to induce a self-myofascial release of tissue stiffness, adhesions, scar tissue, or spasms, the term SMFR for the beneficial outcomes reported is misleading. The term SMFR was widely integrated into the vernacular before FR mechanisms were determined. Some evidence suggests SMFR produces local tissue-specific effects, but the term SMFR does not represent the other mechanisms as the term implies (Behm and Wilke 2019). At this time, it may be prudent to change the name SMFR to something to the effect of tool-assisted soft tissue mobilization. It also should be noted that according to studies of time and force dependency, the manual pressure requirement to affect connective tissue plasticity is significant (Schleip 2003). That stated, FR most likely would not produce

enough pressure to release myofascial restrictions (Behm and Wilke 2019). These explorations are of importance, as clarifying and classifying the correct mechanisms by which change occurs in the body is indeed the responsibility of the research community in order to enlighten those involved in this practice of foam rolling.

 KEY POINT

Foam rolling debuted as an educational and therapeutic tool and seemed to help those in the performing arts and eventually the therapy and exercise/athletic communities. The term "self-myofascial release" became synonymous with foam rolling before the research could determine whether this was a legitimate term for this intervention.

POSSIBLE MECHANISMS OF FOAM ROLLING

Mechanical

Potential pathways that can modify soft-tissue stiffness are, first, mechanical, having to do with alterations in the structure or state of fascial tissue, and second, neurophysiological, focusing on afferent signaling from mechanoreceptors (Schleip 2003). With regard to mechanical mechanisms, thixotropic effects demonstrate how the pressure of the roller on fascia decreases viscosity so that it is more fluid in nature (Schleip 2003). This more fluid-like state of the fascia may allow for more movement and thus create an increase in range of movement (ROM), for example. The piezoelectric effect creates a response in the cells responsible for the maintenance of the biomechanical properties of fascia through an electrical charge created by pressure. This assists with discarding old collagen fibers, creating the alignment of new ones, and can have a significant effect in assisting with the outcomes of FR (O'Connell 2003). Another mechanical mechanism could be a cellular response model that suggests because cells are held in a state of constant tension, mechanical loading of the fascia may initiate biochemical processes (Tozzi 2012).

Fascial tissue hydration is another mechanism that results when mechanical load, such as the compression of a foam roller, encourages water to be pushed out of the affected area and then more nutrient dense water rehydrates the fascial tissues. Dehydration can impose increased stiffness in the fascial tissues and thus decrease mobility (Schleip and Müller 2013). Fascial gliding can also help explain some of the outcomes of FR. Krause and colleagues (2019) found an increased fascial gliding in the interface between the fascia lata and the underlying muscle's epimysium from a foam rolling intervention. With regard to the thoracolumbar fascia (TLF), it was found that foam rolling various muscles around the lumbar region produced acute changes in overall mobility of the TLF but not in individual layers (Griefahn et al. 2017). Foam rolling can also increase blood flow by increasing nitric oxide production. This may help reduce inflammation, which may cause stiffness in muscle and fascia (Beardsley and Škarabot 2015). Foam rolling can acutely decrease arterial stiffness and improve vascular endothelial function. These circulatory improvements can assist in removing waste from the body and improve tissue repair and healing (Okamoto et al. 2013).

Neurophysiological

Neurophysiological mechanisms may also account for some of the effects of FR, as explained by manual therapy results (Beardsley and Škarabot 2015). Golgi organs, Ruffini receptors, Pacini corpuscles, and interstitial receptors are sensory nerve endings that are contained in the fascia. These sensory nerve endings are referred to as fascial mechanoreceptors, as they respond to mechanical tension and/or pressure, such as from FR (Schleip 2017). Golgi receptors, found throughout dense proper connective tissue, respond to slow stretch by signaling the central nervous system to relax related muscle fibers. Foam rolling may not stimulate the Golgi tendon organ specifically (found in muscle-tendon junction) due to lack of active muscle contraction because of the receptors' serial arrangement with muscle fiber (Schleip 2003). The Ruffini receptors respond to sustained pressure and lateral stretch and inhibit sympathetic activity to reduce muscle tone. Pacini corpuscles respond to rapid pressure changes and vibration to assist with proprioception as with a vibrating foam roller. Interstitial free nerve endings respond to periosteum stimulation and produce both a withdrawal response to threatening pain and relief of pain through pain desensitization (Schleip 2017). The pressure of FR may reduce pain and thus assist with the beneficial outcomes of FR (e.g., increased ROM), but the intensity should be monitored so as to not produce a withdrawal response.

A global effect of these neurophysiological mechanisms has also been noted. Killen et al. (2019) found that unilateral FR of the hamstring increased contralateral hip flexion passive ROM (PROM) but did not affect muscle strength performance. Monteiro et al. (2019a) illustrated that a single bout (60 s) of hamstring FR increased shoulder extension and flexion PROM. In understanding the global effect of FR, rolling contralateral may be especially useful if postinjury rehabilitation requires immobilization, or ROM interventions cannot be tolerated. Regardless of the mechanisms that may be prevalent in certain conditions, the research regarding the effects of FR in the literature is steadily growing. Although there is a range in study complexity and findings, the research seems to be determined to create equilibrium. These mechanisms will help place the context in which foam rolling and the behavior of fascia coincide.

> **KEY POINT**
>
> Possible other mechanisms that can modify soft-tissue stiffness are mechanical, having to do with alterations in the structure or state of fascial tissue, and neurophysiological, which focuses on afferent signaling from mechanoreceptors in the fascia.

RESEARCH CONTEXTS

There are a vast number of studies specifically on FR that include relevant topics that seek a deeper understanding of human function as well as a quest to assist with best practices. Some of these investigations include the effect of foam rolling on muscle function; pain reduction; ROM at a specific joint; fascial gliding; and performance parameters, such as jump height, peak torque, and sprint speed. The intention of the research is to translate laboratory findings to application for exercise, sport, and therapy. The use of a foam roller requires the participant to use their bodyweight to create pressure and friction between the foam roller and the muscle group being rolled (Fig. 7.28.1, Fig. 7.28.2). The research suggests that FR produces short-term benefits for increasing flexibility, joint ROM, and pressure pain thresholds, as well as reducing declines in muscle performance and the effects of delayed onset muscle soreness and other sources of myofascial pain (Cheatham and Stull 2018).

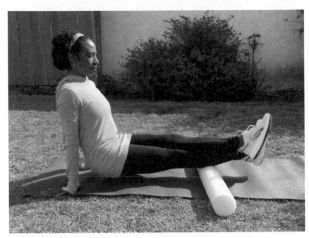

Fig. 7.28.1 Foam rolling for the calf region.

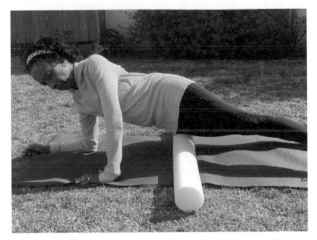

Fig. 7.28.2 Foam rolling the tensor fascia lata muscle.

Flexibility and ROM

With regards to ROM, Monteiro et al. (2019b) concluded that anterior thigh FR resulted in significant acute increases in hip flexion and extension PROM. The higher volume of 120 seconds (vs 60 s) produced the greatest increases in PROM, and this effect appeared to last for 20 minutes. Hall and Smith (2018) concluded that FR over gluteal muscles significantly improved hip adduction PROM. The protocol used was 3 sets of 30 seconds rolling from the posterior superior iliac spine to the gluteal fold, with a 30-second rest between sets. Cheatham and Stull (2018) suggest that FR with active joint ROM may produce greater immediate

effects on flexibility than with no joint motion. This 2-minute intervention on the quadriceps revealed that four active knee bends executed at specific intervals significantly increased passive knee flexion and may be the result of reciprocal inhibition. Do et al. (2018) demonstrated that rolling of the plantar fascia significantly increased lumbar spine and hamstring flexibility.

Pain

The use of foam rollers to address painful myofascial constrictions that may be caused by scar tissue, ischemia-induced muscle spasms, and other conditions is another area of research focus. Myofascial trigger points (MTrPs) are irritable spots within taught bands of skeletal muscle fibers and have been associated with connective tissue (Behm and Wilke 2019). MTrPs can be active or latent in nature, but both can cause negatively altered muscle mechanics and decrease soft-tissue extensibility. Wilke et al. (2018) compared a static hold on the roller on a sensitive latent MTrP (lateral gastrocnemius) to slow rolling of the area. They found the static bout to be more effective in reducing sensitivity. Delayed onset muscle soreness (DOMS) is another pain-evoking condition associated with an alteration to the extracellular matrix (extracellular components of connective tissue), sarcolemma, and intracellular muscle structure (Pearcey et al. 2015). Studies suggest that FR can improve DOMS and help recover from a decline in muscular function. Romero-Moraleda et al. (2017) conducted an FR intervention 48 hours after muscle soreness was induced with drop jumps. The quadriceps were foam rolled simultaneously using short kneading-like motions starting from the most proximal portion of the quadriceps down to just above the patellae and then back to the initial position in one fluid motion. Participants repeated this motion for 1 minute, rested for 30 seconds, and then repeated it again for 5 sets. Participants reported a significant reduction in their pain perception and demonstrated a significant increase in maximum voluntary isometric contraction (MVIC) of the vastus medialis, vastus lateralis, and rectus femoris muscles. Recovery after soreness or fatigue is a valuable component in any training regimen.

Dynamic Performance Measures

In terms of strength, FR as a warm-up generally does not attenuate muscle strength. However, in a maximum repetition strength study, Monteiro et al. (2017) discovered the use of the foam roller directly preceding and between sets of resistance training to failure for 4 sets impeded performance. There was also a dose-dependent factor with declining strength with the longer duration of FR (120 s v. 90 s and 60 s). However, passive rest in the 4-minute rest period between sets yielded the most preservation of strength.

Explosive strength is also another area of investigation. Smith et al. (2018) found that FR alone did not significantly increase vertical jump height (VJ), but it did in combination with dynamic stretching immediately after and 15 minutes later. Kopec et al. (2016) had a similar result but added that in addition to FR having other beneficial physiological effects, FR did not diminish explosive athletic performance. In a recovery-based study where knee extensors were eccentrically loaded (Latella et al. 2018), FR was most effective in restoring pretraining VJ height values 48 to 72 hours later. However, FR immediately after eccentric training and 24 hours later, VJ was maintained around 95% of pretraining jump height (compared with 88% in the control group), suggesting that FR may assist in the loss of explosive performance. In terms of timing of FR, Fleckenstein et al. (2017) found that when FR took place after inducing muscle fatigue, the loss of maximal force production in the lower limb was significantly less compared with a preventative measure of rolling before.

Proprioception

As stated, fascia contains mechanoreceptors that assist with proprioception. David and colleagues (2019) concluded that foam rolling the hamstrings improved knee joint position sense for at least 20 minutes postintervention. However, this was not the case for hip joint position sense or knee joint force sense. Cho and Kim (2016) found that FR for 1 week did increase hip joint position sense. Baseline absolute errors between the studies may be the difference in outcome as well as gender and learning curve. Romero-Franco and colleagues (2019) discovered that after a warm-up of 8 minutes of jogging and 45 seconds of FR to the hamstrings, quadriceps, and calf regions, there was no effect to knee proprioception (or improvement from baseline measures) in a joint position sense test. A stretch sensation study (Krause et al. 2019) indicated that foam rolling the anterior thigh resulted in the perception of stretch shifting to an increased knee flexion angle (an increased degree of stretch of the quadriceps). This may be due to a shift in proprioception presented as changes in perception of stretch or increased

stretch tolerance. This may be from a reduction of muscle/fascial tension and the discomfort associated with that. No study reported a decline in proprioception, and it was suggested that FR may be an effective intervention as part of a warm-up protocol for the other acute benefits it has. Refined proprioception can positively influence performance and may reduce the possibility of acute injury.

KEY POINT

Acute effects of foam rolling have been investigated for several parameters of human movement, performance, and sensory aspects of the body. Foam rolling affects the myofascia in a way that potentiates its features to affect movement and sensory perception.

VARIATIONS AND IMPLEMENTATION

Features and Purpose

Foam rollers vary in length, diameter, density, and material. The selection of roller will depend on the individual's ability and conditioning level as well outcome intention. For example, it may be easier to use a roller 12 inches long than 36 inches long when only rolling one anterior thigh. However, a 36-inch-long roller would be beneficial for lying on the spine lengthwise. In this supine position, a roller 4 inches in diameter may be a more appropriate height because of an individual's movement restrictions. Ease of execution is of utmost importance.

Foam rollers also display various textures—raised surfaces, indented grids, or a combination of the two (Fig. 7.28.3). Cheatham and Stull (2018) found that moderately firm multilevel and grid-pattern rollers produced greater ROM and pain-pressure thresholds than smooth rollers (Fig. 7.28.4). Multilevel rollers are reported to exert higher pressures over smaller contact areas and may produce greater benefits. However, smooth surface rollers tend to reach a broader surface more uniformly, and that may assist better with the dehydration-rehydration mechanism, in addition to acclimating new and deconditioned individuals more appropriately.

Vibrating foam rollers were found to increase an individual's pain tolerance significantly and knee flexion PROM only slightly from that of a nonvibrating roller (Cheatham et al. 2017). However, Lee and colleagues (2018) discovered that vibration rolling did significantly increase knee flexion PROM and isokinetic peak torque

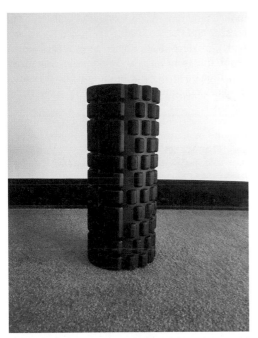

Fig. 7.28.3 A 12-inch-long by 6-inch-diameter combination surface roller.

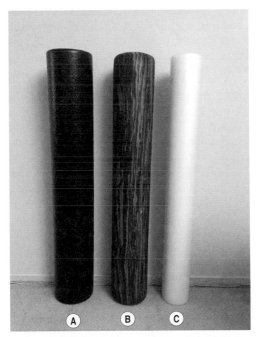

Fig. 7.28.4 Smooth surface foam roller (A) 36 inches long by 6 inches diameter, with firm density; (B) 36 inches long by 6 inches diameter, with low density; and (C) 36 inches long by 4 inches diameter, with moderate density.

and balance. Based on the effect that heat in a therapeutic range has on fascia, the use of a heated roller may increase viscoelasticity and lead to reduced stiffness and more rapid elongation of the tissue. Cold rollers also exist and may be useful for conditions that require cold therapy.

Best Practices

There is no sole consensus on the ideal duration, direction, technique, tempo, volume, and intensity for FR. However, as more research is completed, there will be more rigid parameters depending on the outcome desired. Duration in most studies was generally 60 seconds, but varied from 30 seconds to 120 seconds and up to 5 minutes to test for effect. With regard to rolling direction, several studies had participants start at the distal portion of the muscle and others at the proximal. Techniques also varied, with some studies using a sweeping motion up and back and others using small increments in one direction and then a sweeping motion back to the beginning to repeat again. Some studies used a metronome to set the tempo. Most studies required more than one set of FR before testing, but the range was between one and five sets. The one parameter that was generally the same was intensity—suggesting that the participant only place as much body mass as tolerable on the roller and adjust body position to help with this. It should also be considered that those with greater body weight or less fat mass could produce more force over the tissue.

The question of timing for FR is also part of the discussion. There is a strong consensus in the literature that FR before exercise or sport is beneficial for connective tissue and is not decrement to muscle performance. It has also been suggested that FR can be a part of a cool-down regimen to offset discomfort and encourage recovery. However, if fascial tissue hydration is the goal, it is suggested to roll in a slow, controlled manner with intentional directional changes (Schleip and Müller 2013). Because of the pressure of FR on nerves, blood vessels, and bone, there may be contraindications for several populations. Those with diabetic neuropathy and peripheral artery occlusive disease must not expose affected vessels and nerve tissue to high pressure loads, as sensory and motor disorders may ensue. People with osteoporosis are also cautioned, as pressure on the bones may cause injury (Freiwald et al. 2016).

CONCLUSION

The concept of myofascial release by way of a self-operated tool came before sufficient information was available regarding the behavior of fascia in this practice and also before possible other mechanisms that could explain usage results. There is insufficient evidence to say that release of myofascial restrictions is the primary mechanism for foam rolling. Although there are documented beneficial results from the use of the foam roller, it is clear that there is not a direct transfer of all outcomes from manual therapy to a tool-assisted self-treatment. The conditioning and maintenance of the fascial system is an area of increasing interest, and continuing research is needed to further investigate different variables than in previous research so that fascial conditioning protocol can be refined.

Summary

Foam rolling as a therapeutic tool for both muscle and connective tissue has been around since the 1970s. The term self-myofascial release was made popular as a way to describe a suspected mechanism that produced the results that occurred from FR use. With the expansion in fascial research, explanations regarding the nature and behavior of this tissue, organ, and system revealed possible mechanical and neurophysiological mechanisms for the effect of FR. Relevant research topics include how FR affects flexibility and range of motion, pain sensitivity, dynamic performance measures, and proprioception. Foam rollers are available in varying specifications, and depending on the intent, one may be more appropriate or beneficial over another. Although there has been a vast number of studies using many parameters for testing effects, there is not a single consensus for the exact way to foam roll. This most likely depends on the outcome desired and the research available for that particular situation.

REFERENCES

Beardsley, C., Škarabot, J., 2015. Effects of self-myofascial release: a systematic review. J. Bodyw. Mov. Ther. 19, 747–758.

Behm, D.G., Wilke, J., 2019. Do self-myofascial release devices release myofascia? A narrative review. Sports Med. 49, 1173–1181.

Cheatham, S.W., Stull, K.R., 2018. Comparison of a foam rolling session with active joint motion and without joint motion: a randomized controlled trial. J. Bodyw. Mov. Ther. 22, 707–712.

Cheatham, S.W., Stull, K.R., Kolber, M.J., 2017. Comparison of a vibrating foam roller and a non-vibrating foam roller intervention on knee range of motion and pressure pain threshold: a randomized controlled trial. J. Sport Rehabil. 28, 39–45.

Cho, S., Kim, S., 2016. Immediate effect of stretching and ultrasound on hamstring flexibility and proprioception. J. Phys. Ther. Sci. 28, 1806–1808.

Clark, M., 2001. Integrated Training for the New Millennium. National Academy of Sports Medicine, Thousand Oaks, CA.

David, E., Amasay, T., Ludwig, K., Shapiro, S., 2019. The effect of foam rolling of the hamstrings on proprioception at the knee and hip joints. Int. J. Exerc. Sci. 12, 343–354.

Do, K., Kim, J., Yim, J., 2018. Acute effect of self-myofascial release using a foam roller on the plantar fascia on hamstring and lumbar spine superficial back line flexibility. Phys. Ther. Rehabil. Sci. 7, 35–40.

Educational Council on Osteopathic Principles (ECOP), 2009. Glossary of Osteopathic Terminology. American Association of Colleges of Osteopathic Medicine.

Feldenkrais, M., 2009. Awareness through Movement: Easy-to-do Health Exercises to Improve Your Posture, Vision, Imagination, and Personal Awareness. HarperOne, New York.

Fleckenstein, J., Wilke, J., Vogt, L., Banzer, W., 2017. Preventive and regenerative foam rolling are equally effective in reducing fatigue-related impairments of muscle function following exercise. J. Sports Sci. Med. 16, 474–479.

Freiwald, J., Baumgart, C., Kühnemann, M., Hoppe, M.W., 2016. Foam rolling in sport and therapy – potential benefits and risks. Sports Orthop. Traumatol. 32, 258–266.

Gamboa, J.M., Gallager, S.P., 1996. Developing a comprehensive warm-up and conditioning program for performing artists. Orthop. Phys. Ther. Clin. N. Am. 5, 515–546.

Griefahn, A., Oehlmann, J., Zalpour, C., von Piekartz, H., 2017. Do exercises with the foam roller have a short-term impact on the thoracolumbar fascia? a randomized controlled trial. J. Bodyw. Mov. Ther. 21, 186–193.

Hall, M., Smith, J.C., 2018. The effects of an acute bout of foam rolling on hip range of motion on different tissues. Int. J. Sports Phys. Ther. 13, 652–660.

Killen, B.S., Zelizney, K.L., Ye, X., 2019. Crossover effects of unilateral static stretching and foam rolling on contralateral hamstring flexibility and strength. J. Sport Rehabil. 28, 553–539.

Kopec, T., Bishop, P., Esco, M.R., 2016. Influence of dynamic stretching and foam rolling on vertical jump. Athl. Train Sports Health Care 9, 33–38.

Krause, F., Wilke, J., Niederer, D., Vogt, L., Banzer, W., 2019. Acute effects of foam rolling on passive stiffness, stretch sensation and fascial sliding: a randomized controlled trial. Hum. Mov. Sci. 67, 1–11.

Latella, C., Drinkwater, E.J., Wilsmore, C.C., Bird, S.P., Skein, M., 2018. Foam rolling improves jump performance following eccentric exercise in leg extensors. International Conference of Strength Training 2018. [Poster] Available from: https://www.researchgate.net/publication/329371273_Foam_rolling_improves_jump_performance_following_eccentric_exercise_in_the_leg_extensors.

Lee, C.L., Chu, I.H., Lyu, B.J., Chang, W.D., Chang, N.J., 2018. Comparison of vibration rolling, nonvibration rolling, and static stretching as a warm-up exercise on flexibility, joint proprioception, muscle strength, and balance in young adults. J. Sports Sci. 36, 2575–2582.

Monteiro, E.R., Costa, P.B., Gonçalves Corrêa Neto, V., Hoogenboom, B.J., 2019a. Posterior thigh foam rolling increases knee extension fatigue and passive shoulder range-of-motion. J. Strength Cond. Res. 33, 987–994.

Monteiro, E.R., da Silva Novaes, J., Cavanaugh, M.T., Hoogenboom, B.J., 2019b. Quadriceps foam rolling and rolling massage increases hip flexion and extension passive range-of-motion. J. Bodyw. Mov. Ther. 23, 575–580.

Monteiro, E.R., Vigotsky, A., Škarabot, J., Fernandes Brown, A., 2017. Acute effects of different foam rolling volumes in the interest rest period on maximum repetition performance. Hong Kong Physiother. J. 36, 57–62.

O'Connell, J.A., 2003. Bioelectric responsiveness of fascia: a model for understanding the effects of manipulation. Tech. Orthop. 18, 67–73.

Okamoto, T., Masuhara, M., Ikuta, K., 2013. Acute effects of self-myofascial release using a foam roller on arterial function. J. Strength Cond. Res. 28, 69–73.

Pearcey, G.E.P., Bradbury-Squires, D.J., Kawamoto, J.E., et al., 2015. Foam rolling for delayed-onset muscle soreness and recovery of dynamic performance measures. J. Athl. Train. 50, 5–13.

Remvig, L., Ellis, R.M., Patijn, J., 2008. Myofascial release: an evidence- based treatment approach? Int. Musculoskelet. Med. 30, 29–35.

Romero-Franco, N., Romero-Franco, J., Jiménez-Reyes, P., 2019. Jogging and practical-duration foam-rolling exercises and range of motion, proprioception, and vertical jump in athletes. J. Athl. Train. 54, 1171–1178.

Romero-Moraleda, B., La Touche, R., Lerma-Lara, S., et al. 2017. Neurodynamic mobilization and foam rolling improved delayed-onset muscle soreness in a healthy adult population: a randomized controlled clinical trial. Peer J. 5, e3908.

Schleip, R., 2003. Fascial plasticity-a new neurobiological explanation: part 1. J. Bodyw. Mov. Ther. 7, 11–19.

Schleip, R., 2017. Fascia as a sensory organ: clinical applications. In: Liem, T., Tozzi, P., Chila, A. (Eds.), Fascia in the Osteopathic Field. Pencaitland, East Lothian, Scotland: Handspring Publishing, 59–68.

Schleip, R., Müller, D.G., 2013. Training principles for fascial connective tissues: scientific foundation and suggested practical applications. J. Bodyw. Mov. Ther. 17, 103–115.

Smith, J.C., Pridgeon, B., Hall, M.C., 2018. Acute effect of foam rolling and dynamic stretching on flexibility and jump height. J. Strength Cond. Res. 32, 2209–2215.

Tozzi, P., 2012. Selected fascial aspects of osteopathic practice. J. Bodyw. Mov. Ther. 16, 503–519.

Wilke, J., Vogt, L., Banzer, W., 2018. Immediate effects of self-myofascial release on latent trigger point sensitivity: a randomized, placebo-controlled trial. Biol. Sport 35, 349–354.

The Functional Aspects of Fascia During Human Performance and Sports

Tomasz Zagorski

CHAPTER CONTENTS

WHEEL OF HISTORY

 KEY POINT

Research on fascia has rapidly grown over the years, giving new insights for training practice and revising old concepts. This brings the functional abilities of athletes to a higher level and helps them set new records and provide exciting entertainment for spectators.

Connective tissue (fascia) has long been recognized as integral to the human locomotor system and to human performance and sports. However, since the end of the 20th century, its significance has been further highlighted by scientific research. Conference programs and the scientific literature reveal a growing interest in the application of fascia research to human performance and sports that also reflects our increased appreciation for the complexity of human movement.

Some of the gold standards and training tools used in athletics programs are supported by the findings of this fascia research, others are not. For example, preparatory countermovement or preloading of the tissue, so common in sports routines, is explained by a property of connective tissue known as elastic recoil. When the structures engaged in a specific movement are stretched to create a release (recoil), kinesthetic energy is produced (Sawicki et al. 2009), and this is very efficient in terms of metabolic costs. At the same time, antagonist structures must be engaged to create the stretch.

An example of a global movement involving elastic recoil is a javelin throw. To provide optimal conditions for the throwing movement, the javelin must be drawn far back behind the body, just before the throw, to create pretension and stretch in the tissues. On the other hand, static stretching, also popular in sports, does not affect the elasticity of the fascia. It affects the plasticity of connective tissue, where the application of a steady load leads to long-lasting elongation of the tissue (Kjaer et al. 2009), which may adversely affect power or speed in certain situations.

Dynamic stretching, which involves elastic recoil of fascia, is better supported by the research. In the 1930s, such exercises were popular and recommended, as illustrated by public group gymnastics exercises recorded on old movies. Later on, this kind of movement, also called ballistic stretching, was criticized because of possible damage to muscle tissues. However, sports and performance practice recommend application of both: static and dynamic stretching (Decoster et al. 2005; Fukashiro et al. 2006), and the key is to put them at the correct place in the general training plan. From a sports perspective, the most valuable conclusion we can draw from the research is that fascia can be trained, just like other physiological processes in the body.

NO HUMAN IS LIMITED

The author's experience in long-distance running led to an interest in research on elastic recoil of fascia as it applies to running. Training practice is supported by research demonstrating that pretension of tibialis anterior and stretching of the Achilles tendon has a "catapult effect" in the push-off phase of running. This also explains the power of the "natural" way of running used by many of the African runners who have dominated in most of the important competitions. Other runners who tried this method become equally effective in competitions.

After analyzing the research and progress in results, the question arises, if the "free" kinesthetic energy of elastic recoil could be the key factor (besides physiological preparation) that helped break the 2-hour barrier in marathon runs and similar barriers in other sports (Zagorski 2018). In October 2019 in Vienna, Kenyan Eliud Kipchoge ran a marathon in 1 hour, 59 minutes, and 40 seconds. Watching this historical event convinced me that practical application of the science on fascia could help change current limitations of human performance. It also motivated me to implement scientific results in training and to look to research for answers to my questions about training practice.

WHAT TO TRAIN?

KEY POINT

Top-level performance requires optimal function of the body. The function is determined by the structure and vice versa. In sports we need to adjust the body for specific demands of dominant movement. Starting from releasing the restrictions and proceeding to strengthening the weak elements and fine-tuning the whole myofascial system.

We already know we can train the elastic recoil of fascia. What other qualities can be trained? The answer is: all functions of the fascia in a body's structure and movement. The scope of this chapter does not allow for detailed description of all these aspects, so the focus will be given on the most important things for sports performance. The connective system creates a fascial network throughout the body, and the myofascial part of this system is the most important for efficient movement to happen.

Muscular tissues, fueled by their own energy supply and circulatory system, provide the movement. Fascial tissues provide stability and organization for this movement, supported by the central nervous system. Muscle and fascia work together as myofascial units in groups and chains connected and related to each other. The resilience of a single myofascial unit is determined by the resilience of the fascia, and injuries occur more often to the fascial part of the unit, which significantly decreases performance in sports (Zugel et al. 2018). Most exercises improve the structure of the myofascial units but dynamic jumps and plyometric exercises are especially effective.

The fascial system is a medium for exchange of kinesthetic information and, as such, is considered to be a sensory organ. As mentioned, although muscular tissue gives energy to a movement, fascial tissue provides the precision and fine-tuning of this movement. Human voluntary movement is performed by muscular tissue under conscious control through nerves, which makes movement of single myofascial units precise. But even single units may have structural restrictions, or incorrect functional adaptations, that affect the quality and range of movement.

Seeing the body's movement as of the sum of the movements of all the myofascial units, and being aware that restrictions and adaptations of incorrect movement patterns will arise from the fascial system, can inform the work of sports coaches and therapists. We always start by releasing fascial restrictions and then correct the movement patterns (Earls and Myers 2010). Working with the fascial system includes long-chain coordination to provide the power required in most sports activities, and finally to fine-tune the intranetwork communication.

Work done with athletes and other people using movement for professional purposes requires carefully considered and planned approaches because the margin for error is small. The work must always be coordinated with athletes' training programs, as will be explained later.

RELEASE THE RESTRICTIONS

Releasing fascial restrictions is a first goal in working with an athlete, but not without clinical reasoning and analysis of the athlete's needs. Releasing hamstring restrictions could elongate the step and improve running efficiency. However, it could instead decrease sprinting efficiency and cause the runner to lose a tactical race where sprinting skills decide which place he/she will take. Likewise, changing the range of motion in a golf swing by just 1 or 2 centimeters through fascial release could drive the golf ball greatly off the target.

Such unwanted results are explained by adaptations of the entire fascial system to a single structural change, according to the biotensegrity model (Scarr 2014). To be effective we must apply an individual approach and work with the athlete's training plan, always avoiding significant structural changes just before important competitions (Zagorski 2018). A number of myofascial release approaches can be used effectively, from classical rolfing to myofascial release in water (Zagorski 2014) as well as instrument-assisted techniques.

STRENGTHEN THE WEAK PART

Long-term shortening of one structure leads to structural and functional changes in other (usually opposite) structures. In a balanced system, when something is short, something else has to be long. Addressing long and weak parts is the next step after releasing restrictions, and progression is important here. The incorrect patterns were created over time, so we need to use a wide range of methods to bring the function back. Sometimes it is enough to apply only manually guided soft reeducation of the tissue. Sometimes we need specific corrective exercises, including ones with heavy loads. All this should be integrated into an overall movement pattern using movements that are specific to the client's sports discipline.

FINE-TUNE THE NETWORK

Releasing restrictions and restoring fascial network balance will help many athletes to achieve their optimal performance and can enhance their personal bests. This desirable situation cannot last long, and we need to apply different approaches to maintain it during the season, especially during a competition period. Fascial layers must glide freely between themselves in a frame of optimal movement. We know that repeated extensive load can cause collagen fiber binding and adhesions, so we must prevent this by applying compensatory exercises in directions and planes that differ from the dominant movement pattern.

Another technique that can be applied is active or passive manual myofascial release, including preparatory (warm-up) exercises that create conditions in the tissue that are optimal for performance (Zagorski 2018). There are specific exercises for engaging the fascial component in the muscles and improving communication and coordination of the whole fascial network. An example is stability training: some authors put focus on this training (Elphinston 2013) and some look for controlled instability (Gracovetsky 2007). Valuable insights and practical training tools can be found in the Fascial Fitness concept (Schleip and Muller 2013).

If applied in a planned and logical way, the approaches previously discussed will produce an athlete with an optimal fascial "suit," many of whom we now can see worldwide. More and more athletes are joining this elite group, as sports therapists become more detailed in their approaches to helping athletes improve and gain advantage over others. Even if competitors are closely matched, there can be only one winner. If a winner keeps repeating their success, it is worth looking for the sources of this person's movement skills.

When we watch Michael Phelps swimming, Roger Federer playing tennis, or Usain Bolt running, we can see certain qualities in how they move. There is lightness and grace in their ways of moving, which are still very powerful, in comparison to other competitors. This visible difference is due to efficient use of the fascial system for their specific discipline. Whether it is training or genetics that gives them these skills remains an open question. However, knowing that we can train the fascia (resilience, elasticity, internetwork communication) for improving performance, we can implement this into a general training plan. Understanding the training principles is key to successful application of work on the fascia in sports, as explained briefly below.

THE ART AND SCIENCE OF TRAINING

 KEY POINT

Periodization of training has been applied for more than 60 years with some modifications. It helps to achieve specific training goals in certain time periods and to prepare peak performance in the demanded time (main competition of the year).

Supercompensation

Training is based on supercompensation of physiological processes connected with specific types of performance and on increasing the functional capacity of the body to enable an athlete to perform at a higher level than their baseline (Brezhnev et al. 2011). The training load causes fatigue, which lowers the performance capacity. The resting process rebuilds this capacity to different levels, that is: under baseline, to the baseline or above the baseline. The last one is, desired from the training point of view, a state of supercompensation (see Fig. 7.29.1).

The body always tends to keep its homeostasis, and any stimuli that break it down can cause the natural defense mechanism to improve protective processes, so that the next similar stimulus will not create such great damage (see Fig. 7.29.2). We can use this wisdom of nature in our practice and be inspired by it in our research. In an athlete's training there are several conditions needed to achieve the supercompensation state. The training load (fatigue) must be significant and the recovery period (rest) must be sufficient. The next training load must start from a baseline of functional capacity, ideally from achieved supercompensation.

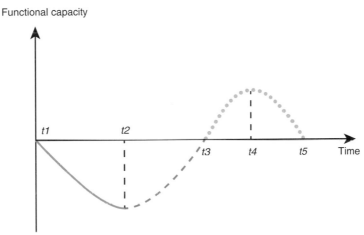

Fig. 7.29.1 Supercompensation as a dynamic regulation of homeostasis: *t1, t3, t5*—baseline of performance ability (homeostasis); *t2*—end of load and recovery starting point; *t3*—beginning of supercompensation; *t4*—maximal supercompensation; *t5*—end of supercompensation (back to baseline).

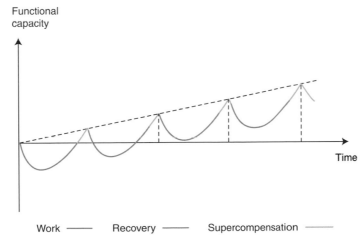

Fig. 7.29.2 Series of supercompensations. If the training starts at the peak of supercompensation and is intensive enough, and the recovery is complete, the body goes to a higher level of functional ability.

If we add the load too early, when the functional capacity is under the baseline, fatigue is greater and overall performance is reduced. This lowers the starting point of the recovery process, and the road to the next supercompensation state is much longer. If this situation is repeated over time, the baseline functional capacity goes down and this may result in overload or overtraining. Different physiological processes have different recovery times and supercompensation phases (Suchanowski 2001), making the training process more complicated. Also, we can see supercompensation in collagen fibers recovery (Magnusson et al. 2010).

Periodization of Training

Athletic training is divided into certain periods of time to create a logical and goal-oriented plan. Classical periodization of training has been known and applied for more than 60 years (Bompa 1994; Zaitsev and Sazanov 2007). We can break it down, starting from the macrocycle (usually 1 or 4 years long), through the mesocycle (1 month long), to the microcycle (5 to 10 days long). To prepare an athlete to achieve maximal performance at the main season's competitions (e.g., Olympic Games), the training plan is created backward, starting from the week of the main competition.

The macrocycle is divided into preparatory, precompetition, competition, and recovery periods, each of which consists of mesocycles with specific training goals. Usually the intensity of training is increased every 3 to 4 weeks and drops in the last week to aid recovery. Similarly, in a microcycle, there is a resting day at the end or after the peak of intensity of training. There are modifications in classical periodization called "block periodization" (Issurin 2008, 2016) or "integrated periodization" (Mujika et al. 2018), which are more precise in training of specific skills in short periods of time and providing multipeaks of performance during the season. All kinds of periodization are used worldwide with good effects. In the next section, the macrocycle and practical aspects of work on fascia will be described, using athletics as an example, and specifically the training of a top-level sprinter. The classical periodization model will be used.

Preparatory Period

If the main competition requires peak performance in, say, August next year, the preparatory period starts at the beginning of November and is 16 to 20 weeks long (February/March). This includes three or four mesocycles.

In most cases, for a sprinter's training, this period includes a subperiod of indoor competitions with intensification of training and applied loads; however, this is not a main goal for the season but a specific kind of training.

The general goal of a preparatory period is to increase the functional capacity of the body in all aspects and to prepare it for more intense and specific loads in the next periods of training. Effectively, it is building a base for the main training. The volume of training is high or very high and the intensity is low to moderate. Coaches and athletes use a wide range of methods in training, and versatile exercises are dominant. This is the best period in which to apply desired structural changes in the body and to create balance in the fascial system by activating any weaker parts. Table 7.29.1 shows an example of microcycle in this period.

Precompetition Period

The goal for this period is to intensify the training loads and to prepare the body for maximal performance in the competition. It is usually made up of two or three or mesocycles in, say, March, April, and May (in this example). Athletes living in colder regions usually travel to warm countries for training. The volume of training is still high but less than in the preparatory period, and the intensity increases. Dominant exercises are targeted. The goals for work on fascia are: maintaining a balanced structure and function by applying compensative exercises and taking special care of the tissues of the most engaged parts of the body. This is the best period in which to develop strategies for the work just before the competition.

Competition Period

During this time, the main goal is to use a functional base developed by previous training to achieve maximal performance, ideally during the main competition of the season. It is three mesocycles long. Usually, after a series of competitions in, say, June and July (for this example), there is a period of training before the main competition called "direct preevent preparation," which aims to achieve the top performance of the year during the competition. The volume of training is low and the intensity is high or very high. Dominant exercises are targeted and specific. Work on fascia focuses on optimizing fascial function and using its advantages for maximal performance effect. This is also a time for testing and adjusting already-developed strategies of the work, just before the competition.

TABLE 7.29.1   Example of Top-Level, Sprinter-Training Microcycle in Preparatory Period— Intervention on Fascia Must Match the Training and Recovery Goals

Day	Training Performed, Hours	Recovery Applied	Fascia Intervention
Monday	General fitness, indoor 2.5 h	Core training	Instrument-assisted self-mobilization
Tuesday	Long sprint, track 3 h	Ice bath	
Wednesday	Gym, 2 h	Core training, massage	Myo-Tone training
Thursday	Short sprint, track 2 h	Ice bath	
Friday	General fitness, gym 2 h	Core training, massage	Instrument-assisted self-mobilization
Saturday	Uphill run, forest 2 h	Massage	
Sunday	Free	Hydrotherapy	Structural bodywork session

Recovery Period

This is the short time after a competition ends and before the next preparation cycle starts. It is very important in terms of restoring physical and mental resources after a demanding session, taking care of any injuries that occurred during the season, and building energy capacity for the next season. It is the best time to create, or start to create, important structural changes in the body through fascial work.

Summary

As has been highlighted in research results, functional aspects of fascia (such as elastic recoil benefit and organized proprioceptive communication through the fascial network) are very important in sports because they meet the demand for detailed work that gives an athlete a slight advantage over their competitors. This provides hope for changing the limitations of human performance and for making sports competitions even more interesting.

Functional aspects of fascia may provide a means for assessing athletes' predispositions and predicting potential for future progress. For athletes who have reached similar levels in specific performance parameters, the level of their skill in using connective tissue could provide an additional advantage; however, this needs to be tested and described by science. Both practice and research results confirm that we can train for many qualities of fascia and thereby improve performance and sports results.

Excellence in training requires experience and applications of new research in order to answer the questions that arise in everyday practice. Applying new fascia research to training modifications and bringing new research ideas back from the practical field are almost as exciting as watching a good sports spectacle.

REFERENCES

Bompa, T., 1994. Theory and Methodology of Training: The Key to Athletic Performance. Kendall/Hunt Publishing, Dubuque, pp. 167–232.

Brezhnev, I., Zaitsev, A., Sazanov, S., 2011. To the analytical theory of the supercompensation phenomenon. Biofizika 56, 342–348.

Decoster, L., Cleland, J., Altieri, C., Russell, P., 2005. The effects of hamstring stretching on range of motion: a systematic literature review. J. Orthop. Sports. Phys. Ther. 35, 377–387.

Earls, J., Myers, T., 2010. Fascial Release for Structural Balance. Lotus Publishing, Chichester, pp. 25–47.

Elphinston, J., 2013. Stability, Sport and Performance Movement: Practical Biomechanics and Systematic Training for Movement Efficacy and Injury Prevention. Lotus Publishing and On Target Publications, Chichester, Aptos, pp. 199–318.

Fukashiro, S., Hay, D.C., Nagano, A., 2006. Bio-mechanical behavior of muscle-tendon complex during dynamic human movements. J. Appl. Biomech. 22, 131–147.

Gracovetsky, S., 2007. Stability or controlled instability? In: Vleeming, A., Mooney, V., Stoeckart, R. (Eds.), Movement, Stability and Lumbopelvic Pain: Integration of Research and Therapy. Elsevier, Edinburgh, pp. 279–294.

Issurin, V., 2008. Block periodization versus traditional training theory: a review. J. Sports Med. Phys. Fitness 48, 65–75.

Issurin, V., 2016. Benefits and limitations of block periodized training approaches to athletes' preparation: a review. Sports Med. 46, 329–338.

Kjaer, M., Langberg, H., Heinemeier, K., et al., 2009. From mechanical loading to collagen synthesis, structural changes and function in human tendon. Scand. J. Med. Sci. Sports 19, 500–510.

Magnusson, S., Langberg, H., Kjaer, M., 2010. The pathogenesis of tendinopathy: balancing the response to loading. Nat. Rev. Rheumatol. 6, 262–268.

Mujika, I., Halson, S., Balague, G., Farrow, D., 2018. An integrated, multifactorial approach to periodization for optimal performance in individual and team sports. Int. J. Sports Physiol. Perform. 13, 538–561.

Sawicki, G., Lewis, C., Ferris, D., 2009. It pays to have a spring in your step. Exerc. Sport Sci. Rev. 37, 130–138.

Scarr, G., 2014. Biotensegrity: The Structural Basis of Life. Handspring Publishing, Pencaitland, East Lothian, pp. 99–108.

Schleip, R., Muller, G., 2013. Training principles for fascial connective tissues: Scientific foundation and suggested practical applications. J. Bodyw. Mov. Ther. 17, 103–115.

Suchanowski, A., 2001. Variability in the dynamic of process of recovery in sports training efficiency control. Akademia Wychowania Fizycznego, Gdansk, pp. 26–45.

Zagorski T. 2014. Work on fascia in water - benefits, possibilities and limitations of application. In: Bilska, M., Golonko, R., Soltan, J. (Eds.), Movement Activities in Disabled Children and Youth. Akademia Wychowania Fizycznego Jozefa Pilsudskiego w Warszawie. Wydzial Wychowania Fizycznego i Sportu w Bialej Podlaskiej, Biala Podlaska, pp. 124–136.

Zagorski, T., 2018. Therapy and recovery of sprinter - Rio de Janeiro 2016 medalist. Lecture, Human in Health and Disease–Health Promotion, Treatment and Rehabilitation Conference, Tarnow.

Zaitsev, A., Sazanov, S., 2007. On the prediction of the supercompensation phase by determining the parameters of the living functional system of the body. Biofizika 52, 727–732.

Zugel, M., Maganaris, C., Wilke, J., et al., 2018. Fascial tissue research in sports medicine: from molecules to tissue adaptation, injury and diagnostics: consensus statement. Br. J. Sports. Med. 52, 1497.

Research Directions

Peter A. Huijing

PART 8

Fascia Research: Methodological Challenges and New Directions

Fascia—Clinical and Fundamental Scientific Research: Considering the Scientific Process and its Potential for Creating Clinical Applications

Peter A. Huijing

CHAPTER CONTENTS

INTRODUCTION

Many of the chapters of this book deal with fascia in relation to many practical aspects of the manual therapies, in the broadest sense of that word.

The chapters within this section (and a few that, for practical reasons, ended up in other sections of the book, see e.g. Chapters 3.1, 3.2, and 5.8) are in some ways quite different. The knowledge described in those chapters is mostly a result of fundamental scientific research, which as it was performed, in most cases, did not have the manual therapies or other application in mind, and initially may not even have had the fascia as the target. An example in case is our own work on force transmission that was aimed initially at studying muscle characteristics, per se, in an effort to understand what determines the physiological length range (or joint angle range) of active and passive force exertion. However, totally unexpected and thought-stimulating results did indicate a new direction of thought and research in which all kinds of fascial structures of the body are to play a major role.

KEY POINT

The enormous differences between conditions of work of scientists and clinicians has to be bridged by mutual respect and discussion.

The clinician works in a totally different world from that described previously. A patient, having a problem, enters the clinic with a request to the therapist to solve that problem. Usually, detailed scientific knowledge is missing to make a personal decision how to best treat the patient. Therefore the therapist has to decide to the best of their knowledge and experience and act almost immediately with a certain therapeutic path.

A scientist has the luxury to simply say about a specific problem, "we don't know" and take no action or defer it to more opportune times. The therapist is not allowed such luxury as action is demanded almost instantly.

Superficially considered, the images of the substance of fascia or other tissues to be treated may seem the same as those on which the scientist builds their hypotheses and, after experimentation, their theories.

However, the two types of roles differ very substantially. The essence of this difference is the systematical testing and confrontation of the theories within science. This is done first by the researcher, and subsequently in the reviewing process of a potential publication by usually very critical expert colleagues.

The therapist will also try to store results of a successful treatment mentally, or in very good cases keep systemized records of the clinic, and are therefore very often a quite personal feature, despite the fact that the schools at which therapists are educated try to generalize such clinical experiences.

Considering such differences, it is not surprising that communication between the two groups is not always an easy process.

THE NEED FOR ONGOING FUNDAMENTAL SCIENTIFIC WORK

 KEY POINT

Despite high level of uncertainties about applicability of results of fundamental scientific work, there is a serious need for it.

Fundamental scientific work is necessary for future developments in fundamental science itself, but also in therapy in general. A problem with fundamental scientific work is that it is impossible to predict which work and which specific results will be highly relevant for practical application in the clinical or other fields in the future. To politicians, science managers, and clinicians, without an open mind, or without a clear understanding of the actual process of scientific advancement, the scientific process described is highly unattractive, because substantial moneys and time need to be spent on projects for which the full outcome is unclear. The only thing that can be tested for is scientific quality, and even that is not always an objective process.

Only in retrospect clarity is provided, as a few relatively small scientific steps ahead are combined into something very new. Depending on the circumstances, this occurs sometimes many decades after the actual

publication (e.g., as in the cases of many historic anatomical discoveries by Vesalius or discovery of the concept of circulation of blood by William Harvey), or in exceptional cases centuries later (e.g., Niels Stensen's 17th-century work on the geometry of pennate muscle). The latter occurs if the seed of new ideas fall on barren ground, because people cling to generally accepted concepts, such as in Stensen's example that nothing, including muscle, can move by itself, because of some internal process, or if some crucial experimental results are known exclusively to a small number of scientists (e.g., the constancy of muscle volume shown in experiments of Jan Swammerdam performed in the 17th century but not published until the 18th century).

Finally, it also becomes clear that a lot of work was performed that did not yield any results for practical application, even though some of it may have advanced general understanding of fundamental principles.

RETROSPECTIVE RESEARCH ANALYZING WHAT IS NEEDED TO ATTAIN POTENTIAL NEW CLINICAL APPLICATIONS IN THE FUTURE

Comroe and Dripps (1976) analyzed and reported crucial sources of the top ten clinical advances in cardiovascular and pulmonary medicine and surgery (e.g., open heart surgery) over a period of 30 years (in the 20th century). Their conclusion was that 41% of over 500 key articles that allowed, or contributed to, these clinical advances in a major way were written by scientists who had no direct interest in disease, and that 62% were the result of basic rather than clinical research. An intuitive feeling for such an awkward-looking process can be obtained from Fig. 8.1.1, showing the conditions of an early recording of ECG. One does not get the impression about this basic research that a major step is taken in fundamental science, with enormous clinical consequences to follow over the next hundred years (Wong 2019).

 KEY POINT

Scientific work, seemingly totally unrelated to application, may yield enormous consequences regarding application of its results.

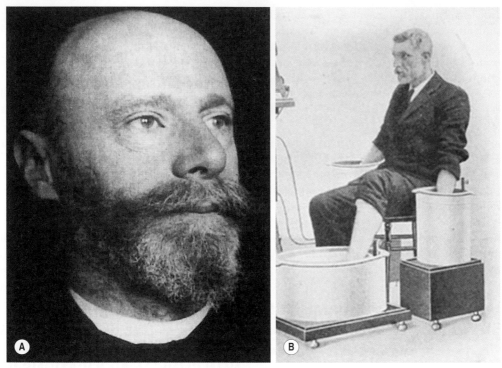

Fig. 8.1.1. A very early recording of an electrocardiogram and its inventor. (A) A portrait of 1924 Nobel Prize winner Willem Einthoven (1860–1927), who invented the string galvanometer consisting of a very thin silver-coated quartz filament placed within a magnetic field that allows very sensitive recordings of very small electric currents. Public domain. (B) Because simple electrodes were not available at that time he used a saline-filled bath as means of making electrical contact with the subject and his voluminous instrument. Initially, electromyography was also measured in a similar way. Public domain.

Comroe and Dripps' results later became the subject of sometimes heated scientific debate (e.g., Smith 1987) that does not always seem fully free of external motives (the competition for limited available resources). Regardless of the proper scientific questions that may be asked concerning this, it is clear that both clinical and fundamental research activity is essential for the advancement of knowledge that may allow changing clinical practice.

This discussion may create the impression that the role of scientists is limited to just creating new knowledge. Even though that is their primary task, scientists also have a moral obligation to be interested in the application and other practical consequences of their work, if the knowledge gathered has reached a level where application is likely. The authors of more fundamentally oriented chapters of this book seem to be fully aware of this.

After contact between clinicians and scientists has been established, difficulties of language will inevitably arise (it should be clear that we do not mean different mother tongues by this, even though that can contribute to the confusion) and need to be overcome through agreement on a common set of ideas and nomenclature before fundamental-clinical collaboration can work to advance knowledge and understanding.

Because both types of workers do that from a different perspective, the exchange of ideas will certainly not be unidirectional but will create potential chances for new insights on both sides. The interactions between clinicians and scientists in the so-called Fascia Research Congresses are good examples of the willingness to create such common conditions and are also one of the major drives for the present book.

> **KEY POINT**
>
> Scientific controversy, as long as it is directed at content rather than persons, is essential for progress.

One factor in science that may be quite puzzling to the nonscientist is scientific controversy. Actually, controversy on content and ideas (rather than on personal preferences) is a major driving force of science and therefore an essential part of it. The intellectual clash of minds is crucial to filtering out confounding information and selecting generally accepted methods and concepts. For that reason we have chosen not to remove all controversy from the content of the chapters. For example, among the scientific authors of this book, ideas about the importance of the continuity of the connective tissues in, for example, a limb may differ quite a bit. Some are convinced that the physiological effects of such continuity are limited to the borders of a fascicle within a muscle, and others think that they have sufficient evidence that intermuscular mechanical interaction is a prominent feature.

CONCLUSIONS

All this means that the scientific (but probably also the clinical) material of this book should not be looked at as a static feature but as knowledge that will be developing continually. In that sense we are certainly not presenting "the truth" as an unchanging character. By incorporating such aspects, this book will not be like most textbooks.

The dynamics of this process also require of both scientists and clinicians that they try to keep up with developments in each other's fields. That is certainly not an easy task, but it remains an essential one. It requires also from both sides that "unwanted" results (deviating from the preconceptions of each profession) should be fully considered in detail and accepted if sufficient evidence is presented.

REFERENCES

Comroe, J.H., Dripps, R.D., 1976. Scientific basis for support of biomedical science. Science 192, 105–111.

Smith, R., 1987. Comroe and Dripps revisited. Br. Med. J. (Clin Res Ed). 295, 1404–1407. Erratum 1988 in: Br. Med. J. (Clin Res Ed) 296, 110.

Wong, S., 2019. How Willem Einthoven gave doctors a window on the heart. New Scientist Health. Available from: https://www.newscientist.com/article/2203921-how-willem-einthoven-gave-doctors-a-window-on-the-heart.

8.2

Imaging: Ultrasound

Yasuo Kawakami and Antonio Stecco

CHAPTER CONTENTS

A SHORT HISTORY

Ultrasonography is now widely used to examine human and animal tissues. For this purpose, brightness-mode (B-mode) ultrasonography is often used. This mode creates two-dimensional images of a tissue section by visualizing the portions where acoustic impedance (tissue density × acoustic velocity) changes (Noce 1990). There are distinct differences in acoustic impedance at the interfaces between adipose and muscle tissues and bones, thereby enabling delineation of their peripheries by ultrasonography. In other words, ultrasonography visualizes fasciae. Ultrasonography was first applied to humans by Howry and Bliss (1952) and used for the purpose of viewing the cross-section of skeletal muscles (Howry 1965). B-mode ultrasonography was then used to measure cross-sectional areas of skeletal muscles by Ikai and Fukunaga (1968). Since then, B-mode ultrasonography has been used to obtain sectional images of skeletal muscles in vivo. Spatial, as well as time, resolution of ultrasonograms has rapidly been improving.

FORM AND FUNCTION OF MUSCLE–TENDON–FASCIAL STRUCTURES REVEALED BY ULTRASONOGRAPHY

When an ultrasonic probe of appropriate frequency (normally between 3–10 MHz, depending on the depth of the muscle) is placed on the skin in a longitudinal direction of the underlying muscle, one can observe hypoechoic striae within the muscle between the horizontal echoes (Fig. 8.2.1a). The former are from echogenic structures between perimysia such as fibro-adipose septa (Fornage 1989), and the latter from the epimysia and aponeuroses. Kawakami et al. (1993) and Narici et al (1996) confirmed that the echo patterns seen represent orientations of fascicles. Fascicle length and angle (with respect to aponeuroses) can be determined by measuring the length of a representative echo within the muscle and its angulation relative to the underlying echo of the aponeurosis (Fig. 8.2.1a). Among the factors affecting the force that a muscle can produce, the length and contractile velocity of its fibers are particularly important. This is because the force exerted by a muscle fiber is

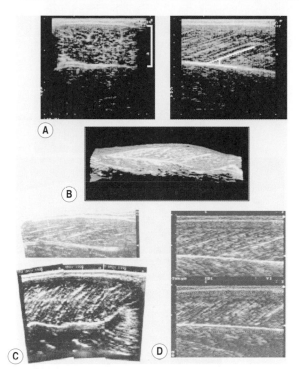

Fig. 8.2.1 (A) Transverse (left panel, lateral-medial) and longitudinal (right panel, distal-proximal) B-mode ultrasound images of the human gastrocnemius medialis muscle. From top to bottom, skin to deep layer. In the right panel, a white line is drawn along a representative echo parallel to fascicle orientation. (B) Three-dimensional reconstruction of ultrasound images of the human gastrocnemius medialis muscle. A part of the soleus muscle is also visualized. (C) B-mode ultrasound images of the triceps brachii muscle (long head) of a normal individual (top panel) and a highly trained bodybuilder (bottom panel). From right to left, distal to proximal. (D) B-mode ultrasound images of the gastrocnemius medialis muscle at rest (top) and during maximal isometric contraction (bottom). From right to left, distal to proximal. (C) Reproduced with permission from Kawakami, Y., Ichinose, Y., Kubo, K., Ito, M., Fukunaga, T., 2000a. Architecture of contracting human muscles and its functional significance. J. Appl. Biomech. 16, 88–97.

sarcomeres in series within a muscle fiber, the ultrasonic measurement of fascicle length will give the force-producing potential of muscle fibers in terms of the force-length relationship (Kawakami et al. 2000b). The disadvantage of ultrasonography may be a relatively limited scan area and two-dimensional, planar information of fascicles and tendinous structures, which in reality are three-dimensional (Scott et al. 1993). These drawbacks can be partly solved by a three-dimensional ultrasound system in which multiple ultrasound images are reconstructed three-dimensionally (Fig. 8.2.1B) (Kawakami et al. 2000a). With this method, homogeneity of the fascicle length over the muscle belly has been found for the medial gastrocnemius muscle in humans (Kawakami et al. 2000a).

HYPERTROPHIC MUSCLES

From ultrasonic observation of individuals with widely varying hypertrophic status of skeletal muscles, Kawakami et al. (2006) found relationships between muscle size and fascicle angles for some limb muscles. Fig. 8.2.1C illustrates longitudinal images of the triceps brachii muscle that shows an outstanding hypertrophic response (Kawakami et al. 1993, 2006). In highly hypertrophied triceps, fascicles are packed curvilinearly, with large angles from the deep aponeurosis. The angulation of fascicles relative to aponeuroses is typically seen in pennate muscles and determines the component of muscle fiber forces in the direction of the line of action of muscle (Huijing et al. 1989). Large variability of fascicle angles suggests different degrees of fiber-tendon force transmission between individuals, and there is some evidence in support of this (Ikegawa et al. 2008).

> ### KEY POINT
> Morphological characteristics and dynamic behavior of fascial structures inside and outside skeletal muscles can be visualized with B-mode ultrasonography.

Fig. 8.2.1D shows longitudinal ultrasonic images of the gastrocnemius medialis muscle at rest and during maximal isometric contraction (Kawakami and Fukunaga 2006). Although this is a fixed-end contraction—that is, the whole muscle-tendon unit length is kept constant—one can clearly observe changes in fascicle orientations by

determined by its length and contraction velocity. Muscle fibers are packed in parallel within fascicles, extending from proximal to distal end of each fascicle in short-fibered muscles such as the triceps surae (Kawakami et al. 2000b). In this case, measurement of the fascicle length can provide information on how muscle fibers develop forces. In this regard there is particular advantage in ultrasonography, in that it enables measurement of fascicle behavior during contraction in real-time. If combined with the information on the number of contraction: fascicles shorten with increasing angles. Contraction thus induces deformation of fascial organization of the muscle. Shortening of fascicles occurs at the expense of elongations of the tendinous structures (Griffiths 1991; Kawakami et al. 1998). During dynamic human movements, this muscle-tendon interaction plays an extremely important role. Kawakami et al. (2002) used ultrasonography to track length changes of the gastrocnemius fascicles during ankle hopping preceded by a countermovement and showed that fascicles contract isometrically when the muscle-tendon unit is being lengthened. In this phase, tendinous structures are lengthened and store elastic energy, which is released during the shortening phase that follows to add to positive mechanical work. A similar mechanism has been found during human walking (Fukunaga et al. 2001).

ULTRASOUND ELASTOGRAPHY

Previous studies have shown that the mechanical properties of tendinous structures, especially that of the aponeuroses, depends on the contractile status (passive or active, static or dynamic, high or low lengths) of fascicles (Kato et al. 2005; Lieber et al. 2000; Sugisaki et al. 2005; Zuurbier and Huijing 1992; Zuurbier et al. 1994). Hence the mechanical behavior of the whole fascial continuum could change during contractions involving dynamic fascicle length changes under varying contraction intensities. If so, the interface between the aponeurosis, tendon, and fascicles could be stressed locally. In the human gastrocnemius muscle, this position corresponds to the distal end of muscle belly where high muscle strains frequently occur (Fig. 8.2.2).

Ultrasound elastography has allowed evaluation of mechanical characteristics of fascial structures, and studies have demonstrated clear anisotropic elasticity of the human deep fascia that changes as a function of intensity of muscle contraction (Fig. 8.2.3). Such mechanical features possibly reflect unique roles of this structure that are linked with underlying muscle contractions (Otsuka et al. 2018, 2019).

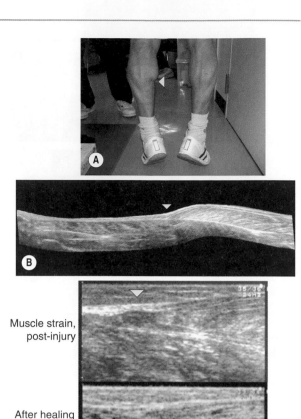

Fig. 8.2.2 (A) Legs of an individual who experienced muscle strain at the distal end (triangle) of muscle belly of the gastrocnemius medialis. (B) Three-dimensional reconstruction of ultrasound images of the calf. Triangles represent the distal end of gastrocnemius belly. (C) B-mode ultrasound images of the distal end of gastrocnemius belly immediately after strain injury (top) and after healing (bottom).

Muscle strain, post-injury

After healing

> ### 🖉 KEY POINT
>
> Human muscle–tendon unit can be viewed mechanically as the composite of actuators (muscle fibers) and springs (tendinous tissues), a group of which systematically connects and interacts with the deep fascia.

STRUCTURES AROUND SKELETAL MUSCLES VISUALIZED AND TESTED BY ULTRASONOGRAPHY

Connective tissue outside of muscle also forms a complex, interconnected network that is increasingly recognized to play an important role in musculoskeletal function. In humans, superficial and deep fasciae are composed of layers of densely woven connective tissue alternating with layers of loose, areolar connective tissue (e.g., Fig. 8.2.4) containing varying amounts of fat (Benjamin 2009; see also Huijing and Langevin 2009).

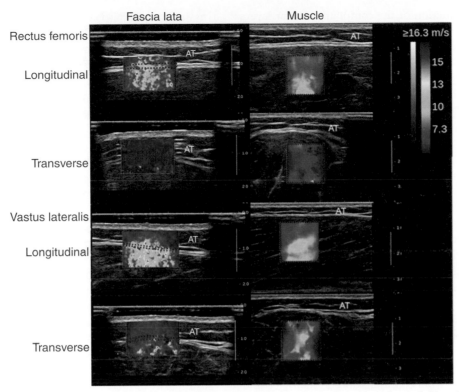

Fig. 8.2.3 Ultrasound elastography color maps within the region of interest of the deep fascia (left) and underlying muscles (longitudinal and transverse) during submaximal voluntary contractions. AT, subcutaneous adipose tissue. Reproduced with permission from Otsuka, S., Shan, X., Kawakami, Y., 2019. Dependence of muscle and deep fascia stiffness on the contraction levels of the quadriceps: An in vivo supersonic shear-imaging study. J. Electromyogr. Kinesiol. 45, 33–40.

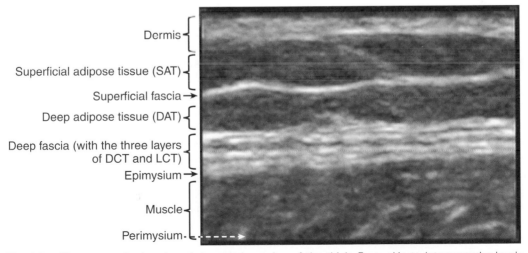

Fig. 8.2.4 Ultrasonography imaging of the anterior region of the thigh. From skin to intramuscular levels structures are indicated within the image. DCT, dense connective tissue; LCT, loose connective tissue.

An important function of the compliant, areolar layers is to allow the dense connective tissue layers to glide past one another (Stecco et al. 2006).

Also for extramuscular tissues, ultrasound elastography is promising as a valuable noninvasive method for analyzing spatial patterns of tissue stiffness *in vivo* (e.g., detection of localized stiffer tissue areas, associated with breast and prostate malignancies). In the original elastography method, successive ultrasound images are acquired while the ultrasound probe compresses the tissue (Ophir et al. 1991; Konofagou and Ophir 1998).

Pathological conditions such as injury, inflammation, scarring, and fibrosis can cause changes in the structure of connective tissue. For example, human subjects with chronic low back pain were found to have increased thickness of perimuscular connective tissue in the lumbar region, compared with subjects without low back pain (Langevin et al. 2009), and a subject with chronic neck pain was found to have a thicker deep fascia (Stecco et al. 2014) compared with control subjects. An altered ultrasound representation of the paratenon, thicker than 1.27 mm, was also found to be a significant indicator of Achilles tendinopathy (Stecco et al. 2015). In addition, in line with the theory of Perez and Roberts (2009), it could also be considered a precursor sign of alterations of the tendon because of the high correlations found with symptoms, severity, and duration. Alteration of the paratenon can exacerbate the pathological morphological changes of the tendon, as compression by extrinsic sources decreases the vascular supply of the tendon.

As paratenon viscoelasticity shapes the dynamic response of mechanoreceptors (Song et al. 2015), it is reasonable to speculate that altered paratenon strains may result in nociception, even without primary tendon tissue involvement. For these reasons, fascial tissue, as paratenon or tendon sheath, are tissue that should be assessed during ultrasonography studies.

Therefore noninvasive measures of connective tissue structure and function, such as ultrasonography, are important for the development of a better understanding of connective tissue physiology and for evaluating connective tissue pathology and effects of treatments.

During ultrasound imaging of biological materials, echoes generated by relatively homogeneous material (e.g., fat-containing areolar connective tissue) produce diffusely scattered signals, whereas echoes generated by interfaces of organized tissues (e.g., dense connective tissue layers) produce more correlated "specular" signals

(Insana et al. 1985; Garra 1993; Kremkau 1998; Lizzi et al. 2006). Dense and areolar connective tissue planes respectively appear as echogenic and echolucent bands in two-dimensional ultrasound images (Langevin et al. 2007). Combined ultrasound and histology examinations of the same tissue in human subjects undergoing surgery showed an excellent concordance between longitudinal echogenic sheets in 3-D renditions of ultrasound images and collagenous sheets seen in 3-D reconstructions of corresponding histological preparations (Fig. 8.2.5). This was confirmed using a method commonly used in geostatistics (Goovaerts 1994).

NEW TECHNIQUES APPLIED TO ANALYSIS OF ULTRASOUND IMAGES

Such geostatistical techniques are used to evaluate structural continuity in the structure of subsurface materials (soil lithology) using ground penetrating radar or soil-boring data (Castrignano et al. 2000; Petrone et al. 2004). In this method, spatial correlations are calculated within a range of distances from each data point in a chosen direction to generate semivariogram plots (customarily termed "variograms"). Parameters such as range, sill, and nugget are used to evaluate the structure of spatial datasets (e.g., smoothness, roughness) in a given direction or plane (Robertson 1987; Goovaerts 1998). For example, laminar structures with high spatial continuity yield highly correlated data in the direction of the laminations. Variogram analyses of ultrasound and histology images showed that rank correlations between serial ultrasound and corresponding histology images were highly correlated if taken parallel to the surface of the skin ($r = 0.79, p < 0.001$) or perpendicular to it ($r = 0.63, p < 0.001$), indicating concordance in spatial structure between the two datasets. Similar results were also found using synthetic deformation vector fields, a semiautomatic approach having showed promising results for the in-vivo study of mobility of the deep fascia layers (Turini et al. 2015; Condino et al. 2015).

In addition to evaluating connective tissue structure, continuous ultrasound recording during dynamic tissue perturbation, also called "dynamic ultrasonography," can be used to evaluate the dynamic mechanical properties of the tissue. Very promising also is ultrasound elasticity imaging, or elastography, a valuable noninvasive method for analyzing spatial patterns of tissue stiffness in vivo (e.g., in detection of localized stiffer tissue areas, associated with

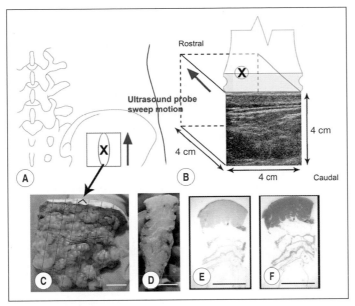

Fig. 8.2.5 Ultrasound evaluation of subcutaneous and perimuscular connective tissue stratification: correspondence between ultrasound and histology in human subject. (A, B) Location and size of ultrasound scan area on the back (X indicates the center of the scanned area in both A and B). (C) Excised tissue sample indicating location of seven serial tissue blocks. (D–F) Fixed tissue block cut transversely with corresponding hematoxylin/eosin (E) and Masson trichrome (F) histological slides. Scale bars, 1 cm.

breast and prostate malignancies). In the original elastography method, successive ultrasound images are acquired while the ultrasound probe compresses the tissue (Ophir et al. 1991; Konofagou and Ophir 1998). Tissue displacement between successive ultrasound frames is calculated using cross-correlation techniques generating a series of displacement images.

Ultrasound is emerging as a useful tool to image and measure the structure and organization of the connective tissue network in normal and pathological conditions (Luomala et al. 2014). A combined evaluation of fascial thickness, with B-mode ultrasonography, and fascial sliding, with dynamic ultrasonography and fascial stiffness, with elastography, can generate reliable data for fascial analysis and facilitate myofascial pain diagnosis.

KEY POINT

Ultrasonography and elastography are helpful in visualizing the structure and organization of the connective tissue network around skeletal muscles and observing dynamic responses of the fascia in normal and pathological conditions.

Summary

Tissue imaging using ultrasound is described for its application to skeletal muscles. B-mode ultrasonography can visualize fascial structures inside and outside skeletal muscles. With this technique, morphological characteristics of muscles (overall size and internal fascicle architecture) can be determined in vivo. Real-time imaging makes it possible to observe muscle fiber (fascicle) length changes during dynamic locomotory activities, which allow one to study how the muscles function for motor performance. Furthermore, the mechanical role of the muscle-tendon unit where muscle fibers act as actuators and tendinous tissues act as springs has been elucidated through recoding fascicle behavior in humans. Recent in-vivo evidence in ultrasound elastography further hints to the notion that the muscle-tendon units should be regarded as a functional entity connected throughout the multilevel fascial system. Muscle-tendon mechanical interaction also has clinical significance in the incidence of injury. Ultrasonography is also helpful in visualizing the structure and organization of the connective tissue network around skeletal muscles in normal and pathological conditions. Ultrasound image processing makes it possible to evaluate mesoscopic fascial structures that have good concordance with histological analyses. Ultrasound allows both imaging and quantification of connective tissue and muscle structure and dynamic responses to local mechanical perturbations. Changes in connective tissue organization and biomechanical behavior may be important components of the pathophysiology of many conditions, including chronic musculoskeletal pain (Langevin and Sherman 2007). Ultrasound-derived techniques, such as those described previously, provide noninvasive tools that can be used as outcome measures in translational studies investigating pathogenic and treatment mechanisms and clinical responses to treatments.

REFERENCES

Benjamin, M. 2009. The fascia of the limbs and back – a review. J. Anat. 214, 1–18.

Castrignano, A., Giugliarini, L., Risaliti, R., Martinelli, N., 2000. Study of spatial relationships among some soil physico-chemical properties of a field in central Italy using multivariate geostatistics. Geoderma 97, 39–60.

Condino, S., Turini, G., Parrini, S., et al., 2015. A semiautomatic method for in vivo three-dimensional quantitative analysis of fascial layers mobility based on 3D ultrasound scans. Int. J. Comput. Assist. Radiol. Surg. 10, 1721–1735.

Fornage, B., 1989. Ultrasonography of Muscles and Tendons. Springer-Verlag, New York, pp. 6–39.

Fukunaga, T., Kubo, K., Kawakami, Y., Fukashiro, S., Kanehisa, H., Maganaris, C.N., 2001. In vivo behaviour of human muscle tendon during walking. Proc. Biol. Sci. 268, 229–233.

Garra, B.S., 1993. In vivo liver and splenic tissue characterization by scattering. In: Ultrasonic Scattering in Biological Tissues. Shung, K.K., Thieme, G.A. (Eds.), CRC Press, Boca Raton, FL, pp. 347–391.

Goovaerts, P., 1994. Study of spatial relationships between two sets of variables using multivariate geostatistics. Geoderma 62, 93–106.

Goovaerts, P., 1998. Geostatistical tools for characterizing the spatial variability of microbiological and physico-chemical soil properties. Biol. Fertil. Soils 27, 315–334.

Griffiths, R.I., 1991. Shortening of muscle fibres during stretch of the active cat medial gastrocnemius muscle: the role of tendon compliance. J. Physiol. 436, 219–236.

Howry, D.H., 1965. A brief atlas of diagnostic ultrasonic radiologic results. Radiol. Clin. North Am. 3, 433–452.

Howry, D.H., Bliss, W.R., 1952. Ultrasonic visualization of soft tissue structures of the body. J. Lab. Clin. Med. 40, 579–592.

Huijing, P.A., Langevin, H.M., 2009. Communication about fascia: history, pitfalls and recommendations. In: Huijing, P.A., Hollander, A.P., Findley, T., Schleip, R. (Eds.), Fascia Research II: Basic Science and Implications for Conventional and Complementary Health Care. Elsevier GmbH, Munich.

Huijing, P.A., van Lookeren Campagne, A.A.H., Koper, J.F., 1989. Muscle architecture and fibre characteristics of rat gastrocnemius and semimembranosus muscles during isometric contractions. Acta Anatom. 135, 46–52.

Ikai, M., Fukunaga, T., 1968. Calculation of muscle strength per unit cross-sectional area of human muscle by means of ultrasonic measurement. Int. Z. Angew. Physiol. 26, 26–32.

Ikegawa, S., Funato, K., Kanehisa, H., Fukunaga, T., Kawakami, Y., 2008. Muscle force per cross-sectional area is inversely related with pennation angle in strength trained athletes. J. Strength Cond. Res. 22, 128–131.

Insana, M.F., Wagner, R.F., Gara, B.S., Brown, D.G., Shawker, T.H. 1985. Analysis of ultrasound image texture via generalized Rician statistics. Proc. Intern. Soc. Opt. Eng. 556, 153–159.

Kato, E., Oda, T., Chino, K., et al. 2005. Musculotendinous factors influencing difference in ankle joint flexibility between women and men. Int. J. Sport Health Sci. 3, 218–225.

Kawakami, Y., Abe, T., Fukunaga, T., 1993. Muscle-fiber pennation angles are greater in hypertrophied than in normal muscles. J. Appl. Physiol. 74, 2740–2744.

Kawakami, Y., Abe, T., Kanehisa, H., Fukunaga, T., 2006. Human skeletal muscle size and architecture: variability and interdependence. Am. J. Hum. Biol. 18, 845–848.

Kawakami, Y., Fukunaga, T., 2006. New insights into in vivo muscle function. Exerc. Sport Sci. Rev. 34, 16–21.

Kawakami, Y., Ichinose, Y., Fukunaga, T., 1998. Architectural and functional features of human triceps surae muscles during contraction. J. Appl. Physiol. 85, 398–404.

Kawakami, Y., Ichinose, Y., Kubo, K., Ito, M., Fukunaga, T., 2000a. Architecture of contracting human muscles and its functional significance. J. Appl. Biomech. 16, 88–97.

Kawakami, Y., Kumagai, K., Huijing, P.A., Hijikata, T., Fukunaga, T., 2000b. The length-force characteristics of human gastrocnemius and soleus muscles in vivo. In: Herzog, W. (Ed.), Skeletal Muscle Mechanics: From Mechanisms to Function. John Wiley & Sons, Chichester, West Sussex, pp. 327-341.

Kawakami, Y., Muraoka, T., Ito, S., Kanehisa, H., Fukunaga, T., 2002. In vivo muscle-fibre behaviour during counter-movement exercise in human reveals significant role for tendon elasticity. J. Physiol. 540, 635–646.

Konofagou, E., Ophir, J., 1998. A new elastographic method for estimation and imaging of lateral displacements, lateral strains, corrected axial strains and Poisson's ratios in tissues. Ultrasound Med. Biol. 24, 1183–1199.

Kremkau, F.W., 1998. Diagnostic ultrasound: principles and instruments. W.B. Saunders, Philadelphia, PA.

Langevin, H.M., Rizzo, D.M., Fox, J.R., et al., 2007. Dynamic morphometric characterization of local connective tissue network structure in humans using ultrasound. BMC Syst. Biol. 1, 25.

Langevin, H.M., Sherman, K.J., 2007. Pathophysiological model for chronic low back pain integrating connective tissue and nervous system mechanisms. Med. Hypotheses 68, 74–80.

Langevin, H.M., Stevens-Tuttle, D., Fox, J.R., et al. (2009). Ultrasound evidence of altered lumbar connective tissue structure in human subjects with chronic low back pain. In: Huijing, P.A., Hollander, A.P., Findley, T., Schleip, R. (Eds.). Fascia Research II: Basic Science and Implications for Conventional and Complementary Health Care. Elsevier GmbH, Munich.

Lieber, R.L., Leonard, M.E., Brown-Maupin, C.G., 2000. Effects of muscle contraction on the load-strain properties of frog aponeurosis and tendon. Cells Tissues Organs 166, 48–54.

Lizzi, F.L., Alam, S.K., Mikaelian, S., Lee, P., Feleppa, E.J., 2006. On the statistics of ultrasonic spectral parameters. Ultrasound Med. Biol. 32, 1671–1685.

Luomala, T., Pihlman, M., Heiskanen, J., Stecco, C., 2014. Case study: Could ultrasound and elastography visualized densified areas inside the deep fascia? J. Bodyw. Mov. Ther. 18, 462–468.

Narici, M.V., Binzoni, T., Hiltbrand, E., Fasel, J., Terrier, F., Cerretelli, P., 1996. In vivo human gastrocnemius architecture with changing joint angle at rest and during graded isometric contraction. J. Physiol. 496, 287–297.

Noce, J.P., 1990. Fundamentals of diagnostic ultrasonography. Biomed. Instrum. Technol. 24, 456–459.

Ophir, J., Cespedes, I., Ponnekanti, H., Yazdi, Y., Li, X., 1991. Elastography: a quantitative method for imaging the elasticity of biological tissues. Ultrason. Imaging 13, 111–134.

Otsuka, S., Shan, X., Kawakami, Y., 2019. Dependence of muscle and deep fascia stiffness on the contraction levels of the quadriceps: an in vivo supersonic shear-imaging study. J. Electromyogr. Kinesiol. 45, 33–40.

Otsuka, S., Yakura, T., Ohmichi, Y., et al., 2018. Site specificity of mechanical and structural properties of human fascia lata and their gender differences: a cadaveric study. J. Biomech. 77, 69–75.

Perez, H.R., Roberts, J., 2009. Flexor tendon sheath as a source of pain in lesser metatarsal overload. J. Am. Podiatr. Med. Assoc. 99, 129–134.

Petrone, R.M., Price, J.S., Carey, S.K., Waddington, J.M., 2004. "Statistical characterization of the spatial variability of soil moisture in a cutover peatland." Hydrol. Process. 18, 41–52.

Robertson, G.P., 1987. Geostatistics in ecology: Interpolating with known variance. Ecology 68, 744–748.

Scott, S.H., Engstrom, C.M., Loeb, G.E., 1993. Morphometry of human thigh muscles. Determination of fascicle architecture by magnetic resonance imaging. J. Anat. 182, 249–257.

Song, Z., Banks, R.W., Bewick, G.S., 2015. Modelling the mech-anoreceptor's dynamic behaviour. J. Anat. 227, 243–254.

Stecco, A., Busoni, F., Stecco, C., et al., 2015. Comparative ultrasonographic evaluation of the Achilles paratenon in symptomatic and asymptomatic subjects: an imaging study. Surg. Radiol. Anat. 37, 281–285.

Stecco, A., Meneghini, A., Stern, R., Stecco, C., Imamura, M., 2014. Ultrasonography in myofascial neck pain: randomized clinical trial for diagnosis and follow-up. Surg. Radiol. Anat. 36, 243–253.

Stecco, C., Porzionato, A., Macchi, V., et al., 2006. Histological characteristics of the deep fascia of the upper limb. Ital. J. Anat. Embryol. 111, 105–110.

Sugisaki, N., Kanehisa, H., Kawakami, Y., Fukunaga, T., 2005. Behavior of aponeurosis and external tendon of the gastrocnemius muscle during dynamic plantar flexion exercise. Int. J. Sport Health Sci. 3, 235–244.

Turini, G., Condino, S., Stecco, A., Ferrari, V., Ferrari, M., Gesi, M., 2015. A 3D sparse motion field filtering for quantitative analysis of fascial layers mobility based on 3D ultrasound scans. Annu. Int. Conf. IEEE Eng. Med. Biol. Soc. 2015, 775–780.

Zuurbier, C.J., Everard, A.J., van der Wees, P., Huijing, P.A., 1994. Length-force characteristics of the aponeurosis in the passive and active muscle condition and in the isolated condition. J. Biomech. 27, 445–453.

Zuurbier, C.J., Huijing, P.A., 1992. Influence of muscle geometry on shortening speed of fibre, aponeurosis and muscle. J. Biomech. 25, 1017–1026.

On the Problems of Oversimplification in Experiments and Modeling of the Body as a Multilevel Organizational Unit

Peter A. Huijing

CHAPTER CONTENTS

INTRODUCTION

For any discipline studying the human or animal body, the following is true: our knowledge simply is not sufficient to deal simultaneously with all aspects of the body, at all levels of organization. As a consequence, specialization is practiced in every discipline.

KEY POINT

In both sciences and clinical work, simplification is necessary, but oversimplification and its potentially serious effects can be dangerous.

Therefore particularly in science, but also in clinical work, working within simplified concepts of the body is essential because of this complexity of the anatomy and physiology of the body.

A special case is the study of movement at the wrist and ankle joints. With the exception of specialized studies focusing on the joints of the hand or foot exclusively, an example of such (over)simplification is the almost universal view used in biomechanical models of, for example, the foot as a rigid structure allowing movement studied in the saggital plane exclusively in the talocrural joint. The argument used, mostly implicitly, is that the errors in estimating the properties of the joints of the foot would be so big that the model would be useless.

To confound the issue further, the reality is that the ankle joint angle (the talocrural joint) is impossible to measure (unless x-ray images are taken, which most often is not practical, nor ethically allowed) and as a consequence the angle between the tibia or fibula and the foot sole is used almost universally in basic science and clinical settings as an estimator of that joint angle.

However, such simplified biomechanical modeling, if it contains major aspects of the subject being investigated, may yield important results that lead to enhanced understanding. It has led to enhanced understanding of energy transport between body segments through the action of bi- or multiarticular muscles (e.g., van Ingen Schenau 2002) and led to practical application: invention and design of the so-called Klap-skate (because of the sounds it makes) that changed international ice skating competition drastically (e.g., Houdijk et al. 2000).

A SERIOUS EXAMPLE OF THE EFFECTS OF OVERSIMPLIFICATION

 KEY POINT

The methods used in analyzing magnetic resonance imaging are not without errors or artifacts, but the images show living tissues and their local strains during in vivo experimentation.

Foot sole angle with the lower leg is not a valid estimator of talocrural joint angle.

As much as simplification is needed in science and the clinic, it also may lead to substantial errors and misunderstanding. It has been shown that movement of the joints with the foot allows the foot sole angle to change, without causing equal changes of the talocrural joint. Work from the Kawakami group shows that this occurs in healthy subjects at high levels of muscular excitation (Iwanuma et al. 2011) but becomes very evident in children afflicted with spastic paresis (Huijing et al. 2013). It was shown that, as a dorsal flexion moment was applied, up to approximately half of the changes of the foot sole angle originated from intrafoot joint movements rather than changes of the talocrural joint angles. The general idea of such a mechanism is illustrated schematically in Fig. 8.3.1A. Panel B of that figure shows an example of analysis of two x-ray images for a child afflicted by spastic cerebral paresis, yielding the result indicated previously. It is obvious that such results may have major implications for clinical application and research in the basic sciences.

DIFFERENT LEVELS OF ORGANIZATION WITHIN THE BODY DISTINGUISHED

1. The intracellular organelles (e.g., nucleus containing the genetic code), endoplasmic reticulum, and mitochondria (also containing some genetic code and many enzymes for metabolism, etc.): within or on such organelles all metabolism and protein synthesis and degradation occurs and intracellular transport is arranged.

2. The intracellular cytoskeleton connects the organelles to the layer delimiting the cell.

3. The cell membrane is an almost-fluid, fatty structure that needs to be maintained by sandwiching it between two stiffer layers of actin molecule on the intracellular face and the basal lamina on the extracellular face (for details see Chapter 3.1, Fig. 3.1.2). This very valuable structure is equipped with molecular chemoreceptors for chemical signaling from the extra- to intracellular space (see also Chapter 8.4) but also with connecting molecules, creating mechanical continuity through the cell membrane via the cytoskeleton to the organelles. Thus, for example, the nucleus may be affected directly mechanically to initiate or enhance protein synthesis.

4. Three levels of fascial organization: (a) The smallest level of organization of fascia. In skeletal muscle this level is very clearly identified as the endomysial tube in which each myofiber is working. (b) The fascial tube containing a bundle of myofibers (fascicle) continuous with their endomysial tubes called perimysium, and (c) the epimysial tube containing the collection of fascicles that are part of one muscle. Note that these intramuscular fascial organizational levels act as a continuum (stroma) that, if stiff enough, acts as a mechanical integrator of force exerted by the myofibers.

5. Different skeletal muscles having similar mechanical effects (synergistic muscles) when exerting force are organized as a muscle group and connected by the shared parts of their epimysial tubes. Note that all nerves, blood vessels, and lymphatics use the pathways of the stroma formed by fascia between muscles and within muscles to get to or from their targets and are, in effect, reinforced by the collagen molecules of the stroma.

6. Muscles with supposedly opposing mechanical effects to the synergistic muscles are grouped with different compartments delimited by intermuscular septa, interosseal membranes, and the general or deep fascia (surrounding the whole body under the superficial fascia with its adipose layers).

7. The skin and superficial fascia (also called general fascia) and its associated adipose layer.

8. If changing joint angles are involved as, for example, in single or double joint experiments within a (mechanically

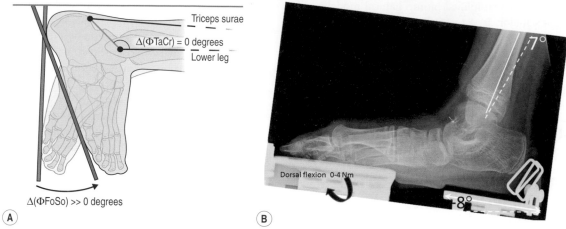

Fig. 8.3.1 Internally deforming the foot allows foot sole rotation without equal talocrural joint angle changes. (A) Superimposed, two positions are shown of the foot sole: (1) while exerting externally no additional moment of on the foot plate (0 Nm) and (2) while exerting a certain dorsal flexion moment. Note that, in this extreme example, the talocrural joint is not changed ($\Delta(\phi TaCr) = 0$), but deformations within the foot allows the foot sole to move and change its angle with the lower leg ($\Delta(\phi FoSo) \gg 0$). Redrawn with permission from Weide, G., 2020. Triceps Surae Hyper-Resistance. Measurements and Morphological Determinants in Children and Adolescents with Spastic Cerebral Palsy. Doctoral dissertation. Vrije Universiteit, Amsterdam. (B) An example of quantitative analysis of two x-ray images of the foot and ankle of a patient: one taken with the foot in a position corresponding to the 0 Nm condition and the second corresponding to the 4 Nm dorsal flexion condition. The muscles are active at quite low levels of excitation (EMG <3% of value during maximal voluntary contraction). The two images were repositioned so that the talus was aligned. This allows visualization of the movement at the talocrural joint and rotation of the foot plate. The image shows the 4 Nm condition with the solid lines indicating the position of the tibia and back part of the foot plate. Superimposed are the dotted lines from the 0 Nm condition, showing the change on talocrural joint to be ≈7 degrees and the foot plate rotation to be ≈8 degrees. (For further details see Huijing et al. 2013.) From Huijing, P. A., Bénard M. R., Jaspers R. T., et al., 2013. Movement within foot and ankle joint in children with spastic cerebral palsy: a 3-dimensional ultrasound analysis of medial gastrocnemius length with correction for effects of foot deformation. BMC Musculoskelet. Disord. 14, 365. Open access. Creative Commons Attribution License (http://creativecommons.org/licenses/by/2.0).

isolated) limb, the variable determining the degree of joint movement is the moment (roughly speaking force times moment arm, both being variable as the function of the joint angle).

9. The whole-body level, for example, looking at the biomechanics of whole-body movement involving multijoint movement and locomotion, or making clinical decisions about possible movement limitations.

> ### KEY POINT
>
> From very simple models a lot can be learned. But the model should not be presented as "realistic" or actually be confused with reality.

Much physiological work in the 19th and 20th centuries was performed on maximally dissected single muscle, and we have learned a great deal from it (e.g., the dependence of muscular force on muscle length [length-force characteristics] and velocity of shortening or lengthening [force-velocity characteristics]). A focus on such work did lead to almost total disregard of fascial tissues and their physiological and morphological role. This disregard is persisting on a large scale, even in the present time, when we are beginning to understand more about the significance of the extracellular matrix. Such knowledge is taking a role next to, as equally important as, the concept of the cell and its function, popular since the late 19th century.

Similarly, most mathematical models of muscle are of Hill type (named after its initiator) and equipped with one contractile element and one series elastic element, as well as one elastic element parallel to the contractile element. This model is ideal if one wants to understand the effects of (visco-) elastic elements in interaction with their contractile element. However, studying interaction by myofascial force transmission is impossible with such models, because in essence the whole muscle is modeled as one giant sarcomere, representing sarcomeres with identical properties.

A MODEL AND EXPERIMENTS DEALING WITH MORE THAN ONE LEVEL OF ORGANIZATION

An exception to this rule is certain finite element models that involve assumptions of mechanical interactions between adjacent structures, thus not allowing them to be independent of each other mechanically. Initially based on a physical model with springs, a particular finite element model (Fig. 8.3.2) was developed by Can Yucesoy and coworkers at Dutch universities (Universiteit Twente and later at Vrije Universiteit) and is presently still being applied at Boağçizi University in Istanbul, Turkey. An important aspect of this model is its built-in assumption that adjacent structures cannot act independently of each other, but only interact. This model has guided our research group (also including Huub Maas, e.g., Maas et al. 2003; Yucesoy et al. 2006) enormously in interpreting and understanding myofascial force transmission, as it allows interaction between adjacent model structures and by design is a multilevel organizational model. A problem for such modeling is the fact that stiffness of intra- and extra-muscular myofascial connections were not known at all and had to be adjusted to fit the experimental results obtained in experimental animals (requiring relatively stiff connections). Compared with the straightforward-type Hill models, there was a price to pay in much increased calculation times (due to reiterations of calculations to accommodate any interactions between structures), even when using commercially available packages of such models.

Note also that the experiments on myofascial force transmission described in Chapter 3.2 involve two levels of organization (4 and 5).

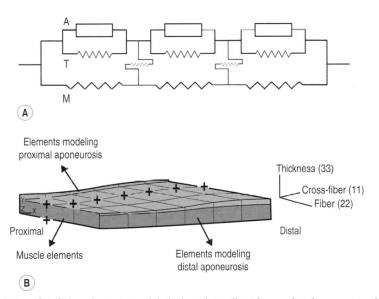

Fig. 8.3.2 Principles of a finite element model designed to allow interaction between serial and parallel arranged elements. (A) Two-dimensional schematic representation of a serial arrangement of muscle elements. The intracellular domain composed of the active contractile elements (A) and intracellular passive cytoskeleton (T), is linked to the ECM domain (M) elastically. Note that the springs representing these elastic connections are loaded (by shearing) in both directions. (B) The finite element model of muscle with extramuscular connections consists of muscle elements (three in series and six in parallel) and aponeurosis elements. The 3D local coordinate system used for the analysis is shown. The nodes of the matrix mesh marked by a "+" sign have extramuscular connections to mechanical ground and the nodes marked by a square have stiffer connections, representing the entrance of the neuromuscular tract into the muscle.

Note that each separate model element can be described, at least schematically, as several type-Hill models arranged in series with each other and with additional parallel elastic elements and bidirectional linear elastic components connecting the two parallel paths (actually representing the effects of shearing of layers). To build a model of muscle and its fascial tissues, several (a finite number, explaining the name of the model type) of such model elements are placed in series with each other to represent a muscle fascicle. Several of those model fascicles are arranged in parallel to arrange the geometrical form of a slice of target muscle. A single slice can be used to model intramuscular myofascial force transmission. Two or more of those slices may be connected to represent inter- and/or extramuscular interactions by myofascial force transmission. Some connections were selected to be stiffer than the rest and are meant to represent the neurovascular tract connected to extramuscular structures.

LIMITATIONS OF EXPERIMENTS ON MYOFASCIAL FORCE TRANSMISSION

Note that the experiments on myofascial force transmission described in Chapter 3.2 involve at least two levels of organization (4 and 5). Such experiments were designed to prove feasibility and effects, as well as its repeatability of epimuscular myofascial force transmission, and thus will also involve conditions differing from in vivo conditions (e.g., maximal or submaximal activation, but always equal activation for several muscle groups)—maximal recruitment, sometimes single muscle lengthening, always without actual joint movement. An example regarding length and position effects: some of the results with very low muscle lengths and high changes in relative position are likely to represent conditions similar to the cramping of human muscle.

Despite such limitations, a very important lesson to be learned from such modeling combined with in situ experiments is that properties known within one of the isolated levels of organization are likely to be modified because of interaction with a higher level of organization. It is also important to realize that, in many manual therapies, if sufficient "hold" can be gotten of the fascial stroma, some of the experimental conditions deviating from normal in vivo conditions may represent or mimic the conditions of the therapy, creating high levels of stress and strain locally. It is conceivable that any therapeutic effects may be dependent on such conditions.

DOES EPIMUSCULAR MYOFASCIAL FORCE TRANSMISSION PLAY A ROLE IN VIVO FOR HEALTHY SUBJECTS?

Considering the limitations of experiments, when involving direct measurements of forces at tendons as indicated previously, the answer cannot be given unequivocally. Therefore it was necessary to perform experiments with the explicit goal to keep muscular length and position changes within the in vivo usual range of lengths. This difficult task was taken up by two independent groups using different experimental techniques: (1) the Yucesoy group at Istanbul using human subjects and magnetic resonance imaging techniques and (2) the Maas group at Amsterdam using measurements of moments at the foot of experimental animals (strictly speaking not in vivo work).

ADVANTAGES AND LIMITATIONS OF THE APPLIED MRI TECHNIQUES

Magnetic resonance imaging (MRI) allows in vivo observations within the muscles. Measuring during movement would be ideal, but that is only possible by averaging MRI signals at specific time intervals during movement repeated for a long time. This makes the imaging process slow. Because the different signals filling any specific time-bin are obtained at very different times, movement of the tissues could produce significant artifacts within images, becoming visible, for example, as images lacking sharpness.

By applying a special technique, an MRI method was applied to *estimate* the position and shapes of voxels in only two images obtained immediately before and after changing the condition of the muscle (e.g., by changing a joint angle). Demons algorithm (Thirion 1998) was used to determine corresponding parts of the images and their displacements. After calculating the strains for each voxel (size: $0.8 \times 0.8 \times 0.8$ mm), principal strains were calculated representing peak local lengthening and shortening (strains) found simultaneously within muscles. As this involves a system of estimation that without doubt makes some errors, the muscle strains were compared with error strains calculated using the same methods for known deformations artificially made on one image. Statistical analysis was used to determine whether the calculated muscle strains were significantly bigger than the errors. The intervention between the images was to change hip and knee angle by placing a support under the belly of the subject. A distinct disadvantage of such intervention is that the table on which the subject is lying has to be moved out and in of the narrow bore of the MRI machine, as this may cause positional artifacts.

KEY POINT

Note that after the foot was moved toward dorsal flexion, MRI analysis showed both lengthening and shortening strains within both synergistic and antagonistic muscles.

Initially (e.g., Yaman et al. 2013), such muscle strains were expressed in a global coordinate system. However, advances were made in the excellent work by Pamuk and colleagues (2016) and Karakuzu and colleagues (2017), combining Demons algorithm with diffusion tensor imaging analyses, the latter method indicating the longitudinal directions of muscle fibers. In this way, estimates of real local muscle fiber strains directly representing altered sarcomere lengths were obtained.

Shortening and lengthening was reported to occur simultaneously along individual fascicles, whereas only lengthening was imposed externally (by changing the joint angle). When analysing the shear strain along fibers it becomes obvious that there is much shearing happening between fascicles. Mean fiber direction strains of different tracts also show nonuniform distribution. Such inhomogeneity of fiber strains is an indication of effects of epimuscular myofascial force transmission.

ADVANTAGES AND LIMITATIONS OF STUDYING MYOFASCIAL FORCE TRANSMISSION BY MEASURING MOMENTS

The Maas group used direct force measurement on muscles and techniques similar to those used previously in animal experimentation regarding myofascial force transmission, but with one important addition. They limited the relative position of the muscle and their muscle tendon-complex length to those corresponding to the healthy in vivo situation (Bernabei et al. 2015). They reported significant mechanical interaction between ankle plantar flexors.

Trying to recognize effects of epimuscular myofascial force transmission at the level of net joint moments is in fact a difficult task. Such effects may be altered, or even become invisible, in the interactions with the higher level of organization. If it should have been easy to recognize, it is likely that some surprising effects would have been noticed. Many experiments on human subjects involve analysis of net joint moments (meaning the summed effect of opposing moments exerted by different muscles at a joint).

In fact there is a widespread opinion that such an analysis is not very difficult. Such opinions stem from the biomechanical approach of considering a joint as a hinge, having a fixed axis. All one needs to do is align the axis of the joint with the axis of the measuring instrument, otherwise the force of compression within the limb will be interpreted as moments. However, the anatomical reality is that joints do not have fixed axes; their axes move to different locations during actual movement or at different joint angles. Nevertheless it is important also at such level of organization to study muscular effects on net joint moments.

I once initiated such work on joint moments in animal experiments, but after some trials gave it up, because after painstaking aligning of axes, one contraction was sufficient to create misalignment. During the defense of Chris Tijs thesis, I was invited to be one of the opponents. And as nothing was mentioned about it in the thesis, I asked him if they had made checks of such alignments, and he answered that they *assumed* the alignment to remain in order. Nevertheless, they used chapter or article titles as "No functionally relevant mechanical effects of epimuscular myofascial connections . . ." (2015b) and "Limited mechanical effects . . ." (2016a, 2016b).

KEY POINT

When measuring net joint moment rather than specific muscle forces, one never knows for sure if effects of myofascial force transmission were not present or simply hidden, unless additional and valid measurements support one or the other conclusion.

The question still remains whether myofascial effects are really not present or just extremely difficult or even impossible to recognize.

In an effort to overcome the limitations of studying at such a high level of organization and involve the level of sarcomeres within muscle fibers, the group studied the length of sarcomeres in isolated soleus muscle fibers (Tijs et al. 2015a).

KEY POINT

Sarcomere length measurements on (always slowly) fixed muscle or within subsequently isolated myofibers are *not* a valid measurement for in vivo sarcomere length.

These fibers were isolated from soleus muscles within a fixed whole limb. The treatment involved in making the fibers accessible is similar to those used in the past in our lab, but previously the sarcomere lengths thus obtained were used exclusively as an intermediate variable to calculating the number of serial sarcomeres so that the multitude of possible artifacts of such treatment is not represented in the final results of the target variable. However, these authors seem to have no limit in their confidence that such (mis-)treated sarcomeres represent their in vivo condition.

Further the Maas group seems to be somewhat inconsistent regarding the significance and relevance of in vivo myofascial force transmission, as in addition to titles indicated previously, they published articles with such titles as: "Mechanical Coupling Between Muscle-Tendon Units Reduces Peak Stresses" (Maas and Fini 2018).

It is clear that the final answer about the in vivo functional significance of myofascial effects has not been given. A lot more work on this difficult problem is indicated, and answering it is quite important. Imagine that in vivo stiffness of myofascial connections under physiological conditions is shown to be insufficient for notable effects intra- and epimuscular myofascial force transmission in healthy people because of the effect that such stiffness is controlled by physiological and molecular biological regulatory mechanisms. In this case it would be extremely important to understand the mechanisms of such control of connective tissues and fascial structures in healthy people; such insight may allow developments of new methods of treatment for those who suffer from pathological conditions in this area. Presently, we know next to nothing about adaptation of these tissues, let alone control mechanisms in this area. It is of extreme importance that a focus is created on research in this field. Obviously that will not be easy.

There is, as far as I know, no difference of opinion among groups of scientists regarding the effectiveness of epimuscular myofascial force transmission exposed to unphysiological conditions, such as lengths and positions of muscles relative to each other and other structures (e.g. Riewald and Delp 1997; Maas and Sandercock 2008; Maas and Huijing 2012).

KEY POINT

The very locally imposed unphysiological stresses and strains by the therapist may form a substantial part of the creation of therapeutic effects.

Fortunately, for the different clinical disciplines involving in vivo manual manipulation of human and animal tissues it is very likely that, if the therapist succeeds in getting hold of the fascia and target connective tissues, the very locally imposed unphysiological stresses and strains form a substantial part of the creation of therapeutic effects.

Summary

Considering the controversy about the in vivo presence of epimuscular myofascial force transmission and limitations of in vivo experimentation, it is probably wisest to postpone final judgment even though the MRI analyses presently gives an edge to the confirmative answer, because it has dealt better with possible artifacts and interactions of levels of organization, exposing or hiding its presence.

Also in manual manipulating therapy, the problems of the difficulties involved in in vivo measurement are present and should be recognized as such. The added dimension there is the manual perception of the therapist. However, the interpretation of such perception is presently still more an art than a science. This makes it more difficult to transfer to a next generation of therapists. Even more efforts should be directed to enhancing scientific research aimed at the clinical practice and its results and mechanisms of the therapy. The institutions educating the therapist should play an important role in this and enhance as much as possible their present levels of such activity. The esteem of such therapies is likely to be enhanced enormously by such activity.

REFERENCES

Bernabei, M., van Dieën, J.H., Baan, G.C., Maas, H., 2015. Significant mechanical interactions at physiological lengths and relative positions of rat plantar flexors. J. Appl. Physiol. 118, 427–436.

Houdijk, H., de Koning, J.J., de Groot, G., Bobbert, M.F., van Ingen Schenau, G.J., 2000. Push-off mechanics in speed skating with conventional skates and klapskates. Med. Sci. Sports Exerc. 32, 635–641,

Huijing, P.A., Bénard M.R., Jaspers R.T., Becher, J.G., 2013. Movement within foot and ankle joint in children with spastic cerebral palsy: a 3-dimensional ultrasound analysis of medial gastrocnemius length with correction for effects of foot deformation. BMC Musculoskelet. Disord. 14, 365

Iwanuma, S., Akagi, R. Hashizume, S., Kanehisa, H., Yanai, T., Kawakami, Y., 2011. Triceps surae muscle–tendon unit length changes as a function of ankle joint angles and contraction levels: the effect of foot arch deformation. J. Biomech. 44, 2579–2583.

Karakuzu, A., Pamuk, U., Ozturk, C., Acar, B., Yucesoy, C.A., 2017. Magnetic resonance and diffusion tensor imaging analyses indicate heterogeneous strains along human medial gastrocnemius fascicles caused by submaximal plantar-flexion activity. J. Biomech. *57*, 69–78.

Maas, H., 2019. Passive Properties of Muscle. Significance of epimuscular myofascial force transmission under passive muscle conditions. J. Appl. Physiol. 126, 1465–1473.

Maas, H., Baan, G.C., Huijing, P.A., Yucesoy, C.A., Koopman, B.H., Grootenboer, H.J., 2003. The relative position of EDL muscle affects the length of sarcomeres within muscle fibers: experimental results and finite-element modeling J. Biomech. Eng. 125, 745–753.

Maas, H., Fini, T. 2018. Mechanical coupling between muscle-tendon units reduces peak stresses. Exerc. Sport Sci. Rev. 46, 26–33.

Maas., H., Huijing, P.A., 2012. Mechanical effect of rat flexor carpi ulnaris muscle after tendon transfer: does it generate a wrist extension moment? J. Appl. Physiol. 112, 607–614.

Maas, H., Sandercock, T.G., 2008. Are skeletal muscles independent actuators? Force transmission from soleus muscle in the cat. J. Appl. Physiol. 104, 1557–1567.

Maas, H., Sandercock, T.G., 2010. Force transmission between synergistic skeletal muscles through connective tissue linkages. J. Biomed. Biotechnol. 2010, 575672.

Pamuk, U., Karakuzu, A., Ozturka, C., Acar, B., Yucesoy, C.A., 2016. Combined magnetic resonance and diffusion tensor imaging analyses provide a powerful tool for in vivo assessment of deformation along human muscle fibers. J. Mech. Behavior Biomed. Mat. 63, 207–219.

Riewald, S.A., Delp, S.L., 1997. The action of the rectus femoris muscle following distal tendon transfer: does it generate knee flexion moment? Dev. Med. Child Neurol. 39, 99–105.

Sandercock, T.G., Maas, H., 2009. Force Summation between muscles: are muscles independent actuators? Med. Sci. Sports Exerc. 41, 184–190.

Tijs, C., van Dieën J.H., Baan G.C., Maas, H., 2016a. Synergistic co-activation increases the extent of mechanical interaction between rat ankle plantar flexors. Front. Physiol. 7, 414.

Tijs, C., van Dieën, J.H., Maas, H., 2015a. Effects of epimuscular myofascial force transmission on sarcomere length of passive muscles in the rat hindlimb. Physiol. Rep. 3, e12608.

Tijs, C., van Dieën, J.H., Maas, H., 2015b. No functionally relevant mechanical effects of epimuscular myofascial connections between rat ankle plantar flexors. J. Exp. Biol. 218, 2935–2941.

Tijs, C., van Dieën, J.H., Maas, H., 2016b. Limited mechanical effects of intermuscular myofascial connections within the intact rat anterior crural compartment. J. Biomech. 49, 2953–2959.

Thirion, J.P., 1998. Image matching as a diffusion process: an analogy with Maxwell's demons. Med. Image Anal. 2, 243–260.

van Ingen Schenau, G.J., Bobbert M.F., van Soest, A.J. 1990 The Unique Action of bi-Articular Muscles in Leg Extensions. In: Winters, I.M., Woo, S.L.Y. (Eds.), Multiple Muscle Systems: Biomechanics and Movement Organization. Springer-Verlag, New York, pp. 639–652.

Weide, G., Huijing, P.A., Becher, J.G., Jaspers, R.T., Harlaar, J., 2020. Foot flexibility confounds the assessment of triceps surae extensibility in children with spastic paresis during typical physical examinations. J. Biomech. 99, 109532.

Yaman, A., Ozturk, C., Huijing, P.A., Yucesoy, C.A., 2013. Magnetic resonance imaging assessment of mechanical interactions between human lower leg muscles in vivo. J. Biomech. Eng. 135, 91003.

Yucesoy, C.A., Maas, H., Koopman, B.H., Grootenboer, H.J., Huijing, P.A., 2006. Mechanisms causing effects of muscle position on proximo-distal muscle force differences in extra-muscular myofascial force transmission. Med. Eng. Phys. 28, 214–226.

Myofascial Force Transmission and Molecular Pathways Involved in Adaptation of Muscle Size

Richard T. Jaspers and Peter A. Huijing

CHAPTER CONTENTS

INTRODUCTION

Skeletal muscle is able to adapt its properties in response to changes in functional demands because of its ability to activate and deactivate molecular systems for protein synthesis and degradation. Adequate functioning of these systems is particularly important in cases of muscle injury, neurological disorders, or chronic diseases associated with loss of muscle mass. With disuse, atrophy is a common adaptation limiting the ability to generate force. Optimizing intervention effects aimed at redressing this requires knowledge of the underlying mechanisms.

Mechanical loading of muscle tissue is a critical stimulus for adaptation of myofiber size. Knowledge of how mechanical loading of the muscle–tendon complex affects the mechanical and molecular environments of myofibers is essential for optimizing the therapeutic treatment of patients with complaints in the muscle-fascia unit. This chapter considers how mechanical loading of this complex activates molecular processes and how fasciae play a role in muscle regeneration and adaptation of muscle size.

MECHANICAL LOADING INDUCES MUSCLE ADAPTATION IN VIVO

The active force that a muscle is able to exert at different lengths depends on the number of sarcomeres arranged in parallel (within the muscle) and those arranged in series (within its myofibers). The more sarcomeres in series (i.e., longer optimum myofiber length), the higher the length range of active force exertion. However, this has no effect on the maximum force a myofiber can exert (at its optimum length). Therefore optimal muscle force is determined by both the number of the myofibers within a muscle and the number and size of myofibrils arranged in parallel within myofibers. The muscle cross-sectional area (A_f) perpendicular to the fiber direction at a standardized mean sarcomere length (e.g., optimum length) provides an estimate of the maximum force a muscle is able to exert.

Both prime parameters, A_f and serial sarcomere number, are highly adaptable in response to changes in mechanical loading of muscle.

Generally, the terms atrophy and hypertrophy refer to decrease or increase of volume of an organ. However, in myology, these terms for adaptation are used specifically for changes in the cross-sectional area of a muscle, whereas adaptation of the serial sarcomere number refers to changes along the myofiber.

How does mechanical loading stimulate adaptation of muscle size? Several in-vivo experiments indicate that mechanical loading–induced adaptation of muscle size is determined by both type and intensity of active contractile activity, as well as the strain applied on the muscle.

TRAINING

Training studies have shown that high-intensity training, particularly consisting of eccentric contractions, most strongly stimulates muscle hypertrophy (Farthing and Chilibeck 2003). In contrast, disuse of muscle as occurs in low gravity conditions or limb suspension causes progressive and severe atrophy (Huijing and Jaspers 2005). Mechanisms causing effects of these types of muscle overload and disuse on muscle remain unreported.

MUSCLE STRAIN

Muscles also adapt their size in response to the length at which they are maintained. Experiments in which rodent muscles were immobilized at high lengths, for periods varying from several days to 4 weeks, have shown a 20% hypertrophy and a 15% increase in the number of sarcomeres in series (Williams and Goldspink 1978). This was effected in such a way that the optimum length of the adapted muscle was brought into an immobilized position. Opposite effects have been reported for muscles that were immobilized in a maximally in-vivo shortened position, yielding 30% to 40% atrophy, and a similar reduction in serial sarcomere numbers (Williams and Goldspink 1978; Heslinga and Huijing 1993). Note that this was found particularly in muscle of a low degree of pennation. Also for this condition, optimal force was reduced substantially and optimum length was attained at the immobilized position (Williams and Goldspink 1978; Heslinga et al. 1995).

From these results, a simple rule has been derived stating that for any muscle adaptation of A_f a serial sarcomere number is regulated in such a way that muscle optimum length is attained at the joint angle at which a muscle is most frequently active (Herring et al. 1984). Although the simple rule seems to be valid for several types of muscles and species, exceptions do exist. It has been suggested that, for some muscles, the length ranges of operation in daily activities differ from those predicted by the simple rule that muscles are operating around their optimum length (Burkholder and Lieber 2001).

Other evidence suggesting that high actual myofiber strain per se does not stimulate hypertrophy and increase of serial sarcomere number is derived from ex-vivo cultures of mature myofibers (see later discussion). This indicates the need for more detailed understanding of mechanisms by which mechanical loading affects the rate of protein synthesis and degradation.

MOLECULAR MECHANISMS OF ADAPTATION OF MUSCLE SIZE

The quantity of proteins constituting the active force–generating apparatus or passive elements within a myofiber is the net result of ongoing processes of simultaneous protein synthesis and degradation, both being modulated in response to mechanical loading, the net results of the two creating the turnover of such proteins.

Protein synthesis involves three types of processes occurring in subsequent order.

MACHINERY FOR PROTEIN SYNTHESIS

Transcription of the Deoxyribonucleic Acid of the Genome

The genetic code itself resides within DNA strings located in the nuclei of the myofiber, but DNA is never applied directly in the synthesis of proteins. First, DNA is "transcribed" (copied) into messenger ribonucleic acid (mRNA) that carries "the recipe" from the DNA. This process is referred to as "transcription." The rate of protein synthesis depends on the quantity of DNA available and on the rate of transcription. Most cells have only one nucleus, which means that the quantity of DNA cannot be regulated. In contrast, myofibers, being the fusion product of many precursor muscle cells, contain a sizable pool of nuclei. In the process of adaptation, this pool may be enlarged or reduced. The former occurs by proliferation of satellite cells (i.e., muscle stem cells resident between the sarcolemma and the basal lamina) that donate additional nuclei to the myofiber.

Activation of satellite cells is important for two reasons: (1) for repair of overload-induced myofiber damage, activation of satellite cells will provide new nuclei to replace degraded ones within the damaged myofiber parts; and (2) the number of nuclei within a myofiber may be the factor limiting the maximal capacity for mRNA transcription (Huijing and Jaspers 2005).

The rate of transcription is determined by the absence or presence of transcription factors that modify DNA molecules such that transcription of genes is facilitated or inhibited.

TRANSLATION OF mRNA

Within the cytoplasm, mRNA binds ribosomes; this complex is used to "translate" mRNA information into a specific sequence of amino acids that constitutes the corresponding protein. The rate of protein synthesis depends also on the rate of translation. This rate is determined by the number of ribosomes per mRNA molecule and by the rate of translation per unit mRNA.

KEY POINT

Messenger RNA brings the "recipe" for protein synthesis into the sarcoplasm.

COMPLETION OF THE PROTEIN SYNTHESIS

The chain of amino acids undergoes posttranslational modifications, which ultimately results in the mature protein. Note that such a protein may be deposited within the myofiber (e.g., contractile proteins) or outside (e.g., muscular proteins that interact with products of fibrocytes to form the specific extracellular matrix at the interface between muscular and connective tissues).

The critical factor determining the overall rate of protein synthesis is the one that is limiting the whole chain of processes.

MACHINERY FOR PROTEIN DEGRADATION

Protein degradation is regulated by activity of proteolytic enzymes and by expression of cofactors leading to altered

expression of these enzymes and their activation. The most important myofiber proteolytic system is the proteasome. Proteins to be degraded are bound to multiple ubiquitin molecules, which marks them for degradation by the proteasome complex (Jackman and Kandaria 2004).

MECHANOCHEMICAL SIGNALING AND MECHANOTRANSDUCTION FOR PROTEIN SYNTHESIS AND DEGRADATION IN MUSCLE

KEY POINT

The quantity of muscular proteins present at any time is determined by the *net* effects of protein synthesis and degradation (there is turnover of muscular material).

Given balanced protein synthesis and degradation, hypertrophy and addition of serial sarcomeres requires either raising protein synthesis rates, or inhibiting degradation rates, or both. This means that mechanical loading triggers intracellular signaling pathways affecting the processes mentioned. To accomplish this, the mechanical load must be sensed and transmitted to the machineries for protein synthesis and degradation.

Myofibers are equipped with sensors via which protein synthesis and degradation are directly and/or indirectly affected (Fig. 8.4.1). Several types of mechanosensors are known: (1) stretch-activated calcium channels within the sarcolemma that open as myofibers are stretched, allowing the influx of calcium into the cytoplasm. Other transmembrane-receptors such as (2) the integrin and (3) dystroglycan complexes (see Chapter 3.1, particularly Fig. 3.1.2, for a schematic view) connect the intracellular cytoskeleton to the extracellular matrix (ECM) that is reinforced by collagen structures within the basal lamina and endomysium. Mechanical loading of such receptors and channels activates enzymes associated with sarcolemma that subsequently elicit cascades of chemical reactions. This mechanochemical signal transduction stimulates muscle gene expression and/or rates of translation (Huijing and Jaspers 2005).

Signaling via these receptors and channels is associated also with increased expression of growth factors that are secreted into the extracellular matrix. These factors

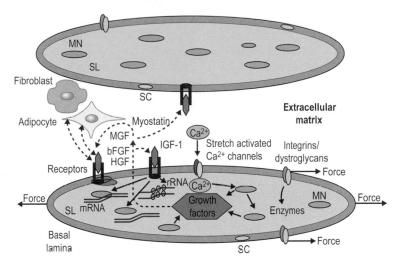

Fig. 8.4.1 Schematic representation of the mechanochemical signaling pathways involved in the regulation of myofiber size. Two adjacent myofibers are shown that are surrounded by their sarcolemma (SL) and a basal lamina. The muscle fibers are anchored to the collagen fiber–reinforced extracellular matrix by the integrin and dystroglycan/sarcoglycan complexes. Mechanical loading is sensed at these complexes at the myotendinous junctions of the myofibers and along the length of the myofiber. Loading of these complexes elicits cascades of signaling molecules (i.e., free radicals and enzymes). Another mechanosensor is the stretch-activated calcium (Ca^{2+}) channel, which allows calcium influx into sarcoplasm. In addition to its role in the contraction, calcium also regulates the activity of particular transcription factors. Transcription factors may alter deoxyribonucleic acid in the myonucleus (MN) and affect the synthesis of muscular proteins directly or indirectly via expression of growth factors, which are released in the interstitial space (i.e., extracellular matrix). Several growth factors have been identified to be expressed within muscle, which likely play a major role in muscle adaptation. Among these are the insulin-like growth factor 1 (IGF-1), mechano-growth factor (MGF), fibroblast growth factor (FGF), hepatocyte growth factor (HGF), and myostatin. Once released, these growth factors can bind to receptors in the membrane of the producing myofiber and stimulate signaling pathways that modulate the rate of transcription of DNA and the rate at which the ribosomal RNA (constituting the body of the ribosome) translates the mRNA into protein. The growth factors may bind to receptors in the membrane of the fiber that release these factors and of its host satellite cells (SC), neighboring myofibers, and/or other cells such as fibroblasts and adipocytes. bFGF, basic fibroblast growth factors.

act on myofibers in which they are produced (autocrine signaling) or on neighboring myofibers and other cells (paracrine signaling).

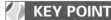

KEY POINT

Growth factors are quite important: autocrine signaling and paracrine signaling play a role in preventing very local changes of myofiber size.

Among many growth factors expressed in muscle, the following play important roles in adaptation of muscle size: (1) insulin-like growth factor 1 (IGF-1), (2) mechano-growth factor (MGF), (3) basic fibroblast

growth factors (bFGF), (4) hepatocyte growth factor (HGF), and (5) myostatin. On overloading muscle in vivo, mRNA expression of these growth factors is increased (Huijing and Jaspers 2005), with the notable exception of myostatin (reduced expression; Heinemeier et al. 2007). Most of these growth factors also play a role in activating satellite cells. Satellite cells are normally quiescent, but exposure to MGF, FGF, or HGF initiates proliferation by cell division (Huijing and Jaspers 2005). In contrast, myostatin inhibits satellite cell proliferation (Huijing and Jaspers 2005). As indicated previously, activation of satellite cells is important. However, some hypertrophy and addition of sarcomeres due to enhanced transcription and/or translation is possible without adding new nuclei (Petrella et al. 2008).

Myostatin and IGF-1 have multiple functions in regulating muscle protein synthesis and degradation. In addition to its role in activation of satellite cells, IGF-1 stimulates transcription of muscle mRNA and its translation into protein (Glass 2005; Jaspers et al. 2008). In addition, IGF-1 reduces expression of the ubiquitin ligases (Glass 2005), inhibiting protein degradation rate. Whereas IGF-1 has strong anabolic effects (protein synthesis), myostatin is its antagonist because of its opposite effects on synthesis and degradation (McFarlane et al. 2006).

An alternative way of mechanical loading of muscle yielding an increase in muscle size is by direct transmission of mechanical loading of transmembrane complexes and transmission via the intracellular cytoskeleton onto myonuclei. Such mechanotransduction will have two effects: (1) release of mRNA and ribosomes attaching to the cytoskeleton and their translocation to the sites where protein synthesis is required (Chicurel et al. 1998) and (2) nuclear deformation or conformational changes of chromatin within myonuclei that may directly affect transcriptional activity (Bloom et al. 1996). Mechanotransduction to the nucleus works almost instantly. However, its relative contribution to protein synthesis and degradation rates compared with mechanochemical pathways is unknown and warrants further investigation.

THE ROLES OF FASCIA IN THE REGULATION OF MYOFIBER SIZE

The continuous fascial stromata within and around muscles constitute the structures mediating any myofascial force transmission (Huijing 2003). In addition to this function, they are likely to play a role also in adaptation of muscle size in a mechanical and biochemical fashion.

Fascia accommodates many different cell types (e.g., fibroblasts, myofibroblasts, adipocytes, endothelial cells, macrophages, and neuronal branches), playing roles in muscle adaptation. Viscoelastic characteristics of the environment of stem cells are a determining factor for differentiation into different types of cells and their mechanical characteristics (Engler et al. 2006). For example, a stiff environment will cause the stem cell to become an osteoblast. Therefore it is expected that the mechanical properties of fascia in and around muscles also affect properties of adult myofibers and other cell types by modulating expression of growth factors and cytokines and their paracrine effects on myofibers.

Apart from control of chemical factors originating from fasciae, substantial effects on muscle adaptation are expected because of epimuscular myofascial force transmission. Epimuscular connections allow force transmission between a muscle and extramuscular connective tissues, as well as between adjacent muscles (Huijing 2003) (see Chapter 3.2). In-situ experiments (e.g., Huijing and Baan 2003) and mathematical modeling (e.g., Yucesoy et al. 2002), but also in-vivo MRI experiments in healthy human subjects (Pamuka et al. 2016; Karakuzu et al. 2017), have indicated that epimuscular force transmission affects local deformations within myofibers (read: local differences in sarcomere length along the length of the myofiber) and active and passive forces generated locally.

This means that a given global strain applied to myofibers is strongly amplified or attenuated locally. Accordingly, it is likely that stimuli for mechano(-chemical) signaling and related atrophy/hypertrophy or adaptation of serial sarcomere numbers are also local, instead of global, events. Therefore fascia and epimuscular force transmission need to be considered as potentially important factors for regulating muscle adaptation.

EX-VIVO CULTURE OF MATURE, SINGLE MYOFIBERS

Testing of hypotheses regarding myofascial connection-induced adaptation of muscle size requires interfering or removing intramuscular and epimuscular connections.

An extreme form of such interference is ex-vivo culture of single mature myofibers. To obtain such preparations myofibers are painstakingly dissected from small fascicles taken from a muscle by cutting away the walls of neighboring endomysial tubes, and thus leaving the target myofiber equipped with intact basal lamina and endomysium (Jaspers et al. 2004). Such preparations allow myofibers to stay alive for up to 3 months and make possible the study of effects on serial sarcomere length distributions independent of myofascial connections, other than their own endomysial tube (Fig. 8.4.2). This also allows studying effects of different components added to the culture medium.

Two weeks' culture of mature myofibers at both high and low length caused dissimilar effects than those reported after in-vivo immobilization of muscles (see previous discussion). This involved myofiber cross-sectional area and serial sarcomere number, as well as expression of IGF-1.

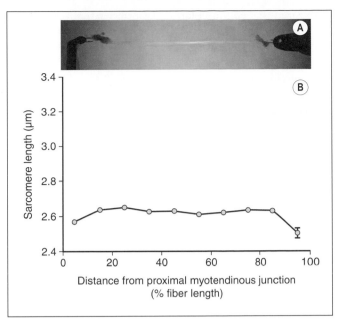

Fig. 8.4.2 Serial distribution of sarcomere lengths within a myofiber. (A) An image of a single myofiber. Myofibers were isolated from *Xenopus laevis* (African claw toad) by dissection using small forceps and scissors, leaving at both ends the myotendinous junctions attached to small pieces of tendon. It can be kept alive outside the body for up to 3 months. Such isolated fibers are still working within their own endomysial tube and used to study adaptive processes that can no longer be affected by the mechanics of neighboring myofibers and the muscular stoma and its connections. (B) Sarcomere lengths measured along the length of a globally strained single myofiber. Using a microscope, lengths of sarcomeres can be measured in this living myofiber. Mean sarcomere length is plotted as function of the location along the myofiber (expressed as normalized distance from its proximal myotendinous junction). Note that near both myotendinous junctions, sarcomeres were shorter (mean length ≈9% over passive sarcomere slack length) than in the middle of the myofibers (length ≈15% over passive slack length). However, the serial sarcomere length distribution is much smaller than calculated for a myofiber working within the mechanical context of a whole muscle, with expected consequences for signaling and processes of adaptation.

KEY POINT

Single living myofibers still equipped with their endomysial tunnel, but devoid of mechanical effects of the rest of the muscular stroma and their extramuscular connections, can contract and exert force but do not adapt their size to the imposed length conditions as in-vivo muscle does.

In contrast to those in-vivo results, these parameters remained unchanged during culture (Jaspers et al. 2004, 2008). One may argue that ex-vivo cultured myofibers may have lost their capability for protein synthesis and adaptation. However, another set of experiments revealed that such preparations show hypertrophy if the culture medium is supplemented with insulin or IGF-1 (Jaspers et al. 2008, 2009). This indicates that the cultured single myofibers still possessed the ability to adapt. Why does a single myofiber cultured at a high global fiber strain not respond to such mechanical loading? Is it removal of intra- and epimuscular myofascial force transmission? Assessing serial sarcomere length distributions, every millimeter along the myofiber length kept at a mean ≈12% over passive sarcomere slack length showed that serial strain distributions are still present with the single myofiber but were limited to between 9% and 15% for lengths over passive sarcomere slack length. This indicates that distributions of strain found do not attain the same magnitude within a living but single myofiber preparation as seen in (1) finite-element modeling (e.g., Yucesoy et al. 2003) for muscle with epimuscular connections, or (2) in-vivo analysis of strains in human muscle fibers, using a combination of diffusion tensor and magnetic resonance imaging (Pamuka et al. 2016; Karakuzu et al. 2017).

Therefore it has been hypothesized that epimuscular connections are crucial for mechano-(chemical) signal transduction in skeletal muscle (Huijing and Jaspers 2005), underlining the potential importance of fascia in the regulation of adaptation of muscle size.

Summary

Mechanical loading has been shown to be a stimulus for adaptation of muscle size. Because mechanical coupling between the myofiber and inter- and extramuscular connective tissue is present, it is hypothesized that fasciae play a role in the regulation of adaptation of muscle size. Variations in local stiffness of the epimuscular fascia are likely to cause local stresses onto the myofiber that is different from the global stress that is accompanied by high strains locally. Such local mechanical effects elicit local biochemical signaling within myofibers, affecting rates of muscle protein synthesis and degradation. These effects may be direct (affecting nuclei) or indirect via enhanced expression of growth factors and cytokines being released into the extracellular matrix and having autocrine and/or paracrine effects there.

In sum, mechanical interaction between epimuscular fascia and myofibers seems to be crucial for the regulation of adaptation of muscle size. This new view on the interaction and communication between muscle and fascia needs to be investigated further in order to make effective use of such mechanisms in training and therapy.

REFERENCES

Bloom, S., Lockard, V.G., Bloom, M., 1996. Intermediate filament-mediated stretch-induced changes in chromatin: a hypothesis for growth initiation in cardiac myocytes. J. Mol. Cell. Cardiol. 28, 2123–2127.

Burkholder, T.J., Lieber, R.L., 2001. Sarcomere length operating range of vertebrate muscles during movement. J. Exp. Biol. 204, 1529–1536.

Chicurel, M.E., Singer, R.H., Meyer, C.J., Ingber, D.E., 1998. Integrin binding and mechanical tension induce movement of mRNA and ribosomes to focal adhesions. Nature 392, 730–733.

Engler, A.J., Sen, S., Sweeney, H.L., Discher, D.E., 2006. Matrix elasticity directs stem cell lineage specification. Cell 126, 677–689.

Farthing, J.P., Chilibeck, P.D., 2003. The effects of eccentric and concentric training at different velocities on muscle hypertrophy. Eur. J. Appl. Physiol. 89, 578–586.

Glass, D.J., 2005. Skeletal muscle hypertrophy and atrophy signaling pathways. Int. J. Biochem. Cell Biol. 37, 1974–1984.

Heinemeier, K.M., Olesen, J.L., Schjerling, P., et al., 2007. Short-term strength training and the expression of myostatin and IGF-I isoforms in rat muscle and tendon: differential effects of specific contraction types. J. Appl. Physiol. 102, 573–581.

Herring, S.W., Grimm, A.F., Grimm, B.R., 1984. Regulation of sarcomere number in skeletal muscle: a comparison of hypotheses. Muscle Nerve 7, 161–173.

Heslinga, J.W., Huijing, P.A., 1993. Muscle length–force characteristics in relation to muscle architecture: a bilateral study of gastrocnemius medialis muscles of unilaterally immobilized rats. Eur. J. Appl. Physiol. Occup. Physiol. 66, 289–298.

Heslinga, J.W., te Kronnie, G., Huijing, P.A., 1995. Growth and immobilization effects on sarcomeres: a comparison between gastrocnemius and soleus muscles of the adult rat. Eur. J. Appl. Physiol. Occup. Physiol. 70, 49–57.

Huijing, P.A., 2003. Muscular force transmission necessitates a multilevel integrative approach to the analysis of function of skeletal muscle. Exerc. Sport Sci. Rev. 31, 167–175.

Huijing, P.A., Baan, G.C., 2003. Myofascial force transmission: muscle relative position and length determine agonist and synergist muscle force. J. Appl. Physiol. 94, 1092–1107.

Huijing, P.A., Jaspers, R.T., 2005. Adaptation of muscle size and myofascial force transmission: a review and some new experimental results. Scand. J. Med. Sci. Sports 15, 349–380.

Jackman, R.W., Kandarian, S.C., 2004. The molecular basis of skeletal muscle atrophy. Am. J. Physiol. Cell Physiol. 287, C834–C843.

Jaspers, R.T., Feenstra, H.M., Verheyen, A.K., van der Laarse, W.J., Huijing, P.A., 2004. Effects of strain on contractile force and number of sarcomeres in series of *Xenopus laevis* single muscle fibres during long-term culture. J. Muscle Res. Cell Motil. 25, 285–296.

Jaspers, R.T., van Beek-Harmsen, B.J., Blankenstein, M.A., Goldspink, G., Huijing, P.A, van der laarse, W.J., 2008. Hypertrophy of mature *Xenopus* muscle fibres in culture induced by synergy of albumin and insulin. Pflugers Arch. 457, 161–170.

Jaspers, R., Van der Laarse, W. J., Krishnan, R., et al., 2009. Differential effects of high strain and insulin-like growth factor 1 on adaptation of muscle fiber size and force. Comparat. Biochem. Physiol. Part A: Molecular & Integrative Physiology, 153(2), S74.

Karakuzu, A., Pamuka, U., Ozturka, C., Acar, B., Yucesoy, C.A., 2017. Magnetic resonance and diffusion tensor imaging analyses indicate heterogeneous strains along human medial gastrocnemius fascicles caused by submaximal plantar-flexion activity. J. Biomech. 57, 69–78

McFarlane, C., Plummer, E., Thomas, M., et al., 2006. Myostatin induces cachexia by activating the ubiquitin proteolytic system through an NF-kappaB-independent,

FoxO1-dependent mechanism. J. Cell Physiol. 209, 501–514.

Pamuka, U., Karakuzua, A. Ozturka, C., Acar, B., Yucesoy, C.A. 2016. Combined magnetic resonance and diffusion tensor imaging analyses provide a powerful tool for in vivo assessment of deformation along human muscle fibers. J. Mech. Behav. Biomed. Mater. 63, 207–219.

Petrella, J.K., Kim, J.S., Mayhew, D.L., Cross, J.M., Bamman, M.M., 2008. Potent myofiber hypertrophy during resistance training in humans is associated with satellite cell-mediated myonuclear addition: a cluster analysis. J. Appl. Physiol. 104, 1736–1742.

Williams, P.E., Goldspink, G., 1978. Changes in sarcomere length and physiological properties in immobilized muscle. J. Anat. 127, 459–468.

Yucesoy, C.A., Koopman, B.H., Baan, G.C., Grootenboer, H.J., Huijing, P.A., 2003. Extramuscular myofascial force transmission: experiments and finite element modeling. Arch. Physiol. Biochem. 111, 377–388.

Yucesoy, C.A., Koopman, B.H., Huijing, P.A., and Grootenboer H.J., 2002. Three-dimensional finite element modeling of skeletal muscle using a two-domain approach: linked fiber-matrix mesh model. J. Biomech. 35, 1253–1262.

Myofascial Effect on Muscle Stem Cell Function and Muscle Regeneration

Mohammad Haroon and Richard T. Jaspers

CHAPTER CONTENTS

INTRODUCTION

Muscle regeneration in response to injury relies on the activation of muscle stem cells (MuSCs), also referred as muscle satellite cells. MuSCs are located within the extracellular matrix (below the endomysium, referred to in this chapter as its niche) on top of the host myofibers (terminally differentiated and multinucleated skeletal muscle cells). Normally, MuSCs are in quiescence but become active upon myofiber injury or mechanical overload (i.e., higher than usual loading). In these conditions, these cells proliferate and generate either committed muscle precursors (myoblasts) or self-renewing daughters. Note that MuSCs are required for myofiber hypertrophy and regeneration (Van der Meer et al. 2011a; Forbes and Rosenthal 2014).

Skeletal muscle regenerative potential declines with age (Conboy et al. 2005; Conboy and Rando 2005), although MuSC numbers per myofiber in aged muscle are only slightly reduced in such conditions (Kadi et al. 2004; van der Meer et al. 2011b).

Upon myofiber damage or exposure to overload, quiescent MuSCs are activated and give rise to a population of proliferating myoblasts expressing the muscle transcription factors MyoD and/or Myf5. Most myoblasts will then exit the cell-division cycle and fuse to repair injured myofibers and regenerate tissue, while a MuSC subpopulation undergoes self-renewal and repopulates its niche (Tidball et al. 1998).

Chemical signals from the local microenvironment (i.e., insulin-like growth factor-1, myostatin, interleukin-6) trigger MuSC activation and control their proliferation and differentiation (von Maltzahn et al. 2012). In addition to biochemical factors, physical characteristics of the MuSC niche are also likely involved in this process. Fibrosis and stiffening of intramuscular connective tissue stroma impairs MuSC activation and differentiation (Thomas et al. 2015). During healthy ageing, wear and tear of skeletal muscle manifests itself as injury and degenerative loss of skeletal muscle mass and strength. This is associated with detrimental changes of the aged MuSC niche that disrupts MuSC quiescence and reduces their capacity for self-renewal and regenerative function (Grounds 1998; Conboy et al. 2003; Ryall et al. 2008; Chakkalakal et al. 2012). Ageing-related reduction in muscle regenerative capacity is due to unfavorable physicochemical MuSC niche properties with detrimental effects on myofiber regeneration, concomitant fibrosis, and further deterioration of niche conditions supporting adequate MuSC proliferation and differentiation.

Optimal conditions for MuSC activation, differentiation, and self-renewal are presently not well understood. It is known that the serum play an important role in MuSC activation (Conboy et al. 2005). Moreover, mechanical loading of skeletal muscle such as occuring during physical exercise will induce expression of growth factors and cytokines within the myofibers (Huijing and Jaspers 2005). Myofibers express growth factors and cytokines upon stretching and under pulsating fluid shear stress (Juffer et al. 2014a; 2014b). Such mechanical loading of skeletal muscle may affect MuSC niche conditions and therefore MuSC proliferation and differentiation. This is conceived to occur in two manners: (1) indirectly by physical loading of myofibers that respond by expressing growth factors and cytokines, or (2) because MuSCs are mechanically linked to the sarcolemma and to the extracellular matrix, active and passive stretch-shortening cycles of myofibers will load the MuSCs (Morrissey et al. 2016; Boers et al. 2018). As MuSCs' cell-delimiting membranes are equipped with mechanosensors, it is likely that they will respond to contractile forces generated by myofibers or to forces externally applied to the myofibers. Later we discuss how interactions of MuSCs and myofascial structures may determine MuSCs functioning and their involvement in muscle regeneration and adaptation.

MECHANICAL LINKAGE OF MUSCLE STEM CELLS TO THEIR NICHE COMPONENTS IN THE EXTRACELLULAR MATRIX

MuSCs are enclosed in their niche between the plasma membrane of the host myofiber (i.e., sarcolemma) and the extracellular matrix consisting of collagen IV (Fig. 8.5.1). Within their cell-delimiting membrane, MuSCs have transmembrane molecular complexes by which they are connected to their surroundings. MuSCs are anchored to the sarcolemma of the host myofiber by so-called adherens junctions, consisting of cadherens and catenin molecules. At their interface with the basal lamina MuSCs are connected via integrins, dystrophin-associated glycoproteins complexes, and syndecans to the collagen fibers of the endomysium surrounding the myofiber (Yin et al. 2013; Dumont et al. 2015). In addition, over its whole periphery, MuSCs are covered with a glycocalyx (Boers et al. 2018), a pericellular meshwork of proteoglycans and glycoproteins connected via core proteins (i.e., syndecans and glypicans) to the intracellular cytoskeleton (Reitsma et al. 2007). MuSCs are coupled mechanically to their surroundings by these different adhesions and are able to exert traction forces onto it, as well as able to sense external forces exerted via its niche.

KEY POINT

Muscle stem cells in their niche are mechanically linked with myofiber and myofascia.

FORCE TRANSMISSION FROM MYOFIBER TO MUSCLE STEM CELL

During movement, myofibers will undergo large length excursions while actively or passively exerting forces generated by its sarcomeres. Such forces are transmitted via cytoskeletal filaments onto extracellular connective tissues via the trans-sarcolemmal complexes, both at the myotendinous junction and along the full periphery of the myofibers (Street 1983; Huijing 1999). It is quite conceivable that because of the anchoring of the MuSCs to sarcolemma and the basal lamina, these cells will undergo tensile strains upon stretch of myofibers and become more aligned with the myofiber (Boers et al. 2018). Recently it has been shown that the forces exerted during myofiber stretch are transmitted to the MuSCs and cause MuSC deformation (Haroon et al. 2021). Local differences in stiffness of the intramuscular connective tissue and effects of epimuscular force transmission, strain of serial sarcomere within myofibers of a muscle is not uniform and the endomysium is exposed to shear forces, as shown by finite element muscle modeling (Yucesoy et al. 2002; Jaspers et al. 2002). MuSCs residing in their niche also experience these shear forces (Haroon et al. 2021) In addition to shearing induced by differences in displacement of sarcomeres within adjacent myofibers, it has been shown that the viscous matrix between myofibers allows displacement of substances. This implies that some fluid shear stress may also act on the MuSC (Evertz et al. 2016).

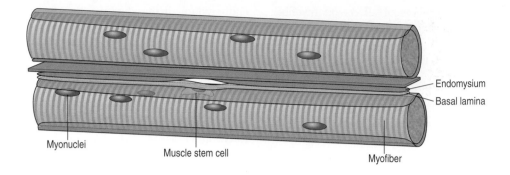

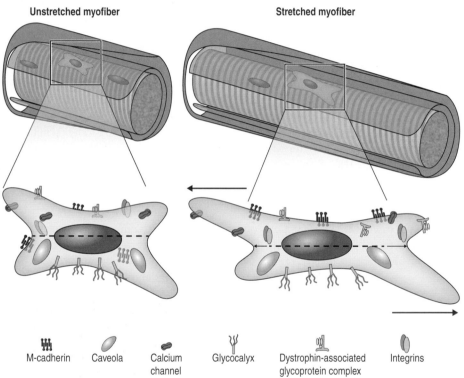

Fig. 8.5.1 Schematic of Muscle Stem Cell in its Niche and Potential Effects of Myofascial Loads on its Orientation and Deformation. Myofibers are postmitotic multinucleated cells that are ensheathed by a basal lamina and endomysium. Along their length, myofibers contain a few muscle stem cells (MuSCs) that have the ability to proliferate and differentiate upon injury or unusual overload. MuSCs are located on their host myofiber in their niche between the sarcolemma and basal lamina. Within their cell-delimiting membranes, MuSCs have transmembrane molecular complexes by which they are connected to their surroundings. MuSCs are anchored to the sarcolemma of the host myofiber by so-called adherens junctions, consisting of cadherens and catenin molecules. At their interface with the basal lamina, MuSCs are connected via integrins, dystrophin-associated glycoprotein complexes, and syndecans to the collagen fibers of the endomysium surrounding the myofiber. It has been proposed that MuSCs will be subjected to mechanical loads and will undergo tensile strain and shear deformation as well as compression via the myofascial linkages. These loads are likely sensed by mechanosensors in the MuSC membrane and induce signaling molecules regulating MuSC fate and function.

KEY POINT

Muscle stem cells are subjected to myofascial forces during muscle stretch shortening.

Another load that may be sensed by MuSCs is pressure. The volume of myofibers remains constant during contractions, a feature discovered by Jan Swammerdam in the 17th century (but unfortunately not published until 1738). Therefore the pressure within the extracellular matrix between the myofibers will increase when a muscle shortens and its myofibers start to bulge. Under these conditions MuSCs are expected to be compressed. Based on this, it is expected that during large movements MuSCs in their niche are loaded simultaneously by diverse mechanical features, creating cues from their niche, causing membrane and cytoskeletal and nuclear deformations.

POTENTIAL EFFECT OF PHYSICAL CUES ON MUSCLE STEM CELL FUNCTION

Mechanical loading of MuSCs may affect their fate and function via several mechanisms. Cyclic stretch of rat MuSCs in culture has shown to stimulate production of nitric oxide (NO) via activation of nitric oxide synthase, which is accompanied by release of hepatocyte growth factors (HGF) into the culture medium (Tatsumi et al. 2002). These data suggest that mechanical loading–induced NO production by MuSCs breaks HGF binding to the carbohydrates within glycocalyx. HGF is known for its stimulatory effect of MuSC proliferation via the C-met receptor in the MuSC membrane (Wozniak et al. 2003). In neuronal and endothelial cells, NO production has been shown to be induced by calcium-induced signaling via stretch-activated ion channels (SACs; Tatsumi 2010). Because the membrane of MuSCs also contain SACs (Yin et al. 2013), it is conceivable that the calcium-mediated signaling is also active in MuSCs. In addition to cyclic tensile stretching, subjecting differentiated myoblasts to pulsating fluid shear stress has shown that this type of loading stimulates the production of NO via the glycocalyx (Juffer et al. 2014a). As MuSCs also express a glycocalyx (Boers et al. 2018), this implies that shear loading could also contribute to HGF signaling. Note that NO has also been suggested to be involved in self-renewal of MuSCs (Buono et al. 2012). Although little is known about the effects of mechanical loading on MuSCs, the observations discussed suggest substantial impact of mechanical loading on gene expression and MuSC function.

 KEY POINT

Muscle stem cells are mechanosensitive.

In addition to responsiveness to external forces applied to MuSCs, MuSCs are also sensitive to the stiffness of their niche. By exerting traction forces, cells in culture are able to sense the stiffness of their substrate (Engler et al. 2006). Culture of MuSCs on substrates with different stiffness has shown that softening of the substrate improves the MuSCs ability to proliferate (Gilbert et al. 2010). With ageing, there is a progressive loss of skeletal muscle myofibers and increased fibrosis causing (local) stiffening of intramuscular connective tissue and myofascia. Such stiffening of intramuscular connective tissue and myofascia can affect MuSC fate and function.

KEY POINT

Myofascia determines MuSC fate and function.

Summary

Muscle regeneration relies on adequate proliferation and differentiation of MuSCs. It is generally acknowledged that MuSC function is regulated by biochemical signaling molecules. In addition to this type of signaling it is conceivable that because of mechanical linkage of MuSCs to their surrounding and myofascial interaction between myofibers, MuSCs are subjected to mechanical loads and deformations and can sense the stiffness of their niche. Because MuSCs are mechanosensitive to mechanical cues, myofascial forces will likely alter gene expression and function of these cells. The myofascial effect on MuSCs and its implications for skeletal muscle regeneration warrant further investigation.

REFERENCES

Boers, H.E., Haroon, M., Le Grand, F., et al., 2018. Mechanosensitivity of aged muscle stem cells. J. Orthop. Res. 36, 632–641.

Buono, R., Vantaggiato, C., Pisa, V., et al., 2012. Nitric oxide sustains long-term skeletal muscle regeneration by regulating fate of satellite cells via signaling pathways requiring Vangl2 and cyclic GMP. Stem Cells 30, 197–209.

Chakkalakal, J.V., Jones, K.M., Basson, M.A., Brack, A.S., 2012. The aged niche disrupts muscle stem cell quiescence. Nature 490, 355–360.

Conboy, I.M., Conboy, M.J., Smythe, G.M., Rando, T.A., 2003. Notch-mediated restoration of regenerative potential to aged muscle. Science 302, 1575–1577.

Conboy, I.M., Conboy, M.J., Wagers, A.J., Girma, E.R., Weissman, I.L., Rando, T.A., 2005. Rejuvenation of aged progenitor cells by exposure to a young systemic environment. Nature 433, 760–764.

Conboy, I.M., Rando, T.A. 2005. Aging, stem cells and tissue regeneration: lessons from muscle. Cell cycle 4, 407–410.

Dumont, N.A., Wang, Y.X., von Maltzahn, J., et al., 2015. Dystrophin expression in muscle stem cells regulates their polarity and asymmetric division. Nat. Med. 21, 1455–1463.

Engler, A.J., Sen, S., Sweeney, H.L., Discher, D.E., 2006. Matrix elasticity directs stem cell lineage specification. Cell 126, 677–689.

Evertz, L.Q., Greising, S.M., Morrow, D.A., Sieck, G.C., Kaufman, K.R., 2016. Analysis of fluid movement in skeletal muscle using fluorescent microspheres. Muscle Nerve 54, 444–450.

Forbes, S.J., Rosenthal, N., 2014. Preparing the ground for tissue regeneration: from mechanism to therapy. Nat. Med. 20, 857–869.

Gilbert, P.M., Havenstrite, K.L., Magnusson, K.E., et al., 2010. Substrate elasticity regulates skeletal muscle stem cell self-renewal in culture. Science 329, 1078–1081.

Grounds, M.D., 1998. Age-associated changes in the response of skeletal muscle cells to exercise and regeneration. Ann. N. Y. Acad. Sci. 854, 78–91.

Haroon, M., Klein-Nulend, J., Bakker, A.D., et al., 2021. Myofiber stretch induces tensile and shear deformation of muscle stem cells in their native niche. Biophys. J. 120, 2665–2678.

Huijing, P., 1999. Muscular force transmission: a unified, dual or multiple system? A review and some explorative experimental results. Arch. Physiol. Biochem. 107, 292–311.

Huijing, P.A., Jaspers, R.T., 2005. Adaptation of muscle size and myofascial force transmission: a review and some new experimental results. Scand. J. Med. Sci. Sports 15, 349–380.

Jaspers, R.T., Brunner, R., Baan, G.C., Huijing, P.A., 2002. Acute effects of intramuscular aponeurotomy and tenotomy on multitendoned rat EDL: Indications for local adaptation of intramuscular connective tissue. Anat. Rec. 266, 123–135.

Juffer, P., Bakker, A.D., Klein-Nulend, J., Jaspers, R.T., 2014a. Mechanical loading by fluid shear stress of myotube glycocalyx stimulates growth factor expression and nitric oxide production. Cell Biochem. Biophys. 69, 411–419.

Juffer, P., Jaspers, R.T., Klein-Nulend, J., Bakker, A.D., 2014b. Mechanically loaded myotubes affect osteoclast formation. Calcif. Tissue Int. 94, 319–326.

Kadi, F., Charifi, N., Denis, C., Lexell, J., 2004. Satellite cells and myonuclei in young and elderly women and men. Muscle Nerve 29, 120–127.

Morrissey, J.B., Cheng, R.Y., Davoudi, S., Gilbert, P.M., 2016. Biomechanical origins of muscle stem cell signal transduction. J. Mol. Biol. 428, 1441–1454.

Reitsma, S., Slaaf, D.W., Vink, H., van Zandvoort, M.A., Oude Egbrink, M.G., 2007. The endothelial glycocalyx: composition, functions, and visualization. Pflügers Archiv. 454, 345–359.

Ryall, J.G., Schertzer, J.D., Lynch, G.S., 2008. Cellular and molecular mechanisms underlying age-related skeletal muscle wasting and weakness. Biogerontology 9, 213–228.

Street, S.F., 1983. Lateral transmission of tension in frog myofibers: a myofibrillar network and transverse cytoskeletal connections are possible transmitters. J. Cell. Physiol. 114, 346–364.

Tatsumi, R., 2010. Mechano-biology of skeletal muscle hypertrophy and regeneration: possible mechanism of stretch-induced activation of resident myogenic stem cells. Anim. Sci. J. 81, 11–20.

Tatsumi, R., Hattori, A., Ikeuchi, Y., Anderson, J.E., Allen, R.E., 2002. Release of hepatocyte growth factor from mechanically stretched skeletal muscle satellite cells and role of pH and nitric oxide. Mol. Biol. Cell 13, 2909–2918.

Thomas, K., Engler, A.J., Meyer, G.A., 2015. Extracellular matrix regulation in the muscle satellite cell niche. Connect. Tissue Res. 56, 1–8.

Tidball, J.G., Lavergne, E., Lau, K.S., Spencer, M.J., Stull, J.T., Wehling, M., 1998. Mechanical loading regulates NOS expression and activity in developing and adult skeletal muscle. Am. J. Physiol. 275, C260–266.

van der Meer, S.F., Jaspers, R.T., Degens, H., 2011a. Is the myonuclear domain size fixed? J. Musculoskelet. Neuronal Interact. 11, 86–297.

van der Meer, S.F., Jaspers, R.T., Jones, D.A., Degens, H., 2011b. Time-course of changes in the myonuclear domain during denervation in young-adult and old rat gastrocnemius muscle. Muscle Nerve 43, 212–222.

von Maltzahn, J., Bentzinger, C.F., Rudnicki, M.A., 2012. Wnt7a-Fzd7 signalling directly activates the Akt/mTOR anabolic growth pathway in skeletal muscle. Nat. Cell Biol. 14, 186–191.

Wozniak, A.C., Pilipowicz, O., Yablonka-Reuveni, Z., et al., 2003. C-Met expression and mechanical activation of satellite cells on cultured muscle fibers. J. Histochem. Cytochem. 51, 1437–1445.

Yin, H., Price, F., Rudnicki, M.A., 2013. Satellite cells and the muscle stem cell niche. Physiol. Rev. 93, 23–67.

Yucesoy, C., Koopman, B., Huijing, P., Grootenboer, H., 2002. Three-dimensional finite element modeling of skeletal muscle using a two-domain approach: linked fiber-matrix mesh model. J. Biomech. 35, 1253–1262.

GLOSSARY

Katja Bartsch and Heike Jäger

A

Actin A globular protein found in all eukaryotic cells, polymerizes to microfilaments; one of the three major components of the cytoskeleton and thin filaments of the contractile apparatus. Actin has an array of functions, including muscle contraction, cell signaling and morphology, vesicle and organelle movement, cell motility, phagocytosis, and cytokinesis.

Adhesions Inflammatory bands of scarlike tissue that form between two surfaces inside the body.

Adhesive capsulitis An inflammatory condition that restricts motion in the shoulder, commonly referred to as "frozen shoulder."

Alpha smooth muscle actin One of six known smooth muscle actin isoforms. In addition to its presence in organ tissue, alpha smooth muscle actin has been identified in myofibroblasts, where it plays an important role in focal adhesion maturation and in cell motility.

Angiogenesis A physiological process involving the growth of new blood vessels from preexisting vessels, for example, in the process of wound healing.

Aponeurosis A thin, flat tendon-like expansion of fascia important in the attachment of muscles to bones.

Apoptosis A morphologic pattern of cell death affecting single cells, marked by formation of cytoplasmic blebs, shrinkage of the cell, condensation of chromatin, and fragmentation of the cell into membrane-bound apoptotic bodies that are eliminated by phagocytosis. It is a mechanism for cell deletion in the regulation of cell populations.

B

Bradykinin A nonapeptide produced by activation of the kinin system in a variety of inflammatory conditions. A potent vasodilator, it also increases vascular permeability, stimulates pain receptors, and causes contraction of a variety of extravascular smooth muscles.

C

Calcitonin gene-related peptide (CGRP) A 37-amino acid polypeptide is formed from the alternative splicing of the calcitonin/CGRP gene and acts as a potent vasodilator and neurotransmitter. Widely distributed in the central and peripheral nervous systems; also present in the adrenal medulla and gastrointestinal tract.

Cell signaling The process by which a cell receives and acts on some external chemical or physical signal, including receiving the information at specific receptors in the plasma membrane, conveying the signal across the plasma membrane into the cell, and subsequently stimulating a specific cellular response.

C-fiber Unmyelinated nerve fiber that conducts action potentials at a velocity of less than 2.5 m/s in humans.

Chondroblasts Immature cartilage cells that produce the cartilaginous matrix.

Chromatin The more readily stainable portion of the cell nucleus, forming a network of nuclear fibrils. Comprised of DNA attached to a protein structure base (primarily histones). Occurs in two states, euchromatin and heterochromatin, with different staining properties, and during cell division coils and folds to form the metaphase chromosomes.

Collagen The most abundant protein in mammals; a major component of fascia, giving it strength and flexibility. At least 14 types exist, each composed of tropocollagen units that share a common triple-helical shape but varying somewhat in composition between types, with the types being localized to different tissues, stages, or functions.

Compartment syndrome Involves the compression of nerves and blood vessels within a fascial compartment, leading to impaired blood flow and muscle and nerve damage. Most common in the lower leg or forearm.

Cytokines A generic term for nonantibody proteins released by one cell population (e.g., primed T lymphocytes) on contact with specific antigens, which act as intercellular mediators, as in the generation of an immune response.

Cytoskeleton The conspicuous internal reinforcement in the cytoplasm of a cell, consisting of tonofibrils, terminal web, or other microfilaments.

D

Deep fascia (or fascia profunda) The dense fibrous fascia that interpenetrates and surrounds the muscles as well as muscle groups.

Differentiated myofibroblast A myofibroblast that expresses alpha smooth muscle actin stress fiber bundles.

Dry needling An invasive procedure in which an acupuncture needle is inserted at myofascial trigger points to inactivate it.

Dupuytren's contracture A thickening and contracture of the palmar fascia.

Dynamometer An instrument for measuring the force of muscular contraction.

E

Ehlers–Danlos syndrome A group of inherited connective tissue disorders, caused by a defect in the synthesis of collagen. Occurs in at least 10 types, varying in severity from mild to life-threatening. Transmitted genetically as autosomal recessive, autosomal dominant, or X linked recessive traits. The major manifestations include hyperextensible skin and joints, easy bruisability, friability of tissues with bleeding and poor wound healing, calcified subcutaneous spheroids, and pseudotumors.

Elastin A scleroprotein, the essential constituent of yellow elastic connective tissue. Brittle when dry, but when moist is flexible and highly extensile.

Electron microscopy An imaging technique using electrons to illuminate and create an image of a specimen. It has much higher magnification and resolving power than a light microscope, with magnifications up to about two million times compared with about 2000 times. Unlike a light microscope, which uses glass lenses to focus light, the electron microscope uses electrostatic and electromagnetic lenses to control the illumination and imaging of the specimen.

Endomysium The fascial layer that sheaths single muscle fibers.

Endotenon A thin fascial membrane within a tendon that invests each collagen fibril and each collagen fiber and envelops the primary, secondary, and tertiary fiber bundles.

Endothelium The layer of epithelial cells that lines the cavities of the heart, the lumina of blood and lymph vessels, and the serous cavities of the body.

Epimysium The fascial layer that envelops an entire muscle.

Epineurium The outermost fascial layer of a peripheral nerve, surrounding the entire nerve and containing its supplying blood vessels and the lymphatic system.

Epitenon A fine, loose connective tissue sheath covering a tendon over its entire length.

Extracellular matrix A three-dimensional network of extracellular macromolecules dissolved in water that surrounds the cells in connective tissues.

F

Fascia Depending on the context, two different definitions are recommended: (1) "A fascia" is a sheath, a sheet, or any other dissectible aggregations of connective tissue that forms beneath the skin to attach, enclose, and separate muscles and other internal organs. (2) "The fascial system" consists of the three-dimensional continuum of soft, collagen-containing, loose and dense fibrous connective tissues that permeate the body. It incorporates elements such as adipose tissue, adventitiae and neurovascular sheaths, aponeuroses, deep and superficial fasciae, epineurium, joint capsules, ligaments, membranes, meninges, myofascial expansions, periostea, retinacula, septa, tendons, visceral fasciae, and all the intramuscular and intermuscular connective tissues, including endo-/peri-/epimysium. The fascial system surrounds, interweaves between, and interpenetrates all organs, muscles, bones, and nerve fibers, endowing the body with a functional structure, and providing an environment that enables all body systems to operate in an integrated manner.

Fasciacytes Fibroblast-like cells that are specialized for hyaluronan synthesis and form small clusters along the surface of each fascial sublayer.

Fascial distortion model (FDM) A diagnostic and treatment system for fascial distortions developed by Stephen Typaldos (see Chapter 7.15).

Fasciotomy A surgical incision or transection of fascia, often performed to release pressure in compartment syndrome.

Fibroblasts Flat, elongated fascial cells with cytoplasmic processes at each end and a flat, oval, vesicular nucleus. Fibroblasts form the fibrous tissues in the body, including tendons, aponeuroses, and supporting and binding tissues of all sorts.

Fibronexus An adhesion in a myofibroblast that links actin across the cell membrane to molecules in the extracellular matrix-like fibronectin and collagen.

Fibrosis The formation of fibrous tissue, as in repair or replacement of parenchymatous elements.

G

Gap junctions Direct connections between the cytoplasms of two cells, allowing various molecules and ions to pass, for example, most sugars, amino acids, nucleotides, vitamins, hormones, and cyclic AMP. A gap junction channel is composed of two connexons (or hemichannels), which connect across the intercellular space. In electrically excitable tissues, these gap junctions serve to transmit electrical impulses via ionic currents and are known as electronic synapses.

Glycosaminoglycans (or mucopolysaccharides) High-molecular-weight linear heteropolysaccharides having disaccharide-repeating units containing an *N*-acetylhexosamine and a hexose or hexuronic acid; either or both residues may be sulfated. This class of compounds includes the chondroitin sulfates, dermatan sulfates, heparan sulfate and heparin, keratan sulfates, and hyaluronic acid. All except heparin occur in proteoglycans that consist of glycosaminoglycans covalently linked to a protein.

Golgi receptors Mechanosensory receptors found in dense proper fascia, in ligaments (Golgi end organs), in joint capsules, and around myotendinous junctions (Golgi tendon organs).

H

Homeostasis A state of internal balance. The tendency of living organisms to keep the internal conditions the same despite changes in the external conditions.

Hyaluronan A glycosaminoglycan; part of the extracellular matrix of synovial fluid, vitreous humor, cartilage, blood vessels, skin, and the umbilical cord. Along with lubricin, it maintains viscosity of the extracellular matrix, allowing for necessary lubrication of certain tissues.

Hypermobility (or laxity) A greater than normal range of motion in a joint, which may occur naturally in otherwise normal persons or may be a sign of joint instability.

Hypertonia Excessive tone of the skeletal muscles that increases their resistance to passive stretching.

Hypertrophy The enlargement or overgrowth of an organ or part due to an increase in size of its constituent cells.

Hypocapnia A deficiency of carbon dioxide in the blood, resulting from hyperventilation and eventually leading to alkalosis.

Hysteresis A property of systems that do not instantly react to the forces applied to them, but react slowly, or do not return completely to their original state.

I

Immunoassay A biochemical test that measures the concentration of a substance in solution, using an antigen/antibody reaction.

Immunofluorescence A technique that uses fluorescent dye-labeled antibodies to visualize subcellular distribution of biomolecules of interest.

Integrins Refers to any of a family of heterodimeric cell-adhesion receptors, consisting of two noncovalently linked polypeptide chains, designated α and β, that mediate cell-to-cell and cell-to-extracellular matrix interactions.

Interoception The perception of internal body states. This includes—but is not limited to—visceroception and relates to physiological tissues that transmit signals to the central nervous system about the current state of the body.

Interstitial fluid The extracellular fluid that bathes the cells of most tissues but that is not within the confines of the blood or lymph vessels and is not a transcellular fluid. Formed by filtration through the blood capillaries and drained away as lymph. It is the extracellular fluid volume minus the lymph volume, the plasma volume, and the transcellular fluid volume.

L

Laminin An adhesive glycoprotein component of the basement membrane. It binds to heparan sulfate, type IV collagen, and specific cell-surface receptors and is involved in the attachment of epithelial cells to underlying connective tissue.

Ligament A band of fascia that connects bones or supports viscera. Some are distinct fibrous structures; some are folds of fascia or of indurated peritoneum; others are relics of fetal vessels or organs.

M

Mechanoreceptors Sensory receptors that respond to mechanical pressure, deformation, or proprioception.

Mechanotransduction The mechanism by which cells convert a mechanical stimulus into chemical activity.

Mepyramine An antihistaminic pharmacological substance that is frequently used as an in-vitro contractile agent for tissues containing myofibroblasts.

Meridian A concept in traditional Chinese medicine (TCM) of invisible energy pathways running through the body.

Microdialysis A diagnostic technique that uses an ultrafine needle to biopsy the chemical components of the fluid in the extracellular space of tissues.

Morphogenesis The evolution and development of form, as in the development of the shape of a particular organ or part of the body.

Myofascial pain syndrome A chronic musculoskeletal pain disorder associated with local or referred pain, decreased range of motion, autonomic phenomena, local twitch response in the affected muscle, and muscle weakness without atrophy.

Myofibroblasts Differentiated fibroblasts that combine the features of both fibroblasts and smooth muscle cells. Because of their expression of stress fiber bundles containing alpha smooth muscle actin and because of strengthened adhesion sites on their membrane, these cells possess a much higher contractile potential than normal fibroblasts.

Myosin The most abundant protein in muscle, occurring chiefly in the A band. Along with actin, it is responsible for the contraction and relaxation of muscle. Myosin uses ATP hydrolysis to generate force and to "walk" along the filament. It is the main constituent of the thick filaments of muscle fibers.

N

Neuropathy A functional disturbance or pathological change in the peripheral nervous system.

Neuroplasticity The changes that occur in the organization of the brain as a result of experience.

Nociceptors A sensory neuron that responds to potentially damaging stimuli by sending "possible threat" signals to the central nervous system. They can be activated by physical, mechanical, thermal, electrical, or chemical stimuli.

O

Osteoblasts Cells that arise from fibroblasts and are associated with the production of bone.

Oxytocin A nonapeptide secreted by the magnocellular neurons of the hypothalamus and stored in the neurohypophysis along with vasopressin. It promotes uterine contractions and milk ejection, contributes to the second stage of labor, and is released during orgasm in both sexes. In the brain, oxytocin regulates circadian homeostasis, such as body temperature, activity level, and wakefulness. It is involved in social recognition, bonding, and trust formation.

P

Pacinian corpuscles Lamellar or lamellated large encapsulated nerve endings located in fascia that are sensitive to vibration and acceleration of movement. They require dynamically changing stimuli and do not respond to static pressure.

Perimysium The fascial membrane that groups individual muscle fibers (between 10 to 100+) into bundles or fascicles.

Perineurium An intermediate layer of fascia in a peripheral nerve, surrounding each bundle (fasciculus) of nerve fibers.

Periosteum A layer of dense fascia surrounding most bones.

Piezoelectric The ability of some materials to generate an electric potential in response to applied mechanical stress.

Plantar fasciitis An inflammatory condition of the plantar fascia.

Plantar fibromatosis The formation of fibrous, tumor-like nodules arising from the deep layer of the plantar fascia, manifested as single or multiple nodular swellings, sometimes accompanied by pain but usually unassociated with contractures.

Prestress Endogenous tension.

Procollagen The precursor molecule of collagen, synthesized in the fibroblast, osteoblast, etc., and cleaved to form collagen extracellularly.

Prolotherapy (or RIT, regenerative injection therapy) An injection therapy used to treat chronic ligament, joint, capsule, fascial, and tendinous injuries to promote nonsurgical soft tissue repair and to relieve pain.

Proprioception Perception mediated by sensory nerve endings found in muscles and fascia, which give information concerning movement and position of the body.

Proteoglycans Heavily glycosylated glycoproteins that are found in the extracellular matrix of fascia, composed mainly of polysaccharide chains, particularly glycosaminoglycans, as well as minor protein components that form large complexes, both to other proteoglycans, to hyaluronan, and to fibrous matrix proteins (such as collagen).

Protomyofibroblasts Develop from fibroblasts under mechanical tension. They form cytoplasmic actin-containing stress fibers that terminate in fibronexus adhesion complexes.

R

Reticular fibers Fascial fibers composed of collagen type III that form the reticular framework of lymphoid and myeloid tissue and also occur in the interstitial tissue of glandular organs, the papillary layer of the skin, and elsewhere.

Retinaculum A thickened band of fascia that retains an organ or tissue in place.

Ruffini endings Types of lamellated corpuscle that are slowly adapting receptors for sensations of continuous pressure.

S

Sarcoplasmic reticulum A special form of a granular reticulum found in the sarcoplasm of striated muscle and comprising a system of smooth-surfaced tubules forming a plexus around each myofibril.

Sclerosis An induration or hardening caused by inflammation, fascial thickening, or disease of the interstitial fluid.

Serotonin A monoamine vasoconstrictor, synthesized in the intestinal chromaffin cells or in central or peripheral neurons and found in high concentrations in many body tissues, including the intestinal mucosa, pineal body, and central nervous system.

Shear motion A deformation of a tissue in which parallel arranged sublayers (or subsections) of this tissue are moving in opposite directions relative to each other along their common axis.

Stiffness A material's resistance to external deformation.

Substance P An undecapeptide that functions as a neurotransmitter and as a neuromodulator and belongs to the tachykinin neuropeptide family.

Super-compensation An increase in performance capacity beyond the pretraining baseline level of performance.

Superficial fascia Comprised mainly of loose areolar connective tissue and adipose. In addition to its subcutaneous presence, this type of fascia surrounds organs, glands, and neurovascular bundles and is found at many other locations.

Surface electromyography A technique in which electrodes are placed on (not into) the skin overlying a muscle to detect the electrical activity of the muscle.

T

Telocytes Specialized connective tissue cells with long extensions called telopodes, which allow for intercellular communication.

Tendon A fibrous cord of fascia by which a muscle is attached to the skeleton.

Tendon sheath A membranous sleeve that envelops the tendon and creates a lubricated low-friction environment for easy movement.

Tensegrity A structural principle that uses isolated components in compression inside a net of continuous tension.

Transdifferentiation A biological process that occurs when a non-stem cell transforms into a different type of cell, or when an already differentiated stem cell creates cells outside its already established differentiation.

Transforming growth factor Two classes that are structurally or genetically not related to one another. TGF-α binds the epidermal growth factor receptor and also stimulates growth of microvascular endothelial cells. TGF-β exists in several subtypes, all of which are found in hematopoietic tissue, stimulate wound healing, and in vitro are antagonists of lymphopoiesis and myelopoiesis.

Trigger point Palpable as localized hardening in the muscle; pain evoked by pressure on the tender spot is recognized as being familiar by the patient, local twitch response is possible; limitation of stretch range of motion, and some weakness of that muscle.

Tropocollagen The basic structural unit of collagen; a helical structure consisting of three polypeptide chains, each chain composed of about a thousand amino acids coiled around each other to form a spiral and stabilized by inter- and intra-chain covalent bonds.

Tropoelastin The precursor of elastin.

Tropomyosin Along with troponin, regulates the shortening of the muscle protein filaments actin and myosin. In the absence of nerve impulses to muscle fibers, tropomyosin blocks interaction between myosin cross-bridges and actin filaments.

Tumor microenvironment (TME) Environment surrounding a tumor, including fibroblasts, extracellular matrix (ECM), cytokines, blood vessels, immune cells, hormones, and other components. In contrast to the normal tissue environment, the TME generally promotes the growth of cancer.

U

Ultrasound elastography A noninvasive imaging method to measure stiffness or strain of soft tissue or to provide images of tissue morphology or other biomechanical information.

V

Vimentin filaments Intermediate filaments of the cytoskeleton that are responsible for maintaining cell integrity. They act as cytoskeletal support structures, play a role in mitosis, and are clustered particularly around the nucleus, probably helping to control its location.

Vinculin A protein found in muscle, fibroblasts, and epithelial cells that binds actin and appears to mediate attachment of actin filaments to integral proteins of the plasma membrane.

Viscoelastic Describes materials that exhibit both viscous and elastic characteristics when undergoing plastic deformation. Viscous materials, like honey, resist shear flow and strain linearly with time when a stress is applied. Elastic materials strain instantaneously when stretched and just as quickly return to their original state once the stress is removed. Viscoelastic materials have elements of both of these properties and, as such, exhibit time-dependent strain.

W

Wolff's law The theory developed by 19th-century anatomist/surgeon Julius Wolff stating that bone in a healthy person or animal will adapt to the loads it is placed under. If loading on a particular bone increases, the bone will remodel itself over time to become stronger to resist that sort of loading. The converse is also true, that is, if the loading on a bone decreases, the bone will become weaker because of turnover as it is less metabolically costly to maintain and there is no stimulus for continued remodeling required to maintain bone mass.

INDEX

Page numbers followed by *b* indicate boxes, *f* indicate figures and *t* indicate tables.